JAYNE ELLIS

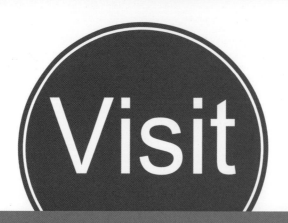

Sixth Edition

Jubb, Kennedy, and Palmer's
Pathology of
DOMESTIC
ANIMALS

Volume 2

Sixth Edition

Jubb, Kennedy, and Palmer's

Pathology of

DOMESTIC
ANIMALS

Volume 2

EDITED BY:

M. GRANT MAXIE, DVM, PHD, DIPLOMATE ACVP
Co-Executive Director, Laboratory Service Division
Director, Animal Health Laboratory
University of Guelph
Guelph, Ontario
Canada

ELSEVIER

ELSEVIER

3251 Riverport Lane
St. Louis, Missouri 63043

JUBB, KENNEDY, AND PALMER'S PATHOLOGY OF DOMESTIC ANIMALS, SIXTH EDITION

ISBN: 978-0-7020-5322-1 (3 VOLUME SET)
978-0-7020-5317-7 (VOLUME 1)
978-0-7020-5318-4 (VOLUME 2)
978-0-7020-5319-1 (VOLUME 3)

Notices

Knowledge and best practice in this field are constantly changing. As new research and experience broaden our understanding, changes in research methods, professional practices, or medical treatment may become necessary.

Practitioners and researchers must always rely on their own experience and knowledge in evaluating and using any information, methods, compounds, or experiments described herein. In using such information or methods they should be mindful of their own safety and the safety of others, including parties for whom they have a professional responsibility.

With respect to any drug or pharmaceutical products identified, readers are advised to check the most current information provided (i) on procedures featured or (ii) by the manufacturer of each product to be administered, to verify the recommended dose or formula, the method and duration of administration, and contraindications. It is the responsibility of practitioners, relying on their own experience and knowledge of their patients, to make diagnoses, to determine dosages and the best treatment for each individual patient, and to take all appropriate safety precautions.

To the fullest extent of the law, neither the Publisher nor the authors, contributors, or editors, assume any liability for any injury and/or damage to persons or property as a matter of products liability, negligence or otherwise, or from any use or operation of any methods, products, instructions, or ideas contained in the material herein.

Previous editions copyrighted 2007, 1993, 1985, 1970, 1963

Library of Congress Cataloging-in-Publication Data

Jubb, Kennedy, and Palmer's pathology of domestic animals / edited by M. Grant Maxie.—Sixth edition.
    p. ; cm.
  title: Pathology of domestic animals
  Includes bibliographical references and index.
  ISBN 978-0-7020-5322-1 (3 vol. set : alk. paper)—ISBN 978-0-7020-5317-7 (v. 1 : alk. paper)—ISBN 978-0-7020-5318-4 (v. 2 : alk. paper)—ISBN 978-0-7020-5319-1 (v. 3 : alk. paper)
  I. Maxie, M. Grant, editor.   II. Title: Pathology of domestic animals.
  [DNLM: 1. Pathology, Veterinary.   2. Animals, Domestic.   SF 769]
  SF769.P345 2016
  636.089'607—dc23
                                                                        2015009121

Vice President and Publisher: Loren Wilson
Content Strategy Director: Penny Rudolph
Content Development Manager: Jolynn Gower
Content Development Specialist: Brandi Graham
Content Coordinator: Kayla Mugle

Publishing Services Managers: Anne Altepeter and Patricia Tannian
Senior Project Manager: Sharon Corell
Project Manager: Louise King
Designer: Brian Salisbury

Printed in China

Last digit is the print number: 9 8 7 6 5 4 3 2

Contributors

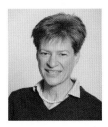

Dorothee Bienzle, DVM, PhD, Diplomate ACVP
Professor
Department of Pathobiology
Ontario Veterinary College
University of Guelph
Pathobiology
University of Guelph
Guelph, Ontario
Canada
Hematopoietic system

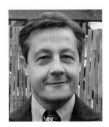

Carlo Cantile, DVM, PhD
Professor of Veterinary Pathology
Department of Veterinary Science
University of Pisa
Pisa, Italy
Nervous system

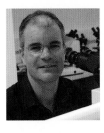

Jeff L. Caswell, DVM, DVSc, PhD, Diplomate ACVP
Professor
Department of Pathobiology
Ontario Veterinary College
University of Guelph
Guelph, Ontario
Canada
Respiratory system

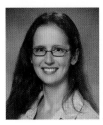

Rachel E. Cianciolo, VMD, PhD, Diplomate ACVP
Assistant Professor
Co-Director, International Veterinary
  Renal Pathology Service
Department of Veterinary Biosciences
College of Veterinary Medicine
The Ohio State University
Columbus, Ohio
USA
Urinary system

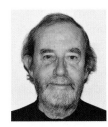

Barry J. Cooper, BVSc, PhD, Diplomate ACVP
Professor Emeritus of Pathology
Department of Biomedical Sciences
Cornell University
Ithaca, New York
USA
Muscle and tendon

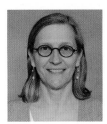

Linden E. Craig, DVM, PhD, Diplomate ACVP
Department of Biomedical and
  Diagnostic Sciences
University of Tennessee College of
  Veterinary Medicine
Knoxville, Tennessee
USA
Bones and joints

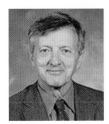

John M. Cullen, VMD, PhD, Diplomate ACVP
Professor
Department of Population Health and
  Pathobiology
College of Veterinary Medicine
North Carolina State University
Raleigh, North Carolina
USA
Liver and biliary system

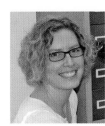

Keren E. Dittmer, BVSc, PhD, Diplomate ACVP
Institute of Veterinary, Animal, and
  Biomedical Sciences
Massey University
Palmerston North, Manawatu
New Zealand
Bones and joints

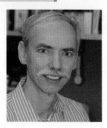

Robert A. Foster, BVSc, PhD, MACVSc, Diplomate ACVP
Professor
Department of Pathobiology
Ontario Veterinary College
University of Guelph
Guelph, Ontario
Canada
Female genital system
Male genital system

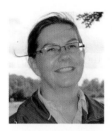

Andrea Gröne, DVM, PhD, Diplomate ACVP, Diplomate ECVP
Professor
Faculty of Veterinary Medicine
Department of Pathobiology
Utrecht University
Utrecht, The Netherlands
Endocrine glands

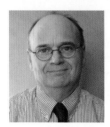

Jesse M. Hostetter, DVM, PhD, Diplomate ACVP
Associate Professor
Department of Veterinary Pathology
College of Veterinary Medicine
Iowa State University
Ames, Iowa
USA
Alimentary system

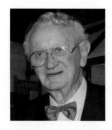

Kenneth V. F. Jubb†
Emeritus Professor
Faculty of Veterinary and Agricultural
    Sciences
University of Melbourne
Melbourne, Victoria, Australia
Pancreas

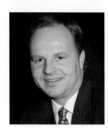

Matti Kiupel, Dr med vet habil, PhD, Diplomate ACVP
Professor
Department of Pathobiology and
    Diagnostic Investigation
College of Veterinary Medicine
Michigan State University
East Lansing, Michigan
USA
Hematopoietic system

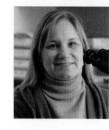

Elizabeth A. Mauldin, DVM, Diplomate ACVP, Diplomate ACVD
Associate Professor
Department of Pathobiology
School of Veterinary Medicine
University of Pennsylvania
Philadelphia, Pennsylvania
USA
Integumentary system

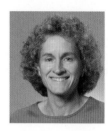

M. Grant Maxie, DVM, PhD, Diplomate ACVP
Co-Executive Director, Laboratory
    Service Division
Director, Animal Health Laboratory
University of Guelph
Guelph, Ontario
Canada
Introduction to the diagnostic process

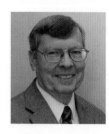

Margaret A. Miller, DVM, PhD, Diplomate ACVP
Professor
Department of Comparative
    Pathobiology
Purdue University
West Lafayette, Indiana
USA
Introduction to the diagnostic process

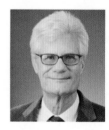

F. Charles Mohr, DVM, PhD, Diplomate ACVP
Professor of Clinical Anatomic
    Pathology
Department of Veterinary Pathology,
    Microbiology, and Immunology
School of Veterinary Medicine
University of California
Davis, California
USA
Urinary system

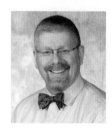

Bradley L. Njaa, DVM, MVSc, Diplomate ACVP
Anatomic Pathologist III
IDEXX Laboratories, Inc.
Professor (Adjunct)
Department of Veterinary Pathobiology
Oklahoma State University
Stillwater, Oklahoma
USA
Special senses

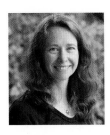

**Jeanine Peters-Kennedy, DVM,
  Diplomate ACVP, Diplomate ACVD**
Assistant Clinical Professor
Department of Biomedical Sciences
College of Veterinary Medicine
Cornell University
Ithaca, New York
USA
Integumentary system

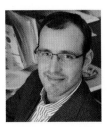

**Brandon L. Plattner, DVM, PhD,
  Diplomate ACVP**
Assistant Professor
Department of Pathobiology
Ontario Veterinary College
University of Guelph
Guelph, Ontario
Canada
Alimentary system

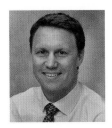

**Nicholas A. Robinson, BVSc (Hons),
  PhD, MACVSc, Diplomate ACVP**
Professor
College of Veterinary Medicine
University of Minnesota
St. Paul, Minnesota
USA
Cardiovascular system

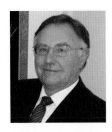

**Wayne F. Robinson, BVSc, MVSc,
  PhD, MACVSc, Diplomate ACVP**
Emeritus Professor
Federation University Australia
Victoria, Australia
Cardiovascular system

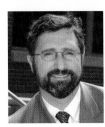

**Thomas J. Rosol, DVM, PhD,
  Diplomate ACVP**
Professor
Department of Veterinary Biosciences
Senior Advisor, Life Sciences,
  Technology Commercialization
  Office
College of Veterinary Medicine
The Ohio State University
Columbus, Ohio
USA
Endocrine glands

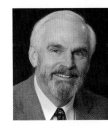

**Donald H. Schlafer, DVM, PhD,
  Diplomate ACVP/ACVM/ACT**
Emeritus Professor
Department of Biomedical Sciences
College of Veterinary Medicine
Cornell University
Ithaca, New York
USA
Female genital system

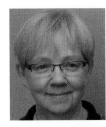

**Margaret J. Stalker, DVM, PhD,
  Diplomate ACVP**
Animal Health Laboratory
Laboratory Services Division
University of Guelph
Guelph, Ontario
Canada
Liver and biliary system

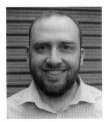

**Andrew W. Stent, BVSc,
  MANZCVS, PhD**
Faculty of Veterinary and Agricultural
  Sciences
University of Melbourne
Melbourne, Victoria
Australia
Pancreas

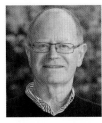

**Keith G. Thompson, BVSc, PhD,
  Diplomate ACVP**
Emeritus Professor
Pathobiology Section
Institute of Veterinary, Animal, and
  Biomedical Sciences
Massey University
Palmerston North, Manawatu
New Zealand
Bones and joints

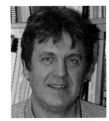

**Francisco A. Uzal, DVM, FRVC, PhD,
  Diplomate ACVP**
California Animal Health and Food
  Safety Laboratory
University of California
San Bernardino, California
USA
Alimentary system

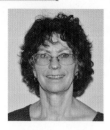

Beth A. Valentine, DVM, PhD, Diplomate ACVP
Professor
Department of Biomedical Sciences
College of Veterinary Medicine
Oregon State University
Corvallis, Oregon
USA
Muscle and tendon

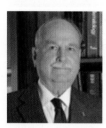

V.E.O. (Ted) Valli, DVM, PhD, Diplomate ACVP
Professor Emeritus
Department of Pathobiology
College of Veterinary Medicine
University of Illinois at
    Urbana-Champaign
Champaign, Illinois
USA
Hematopoietic system

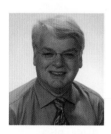

Brian P. Wilcock, DVM, PhD
Histovet Surgical Pathology
Guelph, Ontario
Canada
Special senses

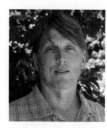

Kurt J. Williams, DVM, PhD, Diplomate ACVP
Department of Pathobiology and
    Diagnostic Investigation
College of Veterinary Medicine
Michigan State University
East Lansing, Michigan
USA
Respiratory system

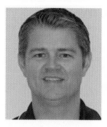

R. Darren Wood, DVM, DVSc, Diplomate ACVP
Associate Professor
Department of Pathobiology
Ontario Veterinary College
University of Guelph
Guelph, Ontario
Canada
Hematopoietic system

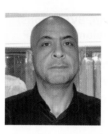

Sameh Youssef, BVSc, PhD, DVSc, Diplomate ACVP
Professor
Department of Pathology
Alexandria Veterinary College
Alexandria University
Alexandria, Egypt
Nervous system

Preface

In this sixth edition of *Pathology of Domestic Animals*, we continue the long tradition of surveying the literature and updating the information in this reference textbook in light of our own practical experience in the pathology of the major domestic mammals. True to the spirit of the first edition, this text is designed to explain the pathogenesis of common and not-so-common diseases, define the distinguishing features of these various conditions, and put them in a context relevant to both students and working pathologists. Knowledge has been generated incrementally since the publication of the fifth edition, particularly with respect to improved understanding of pathogenesis at the molecular level, as well as through the use of improved diagnostic tools, including the frontier of whole genome sequencing. My thanks to the contributors to this edition for their rigorous perusal of the literature in their areas of interest, for their addition of insightful information to their chapters, and for their inclusion of many new figures.

NEW TO THE SIXTH EDITION

The most noticeable, and I think very welcome, change in the sixth edition is the addition of full-color figures throughout the text. Nearly all of the images from prior editions have been replaced. These new images clearly depict the diagnostic features of hundreds of conditions.

We have also added a new chapter, "Introduction to the Diagnostic Process," to the usual lineup of chapters in these 3 volumes. The goal of this new chapter is to illustrate the whole-animal perspective and detail the approaches to systemic, multi-system, and polymicrobial disease.

The complete index is again printed in each volume as an aid to readers. "Further reading" lists have been pruned in the print book to save space. All references are available on any electronic version of the text as well as on the companion website that accompanies the purchase of any print book. These online references link to abstracts on PubMed.com.

COMPANION WEBSITE

In addition to updating the graphic design of these volumes, the print version of *Pathology of Domestic Animals* now has a companion website, accessible at:
PathologyofDomesticAnimals.com

Included on the companion website are:
- A complete image collection, including 325 bonus, electronic-only figures that have been called out in the text. These figures are identified in the printed version as "eFigs."
- An expanded list of useful references, each linked to the original abstract on PubMed.com.

I hope that we have captured significant changes and have synthesized this new knowledge to provide a balanced overview of all topics covered. Keeping pace with evolving agents and their changing impacts is a never-ending challenge. We have used current anatomical and microbial terminology, based on internationally accepted reference sources, such as the Universal Virus Database of the International Committee on Taxonomy of Viruses (http://www.ncbi.nlm.nih.gov/ICTVdb/index.htm). Microbial taxonomy is, of course, continually evolving, and classifications and names of organisms can be expected to be updated as newer phylogenetic analyses are reported. Debate continues, for example, over the taxonomy of *Chlamydophila/Chlamydia* spp. And change will continue.

We have attempted to contact all contributors of figures from previous editions and from various archives and apologize to any whom we were unable to contact or who were overlooked. If any individual recognizes an image as one of his/her own or as belonging to a colleague, we would be happy to correct the attribution in a future printing.

Acknowledgments

My thanks to Elsevier for their help and support throughout this project, beginning in the United Kingdom with Robert Edwards and Carole McMurray, and more recently in the United States, with Penny Rudolph, content strategy director; Brandi Graham, content development specialist; Sharon Corell, senior project manager; Louise King, project manager, and the entire behind-the-scenes production team.

Grant Maxie
Guelph, Ontario, 2015

*These volumes are dedicated to Drs. Kenneth V.F. Jubb (1928-2013)[1],
Peter C. Kennedy (1923-2006)[2], and Nigel C. Palmer,
and to my family—Laura, Kevin, and Andrea.*

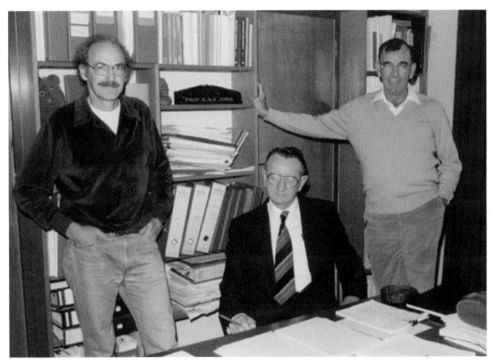

Drs. Palmer, Jubb, and Kennedy while working on the third edition in Melbourne, 1983. (Courtesy, University of Melbourne.)

[1]http://www.vet.unimelb.edu.au/news/2013/memorial.html
[2]http://senate.universityofcalifornia.edu/inmemoriam/peterckennedy.htm

Contents

[†]Deceased

CHAPTER 1

Alimentary System

Francisco A. Uzal • Brandon L. Plattner • Jesse M. Hostetter

ACKNOWLEDGMENTS

We gratefully acknowledge the contributions of all previous authors of this chapter, including Drs. Ken Jubb, Peter Kennedy, Nigel Palmer, Ian Barker, Corrie Brown, and Dale Baker.

ORAL CAVITY

Examination of the oral cavity should be standard procedure during any postmortem examination. To obtain a clear view of the mucous membranes of the buccal and oral cavities, teeth, tongue, gums, and tonsils, it is essential to split the mandibular symphysis and separate the mandibles as far as possible. A thorough examination of all structures will reveal not only local lesions, but often those that may be due to systemic disease. Lesions may be associated with congenital anomalies (genetic and nongenetic); trauma (physical and chemical); bacterial, mycotic, viral, and parasitic infections; metabolic and toxic diseases; and immune-mediated, dysplastic, or neoplastic disease. The poor physical condition of an animal may be directly related to oral lesions that result in difficulties of prehension, mastication, or swallowing of food.

Congenital anomalies

Congenital anomalies may occur as heritable conditions or be the result of nongenetic factors, including toxicity and infectious agents. The development of normal face, jaws, and the oral cavity requires the integration of many embryonic processes, most importantly the frontonasal, maxillary, and mandibular processes. The complexity and duration of this development may lead to a great variety of aberrations. These are usually expressed in the newborn in the form of *clefts resulting from failures of integrated growth and fusion of these processes.* A common failure of fusion is that of the maxillary processes to the frontonasal process. This may leave facial fissures, cleft lip (harelip, cheiloschisis) and unilateral or bilateral primary cleft palate involving the area rostral to the incisive papilla.

Facial clefts may involve the skin only, or the deeper tissues as well. They are variously located, and not all are obviously related to normal lines of fusion. All are rare. The most common is a complete cleft from one angle of the mouth to the ear of that side. This results from failure of fusion of the lateral portions of the maxillary and mandibular processes. A defect extending from a cleft lip to the eye results from failure

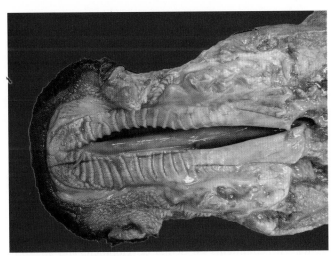

Figure 1-1 Secondary cleft palate exposing the nasal cavity in a calf. (Courtesy J. Caswell.)

of fusion of the maxillary and frontonasal processes, which may be a superficial defect with failure of closure of the naso-lacrimal duct.

Primary cleft palate (harelip, cheiloschisis) includes developmental anomalies of the upper lips rostral to the nasal septum, columella, and premaxilla. They may be unilateral or bilateral and superficial or extend into the nostril. The defect arises from incomplete fusion of the frontonasal process with the maxillary processes.

Secondary cleft palate (cleft palate, palatoschisis) (Fig. 1-1) is often associated with primary cleft palate. The normal hard palate is formed, except for a small rostral contribution from the frontonasal process, and by the bilateral ingrowth of the lateral palatine shelves from the maxillary processes. At the midline, they fuse with each other and with the nasal septum, and undergo intramembranous ossification, except in their caudal part, which becomes the soft palate. Inadequate growth of the palatine shelves leaves a central defect, in either or both of the hard and soft palates, which communicates between the oral and nasal cavities. Other manifestations of disordered palato-genesis include unilateral defects in the soft palate; bilateral hypoplasia of the soft palate; or dorsal displacement of the soft palate, with excess soft tissue on the caudal portion. Affected animals have difficulty sucking, may have nasal regurgitation, and usually die within the first few days of life from aspiration pneumonia. In dogs, malformation of the soft palate has also been associated with alterations in the tympanic bulla and middle ear dysfunction.

Cleft palates have been reported in most species of domestic animals. In one extensive survey of Thoroughbred foals, 4% of congenital defects were secondary cleft palates. Most of these foals had a complete cleft of the hard palate; a few had clefts or hypoplasia of the soft palate only. In calves, cleft palate is one of the most common anomalies, but is very uncommon in sheep. Primary cleft palate is less common than secondary cleft palate in swine, although the two anomalies often occur together. In dogs and cats, cleft palate is often associated with certain breeds, suggesting that these are heritable traits.

The etiology of cleft palate is usually unknown, but examples of *hereditary causes*, maternal ingestion of certain *drugs*, or maternal consumption of *teratogenic plants* during pregnancy have been demonstrated. Secondary cleft palate and arthrogryposis frequently occur together in Charolais calves, and appear to be hereditary (probably simple autosomal recessive), as in Hereford cattle. Cleft palate in lambs may be genetic in origin, but also is associated with the ingestion of *Veratrum californicum*. Secondary cleft palates have been induced experimentally in newborn pigs by feeding gilts seeds or plants of poison hemlock (*Conium maculatum*) during gestational days 30-45. Both tree tobacco (*Nicotiana glauca*) in the western United States and tobacco stalks (*N. tabacum*) when fed to gilts early in pregnancy can induce a high incidence of cleft palate and arthrogryposis in newborn pigs. Piperidine alkaloids (coniine, coniceine, and anabasine) in hemlock and tobacco plants are responsible for the teratogenic effects of these plants. Lupines (*Lupinus formosus, L. arbustus*) produce piperidine alkaloids, including the teratogen ammodendrine, which can cause cleft palate and arthrogryposis (crooked calf disease) in calves born of dams fed the lupine at days 40-50 of gestation. Palatoschisis in piglets has also been associated with consumption of feed contaminated with *Crotalaria retusa* seed by sows during gestation. Primary and secondary cleft palate of German Boxer dogs appear to be hereditary, probably because of a single autosomal recessive gene. A single autosomal recessive gene has been associated with cleft palate in Pyrenees Shepherd dogs. Secondary cleft palate occurs in Siamese and Abyssinian cats and is likely hereditary. Griseofulvin treatment of the pregnant queen and mare will result in palatoschisis in the offspring. The defect has also been reported in both parts of the doubled face in diprosopus cats.

Anomalies in the growth of jaws are quite common. **Brachygnathia superior,** *shortness of the maxillae,* is an inherited breed characteristic among dogs and swine. It has been reported in the Large White or Yorkshire breed. The condition is progressive with age, resulting in malapposition of the incisor and cheek teeth, which interferes with prehension and mastication. In swine, brachygnathia superior may be confused with atrophic rhinitis. In Angus and Jersey cattle, brachygnathia superior occurs as a hereditary trait. In any species, it may be associated with chondrodysplasia and is also present with other facial defects.

Brachygnathia inferior or micrognathia, *shortness of the mandibles,* may be a mild to lethal defect in cattle and sheep and is a breed characteristic of long-nosed dogs. Brachygnathia inferior is a common defect in calves. It is inherited, probably as a simple autosomal recessive trait. There is a higher incidence in males. This condition in calves has been associated with cerebellar hypoplasia. In Aberdeen Angus cattle, the defect may occur concurrently with cerebellar hypoplasia, and with osteopetrosis in this and other breeds (see Vol. 1, Bones and joints). In Merino sheep, brachygnathia is associated with a cardiomegaly and renal hypoplasia syndrome that has an autosomal recessive inheritance pattern. Transplacental infection with Schmallenberg virus, an orthobunyavirus, will lead to brachygnathia among other congenital malformations in lambs and calves. Mild brachygnathia inferior, termed *parrot mouth,* is a common conformational defect in horses.

Prognathism refers to *abnormal prolongation of the mandibles.* It is rather common, especially in sheep. It may develop with recovery from calcium deficiency in this species (see Vol. 1, Bones and joints). The malformation is relative, and it is not always easy to determine whether the jaw is absolutely long or merely apparently so, relative to a mild brachygnathia superior.

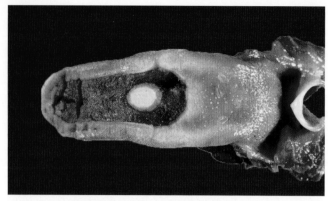

Figure 1-2 Epitheliogenesis imperfecta of the tongue of a pig. (Courtesy Noah's Arkives.)

Agnathia is a mandibulofacial malformation characterized by *absence of the lower jaw*, caused by failure of development of the first branchial arch and associated structures. The defect is one of the most common anomalies in lambs but is rare in cattle. Associated malformations in lambs may include ateloprosopia (incomplete development of the face), microglossia or aglossia, and atresia of the oropharynx. Concurrent anomalies affecting other body systems also may be evident.

A lethal glossopharyngeal hereditary defect, termed **bird tongue** and caused by a simple autosomal recessive gene, has been reported in dogs. Affected pups have a narrow tongue, especially the rostral half, where the margins are folded medially onto the dorsal surface. The pups are unable to swallow. The muscle fibers of the affected tongues are normal histologically. In dogs, there is a congenital defect leading to a thickened short lingual frenulum called **ankyloglossia**. This lesion may be most pronounced at the rostral tongue, and the tip of the tongue may be notched. **Hypertrophy of the tongue** occurs as a congenital anomaly in pigs.

Epitheliogenesis imperfecta is an anomaly that causes *widespread defects in cutaneous epithelium, and also affects the epithelial lining of the oral cavity, especially the tongue* (Fig. 1-2) (see Vol. 1, Integumentary system). The condition is characterized by irregular, well-demarcated, red areas from which the epithelium of the oral mucosa is absent. Histologically, these consist of abruptly defective areas in the squamous mucosa with inflammation of the submucosal connective tissues. The anomaly occurs in most species and is inherited as a simple autosomal recessive character in cattle, horses, and pigs; the mode of inheritance is unknown in the other species. There are several hereditary skin conditions in animals, such as epidermolysis bullosa simplex in Collie dogs, ovine epidermolysis bullosa in Suffolk and South Dorset Down sheep, and familial acantholysis of Aberdeen Angus calves, which have minor involvement of the lips and oral mucosa (see Vol. 1, Integumentary system).

Further reading

Herder V, et al. Salient features of domestic ruminants infected with the emerging so-called Schmallenberg virus in Germany. Vet Pathol 2012;49:588-591.

Kemp C, et al. Cleft lip and/or palate with monogenic autosomal recessive transmission in Pyrenees Shepherd dogs. Cleft Palate Craniofac J 2009;46:81-88.

Noden DM, de Lahunta A. The Embryology of Domestic Animals. Developmental Mechanisms and Malformations. Baltimore: Williams & Wilkins; 1985. p. 187-195.

Shariflou M, et. al. Brachygnathia, cardiomegaly and renal hypoplasia syndrome (BCRHS) in Merino sheep maps to a 1.1-megabase region on ovine chromosome OAR2. Anim Gen 2012;44:231-233.

Temizsoylu MD, Avki S. Complete ventral ankyloglossia in three related dogs. J Am Vet Med Assoc 2003;223:1443-1445.

White R, et al. Soft palate hypoplasia and concurrent middle ear pathology in six dogs. J Small Anim Pract 2009;50:364-372.

Diseases of teeth and dental tissues

Dental disease is common and often is a factor that limits the useful life-span of the animal, especially sheep. Evaluation of dental disease necessitates a thorough examination of the oral cavity. The comments on dental development and anatomy are intended to provide a brief overview and assist the understanding of dental disease.

Teeth develop from a band of ectoderm deep to the mucosal epithelium that spans the length of the gingiva. This ectodermal band is called the *dental lamina*. In the initial stage of tooth development, neural crest cells beneath the dental laminae induce multiple nodular thickenings along the length of the dental lamina. These are the *tooth buds*. Next, ectomesenchymal cells aggregate at the base of each tooth bud. The tooth bud then becomes a bell-shaped structure that grows down over the ectomesenchymal cells and becomes the *enamel organ*, which will give rise to enamel-producing *ameloblasts*. The ectomesenchyme below the enamel organ develops into the *dental papilla*, which will give rise to dentin-producing *odontoblasts* and also the tooth pulp. Ectomesenchyme cells also move around the periphery of the enamel organ to form a limiting sac called the *dental follicle* or *dental sac*. The dental sac will ultimately give rise to cementum-producing cells (*cementoblasts*), the periodontal ligament, and alveolar bone.

The cells of the enamel organ differentiate into 3 layers: outer epithelium, stellate reticulum, and inner epithelium. The *cervical loop* forms where the outer and inner epithelium of the enamel organ join. As the enamel organ develops, the dental lamina begins to disintegrate, leaving the tooth separate from the overlying oral mucosa. Remnants of the dental lamina can persist and give rise to dental cysts or neoplasms.

Hard tissues (dentin and enamel) are deposited on the developing tooth. The *inner enamel epithelium* of the enamel organ induces differentiation of odontoblasts from the ectomesenchyme of the dental papilla. Odontoblasts produce *dentin*, which in turn induces differentiation and enamel formation by the ameloblasts of the inner enamel epithelium. Thus formation of dentin is essential for the formation of enamel. These inductive interactions of epithelium and ectomesenchyme are considered important in the histodifferentiation of some tumors of dental tissues.

The crown of the tooth will ultimately be shaped by the inner enamel epithelium. The shape of the tooth roots will be determined by the cervical loop through epithelial extensions called *Hertwig's epithelial root sheath (HERS)*. The HERS guides the formation of the developing root by inciting differentiation of odontoblasts from the dental papilla. Typically the HERS will disintegrate after it initiates dentin formation. As the HERS fragments, it allows ectomesenchymal cells from the dental sac to contact the root dentin, differentiate into cementoblasts, and deposit cementum on the dentin of the root. Remnants of the HERS can persist and are called *epithelial rests of Malassez*. They persist in the periodontal ligament, and may give rise to tumors or cysts. They may be important in the induction or repair of cementum, and in periodontal reattachment following injury. In pigs and sheep, the rests may be incorporated into the junctional epithelium as it migrates apically in chronic periodontal disease. HERS cells of the root sheath that adhere to the dentin can produce *enamel pearls*.

As tooth development progresses, the crown of the tooth is covered by enamel, whereas the roots are covered by cementum. Dentin is present throughout the tooth. Fibroblasts in the dental follicle (sac) generate collagen that forms the *periodontal ligament*. The collagen of the periodontal ligament is intertwined with the cementum of the root surface and extends to the adjacent alveolar bone along the length of the root. The periodontal ligament is continually modified and reshaped with orientation of fibers in different directions during the life of the tooth.

The tooth will begin erupting while the roots are still developing. The mechanisms of tooth eruption are not fully understood. It is likely that the dental follicle plays a critical role in alveolar bone resorption and remodeling needed to allow the tooth to erupt. The inner enamel epithelium merges with the cells of the overlying stratum intermedium and the outer enamel epithelium to form the *reduced enamel epithelium*. This protects the enamel of the formed tooth before eruption. The reduced enamel epithelium will fuse with the mucosal epithelium as the tooth erupts, and after eruption a portion of the reduced enamel epithelium will persist along the gingival margin of the tooth as *junctional epithelium*. The process of tooth development is similar for *deciduous* and permanent teeth. Tooth germ for permanent teeth begins to develop along with the deciduous teeth. However, the permanent tooth germ is held dormant until later in life when the permanent teeth proceed with development and the deciduous teeth are lost.

There are important differences between the **brachydont teeth** of humans, carnivores, and swine, in which the enamel is restricted to the tooth crown, and the **hypsodont teeth** of herbivores. In hypsodont teeth, enamel extends far down on the roots, and is invaginated into the dentin to form *infundibula*. Also, the hypsodont teeth of herbivores, except the mandibular premolars of ruminants, are covered by cementum, which more or less fills the infundibula. Exceptions to these rules are provided by the tusks of boars, which are hypsodont, but not covered by cementum, and by ruminant incisors, which are brachydont but do have enamel covering part of the root dentin and cementum covering the root enamel.

The 3 hard tissues of teeth are dentin, enamel, and cementum. **Dentin** is light yellow and constitutes most of the tooth. It consists of ~35% organic matter and ~65% mineral. Thus its composition is similar to that of bone, and like bone, it contains type I collagen. Dentin is produced by columnar cells with basal nuclei called *odontoblasts*, which differentiate from ectomesenchyme of the dental papilla. It is formed as unmineralized predentin. The odontoblasts move away from the dentin-enamel junction, gradually encroaching on the pulp cavity as they produce dentin. Each odontoblast has a process extending into the dentin, encased in a dentinal tubule, which arborizes at the dentin-enamel junction. The process also anastomoses with the processes of other odontoblasts.

Dentinal tubules are visible in histologic sections, but the anastomoses are not. Except for the processes, and nerve endings in the dentinal tubules near the pulp, dentin is acellular.

Normal dentin contains incremental or *imbrication lines of von Ebner*, which are fine basophilic lines running at right angles to the dentinal tubules. They represent normal variations in the structure and mineralization of dentin. Sublethal injury caused by certain infections, metabolic stresses, or toxic states may injure the odontoblasts, which then produce accentuated incremental lines known as the *contour lines of Owen*. Sometimes irregular zones of unmineralized or poorly mineralized dentin form between foci of normal mineralization. These are zones of *interglobular dentin*, which may be caused by hypophosphatemia.

There are 3 types of dentin. *Primary dentin* is produced by odontoblasts before tooth eruption. *Secondary dentin* is produced after root formation is complete by odontoblasts that remain active throughout life. Generation of secondary dentin is much slower than primary dentin. *Tertiary dentin* is produced in response to injury to the tooth. Tertiary dentin is called *reactionary* when it is produced by pre-existing odontoblasts. *Reparative dentin* is another type of tertiary dentin that is produced by newly differentiated odontoblasts. Reparative dentin may resemble bone and is sometimes called *osteodentin*. *Sclerotic (transparent) dentin* is formed when dentinal tubules are occluded by calcium salts. The junctions between primary, secondary, and reparative dentin are usually demarcated by basophilic lines.

Enamel has ~5% organic matter and ~95% mineral. It is produced by the tall columnar *ameloblasts* of the inner enamel epithelium. Enamel is produced in the form of prisms or rods, cemented together by a matrix. Mineralization begins as soon as it is formed and is a 2-stage process, somewhat similar to that in bone, but much more rapid. The cells of the inner enamel epithelium also move away from the dentin-enamel junction as the tooth is formed, but unlike odontoblasts, they do not have processes. Formation of enamel ends before tooth eruption. Enamel is hard, dense, brittle, and permeable, and is translucent and white. Mature enamel is not present in demineralized sections, but some of the matrix of immature enamel may be visible near ameloblasts of developing teeth.

Ameloblasts are very sensitive to environmental changes. Normal enamel contains *incremental lines of Retzius*, which are analogous to the incremental lines of von Ebner in dentin, and also reflect variations in structure and mineralization. The incremental lines are accentuated during periods of metabolic stress. More severe injury, as in fluorosis, or infections by some viruses can produce focal **hypoplasia or aplasia of enamel.** The *reduced enamel epithelium* protects the enamel of the formed tooth before eruption. Degeneration of this protective layer permits connective tissue to contact the enamel, and there may be resorption of enamel or deposition of a layer of cementum on it. This normally occurs during odontogenesis in horses.

Cementum is an avascular, bone-like substance, produced by *cementoblasts*; it contains ~55% organic and ~45% inorganic matter. In general the dentin of brachydont teeth is covered by cementum wherever it is not covered by enamel. When dentin formation has begun in the root, degeneration of Hertwig's epithelial root sheath begins and permits mesenchymal cells from the dental sac to contact dentin. They differentiate into cementoblasts, which produce *cementoid*, and later mineralize it. Some layers of cementum do not contain cells (acellular cementum), but in other layers, *cementocytes* are enclosed in lacunae. Sharpey's fibers from alveolar bone are embedded in the cementum. Cementum is more resistant to resorption than is bone, and unlike bone, normally is not resorbed and replaced as it ages; instead a new layer of cementum is deposited on top of the old layer. In some pathologic conditions, cementum is resorbed; subsequently, cellular or acellular cementum is deposited, and more or less repairs the defect.

Hypercementosis is abnormal thickening of cementum and may involve part or all of one or many teeth. When extra cementum improves the functional properties of teeth, it is called *cementum hypertrophy*; if not, it is called *cementum hyperplasia*. Extensive hyperplasia is often associated with chronic inflammation of the dental root.

The **periodontal ligament** is derived from the dental follicle. It is well vascularized and very cellular containing fibroblasts, cementoblasts, undifferentiated mesenchymal cells, and epithelial cells. The periodontal ligament contains type I collagen fibers with complex orientation. The **periodontium** comprises the periodontal ligament, gingival lamina propria, cementum, and alveolar bone. The ligament supports the tooth and adjusts to its movement during growth. It is well supplied with nerves and lymphatics, which drain into alveolar bone. The periodontal ligament is also a source of the cells that remodel alveolar bone and, in disease, cementum.

Epithelial rests of Malassez are present in the periodontal ligament and are particularly numerous in the incisor region of sheep. In all species, they may proliferate and become cystic when there is inflammation of the periodontium. The periodontium is also a site of origin of tumors. The periodontal ligament is normally visible in radiographs as a radiolucent line between tooth and alveolar bone. In prolonged hyperparathyroidism, alveolar bone is resorbed, and the ligament is no longer outlined radiographically, a change referred to as *loss of the lamina dura*.

Developmental anomalies of teeth

Anodontia, *absence of teeth*, is inherited in calves, probably as a sex-linked recessive trait in males, and is associated with skin defects. **Oligodontia,** *fewer teeth than normal*, occurs sporadically in horses, cats, and dogs, and also as an inherited trait in dogs. In brachycephalic breeds, the cheek teeth are deficient; in toy breeds, the incisors are deficient. *Pseudo-oligodontia* and *pseudoanodontia* result from failed eruption. Delayed eruption of permanent teeth occurs in Lhasa Apso and Shih Tzu dogs. *X-linked hypohidrotic ectodermal dysplasia* is a heritable condition in dogs that also has been reported in horses, humans, mice, and cattle. In affected individuals, structures of ectodermal origin may be absent or abnormally formed, including teeth.

Polyodontia, *excessive teeth*, occurs in brachycephalic dogs; the incisors are involved, and the defect is probably related to breeding for broad muzzles. A high incidence of canine polyodontia, involving particularly an extra maxillary premolar, is reported from the Netherlands. Polyodontia also occurs in horses and cats, involving either incisors or cheek teeth (molars and premolars). **Pseudopolyodontia** *is retention of deciduous teeth after eruption of the permanent dentition*. It occurs in horses, cats, and dogs, especially in the miniature breeds. Retention of deciduous teeth can be problematic as it may lead to malocclusion.

Heterotopic polyodontia *is an extra tooth, or teeth, outside the dental arcades*. The best-known example is the *ear tooth of horses*, which develops in a branchiogenic cyst. The cysts originate from failure of closure of the first branchial cleft, or from the inclusion of cellular rests in this area. They are lined by a stratified mucous or cutaneous-type epithelium, and may contain one or more teeth, either loosely attached in the cyst wall or deeply embedded in the petrous temporal bone. The tooth is derived from misplaced tooth germ of the first branchial arch, which is displaced toward the ear with the first branchial cleft. The cysts eventually form in the parotid region near the ear and may fistulate to the exterior. They are occasionally bilateral. Rarely the tooth may form a pedunculated mass enclosed by skin, and attached by a pedicle to the skin of the head. Heterotopic polyodontia also occurs in cattle, dogs, pigs, and sheep.

Developmentally **misshapen teeth** are classified as **geminous** (dichotomous) when there is a single root and partially or completely separate crowns; **fused** when the dentin of 2 teeth is confluent; and **concrescent** when the dentin is separate but the roots are joined by cementum. Gemination represents the embryologic partial division of a tooth primordium. It occurs in dogs, usually involving the incisors, and the affected tooth usually has a groove dividing the crowns, whose pulp chambers can be seen radiographically to merge in a common root. Misshapen teeth and missing teeth have also been reported in dogs as an X-linked recessive trait of ectodermal dysplasia. Fusion and concrescence represent the joining of 2 adjacent tooth primordia, one of which may be supernumerary. *Malformation and malpositioning of teeth* accompany abnormalities of the jaw bones. Aberdeen Angus and Hereford calves with congenital osteopetrosis have brachygnathia inferior, malformed mandibles, and impacted cheek teeth. Impacted molars occur as an inherited lethal defect in Shorthorns; an association with osteopetrosis apparently has not been investigated in this breed.

Odontogenic cysts are epithelium-lined cysts derived from epithelium associated with tooth development. This includes rests of Malassez, cell rests of dental laminae, reduced enamel epithelium, or malformed enamel organs. By definition, **dentigerous cysts** are *cysts that contain part or all of a tooth*. Dentigerous cysts usually are associated with permanent teeth. The cyst often forms over the developing tooth and the affected tooth then erupts into the preformed cysts. Dentigerous cysts enclose at least the crown of the tooth, but may include it all. Of the odontogenic cysts, all except those derived from cell rests of Malassez are potentially dentigerous (the rests of Malassez are the probable source of periodontal cysts). Dentigerous cysts originating in malformed enamel organs usually include malformed teeth. Teeth in cysts of reduced enamel epithelium or rests of dental laminae are also often abnormal. The most common forms of odontogenic dentigerous cysts in animals are those involving the *vestigial wolf teeth* of horses and the *vestigial canines*, especially of mares. The smaller cysts appear as tumors of the gums, whereas some of the larger ones may cause swelling of the jaw or adjacent maxillary sinus. In dogs, brachycephalic breeds often develop dentigerous cysts, which can be bilateral. The first premolar is often affected. Dentigerous cysts of animals are not as destructive as those in humans, in which species they are regarded as the most common benign destructive lesion of the skeleton. In dogs, a cyst that resembles *odontogenic keratocyst* of humans has been reported. This cyst is lined by keratinized epithelium and has a high rate of reoccurrence after removal.

The ear tooth of horses is probably the most common nonodontogenic dentigerous cyst. Occasionally true dentigerous cysts form when normal tooth eruption fails or when there is maleruption resulting from odontodystrophy. Tooth eruption can be interrupted by trauma, including fractures to the mandible and maxilla.

Cystic dental inclusions about vestigial supernumerary teeth also occur in juxtamolar positions in cattle, but are insignificant. These too may be dentigerous, or they may be primordial cysts developed before the stage of enamel formation, and hence contain no mineralized tooth structures. Either type of cyst may give rise to ameloblastomas.

A high incidence of dentigerous cysts involving incisors occurs in some sheep flocks in Scotland, Australia, and New Zealand. A congenital disease involving the jaws and teeth of calves in Germany (*odontodysplasia cystica congenita*) is characterized by massive fibro-osseous enlargement of the maxillae and horizontal rami of the mandibles. Some teeth are malformed, misshapen, or absent. Cystic spaces in the jaws are lined by fibrous tissue or epithelium, the latter probably derived from enamel organs. The dental changes are thought to be secondary to those in bone. Most affected calves are aborted or stillborn, and many have ascites and hydrocephalus. The disease may be caused by environmental influences.

The permanent teeth are unique in that they continue to develop for a long time after birth. Thus, inflammatory and metabolic disease of postnatal life, for instance canine distemper virus infection (Fig. 1-3A), can produce hypoplasia of dentin and enamel. Hypoplasia of the enamel of deciduous teeth occurs in some calves with intrauterine bovine viral diarrhea virus infection (Fig. 1-3B). It has also been described in calves and pigs following irradiation of the dam during gestation. Dysplastic proliferation of dentin and enamel involving mandibular premolars and molars has been seen in young uremic dogs. Extreme fragility of deciduous teeth is a feature of *bovine osteogenesis imperfecta* (see Vol. 1, Bones and joints). Dental dysplasia, characterized by normal dentin, absence of enamel matrix, and excess irregular cementum, was described in a foal with epitheliogenesis imperfecta involving the oral mucosa.

Degenerative conditions of teeth and dental tissue

Pigmentation of the teeth. Normal enamel is white and shiny, but normal cementum is off-white to light yellow, and normal dentin is slightly darker yellow. Depending on the tooth, or the part of the tooth being examined, the normal color may be any one of these. Normal enamel is never discolored. Hypoplastic enamel of chronic fluorosis is discolored yellow through brown to almost black. Discoloration of brachydont teeth results from pigmentation of dentin, which is then visible through the semitransparent enamel, or pigmentation of the cementum of the root. Dentin may be colored red-brown by pulpal hemorrhages or inflammation, gray-green in putrid pulpitis, and yellow in icterus. *Amelogenesis imperfecta* is a disorder of enamel formation that leads to inadequate mineralization of enamel and usually yellow discoloration of teeth. This condition has been reported in cattle and in Standard Poodle dogs. *Congenital erythropoietic porphyria* of calves, cats, and swine discolors the dentin red in young animals (pink tooth) and darker brown in adults, although in swine, the discoloration may disappear with aging.

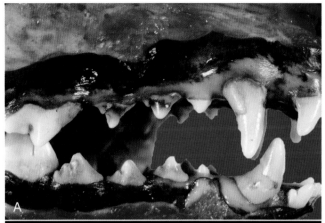
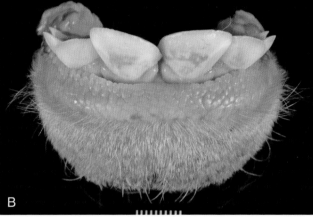

Figure 1-3 Enamel hypoplasia. A. A sequel to canine distemper virus infection in a dog. **B.** Subsequent to intrauterine infection by bovine viral diarrhea virus in a calf. (Courtesy Noah's Arkives.)

Yellow to brown discoloration of teeth, and bright yellow fluorescence in ultraviolet light, caused by deposition of *tetracycline* antibiotics in mineralizing dentin, enamel, and probably cementum, occurs in all species. Treatment of the pregnant dam may cause staining of deciduous teeth in the offspring. Tetracyclines are toxic to ameloblasts in late differentiation and early secretory stages and, at high dose rates, may produce enamel hypoplasia. Black discoloration of ruminant cheek teeth is extremely common, and is caused by impregnation of mineral salts with chlorophyll and porphyrin pigments from herbage.

Dental attrition. *Dental attrition is loss of tooth structure caused by mastication.* The mature conformation of teeth is largely the outcome of opposed growth and wear, and the degree of wear depends on the type of tooth, the species of animal, and the material chewed. Wear is most evident in herbivores, and irregularities of wear are perhaps the most common dental abnormalities, especially in horses. In general, with normal occlusion and use, the extraalveolar portion of the tooth does not shorten. Its length is maintained initially by growth, the period of growth depending on the species, then by hypertrophy of the root cementum and/or dentin and by proliferation of alveolar bone, which serves to push the tooth out. Finally, senile atrophy of the alveolar processes and gingival recession may maintain or increase the length of the clinical crown. Cementum hypertrophy and alveolar atrophy may also result in loss of teeth in senility, or, if combined with subnormal wear, produce teeth that in old age are excessively

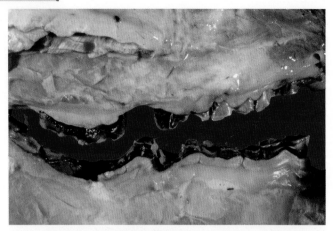

Figure 1-4 **Irregular wear** of the teeth of a horse.

long. Normal wear of the complicated cheek teeth (premolars and molars) of horses and cattle causes smoothing of the occlusal surfaces. As soon as wear of enamel exposes the dentin, which, being softer, wears more rapidly, secondary or tertiary dentin is deposited to protect the pulp. In time, this may fill the pulp cavity and cause death of the tooth. Abnormalities of wear are most common in herbivores (Fig. 1-4). Excessive wear of the deciduous and permanent central incisors occurs in certain sheep flocks in New Zealand. The wear is intermittent and may be severe enough to expose the pulp cavity. The cause is unknown but may be related to delayed eruption of adjacent teeth, leading to increased use of the affected pairs.

Subnormal wear, caused by loss of the opposing tooth, occurs in oligodontia, abnormal spacing of adjacent teeth, and acquired loss of teeth; it results in *abnormal lengthening.* Such elongated teeth may grow against the opposing gum or, if deviated, into an adjacent soft structure such as cheek or lip. These teeth usually wear in abnormal places because complete loss of antagonism is unusual, and, because the upper and lower arcades do not coincide exactly, the coincidence is further reduced by the displacement of chewing.

Abnormal wear resulting from abnormal chewing is caused by voluntary (as in painful conditions) or mechanical impairment of jaw movement. Incomplete longitudinal alignment of the molar arcades allows irregular wear and hook formation on the first and last cheek teeth. Lateral movements of the jaws without the normal rotary grinding movements allow the ridges of the teeth of herbivores to become accentuated. Steep angulation of the occlusal surfaces results from inadequate lateral movement of the jaws, and sharp edges form on the buccal aspect of the maxillary teeth and the lingual aspect of the mandibular teeth. This may be unilateral when the animal chews with only one side of its mouth, the other side then being affected. The teeth wear progressively sharper, and can result in the teeth passing each other like shear blades; hence the term **shear mouth.** Subnormal resistance to wear on the part of the molar teeth is common, and results in **wave mouth** (weave mouth) or **step mouth,** in which successive teeth in an arcade wear at different rates. The wave or step form of the antagonistic arcade is reversed, so that the teeth of the 2 arcades interdigitate. This pattern of attrition is caused by variation in the hardness of opposing teeth, and is usually caused by intermittent odontodystrophy. Opposing teeth of the upper and lower jaws do not develop at the same time;

thus discontinuous nutritional deficiencies often result in unequal wear. Certain vices, such as crib biting, also produce abnormal wear. In severely worn ruminant incisors, a central black core may be visible, which is secondary dentin deposited in the pulp cavity. It is not carious, but stains darker than the surrounding primary dentin.

Odontodystrophies. *Odontodystrophies are diseases of teeth caused by nutritional, metabolic, and toxic insults.* They are manifest by changes in the hard tissues of the teeth and their supporting structures and often occur during the period of tooth development. Lesions of enamel and dentin are emphasized here. The most prominent effects of odontodystrophies appear in enamel, and lesions of enamel are most significant because they are irreparable.

Formation of enamel occurs in a set pattern. It begins at the occlusal surface and progresses toward the root. Mineral maturation occurs in the same sequence, but for each level, it begins at the dentin-enamel junction and moves toward the ameloblast. Deleterious influences have their most severe effects on those ameloblasts that are forming and mineralizing enamel. Depending on the severity on the insult, ameloblasts may produce no enamel, a little enamel, or poorly mineralized enamel. Removal of the insult permits those ameloblasts that were not yet active to begin making normal enamel. Thus enamel defects vary in severity from isolated opaque spots or pits on the surface to deep and irregular horizontal indentations. These defects are most clearly seen on the incisor teeth and canine teeth and are usually bilaterally symmetrical. Similar lesions are also produced by infectious agents that injure ameloblasts, such as canine distemper virus and bovine viral diarrhea virus (see Fig. 1-3).

Odontoblasts are susceptible to many of the same influences as ameloblasts, but they can be replenished from the undifferentiated cells of the dental pulp. Thus lesions in actively forming dentin may be repaired, whereas those in enamel are permanent.

Because of their close anatomical association with the bones of the jaws, teeth are very susceptible to disruption in the harmony of growth. This harmonious arrangement is often upset in the odontodystrophies and osteodystrophies, which may lead to malocclusion, anomalous development of teeth, and tooth loss.

Several nutritional and toxic conditions produce odontodystrophy. **Fluorine poisoning** is exemplary (see Vol. 1, Bones and joints). In **vitamin A deficiency,** ameloblasts do not differentiate normally, and their organizing ability is disturbed. As a result, odontoblastic differentiation is abnormal. Several lesions develop, including enamel hypoplasia and hypomineralization, vascularized dentin (osteodentin), and retarded or failed tooth eruption.

Calcium deficiency retards eruption and causes enamel hypoplasia and mild dentin hypoplasia. Teeth formed during the period of deficiency are very susceptible to wear. In sheep, recovery from prolonged calcium deficiency results in malocclusion caused by inferior prognathia. This reflects inadequate maxillary but normal mandibular repair during the recovery phase.

Phosphorus deficiency, combined with vitamin D deficiency, depresses dentin formation slightly, but has virtually no effect on enamel, at least not in sheep. Hypophosphatemia is associated with formation of interglobular dentin in humans. Malocclusion and abnormalities of bite in rachitic sheep are secondary to mandibular deformity.

Severe, experimental **malnutrition** also produces malocclusion. Recovery from malnutrition does not correct the lesion, and in addition, is associated with misshapen, malformed teeth, oligodontia, and polyodontia.

The major **effects of odontodystrophies** in herbivores are *malocclusion*, and/or accelerated *attrition*. Sometimes a high incidence of these abnormalities is attributable to one of the causes previously discussed, but often they are idiopathic.

A syndrome of dental abnormalities of sheep in the North Island of New Zealand is characterized by excessive wear of deciduous teeth, maleruption and excessive wear of permanent teeth, periodontal disease involving permanent teeth, and development of dentigerous cysts involving permanent incisors. Mandibular osteopathy is also present. Animals older than 5 years are culled for dental problems. The odontodystrophy (and osteodystrophy) is possibly caused by deficiencies of calcium and copper, and perhaps other nutrients, such as protein, and energy. This syndrome exemplifies the naturally occurring odontodystrophies, in that it probably has a complex pathogenesis, and is associated with an osteodystrophy. The latter association is to be expected, because bones and teeth are usually susceptible to the same insults.

Although dental lesions are not described, tooth loss caused by periosteal dysplasia and osteopenia occurs in Salers cattle afflicted with hereditary hemochromatosis.

Infectious and inflammatory diseases of teeth and periodontium

The role of viruses in enamel hypoplasia is mentioned previously. Bacterial plaque, along with other tooth-accumulated materials, is discussed here.

Bacterial diseases involving tooth surfaces are caused by the development of supragingival and subgingival **plaque**. *Supragingival plaque* is located on the exposed crown of the tooth and causes dental caries. *Subgingival plaque* is found in the crevicular groove and causes periodontal disease. Tooth enamel is covered by a translucent pellicle, the *acquired enamel pellicle*, which is formed by selective adsorption of complex salivary proteins, and that is essential to the development of supragingival plaque. This is a dense, nonmineralized, bacterial mass, firmly adherent to tooth surfaces, which resists removal by salivary flow and prevents the buffering capacity of saliva from influencing plaque metabolites. Formation of this plaque involves adhesion of bacteria to the pellicle, and adhesion of bacteria to each other, producing a *biofilm*. Initial bacterial binding to the tooth surface is reversible through electrostatic and hydrophobic interactions, but this transitions to permanent receptor mediated binding.

Only organisms with the ability to adhere to the pellicle can initiate the formation of supragingival plaque; those that cannot are removed by oral secretions and mechanical action. Pathologic reduction of salivary flow, or regions of teeth where flow is reduced (interproximal regions and areas of pits or fissures) increases the prevalence of caries in some species.

The bacteria in supragingival plaque are members of the indigenous oral flora and are usually gram-positive aerobes. Most are streptococci and *Actinomyces* spp., which form an organized array on the tooth surface. Some plaque-forming bacteria synthesize extracellular polymers, which constitute the matrix of the plaque and permit adhesion between organisms of the same species. Some utilize polymers derived from host secretions to adhere to the pellicle, whereas others attach to bacteria of a different species that are already fixed to the tooth. Plaque increases in mass with time, and its composition becomes more complex as anaerobic gram-negative bacteria join the streptococci and actinomycetes that initiated plaque formation.

Supragingival plaque is metabolically active. It utilizes dietary carbohydrates to produce the adhesive polymers and the acids needed to demineralize enamel, and as energy sources for maintenance and for production of various enzymes and stimuli for inflammation. Extensive deposits of supragingival plaque are virtually invisible unless treated with a disclosing solution.

Subgingival plaque is less organized than supragingival plaque, and many of the organisms involved are gram-negative anaerobes that are asaccharolytic, weakly adherent, and motile. They derive their nutrients from the crevicular fluid. The flora of subgingival plaque is less well characterized than that of supragingival plaque. Culture results vary with sample collection technique, site of collection, and selectivity of media, and appear to under-represent the flora detected by molecular means in humans. A number of species including *Bacteroides* spp., *Actinomyces* spp., *Porphyromonas* spp., *Tannerella forsythia*, and spirochetes have been associated with gingivitis and periodontal disease in animals.

Dental calculus (*tartar*) *is mineralized supragingival and subgingival plaque*. In supragingival plaque it is formed by the deposition of mineral, mainly from saliva, in dead bacteria. In subgingival plaque, mineral is generated from gingival crevicular fluid. In horses and dogs, calculus is predominantly calcium carbonate. Calculus is often found in old dogs and cats, occasionally in horses and sheep, and rarely in other species. The distribution is often uneven, but it is *usually most abundant next to the orifices of salivary ducts*. Calculus on horses' teeth is chalky and easily removed. In dogs, it is hard, firmly attached, and often discolored. Red-brown to black calculus with a metallic sheen develops in pastured sheep and goats. It usually involves all the incisors, principally on the neck of the buccal surface. Minor amounts are common along the gum-tooth junction of the molar teeth, but occasionally larger (up to 2 cm) hard, black, rounded concretions may protrude from between opposed surfaces of the premolars. A high prevalence of calculus in sheep on the Scottish island of North Ronaldsay was related to their predominantly seaweed diet. Calculus was most severe around the cranial cheek teeth, increased in severity with age, was associated with periodontal disease, and contained large amounts of calcium, magnesium, and phosphorus.

Materia alba, which adheres to teeth, is a mixture of salivary proteins, desquamated epithelial cells, disintegrating leukocytes, and bacteria. The bacteria are not organized, and materia alba is easily removed. It is distinct from dental plaque, and from food debris, which also accumulates between uncleaned teeth.

Dental caries. Dental caries is a disease of the hard tissues of teeth, characterized by *demineralization of the inorganic part and enzymatic degradation of the organic matrix*. **Erosions** of teeth are characterized by removal of hard tissues layer by layer. These definitions permit the inclusion of equine infundibular necrosis as a form of caries (see following sections). Caries is common in horses and sheep but rare in dogs. Cats are commonly subject to caries-like odontoclastic resorptive lesions of uncertain etiopathogenesis.

There are 2 types of caries:

1. **Pit or fissure caries** develops in irregularities or indentations, which trap food and bacteria, usually on the occlusal surface of the tooth. Plaque is not essential for initiation of this form of caries, of which *equine infundibular necrosis* is an example.
2. **Smooth-surface caries** usually occurs on proximal (adjacent) surfaces of teeth, typically just below contact points, or around the neck, and requires dental plaque for its initiation.

The organic acids, principally lactic, which initiate demineralization, are produced by bacterial fermentation of dietary carbohydrates. In smooth-surface caries, plaque produces the acid and maintains a low pH on the surface of the tooth. Progression of lesions depends on various factors such as salivary pH, hardness and resistance to demineralization of enamel, and frequency of access to carbohydrate. Demineralization of enamel often occurs in the subsurface enamel but progresses to caries only with prolonged exposure to acid. Infrequent exposure allows remineralization of enamel between meals. The enzymes that lyse the organic matrix are probably produced by plaque, but may be derived from leukocytes, for which plaque is chemotactic. Carious enamel loses its sheen and becomes dull, white, and pocked. When dentin is exposed, it becomes brown or black. Dentin is softer and more readily demineralized than enamel, and a pinpoint lesion in enamel may lead to a large defect when the carious process reaches the dentin. Enamel loss to caries is permanent, whereas odontoblasts at the pulp/dentin junction can generate tertiary dentin in response to dentin damage and loss. Nerve endings have not been identified at the enamel-dentin junction, and the pain of caries is thought to be caused by chemical or pressure changes in the dentinal tubules. Neuropeptides, including substance P, are generated in the pulp and may enhance pain during caries. Spread of infection along the dental tubules to the pulp cavity may result in formation of reparative dentin, pulpitis, or periapical inflammation and tooth loss.

In **horses, infundibular necrosis** is the most common form of caries. It develops most often on the occlusal surface of the maxillary first molar. The enamel invaginations (infundibula) in the cheek teeth of horses are normally filled with cementum before the teeth erupt. Filling proceeds from the occlusal surface toward the apex, but often is not completed before eruption. At this time the blood supply is cut off, and ischemic necrosis of any residual cementogenic tissue in the infundibula occurs (Fig. 1-5A). The deficiency of cementum is called *hypoplasia.*

Teeth with incompletely filled infundibula may accumulate food material and bacteria. This can lead to bacterial fermentation and lactic acid production that demineralizes the cementum over the infundibulum (Fig. 1-5B). In some animals, the cavitated area expands to involve all the cementum and the adjacent enamel and dentin. This may result in coalescence of adjacent infundibulum and creation of a large defect in the occlusal surface. Decay of the mineralized tissues and coalescence of infundibula may progress to fracture of the tooth, root abscess, and empyema of the paranasal sinuses. The incidence of infundibular necrosis increases with age, and 80-100% of horses older than 12 years may have the lesion. Most are without signs, and in most, the lesion does not progress. Inflammation of the dental pulp, in horses and in other species, may result from direct expansion of caries from penetration of bacteria and bacterial degradation products along

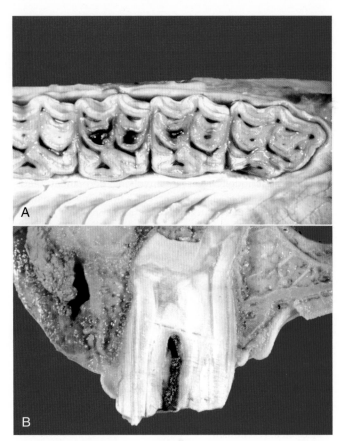

Figure 1-5 A. Infundibular necrosis of first and second maxillary molars in a horse. Necrosis is confined to cement lakes. **B.** Section through (**A**) showing black discoloration of infundibulum.

the dentinal tubules. Production of reparative dentin in the pulp cavity is expected. Horses may also develop *peripheral caries* outside of the infundibulum. This typically occurs in the caudal cheek teeth and leads to loss of cementum that may contribute to irregular wear and periodontal disease.

In **sheep,** the proximal surfaces of mandibular teeth are usually affected by caries, which is commonly accompanied by periodontitis. Erosions of the neck region of the deciduous teeth occurred in sheep in New Zealand. The lesions were mainly located apical to the enamel-dentin junction on the labial or lingual surface. They did not seem to be related to the usual causes of localized tooth destruction.

Cattle develop loss of dentin just below the crown of incisor teeth at increasing frequency with age. This usually follows recession of the gingiva, and is not considered to be a form of caries, but proteolytic digestion of dentin by chyme in an alkaline pH.

In **dogs,** caries most commonly involves the fourth premolar and the first and second molars. Although relatively uncommon, when caries occurs, defects are often multiple and advanced, leading to therapeutic extraction.

Cats, whose teeth do not have centers where food can collect, very commonly develop multiple caries-like **odontoclastic resorptive lesions,** initially involving the subgingival neck or upper root, most often of cheek teeth, and increasing in prevalence with age. This is not a true caries lesion. Odontoclasts are similar to osteoclasts and participate in absorption of roots of deciduous teeth. For reasons that are not entirely clear, they are recruited or form at the tooth and begin to resorb enamel and eventually dentin. A reddened swollen area of gingiva or granulation tissue often lies over the lesion, which may be on the labial or buccal aspect, and frequently is painful to touch. The resorptive lesions begin as shallow defects in the cementum, lined by odontoclasts, facing a somewhat disorganized periodontal ligament. They progress into the underlying dentin, and, with time, into the root canal. Either or both coronal and apical extension of lesions may occur. Extension of the process coronally more superficially undermines the enamel, which is resorbed or breaks off, causing destruction or loss of the crown. Extension of the dentinal lesion apically leads to resorption of the root. Remnants of the root may persist, often overgrown by gingiva, following loss of the crown. Conversely, destruction primarily of the root may result in obliteration of the periodontal ligament, resorption of adjacent alveolar bone, but with odontoalveolar ankylosis by reparative hard tissues, retaining the crown in the dental arcade. In addition to the odontoclasts that line the resorbing cementum or dentinal surfaces of the lesion, more advanced defects contain a mixed leukocyte population, macrophages, and disordered granulation tissue. Repair is often superimposed, with cementoblastic or osteoblastic cells producing new mineralized tissue of varied osteoid, bone, cementum, or osteodentin morphology. Pulpitis may occur in the affected root canal, and reparative dentin may be deposited there. The prevalence of such lesions has increased markedly in the past 40 years, suggesting an association with changes in form of diet, but the lesion is idiopathic, with no clear relationship to periodontitis, mechanical trauma, viral infections, or nutritional or metabolic disturbances. A number of factors have been proposed to be involved with feline resorptive lesions, including local inflammatory mediators, increased vitamin D intake, and local pH.

Pulpitis. The dental pulp is derived from the dental papilla. It is surrounded by odontoblasts and dentin, except at the apical foramen, through which vessels and nerves pass. Pulp is a loose syncytium of stellate fibroblasts, and contains histiocytes and undifferentiated mesenchymal cells. The latter are odontoblastic precursors.

The apical foramen is located at the apex of the root and is where blood vessels and nerves enter the tooth. The apical foramen is narrow, and this predisposes to vascular occlusion, ischemic necrosis of the pulp, and death of the tooth. Production of abundant secondary dentin and reparative dentin can cause occlusion, but the usual cause is inflammation. Normally, pulp is the only vascular tissue of the tooth, and, along with the periodontium, the only site of conventional inflammation. *Pulpitis is always related to infection*, the effect of bacteria or their products entering through the surface of fractured teeth, carious perforations (especially in teeth with enamel defects), perforations resulting from abnormal wear or trimming, from periodontitis, and possibly hematogenously. In herbivores, in which the pulp is divided by enamel foldings, inflammation is usually limited to one division, and is usually purulent. Very mild pulpitis may heal, but usually it terminates in tooth necrosis, periapical abscessation, perhaps with fistula formation, osteomyelitis, or gangrene as inflammation of the pulp extends to the periodontium and the jaws.

Periapical abscess and osteomyelitis of the jaws are complications of pulpitis that may follow clipping the tusks ("needle teeth") of piglets. Trimming of the incisor teeth of sheep to avoid the effects of broken mouth often exposes the pulp cavity, but the pulpitis that ensues is rarely chronic.

The exposed pulp canal is healed in 30-50 days by deposition of reparative dentin and secondary dentin. Similar healing presumably occurs in most piglets. Maxillary (malar) abscess of dogs involves the periapical tissues usually of the carnassial tooth, and may cause a discharging sinus beneath the eye. The pathogenesis of the abscess is obscure, but it may be a sequel to crown fractures or to pressure necrosis of periapical tissues. Some chronic inflammations of the pulp become slowly expansive spherical granulomas about the root apex (root granulomas). Occasionally these granulomas are enclosed by an epithelial cyst (periodontal cyst) derived from cell rests of Malassez. The epithelium contains plasma cells, and the combination may have a protective role in periapical sepsis.

Periodontal disease. Periodontal disease is the *most common dental disease of dogs and sheep*, and an important problem in other ruminants, horses, and cats. Although there are minor differences among species, in general, periodontal disease *begins as gingivitis associated with subgingival plaque*, and may progress through gingival recession and loss of alveolar bone to chronic periodontitis and exfoliation of teeth.

The gingival sulcus, or crevice, is an invagination formed by the gingiva as it joins with the tooth surface at the time of eruption. Clinically normal animals have a few lymphocytes, plasma cells, and macrophages under the crevicular epithelium of the gingiva, which forms the outer wall of the crevice. Low numbers of lymphocytes, plasma cells, and macrophages are also present under the junctional epithelium, which is apposed to the enamel of the tooth.

Clinical **gingivitis** is usually initiated by accumulation of plaque in the crevice, but may be associated with impaction of feed, especially seeds, between teeth. Gingivitis is initially characterized by increased numbers of leukocytes and fluid in the gingival crevice, and then by acute exudative inflammation and accumulation of neutrophils, plasma cells, lymphocytes, and macrophages in the marginal gingiva. If the disease progresses, marked loss of gingival collagen fibers, which hold the gingiva to the adjacent tooth, occurs in a few days. This is probably related to the activity of prostaglandins and matrix metalloproteinases generated in inflamed tissue, or possibly enzymes from plaque bacteria, such as *Porphyromonas gingivalis*, which also produce enzymes (gingipains) thought to damage junctional epithelium. *Porphyromonas* spp. are implicated as obligate pathogens for canine gingivitis, and as probable participants in feline gingivitis/periodontitis. Grossly the gingiva is red and swollen because of the hyperemia and edema of inflammation. Acute gingivitis may become quiescent, with lymphocyte aggregations beneath the junctional epithelium. Halitosis is associated with gingivitis in small animals.

Continuation and exacerbations of the inflammation cause apical recession of the tooth-gingiva junction, and resorption of alveolar bone (Fig. 1-6). Alterations in the periodontal flora may be responsible for these exacerbations. A major part of chronic periodontal disease is *resorption of alveolar bone*, which modifies the attachment site of the periodontal ligament. If concomitant bone loss precedes gingival recession, the sulcus is deepened to form a periodontal pocket, which is lined by transformed junctional "pocket" epithelium, and becomes the site of chronic active inflammation. When gingival recession precedes loss of alveolar bone and gingival collagen, pockets do not form, but tooth roots are exposed. In either case, destruction of the periodontium and periodontal ligament,

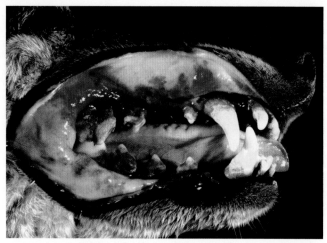

Figure 1-6 Marked gingival recession with exposure of roots of the molar teeth in advanced **periodontal disease** in a dog.

and resorption of alveolar bone, cementum, and root dentin, *lead to exfoliation of teeth.*

Gingivitis is common in **dogs.** Usually it is proliferative, the gingiva being replaced by collagen-poor, highly vascular granulation tissue, which appears as a red, rolled edge next to the tooth. In dogs, gingival pocket formation is quite unpredictable and may be present on one root of a tooth and absent on the other. Bone loss in dogs is often more severe at the bifurcation of two-rooted teeth than in interproximal areas (gingiva between teeth). Resorption of bone is associated with osteitis as the inflammation extends from the periodontium into alveolar bone. In dogs, the premolars and, to a lesser extent, the first molars and central incisors are most severely affected, whereas the second molars and mandibular canines are quite resistant.

Gingivitis is among the most common veterinary problems in **cats.** In general, it resembles that in dogs. Gingivitis in cats is also associated with the feline stomatitis/glossitis complex addressed in the following sections.

In **sheep,** periodontal disease may involve all teeth, but the effects are most severe on the incisors, and periodontal disease is a major cause of premature exfoliation. Sheep develop acute gingivitis during tooth eruption, in association with accumulation of subgingival plaque around the tooth. In some sheep, chronic gingivitis involving the lingual aspect of the incisors ensues, and on farms with a high incidence of broken mouth (lengthening of the incisor crown, forward protrusion, and loosening of the teeth), this progresses to chronic active periodontal disease.

Cara inchada (swollen face) is an epidemic periodontitis of **cattle,** formerly common in the west-central part of Brazil. Animals of 2-14 months were mostly affected, and herd prevalences of more than 50% were recorded. When progressive, cara inchada causes loss of teeth, leading to malnutrition. It is associated with dental eruption, and ingestion of forage thought to contain low levels of antibiotics derived from soil actinomycetes that permit colonization of the periodontal space by a variety of gram-negative bacteria, including *Prevotella* (*Bacteroides*) *melaninogenica.*

Severe periodontitis and tooth loss are an important part of the syndrome associated with *bovine leukocyte adhesion deficiency.*

The sequelae of suppurative periodontitis are many, being mainly variations on a theme of *osteomyelitis.* The osteomyelitis of actinomycosis is discussed in Vol. 1, Bones and joints. If the mandible is involved, the fistula usually develops on the ventral margin. If the maxillary molars are involved, fistulation may occur into the maxillary sinus. If the premolars are involved, fistulation may develop into the nasal cavity or externally. In dogs, involvement of the canine teeth may produce internal or external fistulae, and involvement of the maxillary carnassials usually produces a fistula beneath the eye, and orbital inflammation. Fistulation may be prevented for some time, or permanently, by ossifying periostitis over the involved bone. Fistulae in the upper jaw tend to be persistent. In the lower jaw, they may heal, usually with extensive deposition of new bone. Occasionally, especially in horses, chronic mild periodontitis may be confined by the periodontium, which is, however, expanded by granulation tissue to form a root granuloma. Under the same circumstances, there may be hyperplastic exostosis of the cementum.

Further reading

Booij-Vrieling HE, et al. Increased vitamin D-driven signalling and expression of the vitamin D receptor, MSX2, and RANKL in tooth resorption in cats. Eur J Oral Sci 2010;118:39-46.

D'Astous J. An overview of dentigerous cysts in dogs and cats. Can Vet J 2011;52:905-907.

Di Bello A, et al. Periodontal disease associated with red complex bacteria in dogs. J Small Anim Pract 2014;55:160-163.

Dobereiner J, et al. The etiology of "cara inchada," a bovine epizootic periodontitis in Brazil. Pesq Vet Bras 2004;24:50-56.

Lewis JR, et al. Dental abnormalities associated with X-linked hypohidrotic ectodermal dysplasia in dogs. Orthod Craniofac Res 2010;13:40-47.

Mannerfelt T, et al. Enamel defects in standard poodle dogs in Sweden. Vet Dent 2009;26:213-215.

Miles AEW, Gregson C. Colyer's Variations and Diseases of the Teeth of Animals. Cambridge, UK: Cambridge University Press; 1990.

Muzylak M, et al. The in vitro effect of pH on osteoclasts and bone resorption in the cat: implications for the pathogenesis of FORL. J Cell Physiol 2007;213(1):144-150.

Niemiec B. Veterinary Periodontology. Ames, IA: Wiley-Blackwell; 2013.

Riggio MP, et al. Molecular identification of bacteria associated with canine periodontal disease. Vet Microbiol 2011;150:394-400.

Sacerdote P, Levrini L. Peripheral mechanisms of dental pain: the role of substance P. Mediators Inflamm 2012;2012:95190.

Diseases of the buccal cavity and mucosa
Pigmentation

Melanotic pigmentation is normal and common in most breeds of animals and increases with age. It may be irregular, or the mucosa may be entirely pigmented. Diffuse yellow discoloration may be seen in icterus.

Circulatory disturbances

Examination of the mucous membranes is an essential detail in any clinical or postmortem examination. Pallor may indicate anemia. In cyanosis, the mucosa is dark red-blue. The mucosa are muddy in methemoglobinemia. Acute congestion and cyanosis, associated with ulceration, are common in dogs and sometimes in cats with chronic uremia. Hemorrhages are indicative of septicemia, and larger ones may accompany local inflammation, trauma, and the hemorrhagic diatheses. Petechiae on the ventral surface of the tongue and frenulum in horses are consistent with equine infectious anemia, or other thrombocytopenic or purpuric conditions. The active hyperemia that gives the diffuse pink coloration to the mucosa in diffuse stomatitis disappears immediately at death, so that at autopsy the inflamed mucosa is disappointingly blanched.

Foreign bodies in the oral cavity

The presence of feed in the mouth of a cadaver is abnormal, except in ruminants, which may eructate and have feed in the caudal pharynx at the time of death. In most cases it is attributable to disease, which results in paralysis of deglutition or semiconsciousness. It is common in horses with encephalitis, leukoencephalomalacia, and hepatic encephalopathy. The food in such cases is usually poorly masticated and readily differentiated from that refluxed postmortem. Bones or other large foreign bodies lodged in the pharynx of cattle suggest pica of phosphorus deficiency. They may cause asphyxiation or pressure necrosis in the wall of the pharynx. Large portions of root crops may also lodge in the pharynx. Dogs often have bones and sticks that tend to be wedged across the palate behind the carnassial teeth.

In dogs, **foreign-body stomatitis** occurs, caused by plant fibers, burrs, or quills (Fig. 1-7). In mild cases, gingivitis surrounds the incisors and canine teeth. Small papules or vesicles and shallow ulcers may be evident on the tongue. Plant fibers may protrude from the lesions. Chronic cases are characterized by *exuberant granulomas* associated with lingual ulceration and gingival hyperplasia with plant fibers deeply embedded in these lesions. Long-haired dogs are especially prone to develop this type of lesion when they attempt to remove plant material that is trapped in their hair coat. The granulomas must be differentiated from neoplasms.

Sharp foreign bodies that cause laceration of the mucosa predispose to necrotic and deep stomatitis. Grass seeds and awns frequently impact between the retracted gingival margin and teeth in periodontitis of ruminants and exacerbate the local initial lesion, perhaps predisposing to the development of osteomyelitis. Metallic objects, including wire, may lacerate the oral mucosa, especially in cattle. Horses fed dry triticale hay may develop severe oral ulceration, with masses of awns

embedded in the ulcers. The ulcers vary in size from 1 mm to 5 cm in diameter and are mainly located at the junction of the labial and gingival mucosa adjacent to the upper corner incisors, the lingual frenulum, the sublingual folds, the base of the dorsum of the tongue, and the soft palate. Similar lesions in horses have been associated with contamination of hay by foxtail.

Swine have a diverticulum of the pharynx in the caudal wall immediately above the esophagus, and barley awns and other rough plant fibers occasionally lodge here and penetrate the pharynx. This occurs mainly in young pigs, and death follows pharyngeal cellulitis. Similar problems occur in sheep following improper use of drenching guns, and in cattle injured by balling guns.

Inflammation of the oral cavity

Inflammatory processes of the oral cavity (*stomatitis*) may be diffuse or focal and they may predominantly affect certain regions to produce, if (1) the pharynx is involved, *pharyngitis*; (2) the tongue, *glossitis*; (3) the gums, *gingivitis*; (4) the tonsils, *tonsillitis* (Fig. 1-8); and (5) the soft palate, *angina*. Lesions limited to the mucosa of the oral cavity are termed *superficial stomatitides*. Processes seated in connective tissues of the mouth, the *deep stomatitides*, are usually sequelae to transient superficial lesions.

Superficial stomatitis. Inflammatory changes may be associated with ingestion of irritating chemicals such as caustic or toxic compounds. An example is paraquat, a herbicide that may cause severe erosive stomatitis in dogs. Dogs and cats that chew on the plant *Dieffenbachia* may develop oral erosions and ulcers. Electrical burns are occasionally seen in puppies or kittens that chew through electrical wires. It is often not possible to differentiate the cause of diffuse stomatitis, but an attempt to do so is important because it may indicate a systemic disease state. Viral diseases causing stomatitis will be considered in detail in the section on Infectious and parasitic diseases of the alimentary tract later in this chapter.

Inflammatory disease, localized to the buccal cavity and not part of systemic viral disease, is also common and important. It is generally caused by the indigenous bacterial flora. The oral microbiota ordinarily contains many microbial species,

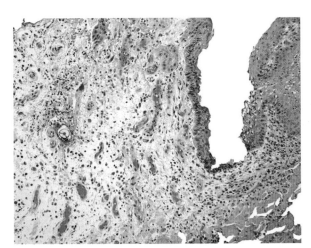

Figure 1-7 Granulomatous reaction to plant material and hair in the tongue of a dog; **foreign-body glossitis**.

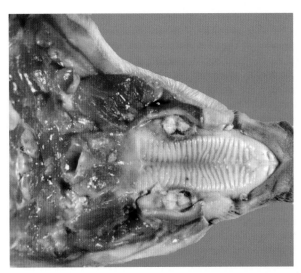

Figure 1-8 Necrotic palatine **tonsillitis** in a pig. (Courtesy Noah's Arkives and A. Doster.)

mainly anaerobes such as *Actinomyces*, *Fusobacterium*, and spirochetes, which exist in balance with each other and in harmony with the host. Disruption of this microfloral balance may lead to stomatitis. The oral mucosa is quite resistant to microbial invasion for several reasons. These include the squamous mucosal lining; antibacterial constituents of saliva such as lysozyme; immunoglobulins, especially immunoglobulin A (IgA), in oral secretions; and the presence of a rich submucosal vascular network and inflammatory cells. Factors altering the balance of indigenous organisms are not well delineated. Systemic illness, stress, and nutritional and hormonal imbalances may alter the microbial population by altering the amount, composition, and pH of saliva. The integrity of the oral epithelium depends on a high rate of epithelial regeneration to balance loss resulting from a high rate of abrasion and desquamation. Rapid epithelial replication promotes quick healing of superficial lesions.

The lamina propria of the oral epithelium is well vascularized, but generally dense and relatively inelastic. For this reason, there is little distention of lymphatics and tissue spaces with fluid exudate, and therefore swelling resulting from edema is not a significant part of stomatitis involving hard palate and gums, with the exception of the gingival margins.

Catarrhal stomatitis. *Catarrhal stomatitis is superficial inflammation of the oral mucosa*, which usually involves the caudal fauces and may be associated with mild gingivitis. It is a common nonspecific lesion, which often develops in the course of debilitating diseases. The mucosae are hyperemic, and the loose texture of the submucosa in the fauces permits development of edema. The swelling is aggravated by edema and hyperplasia of the abundant lymphoid tissues of the soft palate, tonsil, and pharyngeal mucosa. The epithelium accumulates, producing a dull gray mucosal surface. Palatine glands produce excessive mucus. Catarrhal stomatitis resolves with the return of normal oral function.

Thrush, or **oral candidiasis,** occurs most commonly in foals, pigs, and dogs. It involves the proliferation of yeasts and hyphae in the parakeratotic superficial layers of the oral epithelium. It appears grossly as patchy pale-gray pseudomembranous material on the oral mucosa and back of the tongue, and probably reflects alterations in epithelial turnover and oral microbiota (see section on Infectious and parasitic diseases of the alimentary tract, later in this chapter). Mold products of *Stachybotrys alternans* cause catarrhal and necrotizing stomatitis, as well as colitis, if feed is contaminated. Gingivitis and ulceration of the oral mucosa may rarely be associated with infection caused by *Nocardia* spp. in dogs.

Vesicular stomatitides. Stomatitis characterized by the formation of *vesicles* occurs in most species of domestic animals. The vesicles develop as accumulations of serous fluid within the epithelium or between the epithelium and the lamina propria. These may coalesce to form *bullae*, and the elevated epithelium is easily rubbed off during chewing to leave raw eroded patches with bits of epithelium adherent. *The transition from vesicle to erosion occurs rapidly*, so that, in individual animals, vesicles may not be seen. This is especially so in dogs and cats because the oral mucosa is very thin. Because the basal epithelium or basement membrane remains intact, regeneration and healing are complete in a few days unless the local lesions are complicated by bacterial or mycotic infections. However, foci of previous erosion may be identifiable for some months by their slight depression and lack of pigmentation.

Traditionally, vesicular stomatitides in animals were associated with *viral infections*, and these are still important causes. Vesicular stomatitis and foot-and-mouth disease are associated initially with vesicle formation; however, rinderpest, bovine viral diarrhea, and malignant catarrhal fever produce sharply demarcated erosive/ulcerative lesions without initial vesicle formation. *Oral erosions and ulcers in horses, ruminants, and swine should be regarded as indicating one of the vesicular diseases to which the species is susceptible, until proved otherwise* (see section on Infectious and parasitic diseases of the alimentary tract, later in this chapter). Sunburn, photoirritation associated with grazing on celery and related crops, and lesions associated with parvovirus infection in swine may cause lesions of the snout resembling vesicular diseases. Animals exposed to irritant chemicals in feed or bedding may develop vesicles and erosions of the face and oral cavity, for example, toxicity in horses and dogs associated with irritant quassinoids found in wood shavings derived from *Simaroubaceae* species.

Bullous immune skin diseases are recognized with increased frequency, especially in dogs, and some of these have severe oral lesions, which are described here (see also Vol. 1, Integumentary system).

Pemphigus vulgaris is a severe, acute or chronic, vesiculobullous autoimmune disease mediated by autoantibodies to the desmosome protein desmoglein 3, which is involved in joining adjacent epithelial cells to each other. Desmoglein is highly expressed in suprabasal oral epithelium. Pemphigus vulgaris is most common in dogs and cats with rare reports in horses. It is characterized by acantholysis of the epidermis, which results in formation of flaccid bullae and erosions involving mainly mucocutaneous junctions, oral mucosa and, to a lesser extent, skin. Canine pemphigus vulgaris follows a similar pathogenesis to that of humans with overexpression of the proto-oncogene *c-Myc* before acantholysis and bullae formation. *c-Myc* overexpression is likely a consequence of anti-desmoglein 3 antibody binding to its target on basal keratinocytes. Clinically affected dogs and cats have erosions/ulcerations of the oral mucosa and may drool. The oral lesions are generally more prominent than, and precede, the skin lesions. They are most obvious on the dorsal surface of the tongue, which is bright red, with a few scattered pink raised areas representing islands of normal mucosa. The lesions vary greatly in severity and distribution, although the hard palate is often severely ulcerated. Bullae are rarely seen in the oral cavity, because they ulcerate rapidly. Oral pemphigus vulgaris lesions have also been associated with drug reactions in dogs and cats.

Microscopically, the earliest lesion consists of *suprabasilar acantholysis*, which is followed by the formation of clefts. These lead to ulceration of the mucosa. The basal cells of the epidermis remain attached to the basement membrane and form a so-called "row of tombstones." A few neutrophils and eosinophils may infiltrate the epithelium. There is a variable lymphocytic and plasmacytic lichenoid reaction in the propria. *The presence of suprabasilar clefts and bullae caused by acantholysis is considered to be diagnostic of pemphigus vulgaris.* However, extensive erosion and ulceration of the mucosa and secondary bacterial infections frequently obscure these clefts and bullae. Several biopsies from different areas of the oral mucosa may be required to demonstrate the characteristic lesions. A presumptive histologic diagnosis should be supported by direct immunofluorescence tests that show autoantibodies (usually IgG) and complement in the intercellular spaces of stratified squamous epithelium.

Bullous pemphigoid is a term that has been applied generically to superficial autoimmune vesiculobullous or ulcerative disease of mucous membranes (including the oral mucosa) and skin, characterized by subepithelial clefting; acantholysis is not a feature. It has been reported in humans, horses, dogs, and cats. It is now recognized that there is a *complex of autoimmune subepidermal blistering diseases*, varying in their target antigen, clinical manifestations, and prognosis. Those involving the oral cavity of cats and dogs include bullous pemphigoid, mucous membrane (cicatricial) pemphigoid, and canine epidermolysis bullosa acquisita. All are characterized by circulation of IgG and IgE autoantibodies against specific basement membrane antigens. The characteristic microscopic lesions of all are transient subepidermal blisters, which may contain fibrinocellular exudates with variable numbers of neutrophils and eosinophils. Differentiation and diagnosis of each is by the detection of circulating antibody directed at appropriate antigens, using ELISA or immunofluorescent tests, or by identification of immunoglobulin fixed to basement membrane. Paraneoplastic bullous stomatitis characterized by subepithelial clefting has been reported in a horse with a hemangiosarcoma.

Bullous pemphigoid is retained as the name for the second most common of the autoimmune subepidermal blistering disease in dogs and cats. The lesions mainly occur on haired skin, and a minority of cases involve the mucocutaneous junctions or mucosae, including the mouth, which is affected about one-third of the time. Microscopically, there is a rich neutrophilic and eosinophilic dermal infiltrate adjacent to, and sometimes spilling into the subepidermal bullae. The targets for the autoimmune response are epitopes on canine collagen XVII (also called bullous pemphigoid antigen 2 or BPAg2). Collagen XVII is an epithelial transmembrane protein that is a component of the hemidesmosome that joins basal keratinocytes to the lamina densa of the basement membrane.

Mucous membrane pemphigoid is the most common autoimmune subepidermal blistering disease of small animals, causing about half of all cases. Adults are predominantly affected, and among dogs, German Shepherds are overrepresented. The oral mucosa is a common site for lesion development, including gingiva, palate, and tongue. Typically, subepidermal vesicles in mucous membrane pemphigoid are associated with a relatively sparse inflammatory infiltrate. The antigen targeted by autoantibodies is collagen XVII or, in a low number of cases, laminin-5. Basement membrane–fixed immunoglobulin is detected by direct immunofluorescent or immunoperoxidase staining of formalin-fixed paraffin-embedded tissue.

Epidermolysis bullosa acquisita is a rare disease of dogs, representing about 25% of cases of autoimmune basement membrane diseases, with a poor prognosis. The associated autoantibodies are directed against collagen VII, which makes up the anchoring fibrils that join the lamina densa of the basement membrane to the type I collagen of the dermis. The lesions are most common on skin, and advance rapidly to erosions at points of friction, but the oral epithelium often sloughs extensively. Intact subepidermal vesicles may contain no inflammatory cells, or neutrophils may accumulate at the basement membrane, sometimes forming subepidermal microabscesses. The results of serum or cutaneous immunofluorescent tests resemble those in bullous pemphigoid or mucous membrane pemphigoid, but the autoantibodies may be recognized binding to the lower part of the basement membrane.

The oral lesions of pemphigus vulgaris and of the subepidermal blistering diseases must be differentiated from lesions caused by trauma, toxic epidermal necrolysis, drug eruptions, chronic uremia, mucocutaneous candidiasis, and lymphoreticular malignancies.

Feline calicivirus causes mainly a respiratory infection in cats. The disease is complicated by lingual and oropharyngeal ulcers, which start out as vesicles. They are 5-10 mm in diameter, smooth, and well demarcated from the surrounding normal mucosa. They occur mainly on the rostrodorsal and lateral surfaces of the tongue and each side of the midline of the hard palate. The palatine lesions are apparently more severe in cats fed dry food. Microscopically, the earliest lesions consist of foci of pyknotic cells in the stratum corneum and superficial stratum spinosum. They progress to foci of necrosis with vesicle formation and subsequent erosion and ulceration of the mucosa. Regeneration of the oral mucosa in the ulcerated areas generally occurs within 10-12 days. A single layer of squamous epithelial cells extends from the margins of the ulcer beneath a layer of exudate. Active viral replication also takes place in the tonsillar crypt epithelial cells, and virus may be recovered from these areas for weeks postinfection. Viral inclusions have not been observed in oral epithelial cells. The virus is isolated from a high percentage of cats with chronic stomatitis. Concurrent infection with felid herpesvirus 1 may also occur.

Erosive and ulcerative stomatitides. This form of stomatitis is characterized by local epithelial defects of the oral mucosa and nasolabium and is usually associated with acute diffuse stomatitis and pharyngitis. *Erosions* are circumscribed areas of loss of epithelium, which leave the stratum germinativum and basement membrane more or less intact. They are usually associated with acute inflammation in the underlying propria. The erosions vary in size and shape. Although they are often a nonspecific development in a wide variety of conditions, they are also an essential part of a number of important diseases. They heal cleanly and quickly, but if secondarily infected or complicated, may develop into ulcers.

Ulcers, in contrast to erosions, are deeper deficiencies that extend into the substantia propria. They too vary greatly in size and shape; the edges tend to be elevated and ragged, and when they heal, it is with scar formation.

The causes of ulcerative stomatitis are in general those of erosive stomatitis. There are, however, a number of recognized syndromes and specific diseases in which the predominant change is ulceration. Phenylbutazone intoxication in horses may cause oral ulcers in concert with ulcers of the stomach, intestine, and colon; the syndrome is discussed with ischemic diseases of the gut.

Chronic gingivostomatitis—a progressive stomatitis that involves the palatoglossal arches, gingiva, palate, and tongue—is most common in cats, but occurs at a lower frequency in dogs. A number of terms have been used to describe these clinical entities, including *lymphoplasmacytic stomatitis* and *plasma cell gingivitis-stomatitis-pharyngitis*. There are commonalities and differences among the manifestations of these entities, and it is likely that they represent a continuum of disease processes. Two broad categories are described in the following, with the understanding of their overlapping clinical signs, gross and microscopic pathology, and potential etiologies.

Feline ulcerative stomatitis and glossitis or lymphocytic-plasmacytic stomatitis, is an ulcerative and chronic inflammation of the mucosa of the fauces, the angle of the jaws and, less commonly, the hard palate, gingiva, and tongue. Microscopically, there is diffuse inflammation of the oral mucosa and submucosal connective tissues, dominated by lymphocytes and plasma cells. The syndrome is more common in older cats and may accompany periodontitis. The cause is unknown, but is probably multifactorial, involving imbalance in the oral microbiota, with predominance of gram-negative anaerobes and spirochetes, leading to an overall decrease in the microbial diversity at inflammatory lesion sites. Some have reported the isolation of feline calicivirus and felid herpesvirus 1 from more cats with lesions of chronic stomatitis compared with those without, but the role of these viruses in the etiology is unresolved. Feline calicivirus can persist as a sequel to previous disease episodes and in the face of prior vaccination. Feline leukemia virus and feline immunodeficiency virus may predispose some cats to chronic stomatitis because of their immunosuppressive effects, but evidence of infection is not consistently found.

Feline plasma cell gingivitis-pharyngitis or **feline chronic gingivostomatitis** is characterized by raised erythematous, proliferative lesions, mainly in the glossopalatine arches, extending caudally to the palatopharyngeal arch and rostrally to the gingiva. The lesions may involve Eustachian tubes and also can affect the conjunctiva. Histologically the mucosa is hyperplastic and frequently ulcerated, with a marked submucosal inflammatory cell reaction, mainly plasmacytes, including binucleate cells and cells containing Russell bodies. Neutrophils, lymphocytes, and histiocytes are scattered among the plasma cells. Inflammation is most intense at the epidermal-lamina propria junction. Affected cats have elevated polyclonal serum gamma-globulin levels. The polyclonal gammopathy and the plasmacytic, lymphocytic reaction are suggestive of an immune-mediated lesion, and differentiation from mucosally associated lymphoid neoplasia may be challenging. The etiology and the relationship of this syndrome to feline ulcerative stomatitis and glossitis (see previous section) are unclear; the 2 syndromes probably form a continuum, although the plasma cell predominance and the hypergammaglobulinemia attributed to plasma cell gingivitis–stomatitis are distinguishing. Similar stomatitis occurs in dogs.

Eosinophilic ulcer (eosinophilic granuloma, lick granuloma, labial ulcer, rodent ulcer) is a chronic, superficial ulcerative lesion of the mucocutaneous junctions of the lips, and, to a lesser extent, the oral mucosa and skin, in cats of all ages. The cause is unknown. A number of etiologies have been considered, including allergic disease and primary eosinophil dysfunction. The lesions may respond to corticosteroid, oral progestagens, cryosurgery, or radiation therapy, although recurrences are common. Typically, well-demarcated, red-brown, shallow ulcers, often with elevated margins, occur on the *upper lip on either side of the midline*. They are usually a few millimeters wide and several centimeters long. Occasionally, ulcers are present elsewhere in the mouth, such as on the gums, palate, pharynx, and tongue. Skin lesions are located in those areas that are frequently licked, such as the neck, lumbar area, and abdomen. Microscopically, the squamous mucosa is ulcerated, with large areas of necrosis of the underlying connective tissues and accompanied by a marked inflammatory cell reaction. The cellular reaction consists predominantly of neutrophils at the periphery of the ulcers, with plasma cells and mast cells in the lamina propria. Eosinophils and macrophages may not be prominent, especially in the chronic stages of the lesion.

Eosinophilic ulcer is one of the 3 different types of lesions that have been associated with the so-called *eosinophilic granuloma complex*. The other 2 conditions, *eosinophilic plaque* and *linear granuloma*, cause mainly skin lesions, which are different clinically and morphologically from eosinophilic ulcer (see Vol. 1, Integumentary system).

Oral eosinophilic granuloma (collagenolytic granuloma) in dogs occurs as a familial disease in young Siberian Huskies. Sporadic cases have been reported in other breeds, especially Cavalier King Charles Spaniels. Affected dogs have single or multiple firm, often ulcerated, raised plaques, which are covered by yellow-brown exudate, on the *lateral or ventral surfaces of the tongue*. Lesions on the soft palate are less common, and here they tend to be oval to circular ulcers with slightly elevated borders.

Microscopically, *foci of collagenolysis* in the mid and deep zones of the lingual submucosa are surrounded by a mainly granulomatous inflammatory reaction, with macrophages, giant cells, lymphocytes, plasma cells, and mast cells. *Eosinophils* are a constant feature, but their numbers vary from few to many. The lesions are identical to those seen in linear granuloma of cats.

The cause is unknown, although the morphology of the lesion and the response to corticosteroid therapy suggest hypersensitivity. The familial tendency in Siberian huskies indicates that hereditary factors are involved. *Eosinophilic granuloma must be differentiated from oral mast cell tumors*, which also affect the tongue in dogs. Degeneration of collagen fibers is often a feature of mast cell tumors; however, in mastocytoma, the characteristic mixture of mast cells and eosinophils infiltrates the tongue and connective tissues more diffusely. The mast cells may be in various stages of degranulation, and inflammation is minimal or absent in mast cell tumors.

Horses with **eosinophilic epitheliotropic disease** (see Vol. 1, Integumentary system and the later section on Eosinophilic enteritis in cats and horses) may also have eosinophilic stomatitis and lingual ulceration.

Ulcerative stomatitis can be a presenting lesion in *erythema multiforme* in dogs, and must be differentiated from oral epitheliotropic T-cell lymphoma.

In dogs there may be foci of ulceration in the mucosa of the lip or cheek that overlies areas of severe periodontal inflammation. This has been termed **chronic ulcerative stomatitis** or **chronic ulcerative paradental syndrome**.

Feline viral rhinotracheitis is a common upper respiratory tract infection of cats caused by felid herpesvirus 1 (see Vol. 2, Respiratory system). This virus may cause ulcerative lesions in the mouth, especially on the tongue. Rarely, oral and skin ulcers may occur, without evidence of concurrent respiratory tract infection. Microscopically, foci of cytoplasmic vacuolation in squamous epithelium evolve into areas of necrosis and ulceration. The ulcers are often covered by a layer of fibrinocellular exudate. Herpetic inclusions may be present in epithelial cells at the periphery of the ulcers.

Uremia associated with chronic renal disease often causes fetid *ulcerative stomatitis* in dogs, and less commonly in cats. Dirty gray-brown ulcers occur on the gums, lateral surface, and margin of the tongue, and on the inner surface of the lips and cheeks, often adjacent to the openings of salivary ducts. The margins of the ulcers are swollen and hyperemic.

The pathogenesis of the oral lesions in uremia is poorly understood. Elevations in blood and salivary urea in combination with urease-producing bacteria, normally present in the oral microflora, may generate ammonia from salivary urea. Ammonia has a caustic effect on the oral mucous membranes. Experimental antibody production against urease renders some intestinal bacteria nonpathogenic and prevents uremic colitis, providing evidence of the importance of urease. However, there is poor correlation between the levels of blood urea and the development of uremic stomatitis, suggesting other important factors. Uremic vasculitis and impaired microvascular perfusion may contribute to the pathogenesis of uremic stomatitis.

Salivary glucose levels may be elevated in dogs and cats with *diabetes mellitus*, resulting in an imbalance of the oral microflora and predisposing to chronic gingivitis in diabetic animals.

Ulcerative glossitis and stomatitis in **swine** is commonly part of **exudative epidermitis** (greasy pig disease) of preweaning pigs (see Vol. 1, Integumentary system). In addition to the characteristic skin lesions, about a third of the piglets may develop ulcers on the dorsum of the tongue. Erosions and ulcers of the hard palate occur in a small number of piglets. Microscopically, there is ulceration of the squamous mucosa with coagulative necrosis, and vesicle and pustule formation in the superficial epithelium over the rete pegs. A pleocellular inflammatory reaction is evident in the connective tissue below the ulcers.

Further reading

Boutoille F, Hennet P. Maxillary osteomyelitis in two Scottish terrier dogs with chronic ulcerative paradental stomatitis. J Vet Dent 2011;28:96-100.

Buckley L, Nuttall T. Feline eosinophilic granuloma complex(ities): some clinical clarification. J Feline Med Surg 2012;14:471-481.

Favrot C, et al. Isotype determination of circulating autoantibodies in canine autoimmune subepidermal blistering dermatoses. Vet Dermatol 2003;14:23-30.

Lommer MJ. Oral inflammation in small animals. Vet Clin North Am Small Anim Pract 2013;43:555-571.

Lyon KF. Gingivostomatitis. Vet Clin North Am Small Anim Pract 2005;35:891-911.

Nemec A, et al. Erythema multiforme and epitheliotropic T-cell lymphoma in the oral cavity of dogs: 1989 to 2009. J Small Anim Pract 2012;53:445-452.

Olivry T, et al. Diagnosing new autoimmune blistering diseases of dogs. Clin Tech Small Anim Pract 2001;16:225-229.

Williamson L, et al. Upregulation of c-Myc may contribute to the pathogenesis of canine pemphigus vulgaris. Vet Dermatol 2007;18:12-17.

Yang M, et al. Generation and diagnostic application of monoclonal antibodies against Seneca Valley virus. J Vet Diagn Invest 2012;24:42-50.

Deep stomatitides. Lesions of the oral mucosa may permit the entry of pyogenic bacteria, often normal oral flora, into the connective tissues of the submucosa and muscle. Purulent inflammation or cellulitis may develop in the lips, tongue, cheek, soft palate, and pharynx. Abscesses may form and may

fistulate through the mucosa or skin. Abscesses in the wall of the pharynx may result from necrosis of retropharyngeal lymph nodes. Necrotic stomatitis with simple necrosis of the epithelium and lamina propria may be produced by thermal or chemical agencies, but in animals, it is usually caused by *Fusobacterium necrophorum* and other anaerobes.

Fusobacterium necrophorum is the principal cause of **oral necrobacillosis** or **necrotic stomatitis** in animals. It is also associated with necrotizing lesions elsewhere in the upper and lower alimentary tract, and liver. Wherever it occurs, it is usually a secondary invader following previous mucosal damage (Fig. 1-9A). The organism produces a variety of exotoxins and endotoxins; among the latter are leukocidins, hemolysins, and a cytoplasmic toxin, all of which probably enhance the necrotizing ability of the organism. Once established in a suitable focus, *F. necrophorum* proliferates, causing extensive coagulative necrosis.

The best-known form of necrobacillary stomatitis is **calf diphtheria,** an acute necrotizing ulcerative inflammation of the buccal and pharyngeal mucosa, and also of the laryngeal mucosa (**necrotic laryngitis**). The predisposing lesions may include trauma, infectious bovine rhinotracheitis, and papular stomatitis. Necrosis of palatine and pharyngeal tonsils may be seen. The incidence of diphtheria in slaughtered beef cattle may be as high as 1.4%. The same syndrome is rather common in housed lambs as a complication of contagious ecthyma. The infection also may be initiated in the gums about erupting teeth in any species, and by the trauma produced in baby pigs by removing the needle teeth. It is frequently fatal in young animals, in which extension often occurs to other organs. In adults, oral necrobacillosis tends to remain localized to the oral cavity, where it may complicate vesicular and ulcerative stomatitides. It is not unusual, however, for the infection to spread down the alimentary tract.

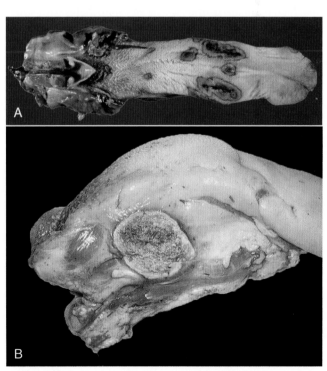

Figure 1-9 A. Necrotic **glossitis and stomatitis** in a dog. **B. Oral necrobacillosis** in a calf. (Courtesy Noah's Arkives.)

The early lesions are large, well-demarcated, yellow-gray, dry areas of necrosis, surrounded by a zone of hyperemia (Fig. 1-9B). They are found on the sides or dorsal groove of the tongue, on the cheeks, gums, palate, and pharynx, especially the recesses beside the larynx. Primary foci may occur in the laryngeal ventricles. Lesions near the larynx often lead to respiratory distress and death may be associated with asphyxia. The necrotic tissue projects slightly above the normal surface, and is friable but adherent and is not easily detached. In time it may slough and leave deep ulcers, which may heal by granulation. The necrotic tissues are histologically structureless and are surrounded at first by a zone of vascular reaction, later by a dense but narrow rim of leukocytes, and finally by thick encapsulating granulation tissue. The bacteria are arranged in long filaments, particularly at the advancing edge of the lesions. The submucosal extension of the lesions may take them deeply into the underlying soft tissues and bone.

Spread from the oral foci occurs down the trachea (causing aspiration pneumonia), down the esophagus, and via blood vessels. Death may occur acutely in septicemia with only multiple small serosal hemorrhages as evidence, or metastases may occur in other tissue. Venous drainage from the face to the vascular sinuses of the meninges may lead to pituitary and cerebral abscessation. A gross diagnosis of oral necrobacillosis is ordinarily possible, but may be confirmed by a smear from the margin of the lesion. The organism is difficult to cultivate because it is a *strict anaerobe.*

Fusobacterium equinum is a recently described bacterial opportunist that is closely related to *F. necrophorum.* It is a component of the normal microbiota of the equine gastrointestinal, reproductive, and respiratory mucosa. *F. equinum* produces a leukotoxin and is associated with necrotizing lesions, including the oral cavity in horses.

Noma (cancrum oris) is a rapidly spreading *pseudomembranous or gangrenous stomatitis;* it is not caused by a specific pathogen but is associated with tissue invasion by the normal oral flora, particularly fusobacteria and spirochetes with widespread local tissue destruction. The predisposing factors are unknown, but they are probably nonspecific and associated with mucosal trauma and debility. The disease, which is occasionally observed in horses, dogs, and monkeys, is in many respects similar to oral necrobacillosis. In the lesions, the spirochetes can be found in large numbers at the advancing margins as well as in peripheral viable tissue. In the deep layers of necrosis, fusiforms predominate, and toward the surface, there is a variety of other organisms, chiefly cocci. The initial lesion is a small tattered ulcer of the cheek or gum, which spreads rapidly and may involve much of the buccal surface of the gums and the mucosa of the cheek. It is intensely fetid and consists of a dirty necrotic pseudomembrane surrounded by a zone of acute inflammation. The necrotic tissue may slough to leave deep ulcers; the cheek may be perforated to leave a gaping defect, or gangrene may supervene.

Actinobacillosis is a disease mainly of cattle, sheep, and pigs, leading to stomatitis, glossitis, lymphadenitis, and sometimes pyogranulomas in the wall of the forestomachs of ruminants. *Actinobacillus lignieresii* is part of the normal oral flora, and in cattle is associated with deep stomatitis.

Actinobacillosis is typically a *disease of soft tissue,* spreading as a *lymphangitis* and usually involving the regional lymph nodes. This distinguishes it from actinomycosis, which causes mostly bone lesions. The tongue is often involved in actinobacillosis, and the chronic condition produces clinical "wooden

tongue." Entry of actinobacilli to the tongue may be gained through traumatic erosions along its sides, but often the primary lesion is in the lingual groove. Here, trapped grass seeds and awns may provoke the initial trauma. Lesions elsewhere in the soft tissue of the mouth may be attributed to disruption of the mucosa by similar types of insults, and eruption of, or abrasion by, teeth.

Microscopically, the lesion is a *pyogranuloma,* centered on a mass of coccobacilli, surrounded by radiating eosinophilic clubs made up of immune complexes (Fig. 1-10). The *club colonies,* in turn, are surrounded by variable numbers of neutrophils, and are invested by macrophages or giant cells. Lymphocytic and plasmacytic infiltrates are present in the surrounding reactive fibrous stroma or granulation tissue. An individual inflammatory focus appears grossly as a nodular, firm, pale, fibrous mass a few millimeters to 1 cm in diameter, containing in the center minute yellow "sulfur" granules, which are the club colonies.

Lymphogenous spread is common. Affected lymphatics are thickened, and nodules are distributed along their course. This distribution is best seen beneath the mucosa of the dorsum and the lateral surface of the tongue and often can be traced through to the pharyngeal lymphoid tissue (Fig. 1-11). Some of these more superficial nodules erode the overlying epithelium, and coalescence may produce quite large ulcers. The most common form of lingual actinobacillosis consists of

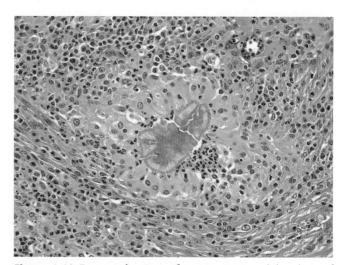

Figure 1-10 Pyogranulomatous focus containing club colony of *Actinobacillus lignieresii* in **actinobacillosis** in a cow.

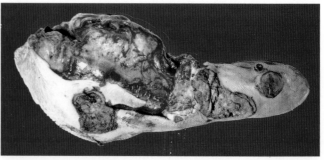

Figure 1-11 Actinobacillosis in a cow. Granulomas bulging on lateral surface of tongue.

granulation tissue in which are embedded many small abscesses surrounded by a dense connective tissue capsule. The epithelium overlying these large granulomas may be intact or ulcerated. Diffuse sclerosing actinobacillosis of the tongue (wooden tongue) is firm because of extensive proliferation of connective tissue, which replaces the muscle fibers. Granulomatous nodules are sparsely scattered in the fibrous stroma.

Although actinobacillosis in cattle is best known as a disease of the tongue, the infection may occur in any of the exposed soft tissues, especially those of mouth and esophagus; occasionally it involves the wall of the forestomachs, the skin, or the lungs. Lesions in these sites resemble those described in the tongue.

Actinobacillosis causes *regional lymphadenitis*. The cut surface of the node reveals small, soft yellow or orange granulomatous masses that project somewhat above the capsular contour and contain "sulfur" granules. There is also sclerosing inflammation of the surrounding tissues, which may cause adhesion to overlying skin or mucous membranes. The retropharyngeal and submaxillary nodes are most often affected, as well as the lymphoid tissues of the submucosa of the soft palate and pharynx. Involvement of the pharynx and the retropharyngeal lymph nodes may cause dyspnea and dysphagia.

Oral actinobacillosis in *swine* causes lesions similar to those in cattle, including glossitis. Actinobacillosis may also occur sporadically or as outbreaks in *sheep*, but in this species the tongue seems to be exempt. The characteristic lesions in sheep occur in the subcutaneous tissue of the head, especially of the cheeks, nose, lips, and submaxillary and throat regions, and on the nasal turbinates. They may also occur on the soft palate and pharynx as complications of wounds received at drenching. The organism has rarely been isolated from horses.

Lesions morphologically similar to actinobacillosis may be caused by a variety of organisms. *Trueperella (Arcanobacterium) pyogenes* may be isolated from lingual ulcers and granulomas in lambs. Microscopic examination of these lesions reveals well-demarcated submucosal granulomas with plant fibers in the center, surrounded by a marked neutrophilic reaction. The organisms most likely gain entry after the mucosa is damaged by hard fibrous plant fibers from the weed lambsleeve sage (*Salvia reflexa*), present in the bedding. *Actinomyces bovis*, a gram-positive filamentous organism, causes pyogranulomatous mandibular and maxillary osteomyelitis in cattle and mastitis in sows. *Actinomyces weissii* has been isolated from dogs with stomatitis/gingivitis. Staphylococci may cause pyogranulomatous lesions (botryomycosis) in any species. Less common causes of similar microscopic lesions include *Nocardia* and the various agents associated with mycetomas (see Vol. 1, Integumentary system).

Oral dermatophilosis—oral infection by *Dermatophilus congolensis*—has been reported in cattle and cats. *D. congolensis* commonly causes exudative dermatitis in a wide variety of species (see Vol. 1, Integumentary system). In cattle, oral dermatophilosis has been associated with *A. bovis* infection. In cats, the organism is uncommonly associated with oral granulomas, especially affecting the tongue and tonsillar crypt. Large numbers of gram-positive, filamentous, branching organisms, with longitudinal and transverse divisions, may be demonstrated in the necrotic centers of submucosal granulomas. The organisms probably enter through damaged mucosa. The lesion must be differentiated from the more common squamous cell carcinomas of the tongue.

Further reading

Hijazin M, et al. *Actinomyces weissii* sp. nov., isolated from dogs. Int J Syst Evol Microbiol 2012;62:1755-1760.

Roberts GL. Fusobacterial infections: an underestimated threat. Br J Biomed Sci 2000;57:156-162.

Tadepallia S, et al. *Fusobacterium equinum* possesses a leukotoxin gene and exhibits leukotoxin activity. Vet Microbiol 2008;127:89-96.

Tan ZL, et al. *Fusobacterium necrophorum* infections: virulence factors, pathogenic mechanism and control measures. Vet Res Commun 1996;20:113-140.

Parasitic diseases of the oral cavity

These are of minor significance. Sarcosporidiosis and cysticercosis occur in the striated muscles of the tongue and produce the same lesions as they do elsewhere (see Vol. 1, Muscle and tendon). *Trichinella spiralis* may be found in muscles of the tongue and mastication. *Gongylonema* spp. are found in the mucosal lining of the tongue, especially in swine allowed to graze, and less commonly in cattle and sheep. They evoke little or no inflammation of the mucosa, but a mild-to-moderate lymphocytic and eosinophilic reaction may be evident in the underlying lamina propria.

The larvae of *Gasterophilus* spp. in the horse and of *Oestrus ovis* in sheep are found attached to the pharyngeal mucosa, where they may cause focal ulceration and incite mild inflammation. The larvae of *G. nasalis* migrate from the lips and invade the gums around and between the teeth and behind the alveolar processes to cause small suppurating pockets.

Halicephalobus gingivalis has been observed in proliferative granulomas of the mandibular gingiva as well as bone, skin, kidney, central nervous system, mammary gland, and eye of horses.

Parasitic leeches of the genus *Myxobdella* may infect the oral cavity of cattle and humans, and *Limnotis nilotica* the oral cavity of dogs, leading to minor dysfunction and hemorrhage. Known colloquially as the "tongue worm," the pentastome *Linguatula serrata* infects the nasal cavity and nasopharynx of dogs and humans.

Nodular and ulcerative glossitis can occur in dogs as an unusual manifestation of canine leishmaniasis caused by *Leishmania infantum*, an endemic zoonotic parasite in southern Europe.

Further reading

Kinde H, et al. *Halicephalobus gingivalis* (*H. deletrix*) infection in two horses in southern California. J Vet Diagn Invest 2000;12:162-165.

Rajaei SM, et al. Oral infestation with leech *Limnatis nilotica* in two mixed-breed dogs. J Small Anim Pract 2013 Dec 10. doi: 10.1111/jsap.12166.

Smith MA. *Gasterophilus pecorum* in the soft palate of a British pony. Vet Rec 2005;156:283-284.

Viegas C, et al. Tongue nodules in canine leishmaniosis—a case report. Parasit Vectors 2012;5:120.

Diseases of the tonsils

The tonsils are normally prominent and protrude slightly from the tonsillar fossa in the dog and cat. In these species, tonsils are compact, fusiform structures with a finely stippled, pale pink mucosal surface. In swine, tonsillar lymphoid tissue is concentrated in the caudal soft palate, and forms a plaque of raised and pitted thickened mucosa. In horses, tonsillar tissues are dispersed over pharyngeal and epiglottic mucosal surfaces and consist of a series of plaques and nodules in the mucosa. In cattle, there are multiple sets of tonsils, including palatine, lingual, soft palate and pharyngeal tonsils. In other species, the tonsils are diffuse. They are subject to the usual conditions involving lymphoid tissue, and undergo progressive atrophy with age.

Tonsils are part of the mucosal-associated lymphoid tissue (MALT) and are constantly exposed to antigenic stimuli, by virtue of their function in immune surveillance in the oropharynx. As a result, they are a site of functional lymphoid hyperplasia and physiologic inflammation. Many bacteria native to the oropharyngeal mucosa probably inhabit the tonsillar crypts. Consequently they may serve as portal of entry for a variety of bacterial agents and viruses. A significant percentage of swine may carry *Erysipelothrix rhusiopathiae* and *Salmonella* spp. in the tonsils, and *Streptococcus suis* type 2 can be cultured from tonsils.

Desquamated epithelium, bacteria, necrotic debris, and neutrophils may normally be present to moderate degree in *tonsillar crypts*. This reaction is exaggerated, and may be associated with ulceration of the crypt and suppuration of involuted tonsillar lymphoid tissue, in certain bacterial infections, causing the formation of visible yellow nodules. Conditions in which such bacterial tonsillitis may occur include pasteurellosis in sheep and pigs, *Actinomyces* and *Tonsillophilus* in tonsils of swine, and necrobacillosis in all species (see Fig. 1-8). In porcine anthrax, hemorrhagic necrotizing tonsillitis is reported.

Prion proteins have been identified in tonsillar tissue of infected animals. *Scrapie*-associated prion protein is consistently detected by immunohistochemistry in the center of primary and secondary lymphoid follicles of sheep with clinical and histologic lesions of scrapie, and this may be a useful antemortem diagnostic approach in this and other prion-associated diseases of animals. The prion protein of chronic wasting disease has been identified in tonsils of elk and deer. The prion protein of bovine spongiform encephalopathy has been shown to accumulate in palatine tonsils 10 months after experimental infection.

The tonsil is the site of primary virus multiplication in pseudorabies (Aujeszky's disease) in swine. The virus causes necrotizing tonsillitis, and intranuclear viral inclusions may be seen in cryptal epithelial cells.

Involution of B-dependent tonsillar lymphoid follicles resulting from viral lymphocytolysis may occur during the early phase of a number of lymphotropic diseases such as feline panleukopenia, canine parvoviral enteritis, canine distemper, bovine viral diarrhea, and swine vesicular disease. Numerous karyorrhectic nuclei, lymphocyte depletion, and prominent histiocytes signal such damage. In distemper, involuted tonsils are susceptible to secondary bacterial invasion and suppuration. Compensatory lymphoid hyperplasia may occur during the postviremic phase of parvoviral infections and distemper. The tonsil often appears to be the preferred organ of viral persistence in a symptomatic carrier infected with feline calicivirus. In porcine circovirus 2 infections (postweaning multisystemic wasting syndrome), involution of lymphoid tissue and accumulation of macrophages and giant cells containing basophilic cytoplasmic circoviral inclusions occur, as they do in other lymphoid organs.

Inflammatory polyps of the tonsils occur infrequently in old dogs. They are flat to pedunculated rubbery masses (1-3 cm in length), attached to the tonsillar sinus, with a smooth to verrucous surface. Histologically, the lesions are composed of mature, sometimes edematous, highly vascularized connective tissue that is covered by squamous epithelial cells. Aggregates of lymphocytes and plasma cells are scattered throughout the connective tissue. The lesions are probably the result of chronic recurrent episodes of subclinical tonsillitis. They are usually asymptomatic but may cause gagging and retching. A tonsillar lymphangiomatous polyp has been reported from a dog.

Tumors, especially lymphosarcomas and squamous cell carcinomas, are common causes of tonsillar enlargement in dogs. Bilaterally enlarged and soft, pale swollen tonsils are usual with lymphosarcoma, and these may become clinically obvious before the development of peripheral lymphadenopathy.

Further reading

Chae C. Postweaning multisystemic wasting syndrome: a review of aetiology, diagnosis and pathology. Vet J 2004;168:41-49.

Miller AD, et al. Tonsillar lymphangiomatous polyp in an adult dog. J Comp Pathol 2008;138:215-217.

Race BL, et al. Levels of abnormal prion protein in deer and elk with chronic wasting disease. Emerg Infect Dis 2007;13:824-830.

Torremorell M, et al. Colonization of suckling pigs by *Streptococcus suis* with particular reference to pathogenic serotype 2 strains. Can J Vet Res 1998;62:21-26.

Wills RW, et al. Porcine reproductive and respiratory syndrome virus: a persistent infection. Vet Microbiol 1997;55:231-240.

Neoplastic and like lesions of the oral cavity

Some of the lumps, bumps, and cysts that develop in and around the oral cavity are malformations, hyperplasias, and neoplasias originating in tooth germ or teeth. Malformations of dental origin have been considered previously under developmental anomalies of teeth. Gingival masses of all types, many of which are of tooth germ origin, are common in dogs, but occur much less frequently in other species. In this discussion we follow revisions in the nomenclature of lesions that formerly were included with epulis, placing those that clearly are of dental origin with other such tumors, and consigning the remainder to hyperplastic and reactive lesions. Prognostic implications for such masses have not changed, despite some reclassification.

Epulis *is a generic clinical term for tumor-like masses on the gingiva.* Epulis has, in the past, been used to describe developmental, inflammatory, and hyperplastic lesions, as well as several neoplastic lesions of tooth germ origin, which are numerous in dogs, and develop occasionally in cats. It has no specific pathologic connotation, and preferably, *the term should not be used in a morphologic diagnosis, except in the context of fibromatous epulis of periodontal ligament origin,* discussed in Tumors of dental tissues, which follows.

In evaluating lesions of the gums and jaws, a potentially confusing element is the nature of the epithelium and of the hard tissues that are often found in the stroma. In interpreting these, it is important to recall the inductive pattern of tooth development. Epithelial remnants from tooth organogenesis occur commonly in the gingiva and the periodontium, and nests of dental epithelium can be found incidentally in any proliferative lesion in this region. Characteristically, dental epithelial cells show reverse polarity, their nuclei being located at the apex of the cell, distal to the basement membrane. Often the cell nests are surrounded by a relatively clear halo that contains a few strands of collagenous tissue. Also, gingival epithelium commonly proliferates extravagantly in response to irritation, and may form complex plexiform patterns. Unless there is neoplastic change; the epithelial component is not of primary significance. Similarly, many stromal masses in the regions of the jaws include mineralized tissues or amorphous, apparently mineralizable tissues, which may develop by metaplasia of fibrous tissue or by de novo cellular differentiation. It is often difficult to determine whether this is bone, cementum, dentin, or their precursors, but in any case this is prognostically irrelevant, as is the abundance of such tissues themselves. *In describing lesions of the gums and jaws, the adjective "peripheral" refers to an origin in the gingiva, whereas "central" implies a deeper origin in the jaw bone.*

The oral and pharyngeal mucosa is a common site of malignant tumors in the dog, as it is in cats. Malignant oral tumors account for ~6% of all canine and ~7% of all feline neoplasms. Large domestic animals have a low prevalence of malignant oral tumors, and when they do occur in ungulates, they are usually relatively nonaggressive.

There are regional geographic differences in the prevalence of certain oral tumors, especially in dogs and cattle. Such differences may be related to the distribution of carcinogens in the environment, and warrant further investigation from the point of view of comparative oncology.

The most common types of malignant oral tumors in dogs and cats are squamous cell carcinoma, fibrosarcoma, and, in dogs only, malignant melanomas. They vary somewhat in their behavior depending on the species in which they occur, and the type and location of the tumor. Dogs and cats with mean ages over about 6 or 7 years of age are mainly affected. The canine population with fibrosarcomas has a mean age of about 8 years. Melanomas in dogs tend to occur in a notably older age class than the other tumors, with the mean of the distribution at about 11-12 years. Typical clinical signs, determined by the location, behavior, and stage of the tumor, are drooling, halitosis, pain, dysphagia, anorexia, weight loss, loose teeth, mandibular fractures, oral bleeding, noisy respiration, coughing, and a change in voice.

Boxers, Cocker Spaniels, German Shorthaired Pointers, Weimaraners, and Golden Retrievers apparently have a higher prevalence of malignant oral tumors than other breeds of dogs, whereas Dachshunds and Beagles apparently have a very low prevalence. The male-to-female ratio has been reported to be as high as 6:1 for melanomas, 3:1 for tonsillar carcinomas, and 2:1 for fibrosarcomas. The ratios have to be interpreted with some caution because they may be partly related to differences in the ratio of males to females in the general population.

All types of malignant oral tumors in dogs and cats tend to progress rapidly, and regardless of the type of malignancy, the prognosis is generally poor, unless the lesion is completely resected early in its clinical course, before metastasis.

Reactive and hyperplastic lesions

Pyogenic granuloma *is a bright red or blue mass on the gums of dogs.* It is composed of extremely vascular granulation tissue covered by gingival epithelium, and is not genuinely granulomatous, despite the name. It ulcerates, is infiltrated by leukocytes, and bleeds easily. The cause is not completely understood. Pyogenic granuloma is probably an exaggerated response to local trauma, irritation, and/or infection. In horses, exuberant granulation tissue of periodontal origin sometimes develops at the site of extracted teeth to produce a tumor-like mass in the dental arcade. Epithelial remnants and proliferative bone may be associated with the granulation tissue in such cases.

Peripheral giant cell granuloma (formerly *giant cell epulis*) occurs in dogs and cats as *gingival masses*, often red, that may be smooth and sessile, or pedunculated. Giant cell granuloma is the second most common gingival tumor in cats after fibromatous epulis. These lesions may not be true granulomas. Very occasionally, similar lesions, described as *central giant cell granulomas*, occur more deeply in the jaw. The gingival epithelium is hyperplastic or ulcerated and extends deeply into the underlying mass, which is well vascularized and often contains hemosiderin-laden cells. Characteristic of the tumor are numerous multinucleated giant cells, with multiple central nuclei and abundant eosinophilic cytoplasm, which are located in a densely cellular stroma. The nature of the giant cells is not fully known, and it is suggested that they may be osteoclastic in origin. Foci of hard tissue, including mineralized osteoid, may be present. Giant cell granulomas are regarded as hyperplastic, and have occurred at the site of tooth extraction.

Fibrous hyperplasia (formerly part of fibrous or fibromatous epulis, *gingival hypertrophy*) is common in dogs, and may be generalized and diffuse, or focal, localized to one or more teeth. When focal, it is a discrete tumor-like mass and, whether local or general, may cover part of the crown (Fig. 1-12). The stromal component of the mass consists of mature fibrous tissue with low cellular density. Foci of hard tissue and epithelial nests may be present. Local enlargement may be promoted by chronic, probably painless, inflammation. It may be associated with periodontal disease. Characteristically there is a band of mononuclear cells, predominantly plasma cells, in the gingival stroma adjacent to the epithelium, which is often hyperplastic, sometimes markedly so. Where the epithelium is ulcerated, neutrophils may be prominent, marginating in vessels, in the stroma, and migrating through the epithelium.

Diffuse fibrous hyperplasia is familial in Boxer dogs, and a more severe overgrowth, termed *hyperplastic gingivitis*, occurs as a recessive inherited disease in Swedish silver foxes. In the foxes, both jaws are affected and the lesion causes

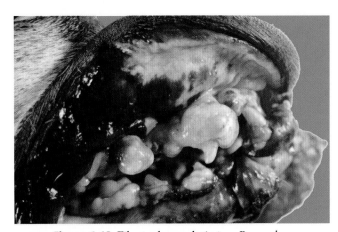

Figure 1-12 Fibrous hyperplasia in a Boxer dog.

displacement and malalignment of teeth, eventually reaching such proportions that the mouth cannot be closed.

Oral papillomatosis

These benign epithelial tumors (*warts*) in dogs, cats, and cattle are caused by papillomaviruses.

In **dogs,** they are caused by canine papillomavirus 1 (CPV1), and mainly occur in young animals, although older dogs in close contact may become infected. The lesions are unsightly, are often multicentric, and may be traumatized and bleed, but only heavy infections that interfere with swallowing or respiration cause other than cosmetic problems.

The virus is host- and fairly site-specific. Injury to the oral mucosa often precedes viral infection. Infection of basal epithelium of the squamous mucosa stimulates increased mitosis, whereas viral genome replicates in the differentiating keratinocytes of the stratum spinosum and granulosum, which degenerate, with viral assembly and expression in superficial squamous layers. The incubation period is generally about 2 months. Spontaneous recovery, mediated by CD4 and CD8 T cells, usually occurs within 1-2 more months, followed by *solid antibody-mediated immunity to reinfection.* The warts first develop as single, smooth papular elevations which are pale or the color of the mucosa. These lesions progress to multiple, proliferative cauliflower-like, firm, white to gray growths (Fig. 1-13). They develop on the lips, gingiva, buccal mucosa, tongue, palate, and walls of the pharynx. The esophagus and the skin of the muzzle also may be involved. Persistent and progressive infections, which may also involve haired skin remote from the mouth, are attributable to immunocompromise of the host, rather than an unusually virulent strain of virus.

The *microscopic structure* of fully developed lesions is typically verrucous, with very thick keratinizing squamous epithelium covering thin, branching, often pedunculated cores of vascularized proprial papillae. There is also marked acanthosis. Individual epithelial cells or small groups in the upper areas of the stratum spinosum and granulosum degenerate (koilocytes), developing koilocytic atypia, with clear cytoplasm around or adjacent to an often somewhat condensed nucleus, and large cytoplasmic granules or inclusions, with loss of intercellular bridges. *Basophilic intranuclear viral inclusions* may be found in cells in the outer spinose layers, but they can be rare; intracytoplasmic inclusions also may be present. Regressing lesions are infiltrated by moderate numbers of T lymphocytes.

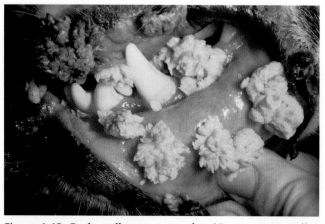

Figure 1-13 Oral papillomatosis in a dog. (Courtesy W.R. Kelly.)

Viral antigen can be demonstrated in nuclei of koilocytes and in intranuclear, but not cytoplasmic, inclusions by specific immunohistochemistry. Electron microscopy reveals intranuclear 50-55 nm viral particles, sometimes forming paracrystalline arrays.

Malignant transformation of infected papillomavirus-infected epithelium to produce squamous cell carcinomas can occur, but its importance in the etiology of canine oral squamous cell carcinomas is unclear. Injections of live CPV1 vaccine into the skin of dogs may result in a spectrum of lesions, including epidermal hyperplasia, papillomas, epidermal cysts, basal cell tumors, and squamous cell carcinomas, and some cutaneous squamous cell carcinomas in dogs contain CPV1 genetic material.

In domestic and wild species of **cats,** oral and cutaneous papillomas and fibropapillomas are very occasionally identified. In the oral cavity they are most common on the ventral aspect of the tongue, and typically they are multifocal, pink, and more sessile than verrucous. Microscopically, raised areas of thickened mucosa are comprised of hyperplastic keratinocytes with occasional fibrovascular stalks. Typical degenerative changes are seen in infected keratinocytes, and papillomavirus antigen can be detected by immunohistochemistry in a high proportion of such cases.

In **cattle,** oral papillomas, caused by bovine papillomavirus 4 (a strain of bovine papillomavirus 3, genus *Xipapillomavirus*), can occur commonly in endemic areas. Their morphology and distribution in the oral cavity are similar to the papillomas of dogs, but because they infect the esophagus and forestomachs extensively, they are considered more fully later in the section on Neoplasia of the esophagus and forestomachs.

Tumors of dental tissues

Tumors of dental tissues are classified either as epithelial (with or without odontogenic ectomesenchyme) or mesenchymal neoplasms, and malformations. Tooth development provides the classic example of epithelial-mesenchymal interactions, and inductive influences appear to be active in some tumors. Familiarity with dental embryology assists an understanding of the origin, appearance, and classification of the tumors discussed later.

Tumors of dental tissues are rare, other than fibromatous epulis of periodontal ligament origin and canine acanthomatous ameloblastomas (acanthomatous epulides). *All are nonmalignant, and infiltrative or expansive.* However, their location predetermines destruction of bone and displacement of teeth, and they are difficult to remove.

Tumors of odontogenic epithelium include the **ameloblastoma,** which is a slowly progressive invasive but nonmetastatic tumor, consisting of proliferating odontogenic epithelium in a fibrous stroma. The proportions of epithelium and stroma vary widely. The terms *adamantinoma* and *enameloblastoma* are obsolete synonyms. These tumors are more common in dogs than in cats and horses, and seem to occur more often in the mandible than the maxilla. Tumors formerly described as ameloblastomas in young cattle are now considered to be ameloblastic fibromas, discussed in the following.

Ameloblastomas occur at any age. They originate from the dental lamina, the outer enamel epithelium, the dental follicle around retained unerupted teeth, the oral epithelium, or odontogenic epithelium in extraoral locations. They are *predominantly intraosseous* and, because of their location, they

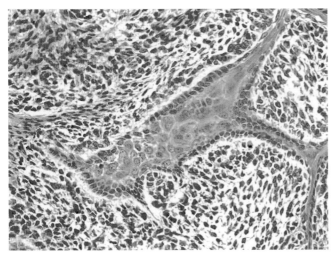

Figure 1-14 Ameloblastoma. Tall enamel-type epithelium. (Courtesy Joint Pathology Center.)

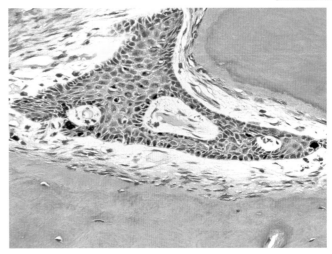

Figure 1-15 Acanthomatous ameloblastoma invading bone of the mandible in a dog.

may destroy large amounts of bone, and extend into the oral cavity or sinuses. Large tumors may undergo central degeneration and become cystic.

Odontogenic epithelium is the criterion for diagnosis of ameloblastoma. Neoplastic odontogenic epithelium has peripheral palisading of epithelial cells. There is typically basilar cytoplasm with an apical nucleus (Fig. 1-14). Odontogenic epithelium may form any one of several patterns. Follicular and plexiform patterns are most common, consisting of discrete islands, or irregular masses and strands of epithelium, respectively. Many tumors contain both patterns. *In both, central masses of cells, often resembling the stellate reticulum of the enamel organ, are surrounded by a single layer of cuboidal or columnar cells that resemble inner enamel epithelium.* Cysts originate from degeneration of the centers of epithelial islands, or from stromal degeneration. Small cysts may coalesce to form grossly evident cavities. Ameloblastomas occasionally undergo keratinization and are termed keratinizing ameloblastomas. In some, stromal osteoid and bone develop, which may be an epithelial inductive effect.

Amyloid-producing odontogenic tumors are rare tumors that occur as unencapsulated gingival masses in dogs and cats. They are characterized by odontogenic epithelium, with deposits of amyloid, and sometimes prominent trabeculae of osteoid/dentinoid. The epithelium may be arranged in strands, nests, or masses and may contain areas of stellate reticulum. Occasionally there is mineralization of epithelium or stroma, in the form of small nodules or amorphous masses. The amyloid also may be nodular or amorphous and may be intermingled with the mineral. Distinguished histologically, but not prognostically, from ameloblastomas by the presence of amyloid, these tumors are cured by surgical excision.

Acanthomatous ameloblastoma (acanthomatous epulis, peripheral ameloblastoma, adamantinoma, basal cell carcinoma) *is a common tumor of odontogenic epithelium arising from the gingiva or epithelial rests of dogs*; it does not occur in other species. It is easily confused clinically with the benign stromal masses found in the canine gingiva, but *it often behaves aggressively*, invading local alveolar bone (Fig. 1-15), causing tooth loss, and recurring in many animals following conservative treatment. Grossly, they are gray-pink papillary to sessile gingival masses in the vicinity of the alveolus (Fig. 1-16).

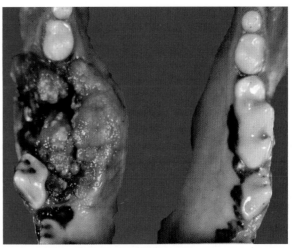

Figure 1-16 Acanthomatous ameloblastoma in a dog. This is an exophytic tumor that is also invading and destroying mandibular bone and displacing teeth. (Courtesy Noah's Arkives.)

Histologically, the tumor is composed of solid sheets, nodules, and anastomosing cords of polyhedral epithelium (acanthocytes) bordered by a row of palisading cuboidal to columnar cells with round to oval nuclei and moderate amounts of cytoplasm. *Prominent intercellular bridges*, the defining feature of the lesion reflected in the name, are present between many of the acanthocytes. The solid sheets/cords of acanthocytic neoplastic cells and prominent intercellular bridges distinguish acanthomatous ameloblastoma from ameloblastoma described previously (Fig. 1-17). In some tumors, intraepithelial cysts contain vacuolated, otherwise structureless, eosinophilic material and cellular debris. These cysts probably form from degenerate epithelium. Small masses of hard tissue may develop in the stroma between the epithelium.

It is sometimes difficult to distinguish an acanthomatous ameloblastoma developing in the gingiva from the epithelial proliferation accompanying gingivitis. Besides the usual prudence required when identifying neoplastic cells in areas of inflammation, other criteria for differentiation include the *predominance of broad sheets of epithelium and the mitotic figures*

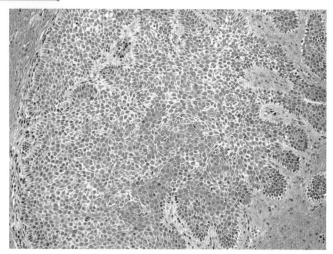

Figure 1-17 Acanthomatous ameloblastoma in a dog, illustrating invasive cords of cells.

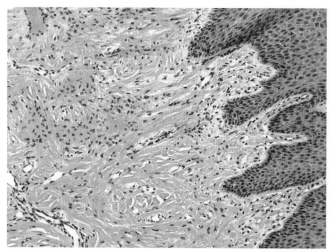

Figure 1-18 Fibromatous epulis of periodontal ligament origin in a dog. Note immature stroma with fusiform mesenchymal cells.

sometimes present in the acanthomatous ameloblastoma. Evidence of invasion of bone is clearly relevant to the diagnosis, care being taken to differentiate alveolar bone from stromal hard tissues.

Some acanthomatous ameloblastomas show characteristics of squamous cell carcinoma when they escape the influence of the subgingival stroma and invade bone, but metastases are not recorded, and complete surgical resection is curative. Squamous cell carcinoma, and occasionally fibrosarcoma or osteosarcoma, has been reported from the site of irradiated acanthomatous ameloblastomas, several months to many years after treatment.

Dental tumors containing both odontogenic epithelium and ectomesenchymal tissue (mixed odontogenic tumors) are rare in domestic animals. The **ameloblastic fibroma** (fibroameloblastoma) occurs in horses, dogs, and cats, often in young animals, but is the *most common odontogenic tumor of cattle,* where it is found in the vicinity of the mandibular incisors of calves. It consists of cords of odontogenic epithelium resembling dental lamina, intimately associated with an ectomesenchymal component consisting of spindle cells resembling dental pulp. Where the epithelium is well differentiated, resembling the enamel organ, it may be associated with enamel and dentin; such variants are termed **ameloblastic fibro-odontomas,** in contrast to ameloblastic fibromas, which contain no mineralized tissue. These tumors generally behave like ameloblastomas, although malignancy has been reported once in a dog.

Feline inductive odontogenic tumor is a rare tumor specific to cats that is most frequent in kittens, where they occur as osteolytic masses in the rostral maxilla, causing tooth loss or facial distortion. They are distinguished by the presence of aggregates of neoplastic odontogenic epithelium partially enveloping somewhat spherical masses of cellular ectomesenchyme, forming structures resembling the cap stage of tooth development, when dental epithelium invests the dental papilla but odontoblasts have not yet differentiated.

Odontomas are malformations (hamartomas) in which fully differentiated dental tissues are represented, and are classified as **complex and compound odontomas.** In *complex odontomas* the tissues are disorganized, and in dogs, cementum is not evident, although it is in horses. In *compound odontomas,*

tooth-like structures (denticles) are present, each containing enamel, dentin, cementum, and pulp, arranged as in a normal tooth. Distinction of the two may be arbitrary. Separate areas of ameloblastic epithelium are not present in complex and compound odontomas. A tumor that contains ameloblastic epithelium and separate areas of complex or compound odontoma is an **odontoameloblastoma.**

Odontomas are usually located in the mandibular or maxillary arch, and are less rare in cattle and horses than in other species. They are connected with existing dental alveoli and are detected when they bulge the contour of the host bone or interfere with other teeth. They may originate from normally or abnormally placed dental lamina as well as from a supernumerary dental lamina.

Fibromatous epulis of periodontal ligament origin *is a peripheral odontogenic neoplasm, indistinguishable clinically from fibrous hyperplasia, and most common in dogs.* Although uncommon, fibromatous epulis is the most frequent epulis in cats. The distinction between fibrous hyperplasia and fibromatous epulis is academic because prognosis following surgical removal is good for both lesions. Fibromatous epulis of periodontal ligament origin is a neoplasm, however, comparable to the rare human tumor called peripheral odontogenic fibroma. Similar tumors occur rarely in cats. Fibromatous epulides of periodontal ligament origin are firm to hard, gray-pink neoplasms, often projecting from between the teeth or from the hard palate near the teeth. Often they are mushroom-shaped and have a smooth, lobulated surface. They are attached to the periosteum, and may displace teeth mechanically, but do not invade bone. Fibromatous epulides are most common around the carnassial and canine teeth of brachycephalic breeds, and usually occur in dogs over about 3 years of age.

Fibromatous epulides of periodontal ligament origin are *stromal tumors* consisting of interwoven bundles of cellular fibroblastic tissue that is often well vascularized (Fig. 1-18). They are distinguished from fibrous hyperplasia by the immaturity of this stroma, which is comprised of small stellate to fusiform fibroblasts dispersed in a dense collagen matrix, and by their tendency to contain less inflammatory tissue and more hard tissue, which may resemble bone, cementum, or dentin. About 60% contain branching cords or islands of

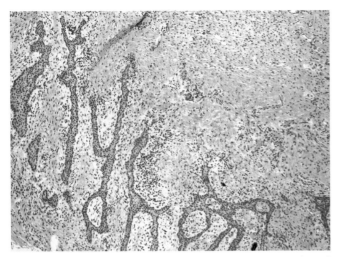

Figure 1-19 Branching cords of epithelium in mesenchymal stroma in a **fibromatous epulis** in a dog.

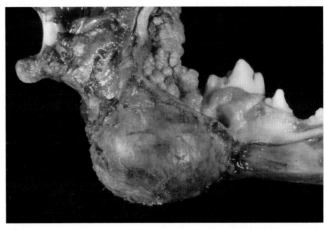

Figure 1-20 Squamous cell carcinoma arising from the gingiva in the caudal lower jaw with invasion of the mandible in a dog. (Courtesy Noah's Arkives.)

epithelium, which may be continuous with the gingiva, or originate in epithelial rests of Malassez. The epithelium is bordered by a row of cuboidal cells somewhat resembling odontogenic epithelium (Fig. 1-19). Although such masses are sometimes categorized as fibromatous or ossifying, depending on the abundance of the hard tissue, there is no prognostic value in this distinction because these are all benign tumors that are cured by excision.

Squamous cell carcinomas

Squamous cell carcinoma (SCC) *is by far the most common oral malignancy of* **cats**, and although there seems to be some geographic variation, it is generally most frequently located on the ventral surface of the tongue, on the midline near the frenulum. The gingiva is the next most common site, and other locations, including the tonsils, are generally much less frequently involved. In the early stages, gingival SCCs are often mistaken for gingivitis. Oral SCCs in cats are generally advanced at presentation. *The tumor is locally invasive,* especially into bone and local soft tissues, but at presentation is less frequently metastatic to regional lymph nodes, and rarely to the lungs, although the survival rate of animals following surgical resection alone is only about 20%. Larger tumors at presentation signal a poorer prognosis. Paraneoplastic hypercalcemia has been reported. Grossly, these tumors are irregular, slightly nodular, red-gray, friable masses, often with an ulcerated surface that bleeds easily. Microscopically the tumor is a conventional SCC in appearance. Infection with feline immunodeficiency virus, feline leukemia virus, or feline sarcoma virus is not clearly a factor in the etiology, which is presumably multifactorial and in some cases may involve exposure to environmental tobacco smoke.

In the **dog,** most studies have found that SCC is second to melanoma in prevalence in the oral cavity. It most frequently involves the tonsils, although the gums are also common sites. Lips, tongue, and other oropharyngeal mucosae are involved much less often. The etiology is likely multifactorial, including epithelial hyperplasia associated with chronic gingivitis, and carcinogens associated with smog and smoke in the case of tonsillar tumors in urban dogs, but, as alluded to previously, infection with canine oral papillomavirus may have a part to play in some cases.

Grossly, tonsillar carcinoma usually appears unilateral. The earliest lesion visible is a small, slightly elevated, granular plaque on the mucosal surface, but it is rarely recognized. In the advanced stages, the affected tonsil is replaced by neoplastic tissue, 2-3 times normal size, nodular, firm and white, and the surface often is ulcerated. There is usually extensive infiltration of the surrounding tissues by microscopically typical SCC. Histologic examination of the grossly unaffected tonsil may also reveal early carcinoma. SCCs originating in the tonsils have a higher metastatic potential than other SCC of the oral cavity of dogs. They often metastasize early to the regional nodes, initially the retropharyngeal nodes, and to the thyroid, with distant metastases to many visceral organs, but especially the lungs, and to bone. Tonsillar SCCs must be differentiated from involvement of the tonsil in lymphosarcoma.

Gingival SCCs may be associated with chronic periodontitis in dogs. It is not always clear whether they have predisposed to periodontitis, or resulted from chronic irritation of the gingiva. It is assumed that some originate in the gingiva and others in subgingival or periodontal epithelial rests. They appear as pink or white nodular masses around the mandibular or maxillary dental arcade, often around canine or carnassial teeth, extending to form larger masses or ulcerative plaques; sometimes they involve adjacent hard palate. Their microscopic appearance is conventional, although the degree of keratinization, and formation of keratin pearls, may be lower than in similar cutaneous tumors. They may often be obscured by chronic active inflammation, as well. They are locally invasive, and may invade bone (Fig. 1-20), maxillary tumors sometimes extending into the sinuses and orbit. However, they are much less likely to have metastasized at presentation than SCC of the tonsil.

In **horses,** SCC are found rarely on the gums and hard palate, possibly arising in chronically irritated hyperplastic alveolar epithelium in cases of chronic periodontitis. They are slow-growing, exceedingly destructive, and metastatic mainly to the regional lymph nodes. Such tumors are large when first observed and may project from the palate or gums as gray extensively ulcerated masses, or appear as craterous ulcers. The large ones are extensively necrotic, and the teeth are lost or loosely embedded in the tumor. These tumors of the maxilla rapidly fill the adjacent sinuses and cause bulging of the face and may extend further, into the nasal, orbital, and cranial cavities. The microscopic appearance of the tumors varies considerably, from well differentiated with keratinization of individual epithelial cells and formation of keratin "pearls," to poorly differentiated with little evidence of keratinization.

In **cattle,** oral SCCs are very rare, with the exception of a few geographic areas where they are associated with oral papillomatosis and ingestion of bracken fern. A similar association is made in the etiology of SCC of the esophagus and forestomachs in cattle, and is considered more fully in that section. There are sporadic reports of this tumor on the lower lip of **sheep.**

Melanomas

Malignant melanomas *are the most common oral tumors in dogs in many parts of the world.* Although cutaneous melanomas are common in gray horses and certain breeds of swine, these species have no tendency to develop oral melanomas, although rare cases are reported. These tumors are also rare in cattle, sheep, and cats.

Most oral melanomas in **dogs** are malignant and highly aggressive neoplasms, and the majority have metastasized by the time they are diagnosed. They arise from melanocytes in the mucosa or superficial stroma, mainly on the gingiva and labia, and less often on the buccal mucosa, palate, tongue, and pharynx. There is variation in the outcomes of studies of sex and breed association. Males have been overrepresented in some studies, but not others. Some consider that melanomas are more common in smaller breeds or in those with a dark hair coat and/or pigmented mucous membranes, such as Scottish and Boston Terriers, black Cocker Spaniels, Dachshunds, Miniature Poodles, and Chow Chows, but not all studies have found size or breed associations. *The degree of pigmentation of these tumors varies considerably, and many are at least partially amelanotic, but there appears to be no relationship between the amount of pigment and biological behavior.* Metastases are usually pigmented, but in some cases the primary tumor is pigmented and the metastases are not, and vice versa.

Symptomatic lesions usually are ~3-4 cm in diameter when discovered. They grow rapidly; necrosis and ulceration are common (Fig. 1-21A), as is invasion of bone by gingival tumors. More than 70% metastasize to the regional lymph nodes. An approximately equal number spread via hematogenous and lymphatic routes to more distant sites, especially the lungs, where they may be evident at autopsy, but too small to be detected radiographically. The median survival time for untreated dogs is reported as 2 months, and survival following treatment is little better, at about 3 months. The median survival time of dogs with no bone, lymph node, or distant involvement detected at diagnosis is about 8 months after surgical resection.

The histologic appearance of melanomas varies greatly, from a fairly well-differentiated heavily pigmented type, to a highly anaplastic amelanotic type. The diagnosis of the latter is often difficult. However, certain features are evident in most of these tumors. *Anaplastic melanocytes show junctional activity,* infiltrating the junction between the basilar epithelial cells and the submucosa (Fig. 1-21B). Round or polyhedral cells with a large nucleus and extensive cytoplasm with well-demarcated borders predominate in some tumors. Others are comprised of spindle-shaped cells with oval nuclei containing small nucleoli. Most frequently there is a characteristic mixture of

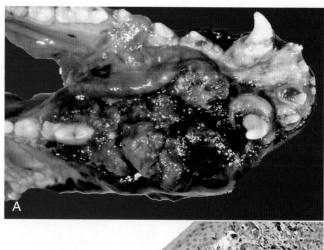

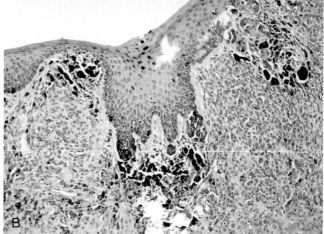

Figure 1-21 A. Malignant melanoma in a dog. (Courtesy Noah's Arkives.) **B.** Junctional activity in oral mucosa adjacent to **melanoma.**

epithelial-like and spindle-shaped cells, which have a marked tendency to form nests supported by a light stroma, extending deep into the submucosa. Multinucleated giant cells also may be present. Osteoid and cartilage have been reported in the stroma of a low number of canine melanomas. Most melanomas have melanin pigment, but detection of this pigment, which also may be concentrated in melanophages, often requires careful examination of individual tumor cells. Cytologic evaluation of melanotic tumors may require bleaching, but any difficulty in interpretation is more likely to involve poorly pigmented variants. They are DOPA-positive (3.4-dihydroxyphenylalanine) in frozen section, and react immunohistochemically (vimentin 100%, melan A >90%). *Melan A is considered sensitive and specific for melanocytes,* differentiating them from melanophages in oral tumors. A panel of immunohistochemical stains that includes melan-A, tyrosinase-related proteins 1 and 2 (TRP-1 and TRP-2), and PNL2 has been shown to be highly accurate for diagnosis of canine oral melanoma.

Most oral melanomas in the dog are malignant. However, a small subset of well-differentiated canine oral melanomas has been associated with prolonged survival times after complete resection. Mitotic index, nuclear atypia and Ki67 have been shown to be useful as prognostic markers for canine oral melanoma.

In **cats,** oropharyngeal malignant melanoma is rare. It occurs in older animals, involves the same regions affected in dogs, resembles the mixed tumor cell phenotype of dogs, and has a short median survival time.

Pigmented basilar epithelial cells are frequently present in superficial areas of the submucosa in a variety of nonneoplastic lesions resulting from irritation to the mucosa. *This so-called "pigmentary incontinence" must be differentiated from malignant melanoma.*

Fibrosarcomas

In **dogs,** fibrosarcoma is the third most common oral malignant tumor, comprising about 15-25% of such lesions, but the most common sarcoma of the oral cavity. It frequently occurs in younger dogs; for example, one report indicated 25% occurred in dogs <5 years of age, and the median age is ~7 years. Larger breeds appear to be predisposed, perhaps especially the Golden Retriever. It occurs mainly on the gums of the maxilla and adjacent palate and the rostral mandible, and less often in the buccal mucosa, lips, and tongue. *Despite a relatively benign histologic appearance in large breeds, it grows rapidly, invading maxillary and mandibular bone in the majority of cases, and frequently recurs after surgical removal.* About 20-35% have metastasized to regional nodes, and pulmonary metastases have occurred in about 10-20% at diagnosis. Median survival times after surgical resection are reported to be near 25 months.

The tumors are solitary gray to red, firm, irregularly shaped to nodular fleshy masses >4 cm in diameter that may ulcerate and become secondarily infected. They are usually fixed to any underlying bone. Microscopically, the submucosa is diffusely infiltrated by densely cellular sheets of pleomorphic fusiform fibroblasts arranged in interwoven bundles with variable, but often relatively small, amounts of collagen. The mitotic index is high in high-grade tumors, and there may be multinucleated giant cells scattered throughout.

In **cats,** this tumor is the second most frequent oropharyngeal malignancy, but it is not common. The gingiva and palate have been reported as sites of predilection by some, but others did not observe any specific location. The tumor resembles that in dogs, and invasion of bone is common.

Mast cell tumors

This tumor occurs occasionally in the oral cavity of middle-aged dogs, and, less frequently, in cats. Most commonly they are found on the lip of dogs, but they may arise in the submucosa of the tongue, gum, and hard palate. The tumor is diagnosed using the same criteria as cutaneous mastocytomas, and *all should be considered potentially malignant,* with metastasis to regional lymph nodes a possibility. Mast cell tumor should be considered in the differential diagnosis of oral lesions resembling granulation tissue or eosinophilic granuloma in dogs and cats. Lymph node metastasis may be higher in oral mast cell tumors compared with the cutaneous counterpart, and metastasis is associated with a poorer prognosis.

Granular cell tumors

This rare tumor occurs in older (mean age 9 years) **dogs,** mainly in the base of the tongue, but also in the gingiva, lips, and palate. Most granular cell tumors are thought to be derived from neuroectodermal precursor cells. They are elevated, usually less than ~2 cm in size, red, and granular or smooth on the mucosal surface. The cut surface is white and firm. Microscopically the mass consists of *large, polyhedral to round epithelioid cells that have abundant acidophilic granular cytoplasm.* The cytoplasmic granules are strongly periodic acid-Schiff–positive, and ultrastructurally are *phagolysosomes.* The nuclei are round to oval, centrally or eccentrically located, and have 1-2 nucleoli. Mitotic figures are rare. The tumor cells have a marked tendency to form nests or cords that are separated by a delicate network of reticulin fibers, although some are arranged as sheets of cells. None of these tumors in dogs have recurred after excision, and there is only one record of metastasis, to thoracic organs. There are a few reports of this tumor in the tonsil, tongue, gingiva, and palate of **cats.** In horses, granular cell tumors are located in the lungs (see Vol. 2, Respiratory system).

Neuroendocrine carcinomas of the oral cavity and pharynx

Neuroendocrine cells of the dispersed neuroendocrine system are present at a low density throughout most levels of the gastrointestinal tract, as well as at other sites, in several mammalian species. In older literature they may be referred to as *Merkel cells.*

Very rarely, they form tumors of the skin and the oral/nasal pharyngeal mucosa in the dog. In the latter site they tend to be pedunculated, and are located on the gums, lips, and pharynx. *Their behavior is aggressive, with metastasis to local nodes and distant sites,* and local recurrence if margins around the resected tumor are not adequate. Histologically, they consist of well-circumscribed, densely packed nests and sheets of polygonal to round cells in the submucosa, resulting in an organoid appearance. The cells have a moderate amount of pale basophilic cytoplasm. The nuclei are pleomorphic, the nuclear membrane is indented, and there are 1-2 centrally located nucleoli. The mitotic index varies from few to 2-3 mitotic figures per high-power field. Multinucleated giant cells are often present. The cells stain negatively with the periodic acid-Schiff stain but have a positive argyrophilic reaction. These are useful features to differentiate this tumor from granular cell tumors. The tumor must also be differentiated from malignant melanoma. Immunohistochemical reactions are usually positive for synaptophysin and neuron-specific enolase, and more variably for chromogranin-A and cytokeratin. Ultrastructurally, the tumor cells contain *cytoplasmic secretory granules characteristic of neuroendocrine cells.*

Plasmacytomas

Extramedullary plasmacytomas are uncommon tumors of the oral mucosa and skin of mainly older dogs (mean age 9-10 years). They arise as primary tumors from plasma cells in the soft tissue, or rarely as metastases from primary osseous myeloma.

This tumor has probably been under-diagnosed in the past, being mistaken for undifferentiated round cell tumor, histiocytic sarcoma, or a variant of dermal lymphoma. In the oral cavity, it has been misdiagnosed as malignant melanoma. Grossly the tumor is a red, lobulated raised mass usually located on the gingiva or lips. It can invade bone, rarely. Plasmacytoma also occurs sporadically in the stomach, colon, and rectum.

Histologically, the tumor is well circumscribed, nonencapsulated, and the overlying mucosa is usually intact, unless it has been traumatized in large tumors. The tumor cells are pleomorphic with variable amounts of amphophilic to basophilic cytoplasm. The nuclei are round to oval and the nuclear membrane is indented. The cells are densely packed into nests and sheets that are divided by scant fibrovascular stroma. Anisokaryosis, binucleated and multinucleated cells are frequently present in the center of the tumor, and the most differentiated plasma cells are usually evident at the periphery. The mitotic index varies widely from one tumor to another. Immunoglobulin, especially IgG, can frequently be demonstrated in the neoplastic cells, and AL amyloid (amyloid immunoglobulin light chain) is occasionally present among the tumor cells. Electron microscopic examination reveals features typical of plasma cells.

In spite of the anaplastic appearance and the presence of mitotic figures, the biological behavior of these tumors is *benign*, and they are cured by simple resection.

Vascular tumors

Lesions variously considered *vascular hamartomas* or *hemangiomas* have been described in the gums of neonatal calves and in the oral cavity of puppies. Hamartomas are focal disorganized overgrowths of mature tissue endogenous to the organ involved. Because of their location, they usually have an inflamed surface, and may resemble, superficially, granulation tissue or pyogenic granuloma. They are pink to red lobulated masses, up to several centimeters in diameter, often pedunculated, on the rostral mandibular gingiva adjacent to the incisors, which may be displaced. They also may be located in the tongue. Microscopically, the tumors consist of irregular thin-walled vascular channels containing erythrocytes or proteinaceous material, and lined by well-differentiated endothelial cells. The vascular spaces are separated by loose fibrous stroma. Vascular hamartomas are benign, but a single hemangiosarcoma in a young calf has been described that involved the palate and gums, as well as distant sites.

Hemangiomas occur rarely in the oral cavity of mature horses, dogs, and cats. Rare hemangiosarcomas have been recorded in the oral cavity of cats and a few dogs, the latter with cutaneous hemangiosarcomas.

Miscellaneous tumors

Various benign and malignant neoplastic and like lesions in the oropharynx have been reported sporadically. In the dog, benign masses include dermoid cysts, histiocytoma, lipoma, lymphangioma, hemangioma, rhabdomyoma, ganglioneuroblastoma, and calcinosis circumscripta (of the tongue). Malignant tumors that have been reported in the oral cavity, mainly in the lip and tongue, are hemangiosarcoma, leiomyosarcoma, histiocytoma, ectopic thyroid carcinoma, hemangiopericytoma, schwannoma, osteosarcoma, rhabdomyosarcoma, and highly malignant undifferentiated tumors.

In cats, benign tumors include hemangioma and fibroxanthoma, and malignant examples are oral and tonsillar lymphosarcoma, schwannoma, and osteosarcoma. Pharyngeal, lingual, and gingival lymphomas have been described in horses. Salivary tumors are described later in the section on salivary glands.

Further reading

Bergin I, et al. Prognostic evaluation of Ki67 threshold value in canine oral melanoma. Vet Pathol 2011;48:41-53.

Bernard H, et al. Classification of papillomaviruses (PVs) based on 189 PV types and proposal of taxonomic amendments. Virology 2010;401:70-79.

de Bruijn N, et al. A clinicopathological study of 52 feline epulides. Vet Pathol 2007;44:161-169.

Desoutter A, et al. Clinical and histologic features of 26 canine peripheral giant cell granulomas (formerly giant cell epulis). Vet Pathol 2012;49:1018-1023.

Fiani N, et al. Clinicopathologic characterization of odontogenic tumors and focal fibrous hyperplasia in dogs: 152 cases (1995-2005). J Am Vet Med Assoc 2011;238:495-500.

Frazier SA, et al. Outcome in dogs with surgically resected oral fibrosarcoma (1997-2008). Vet Comp Oncol 2012;10:33-43.

Hansen D, et al. Intraosseous maxillary hemangioma in an immature Bassett Hound. J Vet Dent 2010;27:234-241.

Head KW, et al. Tumors of the upper alimentary tract. In: Histological Classification of the Tumors of the Alimentary System of Domestic Animals. World Health Organization International Histological Classification of Tumors of Domestic Animals, second series. vol. X. Washington, DC: Armed Forces Institute of Pathology, American Registry of Pathology; 2003. p. 27-45.

Hillman L, et al. Biological behavior of oral and perioral mast cell tumors in dogs: 44 cases (1996-2006). J Am Vet Med Assoc 2010;237:936-942.

Oyamada T, et al. Pathology of canine oral malignant melanoma with cartilage and/or osteoid formation. J Vet Med Sci 2007;69:1155-1161.

Patnaik AK, et al. Neuroendocrine carcinoma of the nasopharynx in a dog. Vet Pathol 2002;39:496-500.

Smedley R, et al. Immunohistochemical diagnosis of canine oral amelanotic melanocytic neoplasms. Vet Pathol 2011;48:32-40.

Smedley R, et al. Prognostic markers for canine melanocytic neoplasms: a comparative review of the literature and goals for future investigation. Vet Pathol 2011;48:54-72.

Smithson CW, et al. Multicentric oral plasmacytoma in 3 dogs. J Vet Dent 2012;29:96-110.

Zaugg N, et al. Detection of novel papillomaviruses in canine mucosal, cutaneous and in situ squamous cell carcinomas. Vet Dermatol 2005;16:290-298.

SALIVARY GLANDS

Salivary glands are a complex set of secretory structures, present both as large discrete glands in the head and cranial neck region, and as an extensive series of submucosal minor salivary glands in the oral cavity, including the tongue, oropharynx and larynx. Gland structure is variable, depending on whether the gland produces serous or mucous secretion, or both. Common *acute reactions* to injury include hypersecretion, necrosis, edema, and inflammation. Gland atrophy, ductular fibrosis and obstruction, and squamous metaplasia may develop following *chronic injury*. *Oncocytic metaplasia* is a benign *age-related* lesion of salivary duct epithelium wherein eosinophilic granular swollen cells (oncocytes) containing abundant cytoplasmic mitochondria replace normal ductal epithelial cells.

The most common conditions of the salivary glands are functional. *Ptyalism* is increased secretion of saliva; *aptyalism* is reduced or absent secretion. Ptyalism is seen as abnormal accumulation of saliva in the mouth, and should be differentiated from failure to swallow. It occurs in a variety of conditions including stomatitis, organophosphate or heavy-metal poisoning, and encephalitis. Aptyalism is less common but may accompany fever, dehydration, and salivary gland disease.

Ptyalism in cattle and horses may be an expression of mycotoxicosis. *Rhizoctonia leguminicola* has a wide geographic distribution, and infestation of legumes is associated with "slobbers syndrome." Mycelial growth on well-cured hay is not grossly visible. Two biologically active alkaloids—*slaframine* and *swainsonine*—are produced by the fungus. Slaframine, a parasympathomimetic alkaloid, is associated with excessive salivation, lacrimation, anorexia, diarrhea, frequent urination, bloat, reduced milk production, and weight loss. No specific lesions have been associated with slaframine toxicosis. Guinea pigs are extremely sensitive to the toxin. Presumptive diagnosis may be based on feeding trials in that species, if chromatographic analysis for slaframine is not readily accessible.

Ptyalism may be associated with *neurointoxication*, particularly those agents that affect the trigeminal nuclei. Known causes include ingestion of *Paspalum destichium* (knotgrass) and *Prosopis glandulosa* (honey mesquite), poisoning with cholinergic stimulants, snake envenomation, neurotropic viruses, especially rabies virus, and in dogs exposure to the toad *Bufo marinus* cause neurologic abnormalities and ptyalism.

Vesicular and ulcerative diseases that affect the oral cavity, such as *foot-and-mouth disease* are usually associated with ptyalism.

Foreign bodies such as plant awns or fiber are occasionally present in the ducts; the parotid duct is more often affected than the submaxillary duct. They invariably cause some degree of inflammation or secondary infection and if the duct epithelium is destroyed, localized cellulitis occurs. **Salivary calculi** (*sialoliths*) may also cause obstruction and inflammation. They are more common in horses than other species; the parotid duct is most commonly affected. Microliths are formed routinely and undergo regular turnover; however, secretory inactivity can cause microliths to accumulate more material, leading to formation of large calculi that may cause obstruction. Calculi in horses are usually single hard white laminated structures composed largely of calcium carbonate; in dogs the composition varies. Many lodge at the orifice and cause some degree of salivary retention, glandular atrophy, and predisposition to infection and further inflammation.

Dilations of the duct are due to stagnation of flow or obstruction resulting from congenital atresia, foreign bodies, calculi, or inflammatory strictures. The dilated ducts appear as fluctuating cords, sometimes with local diverticula. **Ranula** *is the term applied to a smooth, rounded, fluctuant cystic distention of the duct in the floor of the mouth.* The lining epithelium may or may not be intact and cyst contents may be serous fluid or thick tenacious mucus. Rupture of a duct or a gland to an epithelial surface results in a permanent fistula as the continued flow of saliva prevents normal restoration, and the duct epithelium eventually fuses with the surface.

Salivary mucocele or **sialocele** *is an accumulation of salivary secretions in single or multiloculated cavities, not lined by secretory epithelium, in the soft tissues of the mouth or neck.* Sialoceles are often thought to be the result of trauma to the duct, and there may be a history of ranula-like swelling in the mouth. Most sialoceles are subcutaneous and may be large and pendulous, up to 10 cm in diameter. They can be located anywhere from the mandibular symphysis to the middle of the neck, but most are ventrolateral along the midline. They arise most commonly from the sublingual salivary gland, but sialoceles in other locations have been sporadically described.

Pharyngeal sialoceles are uncommon but affected dogs may present with dyspnea. Zygomatic and palatine sialoceles also occur, and can be associated with inflammation and cause exophthalmos and soft palate swelling, respectively. Small sialoceles, seldom exceeding 0.5 cm in size, are occasionally observed on the side of the *bovine tongue*. They presumably result from rupture of the fine tortuous ducts of the dorsal part of the sublingual gland.

The wall is soft, pliable, well-vascularized connective tissue with a glistening lining and the contents are initially mucinous but become progressively inspissated and tenacious. The histologic appearance of sialoceles varies greatly, apparently depending on the stage of development. Centrally there is abundant amorphous amphophilic material with a mixed inflammatory reaction, which may be very mild. Initially, the wall consists of an outer well-vascularized layer of immature connective tissue and an inner layer of loosely arranged fibroblasts. As the sialocele ages, mature fibrous connective tissue forms the wall, plasma cells or lymphocytes are the most numerous inflammatory cells, and the material in the center becomes progressively more basophilic.

Anomalous regression of pharyngeal pouches or clefts results in **pharyngeal (branchial) cysts, sinuses, or fistulae** that can manifest in a variety of ways. The lining of these cysts can vary from squamous to pseudostratified ciliated epithelium; occasionally more than one type of epithelium is observed. Congenital cervical sinuses, cysts and fistulae have been reported in veterinary species. **Thyroglossal duct cysts** have been reported in cats: These are remnants of pharyngeal thyroid primordium, occur directly on the midline, and are readily distinguishable histologically because they are lined by thyroidogenic epithelium.

Sialoadenitis, *inflammation of the salivary glands*, is uncommon, but after malignant neoplasms is the second most frequently diagnosed salivary gland lesion of dogs and cats. The submandibular gland is usually affected. Inflammation of the zygomatic gland in dogs is a cause of retrobulbar abscess. The route of infection is usually via the excretory duct, although it also may be hematogenous or localized trauma. Duct obstruction is due to inflammatory exudate, desquamated epithelial cells, and mucus, which may be expressed from the duct orifice. Partial or complete obstruction of the duct produces secondary atrophic changes in the glands, although there is initial gland enlargement resulting from the combined effects of retained secretion and inflammation. Ducts throughout the gland initially become dilated and inflamed. Acini swell and rupture from retained secretion, and this often leads to marked neutrophilic inflammation. In chronic cases, there is marked glandular atrophy with only remnants of atrophic epithelium embedded within inflamed fibrous connective tissue.

Specific inflammations of the salivary glands in domestic animals are few. Examples include rabies, where there is often focal lysis of acinar cells, mononuclear infiltration and rare Negri bodies in ganglionic neurons; strangles in horses; and distemper in dogs. *Eosinophilic sialoadenitis* may be a component of eosinophilic epitheliotropic syndrome in horses discussed in the section on Eosinophilic enteritis in cats and horses. *Sjögren's-like syndrome* has been diagnosed in cats and dogs, characterized by plasmacytic inflammation of salivary glands. Sialoadenitis can also occur *secondary to squamous metaplasia of interlobular salivary ducts*, which is an early lesion of **vitamin A deficiency**. Exposure to highly chlorinated naphthalenes is now rare, but can lead to hypovitaminosis A and subsequent squamous metaplasia.

Necrotizing sialometaplasia is a distinct and rare disease of dogs, cats and humans. There is characteristic ischemic necrosis of salivary gland lobules with inflammation and squamous metaplasia of the ducts, *features easily and often misinterpreted as malignant transformation*. The cause is thought to be vascular compromise induced by trauma, although immune-mediated destruction of blood vessels or infection have also been hypothesized. The disease is seen in a number of small breed dogs, primarily terriers; the submandibular gland is preferentially affected. Affected dogs are presented in extreme pain with enlarged firm salivary glands. Recurrent vomition is reported, and this is thought to be centrally mediated.

Further reading

Benjamino KP, et al. Pharyngeal mucoceles in dogs: 14 cases. J Am Anim Hosp Assoc 2012;48:31-35.

Cannon MS, et al. Clinical and diagnostic imaging findings in dogs with zygomatic sialadenitis: 11 cases (1990-2009). J Am Vet Med Assoc 2011;239:1211-1218.

Hill BD, et al. Clinical and pathological findings associated with congenital hypovitaminosis A in extensively grazed beef cattle. Aust Vet J 2009;87:94-98.

Nelson LN, et al. Pharyngeal pouch and cleft remnants in the dog and cat: a case series and review. J Am Anim Hosp Assoc 2012;48:105-112.

Spangler WL, Culbertson MR. Salivary gland disease in dogs and cats: 245 cases (1985-1988). J Am Vet Med Assoc 1991;198:465-469.

Trumpatori B, et al. Parotic duct sialolithiasis in a dog. J Am Anim Hosp Assoc 2007;43:45-51.

Neoplasms of salivary glands

Neoplasms of the salivary glands are rare in all species. They have been reported in cattle, sheep, goats, horses, dogs, and cats, but not swine; only in dogs and cats do salivary tumors occur often enough to permit generalization. Tumors are usually unilateral, and they may arise from any salivary gland, but the parotid and mandibular glands are most commonly affected. Neoplasms develop mostly in aged animals and are almost exclusively carcinomas. Cats tend to have more aggressive disease at the time of diagnosis and metastasis to regional nodes and distant sites, especially the lungs, is more common. Adenocarcinomas that have metastasized to the nodes or beyond at diagnosis have a worse prognosis than those with tumor localized to the gland.

The histologic structure of salivary tumors in animals is as diverse as humans, and morphology typically mimics cell types of normal salivary glands. The phenotype of salivary tumors has little bearing on prognosis, with notable exceptions being acinic cell carcinomas, which are tumors of low grade malignancy, and pleomorphic adenomas (or mixed salivary tumor), which have potential for malignant transformation. The most frequent variety is *adenocarcinoma*, and although there are various structural patterns (acinar, ductular, trabecular, solid) sometimes within the same tumor, an acinar or nested arrangement is usually evident somewhere, embedded in an often extensive fibrous stroma.

Mucoepidermoid carcinomas are composed of a combination of squamous epidermoid cells, mucus-producing cells and intermediate cells, which may line cysts, sometimes in a papillary pattern. Cyst rupture initiates a granulomatous response, including giant cells. Tumors with infiltrative peripheral growth pattern are likely to recur locally or metastasize to distant organs.

Acinic cell carcinomas are less common than adenocarcinomas, occurring mainly in dogs and sporadically in the cat, horse, and sheep. An essential criterion for diagnosis of this tumor is the presence of well-differentiated salivary epithelial cells (acinar, intercalated duct, vacuolated, clear or glandular cell subtypes). There is minimal cellular pleomorphism and a low mitotic index. They are at least partially encapsulated masses but often display infiltrative growth along the margins; however, metastases occur only late in course of disease.

Pleomorphic adenomas, or mixed tumors, have been described rarely in the dog, cat, cow, and horse. Analogous to mixed mammary tumors, they are composed of neoplastic myoepithelial and epithelial cells along with myxoid, chondroid, or osseous stromal transformation. They are considered benign, but complete excision is difficult and local recurrence is common. Development of malignant epithelial foci within benign tumors is described and represents malignant transformation (carcinoma in pleomorphic adenoma).

Rarely, other epithelial (myoepithelioma, squamous cell carcinoma, cystadenocarcinoma) and mesenchymal (angiolipoma, fibrous histiocytoma, osteosarcoma, fibrosarcoma) malignancies appear to arise in the salivary glands.

Further reading

Hammer A, et al. Salivary gland neoplasia in the dog and cat: survival times and prognostic factors. J Am Anim Hosp Assoc 2001;37:478-482.

Head KW, et al. Salivary gland tumors. In: Histological Classification of the Tumors of the Alimentary System of Domestic Animals. World Health Organization International Histological Classification of Tumors of Domestic Animals, 2nd series. vol. X. Washington, DC: Armed Forces Institute of Pathology, American Registry of Pathology; 2003. p. 58-72.

Kitshoff AM, et al. Infiltrative angiolipoma of the parotid salivary gland in a dog. J South Afr Vet Assoc 2010;81:258-261.

Smrkovski OA, et al. Carcinoma ex pleomorphic adenoma with sebaceous differentiation in the mandibular salivary gland of a dog. Vet Pathol 2006;43:374-377.

ESOPHAGUS

The esophagus is comprised of an inner circular layer and an outer longitudinal layer of skeletal muscle for much or all of its length. In the pig, there is a short segment near the cardia that is comprised of smooth muscle, and in horses and cats, smooth muscle is found in the distal third of the esophagus. The esophagus is lined by stratified squamous epithelium with a variable number of submucosal mucous glands, depending on the species and location along the esophagus. Esophageal protection against aggressive insults resides mainly in mucus and bicarbonate in salivary secretion and is produced by esophageal submucosal glands.

The esophagus merits particular attention during the examination of animals with inadequate growth rate, cachexia, ptyalism, dysphagia, regurgitation, vomition, and aspiration pneumonia. In ruminants, tympany may be a sequel to esophageal disease. The presence of a *bloat line* in the esophagus at the thoracic inlet may indicate a condition causing increased intra-abdominal pressure such as gastric dilation or ruminal tympany. The squamous mucosa is frequently eroded or ulcerated in viral diseases that cause similar lesions elsewhere in the upper alimentary tract. Conditions of striated muscle, such as nutritional myodegeneration and eosinophilic myositis in the ruminant, or polymyositis, systemic lupus erythematosus, and trypanosomiasis in the dog, involve the esophageal muscle. Envenomation following snake bite may lead to myopathy of the esophageal musculature in dogs. Diseases of the neuromuscular junction, as in myasthenia gravis, and peripheral neuropathies, such as giant axonal neuropathy and polyneuritis, result in esophageal disease.

Anomalies, epithelial metaplasia, and similar lesions

The mucosa of the distal portion of the feline esophagus normally has a herringbone pattern of superficial folds. **Hypertrophy of the smooth muscle** of the distal esophagus, most commonly the inner smooth circular layer, occurs in horses. It is usually found incidentally at autopsy, although some cases also have concurrent terminal ileal muscular hypertrophy. The lesion is considered idiopathic, but potential factors in the pathogenesis include autonomic imbalances or defects in the smooth muscle pacemaker cells normally found at these sites.

Congenital anomalies of the esophagus are very rarely recorded in domestic animals, and their interpretation as such can be difficult because similar defects may develop as sequelae of esophageal trauma or inflammation.

Congenital duplication cysts of the esophagus have been reported in horses and dogs. Esophageal cysts are classified as duplication by 3 essential criteria. The cyst must (1) be located within the esophageal wall, (2) be lined by columnar, squamous, cuboidal, ciliated, or pseudostratified epithelium, and (3) have a double muscle layer in the wall. Esophageal duplication cysts may be clinically silent; however, they manifest as space-occupying lesions if they fill with cellular debris and secretion. Potential complications are associated with compression of adjacent structures or cyst rupture.

Rare **segmental aplasia** of the proximal esophagus may be apparent in the neonate. A short blind pouch communicates with the pharynx, and a thin fibrous band connects it to the distal patent esophagus that follows a normal course to the stomach. Esophageal atresia and congenital esophagorespiratory communications result from anomalies occurring when the respiratory primordium buds from the embryonic foregut.

Esophagorespiratory fistulae without esophageal atresia are also rare in animals. Esophageal fistula formation is likely acquired following foreign body perforation of the esophagus; however, in calves and dogs, some are likely congenital. Short fibrous bands with a narrow epithelial-lined lumen connecting an esophagus of normal diameter with the trachea or bronchus are reported, as are small apertures connecting the lining of esophageal diverticula with the respiratory tree. The lining of such defects changes from stratified squamous to columnar respiratory epithelium in the fistula or wall of the diverticulum. Gastric distention by air in calves, and pneumonia resulting from aspiration, have been associated with esophagorespiratory fistulae.

Esophageal diverticula are irregular outpouchings or herniations of the esophageal mucosa through a defect in the esophageal tunica muscularis. They communicate with the esophagus by variously sized, often slit-like apertures. Most are probably acquired, and they occur most often in the lower cervical esophagus near the thoracic inlet and the distal thoracic esophagus just cranial to the diaphragm. Increased intraluminal pressure associated with foreign bodies, obstruction or stenosis are potential causes of *pulsion diverticula*, in which the mucosa is forced out through the distended or ruptured muscularis. Such diverticula may be large spherical structures with a narrow neck and are most common in the horse and dog. The rare *traction diverticulum* is the result of contraction of a paraesophageal fibrous adhesion, following perforation and inflammation, drawing with it a pouch of esophageal mucosa that is usually small and inconsequential. In contrast to pulsion diverticula, which have a layer of epithelium lining the inner aspect of a wall of fibrous connective tissue, traction diverticula have a wall comprised of all layers of the esophagus. Ingesta and foreign bodies may accumulate in diverticula, causing gradual enlargement with the potential for local esophagitis, ulceration, and perforation or formation of a fistula.

Other rare *anomalies* of the esophageal mucosa include epithelial inclusion cysts and distal esophageal papillae in cattle resembling those of the rumen, and gastric heterotopia.

Hyperkeratosis and hyperplasia of the esophageal epithelium may be signs of vitamin A deficiency or chlorinated naphthalene toxicity, which has been described in herbivores. This is accompanied by squamous metaplasia of mucous glands and ducts of the esophagus and throughout the body. Mild hyperkeratosis may be difficult to assess in herbivores because some degree of keratinization is normal and anorexia or failure to swallow results in loss of the abrasive effect of food passage leading to accumulation of keratinized squames. Parakeratosis and epithelial hyperplasia is indicative of response to epithelial injury (see later section on Esophagitis). In the distal esophagus of pigs, this lesion is often observed concomitant with ulceration of the pars esophagea of the stomach. Esophageal parakeratosis can also occur in pigs with cutaneous parakeratosis caused by zinc deficiency.

Further reading

Adami C, et al. Severe esophageal injuries occurring after general anesthesia in two cats: case report and literature review. J Am Anim Hosp Assoc 2011;47:436-442.

Benders NA, et al. Idiopathic muscular hypertrophy of the oesophagus in the horse: a retrospective study of 31 cases. Equine Vet J 2004;36:46-50.

Gabor LJ, Walshaw R. Esophageal duplication cyst in a dog. Vet Pathol 2008;45:61-62.

Komine M, et al. Megaesophagus in Friesian horses associated with muscular hypertrophy of the caudal esophagus. Vet Pathol 2014;51:979-985.

Nawrocki MA, et al. Fluoroscopic and endoscopic localization of an esophagobronchial fistula in a dog. J Am Anim Hosp Assoc 2003;39:257-261.

Esophagitis

Erosive and ulcerative esophagitis is a common finding associated with viral diseases causing similar lesions in the oropharynx or reticulorumen, including bovine viral diarrhea, rinderpest, bovine papular stomatitis, infectious bovine rhinotracheitis, and feline calicivirus. Epithelial proliferation or granulation tissue during healing of ulcers may result in raised opaque areas at the lesion margin or surface, respectively.

Caustic or irritant chemicals, ionizing radiation, electrochemical reactions (batteries), or heat may cause mucosal injury, the severity of which depends on the nature of the insult and duration of exposure. Mild acute insult may result in reddening of the mucosa. More severe insult results in liquefactive necrosis associated with alkalis, and coagulative necrosis associated with exposure to acids and toxins (paraquat, oak toxicosis) and may result in deep esophageal ulceration and sloughing of the mucosa.

Superficial epithelial damage heals uneventfully, though repeated insult may cause irregular epithelial hyperplasia. Ulcerated mucosa heals by granulation, and raised islands of surviving proliferative epithelium may be observed on the surface. The inflammatory reaction in ulceration frequently involves tunica muscularis and adventitia. Fibrosis and scarring may cause stricture or stenosis, if the original defect involved a significant portion of the esophageal circumference.

Reflux esophagitis occurs because of a loss of functional integrity of the lower esophageal sphincter associated with airway occlusion and increased intra-abdominal pressure, the pharmacologic effects of preanesthetic agents, or abnormality of the hiatus. Esophagitis is due to the action of gastric acid, pepsin, and probably regurgitated bile salts and pancreatic enzymes, on the esophageal mucosa. Reflux esophagitis is most common in dogs and cats as a sequel to surgery involving general anesthesia, although it may follow chronic gastric regurgitation or vomition for any cause (Fig. 1-22). In swine and horses, it may be associated with ulceration of the squamous portion of the stomach. In dogs, it can be associated with hiatus herniation. A high prevalence of apparent gastroesophageal reflux disease in the distal esophagus of premature calves was demonstrated by endoscopy; however, the pathogenesis remains unclear.

Stratified squamous epithelium appears more susceptible to the corrosive effects of gastric secretion than other types of mucosa in the lower gastrointestinal tract. Relatively short duration of exposure to refluxed gastric content is required to induce epithelial damage characterized by hyperemia, linear

erosions, ulcers, or superficial fibrinonecrotic debris. Such damage is most common in the distal esophagus, but in some instances can extend to the pharynx. Epithelial hyperplasia and neutrophilic exocytosis occur in response to mild superficial epithelial necrosis. A consequence of chronic gastroesophageal reflux, well recognized in humans and described in dogs and cats, is columnar and mucous cell metaplasia of the distal esophagus. In humans, the lesion is known as *Barrett esophagus* and is an important risk factor for development of esophageal adenocarcinoma, but this has not been clearly demonstrated in animals.

Hiatus hernia usually involves sliding herniation of all or part of the abdominal esophagus, cardia, and stomach into the thoracic esophagus, rather than periesophageal herniation. It is generally self-reducing, but usually results in lower esophageal sphincter failure and reflux, rather than gastric herniation and obstruction. *Gastroesophageal intussusception* is a rare event, most reported in puppies of large breeds of dogs, and is associated with recurrent vomition that may lead to aspiration pneumonia.

Thrush, or mycotic esophagitis caused by *Candida albicans*, is seen in piglets and weaner swine, and may involve the squamous mucosa of the entire upper alimentary canal. C. *albicans* is an opportunist seen secondary to antibiotic therapy, inanition, or esophageal gastric reflux, and is considered more fully in the later section on Mycotic diseases of the gastrointestinal tract.

Further reading

Gibson CJ, et al. Adenomatous polyp with intestinal metaplasia of the esophagus (Barrett esophagus) in a dog. Vet Pathol 2010;47:116-119.

Guzelbektes H, et al. Prevalence of gastroesophageal reflux disease in premature calves. J Vet Intern Med 2012;26:1051-1055.

Sarosiek J, McCallum RW. Mechanisms of oesophageal mucosal defence. Baillieres Best Pract Res Clin Gastroenterol 2000;14:701-717.

Sivacolundhu RK, et al. Hiatal hernia controversies—a review of pathophysiology and treatment options. Aust Vet J 2002;80:48-53.

Esophageal obstruction, stenosis, and perforation

Esophageal obstruction can have *intrinsic* or *extrinsic* causes, and the lesions are generally obvious. The esophagus proximal to the stenotic area may be dilated, contain retained ingesta, or have evidence of erosion, ulceration or inflammation. *Choke*, or esophageal impaction, is the most common example of *intrinsic obstruction*, and occurs when large or inadequately chewed and lubricated foods, masses of grain or fibrous ingesta, or medically administered boluses lodge in the lumen of the esophagus (Fig. 1-23). Predisposed sites are where the esophagus deviates or is slightly restricted normally: the area overlying the larynx, the thoracic inlet, the base of the heart, and just cranial to the diaphragmatic hiatus.

Complications of obstruction include *pressure necrosis and ulceration of the mucosa*, which may progress to perforation or less commonly development of esophageal diverticula or fistulae. Sharp objects, such as bones, are most likely to cause *perforation*. Severe cellulitis of the periesophageal tissue ensues, and depending on the site of perforation, may involve

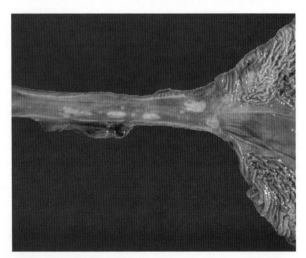

Figure 1-22 **Reflux esophagitis** of the distal esophagus following chronic vomition in a dog.

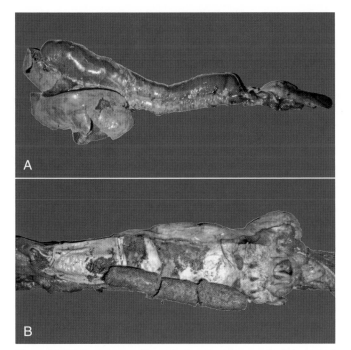

Figure 1-23 Impaction of esophagus in a horse. **A.** Adventitial view. **B.** Open esophagus showing impacted feed.

the mediastinum directly or by extension along fascial planes from the cervical region. Perforation of the thoracic esophagus may lead to pleuritis. Sharp objects, such as needles, quills, grass seeds, and awns, may penetrate and track from the esophagus through adjacent tissues.

Removal or dissolution of an obstruction may allow healing of the segmentally ulcerated esophagus. As for reflux esophagitis, *fibrosis and scarring* of large ulcers may result in narrowing of the lumen, stricture, or stenosis. Although hypertrophy of internal and external muscle layers is seen occasionally in the distal esophagus of cattle and horses (in which species the distal esophageal muscle is normally relatively thick), this change is usually not clearly the result of obstruction. Stenosis rarely is caused by intramural or intraluminal neoplasia, or more commonly by external compression which can be due to enlarged thyroid glands, thymus, and cervical or mediastinal lymph nodes.

The most common causes of external compression and constriction of the esophagus are **vascular ring anomalies** seen in dogs, occasionally in cats, and rarely in other species. *Persistence of the right fourth aortic arch* is the most common of these anomalies, and occurs when the right aortic arch develops instead of the normal left aortic arch. With this condition, the *ligamentum arteriosum* forms a vascular ring around the esophagus, resulting in entrapment and constriction of the esophagus against the trachea. *Other vascular anomalies* that may constrict the esophagus are reported only in the dog and include: persistence of both right and left aortic arches, persistent right ductus arteriosus, aberrant left subclavian artery in association with persistent right aortic arch, and aberrant right subclavian artery arising distal to the left subclavian artery and passing dorsally over the esophagus. The Irish Setter, German Shepherd, German Pinscher, and Boston Terrier are breeds most commonly afflicted with vascular ring anomalies.

Further reading

Feige K, et al. Esophageal obstruction in horses: a retrospective study of 34 cases. Can Vet J 2000;41:207-210.

Manzel J, Distl O. Unusual vascular ring anomaly associated with a persistent right aortic arch and an aberrant left subclavian artery in German pinschers. Vet J 2011;187:352-355.

Thompson HC, et al. Esophageal foreign bodies in dogs: 34 cases (2004-2009). J Vet Emerg Crit Care (San Antonio) 2012;22:253-261.

Dysphagia

Deglutition is a complex and highly coordinated physical act, which may be conveniently divided into three phases—oral, pharyngeal, and esophageal. **Oral dysphagia** occurs because of painful lesions involving the oral cavity and tongue, such as stomatitis, glossitis, and gingivitis, or lesions that impair movement of the tongue or delivery of the bolus to the oropharynx, such as loss of hypoglossal nerve function associated with hydrocephalus, trauma, or myasthenia gravis. Cleft palate can result in nasal regurgitation.

Pharyngeal dysphagia may be associated with painful inflammatory or neoplastic lesions involving the pharynx, tonsils, or retropharyngeal region, which may physically intrude on the pharyngeal space required for swallowing. Encephalitis involving the medulla oblongata and nuclei or tracts of the major cranial nerves involved in pharyngeal contraction and lingual function (V, IX, X, XII) should be carefully examined in cases of pharyngeal dysphagia unexplained by other lesions. Rabies and brain abscess in all species, infectious bovine rhinotracheitis and listeriosis in ruminants, are important central causes of pharyngeal paralysis. Retropharyngeal abscesses or other lesions of the equine guttural pouch may cause peripheral nerve damage and paralysis. Idiopathic myodegeneration, muscular dystrophies, and myasthenia gravis have been reported to impair pharyngeal muscle function.

Cricopharyngeal dysphagia is recognized in dogs as a swallowing disorder of the upper esophageal sphincter characterized by cricopharyngeal muscle **asynchrony** or **achalasia** (failure of the muscle to relax). The cause is unknown but this may be a primary muscular disorder because cricopharyngeal myotomy or myectomy is curative.

Megaesophagus, or *esophageal ectasia*, is recognized as dilation of the esophageal lumen, and is the result of atony and flaccidity of the esophageal muscle (Fig. 1-24). This occurs as the result of segmental or diffuse motor dysfunction of the body of the esophagus, and results in failure of peristaltic propulsion of the food bolus through the lower esophageal sphincter into the stomach. Ingesta accumulates in the esophageal lumen, which may lead to putrefaction and esophagitis in dilated or dependent areas; undigested food is eventually regurgitated. The volume of the dilated thoracic and cervical esophagus may greatly exceed that of the stomach causing ventral displacement of the intrathoracic trachea and heart. Animals with megaesophagus may have signs of malnutrition, including emaciation, dehydration, and osteopenia as well as rhinitis and aspiration pneumonia resulting from regurgitation.

Congenital idiopathic megaesophagus (CIM) is relatively common in dogs; it may improve functionally to some extent with time. CIM has its highest prevalence in Great Danes,

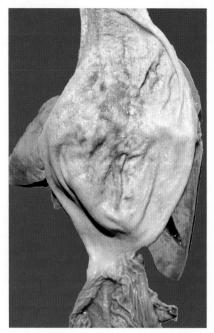

Figure 1-24 Congenital **esophageal dilation** in a dog. The mucosa is eroded, and the capacity of distal esophagus (top) exceeds that of stomach (bottom).

German Shepherds, and Irish Setters. In Miniature Schnauzers, the condition has an inheritance pattern of simple autosomal dominant with incomplete (60%) penetrance. With very rare exceptions, it is not secondary to physical obstruction or failure of the lower esophageal sphincter to open. Motor stimulation to the striated esophageal muscle, despite being carried in the vagus, is not autonomic, and seems intact. There is strong evidence that CIM results from a selective defect in the distension-sensitive afferent autonomic arm of the reflex that coordinates esophageal function.

Idiopathic megaesophagus can develop in *mature dogs,* and based on some studies, this represents the majority of cases. Most cases of idiopathic megaesophagus in dogs are not comparable with humans, in which *esophageal achalasia* is a significant primary motor disorder.

Megaesophagus may be acquired secondary to glycogen storage disease in Lapland dogs, localized or systemic myasthenia gravis, administration of cholinesterase inhibitors, hypoadrenocorticism, canine giant axonal neuropathy, immune-mediated polymyositis, polyradiculoneuritis, canine distemper, systemic lupus erythematosus, lead poisoning, Chagas disease, and snake envenomation.

Megaesophagus in the **cat** may be congenital, and it appears most common in the Siamese breed. The pathogenesis is unclear. Neuronal degeneration or neurogenic atrophy of muscle is not recognized in the esophageal wall. Acquired megaesophagus in cats has been associated with functional pyloric stenosis, hiatus hernia, upper respiratory obstruction/nasopharyngeal polyps, and lead poisoning.

Presumed congenital megaesophagus has been reported in **foals.** Histologic examination of the segmentally dilated proximal esophagus revealed no significant lesions of muscle or ganglia. Aganglionosis has also been implicated in megaesophagus in foals. Megaesophagus also may be acquired in foals; in such cases there is usually ulceration of the distal esophagus, as well as the pars esophagea of the stomach.

Megaesophagus in **cattle** has been described as congenital, or more commonly an acquired lesion associated with hiatus hernia, or pharyngeal trauma presumably causing vagus nerve damage. Megaesophagus is rarely reported in small ruminants.

Further reading

Broekman LE, Kuiper D. Megaesophagus in the horse. A short review of the literature and 18 own cases. Vet Q 2002;24:199-202.

Elliot RC. An anatomical and clinical review of cricopharyngeal achalasia in the dog. J South Afr Vet Assoc 2010;81:75-79.

Evans J, et al. Canine inflammatory myopathies: a clinicopathologic review of 200 cases. J Vet Intern Med 2004;18:679-691.

Mace S, et al. Megaesophagus. Compend Contin Educ Vet 2012;34:E1.

Shelton GD, et al. Risk factors for acquired myasthenia gravis in cats: 105 cases (1986-1998). J Am Vet Med Assoc 2000;216:55-57.

Parasitic diseases of the esophagus

Sarcosporidiosis occurs in the striated esophageal muscle of sheep. Esophageal sarcocysts appear as ovoid white thin-walled nodules ~1 cm long projecting from the esophageal muscle. *Sarcocystis gigantea,* the species producing large esophageal cysts and similar large cysts in skeletal muscle, is spread by cats. Microscopic sarcocysts of other species also may be encountered in esophageal striated muscle of a variety of hosts (see section on protistan infections, and Vol. 1, Muscle and tendon). Sarcocysts in esophageal muscle normally incite little or no local inflammatory reaction and are only of significance in meat inspection. *Eosinophilic myositis* can be observed in the esophageal muscle and, although the cause of this lesion is not certain, it is thought to be associated with rupture of cysts of this parasite.

In horses, **Gasterophilus** spp. larvae may be temporarily attached to the caudal pharyngeal, cranial esophageal or distal esophageal mucosa adjacent to the cardia; ulcers may occur at the sites of attachment.

The larvae of the warble fly **Hypoderma lineatum** reside for some time in the submucosa or adventitia of the bovine esophagus before they migrate to the dermis of the back. Here the small 2-4-mm translucent larvae grow up to 6 times before migrating toward the back of the host, but can cause local hemorrhage and inflammation. Death of first-stage larvae in the esophageal wall following systemic insecticide treatment, for example, can lead to severe acute inflammation in the esophageal submucosa and potentially esophageal obstruction, tympany, and perforation.

Spirurid nematodes of the genus **Gongylonema** may be encountered in the stratified squamous mucosa of the upper alimentary tract, including the esophagus, in ruminants and swine. These white thread-like worms up to 10-15 cm long burrow in the epithelium or propria of the esophagus and produce white or red, blood-filled serpentine tracks (Fig. 1-25). Their presence is inconsequential to the host.

Spirocerca lupi is a spirurid nematode that parasitizes the esophageal wall of Canidae and some other carnivores. It is most common in warm climates where dogs ingest third-stage larvae either via the dung beetle intermediate host or one of several insectivorous vertebrate paratenic hosts such as rodents, chickens, or reptiles. Larvae penetrate the gastric mucosa and migrate along arteries to the aorta, then subintimally to the caudal thoracic area, which they attain within

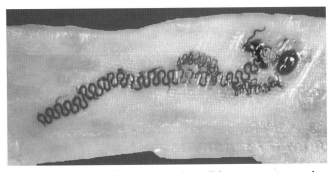

Figure 1-25 Blood-filled tracks and small hematoma in esophageal mucosa caused by **Gongylonema pulchrum** migration in a cow.

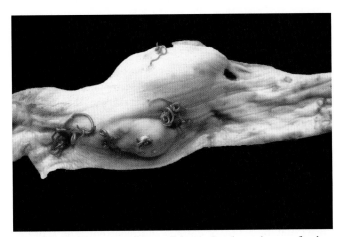

Figure 1-26 *Spirocerca lupi* nodules in distal esophagus of a dog. Worms protrude through fistulae into esophageal lumen. (Courtesy R.G. Thomson.)

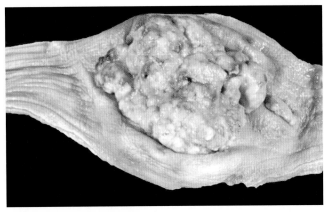

Figure 1-27 Ulcerating **fibrosarcoma** associated with **Spirocerca** granuloma in the distal esophagus of a dog. (Courtesy R.G. Thomson.)

several weeks of infection. Following 2-4 months in a granuloma in the aortic adventitia, worms migrate to the subjacent esophagus where they develop to adulthood. Here the adult nematodes are found within large, thick-walled cystic granulomas in the submucosa of the distal esophagus or gastric cardia. A fistula leading to the esophageal lumen is usually present, through which the tail of the female worm may protrude, and which provides the outlet for ova to the gastrointestinal tract (Fig. 1-26). Larvae that adopt aberrant migratory pathways may be found in granulomas in sites such as the subcutis, bladder, kidney, spinal cord, as well as stomach and intrathoracic locations.

Aortic lesions associated with *Spirocerca* are described in Vol. 3, Cardiovascular system, but include intimal and medial hemorrhage and necrosis with eosinophilic inflammation; intimal roughening with thrombosis; aneurysm with rare aortic rupture; intimal and medial mineralization, and heterotopic bone deposition. The presence of persistent aortic lesions in the dog, even in the absence of esophageal granuloma, is evidence of prior infection with *S. lupi*. Caudal thoracic vertebral body spondylitis occurs in greater than half of cases and is characterized by exostoses or bony spurs arising from the ends of the vertebral bodies. The pathogenesis is unclear, but may by initiated by migrating worms or inflammatory mediators.

In some animals with *S. lupi, mesenchymal neoplasms* develop in the wall of the esophageal granuloma (Fig. 1-27); pulmonary fibrosarcoma has been associated with an ectopic

worm. The granulomas around *S. lupi* contain highly reactive pleomorphic fibroblasts with large open nuclei and numerous mitotic figures. Neoplasms arising from such lesions have cytologic characteristics typical of fibrosarcoma and osteosarcoma, with local tissue invasion, and in many cases, pulmonary metastasis. The carcinogenic stimuli associated with the development of these tumors are unknown. Hypertrophic pulmonary osteopathy is occasionally found in animals with *Spirocerca*-associated sarcoma and, rarely, granuloma.

Further reading

Kirberger RM, et al. *Spirocerca lupi*-associated vertebral changes: a radiologic-pathologic study. Vet Parasitol 2013;195:87-94.

Ranen E, et al. Spirocercosis-associated esophageal sarcomas in dogs. A retrospective study of 17 cases (1997-2003). Vet Parasitol 2004;119:209-221.

Van der Merwe LL, et al. *Spirocerca lupi* infection in the dog: a review. Vet J 2008;176:294-309.

FORESTOMACHS

The rumen represents the central processing unit for ingesta and as such is critical to the animal's well-being. However, because most of this occurs as a chemical process with minimal morphologic correlates, it is an organ that often seems to be overlooked by pathologists. Examination of ruminal contents may provide critical cues with respect to general metabolic states. Overly dry contents are an excellent indicator of dehydration. Voluminous frothy contents occur with primary bloat. Urea toxicity can be detected by an ammoniacal odor and alkaline pH. An odor of cooked turnips or a pungent insecticidal smell is suggestive of organophosphates. In grain overload, contents have a fermentative odor and pH may be <5.0. However, with putrefaction and release of toxic amines into the rumen, pH in cases of acidosis may return to near-normal levels. In these animals, the ruminal epithelium remains adherent to the submucosa despite any intervening postmortem changes, and it is an important clue to mucosal disease. Vagus indigestion, often associated with dysfunction of the esophageal groove, leads to accumulation of large volumes of watery fluid within the forestomachs. The rumen content of animals with *Taxus* spp. toxicity will have an aromatic odor like cedar oil and needles will be present in the ingesta. Recognition of characteristic foliage in rumen content may lead to a diagnosis of poisoning by several different toxic plants, including cyanogenic plants of the genus *Prunus*, oleandrin-containing plants of the genus *Nerium*, and so on. Motor oil, paint flakes, or metallic lead present in the rumen would help to support a diagnosis of lead poisoning. Several other toxic substances can be identified by visual inspection of the ruminal contents.

Dystrophic and hyperplastic changes in the ruminal mucosa

The ruminal mucosa is unique in that it has a stratified squamous epithelium that functions in absorption as well as protection from the vat of fermenting bacteria contained within. Langerhans cells are distributed within the mucosa throughout all compartments of the ovine rumen. T lymphocytes are found individually, and in aggregates, in both intraepithelial and subepithelial locations, with most in the cranial sac and relatively few dorsally.

Ruminal papillae in newborn calves are rudimentary and their subsequent development is dependent on diet, possibly as a consequence of stimulation by insulin-like growth factor-1. The end products of ruminal carbohydrate fermentation, propionate and butyrate, stimulate papillary growth. Papillae can take a variety of shapes, including long and flat, conical, spade-shaped, or hair-like. High-concentrate rations, which provide abundant propionate and butyrate, tend to produce papillae that are club-shaped, clumped (Fig. 1-28), and may be dark. Microscopically, these papillae are covered with epithelium displaying acanthosis, hyperkeratosis, orthokeratosis, and parakeratosis, and hyperpigmentation. Secondary papillae may be hyperplastic as well, creating the clumped appearance or rosette-like configurations. Rumens in animals fed barley rations have similar changes. Hairs from the rachilla of the barley adhere to the mucosa, especially in the interpapillary areas, giving it a distinct matted appearance. These penetrate the mucosa and lamina propria, where they evoke a leukocytic reaction, often causing microabscesses. A diffuse pleocellular reaction is evident in the thickened fibrotic wall.

Roughage also plays a role. When animals receive adequate levels (~15%) of coarse roughage, propionic and butyric acids

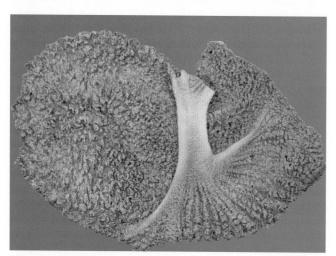

Figure 1-28 Clubbing and adhesion of rumen papillae with parakeratotic epithelium, associated with feeding a high-concentrate ration in a calf. (Courtesy S.S. Diab.)

decrease, whereas acetic acid levels increase, precluding hyperkeratosis and parakeratosis.

Hyperkeratosis of the ruminal epithelium also occurs in calves deficient in vitamin A.

Further reading

Di Giancamillo A, et al. The influence of different fibrous supplements in the diet on ruminal histology and histometry in veal calves. Histol Histopathol 2003;18:727-733.

Liu JH, et al. A high-grain diet causes massive disruption of ruminal epithelial tight junctions in goats. Am J Physiol Regul Integr Comp Physiol 2013;305:R232-241.

Shen Z, et al. Intraruminal infusion of n-butyric acid induces an increase of ruminal papillae size independent of IGF-1 system in castrated bulls. Arch Anim Nutr 2005;59:213-225.

Postmortem change

The ruminal mucosal epithelium usually sloughs within a few hours after death. It separates from the lamina propria in large gray patches, which cover the ingesta when the rumen is opened. *Persistent firm attachment of the ruminal epithelium is abnormal.* This undue adhesion occurs in acute and chronic rumenitis, especially if caused by fungi, and about scars of healed rumenitis. Adhesion may not occur in the early stages of ruminal acidosis.

Dilation of the rumen

Tympanitic distention of the forestomachs (tympany, hoven, bloat) may be acute, or chronic and recurrent. The acute or primary tympany of cattle fed legumes or high-concentrate rations is characterized by foaming of the rumen contents, which prevents gas from being eructated, whereas in chronic or recurrent (secondary) tympany, the gas is free but retained because of some physical or functional defect of eructation.

Primary tympany is also called *frothy bloat*. Foam production in ruminal contents occurs normally. However, the amount of foam produced is small and unstable. There is apparently a delicate balance between profoaming and antifoaming factors in the rumen. These factors are multiple, and there is considerable controversy as to the extent to which each one influences the production of the foamy, viscous ruminal content so characteristic of frothy bloat, the most common cause of rumen distension.

The formation of foam is dependent on *soluble proteins*, especially fraction I proteins, which are present in high levels (up to 4.5%) in bloat-inducing legumes, such as alfalfa and clover, especially in the prebloom stage of growth. Other legumes, notably sainfoin, trefoil, and cicer milk vetch, are not associated with bloat. Soluble proteins, released from chloroplasts, are degraded by the rumen microflora, and they rise to the surface where they are denatured, become insoluble, and stabilize the foam. The optimal pH (isoelectric point) for foam production by soluble proteins ranges from 5.4 to 6.0. *Pectins* are considered to increase viscosity of ruminal fluid and may act as foam-stabilizing agents. Plant lipids may act as antifoaming agents by competing for metal ions with the soluble proteins, thus inhibiting the denaturation of these proteins and resulting in decreased foam production.

Eructation is a complex series of muscular contractions in which gas is forced from the rumen through the cardia and is released through the esophagus. The eructation sequence is initiated by the presence of free gas in the dorsal sac of the rumen. Thus, if ruminal conditions prevent normal contractions from occurring in the reticulorumen or if movement of free gas through the cardia or esophagus is obstructed, bloat occurs. Excessive foam production causes distention of the rumen because it prevents formation of a free gas cap and the clearing of the cardia, which is essential for normal eructation to take place. When foam enters the esophagus, it stimulates the swallowing reflex, which also interferes with normal eructation. Gassy froth accumulates in the rumen as a consequence.

The variation among animals in their susceptibility to bloat may be determined in part by variations in the amount and composition of *saliva*. Saliva apparently has properties that may promote or prevent foaming in the rumen. When secretion of saliva decreases, the viscosity of ruminal contents increases, which in turn promotes foaming. Cows that have high susceptibility to bloating produce less saliva than cows that have low susceptibility. Succulent and high-concentrate feeds reduce salivary secretion, thus increasing viscosity of rumen contents. The composition of saliva also affects foam production in several ways. Combination of salivary bicarbonate with organic acids such as citric, malonic, and succinic, which are present in high levels in legumes, results in the production of large amounts of *carbon dioxide*, enhancing bubble formation. Carbon dioxide accounts for 40-70% of the total gas produced in the rumen.

High and low susceptibility to bloat can be temporarily transferred between animals by exchange of total reticulorumen contents. The understanding of the full role played by these various factors in bloat is incomplete, and other factors may be involved.

Rations high in concentrate and low in roughage not only reduce saliva secretion, but also change the ruminal microflora. They promote the growth of large numbers of encapsulated bacteria, which increase the concentration of polysaccharides, and these, in turn, increase the viscosity, promoting foam. These bacteria are also often mucinolytic and may destroy salivary mucins. Perhaps this explains the more gradual onset of **feedlot bloat**, because it takes time for the ruminal flora to change. Particle size of the grains fed may be one factor in feedlot bloat, with smaller particle size predisposing more to bloat.

The *cause of death* in bloat is probably a combination of physical and metabolic effects. Increased intra-abdominal pressure on the diaphragm inhibits respiration, and adversely affects cardiac function. Hypoxia may be caused by respiratory embarrassment. Increased intra-abdominal pressure also has a marked effect on the hemodynamics of the abdominal viscera, which are compressed, driving blood out of them. The caudal vena cava is also compressed, decreasing venous return to the heart. Distention also affects mucosal permeability and alters vagosympathetic reflexes.

The bloated animal is often found dead and distended with gas; blood exudes from the orifices, and because of the gaseous distention, the carcass often rolls on its back and assumes a sawhorse posture, with forelegs extended forward and rear legs pointing backward. The blood is dark and clots poorly; both features are indicative of death from anoxia. Subcutaneous hemorrhages are prominent in the cranial extremities, which are congested. There is marked edema, congestion, and hemorrhage of the cervical muscles and of the lymph nodes of the head and neck. An inconsistent but suggestive finding

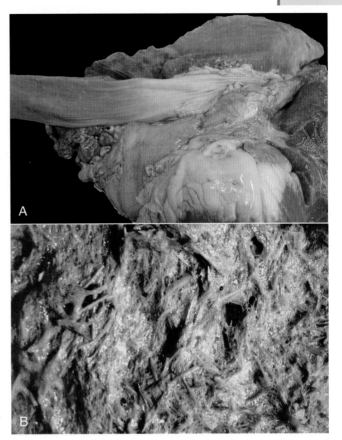

Figure 1-29 A. Bloat line in the esophagus of a cow with ruminal tympany. Congestion of esophagus and connective tissue cranial to thoracic inlet and blanching of esophagus caudal to thoracic inlet. (Courtesy M. Spinato) **B. Frothy bloat** in a cow. Fine bubbles are evident in the rumen content.

is the so-called *bloat line* in the esophageal mucosa (Fig. 1-29A). This lesion is formed because of congestion with petechial and ecchymotic hemorrhages in the mucosa of the cervical esophagus, which changes abruptly or gradually to a pale mucosa at the level of the thoracic inlet. Although the presence of this line is usually considered highly suggestive of bloat, a similar change can apparently be seen in other conditions and some pathologists do not interpret this line as diagnostic for bloat.

The tracheal mucosa is hemorrhagic, especially cranial to the thoracic inlet. Blood clots are frequently seen in the bronchi, and paranasal and frontal sinuses. The lungs are pale and compressed into the cranial thorax by the bulging diaphragm. There is pressure ischemia of the abdominal viscera, especially the liver, though the extreme margins of the hepatic lobes may be congested. Lymph nodes and the muscles of the hind legs are pale.

There may be marked subcutaneous edema, particularly of the vulva, inguinal region, and perineum, and intestines may herniate through the inguinal canals. If the autopsy is done soon after death, the ruminal contents are bulky and foamy (Fig. 1-29B). The foam gradually disappears after death and is usually absent if the autopsy is delayed for 10-12 hours. Inguinal hernia and diaphragmatic rupture may occur after death.

Secondary tympany (free gas or secondary bloat) may be acute, but is generally chronic, with periods of acute exacerbation. It is usually the result of a physical or functional *defect in eructation of gas* produced by normal rumen fermentation. The more common physical problems include internal or external obstructions of the esophagus or esophageal groove by tumor, foreign body, or esophageal stenosis of any cause. Reticular adhesions, abscesses, peritonitis, or tumor masses that interfere with contractions of the forestomach can result in bloat. Functional causes of secondary tympany include organophosphate intoxication, and vagal damage caused by adhesions, lymphosarcomatous infiltrates, or right-sided abomasal displacement and volvulus. Secondary tympany is a component of the syndromes collectively termed *vagus indigestion*. Bloat caused by muscular dystrophy of the diaphragmatic muscles has been described in both Meuse-Rhine-Issel and Holstein-Friesian breeds of cattle.

Secondary tympany, which is sometimes fatal, occurs in *bucket-fed calves*. This may be a persistent problem in some veal calves, which are known as *ruminal drinkers*. They ingest large amounts of milk, which escapes the reticular groove and flows into the rumen, where it putrefies because of digestion by proteolytic bacteria involving transformation of lactose into lactate by lactobacilli causing ruminal and metabolic acidosis. Casein clot formation in the abomasum is partly inhibited. The clinical signs are characterized by inappetence, unthriftiness, recurrent tympany, abdominal distention, and clay-like feces. Because of butyric and lactic acid accumulation in the epithelium of the reticulorumen, ruminal drinking leads to hyperkeratotic parakeratosis and severe reticulorumenitis accompanied by epithelial loss, erosions, and necrosis.

Animals fed rations that have too much indigestible roughage may have recurrent episodes of bloat. Feed must contain adequate portions of protein, starch, and/or sugars, and cellulose to stimulate growth of the cellulolytic microflora. Indigestible roughage accumulates in the rumen and reticulum when the intake of digestible nutrients (starches and sugars) is inadequate. As a result, the forestomachs become dilated, which in turn inhibits reticuloruminal contractions that are required for clearance of the cardia and subsequent eructation.

A postmortem *diagnosis of secondary bloat* is based on autopsy findings, which are similar to those described in primary bloat, but without frothy rumen content, and with the addition of any physical causes of impaired eructation. Postmortem distention of the rumen must not be mistaken for antemortem tympany.

Further reading

Braun U, Gautschi A. Ultrasonographic examination of the forestomachs and the abomasum in ruminal drinker calves. Acta Vet Scand 2013;55:1.

Cheng KJ, et al. A review of bloat in feedlot cattle. J Anim Sci 1998;76:299-308.

Majak W, et al. Pasture management strategies for reducing the risk of legume bloat in cattle. J Anim Sci 1995;73:1493-1498.

Rajan GH, et al. The relative abundance of a salivary protein, bSP30, is correlated with susceptibility to bloat in cattle herds selected for high or low bloat susceptibility. Anim Genet 1996;27:407-414.

Foreign bodies in the forestomachs

Cattle are notoriously lacking in alimentary finesse, a deficiency that allows an amazing variety of foreign bodies,

prehended with the food, to be deposited in the forestomachs. Sheep are largely immune because of their more selective eating habits. Foreign bodies are rarely found in the rumen of goats, despite their reputation for indiscriminate feeding habits. In consequence, a large proportion of adult cattle, and very few goats or sheep, have metallic, wood, or plastic foreign bodies in the rumen and reticulum, but rarely in the omasum.

Spherical masses consisting largely of hair or wool (**trichobezoars**) or plant fibers (**phytobezoars**) may also form in these compartments. Hairballs are most common in younger ruminants, the hair being swallowed after licking, particularly by animals deprived of dietary fiber. They may have some other foreign body as a nucleus and contain a proportion of plant fibers, the whole mass concreted by organic substances and inorganic salts. The same general comments apply to phytobezoars. Being smooth, neither are important unless regurgitated to lodge in the esophagus or passed on to obstruct the reticulo-omasal orifice, the pylorus, or the intestine, which is very infrequent. Otherwise, these bezoars are an incidental finding.

The important foreign bodies are those (such as lead) that cause *intoxication* when dissolved, and those that (being abrasive or sharp) *penetrate the mucosa*. In calves on diets low in roughage, ingestion of wood shavings or straw may lead to diffuse transmural inflammation of the forestomachs and sometimes the abomasum. A mixed bacterial flora containing clostridia and other organisms is responsible, presumably following mucosal trauma. The sequel to penetration by sharp objects in adult cattle is traumatic reticuloperitonitis.

Further reading

Abutarbush SM, Naylor JM. Obstruction of the small intestine by a trichobezoar in cattle: 15 cases (1992-2002). J Am Vet Med Assoc 2006;229:1627-1630.

Farrow CS. Reticular foreign bodies. Causative or coincidence? Vet Clin North Am Food Anim Pract 1999;15:397-408.

Traumatic reticuloperitonitis and its complications

Perforation of the forestomachs by foreign bodies is virtually always caused by a long, thin, and sharp foreign body, usually a *wire or nail*, penetrating the reticular wall. Incomplete perforation is usually inconsequential, although in some cases focal suppurative or granulomatous inflammation develops in the wall of the reticulum, with or without minor overlying peritonitis. There are no adequate answers as to why perforation occurs, but it is probably caused by forceful contraction of the reticulum, and many cases seem to be predisposed by the increased intra-abdominal pressure of late pregnancy and parturition.

The prophylactic use of *magnets* has become common in many herds, and this probably contributes to the marked decrease in fatal cases of traumatic reticuloperitonitis observed over the past few years. Frequently, these magnets are found incidentally in the reticulum, completely covered by metal foreign bodies, including nails and wires, which might otherwise have penetrated the reticular wall. The replacement of baling wire with twine in many parts of the world is another reason for the apparent decline in the prevalence of this disease.

The outcome of complete perforation is common, but variations in the pattern are frequent. The perforation is usually in the cranioventral direction and is followed immediately by *acute local peritonitis*. If the foreign body is short or bent, it may progress no further, and some foreign bodies are apparently withdrawn with the next reticular movement; in such instances, only *chronic local peritonitis* with adhesions develops. The foreign body may advance to perforate the diaphragm and pericardium, resulting in *traumatic pericarditis*.

A ventral penetration may result in subperitoneal and subcutaneous abscess near the xiphoid. Rare perforation of one of the larger regional arteries may result in sudden death from hemorrhage, and sudden death may also occur if there is penetration of the myocardium or rupture of a coronary artery. Septicemia is also a possible but uncommon complication. Penetration of the thoracic cavity may occur without perforation of the pericardium, causing pneumonia and pleuritis. Right lateral deviation of the penetrating agent involves the wall of the abomasum. It is unusual for the liver or spleen to be penetrated, but metastatic abscesses in the liver are common.

As soon as the foreign body penetrates the serosa, local fibrinous peritonitis develops, which later leads to dense adhesion of variable extent between the reticulum and adjacent structures. Further progression of the foreign body is ordinarily slow and produces a canal surrounded by chronic granulation tissue and containing, besides the foreign body, ingesta, purulent exudate, and other detritus. The bacteria commonly active in the tract are *Trueperella (Arcanobacterium) pyogenes*, *Fusobacterium necrophorum*, and a variety of putrefactive types. In many cases, a foreign body cannot be found, perhaps because it has rusted away or been withdrawn into the reticulum.

One of the variants in the usual pattern of migration of the foreign body is penetration of the right side of the reticulum, leading to suppurative inflammation in the grooves between the reticulum, omasum, and abomasum. The acute local peritonitis causes immediate cessation of ruminal movements; however, persistent ruminal atony or irregular motility with gradual onset of bilateral abdominal distention, inappetence, and decreased milk production may ensue. Clinically this is referred to as **vagus indigestion**, which also may be a sequel to abomasal displacement. At autopsy, there are very characteristic changes in the stomachs with this syndrome. The rumen is distended with enough fluid to cause sloshing if the carcass is jolted. There is no ruminal fermentation or normal odor, and bits of unmacerated straw and food particles float on the watery fluid; the more-normal ingesta has sedimented. The omasum can be very large and impacted with dehydrated ingesta. The abomasum may be distended and impacted with dry ingesta, presumably because of functional pyloric stenosis or abomasal stasis.

The question of the importance of vagal nerve damage in the pathogenesis of vagus indigestion remains unresolved. The consensus is that this syndrome is associated with mechanical or functional impairment of outflow of ingesta from the forestomachs or abomasum, but in some cases the primary defect appears to reside in flaccidity of the reticular groove and in degeneration of its muscle and intramuscular nerve plexus. The rumen and reticulum are dependent on intact vagi for normal movement, and a minority of cases of vagus indigestion appears to be associated with damaged nerves. *Vagal*

lesions may be in the pharyngeal and cervical areas, or intrathoracic, such as lymphosarcomatous infiltration, or abdominal. The latter are usually investment of the nerve in adhesions following reticular perforation, or trauma following abomasal volvulus.

In other cases, degeneration of the vagus is not evident. In these, the dysfunction and lesions are more likely to be due to peritonitis and the subsequent abscessation, or adhesions that disrupt the normal tension-receptor activity or cause a pain response that interferes with normal motility of the forestomachs and abomasum.

In **failure of omasal transport** (*type II vagus indigestion*), there is impairment of movement of ingesta from the reticulorumen to the omasum, associated with abscesses adjacent to the reticulo-omasal orifice. There, lesions probably result in mechanical or neural interference to emptying of the reticulorumen.

A *diagnosis* of vagal indigestion at autopsy is ordinarily dependent on evidence of abnormal abomasal, omasal, or reticuloruminal motility, in association with morphologic lesions of the vagus nerves, adhesions, or neoplasms involving the forestomachs and abomasum.

Traumatic pericarditis is a less common sequel now, perhaps because many of the initial penetrations are diagnosed and the foreign body removed surgically, and also because, as explained previously, the cases of traumatic reticuloperitonitis themselves have decreased. The pericardial reaction is copious and fibrinopurulent. There are usually additional lesions of traumatic pneumonia and pleuritis.

Further reading

Braun U. Traumatic pericarditis in cattle: clinical, radiographic and ultrasonographic findings. Vet J 2009;182:176-186.

Rehage J, et al. Evaluation of the pathogenesis of vagus indigestion in cows with traumatic reticuloperitonitis. J Am Vet Med Assoc 1995;207:1607-1611.

Sattler N, et al. Etiology, forms, and prognosis of gastrointestinal dysfunction resembling vagal indigestion occurring after surgical correction of right abomasal displacement. Can Vet J 2000;41: 777-785.

Rumenitis

Inflammatory lesions in the forestomachs occur in a number of *viral, parasitic, mycotic, toxic,* and *nutritional diseases* of the alimentary tract in ruminants. Viral, parasitic, and mycotic rumenitis are described fully in the section on Infectious and parasitic diseases of the alimentary tract, later in this chapter. In neonatal calves, necrosis of ruminal mucosa is an important sequel to bovine herpesvirus 1 infection. *Bovine papular stomatitis* and *contagious ecthyma* may also cause rumen lesions, albeit less frequently. Ruminal erosions and ulcers are present occasionally in cattle with *foot-and-mouth disease, acute bovine viral diarrhea,* or *mucosal disease.* Extensive hemorrhage and ulceration of the reticuloruminal mucosa may be seen in *bluetongue* in sheep and *epizootic hemorrhagic disease* of deer and cattle. Adenoviral infection occasionally causes multifocal fibrinohemorrhagic rumenitis in cattle and deer. *Malignant catarrhal fever* can also produce erosions and ulcers in the rumen of cattle, bison, and wild ungulates. Primary bacterial or mycotic inflammatory lesions of the rumen are uncommon;

they can occur subsequent to chemical rumenitis, primary viral rumenitis, sepsis, or intensive antibiotic treatment.

Mild inflammation of the forestomachs occurs in some young calves fed *milk* from a pail, when, because of laxity of the reticular groove reflex, the milk spills into the rumen and reticulum in large quantity. A similar problem occurs with feeding by stomach tube. Putrefaction in these compartments leads to mild rumenitis, with edema and mild neutrophil infiltration of the mucosa.

Accidental consumption of excessive quantities of *urea*, in the form of nonprotein nitrogen supplement, or fertilizer, in liquid or powder form, results in the production of ammonia in the rumen. The toxic effect is accelerated by urease in soy-based rations, and is based on the production of high blood levels of ammonia. Rumen contents smell ammoniacal when the organ is opened; the content is alkaline (pH 7.5-8); and there may be congestion or coagulative necrosis of the cranioventral wall of the rumen. Elevated ruminal and abomasal pH values (7.0), without specific lesions, have been associated with ingestion of *boron* fertilizer by cattle and goats.

Ingestion of toxic levels of *sulfur* results in chemical rumenitis because of the conversion of sulfur to hydrogen sulfide, and possibly sulfurous acid, in the rumen. Large amounts of yellow sulfur particles are usually found in the rumen and abomasum. Eructation and subsequent inhalation of hydrogen sulfide result in acute alveolitis. Absorption of sulfides from the lungs leads to marked depression of the respiratory and cardiovascular centers in the central nervous system. Affected animals also develop acidosis, probably caused by the absorption of acids, and impaired renal function associated with the direct toxic effects of sulfur metabolites on tubular epithelial cells.

Inflammation of the forestomachs may be associated with certain *plant toxicoses*, mainly in Australia, Africa, and South America. Examples are Kikuyu grass (*Pennisetum clandestinum*), prickly paddy melon (*Cucumis myriocarpus*), and several species of *Bryophyllum*, *Lupinus*, and *Phytolacca*.

Feeding rations deficient in fiber, which is increasingly the case in developed countries, can alter the microflora, predisposing the animals to metabolic disorders or rumenitis. In addition, acute chemical rumenitis develops after overeating on rapidly fermentable carbohydrate, usually grain.

Further reading

Pessoa CR, et al. Pythiosis of the digestive tract in sheep. J Vet Diagn Invest 2012;24:1133-1136.

Rezac DJ, et al. Prevalence, severity, and relationships of lung lesions, liver abnormalities, and rumen health scores measured at slaughter in beef cattle. J Anim Sci 2014;92:2595-2602.

Russell JB, Rychlik JL. Factors that alter rumen microbial ecology. Science 2001;292:1119-1122.

Rumenitis and acidosis caused by carbohydrate overload

Ruminal acidosis and rumenitis associated with ingestion of excess carbohydrate are problems mainly of *intensive beef and dairy production*. Sheep, and especially goats, are also susceptible to this problem. Its importance lies partly in loss of production and partly in mortality because of the acute disease, in which rumenitis is of minor significance and lactic acidosis is the major cause of morbidity and mortality.

Rumenitis assumes significance in subclinical disease or in survivors of acute episodes, by providing a portal for the entry for fungi and *Fusobacterium necrophorum*, which cause secondary infections. These complications are discussed later. Other complications include coexisting primary tympany (frothy bloat), which may be the fatal partner of grain overload in feedlot cattle.

Ruminal acidosis usually follows the *ingestion of excess carbohydrate* in the form of grain, or other fermentable feedstuffs occasionally used, such as root crops, bread, waste baked goods, brewers' waste, and apples. There is wide variation in the amount of carbohydrate necessary to kill an animal, because tolerance to rations high in starch does develop if they are introduced gradually. Sudden increments in the amount of carbohydrate ingested are of more importance than the actual amount. Sudden changes from concentrates with lower energy values to those with higher values may predispose to acidosis. Extreme environmental temperature changes, either hotter or cooler, may result in temporary reductions in feed consumption, and acidosis may develop once such animals return to full feed.

Shortly after the ingestion of a toxic amount of carbohydrate, ruminal pH begins to fall. The decrease in pH during the first few hours is mainly caused by an increase in dissociated volatile fatty acids, not lactic acid. The production of the latter increases after there has been a marked change in the ruminal flora, which is very responsive to the substrate available for fermentation. *In cattle and sheep, the normal pH of ruminal fluid varies between 5.5 and 7.5*, depending on the diet fed.

The gram-negative bacteria that predominate in the normal flora, and the protozoa, are very sensitive to changes in the pH; most die at a pH of 5.0 or less. Once the pH of the ruminal contents starts to fall, streptococci, mainly *Streptococcus bovis*, proliferate rapidly, acting as a major source of lactic acid. When the pH reaches 5.0-4.5, the numbers of streptococci decrease, with a concomitant increase in lactobacilli. The pH of rumen content may fall as low as 4.0-4.5 in fatal cases.

As ruminal pH drops, ruminal atony develops, mainly as the result of an increase in the concentration of the nondissociated volatile fatty acids, lactic, propionic, and butyric. They act on receptors that mediate inhibition of reticuloruminal motility via a vagovagal reflex. Loss of forestomach motility in ruminal acidosis is apparently not dependent on the development of systemic acidosis. There is also cessation of salivary secretion, so that the buffering effect of saliva is absent.

The increase in ruminal organic acids, mainly lactate, causes an increase in ruminal osmotic pressure. This results in movement of fluid from the blood into the rumen, producing bulky and liquid ruminal contents and severe dehydration. Plasma volume is reduced; hemoconcentration, anuria, and circulatory collapse follow. Serum protein levels, urea, inorganic phosphorus, lactate, pyruvate, and liver enzymes are all elevated. The osmotic pressure of the intestinal contents also increases when the ingesta with the high lactate concentrations arrives there. Loss of fluid at this level probably contributes further to the dehydration, and it may also play a significant role in the development of the diarrhea that is commonly seen clinically. In addition to the osmotic effects, there is acidosis caused by the absorption of lactate from the rumen, and possibly from the intestine.

The low ruminal pH is lethal to much of the normal flora and fauna. The protozoa appear to be particularly sensitive, but many types of bacteria are also lost. In those animals that survive the acute phase of ruminal acidosis, recovery is not complete until a normal ruminal flora is re-established through contact with other animals or by transplant of ruminal content from healthy animals. Temporary recovery may be followed by what appears clinically to be a relapse in acidosis, but which is a developing mycotic rumenitis. If treatment of the initial fluid imbalance is delayed, death may occur in a week or so from ischemic renal cortical necrosis.

The **gross findings** in this metabolic disease are not specific, and a practical diagnosis requires knowledge of access to fermentable carbohydrate and a clinically observed circulatory failure. At autopsy, the eyes are sunken, the blood may be thick and dark because of dehydration and hypoxia, and there is general venous congestion. The appearance of the ruminal contents varies with the time interval between ingestion of the carbohydrate and the autopsy. In the early stages, there is a copious amount of porridge-like rumen content, which has a distinct fermentative odor. The amount of grain, corn, or other source of starch varies considerably and is an unreliable indication of acidosis, and the presence of finely ground concentrate may be overlooked. Ruminal pH is only helpful when it is low (<5.0) because it may rise in later stages of the disease. Although the ruminal contents may appear relatively normal in more advanced cases of acidosis, intestinal contents tend to remain very watery. Absence of protozoa is consistent with chemical rumenitis, but is also influenced by the interval between death and the postmortem examination.

The **diagnosis** of ruminal acidosis at autopsy can be difficult. The most suggestive abnormality is the *rumenitis*. It is probably chemical and dependent on the low pH, and is not readily discerned grossly. There may be a slight poorly defined blue discoloration in the ventral sac of the rumen, reticulum, and omasum, visible through the serosa. When the epithelium is detached, the lamina propria may be hyperemic in patches. In some cases, the epithelium appears to have undergone fixation because of low pH and is difficult to peel.

Microscopic examination of the ruminal mucosa is the most reliable way of confirming a diagnosis of chemical rumenitis. The ruminal papillae appear enlarged. There is marked cytoplasmic vacuolation of the epithelial cells, often leading to vesiculation. A mild to marked neutrophilic reaction is evident in the mucosa and submucosa (Fig. 1-30). Focal areas of erosion and ulceration may or may not be present.

Fusobacterium necrophorum is a normal inhabitant of the anaerobic ruminal environment. This bacterium is commonly responsible for complications of ruminal acidosis, producing characteristic lesions in the forestomachs (Fig. 1-31A) and in the liver. Invasion of the wall of the rumen takes advantage of the foothold provided by the superficial necrosis and inflammation of acidosis. Inflammatory changes favor the adherence of *F. necrophorum* to ruminal epithelium.

Necrobacillary rumenitis is common in feedlot cattle, probably a product of mild acidosis following a too-rapid introduction to a high-concentrate ration. It affects the papillated areas of the ventral sac and occasionally the pillars. On the mucosal surface, the early lesions are visible as multiple irregular patches 2-15 cm across, in which the papillae are swollen, dark, slightly mushy, and are matted together by fibrinocellular inflammatory exudate. Affected papillae are necrotic, but ulceration may be delayed if there is ruminal atony and stasis. If the animal recovers from the immediate effects of overeating, the necrotic epithelium sloughs, the ulcer contracts, and

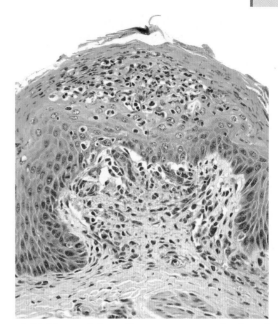

Figure 1-30 Neutrophilic infiltration into superficial epithelium of rumen papilla in **chemical rumenitis** (ruminal acidosis) owing to excess carbohydrate intake.

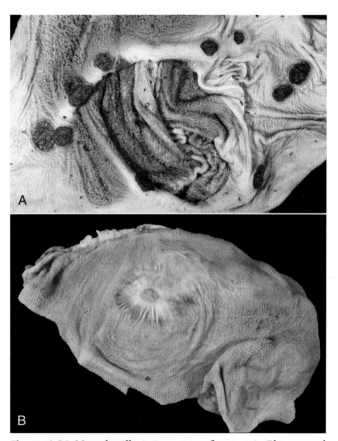

Figure 1-31 Necrobacillosis in rumen of a cow. **A.** Plaques and coalescing areas of necrosis are evident on the mucosa. (Courtesy V. Perez.) **B.** Stellate scarring of incompletely healed **ulcer** in the rumen mucosa in necrobacillary rumenitis.

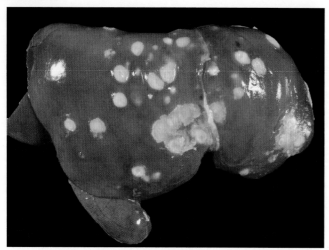

Figure 1-32 Necrobacillosis in the liver of a lamb. Multiple abscesses are present. (Courtesy V. Perez.)

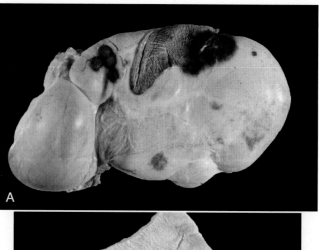

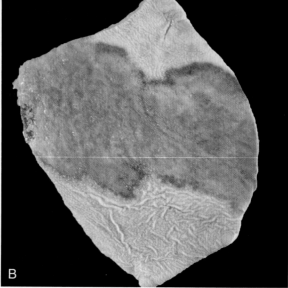

Figure 1-33 Mycotic rumenitis (*Aspergillus* and *Rhizopus*) following acidosis in a cow. **A.** Roughly circular and dark areas of infarction, most of them with a pale center, involving rumen and reticulum. Notice that the spleen is also affected. **B.** Appearance of mucosal surface of rumen; superficial necrosis overlies congested submucosa.

epithelial regeneration begins from the margins. The regenerated epithelium is flat and white, and the papillae do not return completely. A stellate scar often remains, but many of the smaller lesions may disappear completely (Fig. 1-31B). Liver abscesses are the main complication of the *F. necrophorum* rumenitis and the term "*rumenitis-liver abscess complex*" is frequently used to describe this condition. Although the precise mechanism is not fully understood, it is recognized that bacterial emboli are released from the *F. necrophorum*–infected ruminal wall into the portal circulation, followed by bacteria being filtered by the liver, resulting in hepatic infection and abscess formation. *Hepatic lesions* are initially the typical coagulative necrosis of necrobacillosis, but in time they liquefy to form abscesses (Fig. 1-32), and these often persist long after the initial ruminal lesions have cicatrized or disappeared.

It is unusual for ruminal necrobacillosis in cattle to be more than a superficial infection, and although the muscle layers are involved in the inflammation, they are not ordinarily invaded by the organism. However, perforation of the omasal leaves is common. In sheep, the infection is more aggressive, although less frequently observed, than it is in cattle. *Fusobacterium varium* has also been reported to produce liver abscesses associated with rumenitis in sheep.

Mycotic infection should be suspected when inflammation in the wall of the forestomachs extends to the serosa and is *hemorrhagic* and *angiocentric*. The fungi, which, like *F. necrophorum*, are opportunists, are usually zygomycetes of the genera *Mucor*, *Rhizopus*, and *Absidia*, which cannot be differentiated from each other in histologic sections.

Mycotic rumenitis is much more severe and extensive than necrobacillary rumenitis, and is often fatal. *The basis for the lesion is submucosal venular thrombosis caused by fungal invasion,* causing venous infarction of the tissue field involved. The inflammation extends to the peritoneum, causing hemorrhagic and fibrinous peritonitis that mats the omentum to the rumen. In fatal cases, most of the ventral sac and parts of the reticulum, omasum and/or abomasum are involved. The lesions are very striking and suggest on initial inspection that the walls have been massively infarcted, which in part they have (Fig. 1-33A). The margins are well demarcated, usually by a narrow zone of congestive swelling. The affected areas are roughly circular, red to black, sometimes with a pale

central area, thickened to 1 cm or more, firm and leathery. There is acute fibrinohemorrhagic inflammation of the overlying peritoneum, and beneath it in the grooves there is blood-stained, inflammatory edema. The spleen also may be affected.

On the inner surface of the rumen, the lesions are more hemorrhagic than those of necrobacillosis, and more irregular in outline (Fig. 1-33B), and the necrotic epithelium is difficult to detach. Histologically, the rumenitis is characterized by hemorrhagic necrosis of all structures in the wall; by copious fibrinous exudate; and by rather scant leukocytic reaction. *Fungal hyphae* with nonparallel walls are readily visible in the necrotic tissues and the lumina of the thrombosed blood vessels. More chronic cases are characterized by granulomatous inflammation in the deeper parts of the mucosal lesion.

Mycotic rumenitis and **omasitis** may occur in cows that do not have a history of acidosis. It has been suggested that these cases may be a sequel of sepsis, with reflux of abomasal fluid into the forestomachs, and therapy with broad-spectrum antimicrobials acting as predisposing factors for mycotic infections. It can also be a sequel to ruminal damage in survivors of bovine viral diarrhea virus infection.

Metastases sometimes occur in the liver and cause necrotizing thrombophlebitis of the portal radicles visible as small irregular tan areas of infarction surrounded by a deep red margin.

Other conditions that have been associated with ruminal acidosis are *laminitis* and an *encephalopathy* which morphologically resembles the lesions of early polioencephalomalacia (see Vol. 1, Integumentary system; Vol. 1, Nervous system).

Further reading

Foster AP, et al. Hepatitis in a six-month-old lamb with *Fusobacterium varium* infection. Vet Rec 2009;164:98.

Kleen JL, et al. Subacute ruminal acidosis (SARA): a review. J Vet Med A Physiol Pathol Clin Med 2003;50:406-414.

Nagaraja TG, et al. *Fusobacterium necrophorum* infections in animals: pathogenesis and pathogenic mechanisms. Anaerobe 2005;11:239-246.

Tadepalli S, et al. *Fusobacterium necrophorum*: a ruminal bacterium that invades liver to cause abscesses in cattle. Anaerobe 2009;15:36-43.

Parasitic diseases of the forestomachs

Gongylonema spp. occur in the epithelium of the rumen. They appear as described in the esophagus, and are not pathogenic.

More important parasites are the conical **rumen flukes** belonging to the family *Paramphistomatidae*. Although several species of *Paramphistomum* have been described, *Paramphistomum cervi* is probably the most widespread species; *Calicophoron daubneyi* is reported to be common in cattle and sheep in Great Britain. *Paramphistomum* parasites are found in cattle and sheep in warm temperate, subtropical, and tropical regions. These red, plump, droplet-shaped flukes are about the size of the papillae between which they reside in the rumen, where they are usually considered to be mostly non-pathogenic (Fig. 1-34A). However, if present in very high numbers, they can cause rumenoreticulitis, with atrophy of papillae and excessive cornification of the stratum corneum and granulosum (Fig. 1-34B). Loss of condition has been observed in adult cattle with massive ruminal infestation of

Paramphistomum spp. Larval paramphistomes in the duodenum can cause disease. The biology and pathogenicity of paramphistomes are discussed in detail the section on Infectious and parasitic diseases of the alimentary tract, later in this chapter.

Myiasis of the rumen caused by larvae of the **screwworm fly** *Cochliomyia hominivorax* is occasionally a cause of mortality in young calves in South America. The larvae are presumed to be licked from cutaneous wounds and swallowed. They lodge in the rumen and perforate it.

Further reading

Gordon DK, et al. Identification of the rumen fluke, *Calicophoron daubneyi*, in GB livestock: possible implications for liver fluke diagnosis. Vet Parasitol 2013;195:65-71.

Yan H, et al. The mitochondrial genome of *Paramphistomum cervi* (Digenea), the first representative for the family *Paramphistomidae*. PLoS One 2013;8:e71300.

Neoplasia of the esophagus and forestomachs

Neoplasia of the esophagus and reticulorumen is, with the exception of papilloma, rare in domestic animals.

Papillomas of the esophagus in dogs are uncommon and may be associated with oral papilloma. In cattle, papillomata of the esophagus and forestomachs are common in some areas. They are caused by bovine papillomavirus 4 (BPV-4), which infects only squamous mucosa of the mouth, pharynx, esophagus, and forestomachs. Bovine alimentary papillomatosis in healthy immunocompetent animals is usually mild with solitary papillomata, although a minority of infected animals may have multiple lesions. Most are small (<1 cm), broadly pedunculate tapering acuminate masses. They are composed of a number of closely packed fronds of squamous epithelium, each supported by a light core of fibrous stroma, and arising from a common fibrous base. Viral replication and the microscopic changes in infected epithelium are typical, as described earlier for canine oral papillomas, although the characteristic koilocytes and intranuclear inclusions can be sparse. These papillomas are usually rejected by a cell-mediated immune response within approximately 12 months. However, severe

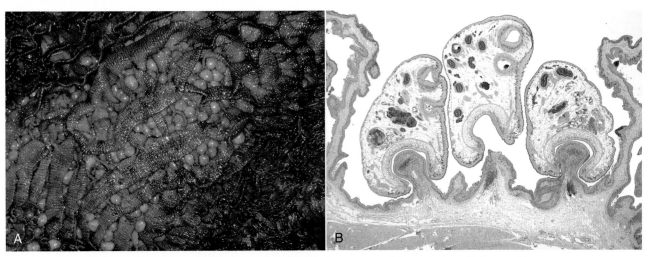

Figure 1-34 A. *Paramphistomum* spp. **flukes** on the mucosa of the reticulum. **B.** *Paramphistomum* spp. **flukes** associated with lymphoplasmacytic reticulitis in cattle.

papillomatosis, often accompanied by development of squamous cell carcinomas (see later) in the same location has been described in the esophagus and forestomachs of bracken fern immunosuppressed, BPV-4 infected cattle in Scotland and England.

Fibropapillomas, limited to the esophagus, esophageal groove and rumen of cattle, are caused by bovine papillomavirus 2 (BPV-2), normally associated with cutaneous papillomas and fibropapillomas. Alimentary fibropapillomas are smooth nodular pearly-white masses, usually about 0.5-1.0 cm in diameter, but occasionally up to 3.0 cm and plaque-like. They are comprised of fibromatous stroma covered by acanthotic epithelium, which occasionally may be ulcerated. No evidence of expression of BPV-2 is found in alimentary fibropapillomas, the viral genome being identified by molecular probes.

Papillomas and fibropapillomas are normally asymptomatic, though large lesions of the reticular groove and esophagus may interfere with eructation and deglutition, causing bloating or loss of condition.

Malignant neoplasms of the esophagus and forestomachs in ruminants are ordinarily extremely rare. However, in several localities, **squamous cell carcinoma** is relatively common in **cattle,** associated with BPV-4–induced papilloma (but not with fibropapilloma because of BPV-2). However, BPV-4 viral antigens or genome are not detected in these carcinomas. An interaction between papillomavirus and ingestion of carcinogens in bracken fern predisposes to the development of squamous cell carcinomas of the esophagus and forestomachs in Scotland and England. Immunocompromise caused by bracken fern intoxication, which is permissive of severe papillomatosis, is also a co-factor in neoplastic transformation to squamous carcinomas. In Brazil and Bolivia, a similar association is made with carcinomas of the oropharynx and esophagus. A high prevalence of carcinoma of the esophagus and forestomachs has also been reported from a single valley in Kenya, in association with papillomata not confirmed as viral, and with a yet undetermined carcinogen apparently ingested with or derived from native forest plants.

Esophageal and ruminal carcinomas are associated with dysphagia or difficult deglutition, ruminal tympany, and apparent abdominal pain with progressive cachexia. Concurrent papillomas, carcinomas, and hemangiomas of the bladder, like those causing enzootic hematuria, but associated with BPV-2, are often found in cattle with esophageal or ruminal cancer. In Scotland, intestinal adenomas or adenocarcinoma also occur in many cases.

Esophageal and ruminal carcinoma may be seen developing from recognizable papillomas; as brown irregular roughened hyperplastic epithelium; or as ulcerated or irregular proliferative fungating lesions. Distal esophagus, reticular groove, and the adjacent ruminal wall are the sites most commonly affected with carcinoma. Microscopically, they are typical squamous cell carcinomas, and invade locally, their scirrhous nature causing induration of the wall of the organ. They may metastasize to local lymph nodes, and to distant sites such as liver and lung.

In **sheep and goats**, alimentary papillomas and squamous cell carcinomas are rare, and little is known of their etiology.

Rarely, **squamous cell carcinomas** also may be encountered in the esophagus of aged cats, where they develop in the mid-thoracic portion, forming proliferative plaques of neoplastic cells that eventually ulcerate and invade the wall of the

esophagus and adjacent mediastinum. In horses, squamous cell carcinoma of the stomach may also involve the adjacent terminal esophagus. Rare squamous cell carcinoma, and adenocarcinomas arising from the esophageal glands, are reported in **dogs.** Invasion of, or metastasis to, the canine esophagus by thyroid, respiratory, and gastric carcinomas is also reported.

Mesenchymal tumors of the esophagus, with the exception of the *Spirocerca*-associated fibrosarcomas and osteosarcomas in dogs, referred to previously in the section on parasitic diseases of the esophagus, are very rare. However, leiomyoma, osteosarcoma, and plasmacytoma have been reported in dogs. Connective tissue tumors of the **ruminant** forestomachs are similarly rare, although fibromas of the reticular groove have been reported. Occasional involvement of the rumen, omasum, and reticulum may occur in cattle with lymphosarcoma, usually also involving the abomasum and more distant sites.

Further reading

Gava A, et al. Bracken fern (*Pteridium aquilinum*) poisoning in cattle in southern Brazil. Vet Hum Toxicol 2002;44:362-365.

Head KW, Else RW. Tumors of the alimentary tract. In: Meuten DJ, editor. Tumors in Domestic Animals. 4th ed. Ames, Iowa: Iowa State University Press; 2002. p. 439-450.

Tsirimonaki E, et al. Extensive papillomatosis of the bovine upper gastrointestinal tract. J Comp Pathol 2003;129:93-99.

STOMACH AND ABOMASUM
Normal form and function

The stomach should be carefully examined in animals of any species with a history of inappetence or anorexia, cachexia, hypoproteinemia, diarrhea, regurgitation, or vomition. Abdominal distention may be associated with gastric dilation or displacement. Hematemesis, melena, or anemia may signify gastric bleeding. Many infectious diseases, with major systemic or alimentary tract signs elsewhere, produce gastric lesions. Systemic states such as uremia and endotoxemia cause characteristic gastric lesions in some species.

The stomach has long been considered to lack a normal bacterial population (microbiota). However, bacteria have been identified in the glandular stomach of healthy animals, including members of the genus *Helicobacter*. In the horse and pig, an obvious smooth white or yellow **esophageal region** is present. It is covered by stratified squamous epithelium, with susceptibility to insult and reparative capacity similar to that of the esophageal lining. Chronic inflammatory infiltrates and lymphoid follicles are normally present in the lamina propria and submucosa of the **cardiac gland mucosa** abutting the esophageal region, especially in the pig. The cardiac gland zone is gray and is particularly well developed in this species, lining the gastric diverticulum, fundus, and about half the body of the stomach. In the dog, cat, and ruminant, cardiac glands are limited to a narrow zone at the cardia or omasal opening. Cardiac glands are branched tubular structures, lined almost exclusively by columnar mucous cells.

The **fundic, or oxyntic, gland acid–secretory mucosa** in the horse and pig is red-brown and slightly irregular but not highly folded. More prominent longitudinally oriented rugae, or plicae, are present in the dog and cat, and in the abomasum of ruminants. Gastric secretion undiluted by ingesta in the dog or cat normally should be pH <3.0. Abomasal content should be pH <3.5-4.0.

Tall columnar mucous cells cover the gastric surface, and line pits or foveolae. The junction of the base of the foveola and the upper portion of the neck of the fundic gland proper is termed the *isthmus*. Cuboidal or low columnar pluripotential stem cells in a narrow zone in this area undergo mitosis. Three lineages are identified: (1) pit (foveolar) cells; (2) parietal cells; and (3) zymogen (chief) cells. Daughter cells of the pit cell lineage differentiate into **foveolar mucous cells,** migrating up on to the gastric surface, where they are lost, probably in about 4-6 days. The neck of the oxyntic gland below the isthmus is lined by pyramidal, peripherally located acid- and intrinsic factor-producing parietal cells. Interspersed are inconspicuous mucous neck cells, mainly in the upper neck and probably stages in the differentiation of chief, and perhaps, parietal cells, and scattered endocrine cells. In the base of the gland the pepsinogen-producing zymogen, or chief, cells are concentrated.

Mucous neck cells, like foveolar mucous cells, contain periodic acid-Schiff–positive mucus. **Parietal cells** differentiate from cells proliferating at the isthmus, and appear to be relatively long-lived, that is, of the order of weeks to months. A complex tubulovesicular/canalicular structure upon which the hydrogen ion-secretory proton pump is inserted opens at the luminal apex of the cell in the secretory state. A number of long-lived enteroendocrine cells, derived from proliferative cells at the isthmus, are recognized in the oxyntic gland, secreting histamine, serotonin, and somatostatin, among other endocrine/paracrine agents. **Endocrine cells** usually abut the basement membrane of the gland, lack exposure to the gland lumen, and have characteristic basal granules. The **chief cells** are apparently long-lived cells, derived from stem cells at the isthmus. Ultrastructurally they have extensive rough endoplasmic reticulum, a prominent Golgi zone, and numerous zymogen granules.

Normally, mitotic figures are not common in cells at the isthmus of fundic glands, and are virtually never seen at any distance from the isthmus. However, the fundic mucosa of newborn ruminants and especially piglets may be relatively poorly differentiated and proliferative. The proliferative compartment, if active, is sensitive to radiomimetic insults, such as cytotoxic agents and parvoviral infection. This is reflected by narrowing of the isthmus and upper neck and attenuation of the epithelium lining the gland.

The **pyloric mucosa** forms a slightly pitted or irregular surface in the distal portion of the stomach; it extends further cranial along the lesser than the greater curvature. The knob-like torus pyloricus at the pylorus of the pig is a normal structure. The tubular glands of the pyloric mucosa open into deep gastric pits that may extend half the thickness of the mucosa. The glands are lined by pale mucous cells, with interspersed endocrine elements, mainly G (gastrin) and D (somatostatin) cells. Scattered parietal cells may be present, especially in glands in the zone intergrading with fundic mucosa.

The stromal elements of the gastric lamina propria are relatively inconspicuous, in fundic mucosa in particular. Normally, a few lymphocytes and plasma cells, and scattered mast cells are present, mainly deep between glands. Occasional lymphocytic nodules or follicles may be present, usually near the muscularis mucosae. Lymphoid infiltrates are more common in antral mucosa. A thick band of amorphous hyalinized connective tissue, sometimes termed the *lamina densa*, is seen sporadically on the luminal aspect of the muscularis

mucosae in the stomach of cats. The cause and significance are unknown.

Hydrolysis of protein in preparation for subsequent intestinal digestion and absorption is accomplished in the stomach by **acid** and by **pepsin,** activated by autocatalysis from pepsinogen at low pH. *Secretion of acid is the function of the oxyntic, or parietal cells*, about one billion of which are present in the stomach of a 20-kg dog. Regulation of the volume and acidity of gastric secretion is physiologically complex and highly integrated, involving neurocrine, endocrine, and paracrine mechanisms.

The *parietal cell secretes hydrochloric acid* in response to stimulation by histamine, acetylcholine, and gastrin. All 3 agonists are probably continuously present and involved in basal acid secretion. However, the effects of acetylcholine and gastrin are largely dependent on concurrent stimulation by the permissive agonist, histamine.

Histamine is a paracrine stimulant, continuously present in the environment of the oxyntic cells, and secreted by mast cells and enterochromaffin-like cells. Occupation of the H_2 histamine receptor on the oxyntic cell causes enhanced generation of cyclic adenosine monophosphate. This in turn stimulates protein kinase cascades culminating in translocation of the proton pump to the apical cell membrane, where acid is secreted.

Acetylcholine, the neurocrine agonist, is released near the oxyntic cell from processes of parasympathetic postganglionic neurons. Its release is enhanced by vagal activity during the central stimulation of the cephalic phase—the Pavlovian response. Gastric distention also stimulates the parietal cell via vagovagal and short intramural reflex pathways. Acetylcholine acting on muscarinic M_3 receptors elevates intracellular Ca^{2+}, which stimulates acid secretion.

Gastrin is released into the bloodstream by G cells, many of which are in the pyloric antrum. Calcium, amino acids, and peptides in ingesta, impinging on G cells, stimulate gastrin release. Vagal stimulation during the cephalic phase, and fundic-pyloric vagovagal reflexes, in concert with local pyloric reflexes, initiated by distention, also cause G cells to release gastrin. Gastrin acts mainly by a receptor-mediated process to release histamine from the enterochromaffin-like cells. Gastrin alone is a weak stimulant of acid production, but it synergizes secretion by oxyntic cells exposed to histamine and acetylcholine. In addition, gastrin has an important trophic effect, increasing the number of parietal and endocrine cells in fundic mucosa. In turn, parietal cell mass seems to impact on chief cell differentiation.

Acid production during the gastric phase of secretion is depressed by the negative-feedback effect of acid in the antrum, through the inhibitory effect of somatostatin on the G cell below pH 3.0. Acid, fat, and hyperosmolal solutions in the proximal small intestine also inhibit acid secretion, perhaps by the mediation of neural reflexes, secretin, gastric-inhibitory polypeptide, epidermal growth factor, transforming growth factor-α, or other enterogastrones. Prostaglandin E_2 also inhibits acid production by parietal cells.

The chief cell is probably susceptible to the same general stimuli for secretion as the parietal cell.

Gastric motility is the outcome of an interaction among myogenic, hormonal, and neuronal factors, the latter two impinging directly or indirectly on smooth muscle. Mediating at least part of the neural component of this control system, by as yet uncertain mechanisms, are the interstitial cells of

Cajal, pacemakers that are variously found between the layers of gastric smooth muscle, or among smooth muscle cells.

Gastric mucosal barrier

The gastric mucosal barrier to acid back-diffusion and auto-digestion resides largely in the *single layer of foveolar and surface mucous cells and its products*. Tight junctions are present between epithelial cells and are critical in maintenance of barrier function. Integrity of the gastric mucosal barrier implies continuity of the mucosal surface epithelium. The capacity of these cells to maintain tight junctions, to migrate rapidly to fill defects, and to secrete mucus, bicarbonate, and a hydrophobic phospholipid surface layer, is central to protecting the gastric mucosa against progressive injury by insults arising in the lumen.

Gastric mucus is freely permeable to hydrogen ions and has little innate buffering capacity, but it resists hydrolysis by intraluminal pepsin, protecting the integrity of the mucosal surface. Mucus forms a layer immediately over the gastric epithelial cells termed the "unstirred mucus layer" and is the first line of defense from injury. This layer consists of a number of different types of mucin, bicarbonate, and phospholipids. Cardiac gland mucosa in the pig, and pyloric mucosa, secrete bicarbonate in considerable quantities, and normally resist acid attack. Fundic surface mucous cells also actively secrete bicarbonate into a thin unstirred layer of surface mucus. Bicarbonate and mucus secretion by mucous cells is stimulated by prostaglandin E_2. Acid is buffered by bicarbonate in the thin unstirred layer of mucus, preventing back-diffusion into the mucosa. In addition, the "alkaline tide" of bicarbonate, released into the gastric interstitial space during the course of acid secretion, further buffers the mucosa against acid back-diffusion.

Prostaglandins, particularly of the E series, ubiquitous in gastric mucosal lamina propria, may have protective effects other than by stimulation of bicarbonate and mucus secretion by mucous cells, and by inhibition of histamine-stimulated acid secretion by parietal cells. They cause proliferation, resulting in an increased mass of foveolar mucous epithelium. They may promote incorporation of surfactant molecules into the apical cell membrane of surface mucous cells, increasing its hydrophobicity and imparting greater resistance to water-soluble insults. They also may be involved in gastric mucosal cytoprotection by sulfhydryl compounds, which may neutralize free radicals and other toxic metabolites.

Prostaglandins and basal nitric oxide production cause vasodilation and increased blood flow, in addition to inhibiting acid secretion by parietal cells, and promoting bicarbonate secretion by foveolar mucous cells. Bicarbonate in the local circulation, resulting from the alkaline tide generated by acid secretion in glands deeper in the mucosa, is probably important in buffering the superficial lamina propria against back-diffusion of acid; adequate blood flow flushes injurious free radicals from the vicinity of surface cells. Experimentally, high blood flow is protective against many mucosal insults, whereas ischemia is ulcerogenic.

Epidermal growth factor, originating in salivary glands, and transforming growth factor-α, produced locally in the gastric mucosa, also appear protective, in that they may promote cell proliferation and migration to fill defects, and suppress acid production. Bombesin is probably protective through stimulation of gastrin-mediated nitric oxide release, promoting gastric mucosal blood flow. The gastric microvascular network is also important in maintaining barrier function through maintenance of adequate oxygenation to the surface and glandular epithelium and in regulation of inflammation.

Further reading

Cryer B. Mucosal defense and repair. Role of prostaglandins in the stomach and duodenum. Gastroenterol Clin North Am 2001;30:877-894.

Guilford WG, Strombeck DR. Gastric structure and function. In: Guilford WG, et al., editors. Strombeck's Small Animal Gastroenterology. 3rd ed. Philadelphia: WB Saunders; 1996. p. 239-255.

Hall JA, et al. Gastric motility in dogs. Part I. Normal gastric function. Compend Contin Educ Pract Vet 1988;10:1282-1293.

Hooda S, et al. Current state of knowledge: the canine gastrointestinal microbiome. Anim Health Res Rev 2012;13:78-88.

Laine L et al. Gastric mucosal defense and cytoprotection: bench to bedside. Gastroenterol 2008;135:41-60.

Prokopiw I, et al. The microvascular anatomy of the canine stomach. Gastroenterol 1991;100:638-647.

Tarnawski A, et al. The mechanisms of gastric mucosal injury: focus on microvascular endothelium as a key target. Curr Med Chem 2012;19:4-15.

Wallace JL, Bell CJ. Gastromucosal defense. Curr Opin Gastroenterol 1996;12:503-511.

Wallace JL, Miller MJS. Nitric oxide in mucosal defense: a little goes a long way. Gastroenterol 2000;119:512-520.

Yao X, Forte JG. Cell biology of acid secretion by the parietal cell. Annu Rev Physiol 2003;65:103-131.

Response of the gastric mucosa to injury

Restitution of acute erosive physical or chemical trauma to the mucosal surface is by rapid (minutes to hours) immigration of surviving attenuated surface and foveolar cells. Under the initial control of transforming growth factor-β and later influenced by epidermal growth factor, repair by proliferation of cells in the isthmus follows, if the erosive lesion is superficial and spares the progenitor cells. The "sonic hedgehog" protein is secreted by parietal cells and has been shown to be important in epithelial cell differentiation and gastric wound repair in animal models. A cap of mucus, exfoliated epithelium, and fibrin over a mucosal defect may form a protective barrier conducive to effective restitution of the mucosal epithelium. An acute inflammatory reaction demarcates severely eroded or superficially necrotic mucosa, and hemorrhage may be evident on the surface and in adjacent mucosa. Mitoses become common in the upper gland. After a gastric insult, mucosal blood flow rapidly increases. This is protective by aiding in dilution and removal of back-diffusing acid and injurious substances from the mucosa.

During the early phase of repair, cells lining shallow foveolae and covering the surface are basophilic, poorly differentiated, and flattened, cuboidal, or low columnar. Sites of epithelial exfoliation and neutrophil transmigration or effusion into the lumen may be evident. Congestion, edema, mild neutrophilia, and fibroplasia are seen in the superficial lamina propria. The evolution and repair of gastric ulceration, to which erosion may be antecedent, are discussed later. The progenitor cells of the fundic mucosa have the potential to produce tall columnar mucous cells of the foveolar or surface type, to produce mucous neck cells, and by further differentiation, to evolve into parietal cells.

Atrophy of parietal cell mass without extensive mucous cell hyperplasia occurs in animals, particularly ruminants, which have signs of gastrointestinal disease, including *inappetence*. The change is not evident grossly. Microscopically, fewer parietal cells are seen in the upper neck of fundic glands, and often in the depth of the gland. This is accompanied by epithelial proliferation, indicated by moderate numbers of mitotic figures at the isthmus and in the neck of the gland. Mucous neck cells become the predominant cell in the upper gland. In extreme cases mucous neck cells are present to the base of glands, and *achlorhydria* occurs. Similar findings occur in animals with a wide variety of syndromes involving loss of appetite. Starvation of moderate duration does not produce comparable lesions. This lesion may be the result of *reduced trophic stimulation of the fundic mucosa*, and is not to be confused with atrophic gastritis, in which loss of parietal cell mass and atrophy of mucosal thickness are accompanied by usually chronic inflammation.

Mucous metaplasia and hyperplasia of glands in the fundic stomach in all species are associated with *chronic inflammation* of the mucosa. As the lesion evolves, parietal cells seem to be lost at an accelerated rate because they are only present in the basal portion of the glands, and they appear to be progressively displaced from above by hyperplastic mucous cells. Mitotic figures may be numerous throughout the neck of the gland, which elongates. The metaplastic epithelium in early lesions tends to resemble mucous neck cells. In established lesions, columnar mucous cells with regular nuclear polarity, similar to foveolar mucous cells, may be present. When inflammatory infiltrates are local, the mucous change is limited to a few surrounding glands. More diffuse inflammation is associated with the development of widespread epithelial mucous metaplasia. Focal or diffuse, superficial or mucosal, proprial infiltrates of plasma cells and lymphocytes are typical. Often, neutrophils, eosinophils, and Russell-body cells will be present in the lamina propria, and lymphocytes may be between epithelial cells in glands. Globule leukocytes may be present in the epithelium of glands, especially in the parasitized abomasum.

This mucous metaplasia, hyperplasia, and chronic inflammation is associated with a *variety of causes*, including chronic traumatic insults, such as those caused by implanted foreign bodies, as well as in the abomasa of ruminants infected with lentiviruses. The specific agency most commonly recognized is *gastric parasitism by nematodes* such as *Ostertagia* spp., *Trichostrongylus axei*, *Hyostrongylus* spp., and *Ollulanus tricuspis*, where the distribution of the lesion is often closely related to the physical presence of nematodes and to the interstitial inflammatory reaction that they incite. Mucous metaplasia and hyperplasia are also typically present around the healing margins of chronic ulcers, perhaps in response to local inflammation.

The mucosa affected in these circumstances is grossly thickened, as on the overhanging margin of an ulcer, or in an *Ostertagia* "nodule," with a pebbled or convoluted surface if the lesion is widespread. Gastric rugae or plicae are thickened, partially as a result of mucosal hypertrophy, perhaps with submucosal edema. The surface of the stomach is usually paler than normal in affected areas; however, local congestion or hyperemia may be evident. Although the surface may be glistening, profuse mucus secretion is not usually obvious. *Achlorhydria* is the consequence of widespread change of this type. Mucous metaplasia and hyperplasia are differentiated from fundic atrophy associated with the loss of appetite on the basis of the degree of mucous cell hyperplasia and differentiation, and the presence of inflammatory cells.

The cause and functional significance of gastric mucous metaplasia are unclear. Parietal cells are important for epithelial homeostasis and their loss during chronic inflammation may contribute to epithelial dysregulation and mucous metaplasia.

Presumably loss of parietal cells and hyperplasia of mucous neck cells is partly a response to soluble local immune-mediated stimuli or products of inflammation because it is localized in the vicinity of glands containing larvae in gastric parasitism, but, as a general phenomenon, seems independent of parasite-specific factors. Tumor necrosis factor-α, interleukin-1, and interferon-γ are candidate cytokines involved in inflammatory mucous metaplasia of the fundic stomach. In vitro, interleukin-1β and tumor necrosis factor-α inhibit acid secretion by isolated parietal cells, and tumor necrosis factor-α induces apoptosis of parietal cells. Replacement of parietal cells by mucous neck cells, or an apparently more fully differentiated mucous cell in chronic gastritis, may be a protective response. It may eliminate the threat of local acid corrosion, and promote the transfer into the lumen of protective soluble factors such as lysozyme and IgA or its analogues. In animal models, gastric mucous metaplasia has been identified as an early event in the progression to gastric neoplasia.

Achlorhydria ensues in severe chronic gastritis and mucous metaplasia. The pH of gastric secretion approaches or exceeds neutrality under some circumstances, as sodium ion replaces hydrogen ion in gastric content and bicarbonate is secreted. With diminished gastric acid concentration, progressive microbial colonization of the stomach and upper intestine ensues. Parietal cell atrophy and replacement by mucous neck cells in ruminants with anorexia caused by enteric disease may predispose to mycotic invasion of the mucosa if it is physically disrupted. However, mucous metaplasia and hyperplasia, as seen in chronic gastritis or conditions like ostertagiosis, do not seem to render the mucosa prone to mycosis. Loss of the hydrolytic effects of acid and pepsin, in achlorhydria, seems to have little effect on digestion of protein and uptake of nitrogen, at least in animals with ostertagiosis, and the effect on protein digestion of atrophic gastritis in humans appears to be minimal. Rather, at least in parasitic gastritis, inappetence diminishes nutrient intake on the one hand, whereas mucosal permeability permits protein loss through the mucosa (protein-losing gastropathy); together, these impact on the nitrogen economy of the animal to cause reduced productive efficiency, or loss of body condition, depending on whether the animal enters negative nitrogen balance or not.

Evaluation of *gastric biopsies* is governed by the same caveats discussed in the section on interpretation of intestinal and colonic biopsies. Rapid fixation of gastric biopsies is paramount. Gastritis, and the pathogenesis of gastrointestinal parasitism, are discussed later in this chapter.

Further reading

Bhowmik A, et al. Regulation of restitution after superficial injury in isolated guinea pig gastric mucosa. APMIS 2004;112: 225-232.

Jones MK, et al. Gastrointestinal mucosal regeneration: role of growth factors. Front Biosci 1999;4:D303-D309.

Liu Z, et al. IFNγ contributes to the development of gastric epithelial cell metaplasia in Huntingtin interacting protein 1 related (Hip1r)-deficient mice Lab Invest 2012;92:1045-1057.

Neu B, et al. TNF-alpha induces apoptosis of parietal cells. Biochem Pharmacol 2003;65:1755-1760.

Simpson HV. Pathophysiology of abomasal parasitism: is the host or parasite responsible? Vet J 2000;160:177-191.

Wallace JL, Granger DN. The cellular and molecular basis of gastric mucosal defense. FASEB J 1996;10:731-740.

Xiao C. Sonic Hedgehog contributes to gastric mucosal restitution after injury. Lab Invest 2013;93:96-111.

Pyloric stenosis

Pyloric stenosis is a functional and sometimes anatomic problem, which in part represents probably the only *anomaly* of the stomach recognized in animals. Pyloric stenosis can be congenital or acquired. It is relatively common in dogs, and rare in cats and horses.

Recurrent vomition and poor growth in recently weaned animals suggest the clinical diagnosis of a *congenital* lesion. Contrast radiographic studies will confirm *delayed gastric emptying*. There is limited critical functional information on congenital stenosis. An analogous condition in humans is associated with a lack of the interstitial cells of Cajal, but this association has not been clearly demonstrated in domestic animals, nor have morphological or significant immunohistochemical neural abnormalities been identified. In some dogs there may be hypertrophy of pyloric smooth muscle, which appears grossly thickened. Tonic stenosis of the pyloric sphincter may occur in dogs, perhaps because of alterations of the myenteric plexus or gastrin excess. Hypertrophy of the pyloric smooth muscle and stenosis has been reported in Siamese cats. An association with esophageal dilation has been made in the cat. Congenital pyloric stenosis in a foal was associated with signs of abdominal pain and reluctance to consume solid feed. In all species, the clinical problem is usually abolished by pyloromyotomy.

Physical causes of acquired pyloric stenosis or obstruction include: ulceration, granulation, and stricture of the pyloric canal in any species; foreign bodies; as a complication of polyps and tumors in the area; and chronic hypertrophic pyloric gastropathy in dogs.

Chronic hypertrophic pyloric gastropathy is the term coined for a syndrome of pyloric obstruction in dogs, associated with *mucosal hypertrophy, hypertrophy of circular smooth muscle, or a combination of the two*. Mucosal hypertrophy alone is the most common lesion; muscular hypertrophy alone is the least common, although some degree of muscular hypertrophy is seen in about half the cases. Affected animals are typically of small breeds, and those middle-aged or older. Males outnumber females. The pathogenesis is speculative, and it is not clear whether muscular hypertrophy is primary, as it seems to be in some cases, or whether it is secondary, in response to obstruction related to excess mucosa. Because mucosal and muscular lesions can be present independently, they may have separate causes. The mucosal hypertrophy has features in common with hypertrophic gastritis, described elsewhere. The cardinal presenting sign is *chronic intermittent vomition*, perhaps with weight loss, and with gastric distention in a few cases. Gross examination, by gastroscopy, at gastrotomy, or autopsy, in most cases reveals *enlarged mucosal folds* surrounding and obstructing the pyloric canal. This reflects

hypertrophy of glands, which may involve foveolar or deeper glandular elements alone, or in combination, perhaps with cystic dilation of deeper portions of glands. There is usually a concomitant chronic inflammatory infiltrate in the mucosa and occasionally submucosa, and small erosions of the mucosal surface may occur. If there is muscular hypertrophy, this is reflected on the cut surface of the pylorus by irregular firm thickening of the circular muscle. Microscopically, smooth-muscle fibers in affected fascicles are irregularly hypertrophic. Recognition of smooth-muscle hypertrophy requires a full-thickness biopsy, which will not be obtained by endoscopy.

Further reading

Abel RM, et al. A quantitative study of the neural changes underlying pyloric stenosis in dogs. Anat Histol Embryol 2002;31:139-143.

Sikes RI, et al. Chronic hypertrophic pyloric gastropathy: a review of 16 cases. J Am Anim Hosp Assoc 1986;22:99-104.

Syrcle JA, et al. Treatment of pyloric stenosis in a cat via pylorectomy and gastroduodenostomy (Billroth I procedure). J Am Vet Med Assoc 2013;242:792-797.

Walter MC, Matthiesen DT. Acquired antral pyloric hypertrophy in the dog. Vet Clin North Am Small Anim Pract 1993;23:547-554.

Gastric dilation and displacement

Gastric dilation in the horse is often *secondary* to obstruction of the stomach, small bowel, or of colic with ileus, and is also part of the syndrome "grass sickness," discussed elsewhere in this chapter. Ingestion of *Datura* sp. seeds, which contain a parasympatholytic alkaloid, can also cause ileus, leading to gastric dilation. *Primary gastric dilation* in horses is a sequel to consumption of excess fermentable carbohydrate, sudden access to lush pasture, or excessive intake of water. Dilation associated with intake of fermentable feed is likely analogous to grain overload in cattle. Ingesta may swell through absorption of saliva and gastric secretion. Evolution of gas and organic acids, including lactic acid, by bacterial fermentation of carbohydrate, occurs in the cranial portion of the stomach. An influx of water follows as the result of increased osmotic pressure in the stomach, contributing to increased distension and to systemic dehydration. Animals surviving for any time with acute gastric dilation of this type may develop laminitis.

Gastric rupture may follow primary or secondary dilation of the equine stomach; it may be idiopathic, in that no clear cause is identified. Gastric rupture is diagnosed in ~5% of horses with colic admitted to veterinary hospitals. Rupture usually occurs along the greater curvature, parallel to the omental attachment, releasing gastric content into the omental bursa or the abdominal cavity. Death ensues acutely as the result of shock and peritonitis. The margins of the laceration show evidence of antemortem hemorrhage, which differentiates the lesion from postmortem rupture of a dilated stomach. There also may be congestion of the cervical esophagus and blanching of the thoracic esophagus, producing a prominent *bloat line*. This, and compression atelectasis of the lungs in some cases, attests to the tremendous increase in intra-abdominal and intrathoracic pressure exerted by the dilated stomach before rupture. **Perforation**, as distinct from rupture, of the stomach in the horse is rare, and is associated with parasitism, gastric ulcer, or neoplasia.

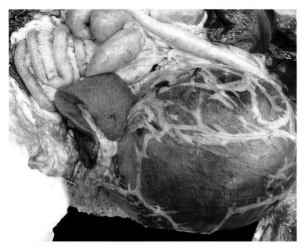

Figure 1-35 Gastric volvulus in a dog. The stomach has undergone venous infarction as a result of strangulation of its vascular outflow, and is extremely distended and congested. (Courtesy J. Smith.)

Gastric dilation and volvulus (Fig. 1-35) occur relatively commonly in dogs, and uncommonly in cats. In **dogs,** gastric dilation and volvulus are usually problems associated with eating, and probably aerophagia, especially in the *deep-chested breeds,* such as Great Danes, St. Bernards, Irish Setters, Wolfhounds, Borzois, and Bloodhounds. Predisposing factors are controversial but may include: increased laxity of the hepatogastric ligament; prior splenectomy; a diet of small food particles; recent kenneling; having a raised feed bowl; and infection with the nasal mite *Pneumonyssoides caninum,* which causes "reversed sneezing."

The gas that contributes to the development of dilation is probably the result of aerophagia, and possibly the evolution of carbon dioxide by physiologic mechanisms. Inability to relieve the accumulation of food, fluid, and gas in the stomach causes the organ to dilate and alter its intra-abdominal position, so that its long axis rotates from a transverse left-right orientation to one paralleling that of the abdomen. In simple dilation, the esophagus is not physically completely occluded, the spleen remains on the left side, and the duodenum is only slightly displaced dorsally and toward the midline. Repeated episodes of gastric dilation probably compromise splenic venous return during periods when the stomach is distended, and eventually lead to episodes of splenic ischemia and segmental infarcts.

For reasons that are unclear, gastric dilation may be converted to gastric volvulus. The stomach rotates about the esophagus in a clockwise direction, as viewed from the caudal aspect. The greater curvature of the distended organ moves ventrally and caudally, and then rotates dorsally and to the right. This forces the pylorus and terminal duodenum cranially to the right and clockwise around the esophagus. Ultimately they lie to the left of midline across and ventral to the esophagus, compressed between the esophagus and the dilated stomach. Depending on the degree of volvulus, the *spleen,* which follows the gastrosplenic ligament, usually ends up lying in a right-ventral position, between the stomach and liver or diaphragm. It is bent into a V shape by tension on its ligaments, becomes extremely congested, and may undergo torsion, infarction, and rupture. The esophagus becomes completely occluded in volvulus, which may involve rotation of up to 270-360°. Venous infarction of the gastric mucosa ensues, as volvulus progressively constricts outflow of blood from the stomach. The mucosa, and usually the full thickness of the gastric wall, is edematous and dark red to black, and there is bloody content in the lumen of the stomach. Ischemic mucosa becomes necrotic, and the stomach may rupture. Hemoperitoneum may occur as a result of avulsion of gastric blood vessels.

Obstruction of veins by volvulus, and pressure exerted by the distended stomach, result in decreased venous return via the portal vein and caudal vena cava, causing reduced perfusion of intra-abdominal organs, reduced cardiac output, and *circulatory shock.* Increased intra-abdominal pressure impinges on the diaphragm and compromises respiration. A variety of acid-base and electrolyte abnormalities ensue in dogs with gastric dilation and volvulus, contributing to the physiologically precarious state. Cardiac arrhythmias as a sequel to gastric dilation and volvulus have been associated with putative release of *myocardial depressant factor* from an ischemic pancreas, and with myocardial necrosis, resulting from ischemia. Death is inevitable in dogs with acute gastric volvulus that are not treated early. Rare cases of chronic gastric volvulus are reported, with fixation of the spleen in the right side of the abdomen by omental adhesions.

In **swine,** gastric volvulus is a cause of sudden death in *adult sows,* perhaps with a brief premonitory period of anorexia, abdominal distention, dyspnea, and drooling. It is associated with excitement in anticipation of feeding among pigs that are fed at regular, often long, intervals, and may be a sequel to unduly rapid ingestion of feed, water, and air. The twist may occur in either direction about the long axis of the stomach, although clockwise torsion predominates.

Abomasal displacement and volvulus is a common clinical problem in high-producing, intensively managed dairy **cattle,** particularly around the time of parturition, but it also occurs in animals that are predominantly pasture fed. *The displacement is usually ventral and to the left of the rumen.* Many affected animals have concurrent problems, including ketosis, hypocalcemia, metritis, and retained placenta. Affected abomasa have decreased sensitivity to acetylcholine, and abomasal atony has been implicated as a prerequisite to displacement. Alterations in the enteric nervous system in the abomasum, including substance P levels, may also play a role. Evolution of gas in the abomasum is directly related to the amount of concentrate in the ration. Left displacement of the gas-filled abomasum is amenable to treatment, and is rarely encountered at autopsy. Handling of an affected animal postmortem may correct displacements in any case. Other than possible scarring of the lesser omentum, the abomasum may be unremarkable. *Abomasal fistulae,* draining in the right paramedian area, may ensue if, during abomasopexy to prevent recurrent displacement, nonabsorbable sutures fixing the abomasum to the abdominal wall penetrate the abomasal mucosa.

Simple right displacement, which accounts for ~15% of abomasal displacements, is probably caused by similar agencies. However, right displacement may be complicated in about 20% of cases by progression to abomasal volvulus, which is clinically serious.

Abomasal volvulus is probably the sequel to rotation of a loop formed by a distended abomasum and attached omasum and duodenum. The volvulus is counterclockwise about a

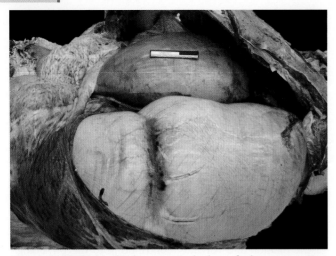

Figure 1-36 Right displacement/volvulus of abomasum. Distended and hemorrhagic abomasum is dorsal to the distended rumen located along the ventral body wall bovine. (Courtesy M. Yaeger.)

transverse axis through the lesser omentum, when viewed from the right side.

Rotation, buoyed by the gas-filled body of the abomasum, may be in the sagittal plane. With a 360° volvulus, the pylorus ends in the cranial right portion of the abdomen dorsal to the twisted omasum, with the duodenum trapped medial to the omasum and lateral to the partially rotated reticulum (Fig. 1-36). Alternative modes of displacement and rotation are possible, but all may end in this relationship.

Obstruction of duodenal outflow in volvulus results in sequestration of chloride in the abomasal content and the development of *metabolic alkalosis*. Severe volvulus causes obstruction of blood vessels at the neck of the omasum, as well as causing trauma to the vagus nerves in the region. The abomasum becomes distended with blood-stained fluid and gas. Venous infarction of the deeply congested mucosa may result in ultimate *abomasal rupture*, often near the omaso-abomasal orifice, and peritonitis. Damage to the vagal branches may prohibit return of normal abomasal motility in animals successfully withstanding surgery, resulting in vagus indigestion. Cases of abomasal volvulus are also occasionally reported in preruminant calves; these are usually fatal.

Sarcina-like bacteria have been associated with abomasal diseases in **lambs and calves.** Pathologic findings include various combinations of abomasal bloat, hemorrhage, and ulcers.

Gastroesophageal intussusception, gastroduodenal intussusception, and **pylorogastric intussusception** are uncommon displacements, involving the stomach of dogs with signs of upper alimentary tract obstruction that require surgical correction.

Further reading

Applewhite AA, et al. Pylorogastric intussusception in the dog: a case report and literature review. J Am Anim Hosp Assoc 2001;37:238-243.

Bird AR, et al. The clinical and pathological features of gastric impaction in twelve horses. Equine Vet J Suppl 2012;43:105-110.

Doll K, et al. New aspects in the pathogenesis of abomasal displacement Vet J 2009;181:90-96.

Edwards GT, et al. *Sarcina*-like bacteria associated with bloat in young lambs and calves. Vet Rec 2008;163:391-393.

Geishauser T, et al. Metabolic aspects in the etiology of displaced abomasum. Vet Clin North Am Food Anim Pract 2000;16:255-265.

Glickman LT, et al. Non-dietary risk factors for gastric dilatation-volvulus in large and giant breed dogs. J Am Vet Med Assoc 2000;217:1492-1499.

Horne WA, et al. Effects of gastric distension-volvulus on coronary blood flow and myocardial oxygen consumption in the dog. Am J Vet Res 1985;46:98-104.

Sartor AJ, et al. Association between previous splenectomy and gastric dilatation-volvulus in dogs: 453 cases (2004-2009). J Am Vet Med Assoc 2013;242:1381-1384.

Van Winden SC, Kuiper R. Left displacement of the abomasum in dairy cattle: recent developments in epidemiological and etiological aspects. Vet Res 2003;34:47-56.

Gastric foreign bodies and impaction

A variety of **foreign bodies** may be encountered in the stomach and in the abomasum. Most are incidental findings, or at worst, associated with vomition, mild acute or chronic gastritis, or occasionally with ulceration. *Trichobezoars* (hairballs) are often found in the stomach of long-haired cats, and in calves reared on diets low in roughage, where most are in the rumen, with a few in the abomasum. *Phytobezoars* (nondigestible plant material) and *trichophytobezoars* have been implicated as the cause of pyloric obstruction and death in young lambs on pasture and, in some regions, in cattle grazing fibrous plants. *Fine sand* may accumulate in the abomasum in considerable amounts, usually with no detrimental effect.

Gastric impaction by inspissated content in horses is related to factors such as consumption of fibrous roughage and persimmons, inadequate water intake, and poor mastication. It may cause anorexia, mild colic, and loss of body condition, and is to be differentiated clinically and at autopsy from gastric impaction secondary to pyrrolizidine alkaloid poisoning, from dilation secondary to intestinal obstruction, and from primary gastric dilation.

Primary abomasal impaction in cattle may result from restricted water intake and coarse, high-roughage feed, such as wheat stubble or straw. Secondary abomasal impaction may follow pyloric stenosis, physical or functional, of any cause. It is perhaps most common as a functional abomasal stasis in one of the manifestations of *vagus indigestion*. Loss of abomasal motility may be the product of intrathoracic inflammatory or neoplastic vagal lesions; vagal involvement in adhesions following traumatic reticuloperitonitis; vagal trauma in surgically corrected abomasal volvulus; adhesions of the abomasum and omasum that may physically impair motility; or systemic disease that causes abomasal stasis.

The abomasum is impacted with thick porridge-like or inspissated coarse fibrous digesta, despite an apparently patent pylorus. **Abomasal rupture** may ensue, particularly in primary impaction associated with coarse feed, resulting in diffuse peritonitis. Most commonly, the laceration is near the omasal-abomasal orifice, but it may be elsewhere. Omasal dilation and ruminal distention are also found in many of these cases; omasa usually contain inspissated digesta, while rumen content tends to be fluid. Metabolic derangement owing to sequestration of chloride in the rumen following regurgitation from the obstructed abomasum, and hypokalemia resulting from decreased intake in feed in the face of continued normal renal excretion, place these animals in perilous physiologic circumstances, often before inanition becomes a significant factor.

A syndrome known clinically as **abomasal dilation and emptying defect** occurs in Suffolk and Hampshire **sheep**. The animals develop chronic inappetence and weight loss, and at autopsy they have a markedly distended abomasum containing digesta resembling rumen contents. No morphologic gross or microscopic lesions of the stomach, vagus nerve, or other organs have been found, except scattered chromatolytic and necrotic neurons in the celiacomesenteric autonomic ganglion. The cause is unknown, but it is suggested that it may be an acquired dysautonomia, possibly toxic, requiring a genetic predisposition for expression. Although rumen chloride levels are elevated, few animals become hypochloremic and alkalotic, as do cattle with abomasal impaction.

Further reading

Bird A, et al. The clinical and pathological features of gastric impaction in twelve horses. Equine Vet J Suppl 2012;43:105-110.

Kuiper R, Breukink HJ. Secondary indigestion as a cause of functional pyloric stenosis in the cow. Vet Rec 1986;119:404-406.

Melendez P, et al. An outbreak of sand impaction in postpartum dairy cows. Can Vet J 2007;48:1067-1070.

Pruden SJ, et al. Abomasal emptying defect of sheep may be an acquired form of dysautonomia. Vet Pathol 2004;41:164-169.

Wittek T, et al. Abomasal impaction in Holstein-Friesian cows: 80 cases (1980-2003). J Am Vet Med Assoc 2005;227:287-291.

Circulatory disturbances

Edema of the gastric rugae occurs with hypoproteinemia in any species, in portal hypertension, and is found in the abomasum of cattle poisoned by arsenic, sheep ingesting tannic acid, and both cattle and sheep with ostertagiasis. Edema fluid collects in the submucosa of the folds, and is particularly obvious in the normally thin abomasal plicae. Edema may contribute to the thickening of rugae seen in gastritis. Edema of the submucosa of the stomach is a common and important lesion in edema disease of swine. It is best appreciated by making several slices through the serosa and external muscle to the submucosa on the greater curvature over the body of the stomach. Edema disease is considered fully in the later section on Infectious and parasitic diseases of the alimentary tract.

Hyperemia of the gastric mucosa occurs with ingestion of chemicals, which usually also cause superficial erosion and necrosis, discussed later under chemical gastritis. Focal hyperemia may be related to local irritation of the mucosa by foreign bodies, and with focal acute viral lesions of the abomasum in cattle. **Congestion** of the mucosa can occur in conditions causing portal hypertension, including cirrhosis and shock in the dog.

Uremic gastritis, seen as severe congestion and hemorrhage of the body of the stomach, associated with signs of hematemesis and melena, is found in some dogs, and occasionally in cats and horses, with renal disease. In such animals, the mucosa is thickened and deep red-black. There may be granular material typical of mineral within the mucosa. Lesions vary in severity from case to case, and premonitory changes without severe hemorrhage and necrosis are present in animals euthanized earlier in the course of disease. Gastric ulceration may occur,

but is not common. In such dogs there may be no gross gastric lesion, or variable edema and thickening of rugal mucosa, perhaps with focal ulceration, is evident.

Microscopically, in dogs, the lamina propria between glands is edematous, and there are increased mast cells. Deposits of basophilic ground substance and mineral are found, especially on the basement membrane of vessels and glands, or on collagen fibrils and in degenerate smooth muscle. These changes occur particularly in the middle and deeper portions of the mucosa. Parietal cells in this area are usually mineralized as well. More extensive mineral deposition also involves the muscular coats and arterioles of the submucosa and serosa. Such vessels also show evidence of endothelial damage, medial necrosis, and, in some cases, thrombosis. Severe mucosal congestion, edema, and necrosis are possibly related to ischemia secondary to the vascular lesions, although perhaps not directly associated with arterial thrombosis and obstruction, which is often not readily found. In cats with uremic gastropathy, gastric fibrosis and mineralization occur, but not gastric ulceration, edema, or vascular fibrinoid change.

The cause of the vascular lesions associated with uremia is incompletely understood. Mineral deposition is probably the product of altered systemic metabolism of calcium in renal failure, perhaps coupled with the local microenvironment resulting from bicarbonate moving across the basal border of secreting parietal cells. Membrane lesions in metabolically compromised parietal cells may also act as foci of mineral deposition (see Vol. 2, Urinary system, for a discussion of uremia). Metabolic acidosis and inflammatory cytokines including tumor necrosis factor-α may also promote vascular mineralization. Mineralization is also a feature of vitamin D intoxication.

Gastric venous infarction is a common lesion in swine, and is also encountered in ruminants and horses. It is related to endothelial damage and thrombosis in venules, usually associated with *endotoxemia or other bacterial or toxic damage*. Salmonellosis and *Escherichia coli* septicemia in all species, and in addition, in swine, postweaning coliform gastroenteritis, erysipelas, swine dysentery, and Glasser's disease are associated with the lesion. Porcine dermatopathy and nephropathy syndrome has also been associated with gastric infarction. The fundic mucosa is bright red or deep red-black and may have excess mucus or perhaps fibrin on the surface. Occasionally the superficial mucosa is obviously necrotic, adopting a yellow-brown caseous appearance, and may lift off with the ingesta. In section there is thrombosis of venules in the mucosa and often at the mucosal-submucosal junction, usually with prominent fibrin plugs. Thrombosed capillaries and venules may be present at any level of the mucosa, along the base of the ischemic zone of superficial coagulative necrosis, with local hemorrhage and edema. There may be an acute inflammatory reaction delineating the necrotic area in the mucosa. Sometimes the full thickness of the gastric mucosa, focally or diffusely, may be necrotic.

Further reading

Al-Aly Z. Vascular calcification in uremia: what is new and where are we going? Adv Chronic Kidney Dis 2008;15:413-419.

McLeland SM, et al. Relationship among serum creatinine, serum gastrin, calcium-phosphorus product, and uremic gastropathy in cats with chronic kidney disease. J Vet Intern Med 2014;28:827-837.

Peters RM, et al. Histopathologic features of canine uremic gastropathy: a retrospective study. J Vet Intern Med 2005;19:315-320.

Gastritis

Gastritis is a term used clinically as a presumptive diagnosis for those cases of vomiting that are thought to arise from gastric irritation rather than disease elsewhere. In pathology, the term is often used with equal imprecision, referring to a wide range of gastric injury in which histologic criteria of inflammation may not be particularly prominent. Under the broad umbrella of gastritis fall several different types of lesions: gastric mucosal necrosis, erosion or ulceration caused by mechanical, chemical, or ischemic insults, among which is uremic gastritis, described earlier; true gastritis, in which the lamina propria contains the leukocytic and vascular changes characteristic of inflammation; and finally, lesions of gastric mucosal atrophy, fibrosis, and lymphofollicular hyperplasia that arguably are the residual lesions of previous active inflammatory disease.

Chemical gastritis or abomasitis, reflected in diffuse gastric congestion, hemorrhage, necrosis, and ulceration, may be induced by chemicals such as arsenic, thallium, formalin, bronopol, steroidal and nonsteroidal anti-inflammatory drugs (NSAIDs), phosphatic fertilizers, and by the toxic principle in bitterweed (*Hymenoxon odorata*). **Blister beetle (*Epicauta* spp.) intoxication in horses,** induced by the *cantharidin* contained in these insects, may cause necrosis and ulceration of the distal esophagus and pars esophagea, and intense hyperemia of the glandular mucosa of the stomach, and in some cases gastric ulcers and rupture. In addition, enterocolitis, nephrosis, hemorrhages of the urinary bladder, and myocardial hemorrhage and necrosis are reported with regularity in blister beetle toxicosis. **Zinc** may cause acute mortality, in which the mucosa of the abomasum and duodenum is a distinctive lime green and necrotic, with an underlying congested, edematous submucosa. Microscopically, radiating crystals are evident in the necrotic tissue. Subacute zinc intoxication may be reflected in abomasal damage characterized by exfoliation of glandular epithelium, ablation of glands in some areas, and reparative proliferation of mucous neck cells, in addition to fibrosing pancreatitis and mild nephrosis. In sheep, type-A trichothecene **mycotoxin** has been associated with rumenitis and abomasal ulceration in acute toxicity. **Mechanical gastritis** is most commonly seen in dogs after ingestion of coarse foreign materials and in cats with hairballs. The lesion is discovered as an incidental finding when careful clinicians biopsy the stomach via endoscopy when making the diagnosis of gastric foreign body, or at the time of surgical removal of that foreign material. Hairballs in the abomasum of ruminants are associated with lack of roughage in young animals, but virtually never with disease.

Eosinophilic infiltrates occur in the squamous stomach of horses with an eosinophilic epitheliotropic syndrome, discussed in the later section on eosinophilic enteritis in horses, and with dermatitis.

The majority of examples of genuine gastritis are seen in dogs and cats with more generalized gastrointestinal inflammatory disease, such as food allergy or idiopathic inflammatory bowel disease, and is discussed further with those topics (see later section on Idiopathic inflammatory bowel disease).

Infectious agents in small animals appear to be minor causes of gastritis, when compared with chemical, mechanical, or idiopathic insults. Following the discovery of *Helicobacter pylori* as a major cause of gastric ulceration in humans, there was a flurry of activity to document its significance as a cause of gastritis and/or gastric ulceration in other monogastric species. The picture that has emerged is a confusing one because of substantial flux in the taxonomy of the various gastric spiral organisms, and because of the existence of many different species of *Helicobacter* (only some of which have been successfully cultivated). At least 20 different *Helicobacter* species, distinguished by mRNA sequencing, have been reported from various mammalian species. It is safe to say that probably all mammals have one or more species of *Helicobacter* as part of the normal gastric flora, and thus determining a causal relationship between *Helicobacter* and gastric disease has proved very difficult.

Helicobacter pylori is a common cause of acute and chronic gastritis affecting antrum, corpus, or both, in humans and in other primates. In humans it is the leading cause of chronic peptic ulcers. This may progress in some cases to gastric mucosal atrophy, with loss of antral and/or oxyntic glands. Chronic *Helicobacter* infection in humans also significantly increases the risk for the development of gastric carcinoma and lymphoma. On the other hand, *H. pylori* appears to be a very uncommon infection in other species, and has never been proved to cause disease in nonprimates. Among nonprimates, the most convincing evidence for clinically significant gastric *Helicobacter* infection is in **ferrets**. Although virtually all adult ferrets have *H. mustelae* as part of the normal gastric flora, heavily colonized ferrets develop diffuse lymphocytic-plasmacytic gastritis with lymphofollicular hyperplasia and sometimes with erosions. Progression to neoplasia has not been documented. *H. heilmannii* has been incriminated in development of gastric lymphoma in cats.

The role of Helicobacter in the development of gastritis or gastric ulceration in other species remains uncertain. Claims for the significance of *Helicobacter acinonychis* as a cause for gastritis in captive cheetahs remain unproved, in that antibiotic treatment improves the clinical disease but does not eradicate the gastric *Helicobacter* infection. Furthermore, wild cheetahs have the same *Helicobacter* colonization, but not the gastritis. In dogs and cats, it is routine to see various spiral organisms colonizing the gastric surface and within canaliculi in parietal cells in normal animals and in those with gastrointestinal disease. Depending on detection methods, the prevalence of colonization is at least 50% and may be nearly universal in adults. The prevalence of such colonization as determined by direct visualization or by culture is as high in clinically healthy animals as in those with clinical signs of gastritis. On the other hand, there are several studies claiming that dogs or cats with natural or experimental *Helicobacter* infection have a higher prevalence of mucosal mononuclear leukocytes and mucosal lymphoid follicles, and faster mucosal turnover, than is seen in animals in which *Helicobacter* infection could not be demonstrated. The problem is that the modest histologic changes have not been correlated with the development of clinical disease. The changes described resemble the kind of changes seen elsewhere in the intestinal tract with, for example, acquisition of the normal flora by germfree animals, or even as part of normal immunologic maturation of the gastrointestinal tract. Improvement in clinical signs following antibiotic therapy appropriate for the elimination of *Helicobacter* has not been documented convincingly.

Chlamydophila *(Chlamydia)* have been recognized in surface mucous cells of otherwise normal fundic mucosa in cats with no signs of disease. Experimental infection produced conjunctivitis and respiratory disease, but only mild gastritis.

Gastric mucosal hypertrophy is a lesion within the stomach of dogs that may be focal or diffuse. The **focal lesion** is much more prevalent, occurring as an intraluminal papillary proliferation of pyloric antral mucosa causing clinical signs of pyloric obstruction. The proliferation is mostly by mucus-containing cells of the mucosal surface and foveolae, forming papillary projections supported by a lamina propria that is either normal or that contains an increase in plasma cells and eosinophils. The significance of the eosinophilic inflammation in causing the regional mucosal hypertrophy is unknown, but many examples do not have any change in mucosal leukocytes. Surgical excision is curative. The diagnosis is usually obvious on the basis of endoscopic examination. Endoscopic biopsies may or may not permit the diagnosis, depending on the depth of mucosa captured by the biopsy forceps. The key to the diagnosis in an endoscopic biopsy is that the entire depth of the sample is taken up by surface epithelium and foveolae, whereas in a normal stomach a biopsy of similar size would capture at least some of the deeper gastric pyloric glands.

Diffuse gastric mucosal hypertrophy (chronic hypertrophic gastritis) of dogs, similar in many respects to Ménétrier's disease in humans, is rare. Vomition and weight loss, in some cases associated with inappetence or diarrhea, are described in the history. The characteristic lesion is marked gastric rugal hypertrophy involving part or most of the fundic gland mucosa in the body of the stomach. Grossly thickened folds of mucosa over an area 4-10 cm in diameter are thrown up in a convoluted pattern that may resemble cerebral gyri.

Microscopically, these areas are composed of hypertrophic/hyperplastic mucosa that may or may not include secondary folds of muscularis mucosae and submucosa. Findings are variable in the few cases reported. There may be foveolar and glandular epithelial hyperplasia with progressive or total loss of parietal cells, which are replaced by mucous cells of various degrees of differentiation. Marked cystic dilation of mucous glands may occur, which may be evident grossly. Mononuclear cells infiltrate the lamina propria between glands and near the muscularis mucosae, and the propria may be edematous, especially superficially. If the gross appearance of the mucosa in animals with hypertrophic gastritis is not seen by endoscopy or at surgery, biopsies that do not sample the full thickness of the mucosa may be misdiagnosed as chronic superficial or diffuse gastritis.

The cause of chronic hypertrophic gastritis is unknown, but in part it may be mediated by immune events in the mucosa. The condition in humans is associated with protein-losing gastropathy. Significantly, chronic gastritis and chronic hypertrophic gastritis have been reported in the Basenji, a breed of dog in which a syndrome of protein-losing gastroenteritis and diarrhea is well recognized (see later section on Idiopathic inflammatory bowel disease).

Hypertrophic antritis, producing a thickened, sometimes convoluted, mucosa in the antrum, is part of the syndrome of chronic hypertrophic pyloric gastropathy, associated with pyloric stenosis in dogs, considered earlier. Etiologic factors are unknown.

Braxy, or bradsot, is an acute abomasitis of sheep and, less commonly, calves, caused by infection with *Clostridium septicum* (Fig. 1-37). It is a sporadic disease of young animals,

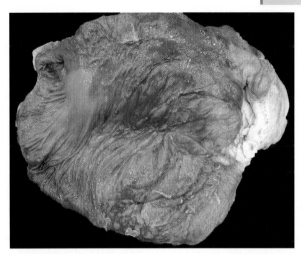

Figure 1-37 Braxy-like **clostridial abomasitis** (*Clostridium septicum*) in a calf. (Courtesy J. Haynes.)

usually occurring in temperate climates of the world. The factors initiating bacterial invasion are unknown, although local tissue damage in the abomasum is implicated. Cold weather is usually associated with the disease, but it is difficult to imagine feed being cold enough, by the time it reaches the abomasum, to cause significant mucosal trauma or hypothermia and necrosis. Production of exotoxin by *C. septicum* causes the signs and death, which usually ensues quickly. A similar gastritis has been associated with *C. sordellii* infection.

At autopsy, there may be blood-tinged abdominal fluid and the serosa of the abomasum may be congested or fibrincovered. Mucosal lesions may be diffuse, or involve demarcated foci of variable size and shape. Abomasal folds may be thickened, reddened, and occasionally hemorrhagic or necrotic. Most notable is the presence of extensive gelatinous edema and emphysema in the submucosa. Diffuse edema, and extensive areas of suppurative infiltrate demarcating areas of coagulative necrosis, with prominent pockets of emphysema, are evident in tissue sections. These involve mainly submucosa, and extend into adjacent mucosa and external muscle. There may be venous thrombosis and hemorrhage. Gram-positive bacilli are usually evident as individuals or colonies in affected tissue.

C. perfringens type A has been associated with a syndrome of **tympany, abomasitis, and abomasal ulceration in calves** in the western United States. However, the role of this pathogen in development of abomasal inflammation and ulceration is not completely understood. Animals have abdominal tympany and pain, depression, or may die suddenly. Grossly, there is variable congestion, hemorrhage, erosion, and ulceration of the abomasal mucosa, usually in the fundic area. Circular or linear perforating ulcers may develop. In association with the expected microscopic changes in erosion or ulceration, there is exfoliation and necrosis of mucosal epithelium, edema of the submucosa, dilation and thrombosis of submucosal lymphatics, and mild acute inflammatory infiltrates in the submucosa. Gram-positive bacilli may be on the mucosal surface, or in inflamed submucosa. Proliferation of *C. perfringens* in the rumen of calves with overflow of milk from the reticular groove is believed to promote colonization of the abomasum, and production of necrotizing exotoxin. Disease has also been associated with overeating, contaminated colostrum, and decreased gut motility. In both calves and lambs, clostridial gastritis may be preceded by the development of superficial peptic micro-ulcers, which subsequently become colonized and progress to typical clostridial lesions.

Abomasitis associated with viral infection occurs in a number of the systemic viral diseases affecting the gastrointestinal tract, including infectious bovine rhinotracheitis in calves and, rarely, older animals, herpesviral infections of small ruminants, bovine viral diarrhea, rinderpest, malignant catarrhal fever, and bluetongue. Abomasal lesions are rarely the sole manifestation of these diseases, but form part of a picture at necropsy that may suggest an etiologic diagnosis. The appearance and pathogenesis of abomasitis in these diseases vary with the conditions (see Infectious and parasitic diseases of the alimentary tract, later in this chapter).

Mycotic gastritis or abomasitis is a sporadic problem almost invariably secondary to insults that cause achlorhydria, focal atrophy, necrosis, or ulceration under conditions in which mycotic colonization can occur. Compromised resistance, perhaps associated with endotoxemia, septicemia, endogenous or exogenous steroids, neoplasia, lympholytic viral disease, and altered gastrointestinal flora caused by antibiotic therapy, may further promote mycosis. Fungal hyphae attaining the submucosa typically invade venules and arterioles, causing *thrombosis and hemorrhagic infarction*. The agents involved are usually zygomycetes (phycomycetes) such as *Rhizopus*, *Absidia*, or *Mucor*; rarely, *Aspergillus* may be implicated. The lesions are areas of necrosis, with an intensely congested or hemorrhagic periphery, ranging in diameter from 1 to 2 cm, to confluence over much of the body of the stomach (Fig. 1-38A). Affected mucosa is thickened, red or pale in the necrotic zone, and may be covered by hemorrhage. Edema and hemorrhage are evident in the submucosa. The lesion may penetrate to the serosa, where it is typically seen as a roughly circular area of hemorrhage in the external muscle and subserosa. *Hyphae*, usually broad and nonseptate zygomycotic in type, are present in sections of the necrotic mucosa, submucosa, and invading vessels, where they initiate thrombosis (Fig. 1-38B). *Candidiasis* of the pars esophagea may occur in swine, often in association with preulcerative epithelial hyperplasia and parakeratosis. For an overview of mycosis of the digestive system, and its sequelae, see the later section on Infectious and parasitic diseases of the alimentary tract.

Parasitic gastritis is often subclinical in **dogs and cats**, but in a small number of animals can be associated with vomiting and mucosal ulceration. Members of the genera *Physaloptera* and *Gnathostoma* are found in dogs, where the former cause focal ulceration and the latter are the cause of submucosal inflammatory cysts containing suppurative exudate and worms. In cats, *Physaloptera* spp. may attach to mucosal ulcers, whereas *Gnathostoma* spp. and *Cylicospirura felineus* are found in nodules in the gastric wall. *Ollulanus tricuspis* is found on the mucosa of the stomach in cats, where it may cause mild to, rarely, severe chronic gastritis. *Cryptosporidium* infection of the gastric mucosa occurs rarely in cats and dogs, with uncertain significance.

In **horses,** *Draschia megastoma* is found in inflammatory nodules in the submucosa of the cardiac zone, especially along the margo plicatus. The nodules can be several centimeters in diameter and contain necrotic debris and worms. *Habronema muscae* and *H. majus* are found in the mucosa and have been associated with mild ulceration. *Trichostrongylus axei* may cause chronic gastritis in the horse. Bots of the genus

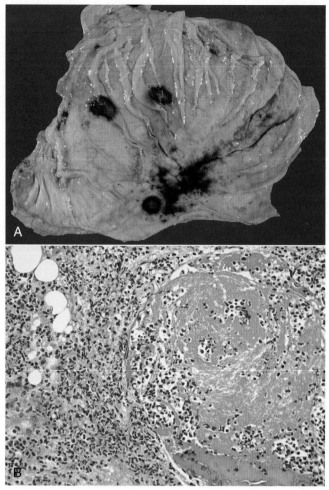

Figure 1-38 Mycotic abomasitis in a calf. A. Focal lesions are surrounded by deep red areas of infarction and hemorrhage as the result of thrombosis of mucosal and submucosal vessels. **B. Thrombosis** of a venule in submucosa of abomasum resulting from hyphal invasion.

Gasterophilus are found attached to small erosions and ulcers in the esophageal and glandular mucosa, which very rarely become complicated or perforate.

In **swine,** the spirurids *Ascarops* spp., *Physocephalus* spp., and *Simondsia* spp. are associated with mild gastritis in heavy infections. *Gnathostoma* may be embedded in inflammatory cysts in the submucosa. *Ollulanus tricuspis* may be encountered. *Hyostrongylus rubidus* can cause chronic gastritis and wasting in pigs.

In **cattle, sheep,** and **goats,** members of the genera *Haemonchus* and *Mecistocirrus* are large abomasal blood-sucking trichostrongyles, capable of causing severe anemia and hypoproteinemia. *Ostertagia* spp. and related genera, including *Camelostrongylus, Teladorsagia, Marshallagia,* and *Trichostrongylus axei,* in various ruminants, cause chronic abomasitis with mucous metaplasia, achlorhydria, diarrhea, and plasma protein loss. *Cryptosporidium andersoni* occasionally causes subclinical abomasitis in cattle, associated with elongation of the gastric glands, hyperplasia of the epithelium in the gland isthmus, attenuation of epithelium lining the neck of fundic glands, and dilation of glands. The small basophilic organisms are present on the surface of epithelium from the base of glands to the mucosal surface. Large schizonts of an incompletely characterized coccidia in sheep and goats form pinpoint pale foci in the abomasal mucosa. The name *Eimeria (Globidium) gilruthi* has been applied. Infection has been associated with elongation of the gastric glands with hyperplasia of the mucous neck cells, and decreased numbers of parietal cells. Gastric parasitism is considered more fully in the later section on Infectious and parasitic diseases of the alimentary tract.

Further reading

Bridgeford E, et al. Gastric *Helicobacter* species as a cause of feline gastric lymphoma: a viable hypothesis. Vet Immunol Immunopathol 2008;123:106-113.

Esteves MI, et al. *Helicobacter pylori* gastritis in cats with long-term natural infection as a model of human disease. Am J Pathol 2000;156:709-721.

Hermanns W, et al. *Helicobacter*-like organisms: histopathological examination of gastric biopsies from dogs and cats. J Comp Pathol 1995;112:307-318.

Maratea KA, et al. Abomasal coccidiosis associated with proliferative abomasitis in a sheep. J Vet Diagn Invest 2007;19:118-121.

Masuno K, Miller MA. Morphological and immunohistochemical features of *Cryptosporidium andersoni* in cattle. Vet Pathol 2006;43:202-207.

Songer JG, Miskimins DW. Clostridial abomasitis in calves: case report and review of the literature. Anaerobe 2005;11:290-294.

Takemura L, et al. *Helicobacter* spp. in cats: association between infecting species and epithelial proliferation within the gastric lamina propria. J Comp Pathol 2009;141:127-134.

Yoshiuchi R, et al. Survey and molecular characterization of *Cryptosporidium* and *Giardia* spp. in owned companion animal, dogs and cats, in Japan. Vet Parasitol 2010;174:313-316.

Gastroduodenal ulceration

Gastroduodenal ulcer produces signs much less often in animals than in humans. The pathogenesis of **peptic ulcer** in both humans and animals in general seems to resolve into a relative imbalance between the necrotizing effects of gastric acid and pepsin on one hand, and the ability of the mucosa to maintain its integrity on the other. Impairment of mucosal integrity in the face of normal acid secretion is probably the predominant mechanism, although there are clear instances when hypersecretion of acid is causative.

Factors implicated in hypersecretion of acid include abnormally high basal secretion, possibly associated with an expanded parietal cell mass, perhaps the result of increased trophic stimulation by gastrin. Gastrinomas cause *Zollinger-Ellison syndrome*, characterized by elevated gastric acid secretion and severe gastroduodenal ulceration. Increased histamine levels associated with mastocytosis or mastocytoma also cause acid hypersecretion and ulceration.

Ulceration caused by compromise of mucosal protective mechanisms is attributed to *nonsteroidal anti-inflammatory drugs* (NSAIDs), such as aspirin, phenylbutazone, and indomethacin. Orally administered NSAIDs that are weak organic acids, such as aspirin, have a direct deleterious effect on the stomach. Active bicarbonate secretion is responsible for a pH gradient from acid in the lumen to near neutrality at the epithelial cell surface. Stimulation of this bicarbonate secretion is induced by prostaglandin E_2 and nitric oxide. Inhibition of bicarbonate secretion occurs in the presence of atropine and various NSAIDs. Decreased prostaglandin is due to NSAID inhibition of cyclooxygenase (COX). Additionally, NSAIDs (except aspirin) may promote gastric hypermotility. Hypermotility is associated with altered microvascular blood flow and decreased mucosal response to injury. This is especially true in the gastric folds. Phenylbutazone may also have a direct toxic effect on vascular endothelium in the mucosa, which also compromises circulation and predisposes to ulceration.

In humans, gastritis associated with *Helicobacter pylori* infection, and duodenal colonization with this agent, are associated with development of duodenal ulcer. *Helicobacter*-associated gastritis extending cranially in the stomach is associated with gastric ulcer. Similar associations between *Helicobacter* infection, gastritis, and peptic ulcer have not been demonstrated convincingly in domestic animals.

Reflux of duodenal contents containing bile salts has been implicated in the induction of gastritis and gastric ulcer. Under some experimental conditions, acid back-diffusion into the gastric mucosa, and morphologic damage, have been caused by the application of bile salts. The effects are dependent on the pK_a of the bile salt, which must be soluble at acid pH, and on the concentration of hydrogen ion. Lipid solubility of bile salts, and associated damage to surface cell membranes, may mediate these effects. Alcohols, also lipid-soluble compounds, alter permeability of gastric mucosa and permit back-diffusion of acid. Lysolecithin, formed when pancreatic lipase hydrolyzes lecithin in bile, increases gastric mucosal permeability too.

Glucocorticoids and stress have been implicated in the genesis of ulcer, although the role of steroids is controversial. Experimentally, gastroduodenal hemorrhage and ulceration occur in some species of animals stressed by restraint or social factors, and they are a feature of "trap death syndrome" in small mammals. Severe gastric hemorrhage or ulceration may occur following neurosurgery, trauma to the spinal cord, and burns, and it is considered by some to be stress related. Administration of methylprednisolone sodium succinate to dogs was clearly acutely ulcerogenic. However, some experimental studies have demonstrated that glucocorticoids released during stress are more gastroprotective than ulcerogenic, although the rate of healing in pre-existing ulcers was decreased in the presence of steroids.

Reduced mucosal perfusion or ischemia may be a principal factor interacting in stress-associated ulceration, and in that initiated by other modalities, discussed previously. Reduced blood flow to the mucosa in local areas, under a number of circumstances, precedes mucosal hemorrhage or erosion. Ischemia will result in hypoxemic compromise of surface mucous cells. In combination with the effects of other insults, this may initiate mucosal permeability and back-diffusion of acid. Neutralization by blood-borne bicarbonate of acid diffusing into the mucosa also may be reduced in ischemia. Mucosal ischemia may result from reduction in local prostaglandin (as in NSAID administration) or nitric oxide concentration, thrombosis, as well as local or systemic hypotension. Ischemia may be more significant in the induction of fundic, rather than antral, ulcers.

Whatever the cause, the results of a breach of the gastric glandular mucosa have the potential to follow a **common pathway to ulceration** in all species. Acute superficial lesions, such as those associated with stress or following administration of aspirin, are often seen as areas of reddening and hemorrhage, especially along the margins of rugae in the fundic mucosa. Acid treatment of hemoglobin gives blood on the surface or in the gastric lumen a red-brown or black color. In some instances, melena, presumably the result of a recent episode of gastric bleeding, may be present in the lower intestine, with minimal gross evidence of hemorrhage or ulceration in the stomach. The microscopic lesion associated with hemorrhage of this type is often subtle; bleeding seemingly results from diapedesis, with minimal mucosal damage. Usually there is superficial erosion of the mucosa, often difficult to differentiate from autolysis, with granules of brown acid hematin in debris on the surface. Inflammation is usually absent. Evidence for healing mild gastric erosion is the presence of basophilic, poorly differentiated, flattened, cuboidal or low columnar cells on the mucosal surface, with mitotic cells in the upper neck of the glands.

Lesions of any genesis proceeding to gastric ulcer do so by progressive, often rapid, *coagulative necrosis of the gastric wall*. Ulcers vary in microscopic appearance depending on their aggression, and the point in their development at which they are intercepted. Acute gastric lesions appear as erosions with superficial eosinophilic necrotic debris and loss of mucosal architecture to the depths of the foveolae, or as a depression in the mucosal surface with necrotic debris at the base. Necrosis usually extends rapidly to the muscularis mucosae, causing ulceration. Once the superficial portion of the mucosa is destroyed, natural local buffering is lost, and the proliferative compartment of the gland, which is near the surface, is obliterated, preventing a local epithelial regenerative response. Ulcers attaining the submucosa impinge on arterioles of increasing diameter, multiplying the risk of significant *gastric hemorrhage*. The ulcer may progress through the muscularis and serosa, culminating in *perforation* of the gastric wall. Severe gastric hemorrhage or perforation are relatively common sequelae of gastroduodenal ulceration in domestic animals.

Ulcers that come into equilibrium with *reparative processes* may do so at any level of the gastric wall below the mucosa, but usually at the submucosa. Subacute to chronic ulcers have a base and sides composed of granulation tissue of variable thickness and maturity, infiltrated by a mixed inflammatory cell population, and overlain by a usually thin layer of necrotic debris. Chronic ulcers wax and wane. Depending on the relative dominance of reparative processes and aggressive ulceration, the layer of granulation tissue may be thick and mature, or thinner, less mature, and with superficial evidence of recent necrosis. There is mucous metaplasia and hyperplasia in glands at the periphery of the ulcer, which, with time, overhang the edge of the lesion, whence epithelial cells may gradually migrate across, closing the defect. Restitution of mucosal integrity is a complex process that is promoted by local activity of cytokines and growth factors such as transforming growth factor-β, vascular endothelial growth factor, basic fibroblast growth factor, epidermal growth factor, interleukins-1β and -2, and interferon-γ. Secretion of growth factors is a coordinated response by gastric epithelium and mesenchymal cells. Angiogenesis, also driven by cytokines and growth factors within the healing ulcer and granulation bed, is important for restoration of the mucosal microvasculature. The mucosa of healed ulcers, even in the fundic zone, is comprised of mucous glands. Excessive scarring of healed ulcers located near the pylorus may lead to pyloric obstruction in any species.

Duodenal ulcers, which usually occur proximal to the opening of the pancreatic and bile ducts, resemble gastric ulcers in their microscopic appearance (allowing for their intestinal location), evolution, and sequelae.

Peptic ulcer in dogs is reported relatively infrequently in the literature. Signs associated with peptic ulcer include variable appetite, abdominal pain, vomition, melena, and anemia. Ulcers, a few millimeters to 3-4 cm in diameter, are found most commonly in the pyloric antrum or proximal duodenum. The gross and microscopic appearance of ulcers varies with their aggressiveness and duration, as previously described. Thrombosed arterioles and venules cut by the ulcerative process are often seen, and should be sought in the bed of gastric and duodenal lesions associated with anemia or obvious hemorrhage.

Perforation of gastric or duodenal ulcers may lead to massive hemorrhage or release of gastric contents into the abdomen. Perforating duodenal ulcer may instigate pancreatitis. Some ulcers perforate silently, the serosal lesion healing by granulation, or adhesion by, and fibroplasia in, the omentum. The irritant nature of gastric contents released in these circumstances may lead to chronic inflammation, granulation, and thickening of the serosa, even when previous perforation cannot be appreciated. A search for microscopic particles of food such as plant material or muscle fibers in the serosal inflammatory response confirms perforation in this circumstance. Chronic peptic ulcers with thickened mucosal margins, scirrhous bases, and perhaps serosal thickening associated with perforation or near perforation, must be differentiated from gastric adenocarcinoma in the dog.

Syndromes resulting from hypersecretion of acid occur in dogs. *Mastocytoma is associated with peptic ulcer*, presumably owing to histamine-stimulated acid hypersecretion and microvascular effects. The tumor and mastocytosis do not involve the stomach directly, and ulcers may occur in animals with solitary skin tumors. In one series of 24 dogs with recurrent or metastatic mastocytoma, gastric and duodenal erosions or ulcers, frequently multiple, were present in 20. In many cases such lesions are clinically silent, and they should be looked for at autopsy in animals with mastocytoma. Mast cell tumors have rarely been associated with gastric ulceration in the cow, and in the cat, where gastric ulcer is very uncommon.

Zollinger-Ellison syndrome, *peptic ulcer caused by gastrin-secreting pancreatic islet cell tumors or gastrinomas*, has been reported in a few dogs and fewer cats. The history usually includes inappetence, vomition, weight loss, and possibly diarrhea or melena. Reflux esophagitis and gastric or duodenal ulcer are present in most cases. Small nodular masses histologically confirmed as islet cell tumors may be found in the pancreas, and in most animals, metastases to the liver, spleen, or hepatic lymph nodes are present.

Firm diagnosis rests on demonstration of elevated serum gastrin levels by radioimmunoassay; by identification of gastrin-bearing cells in fixed or frozen tumor tissue by immunohistochemistry; or by demonstration of gastrin in extracts of frozen tumor.

The microscopic appearance of these islet cell tumors is not diagnostic for gastrinoma, nor is the ultrastructural appearance of tumor cells necessarily characteristic of the G cell. Pancreatic islet cell neoplasms may be difficult to find, and should be sought assiduously in suspect cases.

The cause in dogs of gastroduodenal ulcer possibly associated with decreased resistance to back-diffusion of acid is less clear. Hepatic disease is often present in dogs with gastric ulcer, but the basis for a causal association is obscure. Some ulcers are associated with administration of **glucocorticoids** in high doses as anti-inflammatory, immunosuppressive, or antineoplastic therapy. **Nonsteroidal anti-inflammatory drugs** such as aspirin, naproxen, indomethacin, ibuprofen, flunixin meglumine, and piroxicam, sometimes given in excessive quantity, are also associated with spontaneous ulcers. Gastric hemorrhage and gastroduodenal ulceration are occasionally seen in dogs following **trauma or major surgery**. A syndrome of gastric hemorrhage, pancreatitis, and colonic ulceration and perforation is recognized in dogs following **spinal trauma**. The pathogenesis of this problem is obscure and undoubtedly complex.

Abomasal ulcers in cattle are common (Fig. 1-39); duodenal ulcer is rarely encountered in this species. Acute ulcers or erosions considered to be the result of stress are frequently seen incidentally in animals, of any age, dying of a variety of causes. They are usually present as linear areas of brown or black hemorrhage or erosion along the margins of abomasal rugae, or as punctate hemorrhages and erosions scattered over the mucosa, especially of the fundus.

Ulcers may be present anywhere in the abomasum. They are common in the pyloric region in cattle, and especially at the torus pyloricus in veal calves, but they may scallop or perforate abomasal rugae and excavate the mucosa in the fundus as well. Often more than one ulcer is present.

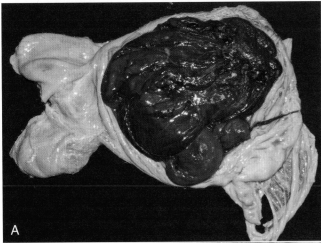

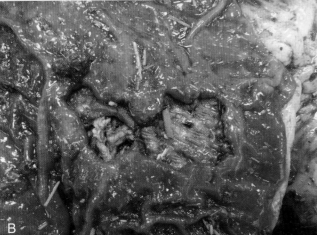

Figure 1-39 Perforated abomasal ulcer in a calf. A. Abomasal lumen filled with blood as a result of an abomasal ulcer (**B**). (Courtesy J. Caswell.)

The causes of abomasal ulcer are usually unclear, but they are most common in young calves, dairy cows, and feedlot animals. Viral agents including bovine viral diarrhea virus and malignant catarrhal fever virus are associated with abomasal ulcers. Abomasal ulcer occurred in about 34% of feedlot cattle in one study, with about half the cases symptomatic, whereas there are reports of over 6% of European dairy cows slaughtered with evidence of active or previous abomasal ulcers. A very high proportion, often in excess of 50%, of veal calves may have abomasal ulcers at slaughter. Ulcers often appear to be subclinical, and apparently without effect on growth or performance. However, about one-third of suckling calves dying under 4 months of age in western Canada had perforating abomasal ulcers. They were often associated with hairballs, which, it was concluded, were probably not causal. Mineral deficiencies, including copper and selenium, have been associated with abomasal ulcers in calves.

Ulcers often seem to occur under *stressful circumstances*, as in recently weaned and veal calves, postparturient cows, animals with concurrent disease such as abomasal displacement or mastitis, or after transportation. Lactic acid and histamine entering the abomasum from the forestomachs in animals poorly adapted to high-concentrate rations may contribute to mucosal damage. In veal calves, consumption of straw, shavings, or other roughage has been associated with an increased prevalence of ulcers, and there appears to be an increase in thickness and altered mucus production in the pyloric mucosa. Abomasal ulcers in range calves in western North America have been associated with *Clostridium perfringens* gastritis, consumption of roughage at pasture, and possibly copper deficiency. Perforating abomasal ulcers may develop in calves secondary to mycotic infection. Abomasal stasis may play a part in animals with physical or physiological abomasal obstruction or displacement. Ulceration of the abomasal mucosa infiltrated by lymphosarcoma will occur, and it may occur as a sequel to ingestion of toxins such as arsenic.

The presenting sign in many cases of abomasal ulceration is *melena*. Hemorrhage causing exsanguination, or perforation and septic peritonitis, is the usual cause of death resulting from abomasal ulcers. Bleeding abomasal ulcer should be looked for in cattle with melena or anemia, and perforating abomasal ulcer in animals presented with septic peritonitis, especially if digesta is in the abdominal cavity. Perforation may occur into the omental bursa, localizing contamination, and occasionally, points of perforation will be adherent to the abdominal wall, or occluded by superficially adherent omentum.

Gastric ulcers in swine are usually restricted to the *pars esophagea*; in a small proportion of affected pigs, lesions extend into the contiguous esophagus. Rarely are significant ulcers of the cardiac, fundic, or pyloric mucosa encountered in swine, sometimes in association with ulcer of the pars esophagea, occasionally with gastric parasitism or systemic disease. Venous infarcts in the body of the stomach in swine are not to be confused with gastric ulcer.

Under conditions of modern pig husbandry, the prevalence of ulcer and associated abnormalities of the pars esophagea is high. Weaned growers and feeders are commonly affected. Most lesions are subclinical; however, some prove fatal. Pigs die without premonition, or with a short history that may include anemia, weakness, inappetence, vomition, and melena. Other animals are affected chronically, with signs of anorexia, intermittent melena, and weight loss that may culminate in death or slow recovery with runting.

There is little disagreement over the morphology of ulceration of the pars esophagea, although its etiopathogenesis has been controversial. Many factors have been implicated in the etiology. Stressful husbandry practices have been considered to contribute to development of ulcer, although glucocorticoid administration results in lesions of the fundus, not pars esophagea, in pigs. Environment has been identified as a factor, for example, pigs held on slatted floors have a higher incidence of nonglandular ulcers than pigs on solid or straw flooring. High dietary copper levels, feeding of whey, starchy diets low in protein, high levels of dietary unsaturated fatty acids, and microbial production of short-chain fatty acids have been associated with the development of ulcers. Experimental infection with *Ascaris suum* has been associated with ulcer, but natural infection is not considered causally associated. Although an association between the presence of *Helicobacter heilmannii* and ulceration has been proposed in pigs, this has not been strongly substantiated, and gastric ulcers in pigs involve squamous, rather than glandular, mucosa. Experimentally in gnotobiotic pigs, *H. heilmannii* has been shown to induce ulcers in the squamous portion of the stomach of pigs fed a ration high in carbohydrate. Experimentally, factors stimulating acid secretion, especially histamine, consistently cause ulcers of the pars esophagea, suggesting that gastric acidity may play an etiologic role. Repeatedly, *finely ground rations have been found to be ulcerogenic*, and this may be the single most important predisposing factor.

Squamous epithelium has no innate buffering capacity, and it is highly susceptible to attack by gastric acid, pepsin, and refluxed bile, as occurs in reflux esophagitis. Similar events may initiate ulceration of the pars esophagea. Swine with gastric ulcers usually have abnormally fluid stomach contents. Feeding of finely divided rations and prolonged fasting are associated experimentally with increased water in stomach content. Normally there is a declining gradient of pH from esophagus to pylorus in stomach ingesta. Abnormally fluid gastric content fails to partition properly, and the pH gradient from esophagus to pylorus is not established. Relatively low pH occurs at the esophageal end of the stomach, where hydrochloric acid, pepsin, and refluxed bile, along with short-chain fatty acids produced by microbial fermentation of carbohydrate, synergistically attack the squamous mucosa. Meanwhile, the pH at the pylorus is higher than normal. Under conditions of prolonged gastric distention and relatively high antral pH, gastrin-stimulated acid secretion may be excessive, promoting that insult.

Lesions of the pars esophagea may involve only a small part, or virtually all of the gastric squamous mucosa. The lesion evolves through parakeratosis, to fissuring and erosion, with ultimate ulceration in severe cases. All stages in this progression will be encountered at autopsy in pigs. The epithelium of the pars esophagea often appears yellow and is thickened, irregular, roughened, and may flake or peel off readily. *Candida* may be present over the epithelial surface, with hyphae invading the parakeratotic epithelium, perhaps because of favorable cystine or glycogen levels. Rete pegs and proprial papillae are elongate.

Erosion of the epithelium progresses to ulceration and exposure of papillae and deeper propria, which bleed as small vessels are disrupted. Such lesions begin as fissures in the hyperplastic parakeratotic epithelium, but advance to ulcerate

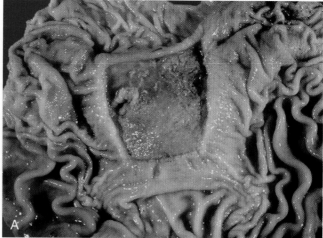

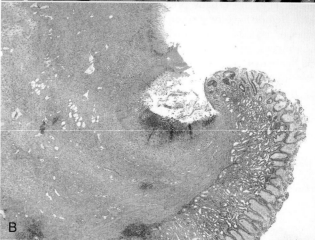

Figure 1-40 Ulceration of the pars esophagea in a pig. **A.** Gross image showing ulceration of squamous mucosa. (Courtesy Noah's Arkives.) **B.** Cardiac glandular mucosa overhangs the margin of the ulcer, the floor of which is at the bottom. (Courtesy E. Whitley.)

the entire pars esophagea. They usually spare only a microscopically visible margin of squamous epithelium adjacent to the cardiac gland mucosa. Ulcers of the pars esophagea, like peptic ulcer, have a floor of necrotic debris overlying exposed connective tissue (Fig. 1-40). Depending on the stage and aggression of the ulcer, there may be a well-developed inflammatory margin to the necrosis and a bed of granulation tissue. *Fatal gastric hemorrhage* often occurs.

Grossly, fully developed ulceration of the pars esophagea is apparent as a punched-out lesion with elevated rolled edges, obliterating the entire pars esophagea and obscuring the esophageal opening (see Fig. 1-40). The floor of the ulcer may be so smooth that it is misinterpreted as normal. Pigs with gastric ulcer at any stage of evolution tend to have fluid content in the stomach. Those with hemorrhagic ulcer may have red-brown gastric content, or massive hemorrhage into the stomach with large blood clots in the lumen, and smaller clots adherent to the base of the ulcer and its exposed bleeding points. Melenic content will often be present in the intestine, and the colon may contain firm black pelleted feces. The carcasses of animals that exsanguinate with gastric ulcer are very pale. Blood in the intestine associated with gastric ulcer in pigs must be differentiated from mesenteric volvulus and from proliferative hemorrhagic enteropathy associated with *Lawsonia*. A few pigs with parakeratosis, erosion, and ulceration of the pars esophagea have esophageal lesions suggestive of gastric reflux.

Gastric ulcers in some pigs resolve by granulation, and they may become re-epithelialized. Such lesions usually become scirrhous, puckered, and contracted as the ulcer closes from the periphery, and scarring may be visible from the serosa. In these circumstances, stenotic occlusion of the esophageal opening into the stomach may occur, and pigs with this problem can develop muscular hypertrophy of the distal esophagus.

In **horses,** *ulcers in the stomach of foals and adults* are often found at autopsy incidental to some other disease process. Gastric ulcer as a clinical entity is less commonly recognized, although a syndrome of abdominal pain, sometimes associated with gastric reflux, has been described in foals, and gastric ulcers are associated with colic in older horses. Ulcers are common in foals under 4 months of age; about half of a group of foals without signs of gastric disease had ulcers visible by endoscopy. Ulcers have been detected endoscopically in >65% of performance horses, in training, racing, or on endurance rides. They are often multiple, and although most frequent in the esophageal region, they can simultaneously involve all 4 mucosal zones of the stomach, and the duodenum, with no relationship apparent in the pattern of distribution. COX expression is altered in ulcers of the squamous regions, with decrease in COX1 and increase in COX2 expression; COX2 may be important in the healing response.

Ulcers of the *esophageal zone* are common. They are usually most severe at or adjacent to the margo plicatus, involving the edge of the squamous epithelium. They are often large and irregular in shape. There may be extensive fissuring, erosion, and ulceration of the squamous mucosa on the remainder of the pars esophagea, and in the esophagus, sometimes nearly to the pharynx, in foals with reflux. Often islands of thickened white proliferative mucosa are scattered as plaques on a predominantly ulcerated mucosa (Fig. 1-41). Microscopically, there is epithelial hypertrophy and hyperplasia in response to insult, marked in some islands of surviving mucosa, with prominent rete pegs and edematous proprial papillae. Parakeratotic hyperkeratosis is also an early lesion. Lesions then grade through increasing degrees of epithelial erosion to

ulceration, with evolution of the ulcer and ulcer bed, as described earlier in swine. In a low number of horses, glandular metaplasia has been observed in the ulcer bed.

Ulcers in the secretory stomach are less common. These ulcers are also often large and multiple, although a full range from focal punctate to extensive deep lesions may be seen.

Perforation may occur at any site of ulceration, and in one series represented 1% of 600 autopsies on foals. Some foals may exsanguinate because of bleeding ulcers, and occasionally clotted blood will fill the stomach, forming a cast.

Pyloric and duodenal stenosis have been associated with healing ulcers in horses. Ulcerative lesions involving the circumference, or the antimesenteric mucosa, of the proximal duodenum have been associated with gastric ulcers in foals, and duodenal stricture may represent a more chronic phase of this process. Severe esophagitis occurs in foals with ulcer and gastric reflux.

Many cases of gastric ulcers in horses are associated with enteric disease, colonic impaction, ileus, surgery, or other circumstances that can be considered stressful or could cause gastroduodenal reflux. Ulcers are common in horses held in stalls, and alternating periods of feeding and feed deprivation have been shown to induce ulceration of the gastric squamous epithelial mucosa. The pathogenesis of ulceration in the pars esophagea in horses probably resembles that in swine. Abnormally fluid content associated with feeding patterns and feedstuffs is permissive of acid, pepsin, and bile reflux to the cranial part of the stomach, where, at pH levels <4.0, volatile fatty acids generated locally may predispose further to damage to the squamous mucosa. A diet of bromegrass hay has been implicated in causing lower gastric pH, and thus facilitating ulcer formation. Exercise increases intra-abdominal pressure, resulting in gastric compression and reflux of acidic content into the cranial stomach, possibly contributing to ulceration associated with intensive training.

It is unclear whether the *ulcerative duodenitis* seen in some cases is a product of peptic ulceration, or whether it represents a process such as "proximal enteritis," which in turn results in stricture, gastric reflux, and ulceration. Administration of NSAIDs is commonly associated with gastroduodenal ulcers, and lesions of the glandular stomach, squamous stomach, and pylorus, among other lesions, have been induced in horses intoxicated with phenylbutazone.

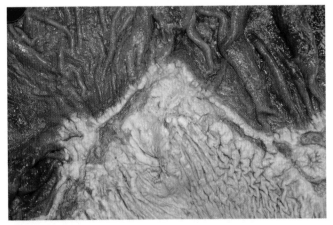

Figure 1-41 Multiple confluent areas of **ulceration** of the squamous mucosa of the stomach of a horse, with surviving hyperplastic mucosa bordering ulcerated areas.

Further reading

Argenzio RA. Comparative pathophysiology of nonglandular ulcer disease: a review of experimental studies. Equine Vet J Suppl 1999;29:19-23.

Arroyo LG, et al. Potential role of *Clostridium difficile* as a cause of duodenitis-proximal jejunitis in horses. J Med Microbiol 2006;55:605-608.

Braun U, et al. Bleeding abomasal ulcers in dairy cows. Vet Rec 1991;129:279-284.

Cariou M, et al. Spontaneous gastroduodenal perforations in dogs: a retrospective study of 15 cases. Vet Rec 2009;165:436-441.

Doster AR. Porcine gastric ulcer. Vet Clin North Am Food Anim Pract 2000;16:163-174.

Kopinski JS, McKenzie RA. Oesophagogastric ulceration in pigs: a visual morphological scoring guide. Aust Vet J 2007;85:356-361.

Liptak JM, et al. Gastroduodenal ulceration in cats: eight cases and a review of the literature. J Feline Med Surg 2002;4:27-42.

Marshall TS. Abomasal ulceration and tympany of calves. Vet Clin North Am Food Anim Pract 2009;25:209-220.

Martineau H, et al. Pathology of gastritis and gastric ulceration in the horse. Part 1: range of lesions present in 21 mature individuals. Equine Vet J 2009;41:638-644.

Neiger R, et al. Gastric mucosal lesions in dogs with acute intervertebral disc disease: characterization and effects of omeprazole or misoprostol. J Vet Intern Med 2000;14:33-36.

Satoh H, et al. Role of dietary fibres, intestinal hypermotility and leukotrienes in the pathogenesis of NSAID-induced small intestinal ulcers in cats. Gut 2009;58:1590-1596.

Sinha M, et al. Current perspectives in NSAID-induced gastropathy. Mediators Inflamm 2013;2013:258209.

Takeuchi K. Pathogenesis of NSAID-induced gastric damage: importance of cyclooxygenase inhibition and gastric hypermotility. World J Gastroenterol 2012;18:2147-2160.

Tarnawski A. Cellular and molecular mechanisms of gastrointestinal ulcer healing. Dig Dis Sci 2005;50 Suppl 1:S24-S33.

INTESTINE

Normal form and function

The microtopography of the **small bowel** is extensively modified to increase its surface area by *spiral mucosal folds* in some species, and by **villi** projecting into the lumen. The villi, projections of lamina propria covered by a layer of epithelium one cell thick, expand the absorptive surface of the small bowel 7-14 fold. In most species, villi are tallest in the duodenum, and decline somewhat in height toward the ileum. The length and shape of villi in normal animals vary with the species, age, intestinal microflora, and immune status. In general, villi in dogs, cats, neonatal piglets, and ruminants tend to be tall and cylindrical; those in horses and in young ruminants tend to be moderately tall and cylindrical; villi in weaned ruminants and swine may be cylindrical, leaf- or tongue-shaped, or rarely ridge-like, with their broad surface at right angles to the long axis of the gut. Villus length typically declines somewhat after weaning.

Opening to the mucosal surface around the base of each villus are several *crypts of Lieberkühn*. Depending on the species and their proliferative status, crypts are straight or somewhat coiled and lined by a single layer of epithelium. The progenitor compartment of the enteric epithelium resides here, producing cells that differentiate and move up on to the surface of villi, mainly as absorptive enterocytes, ultimately to be extruded as effete cells from the tips of villi. Sloughed cells contribute to the enzyme content and complexity of the intestinal luminal content.

Stem cells are found near or at the base of the crypts, depending on species and the position in the gastrointestinal tract, and they give rise to rapid-cycling transit-amplifying cells, which eventually differentiate into 1 of *4 main lineages of cells*, which undergo continuous cycles of renewal: *Paneth cells, goblet cells, neuroendocrine cells, and enterocytes.*

Paneth cells, a population of enigmatic cells turning over slowly (~20 days) in the base of the crypts in small intestine, are most obvious in horses among the domestic animals. They are not found in dogs, cats, or swine, nor prominent in the intestine of ruminants. Conspicuous eosinophilic secretory granules are present in their apical cytoplasm, and these contain a number of *antimicrobial proteins and peptides* including lysozyme, phospholipase, DNAse, ribonuclease, and alpha-defensins. These molecules are now known to be key mediators of homeostasis, host-microbe interactions, innate immune defense, and regulation of epithelial stem cells and the regenerative response of injured intestinal epithelium.

Oligomucous cells are relatively intermediate cells which differentiate into mature **goblet cells**. Both are present in epithelium of crypts and villi, with variable prevalence and distribution at various levels of the intestine, and in the different species. They have basal nuclei with distended apical theca–containing mucin granules. These cells synthesize and secrete by exocytosis bioactive molecules such as mucins, which are components of *mucus*. **Intestinal mucus** provides lubrication and frontline host defense against irritants and microbes while allowing nutrient transport. Mucus also contains *trefoil factor*, which is produced by goblet cells and promotes epithelial restitution after injury; *lysozyme* and *defensins* produced by Paneth cells; *resistin-like molecule β* (RELMβ) produced by goblet cells is involved in immunoregulation and homeostasis; and *immunoglobulin A* secreted by epithelial cells. Goblet cell hyperplasia and mucus secretion are promoted in the acute phase by a variety of noxious stimuli, inflammatory mediators, and by cell-mediated immune events in the gut, whereas chronic infections can result in depletion of goblet cells and alteration of mucus layers.

Enteroendocrine cells comprise a heterogeneous population of approximately 16 amine- or peptide-secreting endocrine/paracrine cells, representing about 1% of the epithelial cell population. Formerly classified by the ultrastructural appearance of their secretory vesicles, subtypes of enteroendocrine cells are now classified based on the contents of their secretory vesicles and are named by letters. Serotonin, somatostatin, cholecystokinin, peptide YY, glucagon-like peptides, and secretin are produced by specialized EC, D, I, L, and S cells in the gastrointestinal tract and these molecules are involved in regulation of intestinal motility and peristalsis, secretions, visceral sensations, and appetite. Immunohistochemistry studies have demonstrated that enteroendocrine cells stain positively for chromogranin A. With the exception of carcinoid tumors of serotonin-secreting cell origin, and rare functional neoplasms of other enteroendocrine cells in humans, the pathologic implications of this class of cells are still poorly defined.

Poorly differentiated **enterocytes** undergo rapid amplification division and these cells are cuboidal or low columnar with relatively few, short microvilli. Daughter cells differentiate and move into the functional compartment of absorptive enterocytes lining the villus. Undifferentiated crypt epithelial cells also secrete electrolytes and water. Mature **enterocytes** are responsible for the final digestion and absorption of nutrients, electrolytes, and water, and are by far the predominant epithelial cell type in the intestine. They are normally tall columnar cells, polygonal in cross-section, with regular basal nuclear polarity. A tight junction, which is permissive to small molecule and water transport, joins the apical margins of adjacent cells. The barrier to transepithelial macromolecular movement is essentially maintained even at sites of extrusion of effete enterocytes at the tips of villi. Basal to the tight junction, the lateral cell membranes interdigitate loosely, and a long, narrow potential space exists between enterocytes. The basolateral cell membrane is the site of sodium-potassium–dependent adenosine triphosphatase that drives the sodium pump, and of carrier systems exporting monosaccharides from the cell. Absorptive epithelial cells lie on a basal lamina with which they interact via integrins; they may be involved in communications with the underlying mesenchyme. Immediately beneath the basal lamina lies the sheath of syncytial **myofibroblasts,** alpha-smooth muscle actin-positive cells that mediate information flow between the epithelium and lamina propria through production of growth factors, cytokines, chemokines, prostaglandins, and extracellular matrix molecules. Myofibroblasts are thus involved in growth and tissue repair, tumorigenesis, inflammation, and fibrosis. Myofibroblasts are probably largely responsible for the remarkable plasticity of the villus during adaptive changes including villus atrophy and reconstitution of mucosal 3-dimensional morphology.

The apical surface of normal enterocytes is highly modified into **microvilli,** ~0.5-1.5 μm long and 0.1 μm wide, which are regularly arrayed in close apposition to each other at right angles to the surface of the cell. They are visible as the "brush border" by conventional microscopy. Microvilli increase the surface area of absorptive epithelium by a factor of ~15-40 times. The plasmalemma of microvilli is studded with massive numbers of enzyme molecules, including aminopeptidases and disaccharidases involved in terminal digestion of peptides and carbohydrates. These protrude as minute knob-like structures into the glycocalyx that coats the surface of microvilli.

In neonatal swine and ruminants, vacuolation of absorptive enterocytes is normal, and the nucleus is often also displaced into the apical cytoplasm. In piglets vacuolation is usual in the ileum but not in the duodenum, and seems to be a function of cell age. Such vacuolation should be differentiated from the presence of eosinophilic colostrum present in cytoplasmic vacuoles in the epithelial cells of neonates.

The cytoplasm of absorptive enterocytes is stabilized at the apical border by the filaments of the terminal web. Smooth endoplasmic reticulum is most prominent in the upper half of cells, whereas cisternal elements of rough endoplasmic reticulum are more uniformly distributed. The Golgi zone lies above the nucleus. Free ribosomes and polyribosomes are numerous in differentiating cells of the upper crypt and lower villus, and are relatively fewer in mature absorptive enterocytes.

The complex of endoplasmic membranes and Golgi apparatus is particularly active in handling *absorbed lipid,* which diffuses from micelles at the cell surface through the apical membrane, in the form of long-chain fatty acids or monoglyceride. These are re-esterified to triglyceride, appearing in the smooth endoplasmic reticulum, and are complexed with apoproteins produced in the rough endoplasmic reticulum to be excreted via the Golgi apparatus through the basolateral cell membrane as *chylomicrons.* Chylomicrons enter the extracellular space and leave the villus via the lacteal.

The **lamina propria** supports the epithelium of the small intestinal mucosa. It is composed of loose fibrous tissue within which blood vessels, smooth-muscle, inflammatory, and immune cells are interspersed. In addition to functioning in defense against microorganisms, *macrophages* phagocytose inert particulate matter reaching the lamina propria from the lumen. Bile pigment, perhaps derived from meconium, can be seen in macrophages in the tips of villi in neonates. Macrophages also phagocytose iron and may play a role in iron homeostasis. Apoptotic bodies, ceroid, and hemosiderin also may be observed in lamina proprial macrophages. This can be prominent in horses and is thought to represent detritus from apoptosis of upwardly migrating subepithelial myofibroblasts, and should not be mistaken for foci of necrosis.

Lymphocytes, neutrophils, and eosinophils are scattered in the lamina propria of villi and between crypts. Eosinophils are especially common in the intestine of ruminants and horses, with no specific pathologic connotation; they are highly variable in the intestine of small animals. Intraepithelial lymphocytes are frequently observed along villi and less commonly along crypts. Globule leukocytes may be found in the epithelium of crypts and low on villi, or sometimes in the lamina propria between crypts. Plasma cells are normally not numerous in villi, but are concentrated in the lamina propria between the upper portions of crypts.

The **vascular supply to the small intestinal mucosa** arises in submucosal arteries that give off arterioles at right angles, some of which send branches to a capillary plexus around crypts of Lieberkühn. Most arterioles arborize near the villus tip into a dense capillary plexus, which lies immediately beneath the basal lamina of the epithelium. Mucosal capillaries have fenestrations facing the basal lamina, which may be more permeable than the remainder of the endothelium. One or more venules drain blood from the capillaries in villi and between crypts, and flow into larger veins in the submucosa, which drain into mesenteric veins and the hepatic portal circulation. The *lacteal,* or central lymphatic vessel of the villus, is sufficiently permeable to permit the entry of macromolecules and chylomicrons, and is the main route of lipid transport from the villus.

The **cecum and colon** vary widely in anatomy and size among domestic animals, depending largely upon the significance of hindgut microbial carbohydrate fermentation. *Production of volatile fatty acids* from carbohydrate by colonic flora occurs in all species. This is a primary source of energy in the horse; it is significant in swine and ruminants as well. Extensive movement of electrolytes and water occurs across the colonic wall. In the horse, a volume of fluid approaching that of the extracellular fluid space may be in the large bowel, which must maintain a fluid medium for microbial fermentation; daily fluid absorption from the hindgut may exceed the extracellular fluid volume. *Absorption of electrolytes and water,* an electrolyte-conserving mechanism, is probably the major function of the colon in dogs and cats, and of the distal colon of herbivores.

The mucosa of the cecum and colon in all domestic mammalian species lacks villi, although there are ridges or folds on the mucosal surface. **Colonic glands,** or crypts, are straight tubular structures. The architecture of colonic glands and their cell population resembles that of small intestinal crypts. *Epithelial cells* differentiate progressively from stem cells deep in the glands to a single layer of columnar absorptive epithelial cells with basal nuclei that line the mucosal surface. Hindgut epithelial cells generally have sparse and irregular microvilli in comparison with those of the small bowel. Numerous glycoprotein-laden vesicles are observed in the apical cytoplasm of epithelial cells in most species. *Oligomucous cells,* also derived from basal stem cells, form a second proliferative population in the lower half of the colonic gland. Well-differentiated *goblet cells* are usually present in the upper half of colonic glands and on the surface. Goblet cells are present in variable numbers, depending on the species and a variety of other factors. *Enteroendocrine cells* of about a half-dozen types have been recognized, and are scattered in the cell column lining glands in the large bowel. *Paneth cells* are not found in normal colon; however, Paneth cell metaplasia has been proposed as a preneoplastic lesion in development of colonic epithelial neoplasia in humans.

The **lamina propria** of the colon is minimal between closely packed glands and contains a cell population similar to that in the small bowel. Normally, relatively few inflammatory and immune cells are present in the superficial mucosa in small animals and young herbivores; most plasma cells and lymphocytes are between deeper portions of glands. Older herbivores, especially horses, may have heavier superficial proprial inflammatory infiltrates, and macrophages containing phagocytosed debris may be present below the surface epithelium. In the equine colon, terminal arterioles entering the mucosa branch at right angles from the submucosal plexus. Capillaries ramify to surround colonic glands, and form an anastomosing network at the luminal surface, whereas sparsely distributed venules drain the superficial capillary plexus.

The connective tissue of the **submucosa** lies between the mucosa and the **external muscle** of the gut, which is formed by fascicles of smooth muscle cells arranged as inner circular and outer longitudinal layers. An extensive **enteric nervous system** with submucosal (Meissner's), and myenteric (Auerbach's) plexuses marked by ganglia, modulates external autonomic neural regulation and coordinates gastrointestinal motility and function. The neurons of the enteric system equal in number those in the spinal cord, and their ramifications sense and influence epithelial absorption and secretion, local endocrine/paracrine secretion, blood flow, immune events, and motility in the gut. Secretomotor neuron branches extend to individual crypts of Lieberkühn, where they stimulate secretion of electrolyte, water, and mucus. Excitatory and inhibitory effects are mediated by acetylcholine and by amine and peptide neurotransmitters such as substance P, adenosine triphosphate, and vasoactive intestinal peptide, which in some cases are also produced by endocrine cells of the gut and pancreas. *Myofibroblastic pacemaker cells of the intestine*, known as **interstitial cells of Cajal**, are distributed throughout the intestinal musculature, integrated with the extrinsic and enteric nervous systems. Abnormalities of these cells are thought to lead to disorders of motility, and to gastrointestinal stromal tumors, a specific entity described in dogs, horses, and cats. Disorders of motility associated with enteric neural lesions, such as the dysautonomias and grass sickness, are discussed in the later section on intestinal obstruction.

Interpretation of intestinal and colonic biopsies is often subjective, unless objective diagnostic criteria can be met, including recognition of an etiologic agent, a specific cell type, a characteristic pattern of inflammation or anatomic abnormality such as lymphangiectasia, or cytologic and morphologic abnormalities indicating malignancy.

There are significant variations in the microscopic morphology of the gut with age; between species and among individuals of a species; at different levels of the small and large intestine within species and within the same individual; and as a result of factors influencing mucosal cell trafficking in health and disease. Limited morphometric data are available in domestic animals, and interpretation is limited by the lack of standardized quantitative criteria defining morphological features during health and disease. Until more such information is available, and its application is validated, particularly in the diagnosis of inflammatory bowel disease, pathologists do well to expand their experience of intestinal morphology by close examination of tissues from animals in which gastro-

intestinal disease is not indicated clinically, and to view critically their reliability in diagnosing such entities.

Biopsy interpretation is enhanced by increasing size and number of specimens, full-thickness sampling, careful tissue handling including minimizing trauma, rapid fixation, and optimal orientation. Sacrificing any of these attributes increases the subjectivity with which a biopsy is interpreted; hence exquisite care must be taken in tissue handling to reduce traumatic artefact and to optimize orientation. Clinicians and pathologists dealing with endoscopic, capsule, and forceps biopsies must remember the limitations in interpretation imposed by small sample size, fragmentation, unfavorable sample orientation, and failure to sample the deep mucosa, submucosa and muscularis. These costs are offset to some degree by the opportunity to obtain a greater number of samples than may be possible by other means, at arguably lower risk and cost, and possibly more focused on a lesion by direct endoscopic examination.

Further reading

Clevers HC, Bevins CL. Paneth cells: maestros of the small intestinal crypts. Annu Rev Physiol 2013;75:289-311.

Day MJ, et al. Histopathological standards for the diagnosis of gastrointestinal inflammation in endoscopic biopsy samples from the dog and cat: A report from the World Small Animal Veterinary Association Gastrointestinal Standardization Group. J Comp Pathol 2008;138(suppl):S1-S43.

Gunawardene AR, et al. Classification and functions of enteroendocrine cells of the lower gastrointestinal tract. Int J Exp Pathol 2011;92:219-231.

Jergens AE, et al. Design of a simplified histopathologic model for gastrointestinal inflammation in dogs. Vet Pathol 2014;51:946-950.

Kim YS, Ho SB. Intestinal goblet cells and mucins in health and disease: recent insights and progress. Curr Gasteroenterol Rep 2010;12:319-330.

Mansell J, Willard MD. Biopsy of the gastrointestinal tract. Vet Clin North Am Small Anim Pract 2003;33:1099-1116.

Ouellette AJ. Defensin-mediated innate immunity in the small intestine. Best Pract Res Clin Gastroenterol 2004;18:405-419.

Roth S, et al. Paneth cells in intestinal homeostasis and tissue injury. PLOS One 2012;7:e38965.

Thomson AB, et al. Small bowel review: normal physiology, Parts 1 and 2. Dig Dis Sci 2003;48:1546-1564, 1565-1581.

Immune elements and the gastrointestinal mucosal barrier

The gastrointestinal tract is presented continually with antigens in food, allergens, toxins, viruses, commensal and pathogenic bacteria and their products, and parasites with their excretions and secretions. The epithelial barrier of the gut is only one-cell thick and has enormous surface area; the enteric mucosal surface of the average human is about 400 m². Therefore, it is not surprising that the epithelium and associated lymphoid and inflammatory cells in the mucosa and submucosa are components of a complex system for excluding, blocking, sampling, tolerating, or neutralizing and eliminating antigens or potential pathogens. Intestinal immune elements are sparse and quiescent at birth; immune activity in the gut is probably stimulated in response to colonization by normal bacterial flora beginning in the early neonatal period. In the mature animal, *lymphoid tissue is estimated to comprise 25% of the intestinal mucosal mass,* and to exceed that of the spleen in volume.

Elements of gastrointestinal mucosal defense are diverse, and include the volume of fluid secretion and peristalsis for dilution and flushing of contents, respectively, and gastric and bile acids and pancreatic secretions that break down ingested antigens. The indigenous microflora competitively inhibit or actively exclude intruding bacteria. Mucins on the luminal surface form a secretory barrier, and retain trefoil factor, antibody and soluble components of innate resistance, including those produced by Paneth cells. The epithelium provides a physical barrier, participates in innate resistance by production of proinflammatory cytokines, enables passive immunity by antibody uptake in the neonate, and contributes to active immunity by antigen uptake and presentation. Intraepithelial lymphocytes are an important first line of defense against pathogens and are recognized to play a significant role in epithelial barrier homeostasis. Soluble antibody in plasma and interstitial fluid neutralizes antigens penetrating the mucosal barrier and contributes to opsonization/phagocytosis, as do endogenous components of the innate immune system, such as complement. The organized elements of the mucosal immune system, Peyer's patches, and other mucosal lymphoid follicles, are sites for induction of intestinal immune responses, generating antigen-activated B and T cells that ultimately home back to the mucosa where they reside along with populations of macrophages and dendritic cells. Regional lymph nodes receive and trap free and phagocytosed antigens, and antigen-presenting cells activate more B and T cells, promoting mucosal and systemic immunity.

The **epithelial cell** of the neonate is uniquely capable of uptake and transport of macromolecules from the intestinal lumen to the basolateral cell surface. In all species of domestic animals, **colostral transfer of immunoglobulins** by this route provides the neonate with passive humoral immunity during the early postnatal period. The period of active uptake of macromolecules is short, usually only 24-48 hours in ungulates, and "closure" precludes further bulk transport of macromolecules.

Although bulk transport does not occur in mature animals, nutritionally inconsequential amounts of macromolecules continue to be transferred by enterocytes. Such molecules must escape both intraluminal hydrolysis and intracellular lysosomal degradation to permit their export from the cell. Fully differentiated small intestinal absorptive epithelial cells express major histocompatibility complex class II molecules on their basolateral membranes, and are capable of presenting antigen directly to T cells. Additionally, enterocytes detect pathogen-associated molecular patterns of bacteria and viruses via *pattern recognition molecules,* including surface toll-like receptors and cytosolic nucleotide-binding oligomerization domain (Nod) molecules for activation of cellular production of proinflammatory or immunomodulatory cytokines.

Intestinal intraepithelial T lymphocytes form a large population strategically located between the basolateral surfaces of epithelial cells and may comprise up to 10-20% of the cells within the epithelial layer. They are more numerous in the small intestine than the large intestine. In domestic animals they are comprised mainly of T cells uniquely expressing the homodimeric form of CD8α; most of these express the γδ T-cell receptor as opposed to the αβ T-cell receptor, especially in the small intestine. They function as a front line of defense, as part of the innate immune response to bacterial and plant

products such as amylamines, and to damaged enterocytes. They also presumably participate in the adaptive response, responding to antigens entering from the lumen and in tumor surveillance. Some may kill compromised epithelial cells. Most, but not all, intraepithelial lymphocytes appear to originate in Peyer's patches.

Globule leukocytes are visible in hematoxylin and eosin-stained tissue sections as *mononuclear cells with large eosinophilic cytoplasmic granules,* in the epithelium of the crypt and lower villus, and sometimes in the lamina propria. They have been associated with parasitism, but their function remains poorly understood and their origin uncertain with some evidence suggesting they originate from *mast cells* or *large granular lymphocytes.*

The **aggregated lymphoid follicles,** or **Peyer's patches,** are scattered in the mucosa of the small intestine, and lymphoglandular complexes or solitary proprial lymphoid nodules may be grossly visible throughout the colonic mucosa. Peyer's patches are present throughout the length of the small intestine in all species, although they tend to be larger distally. They are grossly visible, usually as oval or elongate structures up to several centimeters wide, thickening the antimesenteric wall of the intestine. They may project slightly above the mucosal surface, or appear as cupped depressions that must not be mistaken for ulcers, especially in dogs. In neonates of some species, including swine, they may be poorly developed and not visible grossly. **Continuous Peyer's patches** are found in the distal ileum of calves, lambs, and piglets and develop during late gestation, as opposed to upper intestinal lymphoid tissue, which is dependent on colonization of the gut for postgestational development. They are similar morphologically but apparently functionally distinct from other gut-associated lymphoid tissue. Their role as a primary site of B-cell generation remains controversial and, given that they involute as the animal matures, they likely play an important role in host defense during early life.

Peyer's patches are comprised of *follicular aggregates of B lymphocytes surrounded by aggregates of T lymphocytes* in the submucosa, underlying a discontinuous muscularis mucosae. Overlying the lymphoid follicles is a mixed population of T and B lymphocytes and dendritic cells extending into the lamina propria in rounded mucosal projections known as *subepithelial domes,* which lie between villi. Cell populations of Peyer's patches in newborns and gnotobiotes of most species tend to be sparser than those in older or bacterially colonized animals, although those in neonatal calves appear relatively well developed.

Membranous or microfold cells, **M cells,** are flattened cells lacking a brush border found interspersed among the follicle-associated epithelium overlying the subepithelial dome region, which separates the epithelium from the submucosal Peyer's patches and intestinal lymphoid follicles. Within the dome region are populations of dendritic cell subsets, which probably play a major role in initiation of mucosal immunity. M cells actively sample and transport particulate matter and macromolecules from the lumen to their basolateral membrane pocket where they interact with cells of the underlying mucosal immune system to facilitate mucosal immune responses. Despite, or perhaps because of, its role in adaptive immunity, the M cell is exploited as a likely portal of entry to the mucosa by certain pathogenic bacteria, including *Mycobacteria, Salmonella, Yersinia,* and *Listeria* in some species, and for some viruses. Neutrophils are seen transmigrating the epithelium of the dome, and are found in the lumen over the dome, in enteric bacterial infections of calves in particular.

B and T lymphoblasts gain access to Peyer's patches via specific receptors in permeable *postcapillary venules*. The major cell population in Peyer's patches appear to be B lymphocytes committed mainly to IgA production, whereas among the T cells is a large proportion of T helper cell precursors. Lamina proprial T cells are mixed CD4+ and CD8+, are most numerous between upper crypts and villi, and are likely antigen-activated cells. Cytokine production by activated T lymphocytes is complex and multifactorial, and this plays a significant role in promotion of inflammation and tolerance, particularly toward commensal organisms (covered in more detail later).

Antigen is processed and presented to lymphocytes in Peyer's patches and mesenteric lymph nodes largely by **dendritic cells** trafficking from the mucosa where they initially acquire antigen. Dendritic cells compose 10-15% of leukocytes in the lamina propria and in neonatal calves, are more numerous in the ileum compared with jejunum. Dendritic cells acquire antigen by interactions with intestinal epithelial cells or M cells, and can also directly sample luminal contents by extending their dendrites between enterocytes. The cytokine context within which dendritic cells function is also important and contributes greatly to the differential capacity of dendritic cells to initiate and regulate host immune responses. **Macrophages** are more common in the lamina propria than in Peyer's patches. Macrophages are involved in mucosal protection by phagocytosis and/or killing of invading pathogens such as *Mycobacterium avium* subspecies *paratuberculosis* and *Histoplasma capsulatum*, regulation of inflammatory responses, and as scavengers of dead cells or foreign debris. Macrophages also sequester iron, inhibiting bacterial metabolism. Macrophages in colonic lamina propria are highly phagocytic, but have a low ability to activate T cells and promote T-cell–mediated immune responses.

IgA-producing lymphocytes leave the Peyer's patches or other mucosal-associated lymphoid tissues and home to mucosal surfaces, including the intestinal tract, respiratory tract, mammary gland, and salivary glands. In the lamina propria of the intestine, they differentiate into IgA-secretory plasma cells and localize adjacent to upper crypt epithelium. Dimeric IgA is transported via the polymeric Ig receptor from the basolateral border of columnar crypt epithelial cells onto the apical surface of epithelial cells. IgA-secreting cells are the predominant class of plasma cell in the lamina propria in most species. However, **IgM-secreting plasma cells** are prevalent in young calves, swine, and dogs; locally induced IgA class switching may actually occur in the lamina propria. IgM secretion is also facilitated by polymeric Ig receptor, and this may be significant in the young piglet and calf. Although IgA and IgM are secreted, IgG1 is the major antibody class in intestinal secretion of cattle and it appears to be selectively secreted by the gut and in the bile of that species.

The functions of IgA in the gut lumen are many and include blocking attachment of bacteria and viruses to epithelial cells, promoting pathogen clearance, neutralizing intraluminal toxins, maintenance of homeostasis, facilitation of antigen sampling, limiting absorption of food or microorganism-derived antigens, and promotion of tolerance. Secretion of IgA complexed with antigen into the bile by hepatocytes may be a significant means of clearing the circulation of antigen absorbed from the gut. IgA deficiency is reported in Beagle,

German Shepherd, and Shar-Pei dogs, where it may be associated with increased susceptibility to intestinal and respiratory disease.

IgG-producing plasma cells are relatively uncommon in the intestinal lamina propria in species other than ruminants. However, locally produced and systemically circulating IgG may assume significance when vascular permeability and inflammation occur because of its ability to fix complement, facilitate antibody-dependent cell-mediated cytotoxicity, and to opsonize. **IgE-producing plasma cells** are present in the lamina propria in small numbers in most species. IgE is implicated in immune responses during intestinal parasitism. Its significance may be in IgE-dependent cytotoxicity by eosinophils, mast cells, and basophils, as well as in mediating immediate (type I) hypersensitivity reactions in the mucosa.

Intestinal mucosal mast cells differ histochemically and physiologically from mast cells in most other tissues. They are less demonstrable using standard stains after formalin fixation as are connective tissue mast cells from other tissues; they stain well in tissue fixed in basic lead acetate or Carnoy's fluid. In contrast to connective tissue mast cells they contain tryptase but not chymase, and their granules are few, and variably electron-dense by electron microscopy. Proliferation of intestinal mast cells is T-cell–dependent and occurs during some parasitic and bacterial infections. Histamine, serotonin, and other mediators released by mast cells have many and complex effects on vascular tone and permeability; on motility, chemotaxis, and effector function of leukocytes; on immune-active cells; and possibly on mucus release. Mast cells interact with the enteric nervous system, sensing antigen with their IgE immune probe, and communicating with the sensory arm of the enteric nervous system by degranulation, releasing stimulatory soluble mediators. They undoubtedly play a central role in regulation of physiologic, immune, and inflammatory processes in the gut.

Intestinal **eosinophils** probably do not differ functionally from eosinophils in other sites as cytotoxic effector cells and modulators of local inflammation, particularly during intestinal parasitism, immune-mediated, or hypersensitivity reactions.

Immunoinflammatory events in the large bowel are less well understood than those in the small intestine; presumably similar principles prevail. **Lymphoglandular complexes** consist of submucosal follicular lymphoid aggregates penetrated by glands extending from the mucosa, and presumably facilitate contact of surface epithelium of the large bowel with underlying lymphoid tissue. These occur in the cecum and proximal colon of the dog; in the colon of swine; at the cecocolic junction, proximal spiral colon, and terminal rectum of ruminants. **Solitary mucosal lymphoid nodules,** normally without penetrating glands, and generally restricted to the lamina propria and superficial submucosa, are also scattered throughout the cecum and colon in all species.

Further reading

Acheson DWK, Luccioli S. Mucosal immune response. Best Pract Res Clin Gastroenterol 2004;18:387-404.

Bilsborough J, Viney J. Gastrointestinal dendritic cells play a role in immunity, tolerance, and disease. Gastroenterol 2004;127:300-309.

Butler JE, Sinkora M. The enigma of the lower gut-associated lymphoid tissue (GALT). J Leukoc Biol 2013;94:259-270.

Fries PN, Griebel PJ. Mucosal dendritic cell diversity in the gastrointestinal tract. Cell Tissue Res 2011;343:33-41.

Kunisawa J, et al. Intraepithelial lymphocytes: their shared and divergent immunological behaviors in the small and large intestine. Immun Rev 2007;215:136-153.

Lelouard H, et al. Peyers patch dendritic cells sample antigens by extending dendrites through M cell-specific transcellular pores. Gastroenterol 2012;142:592-601.

Pickard KM, et al. Immune responses. Best Pract Res Clin Gastroenterol 2004;18:271-285.

Santaolalla R, Abreu MT. Innate immunity in the small intestine. Curr Opin Gastroenterol 2012;28:124-129.

Smith PD, et al. Intestinal macrophages and response to microbial encroachment. Mucosal Immunol 2011;4:31-42.

Gastrointestinal microbiota

After birth, no part of the gastrointestinal tract is sterile. Hundreds of species of microorganisms including mostly anaerobic bacteria but also archaea, eukaryotes, and viruses, many of them unidentified, inhabit the stomach and intestine, forming an ecosystem of enormous complexity. Known to be important during inflammatory intestinal disease, the microbiota also provide an array of biochemical and metabolic activities important for normal host physiology and homeostasis, including: facilitation of metabolism of indigestible compounds; synthesis of essential vitamins; required for development of intestinal epithelium and immune system; and protection from invasion of opportunistic pathogens. The microbiota thus contribute prominently to homeostasis, regulated inflammation during host defense, and dysregulated inflammation during autoimmunity.

Generally, bacterial populations are least in the stomach and upper small intestine of ruminants and carnivores, being limited by the acid gastric environment and by peristalsis. The anaerobes and facultative anaerobes increase to ~10^7 per gram of content in the lower small intestine, and total bacterial populations >10^{10} or 10^{11} per gram of content are present in the cecum and colon. Prominent among colonic bacteria are coliforms, *Lactobacillus*, and strict anaerobes, including *Bacteroides, Fusobacterium, Clostridium, Eubacterium, Bifidobacterium*, and *Peptostreptococcus*. Spirochetes are found in swine and dogs. Anaerobic bacteria outnumber facultative anaerobes by a thousand-fold in the large bowel.

The complex ecology of the gut flora imparts upon it considerable stability. It is relatively resistant to the intrusion of new inhabitants and this is one of the major factors protecting against the establishment of pathogenic bacteria. It is no coincidence that bacterial diarrhea occurs most commonly in the neonate with a poorly established flora, or after changes in husbandry or antibiotic therapy, which may disturb the enteric bacterial population. *The normal flora acts as a barrier to colonization by pathogens through several means*, including secretion of host defense peptides such as colicins and bacteriocins. Short-chain fatty acids, particularly butyrate, generated by these microbes during carbohydrate metabolism are significant energy sources and trophic factors for colonocytes and are highly detrimental to members of the *Enterobacteriaceae* and therefore contribute to colonic barrier health in general. Competition for energy, and the effect of metabolites other than short-chain fatty acids produced by the native flora, also militate establishment of invasion by exogenous bacteria.

Normal flora are known to be important for development of the mucus layer properties, mucosal lymphoid structures, modulation of immune cell differentiation and regulation of cytokine and chemokine production in the gut. *Host factors influencing gut flora include composition of the diet; peristalsis*, which continually flushes the small intestine of a large proportion of its bacterial population; lysozyme; lactoferrin; gastric acidity if unbuffered or undiluted; and, in the abomasum of suckling calves, perhaps a lactoperoxidase-thiocyanide-hydrogen peroxide system. Mucosal epithelial maturation is influenced by the microbiota: germfree animals have longer and thinner villi, less-developed proprial vascular network and shallow crypts with fewer proliferating stem cells, compared with conventional animals. The quantity and quality of IgA secretion plays an important role in shaping both composition and function of the gut microbiome.

The use of probiotics, deliberate oral administration of specific microbial cultures, has been shown to improve body weight gain and decrease diarrhea in newborn calves and pigs, as well as to protect adult animals from colonization with certain pathogens, including *Escherichia coli* O157:H7 and some *Salmonella* spp.

Further reading

Kamada N, Nunez G. Role of the gut microbiota in the development and function of lymphoid cells. J Immunol 2013;190:1389-1395.

McCracken VJ, Lorenz RG. The gastrointestinal ecosystem: a precarious alliance among epithelium, immunity and microbiota. Cell Microbiol 2001;3:1-11.

Nyangale EP, et al. Gut microbial activity, implications for health and disease: the potential role of metabolite analysis. J Proteome Res 2012;11:5573-5585.

Sommer F, Backhed F. The gut microbiota - masters of host development and physiology. Nat Rev Microbiol 2013;11:227-238.

Electrolyte and water transport in the intestine

Water movement in the bowel is passive, following osmotically the transport of electrolyte and nutrient solutes. The small intestinal mucosa is highly permeable to the passive movement of small ions and water and is therefore considered leaky, despite the presence of tight junctions along the apical margins of absorptive enterocytes. This ensures that the content of the small bowel is approximately isosmolal with the interstitial fluid space. The permeability of junctional complexes appears to be sensitive to Starling forces, influenced by intravascular hydrostatic and oncotic pressure, so that fluid and solute actively absorbed may leak back into the lumen, thus modulating net absorption by the mucosa. Water is secreted into the gut with digestive juices and is almost entirely resorbed in the small and large intestine; aquaporins, transmembrane water channel proteins, are important in the rapid passage of water across cell membranes.

Sodium absorption takes place by a number of active transcellular mechanisms, which vary in importance at different levels of the gut, and with the physiologic circumstance. Fundamentally, Na^+ absorption depends on electrochemical forces established by the adenosine triphosphate-dependent Na^+ pump on the basolateral cell membrane of the absorptive enterocyte. This pump moves Na^+ up a concentration gradient from the cell into the lateral intercellular space. The concentration of solute, especially Na$^+$, in the lateral intercellular space, causes water to follow from the intestinal lumen. Because cell membranes and junctional complexes are highly permeable to water, movement is rapid via both transcellular and paracellular routes, and differences in osmotic pressure between lumen and lateral intercellular space are small. Absorbed solute and water in isotonic proportions move into the interstitium of the villus, where, within a few micrometers, they encounter a subepithelial capillary or lacteal. The tight junctions also appear to become permeable during sodium ion and nutrient cotransport across the apical cell membrane, resulting in solvent drag of large nutrient molecules into the lateral intercellular space.

The colon of carnivores, the spiral colon of ruminants and swine, and the small colon of the horse play an important role in reducing the volume of electrolyte and water lost in the feces. In contrast to the small intestine, *the colonic epithelium is relatively restrictive to the free movement of sodium and chloride*, although not to potassium. Therefore it is capable of maintaining differences in osmotic pressure, ionic composition, and electrical potential between luminal and proprial surfaces, which make it more efficient than the small bowel in absorbing some electrolytes and water. Ultimately, fecal water may be hypotonic with respect to plasma. Absorption of volatile fatty acids also accounts for considerable water absorption from the colon. Potassium increases in concentration in colonic content as sodium concentration declines; this is due to an active secretory process and a passive response to transepithelial electrochemical gradients.

Under some conditions, the mucosa of the small and large intestine also *secretes chloride, potassium, bicarbonate*, and *water*. This process can be a function of both surface and crypt cells, and is important in some pathologic states; however, it is also physiologic and segmental, maintaining the fluidity and buffering capacity of the intestinal content.

Solute movement across the intestinal epithelium is regulated by a number of *hormones and neurotransmitters*, which act through intracellular second messengers. Activation of adenylate cyclase and guanylate cyclase as well as increased intracellular Ca^{2+} all result in reduction of Na$^+$ absorption by enterocytes and promotion of Cl$^-$ secretion in crypt cells. Some products of intrinsic and extrinsic neurons, such as vasoactive intestinal polypeptide and acetylcholine, may stimulate secretion, whereas others, such as somatostatin and norepinephrine, are absorptive or antisecretory. Local paracrine effects are mediated by the products of enteroendocrine cells, such as somatostatin, neurotensin, and serotonin. Guanylin is a peptide secreted from epithelial cells that stimulates local fluid secretion. Mesenchymal elements in the lamina propria, including myofibroblasts, lymphocytes, mast cells, macrophages, and other inflammatory and connective tissue cells, also produce locally active substances with a direct or indirect effect on epithelial function. Circulating hormones also influence mucosal function: aldosterone and glucocorticoids enhance Na$^+$ absorption by the colon, and the latter may inhibit local production of eicosanoids.

Immunoinflammatory events are thus integrated with the systemic and local neural and hormonal regulation of intestinal absorption and secretion. Dysfunctions of absorption and secretion will be considered in the later section on the pathogenesis of diarrhea.

Further reading

Laforenza U. Water channel proteins in the gastrointestinal tract. Mol Aspects Med 2012;33:642-650.

Masyuk AI, et al. Water transport by epithelia of the digestive tract. Gastroenterol 2002;122:545-562.

Nakazato M. Guanylin family: new intestinal peptides regulating electrolyte and water homeostasis. J Gastroenterol 2001;36:219-225.

Seidler U, et al. Recent advances in the molecular and functional characterization of acid/base and electrolyte transporters in the basolateral membranes of gastric and duodenal epithelial cells. Acta Physiol (Oxf) 2011;201:3-20.

Epithelial renewal in health and disease
Small intestine

The intestinal surface is lined by a population of cells ultimately derived from *stem cells* that are present at or near the base of crypts or glands, but with its proximate source in amplifier populations of undifferentiated columnar or oligomucous cells in the lower half of the crypts. These cells lose their ability to undergo mitosis, and differentiate into *goblet cells* and *absorptive enterocytes* as they move from the crypt to the villus. In most species, they are *shed from the tips of villi* in 2-8 days; apoptosis is a minor contributor to physiological enterocyte loss. Generally cells are shed more quickly in the ileum than in the duodenum; this is perhaps related to reduced height of villi in the distal small intestine of most species.

The mass and topography of the mucosa are quite stable, the result of a dynamic equilibrium between the rate of movement of cells from crypts to villi, and the rate at which they are lost from villar tips. This steady state is influenced by interaction of the microflora with the epithelium, cell cycle regulators, and other mediators including transforming growth factor-β, glucagon-like peptide 2, and urokinase, which may facilitate cell shedding.

In young animals, the intestine grows by generation of new crypts followed by generation of new villi. As the bowel attains mature size, the number of villi and crypts apparently stabilizes; however, some adaptive variation in the ratio of crypts to villi may occur. Adaptive responses to a variety of factors alter the size and rate of turnover of the proliferative and functional epithelial cell populations and thus the microtopography of the gut. The appearance of the small intestinal mucosa is essentially a compromise achieved by equilibrium between the rates of cell production and loss. At one extreme is the intestine of germ-free animals characterized by short crypts containing a small proliferative compartment, and tall villi with a low rate of cell loss supporting a large functional compartment. At the other end of the spectrum is the intestine of an animal with severe intestinal helminthosis characterized by long crypts, shortened villi, few functional enterocytes, and a high rate of cell loss, reflecting an increased proliferative compartment.

Although quantitative description of epithelial kinetics is possible experimentally, in the diagnostic situation it is necessary to make a subjective or semiquantitative assessment of the status of the proliferative and functional compartments in tissue sections. The size of the proliferative compartment is reflected in the length and diameter of the crypts, and in the location of the uppermost mitotic cell. The prevalence of mitotic figures can be assessed subjectively; however, beyond calculating a mitotic index, no inferences can be drawn about the proportion of the crypt cell population that is replicating or the duration of the cell cycle.

The *degree of differentiation*, and hence functional status of enterocytes on villi, can be inferred from their appearance. Cytoplasmic basophilia; loss of regular basal nuclear polarity; low columnar, cuboidal, or squamous shape; and an ill-defined brush border all indicate a poorly differentiated population of surface enterocytes and suggest an increased rate of turnover. *Fasting* causes atrophy and reduction of mucosal epithelial mass caused by prolongation of the postmitotic phase of proliferative cells. Villi do not directly atrophy; however, surface enterocytes persist longer and are lost from the villus more slowly. Fasting-induced atrophy is immediately reversed by refeeding. *Weaning* has similar effects on the microtopography of the intestine, which is observed as marked reduction in height of villi in most species.

Restoration of epithelial integrity is dependent on a finely regulated balance of migration, proliferation, and differentiation of adjacent epithelial cells, which are ultimately mediated by local growth factors, cytokines, dietary factors, and especially by trefoil factors present in mucus.

Following minor loss of mucosal enterocytes, restitution occurs by *lateral migration of adjacent intact epithelial cells* within minutes. If epithelium on villi is obliterated, for instance by transient ischemia or by viral cytolysis, the villus core contracts because of myofibroblast activity mediated by the enteric nervous system, and stromal elements rapidly undergo apoptosis. Surviving epithelial cells become flattened and migrate across the denuded surface. Proliferation of epithelial cells then occurs and *regeneration of the mucosa* follows in hours to days after injury. Last, *maturation and differentiation* of cells occurs as the 3-dimensional architecture is restored within a few days. A bed of granulation tissue forms at the base of extensive mucosal ulcers, and with time (weeks to months) this may become covered by a neomucosa, with crypts and villi following immigration of epithelial cells from the periphery of the lesion. A similar process repairs the mucosal gap in healing intestinal anastomoses.

Villus atrophy

Atrophy of villi is a common pathologic change in the intestine of domestic animals. It results in malabsorption of nutrients, and can be associated with loss of plasma protein into the gut. Villus atrophy can be categorized histomorphologically into 2 broad types based on the appearance of the crypts, recognition of which has implications with respect to pathogenesis and prognosis. The first category includes intestine with apparently normal or hypertrophic crypts, and the second category is characterized by some evidence of damage to the proliferative compartment. Recognition, evolution, and interpretation of each category are considered later.

Villus atrophy with an intact or hypertrophic proliferative compartment takes 2 forms in domestic animals. A **primary increase in rate of loss of epithelium** from the surface of villi is one mechanism initiating such a lesion. This is the major mechanism involved in a number of important viral infections including coronavirus and rotavirus; of coccidial infections, which damage surface enterocytes predominantly; of some enteroinvasive bacteria; of transient ischemia, in which the effect is limited to the functional compartment; and, in some circumstances, of necrotizing toxins released by clostridia in the lumen of the bowel. The effect of these agents is increased loss of surface epithelium over a relatively short period of time, although sparing the proliferative compartment in crypts. Villi contract and become shortened as the size of the functional compartment is diminished. If the animal survives the metabolic sequelae of malabsorption that results from the damage to surface cells, *compensatory expansion of the proliferative compartment in crypts* permits complete recovery. Epithelial cells emerging and differentiating from crypt stem cells result in recovery of normal mucosal topography and full function within a few days.

The microscopic appearance of the mucosa depends partly on the number of functional cells lost, which determines the initial degree of villus atrophy, and partly on the amount of regeneration that has occurred when the gut is examined. During early phases of injury, damaged epithelial cells exfoliate into the gut lumen and villi are shortened and blunted; alternatively, villi are more or less of normal length, but appear somewhat pointed. Atrophic villi are subsequently covered by poorly differentiated low columnar, cuboidal, or squamous cells and there may be fusion of the lateral surfaces or tips of villi in some areas. In severe atrophy there may be mild erosion if inadequate epithelium is available to cover the mucosal surface area. In the acute phase, crypts appear normal, but within 12-24 hours proliferative activity is noticeably increased and crypts enlarge in diameter and length to accommodate more mitotic cells. Mitotic cells are poorly differentiated and crowded, have increased basophilia, and sometimes mitotic figures are observed close to the mucosal surface. The lamina propria may appear hypercellular; perhaps this is due to contraction of the lamina propria or mild mononuclear cell infiltrate. As regeneration progresses, the length of villi and differentiation of lining epithelial cells increases, and proliferation gradually subsides.

Atrophy of villi and hypertrophy of crypts is also associated with **chronic or persistent processes** such as nematode parasitism; chronic coccidial infection; giardiasis in some species; response to some dietary components such as soybean protein in calves, kidney bean protein in pigs, and wheat in dogs; idiopathic or specific granulomatous enteritis such as Johne's disease and histoplasmosis; and chronic inflammatory bowel disease. Epithelial kinetics have not been thoroughly investigated in most of these situations in domestic animals; however, these have in common chronic antigenic exposure, parasitism, or a persistent infectious process, which are usually associated with significant infiltration of inflammatory cells. Where the cause can be eliminated, the lesion usually remits, implying that active host-pathogen interaction is required for its induction and maintenance. The situation is analogous to celiac disease in humans, which is a dietary gluten–specific T helper-1 lymphocyte immune-mediated response resulting in production of interferon-γ, among other cytokines. Some experimental evidence has implicated nitric oxide, interleukin-12, interferon-γ, and tumor necrosis factor-α in the pathogenesis of villus atrophy; however, the source and effect of these molecules remain uncertain.

Immune reactions in the gut are associated with increased epithelial cell proliferation; however, hypertrophy of the proliferative compartment in these conditions *precedes* the development of villus atrophy, and *is not a response to it*. Local stimulation of the proliferative compartment and perhaps the associated myofibroblast sheath is likely mediated by nitric oxide or cytokines produced by activated T lymphocytes in the mucosa. Epithelial cells leaving these crypts usually do not differentiate fully and often exfoliate prematurely, low on the villus or near the crypt opening. Coupled with normal shedding of pre-existing enterocytes, this contributes further to atrophy of villi over a period of several days. Epithelial cells that reach the surface also do not differentiate fully, are rapidly lost into the gut lumen, or undergo mucous metaplasia.

Microscopically, hypertrophy of crypts is the early and outstanding change in this lesion, and is consistently present. In its milder forms, the lesion may be better characterized by elongate crypts than by obvious atrophy of villi. The proliferative compartment is expanded and active, mitotic figures are numerous, and goblet cell hyperplasia may also occur. Elongation of crypts may be so extensive that even with severe atrophy of villi the total mucosal thickness will not be much reduced from normal. Close observation may reveal poorly differentiated enterocytes exfoliating prematurely from inter-crypt ridges on the mucosal surface, or from buttress-like folds around the base of stubby villi. The lamina propria has a prominent population of lymphocytes, plasma cells, and associated inflammatory cells; intraepithelial lymphocytes are common. The etiologic agent may be evident, removal of which, where possible, usually results in a return to "normal" within days or weeks.

However it is induced, atrophy of villi with hypertrophy of crypts results in local malabsorption of nutrients and water. Poorly differentiated surface epithelial cells may secrete electrolytes and water, and increased epithelial turnover may contribute to enteric loss of endogenous protein. Proprial inflammation and microerosion of the mucosa may also contribute to effusion of tissue fluid.

Villus atrophy associated with damage to the proliferative compartment is also commonly seen in domestic animals. This form is the sequel to insults that cause necrosis of cells in crypts, or impair their mitotic capacity. Agents that cause these lesions usually have a propensity for damaging actively proliferating cells in any tissue. Because ionizing radiation was recognized early as a cause of such lesions, they are generally often termed *radiomimetic*. Other agents inducing similar lesions include cytotoxic chemicals and mitotic poisons, such as chemotherapeutic agents, T-2 mycotoxin, and pyrrolizidine alkaloids in large doses; viruses that infect proliferating cells, particularly the parvoviruses, and bovine viral diarrhea virus. Ischemia of sufficient duration to cause necrosis of some or all cells lining the crypts also causes this lesion.

The microscopic appearance of affected mucosa depends on the severity and extent of the insult, and the interval since it occurred. The primary event is damage to the proliferative compartment, and, except in ischemia, lesions will be evident in crypts well before significant atrophy of villi occurs. Individual necrotic epithelial cells and neutrophils may be present in the dilated lumen of damaged crypts. With severe damage to crypts, remaining epithelial cells become extremely flattened in an attempt to maintain the integrity of the crypt lining. Following the radiomimetic injury, irregular epithelial cells with large nuclei and nucleoli may be observed within crypts and will migrate onto the surface.

Pre-existing surface epithelial cells are shed from villar tips at an apparently normal rate, even though few or no new cells emerge from crypts. Villi eventually become atrophic or collapse as the surface cell population shrinks. If the majority of crypt cells are damaged, crypts stripped of epithelium collapse or "drop out," perhaps leaving a few scattered cystic remnants, lined by attenuated epithelial cells in the deeper lamina propria. The overlying surface may be eroded, or covered by squamous epithelial cells derived from surviving crypts. The mucosa may eventually ulcerate, to be eventually lined by granulation tissue. Crypts that have not been severely damaged will undergo hypertrophy within several days of the original insult, as compensatory hyperplasia of the remnant crypt epithelial cells occurs. In viral diseases, the severity and histologic appearance of the lesion often vary considerably at different sites in the gut, and even within an individual tissue section. Lesions caused by ischemia tend to be uniform in severity but may be localized; acute or subacute lesions are often hemorrhagic, especially if there has been re-establishment of blood flow.

Extensive crypt cell necrosis, erosion, or ulceration lead to severe malabsorption and effusion of tissue fluid and hemorrhage. The mucosa is susceptible to invasion by the enteric flora, sometimes including fungi. Local ulceration may contribute further to persistent fluid and plasma loss, and if circumferential, to eventual stricture formation and stenosis. Small ulcers in areas where a few crypts have dropped out will heal as epithelial cells from adjacent crypts migrate to repair the denuded surface; however, crypts may take longer to regenerate, so local villus atrophy will persist.

Large intestine

Epithelial turnover in the cecum and colon is fundamentally similar to that in the small intestine, though villi are not present on the surface. Epithelial cells lose the ability to divide after leaving the proliferative compartment in the lower part of the gland. In the upper portion of the gland, they differentiate into goblet cells or columnar absorptive cells that emerge and migrate over the surface. Cells are subsequently lost into the lumen, probably within about 4-8 days of being produced, although no studies of colonic epithelial turnover have been made in domestic animals. Colonic epithelial cell proliferation is experimentally reduced by fasting and restored by refeeding. Physical colonic distention and certain types of dietary fiber also appear to induce colonic epithelial cell proliferation. Compared with conventional animals, the colon of gnotobiotic animals has fewer proliferative cells, mostly limited to the lower portion of the glands.

Following insult and exfoliation of surface epithelial cells, restitution of the epithelial integrity in the large bowel resembles that in the small bowel. Within a few minutes of injury, surviving surface epithelial cells and cells emerging from crypts become attenuated and migrate at a rate of several micrometers per minute to cover mucosal defects. Ulcers, surgical incisions, or anastomotic sites in the colon heal by immigration of a single layer of epithelium from the periphery of the defect, with gradual differentiation of crypts, and eventual restitution of normal mucosal architecture. Depending on the type of anastomosis in the horse, epithelial cells may take >2 weeks to bridge the granulation tissue in the mucosal gap, and full restoration of mucosal architecture may require ~2 months.

Microscopic lesions in the large bowel associated with increased epithelial turnover can be induced by alterations in the replication rate of both surface and glandular epithelium. The number of goblet cells on the surface and in the upper portion of glands is often diminished. Epithelial cells in these areas appear poorly differentiated, have increased cytoplasmic basophilia and morphologically may be of low columnar, cuboidal, or squamous type. In severe diseases, erosion of the surface is present. The proliferative compartment in the gland may hypertrophy, causing glands to elongate and dilate. Mitotically active cells are increased in number and distributed over a greater proportion of the glands' length. In some acute or chronic inflammatory conditions of the lamina propria, goblet-cell hyperplasia may occur. It is uncertain whether this is caused by primary damage to surface epithelium, or by local cell-mediated immune effects on the proliferative compartment, as occurs in the small intestine in celiac disease of humans.

The *proliferative compartment* in the cecal and colonic glands is damaged by the same insults that attack cells in crypts of the small bowel, although the lesions in large bowel tend to be comparatively less severe. This is perhaps because a lower proportion of the proliferative compartment in the colon is in mitosis at the time of maximum availability of drug or virus. Additional agents that damage the proliferative compartment in the colon include bovine and canine coronaviruses, and several species of coccidia in ruminants, which develop in the epithelial cells lining colonic glands.

The *evolution and sequelae of lesions* resulting from damage to proliferative epithelial cells in the colon are similar to those in small bowel: dilation of crypts, accumulation of necrotic debris within crypts, and/or attenuation of the lining epithelium. Severe lesions will lead to loss of glands, erosion, and ulceration of the mucosa; hemorrhage; stricture and stenosis may ensue. Following milder damage that spares some stem cells in each gland, the mucosa has the potential to recover fully after a period of reparative hyperplasia.

Further reading

Burrin DG, et al. Glucagon-like peptide-2 function in domestic animals. Domest Anim Endocrinol 2003;24:103-122.

Denham JM, Hill ID. Celiac disease and autoimmunity: Review and controversies. Curr Allergy Asthma Rep 2013;13:347-353.

Gordon JI, et al. Epithelial cell growth and differentiation. III. Promoting diversity in the intestine: conversations between the microflora, epithelium, and diffuse GALT. Am J Physiol 1997;273:G565-G570.

Ierna MX, et al. Transmembrane TNF alpha is required for enteropathy and is sufficient to promote parasite expulsion in gastrointestinal helminth infection. Infect Immun 2009;77:3879-3885.

Moon HW. Comparative histopathology of intestinal infections. Adv Exp Med Biol 1997;412:1-19.

Scales HE, et al. Effect of inducible costimulator blockade on the pathological and protective immune responses induced by the gastrointestinal helminth *Trichinella spiralis*. Eur J Immunol 2004;34:2854-2862.

Vereecke L, et al. Enterocyte death and intestinal barrier maintenance in homeostasis and disease. Trends Mol Med 2011;17:584-593.

Pathophysiology of enteric disease

Protein-energy malnutrition caused by inadequate intake of feed or deficiencies in quantity or quality of nutrients is a well-recognized co-morbidity factor in many diseases. In its most severe forms, this results in *depletion of fat and muscle mass*, emaciation, and ultimately death by starvation. Importantly, protein-energy malnutrition is a common cause of secondary immune deficiency and is thus associated with increased susceptibility to infections.

Inappetence or **anorexia** are commonly associated with gastrointestinal diseases. Appetite is modulated by a complex and incompletely understood meshwork of neurologic, neuroendocrine, and systemic cytokine inputs impacting centrally on satiety. The potential for physical impairment of gastrointestinal function to affect appetite seems relatively obvious. Less apparent but highly significant are effects on appetite of chronic inflammatory or neoplastic diseases affecting the alimentary system or distant sites. Proinflammatory cytokines, such as tumor necrosis factor-α and interleukin-1 associated with chronic inflammation and neoplasia, are probably strategic mediators in the complex metabolic puzzle that is **cachexia**. *Ghrelin* is a stomach-derived hormone known to be an important mediator of cachexia, and although the mechanisms remain unclear, ghrelin may function directly by stimulating appetite centrally and indirectly by attenuating inflammation or altering lipid and muscle metabolism to limit cachexia.

Protein-energy malnutrition must be differentiated from the effects of endogenous conditions, resulting in malassimilation or protein-losing enteropathy, from cachexia induced by chronic inflammatory and neoplastic disease, and from other conditions resulting in recumbency.

In neonates, several factors predispose to death by starvation within the first few weeks of life. These include fetal malnutrition with poor fat depots at birth; increased energy demands caused by cold and exposure; and postpartum hyponutrition. Piglets are born with negligible fat reserves and die quickly of hypoglycemia if not fed adequately. Neonatal ruminants usually have fat depots sufficient to compensate for longer periods of inanition (2-4 days for lambs; 6-10 days for calves), if the quality and quantity of milk is sufficient, and cold stress is not severe.

In animals that die of inanition, muscle mass is reduced because of mobilization of amino acids for gluconeogenesis. Fat in the bone marrow, coronary groove, on the pericardial sac, and around the kidneys is completely depleted, and has the gelatinous clear pink appearance of **serous atrophy**. The liver may appear small, with sharp margins, presumably because of reduced trophic stimuli. A diagnosis of starvation is supported by a history of conditions compatible with reduced quantity or quality of feed, and by ruling out other conditions causing protein loss.

Malassimilation

Digestion and assimilation of nutrients have an *intraluminal phase* mediated by biliary and pancreatic secretions, and an *epithelial phase* carried out by enzyme systems on the surface and in the cytoplasm of absorptive enterocytes. The final step is delivery of the nutrient by the enterocyte to the interstitial fluid, and its uptake into the blood or lymph.

Exocrine pancreatic insufficiency *is the major cause of intraluminal maldigestion*, and is usually the result of juvenile pancreatic atrophy in dogs, or of pancreatic fibrosis and atrophy following repeated episodes of pancreatic necrosis (see Vol. 2, Pancreas). It is occasionally seen in cats. This condition may be complicated by bacterial overgrowth of the small intestine. Bile salt deficiency is rarely seen as a cause of intraluminal maldigestion in domestic animals.

The **epithelial phase of assimilation** *is impaired by loss of functional epithelial surface area*. This occurs with *villus atrophy*, or less commonly in short-bowel syndrome following intestinal resection in which >75-85% of the small bowel has been removed. This phase of assimilation is dependent on enzyme systems, which vary in domestic animals. Neonates and ruminants have low levels of maltase; ruminants lack sucrase. In most species, lactase levels decline with age, and malabsorption in dogs has been attributed to low levels of lactase. The poorly differentiated surface epithelium present on atrophic villi may lack the full complement of enzymes on the brush border and in the cytoplasm necessary for nutrient digestion and assimilation. Lectins present in uncooked beans attach to and damage microvilli on enterocytes, which may explain the malabsorption and diarrhea associated with their use in feeds; lectins also promote bacterial adhesion and overgrowth in the small intestine. A heritable syndrome of *gluten-sensitive enteropathy* is reported in Irish Setter dogs, and is characterized by villus atrophy, increased intraepithelial lymphocytes, and abnormal levels of mucosal microvillar hydrolases. *Cobalamin malabsorption* has been described as a hereditary defect in Beagles, Australian Shepherd Dogs, Chinese Shar-Peis, Giant Schnauzers, and Border Collies, resulting in anemia and failure to thrive. Delivery of nutrients, especially lipid, to the circulation, may be impaired in lymphangiectasia. The pathogenesis of malabsorption of the major classes of nutrients will be considered briefly.

Assimilation of fat is susceptible to interference at all 3 phases of digestion and absorption. Lipolysis is impaired if insufficient lipase is available. Mostly this is a result of pancreatic atrophy or fibrosis; however, it also may be due to failure by atrophic intestinal mucosa to release the cholecystokinin necessary to stimulate pancreatic secretions. Reduced surface area for lipid uptake also may contribute to malabsorption of fat. The availability of bile salts is reduced in intrahepatic cholestasis, biliary obstruction, or by depletion resulting from reduced ileal absorption following resection or atrophy. Thus fatty acid and monoglyceride are not emulsified and are therefore not as accessible to absorptive enterocytes. Poorly differentiated enterocytes may be less able than normal epithelium to re-esterify long-chain fatty acids to triglyceride and to produce chylomicrons for export from the cell. Obstructed lymphatic drainage in lymphangiectasia, granulomatous enteritis, and intestinal lymphosarcoma contributes to reduced flow of chylomicrons to the systemic circulation.

Malabsorption of lipids may cause *steatorrhea* (excess fat in the feces), and this is seen in monogastric animals, especially dogs. Severe fat malabsorption may result in deficiencies of fat-soluble vitamins. Malabsorption of calcium, magnesium, and zinc occurs when these minerals are sequestered in soaps formed by combination with malabsorbed luminal fatty acids. Increased absorption of oxalate predisposing to nephrolithiasis may be a sequel to reduced concentrations of calcium in the lumen because of soap formation. Malabsorbed lipid may cause *colonic diarrhea*, by mechanisms that will be discussed subsequently.

Maldigestion of polysaccharides occurs if levels of pancreatic amylase are reduced; this is most commonly encountered in dogs with severe loss of functional exocrine pancreatic tissue. Ruminants normally lack significant amounts of pancreatic amylase and digest starch poorly in the small intestine. Mucosal oligosaccharidase deficiency occurs in villus atrophy, because poorly differentiated enterocytes have a reduced complement of oligosaccharidases. This results in impaired membrane digestion of disaccharide and malabsorption of carbohydrate. The osmotic effect of malabsorbed disaccharide in the small intestine is an important component of neonatal diarrhea caused by rotavirus and coronavirus, or other conditions in which there is extensive villus atrophy in the small intestine.

Protein maldigestion occurs if pancreatic protease activity is decreased to ~10% of normal, as may occur with exocrine pancreatic insufficiency. Loss of gastric proteolytic activity is of little nutritional significance. In conditions with villus atrophy, reduced mucosal surface area and poor differentiation of enterocytes result in malabsorption of small peptides and particularly of amino acids by mechanisms similar to those involved in carbohydrate malabsorption.

Further reading

Argiles JM, et al. Cytokines in the pathogenesis of cancer cachexia. Curr Opin Clin Nutr Metab Care 2003;6:401-406.

Garden OA, et al. Inheritance of gluten-sensitive enteropathy in Irish Setters. Am J Vet Res 2000;61:462-468.

Guillory B, et al. The role of ghrelin in anorexia-cachexia syndromes. Vitam Horm 2013;92:61-106.

Krawinkel MB. Interaction of nutrition and infections globally: an overview. Ann Nutr Metab 2012;61(Suppl.):39-45.

Marcos A, et al. Changes in the immune system are conditioned by nutrition. Eur J Clin Nutr 2003;57(Suppl. 1):S66-S69.

Oetzel GR, Berger LL. Protein-energy malnutrition in domestic ruminants. Part I. Predisposing factors and pathophysiology. Part II. Diagnosis, treatment and prevention. Compend Contin Educ Pract Vet 1985;7:S672-S680. 1986;8:S16-S22.

Diarrhea

Diarrhea is the presence of water in feces in relative excess in proportion to fecal dry matter. Diarrhea usually reflects increased absolute fecal loss of water, but may not, if absolute fecal dry-matter excretion is markedly reduced. Loss of solute and water in diarrhea may lead to *severe electrolyte depletion, acid-base imbalance, and dehydration*, which are life-threatening if not corrected.

Large volumes of fluid derived from ingesta, and from gastric, pancreatic, biliary, and enteric secretions, enter the small bowel; in addition, considerable passive movement of water occurs into the upper small bowel from the circulation in response to osmotic effects. Overall, the bulk of the fluid entering the small intestine is absorbed by the enterocytes, so that the volume leaving the ileum and entering the colon is but a small fraction of the total fluid flux through the small bowel. The large size of this flux implies that relatively small perturbations in unidirectional movement of electrolyte and water in the small intestine may have significant effects on the net movement of fluid.

The colon, in addition to its fermentative function, has the ultimate responsibility to minimize fecal water loss by conserving electrolyte and water by absorption from the digesta. It has a finite capacity for absorption, and if this is exceeded by the rate at which content enters from the small bowel, diarrhea occurs. This is important in so-called *small-bowel diarrhea*, where the lesion is in the small intestine. Because the colon has reserve absorptive capacity, the excess volume entering from the ileum must be considerable for diarrhea to occur. The large capacity and fermentative function of the equine colon may mitigate to some extent the expression of small-bowel diarrhea in mature horses. *Large-bowel diarrhea*, on the other hand, reflects an intrinsically reduced capacity of the colon to handle even normal volumes of fluid and electrolyte presented to it by the small intestine.

Small-bowel diarrhea is classified as secretory, malabsorptive, or effusive; however, these mechanisms are not mutually exclusive and are often seen as overlapping syndromes. Small-bowel diarrhea is characterized by *infrequent passage of large amounts of fluid feces.*

Secretory diarrhea is due to an excess of secretion over absorption of fluid, resulting from derangement of normal secretory and absorptive mechanisms. It is best exemplified by the effects of *diarrheagenic bacterial enterotoxins. Vibrio cholerae* and *Escherichia coli* are the most important sources of such toxins, though only the latter occurs in domestic animals; some *Salmonella* serotypes, *Yersinia enterocolitica*, and *Shigella* also produce enterotoxin. Cholera and heat-labile *E. coli* enterotoxin act through the mediation of cyclic adenosine monophosphate (cAMP). Toxin-stimulated cAMP shuts down sodium chloride cotransport at the luminal cell membrane of enterocytes, reducing passive water absorption. Meanwhile, cAMP-stimulated chloride secretion is promoted, and water follows. The resultant increase in secretion and decrease in absorption increase the solute and water load passing from the small bowel to the colon. Heat-stable *E. coli* and *Y. enterocolitica* enterotoxins stimulate cyclic guanosine monophosphate-mediated secretion by the mucosa.

In addition to bacterial enterotoxins, other factors may cause or contribute to secretory diarrhea. Prostaglandins, other eicosanoids, histamine, kinins, and various other cytokines directly or indirectly stimulate secretion, often by local stimulation of enteric nervous reflexes, and they may contribute to diarrhea in inflammatory bowel disease. Vasoactive intestinal polypeptide secreted by pancreatic islet cell tumors causes severe diarrhea in humans with such tumors; this neurotransmitter causes active chloride and bicarbonate secretion, and is probably the final mediator in secretion stimulated by the enteric nervous system. Other circulating agents are directly or indirectly diarrheagenic: calcitonin secreted by thyroid C-cell tumors; serotonin, bradykinin or substance P secreted by carcinoids; histamine secreted by mast cell tumors; gastrin secreted by gastrinomas. Peptide YY is secreted by enteroendocrine cells of the gut and is known to inhibit intestinal secretion and promote absorption; altered peptide YY secretion has been observed in a variety of gastrointestinal diseases in humans and some domestic animal species.

Malabsorptive diarrhea *commonly results from villus atrophy no matter what the cause*, and is exemplified by osmotic retention of water in the gut lumen by poorly absorbed magnesium sulfate, used therapeutically as a laxative. Electrolyte and nutrient solute are malabsorbed as the result of reduced villus and microvillus surface area, and along with osmotically associated water are retained in the lumen of the bowel and then passed into the colon. A secretory component probably contributes to diarrhea caused by villus atrophy, at least in transmissible gastroenteritis in pigs. In this scenario the villus limb of the postulated crypt-villus fluid circuit is diminished or missing, so fluid secreted by the crypts may not be absorbed and poorly differentiated cells emerging on to the intestinal surface from crypts may also retain some secretory capacity. Malabsorptive diarrhea also occurs in *short-bowel syndrome* caused by reduced absorptive surface.

Increased permeability of the mucosa may contribute to diarrhea by permitting increased retrograde movement of solute and fluid from the *lateral intercellular space* to the lumen, or by facilitating transudation of tissue fluid. **Filtration secretion** is characterized by increased protein-rich fluid movement via the *paracellular route* across the mucosa into the intestinal lumen, which is driven by alterations in the interstitial and vascular pressure gradients. Elevated hydrostatic pressure, or decreased plasma oncotic pressure in the villus, alters Starling forces, permitting leakage of interstitial fluid and large protein molecules. Portal hypertension, right-sided heart failure, hypoalbuminemia, and expansion of plasma volume establish such conditions. Effusion also may be associated with lymphangiectasia, inflammation or edema of the lamina propria, increased vascular permeability, and enteric plasma protein loss. Increased rate of epithelial loss and transient microerosions may provide further potential sites for effusion of interstitial fluid. Extensive necrosis of the epithelium and vascular damage in the mucosa cause more severe malabsorption and effusion of tissue fluid and blood, evident grossly as fibrin and hemorrhage in the lumen.

Large-bowel diarrhea *is due to a reduction in the innate capability of the colon to absorb the solute and fluid presented by the more proximal bowel.* A reduction in net absorption by the colon that is relatively small in absolute terms may be sufficient to cause diarrhea. Large-bowel diarrhea is characterized by *frequent passage of small amounts of fluid feces*, perhaps with mucus and blood. The colonic mucosa is not as leaky as the small intestinal mucosa because of the nature of the tight junctions between epithelial cells. As a result it is relatively resistant to alterations in permeability owing to increased hydrostatic pressure in the propria, in comparison with the small intestine.

When normal enterohepatic circulation of bile acids is interrupted by ileal damage or resection, *excess dihydroxy bile acids* enter the colon where they stimulate colonic epithelial cells to secrete fluid and electrolytes through calcium and cAMP-dependent mechanisms, resulting in diarrhea. *Fatty acids* enter the colon in increased quantities in steatorrhea resulting from bile salt depletion, where they cause diarrhea by altering mucosal permeability and stimulating fluid secretion from colonic epithelium. This is also the mode of action some laxatives such as castor oil, which contains the hydroxy fatty acid ricinoleic acid.

Although colonic secretion stimulated by bacterial enterotoxin is not clearly implicated in diarrhea, alterations in the flora of the large bowel may be detrimental to normal function. Short-chain fatty acids, especially butyric acid produced by bacterial fermentation in the lumen, regulate colonic epithelial cell growth and differentiation and are linked to electrolyte and fluid absorption in the colon. Reduced production or absorption of short chain fatty acids secondary to *imbalance of the bacterial flora* in the cecum and colon may explain some instances of wasting and diarrhea in horses in which no morphologic abnormality of the mucosa can be found.

Osmotic overload of the large bowel results from the delivery by the small bowel of a large volume of fermentable substrate. This is usually caused by malabsorption in the small intestine, but may result from excessive intake. Carbohydrate is the only nutrient of significance in initiating *colonic osmotic overload*, as bacterial fermentation of carbohydrate results in the generation of excess short-chain fatty acid. This is rapidly absorbed and buffered in the colon under normal circumstances; however, a heavy carbohydrate load may overwhelm the colonic buffering capacity, and cause reduced pH. The result is an *altered gut flora* in which there is overgrowth of organisms producing lactic acid, further contributing to acidification and increased mucosal permeability. Loss of water and solute into the lumen along the osmotic gradient generated by lactic acid in the lumen leads to diarrhea.

Increased intestinal motility probably does not have a primary role in the pathogenesis of diarrhea in domestic animals. Often the small intestine of animals with diarrhea is flaccid and fluid-filled, rather than hypermotile. Increased colonic motor activity is often segmental and antiperistaltic, and probably unrelated to increased transit. Hypermotility, if it does occur, may be in response to, rather than a cause of, increased volumes of fluid in the gut.

Further reading

Argenzio RA. Neuro-immune pathobiology of infectious enteric disease. Adv Exp Med Biol 1997;412:21-29.

El-Salhy M, et al. The role of peptide YY in gastrointestinal diseases and disorders (review). Int J Mol Med 2013;31:275-282.

Kvietys PR. The gastrointestinal circulation. Colloquium Series on Integrated Systems Physiology: from molecule to function, vol. 2. Morgan and Claypool Life Sciences; 2010. p. 1.

Rao MC, et al. Intestinal water and electrolyte transport in health and disease. Colloquium Series on Integrated Systems Physiology: from molecule to function to disease. Morgan and Claypool Life Sciences; 2012.

Stephen J. The pathogenesis of infectious diarrhea. Can J Gastroenterol 2001;15:669-683.

Protein metabolism in enteric disease

Disorders of protein metabolism attributable to enteric disease are responsible for significant economic loss in the form of reduced weight gain, wool growth, and milk production. Severe derangement resulting in negative nitrogen balance in any species may lead to cachexia, hypoproteinemia, and death.

Decreased protein intake is the most obvious threat to the nitrogen economy, and it is probably the most important in many chronic gastrointestinal diseases. Subclinical inefficiency in production, reduced growth, and emaciation may be the product of various degrees of inappetence, or difficulty in prehension, mastication, and swallowing, or recurrent regurgitation. Low feed quality compounds the effect of reduced feed intake.

Anorexia is *a sharp decline in appetite*, and a common sign of indigestion, obstruction, or systemic disease. In ruminants, loss of appetite to various degrees is an especially important component of the pathogenicity of gastrointestinal parasites, including those infecting the abomasum (*Ostertagia*), small intestine (*Trichostrongylus*), and large bowel (*Oesophagostomum*). Interactions among cholecystokinin, parasympathetic efferent and afferent reflexes, and systemic or gastric leptins appear to mediate satiety; however, their mechanisms in health and disease remain unclear.

Malabsorption of peptides and amino acids may occur locally in the small intestine as a result of significant *villus atrophy*. However, unless the lesion is widespread or low in the small bowel, net absorption of nitrogen over the length of the small intestine will not be reduced because of the compensatory capacity of more distal normal mucosa. Overall, the contribution of malabsorption to disordered nitrogen metabolism appears to be minor in most situations.

Protein-losing gastroenteropathy, increased catabolism and loss of endogenous nitrogen via the gastrointestinal tract, is important in many diseases. Excess endogenous protein entering the intestine is derived mainly from *effusion of plasma protein into the lumen of the bowel* but can also be associated with *increased turnover of cells lining the gut*. Protein-losing enteropathies can be divided into 3 categories according to the mucosal alteration causing protein loss: mucosal ulcerations or erosions leading to secondary protein exudation; nonulcerated mucosa with abnormal permeability; and lymphatic disruption with leakage of protein-rich lymph (see later section on lymphangiectasia).

Plasma protein loss may result from the blood-sucking activity of nematodes such as *Haemonchus*, *Ancylostoma*, and *Bunostomum*, or hemorrhage from sites of trauma in the mucosa caused by the feeding activity of worms such as *Oesophagostomum*, *Chabertia*, and *Strongylus*. Considerable loss of erythrocytes and plasma protein leading to fibrinohemorrhagic enteritis can occur secondary to mucosal erosions or ulcerations caused by ischemia, epithelial cell necrosis, or inflammation associated with bacteria, viruses, and coccidia. Plasma protein can also be lost through transient gaps, or leaks in the mucosa that develop during increased exfoliation of enterocytes into the lumen. With an increased rate of enterocyte turnover seen in villus atrophy, temporary microerosions may develop when flattened enterocytes fail to maintain the integrity of the surface epithelium.

The permeability of tight junctions between epithelial cells may be sufficiently altered to permit transit of plasma protein molecules. **Filtration secretion** occurs when the hydrostatic pressure in the proprial interstitium is elevated in congestive heart failure and portal hypertension; by decreased plasma oncotic pressure; by increased vascular permeability in acute or chronic inflammation; and in lymphatic obstruction or lymphangiectasia. Proinflammatory cytokines such as tumor necrosis factor-α are often prevalent during acute or chronic inflammation and may cause increased paracellular epithelial permeability to large molecules entering the mucosa.

Plasma protein loss into the gut is generally considered nonselective, as albumin, immunoglobulins, clotting factors, and a variety of transport or carrier proteins, including transferrin, ceruloplasmin, and transcortin, are lost equally. The physiologic consequences of protein-losing enteropathy may be observed with increased loss of any of these molecules, but are most frequently related to albumin turnover. Loss of plasma protein into the gut expressed as a proportion of the total body pool will vary in absolute terms; this concept of **fractional catabolic rate** is essential to understanding the kinetics of plasma protein turnover.

In protein-losing enteropathy, albumin turnover may pass through 3 phases. During the first phase, the *fractional catabolic rate increases* along with the absolute amount of protein lost into the bowel. As the size of the circulating pool of albumin shrinks, so does the absolute rate of loss of protein, even though the fractional rate remains the same. During the second phase, the size of the circulating pool stabilizes as the rate of albumin synthesis by the liver increases to match in absolute terms the rate of loss into the gut lumen. The plasma albumin pool is then in a state of *hyperkinetic equilibrium* in which the total pool is smaller, but a higher than normal fractional catabolic rate is compensated by an increased rate of hepatic albumin synthesis. Provided that the amount of albumin lost does not exceed the synthetic capacity of the liver, this equilibrium may persist for a considerable period. In the third phase, *hypoalbuminemia develops* as the fractional catabolic rate exceeds in absolute terms the synthetic capacity of the liver. Alternatively, hypoalbuminemia occurs in the third phase if the rate of synthesis declines because of deficiency in amino acids derived from the diet or by catabolism of other body protein. The hypoalbuminemia in enteric plasma loss may be accompanied by *hyperglobulinemia*, the mechanism of which is not completely clear, but has been associated with underlying or concurrent inflammatory disease stimulating hepatic globulin production in these patients.

The progression and clinical manifestations of protein-losing enteropathy vary with the rate of onset of plasma loss and the fractional catabolic rate. A sudden onset of severe plasma protein loss may cause death during the first phase, before there is time for compensatory synthesis. If the fractional catabolic rate is gradually and only slightly increased, so that compensation occurs with the albumin pool in equilibrium at only a marginally reduced state (perhaps near or within the normal range), subclinical protein loss occurs. Although the fractional catabolic rate is only slightly elevated, the relatively large size of the albumin pool may mean that the absolute loss of protein exceeds that in a hypoalbuminemic animal with a higher fractional catabolic rate, but a smaller albumin pool.

Endogenous protein derived from exfoliated cells of the stomach or upper small intestine during villus atrophy may be digested and absorbed in the lower small intestine. This is dependent on luminal proteolysis by pancreatic enzymes, digestion and absorption that may compensate for any malabsorption caused by the more proximal lesions. The efficiency of protein digestion and absorption is not 100%, so a proportion of this increased endogenous protein is added to the protein escaping digestion in the small bowel, and enters the large intestine. Here, most of this protein may be converted to ammonia by the colonic flora and absorbed. The loss of significant protein from stomach or small intestine may be accompanied by little or no increase in fecal nitrogen excretion, although much of the protein lost from lesions in the colon is ultimately lost in the feces. Ammonia nitrogen absorbed from the colon is converted in the liver mainly to urea, so animals with increased endogenous protein loss into the stomach or small intestine tend to have slightly raised levels of plasma urea, and an elevated rate of urinary urea excretion.

Elevated hepatic synthesis of albumin, resulting from increased turnover of the plasma albumin pool, and increased enteric protein synthesis in support of elevated epithelial turnover in conditions with chronic villus atrophy, is at the expense of anabolic processes elsewhere. Dietary amino acid is diverted preferentially to synthesis of plasma and enteric protein. If protein intake is poor due to inappetence or a low-quality ration, or if the rate of protein loss is high, the animal moves into **negative nitrogen balance.** Catabolism of peripheral protein then assumes an increasingly important role in maintaining the pool of amino acids available for plasma and intestinal protein synthesis. This explains in part the reduced growth rate, decreased muscle mass, and reduced bone matrix in sheep with subclinical or mild parasitism, and the cachexia and osteopenia associated with severe parasitism. These principles probably hold for all syndromes causing enteric loss of endogenous protein in any species.

Loss of enteric protein, and especially plasma, should be suspected in cachectic or hypoproteinemic animals, although diarrhea is not invariably present. *The 2 major routes of occult plasma protein loss are glomerular disease, particularly amyloidosis, and gastrointestinal disease;* exudative skin lesions are a less common source. Anemia and hypoproteinemia may be due to hemorrhage externally or into the gastrointestinal tract. Advanced liver disease may cause hypoalbuminemia, in which case concurrent signs of hepatic failure will likely be observed (see Vol. 2, Liver and biliary system). Inability or reluctance to eat, inadequate nutrition, or starvation also cause emaciation, usually without profound hypoalbuminemia. The cachexia of malignancy also must be differentiated.

When adequately hydrated, the hypoalbuminemic animal shows evidence of subcutaneous, mesenteric, or gastric submucosal edema, perhaps with hydrothorax or ascites. Wasting of muscle mass may be marked if the protein loss has been severe and chronic. Unlike starvation, protein-losing gastroenteropathy may be associated with the presence of internal fat depots because assimilation of energy is not necessarily severely impaired, especially in ruminants.

Anemia

The development of anemia and the kinetics of the erythron following blood loss into the gastrointestinal tract are similar to those of albumin in plasma loss. *Blood loss of any origin, including that caused by hematophagous parasites, may cause anemia.* Erythroid hyperplasia in the marrow or in extramedullary sites may not compensate for the continued erythrocyte loss. Resolution of the hemorrhage results in eventual restoration of normal red cell numbers and an ultimate decline in erythrocyte production. Chronic blood loss may culminate in depletion of iron stores and development of a nonresponsive hypochromic microcytic anemia.

Further reading

Coop RL, Holmes PH. Nutrition and parasite interaction. Int J Parasitol 1996;26:951-962.

Dossin O, Lavoue R. Protein-losing enteropathies in dogs. Vet Clin North Am Small Anim Pract 2011;41:399-418.

Granger DN, et al. The microcirculation and intestinal transport. In: Johnson LR, editor. Physiology of the Gastrointestinal Tract. 2nd ed. New York: Raven Press; 1987. p. 1671-1697.

Guilmeau S, et al. Gastric leptin: a new manager of gastrointestinal function. Curr Opin Pharmacol 2004;4:561-566.

Congenital anomalies of the intestine

Segmental anomalies of the intestine are commonly encountered. In early embryonal life the intestine consists of a simple tube, the lumen of which is lined by epithelial cells of endodermal origin surrounded and supported by an outer layer of connective tissue from the splanchnic ectoderm. As the intestines grow with the developing fetus, they form coiled loops that herniate temporarily through the umbilicus into a peritoneal-lined sac before they are later retracted back into the fetal abdomen. The most plausible cause of segmental defects in intestinal continuity is *ischemia of a segment of gut during early fetal life*, resulting in necrosis of the affected area.

The segmental anomalies of the intestine may vary in degree. **Stenosis** *implies incomplete occlusion or narrowing of the lumen; complete occlusion is referred to as* **atresia.** Atresia is further subdivided into *membrane atresia*, when the obstruction is formed by a simple membrane; *cord atresia*, in which the blind ends of the gut are joined by a cord of connective tissue; and *blind-end atresia*, in which a segment of gut and possibly the corresponding mesentery are missing, leaving two blind ends. All types of segmental anomaly can be produced experimentally by ischemia to a portion of the fetal intestine.

Atresia coli *is the most common segmental anomaly of the intestine in domestic animals.* It is seen particularly in the spiral colon of Holstein calves, and in the large and small colon of foals; it occurs rarely in cats. Atresia coli may be an autosomal recessive trait in Holsteins. A predisposition for male calves has been described, but this is not consistent among studies. An association has been postulated between pressure on the amniotic vesicle during palpation of the embryo for pregnancy diagnosis before 42 days of gestation, and the development of atresia coli in calves; however, the mechanism of this effect is uncertain. **Atresia intestinalis** is less common. **Atresia ilei** is most prevalent in calves, and rare in foals, lambs, piglets, and pups. These lesions prevent normal movement of gut content and meconium and therefore lead to dilation of the proximal segment and progressive abdominal distention, which may become so extensive in an affected fetus to cause dystocia. The bowel distal to the obstruction is small in diameter, and devoid of content other than mucus and exfoliated cells. Animals fail to pass feces after birth.

Atresia ani (*imperforate anus*) *is the overall most common congenital defect of the lower gastrointestinal tract.* It may be seen in all species, but is most often encountered in calves and pigs, in which it is considered to be hereditary. The defect may consist only of failure of perforation of the membrane separating the endodermal hindgut from the ectodermal anal membrane, or both anus and rectum may be atretic. Atresia ani may be an isolated abnormality, but is more commonly associated with other malformations, especially of the distal spinal column (spinal dysraphism, sacral or coccygeal vertebral agenesis), genitourinary tract (rectovaginal fistula, renal agenesis, horseshoe kidney, polycystic kidneys, cryptorchidism, duplication of scrotum or penis), and occasionally with intestinal atresia or agenesis of the colon. Vitamin A deficiency during pregnancy has been associated with increased risk of congenital ano-rectal malformations in several species; this is thought to be related to improper development of the enteric nervous system.

Short colon has been reported in dogs and cats, and is probably the result of abnormal rotation of the midgut and failure to lengthen during fetal life. Clinical signs were subtle and possibly unrelated to the colonic lesion. Affected animals had a shortened colon with the cecum located on the left side of the abdomen. Concurrent anorectal or urogenital abnormalities were observed in some cases. **Anomaly of the colonic mesenteric attachments** has been described and associated with development of colic in a horse, because of distortion and convolution of the large colon.

Congenital colonic aganglionosis, somewhat analogous to Hirschsprung's disease in humans, occurs in *white foals* that are the offspring of "frame overo" spotted parents. The disease has not been convincingly demonstrated in other species of domestic animals. Clinically affected foals, which are predominantly white, develop colic and die generally within 48 hours of birth. Grossly, there is stenosis mainly of the small colon, but the entire colon and rectum may be patent but contracted; the proximal intestine is distended with gas and meconium. Microscopically, *ganglia of the myenteric plexus are absent in the walls of the terminal ileum, cecum, and colon,* although occasional nerve fibers are evident. Except for the few pigmented spots, melanocytes are absent in the skin.

Although several gene mutations can cause intestinal aganglionosis, loss of function mutation of the *endothelin receptor type B gene* are observed in horses, rodents, and humans with this condition. The pathogenesis is thought to involve improper migration of cells of the neural crest, from which cutaneous melanoblasts and the myenteric plexus neurons are derived. A similar condition of megacolon resulting from segmental colonic aganglionosis has been reported in pigs. Megacolon associated with few myenteric ganglion cells in Clydesdale foals is not clearly congenital, and is discussed with intestinal obstruction, as is megacolon in other species.

Intestinal diverticula occur rarely in dogs, cats, and horses. *True diverticula,* congenital lesions involving all layers of the intestinal wall, are distinguished from *pseudodiverticula* resulting from disruption or weakening of the tunica muscularis and not involving all layers of the intestinal wall. They may be incidental, but in horses have been associated with idiopathic muscular hypertrophy or other lesions of the small bowel, including neoplasia. Diverticula can cause impaction, obstruction, intussusception or fistula, and potentially diverticulitis, rupture, and peritonitis.

Persistent Meckel's diverticulum is an uncommon embryonic developmental anomaly occurring mostly along the antimesenteric border of the lower small bowel, mainly in swine and horses. It is derived from the omphalomesenteric (vitelline) duct, which is the stalk of the yolk sac. The vitelline membrane can also persist forming a fibrous ligament or *mesodiverticular band* between the distal small jejunum and the diverticulum or umbilicus. **Multiple persistent vitelline duct cysts,** distinct from Meckel's diverticulum, have been described on the ileal serosa in a dog.

Hypoplasia of the small intestinal mucosa has been reported in foals with failure of passive transfer, and this may represent defective fetal organogenesis.

Further reading

Ablin LW, et al. Intestinal diverticular malformations in dogs and cats. Compend Contin Educ Pract Vet 1991;13:426-430.

Binanti D, et al. Perineal choristoma and atresia ani in 2 female Holstein Friesian calves. Vet Pathol 2013;50:156-158.

Butler Tjaden NE, Trainor PA. The developmental etiology and pathogenesis of Hirschsprung disease. Transl Res 2013;162:1-15.

Furness JB, Poole DP. Involvement of gut neural and endocrine systems in pathological disorders of the digestive tract. J Anim Sci 2012;90:1203-1212.

Wefel S, et al. Small intestinal strangulation caused by a mesodiverticular band and diverticulum on the mesenteric border of the small intestine in a horse. Can Vet J 2011;52:884-887.

Young RL, et al. Atresia coli in the foal—a review of 6 cases. Equine Vet J 1992;24:60-62.

Intestinal obstruction

Acute obstruction typically involves the upper or middle small intestine whereas chronic blockage usually involves the ileum and large bowel. Intestinal obstruction may be the sequel to a physical blockage of the lumen resulting from **stenosis** (narrowing, stricture) caused by an **intrinsic lesion** involving the intestinal wall, **obturation** (occlusion) by an intraluminal mass, or **extrinsic compression.**

Failure of the intestinal circular smooth muscle to contract blocks the peristaltic wave, causing **functional obstruction,** a clinical syndrome of pseudo-obstruction in which there is no physical occlusion of the lumen of the impacted intestine. **Adynamic ileus**, intestinal obstruction resulting from inhibition of bowel motility, is a common sequel to peritonitis and pain. Circulatory embarrassment of a segment of bowel via embolism or venous infarction also causes functional obstruction without a physical blockage. Many intestinal displacements that produce obstruction such as volvulus, strangulation, or intussusception may cause *ischemia*. The term **strangulation obstruction** refers to an event that simultaneously causes ischemia and physically blocks the intestine. Mucosal hypoxia may be a sequel to venous occlusion caused by physical distention of gut proximal to an obstruction; to local pressure caused by an adjacent mass; or to generalized circulatory failure. The pathogenesis and consequences of intestinal ischemia are dealt with later in this chapter.

Proximal to an obstruction there is *accumulation of fluid* derived from ingesta, gastric, biliary, pancreatic, and intrinsic intestinal secretion, and *gas* swallowed or originating from bacterial activity in the gut (Fig. 1-42). Intestinal distention results in luminal sequestration of water and electrolytes and mucosal edema; further fluid secretion into the lumen may be associated with contractile stimuli, and potentially transudation from the peritoneal surface. Upper small-bowel obstruction progresses rapidly to *vomiting* in most species, with dehydration, hypochloremia, hypokalemia, and metabolic alkalosis caused by loss of acid in vomitus and of fluid sequestration in the stomach. If acute complications of ischemia including rupture do not occur, an animal with obstruction succumbs to the *systemic effects of hypovolemia, electrolyte, and acid-base disturbance.*

With obstruction of the lower small intestine or colon, there is usually less pronounced electrolyte and acid-base imbalance because vomition is less severe and absorption of fluid proximal to the obstruction may prevent or delay severe distension and additional fluid secretion. Metabolic acidosis eventually follows however, with dehydration and catabolism of fat and muscle once food consumption and assimilation ceases. In the horse, obstruction or impaction of the cecum or colon in particular often leads to *local ischemia and rupture.*

In obstruction, the outstanding gross alteration in the bowel is distention proximal to the point of blockage, caused by ileus and accumulation of fluid contents and gas. The volume of distention and length of bowel involved is dependent on the location, degree, and duration of obstruction; this may be remarkable with distal lesions such as rectal stricture in pigs, which can cause profound abdominal distention. As distention increases, interference with venous return may develop and the mucosa and submucosa become congested. Devitalization of severely dilated gut or pressure necrosis of the mucosa at the site of lodgment of intraluminal foreign bodies may occur, leading to necrosis, perforation, and peritonitis. Distal to the point of obstruction, the bowel is collapsed and empty.

Stenosis and obturation

Congenital intrinsic obstruction caused by segmental atresia and imperforations is considered under the previous section on congenital anomalies of the intestine. The primary lesions involving the intestinal wall causing **acquired stenosis** include intramural abscesses or hematomas, neoplasms, and fibrosis secondary to ulceration. These lesions can result in partial or complete stenosis and may develop slowly with a course as described for simple chronic obstruction.

Foreign bodies of all kinds are commonly found. Small rounded foreign bodies and even some sharp-edged objects may pass through the intestines uneventfully, but for these and many large foreign bodies the course is unpredictable. Some may reside in the intestine for long periods and produce no disturbance until they act as a nidus for the development of an enterolith. Foreign bodies may cause partial or complete intestinal obstruction and compromise the blood supply by luminal distention, which may progress to edema, necrosis, and possibly perforation. Most obstructions occur in the jejunum, although any segment of bowel can be affected. **Linear foreign bodies** such as strips of cloth or string probably occur more commonly in cats compared with dogs, and once ingested may pass through the intestine. However, if they become immobilized they produce a characteristic lesion. One portion becomes fixed, most commonly around the base of the tongue or by impaction at the pylorus. The free end is then stretched taut distally because of peristalsis, which results in pleating of the distal gut onto the string (Fig. 1-43A). Peristalsis results in progressive mucosal damage (Fig. 1-43B) along the lesser curvature of intestinal loops that may lead eventually to perforation and peritonitis.

Enteroliths (mineral concretions) were historically common in the colon of horses, and are observed more frequently in some areas, such as California and Florida. Aged Arabians, Morgans, American Saddlebreds, and donkeys seem to be overrepresented. The concretions are comprised of *magnesium ammonium phosphate*, the source of which is probably grain, bran, alfalfa, or alkaline water. Colonic pH >6.6 seems to contribute to enterolith formation. The mechanism is not completely clear; however, mineral salts are deposited in concentric lamellae around a central *nidus*—a foreign body such as a nail, wire, stone, or particle of feed. They can vary greatly in size, some weighing as much as 10 kg. Enteroliths are usually smooth and spherical but can be flattened; irregular mineralized masses may also occur, usually centered on a fibrous nidus, such as twine, rope, or netting.

Fiber balls (**phytobezoars** or phytotrichobezoars), which consist largely of plant fibers intermixed with phosphate salts, may be found especially in the colon of horses. They are not as heavy as enteroliths, and are usually round, smooth, and

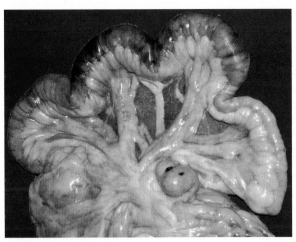

Figure 1-42 Small intestinal obstruction of a dog caused by a foreign body. Dilation is present proximal to the obstruction, with contraction of the empty intestine distally. (Courtesy J. Caswell.)

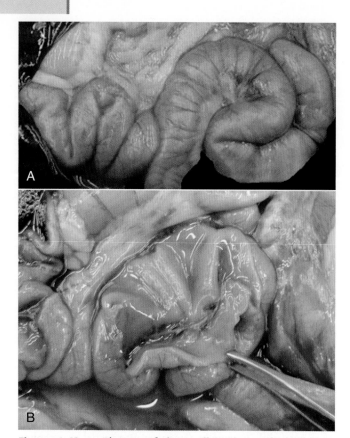

Figure 1-43 A. Pleating of the small intestine of a cat along (B) a **linear foreign body.** (Courtesy A.J. Fales-Williams.)

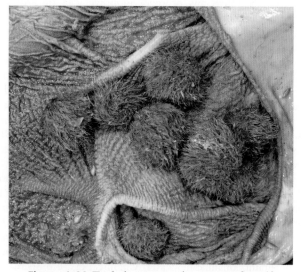

Figure 1-44 Trichobezoars in the rumen of a calf.

moist with a velvety and occasionally convoluted surface. Response to medical therapy and dissolution of phytobezoars has been reported in horses. Hairballs (**trichobezoars**) sometimes occur in dogs, cats, and ruminants; in ruminants they occur mostly in the forestomachs (Fig. 1-44) and abomasum but can also cause *small intestinal obstruction*. Enteroliths and bezoars in horses are often insignificant; apparently they are moved about by peristalsis and are passed in the feces. They may obstruct the gut if they become impacted, usually where

the colon lumen narrows or changes direction, for example, at the pelvic flexure, and the transverse or small colon.

Small intestinal obstruction may be caused by parasites that can form rope-like tangled masses in the lumen. This occurs in pigs and foals infested with large numbers of *ascarid nematodes*. It also occurs rarely in sheep heavily infested with *cestodes*. Impaction of the ileum is the most common cause of small intestinal nonstrangulating obstruction in horses. Feeding of a high-fiber diet, such as coastal Bermuda grass hay, predisposes to this condition. Gravel and sand have been reported as causes of small intestinal obstruction in cattle and dogs, respectively.

Impaction of the colon is a common cause of simple intestinal obstruction. The impaction cause is often feces in dogs and cats. In horses the cause is digesta, fibrous foreign material, sand, or feces and can be complicated by intestinal tympany from fermentation if the obstruction is complete. *Obstipation of the colon* in dogs may result from voluntarily suppressed defecation caused by pain from inflammation or neoplasia involving the prostate gland or anal sacs. Impaction with foreign bodies, such as hair or fine bones in the colon or rectum, or the result of stenosis caused by tumors or strictures, is less common. Colonic obstipation also may be associated with trauma to the pelvic area or spinal cord; it is described in Manx cats because of sacral spinal cord anomalies. **Megacolon** ensues if the obstruction persists; however, in small animals megacolon is frequently idiopathic. Examination of the syndrome in cats reveals no histologic abnormalities and it is suggested that the underlying problem is a disturbance in the activation of smooth-muscle myofilaments.

Impaction of the cecum or colon in horses occur mostly where the lumen narrows at the pelvic flexure and transverse or small colon. Impaction may be precipitated by water deprivation, a dietary change to rough hay or chaff, or poor dentition; recurrent impaction is seen in animals with dental problems. Abnormal motility resulting from altered colonic or cecal peristalsis may explain impaction in the absence of other predisposing causes and is discussed later with pseudo-obstructions of the gut. Ingestion of indigestible *synthetic fibers* has been associated with colonic impaction. In horses grazing poorly covered sandy soils, *sand* may cause chronic colitis and diarrhea or it may sediment, accumulate, and cause impaction at any level of the large or small colon. *Sand impaction* in horses is often associated with concurrent displacement or torsion. Ingestion of large numbers of *acorns and leaves* may also cause impaction of the intestinal tract in ruminants. Rupture of the bowel may occur if impactions are not treated, and the bowel wall becomes ischemic and devitalized.

Cecal rupture in horses occurs as a complication of impaction, or of parturition in mares. Two distinct forms of cecal rupture are described. In type 1, the cecum is filled with firm dehydrated food, whereas in type 2, the cecum is distended with more normal digesta, often with increased amount of fluid. Type 2 is considered a rare complication of general anesthesia or administration of NSAIDs, and is thought to be due to dysfunctional motility.

Extrinsic obstruction

Compression of intestine causing obstruction is rather common and is caused by tumors, abscesses, peritonitis, and fibrous adhesions. **Neoplasms** involve the intestine by extension from adjacent viscera, particularly the pancreas. Many abdominal tumors involve the craniodorsal part of the abdominal cavity and thus cause compression of the duodenum. Peritoneal **adhesions** are common, and fibrous bands may stretch from the wall of the bowel to some fixed point, or between two or more points along the bowel or mesentery. In these cases, obstruction develops gradually as fibrous tissue contracts and restricts or adheres the bowel to itself or other abdominal structures. Large firm masses of **abdominal fat necrosis** cause extrinsic obstruction of small intestine, spiral colon, or descending colon and rectum of cattle. **Pedicles of some tumors,** especially *mesenteric lipomas in older horses,* occasionally entrap loops of intestine causing obstruction and strangulation. Similarly, the **ovarian suspensory ligaments** may entrap the equine colon if the ovary is enlarged because of neoplasia or inflammation. Incarceration in hernias, discussed with other displacements of the bowel, is also a common cause of extrinsic obstruction of the gut.

Functional obstruction

Adynamic (paralytic) ileus is itself not of specific interest to the pathologist but is a rather common condition. It frequently follows abdominal surgery, especially when the intestines are handled roughly or traumatized. It also is associated with peritoneal irritation of any cause, especially peritonitis. It is the result of neurogenic reflexes that interfere with control of the inhibitory neurons of the myenteric plexus. Continual tonic discharge by these neurons inhibits contraction of circular smooth muscle and prevents peristalsis. Grossly, the intestines are distended with a mixture of gas and fluid, and the wall is flaccid. The defect may be segmental, involving short lengths of the intestinal tract, but many such segments may be involved, especially in diffuse peritonitis. Idiopathic gastric or intestinal ileus may be more common in horses during the postparturient period, and acute colic and gastric rupture may occur in this species as a complication.

Pseudo-obstruction, a clinical syndrome described mostly in dogs, in which there is *no physical occlusion of the lumen* of an impacted intestine, may result from segmental or diffuse neuromuscular dysfunction in the gut. In humans, pseudo-obstruction is classified as failure of nervous or muscular components of the intestine. In dogs, fibrosis and cellular infiltration of the tunica muscularis are the most commonly described lesions leading to pseudo-obstruction. In addition to equine congenital aganglionosis discussed previously, pseudo-obstruction associated with neuronal loss or ganglioneuritis involving autonomic ganglia in the gastrointestinal tract, systemic dysautonomia, and intrinsic disease of intestinal smooth muscle are recognized among domestic animals. A segment of contracted or thickened bowel may be noted as a cause of obstruction; in neurogenic disease, the affected bowel is often dilated, flaccid and unable to maintain tone.

Megacolon in Clydesdale foals associated with *hypoganglionosis of the myenteric plexus* has been reported in 4-9 month foals from the United States and Australia. The timing of clinical onset of these cases suggests an acquired condition; however, the common breed suggests a genetic basis for the syndrome. The pathogenesis of the condition remains unknown. Some variation in neuron density of the dorsal colonic myenteric plexus has been reported.

Grass sickness in horses, the prototypic **dysautonomia** in domestic animals, occurs chiefly in parts of the United Kingdom, western Europe, and southern South America where it is known as *mal seco.* The disease more commonly affects young horses with pasture access during the spring season and the gastrointestinal tract is most affected. Grass sickness can occur acutely as colic, tympany, and drooling with rapid progression and is nearly always fatal, usually within 7 days. The condition can also occur as chronic colic of >7 days duration, usually characterized by weight loss or dysphagia. Horses with this form may survive with appropriate management. In acute cases, postmortem findings include gastric and small intestinal distention; often there is esophageal ulceration caused by reflux. In chronic cases gross lesions are often not present except for marked emaciation. There also may be impaction of the colon and cecum by dehydrated ingesta in cases of longer duration. Characteristic histologic lesions are present in the intestinal and extraintestinal autonomic ganglia and include chromatolysis, nuclear eccentricity, and karyorrhexis of nerve cell bodies of both peripheral and central neurons. Neuronophagia and the presence of smooth round eosinophilic bodies or spheroids within or adjacent to perikarya are also recognized. Significant inflammation is not evident. Lesions in several brainstem nuclei have been described, albeit inconsistently. The severity of lesions has been shown to correlate with decreased functional cholinergic responses. Diagnosis can be confirmed in live horses by histological evaluation of nerve cell bodies of the myenteric or submucosal plexus in surgically obtained ileal samples. Examination of the cranial celiaco-mesenteric ganglia, sympathetic thoracic chain, stellate and/or superior cervical ganglia provide confirmation of the diagnosis in dead horses. *Clostridium botulinum* has been suggested to play a role in equine dysautonomia, although this remains unconfirmed and it is not known if the presence of *C botulinum* type C and/or type C neurotoxin represents secondary bacterial overgrowth or the cause of this syndrome.

Feline dysautonomia, or Key-Gaskell syndrome, is an autonomic dysfunction of unknown etiology, most common in the United Kingdom and continental Europe, with sporadic cases reported elsewhere. A similar syndrome has also been reported in a few dogs and a llama. Cats <3 years of age seem to be preferentially affected. Signs include depression, anorexia, reduced lacrimation and salivation, bradycardia, mydriasis, delayed pupillary light reflex, megaesophagus, constipation, or ileal impaction. Diarrhea is reported in some dogs with dysautonomia. The gastrointestinal signs suggest *disordered motility,* and animals often succumb to the effects of regurgitation, inanition, or aspiration pneumonia, among other problems. Cases tend to occur in clusters, suggesting an environmental toxin or infectious agent. As for horses, exposure to *Clostridium botulinum* and type C neurotoxin has been hypothesized, although no conclusive etiologic associations have been made.

Involvement of functions of both sympathetic and parasympathetic divisions of the autonomic nervous system, and of some functions under voluntary control, is reflected in the distribution of neuronal lesions in autonomic ganglia. Cranial nerve nuclei III, V, VII, and XII, ventral horns of the spinal gray matter, and dorsal root ganglia may be involved. Chromatolysis-like lesions of affected neurons seen by light microscopy have a *distinctive ultrastructural appearance* in dysautonomia: autophagocytic vacuoles, dilated cisternae, and complex stacks of smooth endoplasmic membranes are in the cytoplasm of affected cells. Neuronal lesions including neuronal loss may be transient and difficult to confirm histologically.

Intrinsic disease of intestinal smooth muscle may produce a syndrome of **intestinal sclerosis,** resembling progressive systemic sclerosis or *scleroderma* of humans. In dogs the lesions are restricted to the intestinal tract, where there is diffuse dilation of the small and large bowel. Histologically, mononuclear inflammatory cells infiltrate the smooth muscle of the bowel wall; also there is atrophy of myofibers and fibrosis. Fibrosis of the small intestinal submucosa has also been reported in horses, and in some cases there is arteriolosclerosis. The cause is unknown, although geographical clustering of cases is described.

Further reading

Bebchuk TN. Feline gastrointestinal foreign bodies. Vet Clin North Am Small Anim Pract 2002;32:861-880.

Blikslager A. Cecal impaction in horses. Comp Contin Educ Vet 2011;33:E1-E4.

Harkin KR, et al. Dysautonomia in dogs: 65 cases (1993–2000). J Am Vet Med Assoc 2002;220:633-639.

Hassel DM, et al. Dietary risk factors and colonic pH and mineral concentrations in horses with enterolithiasis. J Vet Intern Med 2004;18:346-349.

Hayes G. Gastrointestinal foreign bodies in dogs and cats: a retrospective study of 208 cases. J Small Anim Pract 2009;50:576-583.

Kidder AC, et al. Feline dysautonomia in the Midwestern United States: a retrospective study of nine cases. J Fel Med Surg 2008;10:130-136.

Newton JR, et al. Equine grass sickness: Are we any nearer to answers on cause and prevention after a century of research? Equine Vet J 2010;42:477-481.

Perkins JD, et al. Functional and histopathological evidence of cardiac parasympathetic dysautonomia in equine grass sickness. Vet Rec 2000;146:246-250.

Tabar JJ, Cruz AM. Cecal rupture in foals: 7 cases (1996-2006). Can Vet J 2009;50:65-70.

Wylie CE, Proudman CJ. Equine grass sickness: epidemiology, diagnosis and global distribution. Vet Clin North Am Equine Pract 2009;25:381-399.

Displacements of the intestines

Eventration

Eventration is displacement of a portion of the gut, usually the small intestine, outside the abdominal cavity, and it has been described in most domestic animal species. This is commonly congenital or predisposed by a congenital anomaly, as in schistosomus reflexus, patent umbilicus, and congenital diaphragmatic hernia. Acquired eventrations result from trauma, and therefore are varied. The displaced intestine herniates into the abdominal muscle or subcutis, or it may be completely exteriorized. Vaginal eventration may occasionally occur in females following trauma. Diaphragmatic eventration may occur as a consequence of diaphragmatic rupture or malformation.

Cecal and colonic dilation, tympany, and torsion

In ruminants, cecal dilation and torsion is an uncommon condition. It mainly occurs in animals fed *high-concentrate rations*, but it has been associated with late gestation and ileus from other causes. It usually occurs within 2 months postpartum in cattle. It is rare in other ruminants. About 30% of the carbohydrates in the ration are digested in the cecum of ruminants. Sudden change from a roughage to a grain-based ration results in an increase in the concentration of volatile fatty acids, with only a slight decrease in pH of the cecal contents.

An increase in the concentration of dissociated volatile fatty acids, especially butyric acid, causes atony of the cecum, and dilation follows. Cecal dilation occurs more often in cattle that are not receiving mineral supplements and in one study hypocalcemia was found in 85% of cases of cecal dilation. Although it has been suggested that calcium deficiency may cause cecal dilation, this has not been proved and it is not clear whether hypocalcemia is the cause or a result of cecal dilation. Once the cecum is dilated and distended with watery digesta, various degrees of clockwise or counterclockwise rotation can occur, which may incorporate adjacent terminal ileum or proximal colon.

In horses, cecal and colonic tympany has a similar pathogenesis. Readily fermentable carbohydrate, following a sudden change in feed, results in an increase in volatile fatty acid production, which exceeds the buffering and absorptive capacity of the organ. As the pH drops, and fermentation shifts to production of the less well-absorbed butyric and lactic acids, water is drawn into the lumen by the osmotic effect. The large bowel dilates with fluid digesta and gas, and motility is reduced by the effects of the volatile fatty acids. Severe abdominal distention, compression of intra-abdominal organs, reduced cardiac return caused by postcaval compression, and reduced respiratory capacity resulting from compression of the diaphragm may follow, with attendant severe pain. Death caused by hypovolemia and acidosis may occur before the large bowel ruptures. In recovered horses, laminitis may occur because of absorption of endotoxin through the cecal mucosa, which becomes eroded and permeable as a result of local acidosis.

Displacements of the equine colon

The large colon of the horse is comprised of a loop of capacious bowel joined along its length by the short mesocolon, and folded upon itself at the sternal, pelvic, and diaphragmatic flexures. The loop is only fixed at its base, by the cecum, the transverse colon, and mesenteric root. Its volume and lack of attachment make the large colon prone to displacement or torsion.

Right dorsal displacement of the colon involves displacement of the left segments of the large colon to the right of the cecum. This occurs when the large colon pelvic flexure moves under or around the cecum (clockwise in the standing animal viewed from above), ending up located between the cecum and the right abdominal wall. Consequently, when the carcass is opened from the right side of the body, the left colons are visible first. It presumably results from displacement and wedging of the large colon because of tympany. This displacement is usually preceded by impaction of the pelvic flexure, which then is bent to the left and migrates cranially in the abdomen coming to rest close to the sternum. This is termed *right dorsal displacement with flexion*. Alternatively, the left colon may move in the opposite direction, caudal and to the right of the base of the cecum, with the pelvic flexure again lying at the sternum. This is termed *right dorsal displacement with medial flexion*. Some degree of torsion may also occur, and obstruction, with mild to severe colic, ensues. Surgery is required to correct the displacement.

Left dorsal displacement of the colon, variously known as entrapment of the colon by the nephrosplenic, renosplenic, or phrenicosplenic ligament, or by the suspensory ligament of the spleen, is also encountered as a cause of obstruction and colic in horses (Fig. 1-45). The left dorsal and ventral large

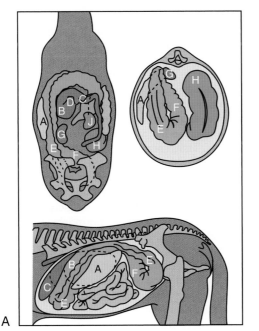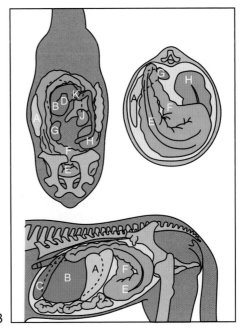

Figure 1-45 A. Left dorsal displacement (nephrosplenic entrapment) of the equine colon. Entrapment with the sternal and diaphragmatic flexures of the colon below the stomach. **B. Entrapment** with the sternal and diaphragmatic flexures displaced dorsal to the stomach. A, spleen; B, stomach; C, liver; D, esophagus; E, left ventral colon; F, left dorsal colon; G, left kidney; H, base of cecum; J, right kidney; K, duodenum. (Reprinted with permission from Livesey MA, et al. Can Vet J 1988;29:135-141.)

colon move laterally and dorsally between the spleen and the left body wall, and become entrapped, with the spleen to the left and below, the suspensory ligament of the spleen below, the left kidney on the medial aspect, and the abdominal wall dorsolaterally. As the colon becomes entrapped it rotates along its axis with the result that the ventral colon lies dorsally and the dorsal colon lies ventrally. The colon caudal to the entrapment may become curved cranially, with the pelvic flexure rotated through 180° because of tension on the taeniae. If the weight of the displaced colon is supported by the nephrosplenic ligament, the spleen may move away from the left body wall. The weight of the colon may also compress the splenic vein causing splenic congestion. Compression of the colon at the point of entrapment can cause impairment of the flow of ingesta, local bruising or edema and partial ischemia of the displaced organ, and results in partial or complete impaction. If the gut remains patent, clinical signs are intermittent. The cecum and small intestine may be distended as a result of the colonic obstruction. The cause of left dorsal displacement is unknown, but may be related to an anatomic predisposition resulting from a large cleft between the spleen and the left kidney.

Colonic volvulus *is one of the most common and grave colic causes in horses.* The loop of large colon, with or without the cecum, may rotate around itself at some point along its length, or around the root of the mesentery. The condition is life-threatening because of severe vascular embarrassment, and is discussed further under the section Intestinal ischemia and infarction.

Internal hernia

This is a displacement of intestine through normal or pathological foramina within the abdominal cavity without the formation of a hernial sac. It is *uncommon.*

Herniation through a natural foramen occurs mainly in horses. In **incarceration in the epiploic foramen**, a portion of small intestine, usually distal jejunum and ileum, may pass down into the omental bursa and become incarcerated, if the normally short and slit-like epiploic foramen of Winslow is dilated for any reason. In these circumstances, the wall of the omental bursa often ruptures.

Omental hernia occurs when a loop of intestine passes through a tear in the greater or lesser omentum. **Mesenteric hernia** is the result of passage of intestine through a tear in the mesentery. These are probably traumatic defects and usually involve the mesentery of the small intestine, but occasionally, that of the colon.

Pelvic hernia occurs in young ruminants, and rarely in other species, following castration. During the operation, excessive traction on the spermatic cord may tear the peritoneal fold of the ductus deferens, which fixes the duct to the pelvic wall. A hiatus is formed between the ductus deferens and the lateral abdominal or pelvic walls through which loops of intestine may become incarcerated.

Gut may also become incarcerated by passing through lacerations in the lateral ligament of the bladder, or through entrapment by the remnant of a persistent urachus, by the gastrosplenic ligament, and by mesodiverticular or vitelloumbilical bands in the horse.

External hernia

External hernia typically consists of a *hernial sac* formed as a pouch of parietal peritoneum; a *covering* of skin and soft tissues; depending on the location of the hernia, a *hernial ring;* and the *hernial contents.* The hernial ring is an opening in the abdominal wall, and this may be acquired, or it may be natural as, for example, the vaginal ring at the inguinal canal. The hernia usually contains a portion of omentum, a freely mobile portion of the intestine and occasionally, other viscera.

Ventral hernia of the abdominal wall occurs uncommonly in horses, rarely in cattle, and exceptionally in other species, except perhaps following blunt trauma or biting injuries in small animals. These hernias through the abdominal musculature into the subcutaneous tissue, may be spontaneous in heavily pregnant females, especially older animals, or be a consequence of blunt trauma, bite wounds, horn injuries, surgical scars, or inflammations, which cause weakening or perforation of the muscle. In pregnant mares, they often occur in the lower flank lateral to the mammae, where there is only a single layer of muscle, the transverse abdominal. They may become very large in herbivores because of the weight of the alimentary viscera and pregnant uterus. The lesion must be differentiated from rupture of the prepubic tendon, and from postmortem rupture of abdominal muscle in bloated animals.

Umbilical hernia is *common* and is often present as a congenital and perhaps inherited defect. It is most frequent in pigs, foals, calves, and pups and depends on persistent patency of the umbilical ring. It is the *most common congenital defect in cattle* and has a hereditary component in the Holstein and probably other breeds. In calves it is also significantly predisposed by umbilical infection. The hernial sac is formed by peritoneum and skin; the contents depend on the size of the ring and of the sac. Incarceration of enclosed intestine is uncommon. Formation of an *enterocutaneous fistula*, a rare complication of umbilical hernia, is seen most frequently in the horse.

Inguinal hernia may evolve to **scrotal hernia** when the herniated viscera pass down the inguinal canal. The internal, or deep, inguinal ring remains patent in intact male animals, but its diameter and the tendency to herniation in the neonate may be inherited. Inguinal hernias are classified as direct or indirect.

In **direct inguinal hernia**, which is less common, abdominal contents pass through the internal inguinal ring and come to rest in a subcutaneous position, through a tear in either the peritoneum or the fascia around the deep inguinal ring. This is most commonly seen in foals and is thought to result from increased intra-abdominal pressure during passage through the birth canal. These direct inguinal hernias often cause necrosis of overlying skin, can become fixed by adhesions and strangulate. They are life threatening.

Indirect inguinal hernias, by contrast, *consist of abdominal contents contained within the tunica vaginalis*. These are by far the *most common form*, occurring as a congenital problem in the young of many species, and as an acquired problem in older animals. Although size of the inguinal rings may be a factor in neonates, there is usually no apparent cause in acquired cases. The herniated viscus passes through the inguinal and vaginal rings within the vaginal sheath, coming to lie in the scrotum inside the cavity of the tunica vaginalis. If the hernia is scrotal, there may be degeneration of the testicles. Routine castration of such animals can lead to eventration through the scrotal incision, and closed castration may cause infarction of the herniated loop of gut.

Congenital inguinal hernia is rare in dogs; West Highland Whites, Pekingese, and Basenjis may be predisposed, and it is more common in males than females. However, overall, inguinal hernia is much more common in female dogs. The bitch differs from females of other species in having a patent inguinal ring and canal, through which the omentum and the uterus may pass. The herniated uterus may become incarcerated when pregnant, or if pyometra develops. In horses, indirect inguinal hernias may rupture through the inguinal canal, coming to rest in a subcutaneous location. These ruptured indirect hernias have a similar prognosis as the direct inguinal hernias described previously.

Femoral hernias develop as an outpouching of peritoneum through the femoral triangle along the course of the femoral artery. They contain omentum and small intestine.

Perineal hernias *occur principally in old male dogs in association with prostatic enlargement and obstipation.* They are precipitated by abdominal straining and are probably predisposed to by weakening of perineal fascia and muscles from some unknown cause, possibly hormonal. They are very unusual in females. Retroperitoneal pelvic fat bulges through a defect between the coccygeus medialis muscle and the cranial border of the anal sphincter. Usually this is the only tissue to prolapse, and the lesion consists, essentially, of a loss of support on one side of the anal ring. Concomitant with the loss of pelvic support the rectum deviates, and the prostate and the bladder may move into the pelvis. Further displacement may occur occasionally and then the latter organs are forced through the ruptured perineal fascia, causing acute urethral obstruction. Perineal hernias are most commonly unilateral, but bilateral hernias may occur.

Diaphragmatic hernias are *common*. The defect in the diaphragm may be congenital, but most often it is acquired, generally as the result of increased abdominal pressure. Although abdominal viscera pass into the thoracic cavity, strangulation of displaced gut is rare. Acquired diaphragmatic hernias are considered more fully in the section Traumatic lesions of the abdomen and peritoneum.

Prepubic hernias occur in small animals, usually associated with severe trauma to the caudal abdomen that produces rupture of the prepubic tendon.

The **sequelae of hernias** depend largely on their location and content, but some generalities apply to all. As long as the hernial contents remain freely movable and reducible, there may be no untoward sequelae. Fixation of the hernial contents (*incarceration*) is a serious development. Incarceration may result from stenosis or tension of the hernial ring, adhesion between the contents and the sac, or distention of the herniated viscus. This distention may be due mainly to mural congestion and edema in any incarcerated viscus, accumulated gas or ingesta in the intestine, urine in a herniated bladder, and fetuses or pus in a herniated uterus. Incarcerated intestine may become obstructed, or undergo ischemic necrosis and perforate, causing peritonitis. Small intestine fixed by incarceration may be predisposed to volvulus.

Further reading

Archer DC, et al. Entrapment of the small intestine in the epiploic foramen in horses: a retrospective analysis of 71 cases recorded between 1991 and 2001. Vet Rec 2004;155:793-797.

Beittenmiller MR, et al. Clinical anatomy and surgical repair of prepubic hernia in dogs and cats. J Am Anim Hosp Assoc 2009;45:284-290.

Braun U, et al. Clinical findings and treatment in cattle with caecal dilatation. BMC Vet Res 2012;8:75.

Jackson C, et al. Congenital diaphragmatic eventration in a stillborn foal. J Vet Diagn Invest 2006;18:412-415.

Sutradhar BC, et al. Comparison between open and closed methods of herniorrhaphy in calves affected with umbilical hernia. J Vet Sci 2009;10:343-347.

The Glass Horse Equine Colic CD. A comprehensive exploration in 3D. ©2001-2014 Science In 3D, Inc. Athens, Georgia. <www.sciencein3d.com>.

Intestinal ischemia and infarction

Inadequate or interrupted circulation of blood to the gut is a common problem, particularly in the horse. Obstruction of the efferent veins, blockage of afferent arteries, and reduced flow through an open circulation cause hypoxic damage to the intestine. Whatever the initiating cause, the effect of hypoxia at the level of the mucosa is similar.

In the **small intestine,** within 5-10 minutes of the onset of ischemia, changes are observed at the tips of villi in tissue sections examined under the light microscope, and lesions are well advanced by 30 minutes. Separation of the epithelium from the basement membrane, beginning at the tip of the villus and progressing toward the base, causes the formation of the so-called Gruenhagen's space. Epithelial cells appear relatively normal, and may separate from the villus in sheets. The core of the villus contracts toward the base. Within 1-3 hours, the villus is almost completely denuded of epithelium, and the mesenchymal core is disintegrating or collapsed and stumpy, with hemorrhage from capillaries. Superficial epithelium may persist for several hours in the crypts of Lieberkühn.

That this lesion is largely a function of hypoxia is indicated by the mitigating effects of intraluminal perfusion of oxygenated saline demonstrated experimentally in dogs and cats. The putative countercurrent exchange of oxygen between the afferent arteriole and efferent venules in the villus, and an associated progressive decline in oxygen tension distally in the villus, may render the tip prone to early damage in hypoxia. Villus smooth-muscle contraction, exacerbating the epithelial exfoliation on the distal villus, may be mediated by sympathetic stimulation in ischemia.

Dissociation and necrosis of cells in the crypts of Lieberkühn begin ~2-4 hours after the initiation of ischemia, and within 4-5 hours the epithelium appears completely necrotic or has sloughed, leaving a mesenchymal ghost of the mucosa. The muscularis mucosae may undergo necrosis, but the muscularis externa remains viable for 6-7 hours. During acute ischemia, there is initial hyperexcitability of muscle in affected areas, followed by progressive loss of contractility, which will fail to recover if ischemia persists beyond 4-6 hours. Mesothelial cells on the serosa undergo necrosis within 30-60 minutes of ischemia, and exfoliate; there is a local acute inflammatory response, which may predispose to the development of adhesions. *The speed with which lesions develop in hypoxia emphasizes the significance of rapid fixation of intestinal mucosa if artifact is to be avoided.* Differentiation between post mortem autolysis and necrosis can be particularly challenging in the intestine. A few useful hints to help determining autolysis versus necrosis include hemolysis of red blood cells, large numbers of rods within blood vessels and tissues not associated with inflammation, gas bubbles in the tissues and desquamation of slabs of epithelial cells.

The **colon** of the dog and horse seems less sensitive to short-term ischemia than the small intestine. Mild morphologic damage, characterized by mild edema, and separation and exfoliation of surface epithelium between crypts, is found after 1 hour. However, by 3-4 hours, crypt epithelium is becoming necrotic, dissociating and exfoliating, and from that point events progress as in the small intestine.

Reperfusion injury, superimposed on the effects of ischemia alone, may enhance the severity of the lesion, if hypoxia is only partial or ischemia is transient, and reflow of blood raises the tissue oxygen tension. Reperfusion injury implies that the effects of the hypoxic episode have not progressed to complete necrosis of the mucosa, and that further damage is possible because of oxygen free radicals and/or cytokines. Hence, there is a relatively short duration of hypoxia, and a concomitant mild-to-intermediate degree of mucosal damage, permissive of this phenomenon. In cases of enteric ischemic disease encountered in veterinary medicine, this threshold may frequently have been crossed by the time that the animal is presented for therapy. In addition, there is evidence that in swine and in horses, where intestinal ischemic events are most common, reperfusion injury is less likely to occur than in other species. Because reperfusion injury may cause necrosis and/or apoptosis, it is almost impossible to differentiate morphologically the changes produced by ischemia from those of reperfusion injury.

Reperfusion injury is the result of the interplay among free-radical–mediated damage to the microvasculature and probably stromal elements and epithelium; neutrophil margination and diapedesis into tissue; complement activation; and release of proinflammatory proteins and cytokines, some of which may have systemic effects.

Free radicals in reperfusion injury are largely generated through xanthine oxidase mechanisms in the intestinal mucosa, and through NADPH oxidase mechanisms in leukocytes, mainly neutrophils, already resident in or recruited to the damaged tissue. Hypoxia stimulates the conversion of xanthine dehydrogenase to xanthine oxidase in epithelial cells. In the presence of xanthine oxidase, hypoxanthine accumulating from adenosine triphosphate degradation in hypoxia is converted to xanthine, and molecular oxygen is reduced, generating hydrogen peroxide, superoxide radical and hydroxyl radical intermediates, which inhibit the accumulation of protective nitric oxide. The hydroxyl radical is likely most significant in damaging proteins and initiating a cascade of lipid peroxidation, resulting in metabolic and structural lesions and culminating in cell death.

The acute inflammatory response that accompanies reperfusion results in production of free radicals by the respiratory burst from neutrophils, release of proteolytic enzymes, and physical impairment of the microcirculation. Reduction in tissue nitric oxide permits dismutation of oxygen free radicals to H_2O_2, which promotes activation of phospholipase, accumulation of proinflammatory mediators, and production of cytokines (tumor necrosis factor-α and -β, interleukins) and adhesion molecules by endothelium. Complement activation is mediated by adhesion molecules, promoting inflammatory events and release of cytokines such as tumor necrosis factor-α and interleukin-1, as well as other cytokines that increase during reperfusion.

Sequelae of ischemia vary with duration and severity of insult. Short-term ischemia (maximally, ~3-4 hours), with preservation of at least the base of the crypts of Lieberkühn, will permit repair, as *cells proliferating in the crypts re-epithelialize the mucosal surface within 1-3 days.* Normal architecture is re-established after up to 1-2 weeks, although necrotic muscularis mucosae is not replaced. Effusion of tissue fluid and

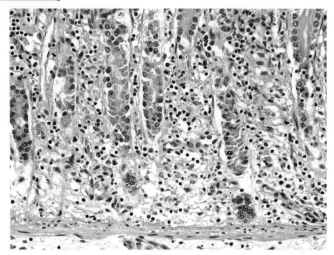

Figure 1-46 Small intestine, sequel to transient ischemia. Hyperplastic basophilic cells populate surviving crypts. A few crypts show degenerate and necrotic epithelium. Inflammatory cells, mostly neutrophils, are infiltrating the lamina propria and crypt lumen.

acute inflammatory cells prevails until epithelium extends to cover the eroded surface fully. Partial damage to the proliferative compartment initially results in dilation of crypts, which are lined by flattened epithelium resembling that seen after radiation injury. If the amplifier population of progenitor cells can be regenerated, hyperplastic basophilic cells will populate crypts until the mucosal architecture is reconstituted (Fig. 1-46).

Ischemic necrosis of the full thickness of the mucosa will be bounded by an acute inflammatory reaction in the submucosa, which, under favorable conditions, evolves into a granulating ulcerated surface. Focal ulcerative lesions may ultimately heal by epithelial migration over the bed of granulation tissue from surviving crypts within the lesion and around the periphery.

Extensive *mucosal ulcers* that form following severe ischemia have little chance of resolution, owing to their large surface area. Chronic ischemic ulcers in the small bowel tend to develop a depressed, fairly clean granulating surface, occasionally with some fibrinous exudate.

Ischemic ulcers in the large bowel, especially of horses, develop a dirty yellow-gray fibrinonecrotic surface. If the animal does not succumb to the effects of malabsorption and protein loss from the defect, or to transmural bacterial invasion, scarring and stricture may occur. The sequelae of ischemia with reflow are mainly seen in strangulated segments of gut that have been reduced without resection, or with inadequate resection, and in some cases of presumed thromboembolic infarction of the equine colon.

Persistent ischemia results in necrosis involving all mural elements. The full thickness of the gut wall ultimately becomes necrotic, green-brown or black, flaccid, and friable.

The *consequences of ischemic lesions* are partly a function of the species, and of the level of bowel affected. Strangulation, volvulus, and similar lesions cause physical obstruction at the site, and ileus proximal to it. Reduced arterial perfusion or thromboembolism causes functional obstruction and ileus. Loss of mucosal integrity results in cessation of electrolyte and water absorption, and ultimately in effusion of tissue fluid and blood into the lumen. Proliferation of anaerobes occurs in the

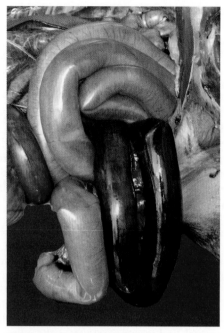

Figure 1-47 Venous infarction of a segment of equine small intestine that has undergone volvulus.

lumen of the stagnant ischemic area, with accumulation of gas, and extreme distention of the closed loop in strangulation obstruction. Toxin production by anaerobes, particularly clostridia, plays a large part in gangrene and ultimate rupture of ischemic gut, as well as having systemic effects. Absorption of endotoxins and exotoxins from the lumen may occur through devitalized mucosa via the portal flow, lymphatic return, or peritoneum. Toxins have a severe detrimental effect on cardiovascular function, contributing to circulatory failure. If death from some other cause does not supervene, transmural invasion by enteric bacteria or perforation of the devitalized wall results in septic peritonitis that is ultimately fatal.

Venous infarction
Obstruction of efferent veins is by far the most common cause of intestinal ischemia. This is a sequel to **incarceration** of herniated loops of bowel; **strangulation** by pedunculated masses, such as lipomas in older horses; **torsion** (twist about the long axis of the viscus); **volvulus** (twist of the intestine on its mesenteric axis); and **intussusception**. In these circumstances, compression of thin-walled veins tends to occur before the influx of arterial blood is obstructed.

In venous infarction, the affected tissue field, often including involved mesentery, becomes intensely edematous, congested, and hemorrhagic, so that the hypoxic bowel wall is thickened and eventually assumes a deep red-black appearance (Fig. 1-47). It has been estimated that 40 liters of fluid may accumulate in the wall of a horse colon that has undergone volvulus. Bloody fluid content and gas distend the lumen of the infarcted segment. As gangrene of the intestinal wall proceeds, the tissue becomes green-black, and septic peritonitis eventually ensues, with or without perforation of the bowel. Advanced venous infarction involves the full thickness of the intestinal wall, and the initiating intestinal accident is commonly evident, except in cases subjected to surgery. Even if a displacement has been reduced, the limits of the infarcted segment are usually relatively sharply demarcated, and the affected bowel remains edematous and hemorrhagic. Microscopically, severe transmural edema, congestion, distention of veins, sometimes venous thrombosis, and hemorrhage are present, initially most severe in the mucosa and submucosa. With time, the full thickness of the mucosa becomes necrotic, and the deeper layers of the muscular wall are also devitalized, with invading enteric flora present throughout. Lesions that have advanced to significant necrosis or effacement of the crypt epithelium are associated with failure of the animal to survive, resulting from either euthanasia on the grounds of the degree of damage, or systemic complications despite correction of the strangulation, or resection.

Displacements of intestine that may progress to incarceration or volvulus with strangulation and infarction have been discussed in the previous section. They are a common cause of colic and mortality in horses.

Mesenteric volvulus (often referred to as "mesenteric torsion") occurs commonly in suckling ruminants and in swine, uncommonly in horses, and rarely in cats and dogs. The abdomen is distended and, upon opening the cavity, tensely dilated deep red-to-black loops of bowel are usually immediately apparent.

In *swine* the mesentery of the small intestine and sometimes the large bowel is involved in a volvulus that is usually counterclockwise, when viewed from the ventrocaudal aspect. In volvulus involving the small and large intestines, the apex of the cecum may be pointing cranial in the cranial left quadrant of the abdomen, reflecting the rotation of ~180°. In swine, mesenteric volvulus may be due to gas production from a highly fermentable substrate in the colon, and its subsequent displacement, with progression to mesenteric volvulus. Mesenteric volvulus is a common cause of sporadic sudden death in swine but may occur as a recurrent problem in a herd. Many cases of *intestinal hemorrhage syndrome* in that species are probably misdiagnosed mesenteric volvulus.

Death caused by mesenteric volvulus is common in suckling or artificially reared *calves and lambs*. In these species, vigorous ingestion of large amounts of feed over a short period may predispose to gas formation in the gut, or perhaps hypermotility, which induces volvulus. Usually only the mucosa of the proximal duodenum and terminal ileum, cecum, and colon is spared from infarction, although occasionally volvulus is restricted to shorter segments of intestine. Similar lesions are occasionally encountered in other species.

In *dogs*, volvulus has been associated with ingestion of large quantities of food, and with exocrine pancreatic insufficiency in German Shepherds. It is occasionally accompanied by gastric volvulus.

Volvulus of various lengths of the small intestine may occur in any species, but is perhaps most prevalent in the horse, where it is a common cause of strangulation obstruction of the bowel.

The large colon of the horse is predisposed to **volvulus** by its lack of mesenteric anchorage, and potential mobility. Although frequently referred to as large colon torsion, this condition is a true volvulus, because the twist involves the mesentery between the ventral and dorsal colon at the level of the ceco-colic mesentery. The volvulus begins with the right ventral colon rotating medially and dorsally (clockwise as seen from behind); the severity of the rotation can vary between 270° and 720°. If the twist exceeds 360°, there is obstruction of the lumen of the colon with subsequent accumulation of gas, ischemia of the majority of dorsal and ventral colon wall

and eventually endotoxemia. Part of the cecum may be incorporated in the volvulus. The equine cecum alone rarely undergoes torsion, and if so, it may be related to hypoplasia of the cecocolic fold. At surgery or autopsy, the usual signs of strangulation obstruction are evident, including dilation and devitalization of the infarcted segment and distension of the cecum if it is not twisted. Postmortem rupture of the diaphragm or abdominal wall may occur because of tympany.

Duodenal sigmoid flexure volvulus is a recently described and unusual lesion of adult dairy cattle. The sigmoid flexure of the duodenum is first displaced in a dorsolateral direction, and then rotates about its omental attachment causing obstruction of the proximal small intestine and the common bile duct. The cause is unknown but this condition has been associated with prior surgical correction of a displaced abomasum.

Intussusception involves the telescoping of one segment of bowel (the intussusceptum) into an outer sheath formed by another, usually distal, segment of gut (the intussuscipiens) (Fig. 1-48). Any level of the gut with sufficient mesenteric mobility may be involved. The naming convention is that the intussusceptum is followed by the intussuscipiens; hence an ileocolic intussusception is a normograde intussusception in which the ileum has invaginated into the colon.

The *cause* is usually not apparent, although linear foreign bodies, heavy parasitism, previous intestinal surgery, enteritis, and intramural lesions such as abscesses and tumors may be associated. It also may be a *terminal, agonal,* or *postmortem event*. The history is that of partial or complete intestinal obstruction, perhaps with bloody feces, and it is most common in young animals.

Intussusception is common in *dogs*, in which most frequently it is ileocolic. It is much less common in cats. Intussusception is also moderately common in lambs, calves, and young horses, where it may involve small intestine, cecum, and colon.

The progressive invagination of the leading edge of the intussusceptum into the distal segment results in the *wall of the intussusception being comprised of 3 layers*: (1) the inner entering, (2) middle returning, segment of invaginated bowel, and (3) the outer wall of the receiving segment of gut. It is

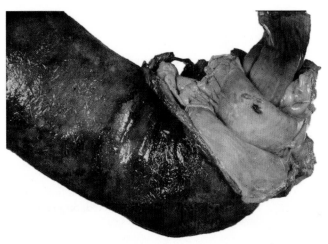

Figure 1-48 Intussusception of the intestine in a dog. Outer intestinal layer has been cut away to expose the edematous and congested infarcted mucosa of the strangulated portion of the intussusception.

limited in length by the increasing tension on the mesentery drawn into the lesion, to ~10-12 cm in small animals, and ~20-30 cm in large animals. This tension along one edge of the gut may cause the mass to become bowed or spiraled.

Tension and compression of mesenteric veins cause the intussusceptum, or a portion of it, to undergo *venous infarction*. It swells with edema and congestion, and the adjacent apposed serosal surfaces become adherent as fibrin and inflammatory cells effuse from the affected bowel. Adhesion quickly renders the intussusception irreducible. Necrosis and gangrene of the invaginated intestine usually develop, but sometimes the intussusceptum sloughs, and the remaining viable segments maintain continuity of the gut, or rarely, form two adjacent blind ends. Intestine cranial to the obstructing intussusception may be dilated, and that distal contracted and devoid of content. If obstruction is chronic or partial, there may be hypertrophy of the smooth muscle of proximal bowel. In horses, chronic ileocecal intussusception involves a relatively short (<10 cm) length of bowel. Incidental terminal, agonal, or postmortem intussusception is recognized by the relative absence of congestion, edema, and adhesion of the involuted segment of gut.

Cecal inversion, and cecocolic intussusception in the horse, with inversion of the cecum into itself, or into the right ventral colon (Fig. 1-49), may result in ischemia of the cecum and possibly part of the involved colon; if partial, ischemia usually involves the more distal cecum. Cecocolic intussusception in horses has been associated with typhlocolitis caused by *Salmonella* spp., cyathostomiasis, or *Anoplocephala perfoliata*.

Segmental ischemic necrosis of the small colon may occur in pregnant or postpartum mares, because of mesenteric tension from intussusception and rectal prolapse of the distal large bowel, or perhaps because of laceration of the mesocolon and associated vessels by the feet of the foal during parturition. Colic, and intestinal obstruction, necrosis, rupture, and peritonitis may follow.

Arterial thromboembolism

Ischemia of the gut caused by arterial thrombosis and embolism is rare in domestic animals other than the horse. Mucosal and occasionally transmural focal or segmental infarctive lesions are seen in *Pasteurella* septicemia in lambs and in *Histophilus somni* bacteremia in cattle. Most cases of embolic disease are associated with bacterial infections that cause softening and lysis of thrombi and facilitate formation of emboli. This is particularly true for the lesions associated with strongyle migrations in horses, in which lesions remain localized unless thrombi induced by the parasite become secondarily infected.

In **horses** it is associated with **endoarteritis,** mainly at the root of the cranial mesenteric circulation, caused by migrating larvae of *Strongylus vulgaris* (see Vol. 3, Cardiovascular system). Effective worm control programs have rendered this problem increasingly rare.

Candidates for a diagnosis of nonstrangulating infarction are animals in which the anatomic distribution of an ischemic lesion is incompatible with volvulus or other strangulation, or physical evidence for incarceration or strangulation obstruction is not present in the surgical history or at autopsy, and there is evidence of verminous arteritis. Careful consideration should be given to the fact that verminous arteritis can be present in horses without embolic intestinal lesions. Therefore the presence of the former does not definitely prove that intestinal infarction was produced by verminous arteritis. Typically, ischemic lesions of this type are limited to the "watersheds" at the periphery of the colic and cecal arterial circulatory fields—the pelvic flexure and the distal cecum—because collateral circulation within these circulatory fields is extensive.

Lesions limited essentially to the mucosa usually appear to be subacute, the result of ischemia of relatively short duration, and are ulcerative or fibrinonecrotic, usually with a hyperemic margin. They may be tens to many hundreds of square centimeters in area.

Transmural lesions represent ischemia of longer duration. Devitalized gray-brown intestine of normal thickness is interpreted to represent arterial obstruction without significant reflow, except along the boundary with viable tissue. Large edematous, congested, or hemorrhagic, full-thickness lesions, physically or anatomically inconsistent with strangulation, are interpreted as severe arterial obstruction, with subsequent reflow either by relief of the obstruction or by way of collaterals. Ischemic damage to vessels of the mucosa, submucosa, and perhaps deeper structures results in hemorrhage and edema when blood flow returns (Fig. 1-50A). Ulcerative or fibrinonecrotic mucosal lesions are probably the result of transient ischemia with subsequent reflow (Fig. 1-50B). Similar lesions may occur after relief of strangulation of short duration, and in NSAID drug toxicosis, salmonellosis, and infections by *C. difficile* or *C. perfringens* type C, all of which involve, in part, mucosal microthrombosis.

Reduced perfusion

Ischemia caused by reduced perfusion of the intestinal vascular bed is a *difficult and uncommon diagnosis*. Circumstances in which it may be expected to occur include severe hypovolemic states, such as *hemorrhagic shock* in the dog, cat, and possibly other species; in animals, particularly dogs, with *disseminated intravascular coagulation* (DIC); in dogs with hepatic disease and *portal hypertension;* in *hypotensive shock* caused by heart failure; and in animals with reduced mesenteric arterial perfusion, mainly horses with severe *verminous endoarteritis.*

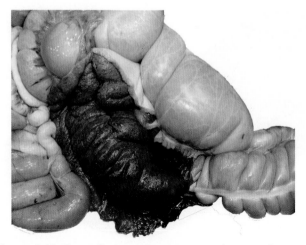

Figure 1-49 Cecocolic intussusception in a horse with severe cyathostomiasis. The cecum has been completely invaginated into the right dorsal colon (open). The cecal mucosa is completely necrotic. (Courtesy M. Anderson.)

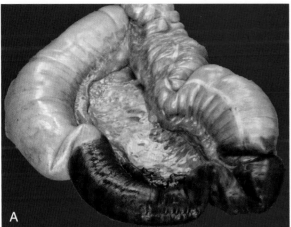

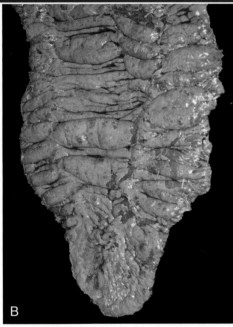

Figure 1-50 **A. Infarction of pelvic flexure** of the large colon of a horse. Hemorrhage and edema of the serosa suggest that arterial thrombosis and infarction have been followed by reperfusion, with extravasation of blood from damaged vessels in the affected tissue. (Courtesy S.S. Diab.) **B.** Mucosa of equine **cecum** that has undergone **ischemic necrosis** resulting from reduced arterial perfusion. Subsequent reflow has occurred and the infarcted mucosa is covered with fibrinonecrotic exudate. Irregular ulcers and exudation are present throughout the mucosa.

In "shock gut" in dogs, and rarely other species, associated terminally with heart failure, hemorrhage, hypovolemia, and DIC, part or all of the mucosa of the small intestine is deeply congested, and the content is hemorrhagic. The pathogenesis of the lesion is related to reflex vasoconstriction in the mucosa and submucosa, shunting of blood away from the mucosa, dilation of mucosal capillaries, and reduction in rate of flow of blood through the villus. Countercurrent transfer of oxygen from the afferent to efferent vessels in the villus aggravates hypoxemia in the villus by increased shunting of oxygen to the efferent venule. Splanchnic pooling of blood, systemic arterial hypotension, and intestinal vasoconstriction occur in endotoxic shock in dogs, causing similar mucosal lesions. Microthrombosis associated with sluggish flow, DIC, and

endotoxemia may contribute to mucosal ischemia by obstructing capillaries in the villi, and mucosal and submucosal venules. Microthrombi in these vessels in association with hemorrhagic mucosal necrosis suggest the possibility of ischemia caused by "slow flow."

Transient or incomplete reduction in perfusion caused by obstruction of the arterial blood supply has a similar effect on the mucosa. The obstruction may be due to *arteriospasm*, perhaps induced by vasoactive mediators such as thromboxane. Mucosa devitalized by hypoxia will become hemorrhagic with continued blood flow. Because the primary problem may not involve a systemic state as complicated as severe shock, the animal may survive long enough to develop an effusive ulcerated or pseudomembranous mucosa, with some prospect of stabilization or repair, if the lesion is not widespread. "Slow flow" caused by reduced arterial perfusion with inadequate collateral flow may be expected to affect the "watershed" of a circulatory field preferentially. In the horse this may be the explanation for mucosal lesions at the pelvic flexure and apex of the cecum in which thromboembolism cannot be implicated, but in which mural thrombi in the cranial mesenteric root could have caused significantly reduced perfusion or flushed vasoconstrictive thromboxane into circulation.

Transient or noninfarctive "slow flow" has been proposed as a cause of intermittent colic resulting from verminous arteritis. It may also play a role in the development of functional obstruction and volvulus in horses with cranial mesenteric arterial lesions.

Ischemia at the periphery of the circulatory field of the caudal mesenteric artery may possibly predispose to rectal perforation in horses. The precarious perfusion of the mucosa at this site may contribute to ischemic ulceration and the development of *rectal stricture in swine*. In many cases this condition appears to be associated with *Salmonella* infection, and it is discussed further with porcine salmonellosis.

Acute acorn poisoning in the horse may cause severe gastrointestinal edema and focal hemorrhage, with infarction and ulceration in the cecum and colon. Microscopic lesions in the small and large intestine are consistent with an ischemic pathogenesis, and microthrombi have been associated with mucosal infarcts in the large bowel as well as in other organs.

Nonsteroidal anti-inflammatory drugs (NSAIDs) cause ulceration of the upper small intestine and colon, as well as oral and gastric ulceration, which seem to be related to ischemia, in horses and dogs. In horses, phenylbutazone, even at therapeutic dosages, can result in ischemic damage to the intestinal mucosa. It may be that intercurrent stress or dehydration contributes to the pathogenesis. The right dorsal colon is affected preferentially, resulting in the term *right dorsal colitis*; lesions in other parts of the colon also occur occasionally. The NSAID-associated lesions are characterized by ischemia, often with marked edema and avascular necrosis. Lesions may be focal, linear, or extensive and segmental, involving the entire circumference of the bowel (Fig. 1-51). Depending on the duration and severity of the lesion, the mucosa may be congested and edematous, with superficial necrosis and fibrin exudation, or extensively eroded and ulcerated, with fibrinonecrotic exudate. Early in the process, superficial epithelial necrosis and progressive mucosal necrosis and inflammation are evident.

Microvascular injury, with subsequent microthrombosis and ischemic ulceration, is considered by some to be the cause of the lesions in the stomach and intestine. This

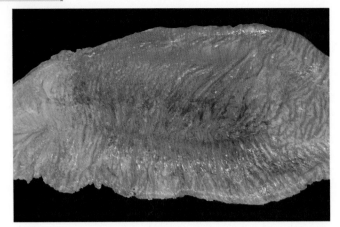

Figure 1-51 Ulcerative colitis in a horse treated heavily with nonsteroidal anti-inflammatory drugs.

may be the result of direct phenylbutazone toxicity to the microvasculature.

Vasoconstriction or depression of other cytoprotective effects, mediated by phenylbutazone inhibition of prostaglandin synthesis, could be the cause of the lesions. Animals may develop diarrhea and hypoproteinemia as a result of the extensive mucosal defects. Minor mucosal lesions may resolve; a sequel to severe colonic damage in horses is colonic stricture.

Lesions in the oral cavity associated with NSAID administration are deep crateriform ulcers, with a clean granulating base. Concurrent with punched-out ulcers in the glandular mucosa, there may be chronic gastritis and atrophy of the mucosa with loss of differentiation of the cells in the fundus. In the upper small intestine, ulcers may be focal, linear, or segmental and annular. Microscopic lesions that may precede ulceration of the small intestine include mild to severe atrophy of villi, epithelial necrosis, mucosal inflammation, and fibrin exudation. Renal papillary necrosis is often concurrent, if animals are dehydrated.

Further reading

Allman DA, Pastori MP. Duodenogastric intussusception with concurrent gastric foreign body in a dog: a case report and literature review. J Am Anim Hosp Assoc 2013;49:64-69.

Bell RJW, Textor JA. Caecal intussusceptions in horses: a New Zealand perspective. Aust Vet J 2010;88:272-276.

Carden DL, Granger DN. Pathophysiology of ischemia–reperfusion injury. J Pathol 2000;190:255-266.

Haglund ULF. Therapeutic potential of intraluminal oxygenation. Critical Care Med 1993;21:S69-S71.

Jones SL, et al. Ultrasonographic findings in horses with right dorsal colitis: five cases (2000–2001). J Am Vet Med Assoc 2003;222:1248-1251.

Levien AS, Baines SJ. Histological examination of the intestine from dogs and cats with intussusception. J Small Anim Pract 2011;52:599-606.

Nelson BB, Brounts SH. Intussusception in horses. Compend Contin Educ Vet 2012;34:E4.

Parfitt JR, Driman DK. Pathological effects of drugs on the gastrointestinal tract: a review. Hum Pathol 2007;38:527-536.

Rotting AK, et al. Effects of phenylbutazone, indomethacin, prostaglandin E$_2$, butyrate, and glutamine on restitution of oxidant-injured

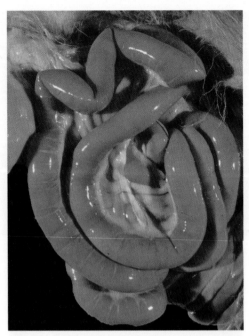

Figure 1-52 Intestinal lipofuscinosis (brown gut), discoloring the small intestine to a tan hue in a dog.

right dorsal colon of horses in vitro. Am J Vet Res 2004;65:1589-1595.

Vogel SR, et al. Duodenal obstruction caused by duodenal sigmoid flexure volvulus in dairy cattle: 29 cases (2006-2010). J Am Vet Med Assoc 2012;241:621-625.

Wong DM, et al. Intestinal ischemia-reperfusion injury in horses: pathogenesis and therapeutics. Compend Contin Educ Vet 2012;34:E5.

Miscellaneous conditions of the intestinal tract

Small intestinal bacterial overgrowth (SIBO) is defined as an absolute increase in small intestinal bacterial numbers. SIBO is a recognized entity in humans occurring *secondary to a number of underlying disorders* including hypochlorhydria, exocrine pancreatic insufficiency, hypomotility, partial small-bowel obstruction, radiation injury, or impairment of systemic and local immunity. The existence of genuine bacterial overgrowth in animals remains controversial. Though cases of "idiopathic SIBO" have been described in young large-breed dogs, many of these have been responsive to antibiotic therapy, which supports a diagnosis of a similar condition **antibiotic-responsive diarrhea** (ARD). This term is more appropriate in cases that respond clinically to antibiotics and where other conditions have been ruled out. Secondary SIBO, however, likely exists in dogs, and this term is best used in cases where such an initiating cause is documented. For SIBO and ARD, histologic examination of intestinal biopsies is often normal, other than the presence of bacterial colonies in mucus on the mucosal surface in some cases.

Intestinal lipofuscinosis (*brown gut*) in dogs is characterized grossly by *tan-brown discoloration of the tunica muscularis* (Fig. 1-52). It may involve any segment of gut, but is most commonly observed in the lower small intestine; the bladder and mesenteric or peripheral lymph nodes also may be affected. Although the lesion may be incidental, it is usually associated with *chronic enteric and/or pancreatic disease.*

Lipofuscinosis is reported in Boxer dogs with histiocytic ulcerative colitis, but a definitive correlation between the two conditions has not been established. Increased prevalence of lipofuscinosis has also been reported in dogs consuming high levels of polyunsaturated fats with a *relative deficiency of vitamin E*, and the condition is prevented by vitamin E supplementation. Any condition, such as exocrine pancreatic insufficiency, causing a reduction in the absorption of fats and fat-soluble vitamins, especially in the presence of polyunsaturated fatty acids in the diet, may predispose to lipofuscinosis.

The microscopic lesions of intestinal lipofuscinosis are gray-to-brown granules in the cytoplasm of smooth-muscle cells in the tunica muscularis; the reason they tend to accumulate here is unknown. The granules stain positive by periodic acid-Schiff and Sudan, are weakly acid-fast with Ziehl-Neelsen, and are mildly fluorescent in paraffin section. The granules, termed *leiomyometaplasts*, are oxidized polymerized phospholipids derived from cell membrane lipid peroxidation, and are highly resistant to further endophagocytic degradation. In Cocker Spaniel dogs affected with the inherited storage disease *generalized ceroid-lipofuscinosis*, intestinal lipofuscinosis is also observed, and is often accompanied by progressive hindlimb paresis and incoordination.

Muscular hypertrophy of the intestine was formerly a common finding in **swine,** but it appears to have diminished in prevalence in most areas. It may be found in apparently healthy animals at slaughter as a uniform thickening of the muscular coats of the *terminal ileum*. The most caudal ileal segment is involved, but it may extend a variable distance forward, usually 25-50 cm. The ileum is thickened and turgid; the lumen is small, the tunica muscularis is markedly thickened and the mucosa is folded. This condition must be differentiated from manifestations of enteropathy associated with *Lawsonia* in swine. *Perforation or rupture* of the intestine may occur in association with feed impaction in the hypertrophic segment; this may be a secondary to formation of pseudodiverticula, or as the result of violent peristalsis through the affected segment. Although the underlying basis remains obscure, it is likely that the muscular hypertrophy is secondary to a functional obstruction of the ileocecal orifice.

Idiopathic muscular hypertrophy of the small intestine also occurs in **horses** (Fig. 1-53). A similar lesion has been associated with *Anoplocephala* sp. tapeworms at the ileocecal orifice; however, this remains uncertain because many cases also show muscular hypertrophy of the *terminal esophagus*. The lesions are similar to those described in swine and the *ileum is the most common site*; however, any segment of the small intestine, and occasionally the large intestine can be affected. Horses with this condition may have chronic mild colic and anorexia or intermittent diarrhea with progressive loss of weight. Diverticula, and perforation or laceration of the thickened intestinal wall, also may occur.

Intestinal smooth-muscle hyperplasia has been described in a goat and, unlike the condition in horses and swine, only the jejunum was affected.

Pseudodiverticulosis of the small intestine is a rare lesion that is sometimes associated with muscular hypertrophy in pigs and horses. Single or multiple saccular dilations lined by intestinal mucosal epithelium are formed secondary to defects in the tunica muscularis and subserosa of the small intestine. Pseudodiverticula are distinguished from true diverticula, which are congenital defects involving all layers of the

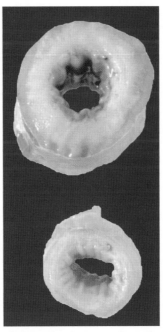

Figure 1-53 Ileal muscular hypertrophy in a horse. Normal equine ileum below.

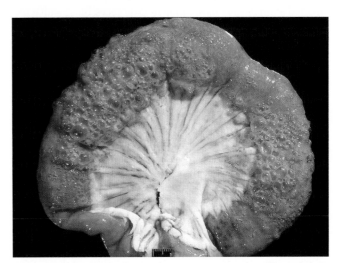

Figure 1-54 Intestinal emphysema in a pig. (Courtesy P. Stromberg.)

intestinal wall, and they tend to follow the pathway of blood vessels and are mainly located adjacent to the mesenteric attachment.

Intestinal emphysema, or *pneumatosis cystoides intestinalis*, is a rare condition found mainly in weaned *pigs*, in which it is usually an incidental finding in slaughtered animals (Fig. 1-54). It is characterized by numerous thin-walled, gas-filled cystic structures, a few millimeters to several centimeters in diameter, within the gut wall and on the serosal surface. These are mainly located in the small intestine, although the large intestine, mesentery, and mesenteric lymph nodes may be involved. Microscopically, the cystic structures appear to be *dilated lymphatics* that are located in the lamina propria, submucosa, muscularis, subserosa, mesentery, and mesenteric lymph nodes. A mixed cellular inflammatory reaction may be evident in the walls of the cysts. Although production of gas by bacteria has been implicated, the cause remains obscure.

Rectal prolapse most commonly occurs in *swine, sheep,* and *cattle.* It may occur in any animal that has *prolonged episodes of tenesmus or excessive coughing increasing abdominal pressure,* and is often associated with colitis or urinary infection or obstruction. In pigs, rectal prolapse occurs as a herd problem when the ration contains *zearalenone,* an estrogenic mycotoxin produced by fungi of the genus *Fusarium.* The toxin causes marked swelling and congestion of the vulva and vaginal mucosa, straining, and eventually vaginal and/or rectal prolapse. *Rectal prolapse in sheep* may be the consequence of ingestion of estrogenic pastures, and is accompanied by other signs of hyperestrogenism (see Vol. 3, Female genital system).

The prolapsed rectum is edematous, congested, and there may be necrosis and ulceration of the everted mucosa. These lesions are ischemic in origin owing to interference with venous blood flow from the prolapsed section. Only the mucosa, or all layers of the bowel, may be involved in the prolapse. In swine surviving slough or amputation of the prolapsed tissue, *rectal stricture* may ensue. Rectal stricture is discussed further in the section on salmonellosis.

Jejunal hematoma (hemorrhagic bowel syndrome, intestinal hematoma) has been described mainly in adult *dairy cattle* in North America, with occasional reports from Europe, the Middle East, and South America. The syndrome is usually characterized clinically by sudden death, although a few affected animals may have blood in their feces, bloat and acute abdominal pain for a short time before death. At postmortem examination, there are one or more short jejunal loops with intramural hemorrhage (Fig. 1-55A). The latter usually distends the intestinal mucosa to the point of complete or partial obstruction of the intestinal lumen (Fig. 1-55B). Intraluminal hemorrhage is also present in some cases. Determination of the primary location of the hemorrhage (intramural versus intraluminal) requires careful dissection, as in the cases of intramural hemorrhage, the compressed and thin intestinal mucosa frequently tears when the intestine is opened, giving the false impression that the blood is intraluminal rather than intramural. *Microscopically,* the interface between the hematoma and nonhematoma portions of the jejunum has an abrupt elevation of the mucosa, and the muscularis mucosa is often split by severe hemorrhage, with one portion adherent to the submucosa and the other to the lamina propria. The elevated mucosa may be completely necrotic or have only necrosis of the surface epithelium. Often, the affected mucosa has moderate to large numbers of large, gram-positive rods on the luminal surface. Because the percentage of gram-positive rods was found to increase with the degree of autolysis, it has been postulated that this bacterial population is a consequence rather than a cause of the condition. The affected mucosa, but also the more normal looking adjacent mucosa, has dilated villus lacteals that are either empty or contain abundant erythrocytes and/or pale eosinophilic, hyalinized material. Occasionally there are small numbers of hemosiderophages in the lamina propria of the affected mucosa. In a few cases, the mucosa may show mild to moderate edema, mild neutrophilic infiltration and small foci of submucosal hemorrhage. Submucosal blood vessels in these areas are usually within normal limits but a small percentage of cases may have mild to moderate vasculopathy with hyaline change of the vessel wall, mild pleocellular perivascular and subintimal inflammatory infiltrates and plump lining endothelium. Focal suppurative peritonitis can rarely be seen in affected areas of the jejunum. The cause of this entity is not known.

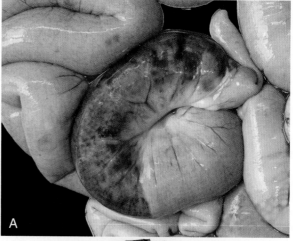

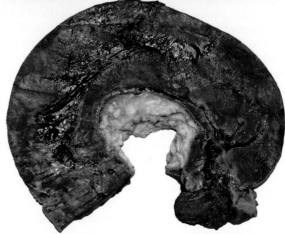

Figure 1-55 Jejunal hematoma (hemorrhagic bowel syndrome) in a dairy cow. A. Serosal view showing hemorrhage in a jejunal loop. **B.** Mucosal view; there is severe intramural hemorrhage with only a narrow remnant of the lumen.

A study of a large number of cases of jejunal hematoma and normal cows did not find a statistically significant relationship between the isolation of *C. perfringens, C. perfringens* type A or the *cpb2* gene and jejunal hematoma, strongly suggesting that *C. perfringens* is not associated with this condition. No association was found between jejunal hematoma and bovine viral diarrhea virus, *Salmonella sp.,* or copper levels.

Intestinal encephalopathy with clinical signs and lesions similar to those traditionally seen in hepatic encephalopathy, has been described in horses without liver disease, but with colic and/or diarrhea preceding neurological signs. Because those horses had hyperammonemia, it was speculated that this was consequence of excessive production and absorption of ammonia in the intestine because of intestinal disease. Intestinal overgrowth of ammonia-producing bacteria may be responsible. An investigation of 13 documented cases of this syndrome did not find any breed, age or sex predisposition, and no specific diet could be found to be associated with these cases. As in cases of hepatic encephalopathy, the most common microscopic finding in the brain of horses with the disease is the presence of Alzheimer type II cells. Laboratory findings include hyperammonemia, metabolic acidosis, and hyperglycemia.

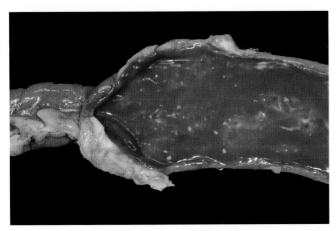

Figure 1-56 Oleander intoxication in a llama. The mucosa of the small intestine is severely hyperemic and hemorrhagic.

Baccharis cordifolia and *B. megapotamica* are found in several South American countries, but most cases of intoxication have been reported in Brazil and Argentina. *Baccharis pteronioides* has been implicated in similar livestock poisoning in the southwestern United States. The numerous toxic principles of these plants include the macrocyclic trichothecene complex of antibiotics. Spontaneous intoxication by *B. cordifolia* causes acute disease in cattle, sheep, and horses; intoxication by *B. megapotamica* has been reported in cattle, buffalo, and sheep. The syndrome produced by both plants is similar and it is characterized clinically by ocular discharge, incoordination, mild bloat, and muscle trembling. Gross findings include dehydration, abundant liquid rumen content, reddening of the mucosa of forestomachs, abomasum and intestine, and edema of the ruminal wall. The main histologic lesions are superficial to full-thickness degeneration and necrosis of the stratified epithelium lining the forestomachs, necrosis of the small intestinal mucosa, hemorrhagic gastroenteritis, and widespread lymphoid necrosis.

Chinaberry tree (*Melia azedarach*) is cultivated worldwide as an ornamental plant which has caused intoxication in pigs, cattle, sheep, goats, and dogs. The toxic principles (melia toxins A1, A2, B1, and B2) are concentrated in the fruit. Pigs seem to be most susceptible. Neurological and/or gastrointestinal clinical signs develop within a few hours of ingestion of the fruits. The former include excitement or depression, convulsions, ataxia, paresis, and coma. Gastrointestinal signs include anorexia, vomiting, constipation or diarrhea, frequently bloody, and colic. *Grossly*, the changes observed in different animal species are similar and include intestinal congestion, yellow discoloration of the liver, and brain congestion. *Microscopically* there is individual cell necrosis randomly distributed throughout the parenchyma or concentrated in the centrilobular zone of the liver, degenerative and necrotic changes in the epithelium of the forestomachs, necrosis of lymphoid tissue and hyaline degeneration and fiber necrosis.

Oleander toxicosis occurs in several mammalian species, including sheep, goats, cattle, camelids, monkeys, equids, and humans. In addition to the main cardiac lesion produced by intoxication with *Nerium oleander*, intestinal changes are frequently observed in several animal species. In horses and ruminants, it is thought that the changes in the alimentary tract are primarily caused by the highly irritant effect of *oleandrin*, the main glycoside present in oleander. However, it is possible that hypoperfusion caused by cardiac failure is a contributing

factor for these changes. In a study of 30 equids referred to a medical teaching hospital with a diagnosis of oleander intoxication, 85% had gastrointestinal signs included colic, diarrhea, gastric reflux, intestinal hyper- or hypo-motility, and abdominal distention. *Gross changes* in the alimentary tract of horses and ruminants with oleander intoxication include hemorrhage (Fig. 1-56), edema and, occasionally, the presence of pseudomembranes in the small intestine. *Histologically*, the most significant changes are hyperemia and hemorrhage of the mucosa in the small and/or large intestine, although neutrophilic and/or pseudomembranous enteritis can be seen in more advanced cases.

Further reading

Adaska JM, et al. Jejunal hematoma in cattle: A retrospective case analysis. J Vet Diagn Invest 2014;26:96-103.

Bohm M, et al. Diagnosis and management of small intestinal bacterial overgrowth. Nutr Clin Practice 2013;28:289-299.

Cortinovis C, Caloni F. Epidemiology of intoxication of domestic animals by plants in Europe. Vet J 2013;197:163-168.

Divers TJ. Metabolic causes of encephalopathy in horses. Vet Clin North Am Eq Pract 2011;27:589-596.

Elhanafy MM. Understanding jejunal hemorrhage syndrome. J Am Vet Med Assoc 2013;243:352-358.

Hall EJ. Antibiotic-responsive diarrhea in small animals. Vet Clin North Am Small Anim Pract 2011;4:273-286.

Renier AC, et al. Oleander toxicosis in equids: 30 cases (1995–2010). J Am Vet Med Assoc 2013;242:540-549.

Stegelmeier BL, et al. *Baccharis pteronioides* toxicity in livestock and hamsters. J Vet Diagn Invest 2009;21:208-213.

Malassimilation and protein-losing syndromes

In dogs, and to a lesser extent in horses, cats, and other species, usually idiopathic syndromes occur, variably signaled by *chronic diarrhea, weight loss, hypoproteinemia,* and *malabsorption. Endoscopic or full-thickness intestinal biopsy, where feasible, is usually necessary to make a diagnosis and establish a prognosis.* These syndromes are typically characterized by abnormal lamina proprial inflammatory infiltrates (eosinophils, lymphocytes, and plasma cells, or granulomatous inflammation), neoplasia, especially lymphosarcoma, or amyloid, and structural alterations, including hyperplasia of the crypts and villus atrophy. Lymphangiectasia may also produce a similar syndrome. Infectious causes of erosion or ulceration need to be considered, but are less common. In dogs, histoplasmosis, protozoal infections (giardiasis, cryptosporidiosis), and sequelae to severe parvoviral infections in animals recovered from the acute phase may cause such a syndrome. Inflammatory bowel disease in dogs and cats can be associated with protein-losing enteropathies where clear evidence of lymphangiectasis is absent. This may be due to alterations in epithelial permeability secondary to chronic mucosal inflammation. In horses, chronic salmonellosis and *Lawsonia* are potential infectious causes of malassimilation and protein loss.

The limitations on the interpretation of biopsies noted in the section on normal form and function of the intestine must be borne in mind. Neoplasia needs to be differentiated from inflammation, amyloidosis, and lymphangiectasia. Rarely, characteristic lesions or an agent may be recognized, implicating an infectious process. If inflammatory bowel disease is recognized, associated or complicating problems, such as

Giardia infection or bacterial overgrowth, should be sought. Associations with the dietary habits and history of the animal also should be investigated because some cases may be associated with inappropriate responses to dietary antigen.

Lymphangiectasia

Lymphangiectasia has been described most commonly in the dog, where it is among the most common causes of malabsorption/protein-losing enteropathy; it has not been reported in cats. Breed predisposition seems limited to Yorkshire Terriers and the Norwegian Lundehund, in which lymphangiectasia is part of a syndrome of protein-losing enteropathy with inflammatory bowel disease and in which gastritis and gastric neoplasia may co-exist. The disorder has also been reported in the horse. Lymphangiectasia is associated with a syndrome variably characterized by *chronic diarrhea, wasting, hypoproteinemia, lymphopenia, hypocalcemia, and hypocholesterolemia.* Peripheral edema, ascites, and hydrothorax result from hypoalbuminemia.

The lesion in the small intestine is *dilation of the lacteals, and often lymphatics* of the submucosa, muscularis, serosa, and mesentery (Fig. 1-57). Villi containing dilated chyle-filled lacteals may stand out grossly as white papillate foci in a thickened, transversely folded edematous mucosa. Serosal and

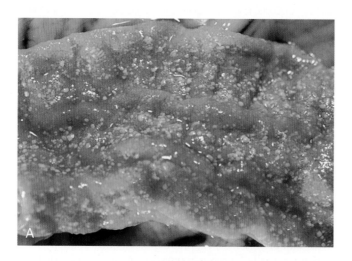

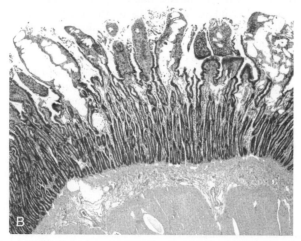

Figure 1-57 Lymphangiectasia in the small intestine of a dog. A. Mucosa, thickened by edema, is thrown into folds. Many villi contain white chyle-filled lacteals. **B.** Lacteals are dilated, and lymphatics in submucosa and muscularis are open.

mesenteric lymphatics may be prominent, white, and dilated. *Nodular white masses* up to 5-10 mm in size may be present on the serosa at the mesenteric border and along lymphatics; rarely, they are found on the liver, diaphragm, other abdominal organs, and pleura.

In section, villi may be of normal length or somewhat blunt or stubby, with some hypertrophy of crypts. The surface epithelium may appear normal or perhaps slightly attenuated, and lateral interepithelial spaces are often dilated. The lacteals in many villi are distended, and lymphatics in deeper portions of the mucosa, submucosa, and muscularis usually are as well. Occasional lipid-laden macrophages are present in and around lacteals and lymphatics; large focal accumulations of lipophages around lymphatics, sometimes with a local granulomatous response to lipid or saponified fat, form the white masses that may be seen grossly. A similar reaction may be present in the draining lymph nodes. The lamina propria is edematous, as are the submucosa and deeper portions of the gut wall. The proprial inflammatory cell population may be normal, or the numbers of lymphocytes, plasma cells, and eosinophils may be increased, as in chronic inflammatory bowel disease. Multiple dilated crypts that are filled with cellular debris (crypt abscesses) can be a microscopic finding associated with lymphangiectasia; however, this is a fairly nonspecific finding. Because dilation of lymphatics may be present in the submucosa and muscularis, multiple full-thickness intestinal biopsies that include duodenal and ileal samples may be more sensitive than endoscopic biopsies for diagnosis of lymphangiectasia.

The cause of lymphangiectasia may be lymphatic obstruction with increased lymphatic pressure that can be primary or acquired. Many cases appear to be acquired and common causes include lamina proprial inflammatory cell infiltrates, intestinal neoplasia (lymphosarcoma), and granulomatous infiltrates obstructing flow in mesenteric lymph nodes. Lesions may be multifocal or diffuse in the intestinal tract. Lipogranulomas along the lymphatic drainage are inconsistent features of lymphangiectasia, and are probably in response to chronic leakage of lipid-laden chyle, rather than a cause of lymphatic obstruction. Usually, no congenital or acquired obstruction of the lymphatic system is obvious, although several dogs with lymphangiectasia have had chylothorax associated with thoracic duct obstruction. Experimental obstruction of mesenteric lymphatics produces hypoproteinemia and lymphangiectasia, but not diarrhea and weight loss, suggesting that *the etiology of the clinical syndrome may be more complex than simple lymphatic obstruction.* Increased vascular permeability associated with chronic inflammatory bowel disease may also contribute to mucosal edema and lymphatic dilation.

Moderate malabsorption of lipid, and plasma protein loss into the gut, causes the signs associated with lymphangiectasia. Malabsorbed lipid may contribute to diarrhea via the effects of fatty acids on colonic secretion. Mucosal permeability associated with increased proprial hydrostatic pressure may cause filtration secretion and contribute to plasma protein loss. It has been proposed that dilated lacteals may rupture, releasing lymph into the lumen of the intestine. Hypocalcemia may be related to loss of the mineral bound to plasma albumin, and perhaps to vitamin D malabsorption, or formation of soaps with malabsorbed lipid in the gut lumen. Hypocholesterolemia is due to lipid malabsorption and effusion of plasma. Lymphopenia is thought to be the result of the loss of lymphocyte-rich lymph into the gut.

Further reading

Dossin O, Lavoué R. Protein-losing enteropathies in dogs. Vet Clin North Am Small Anim Pract 2011;41:399-418.

Kull PA, et al. Clinical, clinicopathologic, radiographic, and ultrasonographic characteristics of intestinal lymphangiectasis in dogs: 17 cases (1996–1998). J Am Vet Med Assoc 2001;219:197-202.

Larson R, et al. Duodenal endoscopic findings and histopathologic confirmation of intestinal lymphangiectasia in dogs. J Vet Intern Med 2012;26:1087-1092.

Santín M. Clinical and subclinical infections with *Cryptosporidium* in animals. N Z Vet J 2013;61:1-10.

Willard M, et al. Intestinal crypt lesions associated with protein-losing enteropathy in the dog. J Vet Intern Med 2000;14:298-307.

Amyloidosis

Amyloid deposition in the small intestine and stomach occasionally may be encountered in animals with systemic amyloidosis. Sometimes the gastrointestinal lesions predominate and contribute to the clinical syndrome. Significant intestinal amyloidosis leads to signs consistent with malabsorption and enteric protein loss. Usually there is no gross indication of the deposition of amyloid in the intestine. However, occasionally focal ulceration or hemorrhage may be noted. In geriatric dogs, amyloid deposits may occur in the intestine, often around blood vessels. Rarely, intestinal amyloid is associated with neoplasia, including intestinal extramedullary plasmacytomas. Microscopically, amyloid is seen beneath the epithelium or throughout the propria in villi, and perhaps around or within vessels in the submucosa (Fig. 1-58). It must not be mistaken for collagen deposition, which is most unusual in these locations, although a band of collagenous material is sometimes present at the base of the mucosa in cats. The pathogenic effects of amyloid in the intestine seem to involve either

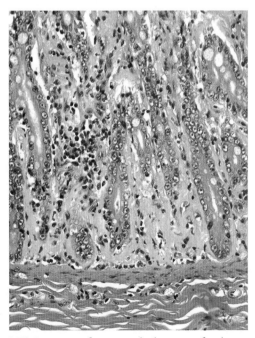

Figure 1-58 Intestine of a cat with deposits of pale amorphous **amyloid** within the deep lamina propria between crypts.

impaired movement of interstitial fluid into lacteals or perhaps increased permeability of capillaries, possibly explaining protein loss into the lumen.

Further reading

Kim DY, et al. Systemic AL amyloidosis associated with multiple myeloma in a horse. Vet Pathol 2005;42:81-84.

Ramos-Vara JA, et al. Intestinal multinodular A lambda-amyloid deposition associated with extramedullary plasmacytoma in three dogs: clinicopathological and immunohistochemical studies. J Comp Pathol 1998;119:239-249.

Tani Y, et al. Amyloid deposits in the gastrointestinal tract of aging dogs. Vet Pathol 1997;34:415-420.

Idiopathic inflammatory bowel disease

Some animals, mainly dogs and cats, but less commonly cattle and horses, showing signs consistent with malabsorption and/or plasma loss into the gut, have microscopic lesions in the mucosa of the small intestine described as *chronic inflammatory bowel disease, lymphocytic-plasmacytic enteritis, filled-villi syndrome,* or *eosinophilic gastroenteritis.* Eosinophilic gastroenteritis in cats and horses is often part of systemic eosinophilic syndromes affecting those species, considered separately in a later section. In dogs, there is no proof that differentiation of eosinophilic gastroenteritis from chronic inflammatory bowel disease is clinically relevant, nor are there clear criteria for such differentiation, so the two will be considered together. In both dogs and cats, idiopathic mucosal colitis and gastritis may be present as components of chronic inflammatory bowel disease, perhaps with predominant signs reflecting gastric or colonic dysfunction; both are considered here. In contrast to the mucosal pattern of inflammation evident in these entities, inflammatory lesions of the large and small intestine of any species that include a significant population of macrophages usually adopt a transmural pattern, and may be associated with a specific etiology (e.g., *Mycobacterium, Histoplasma*) or represent a distinct syndrome (histiocytic ulcerative colitis of Boxers). They are described with transmural granulomatous enteritis and with typhlocolitis.

Inflammatory bowel disease is a clinical syndrome for which it is difficult to develop a valid, objective histologic counterpart, and it should be *considered* by the clinician after alternatives such as food intolerance, motility disorders, and infectious disease have been ruled out. However, the thoroughness of the clinical and laboratory investigation before the use of endoscopic biopsy is influenced by the amount of time and money available to evaluate what are often elusive functional entities. Endoscopic biopsies are often done early, after symptomatic medical therapy has failed to control clinical signs. The microscopic findings commonly associated with inflammatory bowel disease are not specific, and reflect chronic mucosal inflammation resulting from a number of potential etiologies. It is probably not appropriate for a pathologist to issue a diagnosis of inflammatory bowel disease; it is more appropriate simply to list the histologic findings and to indicate that *the changes could be compatible with a clinical diagnosis of that syndrome.*

Regardless of the portion of the gastrointestinal tract under consideration, the histologic abnormalities are grouped under 3 broad headings: (1) *changes in mucosal architecture reflecting active or recent epithelial abnormality;* (2) *increased numbers of*

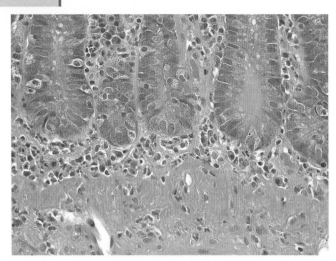

Figure 1-59 Eosinophilic enteritis in a dog. Numerous eosinophils infiltrating the epithelium of small intestinal crypts and adjacent lamina propria. (Courtesy Gastrointestinal Laboratory, Texas A&M University.)

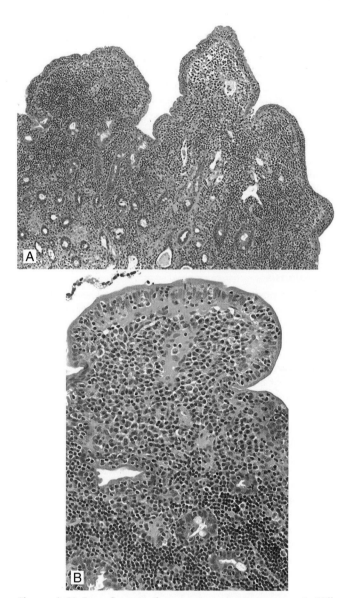

Figure 1-60 Lymphocytic-plasmacytic enteritis in a cat. A. Villi are stumpy, club-shaped, or fused. Excessive mononuclear infiltrate at all levels of the mucosa. **B.** The villi are blunt with cuboidal and attenuated surface epithelium. The lamina propria is heavily infiltrated by lymphocytes and plasma cells and intraepithelial lymphocytes are increased. (Courtesy Gastrointestinal Laboratory, Texas A&M University.)

proprial leukocytes; and (3) *fibrosis within the lamina propria.* Of these, the epithelial changes are the most reliable, yet the least prevalent. Although severe inflammatory changes can be quickly identified, it is often more difficult to objectively identify moderate or mild mucosal inflammation. Subjective impressions of increased numbers of leukocytes within the lamina propria are the least reliable, but are the most widely used criterion for a diagnosis, simply because most biopsy samples do not have any other mucosal abnormalities. The pathologist, faced with substantial pressure to make some kind of diagnosis, may reach for the one observation that cannot be disproved (or proved): too many leukocytes.

In the **small intestine,** the cardinal finding is abnormally intense infiltrates of well-differentiated lymphocytes and plasma cells, and sometimes eosinophils, in the lamina propria of villi, between crypts and perhaps in the submucosa. However, normal intestine contains these types of cells and the distinction between normal and abnormal infiltrates is subjective, based on the position and number of cells in the villus. *A layer of lymphocytes, plasma cells, and perhaps neutrophils or eosinophils more than about 4 cells thick, in the deep mucosa, below the crypts and above the muscularis mucosae, is abnormal* (Fig. 1-59).

Villi may be normal, blunted, or moderately to severely atrophic, and occasionally fusion of villi may be prevalent (Fig. 1-60A). The surface epithelium may appear relatively normal, mucous metaplastic, or low columnar to cuboidal with an indistinct brush border. Intraepithelial lymphocytes may be increased. Detection of increased intraepithelial lymphocytes may aid in diagnosis of chronic mucosal inflammation associated with inflammatory bowel disease. Crypts may be hypertrophic and lined by numerous goblet cells; in other cases goblet cells are less obvious. There may be edema of the lamina propria and dilation of lacteals, suggesting concurrent lymphangiectasia, but usually the edema is not as severe as occurs with that lesion. In this and other conditions with increased inflammatory infiltrates (Fig. 1-60B) or edema in the lamina propria, including lymphangiectasia, crypts may be obstructed and dilated, and contain mucus and a few exfoliated epithelial cells. This has been termed *cystic mucinous*

enteropathy; it is merely a severe variant of lymphocytic-plasmacytic enteritis, and we see no benefit in expanding the nomenclature in an already-confused area. Occasionally, rupture of such crypts will be seen; lakes of mucus, reactive histiocytes, and occasional giant cells are present in the lamina propria (Fig. 1-61). Other distended crypts may contain casts of eosinophilic glycoprotein.

Care should be taken to differentiate chronic inflammatory bowel disease from early intestinal lymphoma (see discussion of Malignant lymphomas). Some suggest that, in the Basenji at least, the former can evolve into the latter. In cats this also can be problematic, where differentiation of lymphocytic enteritis from low-grade lymphoma is a diagnostic challenge.

Idiopathic mucosal colitis is the colonic manifestation of chronic inflammatory bowel disease, and the *commonest form*

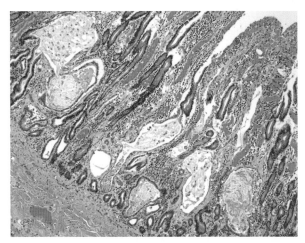

Figure 1-61 Small intestine of a dog with severe lymphoplasmacytic enteritis and chronic diarrhea compatible with **inflammatory bowel disease.** Blunt and occasionally fused villi, mononuclear cells in lamina propria, and elongate, dilated, and mucus-filled crypts. Some distended crypts have ruptured, releasing mucus into lamina propria.

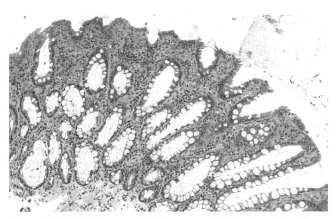

Figure 1-62 Mild acute colitis in a cat with diarrhea. Glands are mildly dilated and contain mucus. The lamina propria is infiltrated by lymphocytes, plasma cells, and low numbers of neutrophils. (Courtesy Gastrointestinal Laboratory, Texas A&M University.)

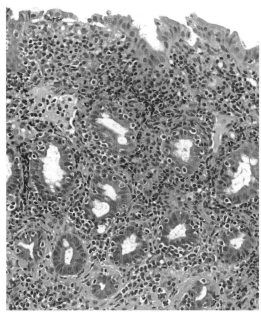

Figure 1-63 Chronic erosive colitis in a cat with chronic diarrhea. The surface epithelium is low cuboidal and ulcerated. The lamina propria contains large numbers of lymphocytes, plasma cells and neutrophils. The number of goblet cells is decreased in the glands. (Courtesy Gastrointestinal Laboratory, Texas A&M University.)

glands dilate and fill with mucus or cell debris. Hyperplastic glands are lined by basophilic enterocytes and goblet cells may be decreased. In some cases, goblet cells may be increased. Inflammatory cells, mainly neutrophils, but perhaps lymphocytes, plasma cells, and eosinophils, may accumulate excessively along the mucosal side of the muscularis mucosae, as in inflammatory disease involving the small intestine. The lesions in mild acute colitis often seem mild in proportion to the severity of the clinical syndrome.

The *spectrum of inflammation* in colitis grades from acute toward an increasingly chronic infiltrate, which, along with edema, separates colonic glands and may accumulate deep in the mucosa between glands and muscularis mucosae (Fig. 1-63). Neutrophils and eosinophils may be scattered among round cells in the propria, and transmigrating surface and glandular epithelium. Globule leukocytes may be prevalent. Accumulation of granulocytes and necrotic debris in the lumen of glands forms so-called *crypt abscesses.*

Greater severity of the lesion is reflected in attenuation and exfoliation of surface epithelium, and the development of *microerosions* on the mucosal surface. Inflammatory cells, mainly neutrophils, and tissue fluid effuse into the lumen through defects in the epithelium. Persistent erosion, or previous erosion in a healed mucosa, is marked by the development of a thin, horizontally arrayed layer of connective tissue in the superficial lamina propria. With increasing chronicity in colitis of mild or moderate degree, there may be deposition within the lamina propria of a collagenous stroma, throughout which inflammatory cells are interspersed, which separates glands abnormally throughout the mucosa. Downgrowth of glands into often-involuted submucosal lymphoid follicles may occur in chronic colitis.

Severe erosion and ulceration are usually associated with local acute inflammation and with a heavy, mainly

of colitis recognized in dogs. It is etiologically nonspecific, occurring as chronic or chronic-active lymphocytic-plasmacytic or eosinophilic mucosal inflammation. *Histiocytic ulcerative colitis* is the distinctive pattern differentiated from it on microscopic grounds, along with rare cases of *Histoplasma* or protothecal colitis.

Mild acute mucosal colitis, reflecting a grossly reddened friable surface visible on endoscopy, is characterized by congestion of superficial capillaries and venules, and proprial edema. Neutrophils infiltrate the superficial lamina propria around vessels, and transmigrate or pass between surface epithelial cells into the lumen. The population of lymphocytes and plasma cells in the lamina propria may not differ from normal, but there is generally a moderate increase in mononuclear cells, and perhaps eosinophils, which are usually rare in the superficial colonic mucosa, between glands (Fig. 1-62). There are often few goblets on the surface and in glands, probably owing to mucous discharge, rather than cell loss. Surface epithelium may be basophilic, low columnar, or cuboidal. Hyperplasia of epithelium in glands may be evident, and mononuclear cell infiltrate in the lamina propria, and often in the submucosa. The ulcerated areas extend usually no further than the muscularis mucosae, and have a base of granulation tissue heavily infiltrated by neutrophils that effuse into the lumen of the bowel. The margin of surviving mucosa may overhang the ulcer. Crypt abscesses may be present in remaining mucosa, and all degrees of erosion and partial ulceration may be present. Idiopathic ulcerative colitis is uncommon, and does not seem as severe as histiocytic ulcerative colitis of Boxers; it rarely comes to autopsy. Severely affected dogs may be cachectic, probably owing in part to enteric loss of plasma protein. The mucosa in ulcerative colitis is usually deep red, swollen, folded, and granular because of edema and cellular infiltrates; the depressions may be punctate or up to several centimeters across, roughly round or oval, irregular or elongate. Their margins may be tattered or puckered. Colonic lymph nodes may be enlarged and edematous.

In *canine colitis*, there is a broad 3-dimensional spectrum: (1) in relative chronicity and density of the inflammatory infiltrate; (2) in the distribution of the infiltrate within the wall of the bowel; and (3) in the severity of the epithelial and mucosal change. Generally, milder lesions of superficial epithelium are associated with mild or moderate mucosal inflammation, which may be acute or chronic. In many cases of mild chronic mucosal colitis, the glands do not appear particularly hyperplastic. However, defective repair in the face of severe or ongoing injury may result in crypts that are tortuous or even nearly horizontal, and papillary hyperplasia of the epithelial surface. Severe erosion and ulceration are usually related to a more intense or heavy chronic inflammatory process, which may be limited to the mucosa, but which can extend into the submucosa. Truly granulomatous colitis is not common; when fully developed, perhaps as a component of regional enteritis involving the ileocecocolic area, or in histiocytic colitis of Boxer dogs considered later, it is ulcerative and transmural. Occasionally, a granulomatous response to barium, or to other foreign material breaching the epithelium, may be observed in the mucosa and submucosa. *Atrophic colitis*, in which the mucosa is markedly thinned, with relatively inactive crypts and modest chronic or chronic-active interstitial inflammation, perhaps with notable interstitial fibrosis, is occasionally encountered.

Gastric changes in dogs or cats with clinically suspected inflammatory bowel disease are challenging to interpret, because of variation in normal microscopic anatomy within the stomach, and because gastric lesions are often patchy. As well, ingestion of chemicals and foreign bodies can create gastric lesions misinterpreted as being those of inflammatory bowel disease.

The stomach has a variety of *normal anatomic features and common background lesions* that have not been proved to have any functional significance. These include a dense band of hyalinized fibrous tissue (*lamina densa*) between the muscularis mucosae and the base of the crypts in cats, lymphoid nodules within the deep lamina propria of both dogs and cats, and a substantial amount of fibrous tissue within the lamina propria of the pyloric antrum. It is not clear whether some of these have any significance as signposts of previous disease. Background lesions that may or may not be correlated with some previous specific stimulus include globule leukocytes in the gastric epithelium of cats, and a combination of gastric proprial fibrosis, glandular atrophy, and glandular nesting within the fundic mucosa. Although we assume (without

proof) that such fibrosis and glandular atrophy are sequelae to previous inflammation or necrosis, such changes have not been correlated with gastric dysfunction or clinical illness.

Unlike the situation in the intestinal and colonic mucosa, *epithelial injury is not as prominent in gastritis in dogs or cats.* It is uncommon to encounter erosion or ulceration as part of gastritis, and acute ulceration associated with chemical or mechanical injury to the stomach has little mucosal cellular infiltrate. It is therefore prudent to distinguish gastric ulceration from gastritis. Lesions compatible with a diagnosis of gastritis include leukocytic infiltrates in the superficial third of the mucosa, mucous metaplasia and hyperplasia in fundic glands, extensive lymphoplasmacytic and/or eosinophilic infiltrates deep in the mucosa, interstitial fibrosis, and associated atrophy of glands. The diagnosis of **gastric mucosal atrophy** must be made with great care because there is substantial difference in mucosal thickness between various portions of the stomach, and even within the same anatomic region.

Most discussions of inflammatory bowel disease assume that the change in mucosal cellularity is primary and that characterization of that cellularity should provide the greatest insight into pathogenesis and therapy. However, assessment of mucosal cellularity is almost entirely subjective and has exceedingly poor interobserver agreement. There are no useful objective reference intervals for small intestinal mucosal cellularity because the range is so broad, and accurate identification of the different cell types is problematic. Characterization of the immunophenotype of lymphocytes in the small intestine has produced variable results that have yet to be usefully associated with the presence or absence of clinical signs.

Attempts to create more *objective grading systems* for the histologic assessment of inflammatory bowel disease have stressed the significance of architectural changes within the surface epithelium and lamina propria rather than relying exclusively on shifts in total or relative leukocyte populations. Such grading criteria include detection of villus or cryptal enterocyte injury (villus fusion, superficial ulceration, enterocyte flattening and basophilia, cryptal hyperplasia), as well as remodeling of mucosal architecture (separation of the crypts from one another or from the muscularis mucosae by edema, fibrosis, and/or leukocytes). However, these schemes still fail to resolve the dilemma of substantial overlap between "normal" and subjectively increased leukocyte numbers in mild inflammatory bowel disease in which there is no epithelial injury or architectural change. The World Small Animal Veterinary Association Gastrointestinal Standardization Group has developed a standardized grading scheme that works toward distinguishing normal from mucosal lesions in each grading criterion.

Skepticism about the utility of estimating leukocyte numbers or identifying shifts in phenotype among mucosal leukocytes may not be so appropriate when looking at colonic and gastric inflammatory disease. Perhaps because of its lesser overall proprial cellularity in comparison with small intestine, or perhaps because of its greater accessibility to biopsy, the colonic mucosa was the first part of the canine intestinal tract to be subjected to morphometric grading of architectural changes and objective leukocyte counting, although application of such data is difficult. In comparison with small intestine, the normal range in leukocyte numbers is narrower and the overall population much smaller in both colon and stomach. This is particularly true of the granulocytes. *The presence of neutrophils within the lamina propria of any part of* the intestine is probably abnormal, and is probably a reliable marker for recent epithelial damage or permeability. Eosinophils have more variation, and often are present in very large numbers throughout the small intestinal mucosa. However, they are very sparse within the superficial half of the canine colonic mucosa, and are infrequent within the gastric mucosa.

Because the normal stomach has relatively few mucosal leukocytes, the pursuit of a diagnosis of gastritis based upon objective assessment of leukocyte numbers may be a credible goal. Although it has been possible, by counting different types of leukocytes identified by routine histology and immunohistochemistry, to establish reference intervals for eosinophils, plasma cells, B cells, and T cells within various parts of the gastric lamina propria of healthy dogs, more than half of the round cells in the normal canine gastric lamina propria could not be precisely identified. Healthy dogs had an 8-fold range in total mucosal cellularity, and the pyloric antrum was 3 times more cellular than the fundic mucosa. Although dogs with clinical signs of gastritis had an objective increase in eosinophils, plasma cells, and/or intraepithelial lymphocytes in many different combinations, it was difficult to correlate clinical severity or response to therapy with cellular or other parameters of gastric mucosal abnormality. There was no significance to whether the inflammation was limited to the superficial third of the mucosa or was found throughout, although the former was more common than the latter. In a second study of idiopathic gastritis, all cases were classified as lymphocytic, and T cells predominated. Eosinophils were not a significant component, and there was no observed regional variation in severity.

The etiopathogenesis of idiopathic inflammatory bowel disease is not understood in any animal species. Similar to humans with IBD, it is likely that multiple factors, including genetics, mucosal immunity, intestinal microbiota, diet, and environment, play a role in pathogenesis. A familial role in dogs is established with enteropathies documented in multiple breeds including Boxers, Basenjis, German Shepherds, and Irish Setters. As molecular techniques to detect intestinal microbes improve, alterations in the intestinal microbial communities in dogs and cats have been detected. Shifts in the major microbial constituents, from gram-positive Firmicutes species to gram-negative proteobacteria in the gut have been noted in healthy animals versus those with intestinal inflammation. These alterations in the composition of the intestinal microbiota have been termed dysbiosis. Dysbiosis correlates with mucosal inflammation and may be a driver of persistent inflammation. Potential pathogens, such as invasive species of E. coli in Boxer dogs and French Bulldogs with granulomatous colitis, have been identified. Diet also appears to be important with a significant percentage of dogs and cats with chronic enteropathy responding favorably to dietary changes. An immunologic basis for this sensitivity is not always determined and adverse food reaction may be better terms than food allergy. In addition to food allergy, adverse food reactions would include food intolerance and intoxications.

The nature of the inflammatory infiltrate suggests that loss of tolerance to dietary antigen or antigens produced by the enteric microflora may be implicated. Similar to humans' defects in regulation of innate immune responses may be an initial component of loss of mucosal tolerance in dog and cats. In dogs with inflammatory bowel disease, innate recognition of commensal bacteria through toll-like receptors has been shown to generate a proinflammatory response typical of invading enteric pathogens. Changes in mucosal dendritic cell phenotype and frequency have been detected in dogs with inflammatory bowel disease, suggesting altered antigen sampling and subsequent adaptive immune responses. The common morphologic changes in the mucosa—cryptal hypertrophy, villus atrophy, and in severe cases, mucous metaplasia of surface enterocytes—may be side-effects of T-cell–mediated activity in the mucosa. Similar lesions occur in humans with celiac disease (gluten-sensitive enteropathy), which is T-cell mediated. Reduced numbers of T-regulatory cells has been identified in dogs which also may play a role in loss of tolerance to luminal antigens, recruitment of inflammatory T-cell populations, and progression of mucosal inflammation.

Lymphocytic-plasmacytic enteritis associated with familial sensitivity to wheat protein has been demonstrated in Irish Setters. An enteropathy in Basenji dogs has similarities to other forms of inflammatory bowel disease. In Basenjis and in the Lundehund, syndromes of hypoalbuminemia, chronic diarrhea, and wasting occur with high prevalence, primarily attributable to lymphocytic-plasmacytic enteritis, with lymphangiectasia in some dogs. In the Basenji chronic gastritis or hypertrophic gastritis may be associated, and malassimilation and plasma protein loss into the gut have been documented. Hypergammaglobulinemia commonly occurs in the late stages of the syndrome in Basenjis, and lymphosarcoma develops in some affected animals. In this sense, the syndrome resembles immunoproliferative small intestinal disease (α-heavy chain disease, or Mediterranean lymphoma), which is a disorder of IgA immunoblasts in humans. IgA plasmacytes do not dominate in the Basenji intestinal mucosa; though high circulating levels of IgA are present, it is not known if they are associated with abnormal α–heavy-chain protein.

In cats, dogs, and horses, submucosal or transmural lymphoplasmacytic infiltrates may signal a precursor to lymphoma, and the infiltrating cell population must be carefully evaluated; a monomorphic population of lymphocytes, blurring of the proprial-epithelial interface by lymphocytic infiltrates, and mitotic activity suggest lymphosarcoma.

Animals with the gray Collie syndrome (cyclic neutropenia) also may have lymphocytic-plasmacytic enteritis (see Vol. 3, Hematopoietic system).

Malabsorptive and syndromes with weight loss have been described in the horse with some similarities to inflammatory bowel disease. The etiologies in the horse are unknown, but it is possible that similar mechanisms described earlier are involved. Multiple forms are described that include lymphoplasmacytic, granulomatous, and eosinophilic.

Further reading

Day M, et al. Histopathological standards for the diagnosis of gastrointestinal inflammation in endoscopic biopsy samples from the dog and cat: a report from the World Small Animal Veterinary Association Gastrointestinal Standardization Group. Comp Pathol 2008;138(Suppl. 1):S1-S43.

Gaschen FP, Merchant SR. Adverse food reactions in dogs and cats. Vet Clin North Am Small Anim Pract 2011;41:361-379.

Junginger J, et al. Canine gut dendritic cells in the steady state and in inflammatory bowel disease. Innate Immun 2014;20:145-160.

Kalck K. Inflammatory bowel disease in horses. Vet Clin North Am Equine Pract 2009;25:303-315.

MacLachlan NJ, et al. Gastroenteritis of basenji dogs. Vet Pathol 1988;25:36-41.

Roth L, et al. Comparisons between endoscopic and histologic evaluation of the gastrointestinal tract in dogs and cats: 75 cases (1984–1987). J Am Vet Med Assoc 1990;196:635-638.

Simpson K, Jergens A. Pitfalls and progress in the diagnosis and management of canine inflammatory bowel disease. Vet Clin North Am Small Anim Pract 2011;41:381-398.

Simpson K, et al. Adherent and invasive *Escherichia coli* is associated with granulomatous colitis in boxer dogs. Infect Immun 2006;74:4778-4792.

Suchodolski J, et al. 16S rRNA gene pyrosequencing reveals bacterial dysbiosis in the duodenum of dogs with idiopathic inflammatory bowel disease. PLoS ONE 2012;7:e39333.

Webb C, Twedt DC. Canine gastritis. Vet Clin North Am Small Anim Pract 2003;33:969-985.

Eosinophilic enteritis in cats and horses

Eosinophilic enteritis in cats is rare, and appears to be one manifestation of a hypereosinophilic syndrome that may involve many organs in middle-aged or older cats. It is much more severe than eosinophilic gastroenteritis in dogs. Diarrhea, sometimes bloody, vomition, loss of appetite, and loss of condition may occur. Clinically, *intestinal thickening*, hepatomegaly and splenomegaly, and enlarged mesenteric lymph nodes may be present, in association with circulating eosinophilia and hyperplasia of the eosinophil series in the marrow.

The postmortem picture reflects the clinical findings. Enlargement of the various organs, including liver, spleen, lymph nodes in many locations, and tan nodularities on the kidneys, is associated with *heavy infiltrates of usually well-differentiated eosinophils*. In the small intestine, the eosinophilic infiltrate may be transmural and is accompanied by grossly visible hypertrophy of the muscle layers (Fig. 1-64). Eosinophilic colitis may occur in some cases. Lymph nodes may have hyperplastic follicles and many mature eosinophils in sinusoids. Alternatively they may vary through eosinophilic lymphadenitis with fibrosis to complete obliteration of normal architecture and replacement by eosinophils in a fibrillar stroma extending through the capsule into surrounding tissue.

Chronic eosinophilic enteritis in horses has been described as part of a distinct *multisystemic epitheliotropic*

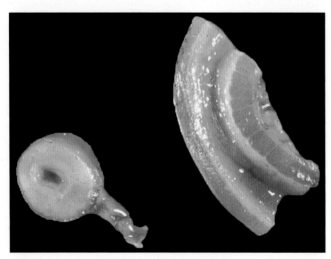

Figure 1-64 Eosinophilic enteritis in a cat. Segmental transmural thickening and hypertrophy of smooth muscle in an area heavily infiltrated by eosinophils. (Courtesy Noah's Arkives.)

syndrome, associated with eosinophilic granulomatous pancreatitis and eosinophilic dermatitis, among other lesions. Affected animals have weight loss, and diarrhea or unformed feces, associated with hypoalbuminemia, suggesting enteric loss of plasma protein. Reduced absorption of glucose occurs, but peripheral eosinophilia is absent. At *autopsy, mucosal and sometimes transmural thickening* may occur at any level of the alimentary tract from esophagus to rectum. Esophageal and gastric squamous mucosa is hyperkeratotic. Thickened mucosa is thrown into turgid transverse folds, or occasionally is fissured and roughened. Focal or diffuse ulcers may be present on the small and large intestine and focal caseous lesions up to 1.5 cm in diameter may be in the submucosa of the gut and common bile duct, as well as in an enlarged fibrotic pancreas.

Microscopically there is diffuse infiltration of the mucosa, submucosa, and often deeper layers of the enteric wall by eosinophils, mast cells, macrophages, lymphocytes, and some plasma cells. Moderate to severe villus atrophy, fibroplasia in the lamina propria, and hypertrophy of the muscularis mucosae occur. Caseous foci in the mucosa and submucosa consist of central masses of eosinophils, sometimes surrounded by macrophages, giant cells, and occasionally fibrous tissue. Eosinophilic interstitial infiltrates and granulomas are described in the biliary and pancreatic ducts, pancreas, salivary glands, capsule, and outer cortex of enlarged firm mesenteric lymph nodes, and near portal tracts in the liver. The skin may be thickened and hyperkeratotic and the limbus of the hoof thickened and ulcerated. The eosinophilic dermatitis is described in Vol. 1, Integumentary system.

Villus atrophy is common, but if large-bowel lesions are absent, there is no diarrhea. Chronic inflammation in the mucosa may explain protein loss and hypoalbuminemia. The cause of this syndrome is unknown. A hypersensitivity response to migrating parasitic larvae has been suggested, as has the possibility that undetected T-cell lymphoma secreting interleukin-5 may be responsible.

Eosinophilic gastroenteritis also occurs in horses apart from the multisystemic eosinophilic syndrome. In addition to eosinophilic inflammation associated with enteric parasitism, idiopathic eosinophilic enteritis has been described as a part of the equine inflammatory bowel disease complex. An uncommon focal form of eosinophilic inflammation of the equine small intestine also has been described. This lesion is characterized by focal infiltration of large numbers of eosinophils and macrophages that are focused on the submucosa and the tunica muscularis. In the lamina propria there is often increased density of lymphocytes, plasma cells, and macrophages with fewer eosinophils. This lesion has been associated with obstruction and colic.

Further reading

Bosseler L, et al. Equine multisystemic eosinophilic epitheliotropic disease: a case report and review of literature. N Z Vet J 2013;61: 177-182.

Mäkinen P, et al. Characterisation of the inflammatory reaction in equine idiopathic focal eosinophilic enteritis and diffuse eosinophilic enteritis. Equine Vet J 2008;40:386-392.

Swain JM, et al. Multifocal eosinophilic enteritis associated with a small intestinal obstruction in a standardbred horse. Vet Rec 2003;152: 648-651.

Granulomatous enteritis

The presence of chronic inflammatory infiltrates, including aggregates of histiocytes, and perhaps giant cells, in the lamina propria is the criterion for a diagnosis of **granulomatous enteritis.** With time, the inflammatory reaction typically follows lymphatics transmurally into the submucosa and through the muscularis to the serosa. The submucosa is usually edematous, and lymphatics are prominent. Granulomas may be present in the submucosa or at intervals along lymphatics. The affected lymph nodes are hyperplastic, usually with prominent sinus histiocytosis. Giant cells may be present in sinusoids, or granulomatous foci of various sizes may be evident. Sinusoids contain numerous neutrophils and perhaps eosinophils, and neutrophils may accumulate in the center of granulomas.

Granulomatous enteritis can potentially occur in *all species.* Johne's disease, other intestinal mycobacterioses, and *Histoplasma* enteritis are specific examples (see later section on Infectious and parasitic diseases of the alimentary tract). Often the cause is not identified.

Transmural granulomatous enteritis is occasionally seen in **dogs** and **cats.** It is generally segmental and perhaps discontinuous in distribution, usually affecting the lower ileum, colon, and draining lymph nodes. Because of the extent of the attendant fibrosis, these lesions may be stenotic, and must be differentiated from invasive carcinoma. In dogs, there may be marked necrosis in the centers of granulomas and considerable fibrosis.

Idiopathic granulomatous enteritis as a cause of wasting and protein-losing enteropathy is most commonly seen as a sporadic problem in **horses.** Depending on the duration of the disease, animals may be markedly cachectic, have subcutaneous edema, especially of dependent areas, and there may be hydrothorax, hydropericardium, and ascites. Lesions in the horse usually affect the small intestine; stomach and large bowel are occasionally also involved. Mesenteric lymph nodes are usually enlarged, edematous, with mottled firm gray areas, fibrotic nodules, or, rarely, caseous or mineralized foci on the cut surface. Granulomatous pale, caseous, or calcified foci may be scattered in the liver.

The *microscopic lesion* may be patchy, regional, or diffuse, and it may be mucosal, or transmural, ultimately gaining the draining lymph nodes. Transmural inflammation is characteristically granulomatous. Villi are mildly to markedly atrophic with hypertrophy of crypts. The epithelium may vary from apparently normal to low columnar or cuboidal with an indistinct brush border. There may be leaks between cells on the surface, or microerosions may be present through which neutrophils and proteinaceous exudate pass into the lumen. The lamina propria is edematous and contains scattered aggregates of histiocytes and perhaps giant cells, or less commonly, more organized granulomatous foci. Neutrophils and eosinophils are distributed diffusely throughout the lamina propria, and may be concentrated in or near granulomatous foci. A heavy population of lymphocytes and plasma cells inhabits the lamina propria, and the infiltrate and edema may separate crypts abnormally from each other.

Further reading

Horn B, et al. Disseminated *Mycobacterium avium* infection in a dog with chronic diarrhea. Aust Vet J 2000;78:320-325.

Schumacher J, et al. Chronic idiopathic inflammatory bowel diseases of the horse. J Vet Intern Med 2000;14:258-265.

Inflammation of the large intestine

For general reactions to injury of the cecal and colonic epithelium, see the earlier section, Epithelial renewal in health and disease.

Ischemia, obliteration of the proliferative epithelium by etiologic agents, severe inflammation, and some luminal toxins are responsible for the development of focal or diffuse ulceration of the large intestine. Inflammatory infiltrates in the lamina propria are classified based on the inflammatory cell phenotype, and may be limited in distribution to the mucosa or be transmural involving all layers of the intestinal wall and frequently the draining lymph nodes. *Typhlitis* and *colitis* may be manifestations of a generalized disease; they may be part of *enterocolitis* involving both small and large intestine, or they may be regional and limited to any specific segment or segments of the intestine. Damaged colonic mucosa may provide the portal of entry for cross-mucosal translocation of bacteria or toxins. Increased mucosal permeability in the colon may permit enteric loss of plasma protein or blood. Intestinal flora dysbacteriosis in hindgut fermenters may compromise uptake of volatile fatty acids and water. In any species, damage to the colonic mucosa may result in malabsorption of electrolytes and water, or altered secretion. Colitis in each of the species is considered in turn.

Colitis cystica profunda, the presence of dilated mucus-filled colonic glands protruding through the muscularis mucosae into the submucosa or tunica muscularis, is uncommon in domestic animals and has been described in pigs, dogs, and goats; the cause is unknown. The lesion may be a sequel to colitis and local damage to the muscularis mucosae, or it may represent herniation into the space left by an involuted submucosal lymphoid follicle. The lesion may be associated with colitis, especially swine dysentery, or it also may be found incidentally.

Typhlocolitis in dogs

Inflammation of the large bowel in dogs is usually associated with frequent *diarrhea*, which is small in volume, mucoid or bloody, and often accompanied by tenesmus. By far the most common form encountered in dogs is **idiopathic mucosal colitis**, considered in the earlier section, Idiopathic inflammatory bowel disease.

Histiocytic ulcerative colitis, or granulomatous colitis, is a distinctive histologic syndrome described mostly in young Boxers and French Bulldogs. This is a chronic transmural ulcerative colitis with nonspecific gross and characteristic histologic lesions. Clinically, there is frequent bloody mucoid diarrhea, anemia, hypoalbuminemia, weight loss, and chronic cachexia. *Grossly*, the colon of dogs with advanced disease is ulcerated, variably thickened, folded, and perhaps dilated and shortened with some segmental or focal areas of scarring and stricture. Lesions on the mucosa vary from patchy punctate red ulcers to more extensive irregular circular or linear coalescing ulcers, with islands of remnant surface mucosa. *Histologic lesions* are unique and include severe mucosal ulceration, goblet cell loss and infiltration of the lamina propria and submucosal layers by many granulocytes and macrophages (Fig. 1-65) containing periodic acid-Schiff positive material. These cells are also found within and surrounding lymphatics of the tunica muscularis and serosal surface. Their presence in draining lymph nodes, along with lymphoid hyperplasia, explains the localized or generalized lymphadenopathy that often accompanies this syndrome. The cecum is

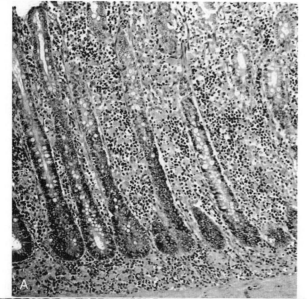

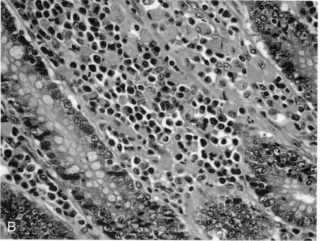

Figure 1-65 Histiocytic ulcerative colitis in a Boxer dog. A. Accumulation of macrophages with abundant cytoplasm throughout mucosa, between base of glands and muscularis mucosae and in submucosa. **B.** Detail of macrophages in mucosa between the crypts.

also involved with similar lesions, although often to a lesser degree.

This condition was long regarded as an idiopathic immune-mediated disease with variable response to empirical therapeutic support. Recent work, however, has elegantly demonstrated the presence of selective intramucosal colonization by invasive strains of *Escherichia coli*. Furthermore, long-term clinical remission has been demonstrated in cases of ulcerative histiocytic colitis of Boxer dogs, with eradication of invasive *E. coli* using appropriate antibacterial therapy. Antibiotic resistance, especially to enrofloxacin, has been correlated with invasive *E. coli* isolated from Boxer dogs with nonresponsive or refractory disease.

Severe acute necrotizing colitis and, less commonly typhlitis leading to *ulceration and perforation* has been associated with functional adrenal cortical tumors or glucocorticoid administration, especially following trauma or surgery involving the spinal cord; gastric ulceration may occur concurrently. The perforations can occur anywhere in the colon, but usually

occur in the antimesenteric border of the left colonic flexure or proximal descending colon. The pathogenesis of these lesions remains unclear.

Ulcerative colitis with perforation has been reported in dogs with **uremia**, but the mechanism is uncertain. Given the frequency of concurrent vascular lesions including arteritis, fibrinoid necrosis, and mineralization, colonic mucosal damage may be related to mucosal ischemia or a variety of toxins, including increased ammonia formed by bacterial urease in the colon. ***Trichuris vulpis***, the *canine* whipworm, causes acute or chronic mucosal colitis or typhlitis; in heavy infestations, there may be significant blood loss because of mucosal damage inflicted by the nematodes. Clinical trichuriasis is generally associated with adult trichurid nematodes extending from the cecum and proximal ascending colon into more distal parts of the large intestine. Ulcerative colitis in dogs is also rarely caused by ***Entamoeba histolytica***. Ulcerative granulomatous transmural colitis is common as an enteric manifestation of infection with ***Histoplasma capsulatum***. The alga ***Prototheca*** is a rare cause of enterocolitis as part of systemic disease in dogs. **Leishmaniasis** in dogs is often a multisystemic disease, but chronic mixed-cell inflammatory infiltration of the colon along with numerous *L. infantum* amastigotes is usually observed. **Canine parvovirus 2** causes colonic damage, but in virtually all cases, there are more severe lesions elsewhere, notably in the small intestine. **Canine coronavirus** has also been implicated as a cause of colonic and small intestinal lesions. ***Brachyspira*** spp. may be present in the canine colon and may be associated with diarrheal disease; however, their role in disease remains controversial. ***Campylobacter*** spp. can be isolated from dogs with and without diarrhea, but has been implicated as a cause of enterocolitis outbreaks in some dog colonies. These conditions are discussed fully in the later section, Infectious and parasitic diseases of the alimentary tract.

Further reading

Craven M, et al. Granulomatous colitis of boxer dogs. Vet Clin North Am Sm Anim Pract 2011;41:433-445.

Duhamel GE. Comparative pathology and pathogenesis of naturally acquired and experimentally induced colonic spirochetosis. An Health Res Rev 2001;2:3-17.

Manchester AC, et al. Association between granulomatous colitis in French bulldogs and invasive *Escherichia coli* and response to fluoroquinolone antimicrobials. J Vet Intern Med 2013;27:56-61.

Simpson KW, et al. Adherent and invasive *Escherichia coli* is associated with granulomatous colitis in boxer dogs. Infect Immun 2006;74: 4778-4792.

Colitis in cats

Colitis in cats is less common compared with dogs. **Idiopathic mucosal colitis**, similar to that described in dogs, also occurs in cats, and is discussed with the previous section on idiopathic inflammatory bowel disease. ***Tritrichomonas foetus*** is associated with persistent large-bowel diarrhea and idiopathic mucosal colitis in cats <1 year of age, and is considered later in this chapter in the section Infectious and parasitic diseases of the alimentary tract.

Feline panleukopenia virus (FPLV) causes colonic lesions in about half of the cases; typical lesions are less widespread or severe compared with small intestinal lesions.

Panleukopenia is considered in the section on Infectious and parasitic diseases of the alimentary tract. **Mycotic colitis** has been reported in cats as a hemorrhagic ulcerative colitis with microvascular thrombosis and mucosal invasion by *Candida*, zygomycetes, or *Aspergillus*; these are probably secondary to colonic damage and leukopenia caused by FPLV. ***Clostridium piliforme*** is reported as a cause of mild mucosal colitis in kittens, also probably occurring primarily in kittens immuno-compromised by FPLV infection. The lesions include focal necrosis, dilation of crypts, exfoliation of epithelial cells, and neutrophilic inflammation. *C. piliforme* was recognized by histology, immunohistochemistry, and ultrastructure.

Necrotic colitis caused by *Entamoeba histolytica* and characterized by severe necrosis of the colon and cecum is described in cats; a similar condition in older cats with no apparent etiologic agent has been described, and is hypothesized to be secondary to ischemia. Transmural acute ulcerative colitis with heavy infiltration of neutrophils is the hallmark of ***Salmonella enterica*** sv. **Typhimurium** infection in cats; this is discussed with salmonellosis in the section on Infectious and parasitic diseases of the alimentary tract. ***Anaerobiospirillum*** sp. is also associated with ileocolitis in cats, is discussed later in the section on Bacterial diseases of the alimentary tract. Ulcerative **colitis** as seen in dogs is apparently very rare in cats. Granulomatous or pyogranulomatous foci in the wall of the colon or ileocecocolic junction associated with **feline infections peritonitis virus** may mimic a neoplasm.

Further reading

De Cock HE, et al. Ileocolitis associated with *Anaerobiospirillum* in cats. J Clin Microbiol 2004;42:2752-2758.

Feinstein RE, Olsson E. Chronic gastroenterocolitis in nine cats. J Vet Diagn Invest 1992;4:293-298.

Typhlocolitis in horses

The diagnosis of acute colitis/typhlocolitis in horses resolves mainly into the differentiation of salmonellosis, intestinal clostridial diseases, and Potomac horse fever (equine monocytic ehrlichiosis). Although acute colitis can be produced in horses by other agents, they are less common and the role of many of them remains not fully understood. Infectious colitis must also be differentiated from the sequelae of intestinal accidents, NSAID intoxication, and thromboembolism involving the large bowel.

Salmonellosis in horses is most frequently associated with ***Salmonella enterica*** ssp. ***enterica*** serovar **Typhimurium**, although other serovars may be associated with sporadic cases of disease. Diarrhea is the main clinical sign of equine salmonellosis.

Equine intestinal clostridial diseases are increasingly well defined. In the past, many of these cases were lumped together in an umbrella category, *colitis X*, a term that was used to refer to severe acute colitis in which all known etiologic agents had been ruled out. This term should no longer be used as it does not describe a specific syndrome but rather a group of diseases in which a final diagnosis cannot be established. *Clostridium perfringens* type C and *Clostridium difficile* (Fig. 1-66) are the most common clostridial species responsible for equine clostridial enteric disease. *C. perfringens* type C occurs most commonly in neonates although disease in older horses occasionally can be seen; diarrhea is a frequent but not consistent clinical

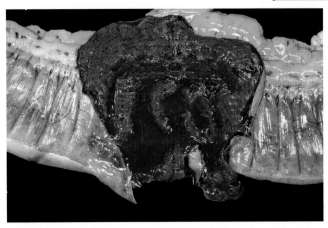

Figure 1-66 Acute necro-hemorrhagic colitis produced by ***Clostridium difficile*** in a horse.

sign, with sudden death the only sign in a few foals. *C. difficile* occurs in horses of any age and it almost invariably produces diarrhea regardless of the age of the affected animal.

Potomac horse fever usually results in diarrhea that does not exceed 10 days in duration; at autopsy there is congestion and ulceration of the mucosa of the large bowel, and enlargement of mesenteric lymph nodes.

Suppurative ulcers involving lymphoid tissue in the cecocolic mucosa, and cecal and colic lymphadenitis, characterize enteric infection with **Rhodococcus equi** in foals.

Other bacterial agents, including ***Clostridium sordellii***, ***Actinobacillus equuli***, and others, have been associated with acute colitis in horses, but definitive evidence of their role in these infections is lacking.

Subacute and chronic diarrhea in horses almost always involves the large intestine, with or without concomitant small-bowel involvement. **Salmonella** and **C. difficile** typhlocolitis must be suspected in such cases. Salmonellosis in horses may have an extremely variable course and pathologic manifestations (see section on Infectious and parasitic diseases of the alimentary tract). **Histoplasmosis** has been reported once in a horse with salmonellosis and ulcerative colitis. Extensive mucosal involvement by **larval cyathostomes and strongyles** and, rarely, ulcerative typhlitis resulting from **anoplocephalid tapeworms,** may also cause chronic diarrhea and wasting; these topics are discussed under specific parasitisms. Co-infection by *Listeria monocytogenes*, *Salmonella enterica* sv Typhimurium, and cyathostomes probably led to granulomatous typhlocolitis in a horse.

Ciliate protozoa may be seen over the colonic mucosa of horses dead of a variety of enteric and nonenteric problems; the protozoa are usually not associated with tissue inflammatory changes and are considered normal inhabitants of the intestine with no proven pathogenic role in enteric disease. Intralesional protozoa, however, have been reported in a horse with diffuse eosinophilic colitis.

Chronic diarrhea and possibly cachexia may also result from persistent ulceration of the cecum or colon caused by **ischemic mucosal lesions**. These may be the product of arterial thromboembolism and slow flow, or less likely, corrected strangulation with reflow. Use of NSAIDs also has been associated with cecal and colonic ulceration and plasma protein loss. *Right dorsal colitis*, in which ulcerative lesions are mostly limited primarily to the right dorsal colon, may be associated with colic, and acute or chronic diarrhea. This syndrome and others associated with the use of NSAIDs are considered with ischemia caused by reduced perfusion (see section on Intestinal ischemia and infarction). The specific cause of extensive ulceration may be difficult to determine. Smaller chronic ulcers and widespread subacute erosion and ulceration are most likely the result of salmonellosis, rather than ischemia. A history of administration of NSAIDs, and the presence of lesions in the renal papilla, mouth, and upper alimentary tract, suggests intoxication by those agents.

Further reading

Arroyo LG, et al. Experimental *Clostridium difficile* enterocolitis in foals. J Vet Intern Med 2004;18:734-738.

Diab SS, et al. Pathology of *Clostridium perfringens* type C enterotoxemia in horses. Vet Pathol 2012;49:255-263.

Diab SS, et al. Pathology and diagnostic criteria of *Clostridium difficile* enteric infection in horses. Vet Pathol 2013;50:1028-1036.

Donaldson MT, Palmer JE. Prevalence of *Clostridium perfringens* enterotoxin and *Clostridium difficile* toxin A in feces of horses with diarrhea and colic. J Am Vet Med Assoc 1999;215:358-361.

Nemeth NM, et al. Granulomatous typhlocolitis, lymphangitis, and lymphadenitis in a horse infected with *Listeria monocytogenes*, *Salmonella* Typhimurium, and cyathostomes. Vet Pathol 2013;50:252-255.

Songer JG, et al. Equine colitis X associated with infection by *Clostridium difficile* NAP1/027. J Vet Diagn Invest 2009;21:377-380.

Typhlocolitis in swine

The differential diagnosis of typhlocolitis in swine mainly revolves around identifying swine dysentery and other spirochetoses, *Salmonella* enterocolitis, and *Lawsonia intracellularis* infection.

Swine dysentery, caused by *Brachyspira hyodysenteriae*, involves only the cecum and spiral colon. It is a catarrhal to mildly fibrinohemorrhagic erosive mucosal typhlocolitis. The colonic content is fluid and usually blood-tinged. A similar but milder disease, **intestinal spirochetosis**, is associated with *B. pilosicoli*, which causes distinctive microscopic lesions as it colonizes the apex of surface epithelium. ***Salmonella* enterocolitis**, mainly resulting from *Salmonella* Typhimurium, is a fibrinous, erosive to focally ulcerative condition, mainly of the cecum and colon, but occasionally involving the small intestine, especially terminal ileum. The intestinal content is fluid but usually not bloody. Mesenteric lymph nodes are prominent. *L. intracellularis* infection is readily recognized by the consistent involvement of the terminal ileum by adenomatosis, with or without hemorrhage, or by necrotic ileitis.

Postweaning colibacillosis is characterized by catarrhal to mild fibrinohemorrhagic enterocolitis in piglets after weaning.

Fibrinohemorrhagic typhlitis is caused by heavy infestations with **Trichuris suis,** especially in weaned pigs with access to pastures and yards. Under similar circumstances, **Eimeria** infection may rarely cause ileotyphlocolitis.

Rectal stricture appears to be a product of ischemic proctitis, probably related in many cases to infection with *Salmonella* Typhimurium.

Clostridium perfringens type C and *C. difficile* are also increasingly important causes of enteritis with occasional typhlocolitis in neonatal piglets. They are both characterized by necrotizing or pseudomembranous inflammation, with

acute stages of *C. difficile* infection being suppurative and marked by characteristic mesocolonic edema. Details of these conditions are discussed in the section on Infectious and parasitic diseases of the alimentary tract.

Typhlocolitis in ruminants

Diagnostic considerations in cattle >2-3 months of age with acute to subacute fibrinohemorrhagic typhlocolitis include salmonellosis, bovine viral diarrhea, coccidiosis, adenoviral infection, and winter dysentery (coronavirus). Lesions of the oral cavity and upper alimentary tract may be expected, but are not necessarily present, in **bovine viral diarrhea** and **rinderpest**. **Bovine coronavirus** causes microscopic lesions in colonic crypts in cattle with **winter dysentery;** mild fibrinous typhlocolitis may be seen grossly. **Salmonellosis** affects all age groups from neonate to adult and may frequently involve both small and large intestine in catarrhal to fibrinohemorrhagic enteritis; mesenteric lymph nodes usually are enlarged. **Coccidiosis** may involve ileum and large intestine. **Bovine adenovirus** infection may cause severe hemorrhagic colitis, with few lesions elsewhere. **Arsenic**, other **heavy metals**, and **oak or acorn poisoning** also may cause hemorrhagic typhlocolitis and dysentery. Rarely, **trichuriasis** causes hemorrhagic mucosal typhlitis in calves.

Chronic fibrinous or ulcerative typhlocolitis may occur in salmonellosis, bovine viral diarrhea, and coccidiosis.

Granulomatous typhlocolitis associated with chronic diarrhea and wasting may occur in **Johne's disease,** concurrently with granulomatous ileitis and mesenteric lymphadenitis. The mucosa of the large bowel in these cases is thickened and rugose. Impressions of affected mucosa or ileocecal lymph node will contain acid-fast bacilli. Johne's disease in sheep and goats is usually associated with wasting, but often not diarrhea. The large bowel may be involved in a minority of cases; the ileum is consistently affected.

In **sheep,** hemorrhagic typhlocolitis may be present in animals with **bluetongue** and **peste des petits ruminants**; it is rarely the only lesion. **Salmonellosis** may cause fibrinohemorrhagic enteritis in lambs and pregnant ewes, and typhlitis caused by **trichuriasis** will occur rarely, although the presence of parasites in small numbers is common in weaners. **Coccidiosis** may be implicated in hemorrhagic ileotyphlocolitis in lambs and kids, although the small intestine is usually more commonly and severely involved. In goats, enterotoxemia caused by *C. perfringens* type D may cause moderate to severe fibrinonecrotic typhlocolitis, which occasionally extends to the terminal small intestine as well. Uremia may cause hemorrhagic lesions associated with vasculitis in the cecum and colon.

Neoplastic and proliferative lesions of the stomach and intestine

Tumors of the lower gastrointestinal tract are *not common* in domestic animals. However, they are relatively prevalent among surgical biopsy submissions from dogs and cats, in sharp contrast to their rarity in horses and food-producing animals. Malignant neoplasms are more common than benign tumors, and excepting lymphosarcoma, *most are carcinomas*. Polyps are generally hyperplastic rather than neoplastic. The exceptions are rectal polyps in dogs, which also can be adenomas or carcinomas. Highly malignant scirrhous adenocarcinomas of the stomach and intestine occur in all species. *Lymphosarcoma* is the most common malignant tumor of mesenchymal origin in most species. It may arise in the gut, although involvement of this area is often part of multicentric disease (see Vol. 3, Hematopoietic system). The third major category of gastrointestinal tumors is *stromal*, mainly phenotypically smooth muscle or undifferentiated.

Elaborate classification schemes have been proposed based on histologic or immunophenotypic characterization with, in many cases, little evidence that they are relevant to the biological behavior of the tumor or its response to therapy. Furthermore, there is often so much variation within these lesions that it is difficult to make them conform to arbitrary categories. However, it is important to recognize the range in appearance inherent in the various neoplasms, so that they may be diagnosed correctly, in a clinically meaningful way.

The 2003 World Health Organization *Histological Classification of Tumors of the Alimentary System of Domestic Animals* lists >50 specific neoplastic entities and >15 additional tumor-like lesions of the lower gastrointestinal tract. *The pragmatic classification of neoplasms and proliferative lesions outlined in Table 1-1 is considerably simpler.* This classification, and the discussion arising from it, is based upon several fundamental principles:

Any classification of neoplasms should be:
- The simplest that is compatible with our current understanding of tumor biology, including therapeutic and prognostic information;

Table • 1-1

Major neoplasms and tumor-like proliferative lesions of the lower gastrointestinal tract of domestic animals[*]

Epithelial
- Benign
  - Papillary adenomatous hyperplasia
  - Gastric pyloric mucosal hypertrophy
  - Canine rectal papillary adenoma
- Malignant
  - Gastrointestinal adenocarcinoma
  - Neuroendocrine carcinoma (carcinoid)
  - Gastric squamous cell carcinoma

Stromal
- Benign
  - Leiomyoma
- Malignant
  - Leiomyosarcoma
  - Gastrointestinal stromal tumor

Round Cell
- Benign
  - Plasmacytoma
- Malignant
  - Malignant lymphoma (lymphosarcoma)
  - Mast cell tumor
  - Malignant plasmacytoma

Neoplasms Metastatic to the Gastrointestinal Tract

[*]Because most of these tumors are histologically and behaviorally similar regardless of where they occur in the lower gastrointestinal tract, where appropriate the tumor name can simply be preceded by the adjective gastric, intestinal, or colonic.

- Based on easily observed and objective features to allow a high degree of interobserver agreement when in use; and
- Easily adaptable in response to new information about significant differences in behavior or response to therapy.

There appears to be no significant difference in the histologic appearance or the biological behavior of the various neoplasms based on their site of origin in the lower gastrointestinal tract, that is, there is no reason to consider colonic adenocarcinomas (or lymphomas) separately from small intestinal or gastric adenocarcinomas. Prefixes such as "gastric" or "colonic" are used as descriptive anatomic terms only to aid in communication of results.

Further reading

Head KW, et al. Tumors of the alimentary tract. In: Meuten DJ, editor. Tumors in Domestic Animals. 4th ed. Ames, IA: Iowa State University Press; 2002. p. 401-482.

Head KW, et al. Histological Classification of the Tumors of the Alimentary System of Domestic Animals. World Health Organization International Histological Classification of Tumors of Domestic Animals, second series, vol. X. Washington, DC: Armed Forces Institute of Pathology, American Registry of Pathology; 2003. p. 1-257.

Gastrointestinal adenocarcinomas

The prevalence and distribution of gastrointestinal adenocarcinomas vary among species. In dogs, gastric carcinomas predominate; small intestinal and colonic carcinomas are relatively uncommon. In contrast, gastric carcinoma is rare in cats, but small intestinal and colonic adenocarcinomas are relatively common. In other species, where they are generally rare, gastrointestinal adenocarcinomas also involve mainly small intestine.

The microscopic appearance is similar, regardless of species or location. A few develop as tubular and papillary proliferations of differentiated columnar epithelial cells projecting into the intestinal lumen. This is perhaps most commonly seen with colonic carcinomas in cats. Such lesions are distinguished from rare papillary adenomatous hyperplasia because *they have at least some invasion into the lamina propria, submucosa, or tunica muscularis.* Such invasion cannot be appreciated with endoscopic biopsies, and these papillary carcinomas sometimes cannot be distinguished from benign adenomatous hyperplasia or papillary adenomas without full-thickness surgical biopsies. This becomes particularly relevant when trying to distinguish the very common rectal papillary adenoma from the occasional, truly malignant, papillary carcinoma arising in the distal colon or rectum of dogs.

The earliest recognizable histologic lesion of gastrointestinal carcinomas, regardless of the location, is local effacement or obliteration of glandular mucosal architecture at the site of origin by proliferating polygonal mucus-producing epithelial cells. These cells infiltrate the lamina propria, and then invade sequentially through the submucosa and tunica muscularis, infiltrating into lymphatics, and sometimes veins. They penetrate the serosa and exfoliate into the peritoneal cavity to establish neoplastic implants on omentum and mesentery. The tumor also spreads early via lymphatic and venous routes, so that even surgical excision on discovery is rarely curative, because it is too late to prevent metastasis.

The microscopic appearance of the invading tumor can be quite variable, and usually more than one histologic subtype occurs within the same neoplasm. There is no proven prognostic or therapeutic significance to the different histologic patterns. *Most are scirrhous, mucus-producing carcinomas* that can create mucus-filled epithelial lakes throughout the intestinal wall, accompanied by what is often a great deal of fibrous stromal proliferation. The degree of cytologic maturation may be high, yet the diagnosis of carcinoma is obvious, given the transmural invasive behavior. Less commonly, the tumor cells invade in a tubular or acinar pattern, which tends to be less scirrhous, or as scattered individual anaplastic epithelial cells, accompanied by a great deal of desmoplastic fibrous tissue, so that recognizing carcinoma (in contrast to stromal malignancy or postinflammatory reactive fibrosis) may be challenging. In almost all cases, however, the tumor cells produce mucus, which may be revealed by periodic acid-Schiff staining. Formation of *signet ring cells* (an epithelial cell with the nucleus displaced to the periphery by a single large clear cytoplasmic vacuole) is relatively common.

The histologic diagnosis is best made with a *full-thickness biopsy.* The submucosal and transmural portions of the tumor are routinely larger and more readily identified as malignancy than the mucosal portion of the tumor, which endoscopic biopsies may not capture.

Alternatively, especially when large deep ulcerative lesions are biopsied endoscopically, only the necrosis, inflammation, and fibrosis that accompany neoplastic cells may be captured. On the other hand, a false-positive diagnosis may be made when attempting to distinguish early carcinoma (especially gastric carcinoma) from dysplastic repair of recent ulceration; in such cases, a full-thickness biopsy to detect invasion is more reliable than the best endoscopic sample.

Adenocarcinoma of the stomach is most frequently reported in **dogs,** usually in animals <10 years of age. It is the most common gastrointestinal adenocarcinoma in dogs, and the most common gastric neoplasm in that species. Males predominate in the population with gastric cancer, and more than half of gastric adenocarcinomas in dogs occur in the pyloric region. Breed predisposition has been reported in multiple breeds including the Tervuren, Bouvier des Flandres, Groenendael, Collie, Standard Poodle, and Norwegian Elkhound. In the Lundehund, there may be a relationship to the chronic gastritis common in that breed, but otherwise no causal association is recognized in dogs.

The antrum and pylorus are common sites for development of gastric adenocarcinoma in the dog. Grossly, some gastric neoplasms appear as nonulcerating, firm thickenings involving most of the gastric wall and causing loss of the normal rugal pattern on the mucosal surface (Fig. 1-67). Others are more localized plaque-like thickenings that tend to obliterate rugae and ulcerate centrally. Ulceration occurs in more than half of canine gastric adenocarcinomas. Surface proliferation or irregularity other than ulceration is very uncommon in gastric carcinoma in dogs. Cut sections through the stomach wall invaded by carcinoma reveal edema and pale, firm fibrous tissue. Induration or plaque-like pale masses may be evident on the serosa, where the pale outline of infiltrated lymphatics may be prominent. Widespread gastric mural fibrosis and thickening, the result of desmoplasia induced by the malignant epithelium, cause *linitis plastica,* the so-called "leather bottle" appearance.

Gastric carcinomas in dogs infiltrate the stomach wall aggressively, invading lymphatics, and usually they have metastasized to the local lymph nodes, and often to distant organs,

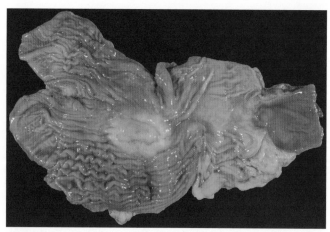

Figure 1-67 Gastric adenocarcinoma in a dog. (Courtesy M. Stalker.)

particularly lung, liver, and adrenal, by the time they are diagnosed.

Rare cases of gastric adenocarcinoma are described in **cats.** They adopt tubular and diffuse patterns, and behave typically, but are so rare that a diagnosis of carcinoma should be made only on a full-thickness surgical biopsy or autopsy specimen. Endoscopic samples suggestive of gastric carcinoma in cats are almost always foci of adenomatous hyperplasia upon further investigation.

Gastric adenocarcinoma in **cattle** is exceptionally uncommon, but when it occurs it resembles similar tumors in other species.

Intestinal adenocarcinomas are uncommon in **dogs;** they occur most frequently in the proximal small intestine and large bowel of animals averaging 8-9 years old. Some investigators have reported a slightly higher prevalence of intestinal carcinomas in males, with a breed predisposition in Boxers, Collies, Poodles, and German Shepherds. Weight loss, persistent vomiting, anorexia, emaciation, and abdominal distention are the most common signs when the tumor is located in the small intestine. Dogs with colorectal tumors have large-bowel diarrhea, tenesmus, hematochezia, and dyschezia. Many dogs with intestinal carcinomas are anemic on account of hemorrhage from ulcerating tumors.

Macroscopically, the tumors appear as gray-white, firm, sometimes annular, stenotic areas that commonly affect the entire thickness of the intestinal wall. These tumors often do not ulcerate, and they usually do not project into the lumen of the gut. Papillary or polypoid intestinal adenocarcinomas do form intraluminal masses, which tend to involve larger segments of the intestine, suggesting horizontal spread. There is dilation of the gut proximal to stenotic and obstructive tumors and there may be hypertrophy of the intestinal muscularis proximal to such neoplasms.

These tumors metastasize widely, mainly via the lymphatics (Fig. 1-68). Involvement of the small intestine leads to metastases mainly in the mesenteric lymph nodes, less commonly to other abdominal nodes, liver, spleen, and lungs. Histologic evidence of metastasis at the time of resection of small intestinal tumors predicts a markedly reduced postsurgical survival time, but even dogs without such evidence may succumb to metastatic disease, albeit with longer survival.

Colonic adenocarcinomas metastasize to colonic, iliac, and other pelvic and abdominal nodes. Metastases also may occur

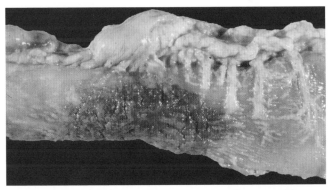

Figure 1-68 Adenocarcinoma of rectum in a dog. Serosal hemorrhage, and plaque-like masses of desmoplastic fibrous tissue and neoplastic cells on the serosa and along serosal lymphatics draining to the mesentery.

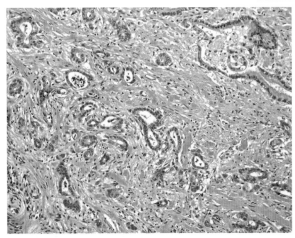

Figure 1-69 Colon adenocarcinoma in a cat.

in most abdominal organs and the lungs. Implantation on serosal surfaces may result in obstruction of omental and diaphragmatic lymphatics, leading to ascites. In a few cases malignant cells may spread retrograde in the lymphatics of the abdomen and pelvic limbs, causing edema of the abdominal wall and legs. Dogs with annular colorectal carcinomas have a much shorter survival period compared to dogs that have a single, pedunculated polypoid tumor in this location. The etiopathogenesis of colonic carcinomas in dogs is uncertain, but there appears to be progression to malignancy from benign adenomatous lesions in at least some instances. Colorectal adenocarcinoma in the dog has been used as a model of human colon cancer with common features in tumorigenesis being identified. β-Catenin and cyclooxygenase-2 are overexpressed in malignant colonic epithelial cells in some cases, as they are in humans. In addition, adenomatous polyposis coli (APC), a protein encoded by the tumor suppressor gene *APC*, is frequently altered in sporadic canine colon adenomas and adenocarcinoma as it is in human colon tumors and changes in this gene may be an early event in tumor development.

In cats, intestinal adenocarcinoma is less prevalent than lymphosarcoma, but it is relatively more prevalent in cats than in dogs. Carcinomas of the intestine are more prevalent in Siamese cats than in other breeds. As in dogs, a higher prevalence of this tumor has been reported in males than females. The mean age of cats with intestinal carcinomas is 10-11 years.

The ileum is the most common site affected, followed by the jejunum. Carcinomas occasionally arise in the large intestine, and when the tumor is located at the ileocecal junction, both the large and small intestine usually are involved. The clinical signs and gross appearance are similar to those in dogs.

The microscopic appearance of intestinal carcinomas in cats is typical (Fig. 1-69), except that osteochondroid metaplasia of the stroma may be a feature. The rare carcinomas involving the large intestine have tended to be papillary, better differentiated, and less scirrhous than carcinomas involving the small intestine.

Intestinal adenocarcinoma is relatively common in **sheep** in New Zealand, the United Kingdom, Scotland, Iceland, Norway, and southeastern Australia; in New Zealand and Australia there is a high prevalence in breeds used for fat lamb production. The cause of the high prevalence is unknown, but may be related to exposure to bracken fern or other unidentified carcinogens. Other associations, such as heavy use of

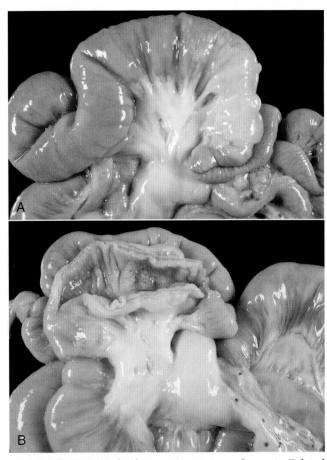

Figure 1-70 Intestinal adenocarcinoma in a sheep. A. Dilated segments in the small intestine. **B.** Cut section of (**A**). (Courtesy K.G. Thompson.)

certain fertilizers, and pastures with the weed *Cynosaurus cristatus*, have been reported from New Zealand. Tumors occur mainly in animals ≥5 years of age. Clinically affected sheep lose weight and have abdominal distention caused by ascites, but most cases are incidental findings at slaughter.

The tumors are usually located in the middle or lower small intestine (Fig. 1-70), rarely in the colon. They are dense, firm, white masses, 0.5 to several centimeters long and up to 1 cm thick, which may form annular constrictive bands at the affected site. Cauliflower-like growths may be evident on the serosal surface. Polyps or plaques may protrude into the lumen, but ulceration of the mucosa is uncommon. The distal edge of the tumor is generally well demarcated. There is dilation of the intestine proximal to the lesion. Metastatic implantations on serosal surfaces are common and these appear as opaque to white plaques or diffusely thickened areas, which must be differentiated from mesothelioma. Obstruction of serosal lymphatics by tumor emboli may lead to ascites. Lung and liver metastases are rare.

Microscopically, the tumor is characterized by solid sheets or nests of well-differentiated to highly anaplastic polyhedral, cuboidal, or columnar epithelial cells that may form irregular acinar structures. They may be distributed singly, or in small aggregates, and are often difficult to detect in the heavy fibrous desmoplastic response. The neoplastic cells infiltrate the bowel wall along lymphatics, vessels, and nerve trunks, through to the serosal surface, whence they spread to the mesenteric lymph nodes. This is apparently followed by retrograde lymphogenous metastasis to the gut wall proximal to the primary tumor. These secondary tumors are particularly responsible for constriction of the gut lumen. Sclerotic masses with anaplastic epithelial cells, many of which are periodic acid-Schiff–positive, are located on the serosal surfaces of the abdominal organs but rarely infiltrate the parenchyma. Argentaffin cells may form part of some intestinal carcinomas, especially in lymph node metastases. Mineralization and osseous metaplasia may develop in the stroma.

Intestinal carcinomas are generally rare in **cattle** (Fig. 1-71), **goats, horses,** and **swine.** In horses, intestinal adenocarcinomas represent <1% of equine neoplasms and are found less frequently than intestinal lymphoma. In cattle, intestinal adenocarcinoma is associated with bracken fern, papillomavirus, and upper alimentary cancer (see section on Neoplasia of the esophagus and forestomachs). Most of these tumors in cattle are **adenomas** and three types are recognized: (1) a sessile plaque; (2) an adenomatous polyp; and (3) a more proliferative adenoma of the ampullae in which the bile and pancreatic ducts open into the duodenum. Intestinal carcinomas are usually an incidental finding at meat inspection. The location, morphology, and routes of metastasis are similar to those described for sheep, except that serosal lesions are less obvious.

Hematogenous spread to the liver, lung, kidney, uterus, and ovaries may occur in cattle.

Further reading

Birchard SJ, et al. Nonlymphoid intestinal neoplasia in 32 dogs and 14 cats. J Am Anim Hosp Assoc 1986;22:533-537.

Church EM, et al. Colorectal adenocarcinoma in dogs: 78 cases (1973–1984). J Am Vet Med Assoc 1987;191:727-730.

Cribb AE. Feline gastrointestinal adenocarcinoma: a review and retrospective study. Can Vet J 1988;29:709-712.

Johnstone AC, et al. Small intestinal carcinoma in cattle. N Z Vet J 1983;31:147-149.

Seim-Wikse T, et al. Breed predisposition to canine gastric carcinoma–a study based on the Norwegian canine cancer register. Acta Vet Scand 2013;55:25.

Taylor SD, et al. Intestinal neoplasia in horses. J Vet Intern Med 2006;20:1429-1436.

Youmans L, et al. Frequent alteration of the tumor suppressor gene APC in sporadic canine colorectal tumors. PLoS ONE 2012;7:e50813.

Adenomatous hyperplasia/papillary adenoma/polyps

Adenomatous hyperplasia occurs as focal papillary or papillotubular proliferation of surface epithelium anywhere in the gastrointestinal tract. In the stomach (Fig. 1-72), it is to be distinguished from chronic hypertrophic pyloric gastropathy, discussed with pyloric obstruction.

The most common site is the distal rectum of middle-aged **dogs,** within 10 cm of the anal-rectal margin. Given a variety of names, such as *adenomatous hyperplasia, papillotubular adenoma, colorectal polyp or adenoma,* and *polypoid carcinoma in situ,* we refer to it as **rectal papillary adenoma.** It occurs in dogs of almost any age, and is usually a single nodule easily managed by adequate surgical excision. Tenesmus, prolapse of the polyp, rectal bleeding following defecation, chronic dyschezia, and diarrhea are the most common signs. Some, but not all, surveys indicate that this tumor is more common in males.

Macroscopically, the tumor is usually sessile or slightly pedunculated, varying from 1 cm to several centimeters in

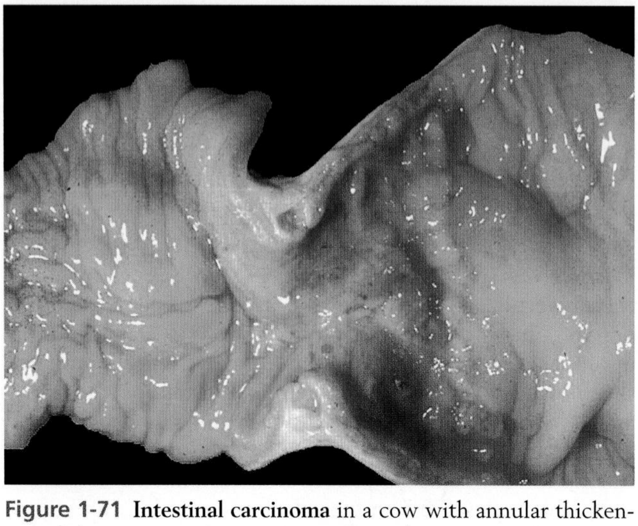

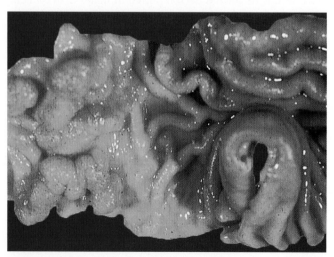

Figure 1-71 Intestinal carcinoma in a cow with annular thickening of the intestine. (Courtesy Noah's Arkives.)

Figure 1-72 Mucosal polyps in the pylorus of a dog. (Courtesy Noah's Arkives.)

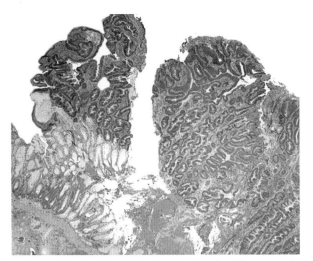

Figure 1-73 **Rectal papillary adenoma** in a dog, showing tubulo-papillary microscopic architecture.

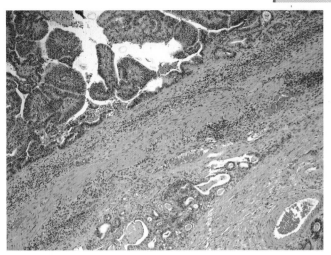

Figure 1-74 **Invasive carcinoma in the colon of a dog.** A polypoid mass is present along the surface and neoplastic cells invade into the underlying submucosa and muscularis.

diameter. It may be firm or friable and hemorrhagic; the mucosal surface is often ulcerated.

Microscopically, the polyp may have a predominantly tubular or papillary growth pattern (Fig. 1-73). In well-oriented specimens the tubular pattern is characterized by branching crypts that are lined by generally well-differentiated columnar-to-cuboidal pseudostratified epithelial cells. The papillary type consists of villus-like projections of proprial connective tissue that are covered by a layer of pseudostratified columnar epithelial cells. There may be cytoplasmic basophilia, loss of nuclear polarity, and prominent nucleoli in epithelium in both types of polyps. The number of mitotic figures varies, often within the same polyp. These tumors often appear to originate in the superficial portion of the crypts, deeper portions of which may remain normal, with tubules or slender papillae of hyperchromatic tumor cells above them. The stalk of the tumor is highly vascular and is continuous with the lamina propria or submucosa of the rectum. The tumors are generally well demarcated from the adjacent normal mucosa. The amount of mucin in the epithelium varies considerably, and it is often absent, especially in more dysplastic cells. Some polyps have a malignant appearance histologically. These are characterized by the presence of anaplastic epithelial cells in situ in the mucosa, and, in some cases, invading the propria and adjacent submucosa (Fig. 1-74).

There is limited information on the *biological behavior* of these tumors. In dogs, adequate surgical removal usually results in complete recovery. Some are interpreted at presentation as carcinoma in situ, based on cytologic characteristics, and deep biopsies and/or complete excision of these polyps are essential to rule out local invasion or infiltration of lymphatics, which should be sought in specimens with epithelial morphology suggesting malignancy. Polyps that are >1 cm in diameter tend to have cells with a more anaplastic appearance, and recurrence is most probable in cases interpreted as carcinoma in situ, those with multiple masses, or those with more diffuse colonic involvement.

In other species, polypoid and adenomatous tumors are uncommon. Benign adenomatous polyps are reported in the stomach and duodenum of **cats,** predominantly middle-aged males of Asian breeds. They are presented with vomition,

hematemesis, and possibly anemia. Excision is curative. These lesions can be confused with papillary adenocarcinomas if sampled only by endoscopic biopsy.

In **cattle,** intestinal polyps are usually an incidental finding, except in those cases in which they are large enough to cause partial obstruction. The tumors are raised, often pedunculated, gray-to-brown masses on the mucosal surface. They may occur singly, in grape-like clusters, or they may be scattered. Microscopically they resemble benign rectal polyps in the dog, but they may be capable of malignant transformation (see earlier in this chapter).

Adenomatous polyps frequently occur in **sheep** with intestinal carcinoma. Hyperplastic polyps occur in the small intestines of **lambs** and **goats** with chronic coccidiosis (see section on Infectious and parasitic diseases of the alimentary tract).

The proliferative lesions caused by *Lawsonia intracellularis* in horses and swine may impart a polypoid appearance to the intestinal mucosa grossly, and microscopically should not be mistaken for adenomatous neoplasia.

Further reading

Igarashi H, et al. Polypoid adenomas secondary to inflammatory colorectal polyps in 2 miniature dachshunds. J Vet Med Sci 2013;75:535-538.

MacDonald JM, et al. Adenomatous polyps of the duodenum in cats: 18 cases (1985–1990). J Am Vet Med Assoc 1993;202:647-651.

Patterson-Kane JC, et al. Small intestinal adenomatous polyposis resulting in protein-losing enteropathy in a horse. Vet Pathol 2000;37:82-85.

Valerius KD, et al. Adenomatous polyps and carcinoma in situ of the canine colon and rectum: 34 cases (1982–1994). J Am Anim Hosp Assoc 1997;33:156-160.

Gastrointestinal neuroendocrine carcinomas (carcinoids)

Carcinoids arise from neuroendocrine cells that are scattered in the mucosa of a wide variety of organs, including the stomach and the intestine. These cells secrete low-molecular-weight polypeptide hormones, such as secretin, somatostatin, and cholecystokinin, or they are part of the amine precursor uptake decarboxylation (APUD) group, producing compounds such as serotonin (5-hydroxytryptamine).

Carcinoid tumors of the gastrointestinal tract are *rare* in domestic animals. They have been reported mainly in aged dogs and very rarely in the cat, cow, and horse. In **dogs,** most carcinoids are located in the duodenum, colon, and rectum, and only rarely in the stomach and lower small intestine. Clinically, they may cause intestinal obstruction, and anemia resulting from ulceration and hemorrhage. Associated diarrhea in some cases can speculatively be attributed to hypersecretion of functional polypeptide hormones. Rectal carcinoids may protrude from the anus and resemble adenomatous polyps.

Macroscopically, carcinoids are usually lobulated, firm, dark-red to cream-colored masses a few millimeters to perhaps 2 cm in diameter. They seem to arise deep in the mucosa, often forming submucosal or subserosal nodules, perhaps with ulceration of overlying mucosa, and infiltrating transmurally and into the mesentery.

Microscopically, carcinoids have a *distinct endocrine appearance.* Round or oval to polyhedral cells have abundant finely granular eosinophilic or vacuolated cytoplasm and vesiculate nuclei with prominent nucleoli. They form nests, ribbons, rosettes, or diffuse sheets in the mucosa, submucosa, and muscularis. A fine vascularized fibrous stroma often divides the tumor masses into pseudoalveolar arrays. Amyloid may be present in intercellular and perivascular spaces. Uninuclear megalocytes and multinucleated giant cells are present occasionally.

A *diagnosis* of carcinoid is based on the endocrine histologic pattern, cytoplasmic argentaffinic and argyrophilic granularity, immunohistochemical identification of specific secretory products, and the typical ultrastructural appearance. The histochemical reactions may be negative, especially in rectal carcinoids, and they also may be lost during fixation in formalin or by autolysis prior to fixation, as may immunohistochemical reactivity. These cells are routinely positive with immunohistochemical staining for neuron-specific enolase and chromogranin, as are most neuroendocrine tumors, and then with one or more of the specific immune probes related to the peptides being produced. An increased concentration of specific secretory products may be detected in circulation.

Electron microscopic examination helps to differentiate carcinoids from intestinal mast cell tumors. Carcinoid cells have dense, round-to-oval, membrane-bound secretory granules in the cytoplasm, which vary in diameter from 75 to 300 nm. They have abundant rough endoplasmic reticulum and the plasma membrane forms interdigitating processes. Carcinoid cells are Schiff-negative and do not show metachromasia with Giemsa stains.

Data on biological behavior of intestinal carcinoids in dogs are limited. Most cases reported have been malignant. There may be extensive invasion of the gut wall and veins, with metastasis, especially to the liver. The few cases that have been described in other species have features similar to those described in dogs.

Goblet cell carcinoids (adenocarcinoids, mucinous carcinoids) are tumors that are most commonly found in the appendix of humans, with features of both carcinoids and adenocarcinomas. There is a single report of such a tumor in the rectum of a dog. Microscopically goblet cell carcinoids have distinct areas of mucinous adenocarcinoma and carcinoid

that may merge. The carcinoid component is most prominent in the primary tumor and the metastases.

Further reading

Albers TM, et al. A poorly differentiated gastric carcinoid in a dog. J Vet Diagn Invest 1998;10:116-118.

Michishita M, et al. Poorly differentiated rectal carcinoid in a cow. Vet Pathol 2007;44:414-417.

Modlin IM, et al. Current status of gastrointestinal carcinoids. Gastroenterol 2005;128:1717-1751.

Sako T, et al. Immunohistochemical evaluation of a malignant intestinal carcinoid in a dog. Vet Pathol 2003;40:212-215.

Gastric squamous cell carcinomas

Squamous cell carcinomas derived from the mucosa of the pars esophagea are the most common gastric tumor in **horses.** They occur predominantly in middle-aged or older animals, which are usually presented in an advanced state, with unexplained anorexia, occasionally dysphagia, and weight loss sometimes progressing rapidly to emaciation. At autopsy there may be peritoneal effusion, and there is usually evidence of the neoplasm as plaques of proliferative or scirrhous tissue on the serosa of the stomach. There also may be peritoneal implants, especially on intestine, testes, omentum, parietal abdominal surfaces, and diaphragm; direct extension to adjacent organs, including liver, spleen, and diaphragm, with progression to the pleural space; and sometimes distant metastases, usually in liver and lung. The appearance of the tumor on serosal surfaces resembles mesothelioma, with smooth creamy plaques or nodules up to 2-4 cm in diameter.

The origin of these lesions is usually a fungating cauliflower-like mass 10-40 cm in diameter, with superficial fissures, projecting above the surface of the pars esophagea (Fig. 1-75). Sometimes these lesions are superficially more ulcerative than proliferative. Necrosis and hemorrhage are evident in the tumor mass, which is usually well demarcated from adjacent normal squamous mucosa. Occasionally the tumor extends into the distal esophagus, and may obstruct it. Microscopically, these neoplasms are typical squamous cell carcinomas, invading in cords or nests of cells through the gastric wall. They

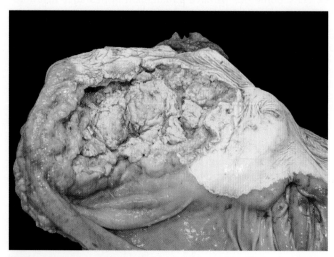

Figure 1-75 Squamous cell carcinoma arising from the gastric squamous mucosa of a horse.

induce desmoplasia, imparting a scirrhous, firm texture and appearance to the thickened gastric wall and to the peritoneal and pleural implants. One such tumor has been reported as a cause of pseudohyperparathyroidism in a horse.

A squamous cell carcinoma is reported arising from the pyloric gland mucosa in a dog.

Further reading

Patnaik AK, Lieberman PH. Gastric squamous cell carcinoma in a dog. Vet Pathol 1980;17:250-253.

Taylor S, et al. Gastric neoplasia in horses. J Vet Intern Med 2009;23:1097-1102.

Malignant lymphomas

Gastrointestinal lymphomas occur in most species and are common in **cats**. These neoplasms may be primary or part of the systemic or multicentric form of the neoplasm (see Vol. 3, Hematopoietic system). Primary lymphoma of the intestine includes cases having malignant lymphocytic infiltrates in the intestine, with or without involvement of the abdominal organs or bone marrow, but with no lesions in the thorax or peripheral sites.

Lymphoma is the most common gastrointestinal neoplasm in companion animals, more prevalent in cats than dogs. It can be segmental within any portion of the gastrointestinal tract, or diffuse. Although the gastrointestinal tract may be involved in advanced multicentric lymphoma in dogs, such cases are rarely submitted for biopsy because the diagnosis has already been made based on lesions elsewhere. Most samples submitted for histologic assessment are from cases suspected of having primary gastrointestinal lymphoma. In cats, almost all cases examined at biopsy are primary within the stomach or intestine.

In both species, spread outside intestine is usually to mesenteric lymph nodes and to liver, and less commonly beyond. In liver, the neoplasm infiltrates in a characteristic portal pattern that should not be mistaken for chronic portal hepatitis or lymphocytic cholangiohepatitis. In lymphoma, the tumor cells often form layers 10-20 deep in the portal tract, and cholangiolar proliferation, fibrosis, and hepatocellular atrophy are absent. In advanced hepatic disease, the cells also surround central veins. Although scattered tumor cells may occur within the sinusoids, a primarily sinusoidal distribution of lymphocytes signals lymphocytic leukemia rather than intestinal lymphoma.

The classification of lymphomas in animals is complex, integrating distribution, histologic and cytologic appearance, and immunophenotype. Most categories are based on lymphomas discovered in lymph nodes or skin; as a group, intestinal lymphomas have received little detailed investigation in this context. Most of the controversy about intestinal lymphoma is related not to its diagnosis, but rather to the relationship (if any) between its classification and subsequent behavior, including response to therapy; currently no clear association is evident.

In **dogs,** intestinal lymphoma can affect animals from adolescence to old age, with a male sex bias. Nonspecific signs of enteric disease and weight loss may be acute or occur over a period of weeks to months. Hypoproteinemia, probably associated with enteric protein loss, occurs in ~30% of affected dogs.

The tumors are located in the small intestine, stomach, and colon in that order of frequency. They are soft-to-firm, cream-colored masses located in the submucosa that may protrude into the gut lumen. The overlying mucosa may be ulcerated. The masses can be nodular to diffuse and several sections of the gut are usually affected. The mesenteric nodes are often enlarged and the liver is frequently involved at the time of presentation.

The majority of primary gastrointestinal lymphomas in dogs are *epitheliotropic T-cell tumors* based on immunohistochemical reactions, the remainder being mixed, B-cell, or indeterminate. Microscopically, in typical cases of epitheliotropic intestinal lymphoma, the mucosal, submucosal, and muscular architecture is effaced by a population of monotypic large lymphocytes with variable nuclear morphology and obvious mitotic activity. The crypts are effaced as they become infiltrated by neoplastic cells. In contrast to cats, alimentary lymphoma in dogs is usually large lymphoblastic type with small cell neoplastic infiltrates being uncommon.

The lesions of *very early lymphoma* are more challenging. They are distinguished from chronic inflammatory bowel disease by the *relatively monotypic lymphocyte population* and the *intraepithelial infiltration of lymphocytes* that obscures the distinction between lamina propria and epithelium. Even with these criteria, differentiation of early neoplastic from inflammatory disease can be problematic because residual plasma cells, eosinophils, and benign lymphocytes of the normal lamina propria persist among the neoplastic lymphocyte population. Similarly, not all cases of intestinal lymphoma exhibit epitheliotropic growth, and there is overlap between neoplastic epithelial invasion and the increase in intraepithelial lymphocytes that is commonly seen with inflammatory disease. The key is not just the presence of the lymphocytes, but the *obliteration of the proprial:epithelial boundary*. Once the lymphoma effaces crypts or invades submucosa, diagnosis should not be problematic, but full-thickness biopsies from several areas of the intestine may help differentiate chronic inflammatory bowel disease from intestinal lymphoma.

Lymphoplasmacytic enteritis in the dog, particularly the Basenji, may represent a prelymphomatous stage similar to immunoproliferative small intestinal disease in humans. The latter is characterized by diffuse lymphoplasmacytic infiltration of the small intestinal mucosa that results in malabsorption, and predisposes to the development of primary enteromesenteric lymphoma.

In **cats,** the situation is substantially more complicated. There are at least three histologic categories of gastrointestinal lymphoma, small cell lymphocytic villus lymphoma, large cell lymphoblastic lymphoma, and large granular cell lymphoma. The small cell lymphomas tend to have a longer clinical course, whereas the lymphoblastic (T- and B-cell) and large granular cell lymphomas are associated with more rapidly progressive disease. The jejunum may be the site of highest incidence of T-cell lymphoma in the cat.

Small cell lymphocytic villus lymphoma is a T-cell lymphoma that typically begins at the base of the villi within the small intestine of old cats, and is the most frequent type of intestinal lymphoma in geriatric cats. Clustering of suspiciously monotypic small hyperchromatic lymphocytes within the lamina propria just at the base of villi is an exceedingly common observation in cats 15 years of age and older. It is not clear whether this is incipient lymphoma or a normal finding. The number of such cells may vary substantially from villus to villus. As these clusters seem to expand, the lymphocytes infiltrate into the overlying epithelium, obliterating the distinction between lamina propria and epithelium. Unlike inflammatory bowel disease, such lesions may be very patchy, and there is no concurrent increase in plasma cells or eosinophils. With time, the lymphocyte population appears to expand throughout the lamina propria and then transmurally. Sixty percent of intestinal T-cell lymphomas have been reported to be epitheliotropic. Microscopically this is demonstrated by increased numbers of intraepithelial lymphocytes within villus and crypt epithelium. The syndrome shares substantial clinical overlap with inflammatory bowel disease in that it is often slowly progressive and it is usually not accompanied by clinical signs related to neoplastic infiltration of liver, spleen, or lymph node, even though there is often microscopic tumor within those organs. The extent of microscopic disease within the intestine is usually much greater than the macroscopic impression at the time of surgery. Determination of T-cell receptor (TCR) rearrangement clonality using PCR has been shown to be an accurate method of diagnosis of small cell lymphoma in cats.

Large cell/lymphoblastic lymphoma, in contrast, is characterized by a rapidly progressing transmural lesion that is usually accompanied by clinically palpable intestinal masses and by markedly enlarged mesenteric lymph nodes. Cats of any age may be affected. Most of these are reported as B-cell tumors, although not all investigators concur, and the majority of these high-grade lymphomas have not been subjected to immunophenotyping. It is likely that the incidence of T-cell lymphoma has been underestimated. B-cell lymphomas have been shown to be most common in the stomach and ileocecocolic junction, whereas T-cell lymphomas are most common in the proximal small intestine, especially the jejunum. The tumor resembles canine lymphomas, in that there is usually transmural effacement of intestinal architecture, and obliteration of the structure of affected mesenteric lymph nodes. Many cases differ from canine lymphomas, however, in having marked cellular pleomorphism. The tumor cells may have fairly abundant cytoplasm, nuclear cleavage, and up to 2-fold anisokaryosis. Descriptive names such as "histiocytic lymphoma" for some of these more anaplastic variants are no longer appropriate because immunophenotyping is available to identify the cells more precisely. Lesions are often sharply segmental and the primary lesion can be completely excised. However, the high prevalence of metastatic disease makes surgical cures rare.

Large granular lymphoma is usually a rapidly progressive intestinal lymphoma of cats. The tumor cells are either T cells or natural killer cells. These are medium-to-large lymphocytes with pleomorphic nuclei with frequent clefting. The distinctive features are the large red cytoplasmic granules, and perforin immunoreactivity. In the presence of cleaved nuclei, the large granules may be mistaken for those of eosinophils, but they are larger, rounder, and are more intensely eosinophilic. The cytologic characteristics have also caused such tumors to be attributed to globule leukocytes in the past. The granular cells are not present as a pure population. They are often intermingled with other lymphocyte types and with macrophages, so these invasive and destructive transmural lesions are sometimes confused with transmural granulomatous disease or mast cell tumors. These tumors progress rapidly, with widespread dissemination and even leukemia, and they may perforate affected areas of intestine.

In the **horse,** alimentary lymphoma is a relatively common tumor; most are attributed to *B lymphocytes*. It occurs mainly in young adults. Affected horses lose condition, likely because of malabsorption and protein loss; in addition they may be anemic, icteric, and have mild intermittent bouts of colic. Diarrhea is inconsistent. Serum albumin often can be decreased, but they are frequently hypergammaglobulinemic. Alimentary lymphoma in horses needs to be differentiated from inflammatory bowel disease.

Macroscopic lesions in horses are usually located in the small intestine, and these are characterized by local to diffuse thickening of the gut wall with prominent rugae on the mucosa. Nodules or plaques with fibrous adhesions may be evident on the serosa. The mesenteric nodes are markedly enlarged. Other nodes may be enlarged, but to a lesser extent. Microscopically, there is diffuse lymphoid infiltration of the lamina propria and submucosa, usually extending transmurally to the serosa. There is marked villus atrophy to the point of complete loss of villi and crypts. Plasmacytoid cells are regularly present in the lamina propria but less numerous in the submucosa. Similar lymphoid cell infiltration involves the mesenteric nodes and the perinodal connective tissue. Other lymph nodes are involved in about half the cases. A plasmacytoid or plasmacytic reaction and occasional giant cells are also present in the nodes. The neoplastic lymphoid cells are probably of B-cell origin and home into the gut-associated lymphoid tissue and the lamina propria of the small intestine.

Epitheliotropic T-cell lymphomas resembling those in dogs, and ulcerating large granular lymphomas caused by T cells, somewhat resembling those described in cats, also occur infrequently in horses. A T-cell lymphoma occurred concurrently with multisystemic eosinophilic epitheliotropic disease in a horse, prompting the suggestion that undetected T-cell lymphoma secreting interleukin-5 may underlie that syndrome. Paraneoplastic eosinophilia has also been associated with intestinal lymphosarcoma in the horse.

In **cattle** and **sheep,** alimentary lymphomas are generally part of the adult multicentric form of the disease, and the intestinal lesions resemble the effacing tumors described in other species. More important in cattle is lymphosarcoma of the abomasum, which is common in adult cattle. Diffuse mucosal and submucosal lymphocytic infiltrates or nodular proliferations may occur. Strategically placed pyloric tumor may cause obstruction. Diffuse lesions, thickening the gastric wall, frequently ulcerate, and hemorrhage from such ulcers, as melena, is a common sign. The lymphoid infiltrates are recognizable as firm gray-white tissue in the submucosa and mucosa. Involvement of abomasal lymph nodes is disproportionately slight.

In **swine,** diffuse gastric lymphosarcoma occurs. The wall of the stomach is thickened by submucosal lymphocytic infiltrates, which sometimes invade the mucosa locally in many areas, producing nodular elevations that may ulcerate. B-cell lymphomas involving the Peyer's patches also have been detected at meat inspection in swine.

Further reading

Coyle KA, Steinberg H. Characterization of lymphocytes in canine gastrointestinal lymphoma. Vet Pathol 2004;41:141-146.

Duckett WM, Matthews HK. Hypereosinophilia in a horse with intestinal lymphosarcoma. Can Vet J 1997;38:719-720.

Kiupel M, et al. Diagnostic algorithm to differentiate lymphoma from inflammation in feline small intestinal biopsy samples. Vet Pathol 2011;48:212-222.

Moore P, et al. Feline gastrointestinal lymphoma: mucosal architecture, immunophenotype, and molecular clonality. Vet Pathol 2012;49:658-668.

Pinkerton ME, et al. Primary epitheliotropic intestinal T-cell lymphoma in a horse. J Vet Diagn Invest 2002;14:150-152.

Pohlman L, et al. Immunophenotypic and histologic classification of 50 cases of feline gastrointestinal lymphoma. Vet Pathol 2009;46:259-268.

Willard M. Alimentary neoplasia in geriatric dogs and cats. Vet Clin North Am Small Anim Pract 2012;42:693-706.

Gastrointestinal mast cell tumors

These tumors are uncommon. They occur in aged dogs, and occasionally in cats, with signs such as vomition, diarrhea, and melena. They are seen in biopsies as invasive round cell tumors that can resemble carcinoids, lymphomas, and gastrointestinal stromal tumors; *definitive diagnosis requires histochemical and possibly immunohistochemical investigations.* Primary mast cell tumors of the gastrointestinal tract are comprised of mucosal mast cells, which differ from connective tissue mast cells, such as those found in skin, in having few granules, which usually do not stain well in formalin-fixed tissue. Abnormal mast cells do not appear in circulation in animals with these tumors.

Mast cell tumors are most commonly seen in stomach, and least common in the colon. Affected areas in the mucosa are tan-colored, firm, thickened, possibly ulcerated, and may be 1 cm to several centimeters in size. The tissue architecture is effaced by a population of granular round cells accompanied by variable numbers of eosinophils. They generally grow in infiltrative cords, but occasionally form endocrine-like packets surrounded by a delicate fibrovascular stroma. There is a wide range in the cytologic appearance. Some tumors are populated by fairly mature mast cells with abundant cytoplasmic granularity easily demonstrated with toluidine blue. Others are populated by anaplastic and pleomorphic round cells or spindle-shaped cells, sometimes with giant nuclei or forming syncytia, in which cytoplasmic granules with metachromatic staining, while present, may be difficult to observe. Those with abundant metachromatic granules must be differentiated from connective tissue mast cell tumors metastatic to the gastrointestinal tract, in which case lesions should be sought in skin and elsewhere. There can be marked variation in the number of eosinophils in the tumor, and they are not definitive because eosinophils are also common in some intestinal lymphomas, and as part of the background cell population in normal lamina propria. In cats, a subset of intestinal mast cell tumors is associated with a significant collagen stroma.

Gastrointestinal mucosal mast cell tumors are differentiated using a suite of histochemical and immunohistochemical characteristics. They have at least a few *metachromatic granules* when stained with toluidine blue, and many tumors have at least some cells that stain with alcian blue. They stain *immunohistochemically positive* for mast cell tryptase and c-KIT (CD117), but negatively for CD3 (distinguishing them from most T-cell lymphomas), cytokeratin (distinguishing them from carcinomas), and chromogranin and synaptophysin (distinguishing them from carcinoids). However, only 33% of feline gastrointestinal mast cell tumors were positive for c-KIT. Gastrointestinal stromal tumors should be positive for c-KIT, but cytology and lack of metachromatic granules when stained with toluidine blue differentiate them.

Ultrastructurally the cytoplasm of gastrointestinal mucosal mast cell tumor cells contains many membrane-bound granules that appear as single or fused vesicles. Fine fibrillar material forms a loose network within these vesicles. A few tumor cells contain electron-dense fibrillar granules or intermediate forms. The crystalline electron-dense granules that are present in connective tissue mast cells, such as those from the skin, are rarely evident.

Metastases occur most often in the mesenteric lymph nodes, followed by the liver, spleen, and, rarely, the lungs. Ulceration of the gastrointestinal mucosa occurs commonly with systemic tissue mast cell tumors in cats and with large cutaneous mastocytomas in dogs, owing to histamine stimulation of acid production by gastric parietal cells. Gastrointestinal ulceration is not a feature of mucosal mast cell tumors of intestinal origin, except perhaps as a result of mucosal effacement by the tumor.

Further reading

Halsey C, et al. Feline intestinal sclerosing mast cell tumour: 50 cases (1997-2008). Vet Comp Oncol 2010;8:72-79.

Mallett C, et al. Immunohistochemical characterization of feline mast cell tumors. Vet Pathol 2013;50:106-109.

Ozaki K, et al. Mast cell tumors of the gastrointestinal tract in 39 dogs. Vet Pathol 2002;39:557-564.

Extramedullary plasmacytomas

Plasmacytomas of the lower gastrointestinal tract are *uncommon neoplasms in dogs*, and rare in cats and other species. They are encountered most frequently in the submucosa of the distal colon and rectum of dogs, where they are associated with signs of large-bowel diarrhea and bleeding.

Histologically they resemble plasmacytomas of the skin, oral cavity, or larynx. The tumor is formed by solid packets of pleomorphic round cells with various degrees of plasmacytoid maturation, especially at the periphery of the tumor. There is frequent nuclear hyperchromasia and convolution. The cells are typically arranged in solid endocrine-like packets of 10-20 cells surrounded by a delicate fibrovascular stroma, and there may be AL amyloid deposition among the tumor cells. A few syncytial plasmacytoid or histiocytic cells may be evident. The majority of the tumor growth is submucosal, with a little bit of overflow into the deep half of the lamina propria. Most tumors have a discrete local growth habit amenable to surgical cure. A small proportion exhibit more aggressive behavior, including invasion of tunica muscularis, and some spread to regional lymph nodes and spleen, perhaps producing a monoclonal gammopathy.

Further reading

Platz SJ, et al. Prognostic value of histopathological grading in canine extramedullary plasmacytomas. Vet Pathol 1999;36:23-27.

Ramos-Vara JA, et al. Intestinal extramedullary plasmacytoma associated with amyloid deposition in three dogs: an ultrastructural and immunoelectron microscopic study. J Ultrastruct Pathol 1998;22:393-400.

Rannou B, et al. Rectal plasmacytoma with intracellular hemosiderin in a dog. Vet Pathol 2009;46:1181-1184.

Intestinal stromal tumors

The intestinal stromal tumors include leiomyoma, leiomyosarcoma, gastrointestinal stromal tumor, and very uncommon examples of almost every other type of stromal neoplasm, including hemangiosarcoma, nerve sheath tumors, fibroma and fibrosarcoma, osteosarcoma, and even lipoma. Ganglioneuromas have been described in dogs, a sow, horse, and a kitten. Other mesenchymal tumors include fibrous histiocytoma in a cow and histiocytic sarcoma in a dog.

Leiomyoma, leiomyosarcoma, and gastrointestinal stromal tumor are considered together, because recognition of the latter prompted re-evaluation of the criteria for diagnosis of leiomyosarcoma; older literature should be read with this in mind. Together, they are more common in dogs than other types of mesenchymal tumors except lymphosarcoma, and they also occur with some frequency in horses. Smooth-muscle tumors occur uncommonly in cats, equally prevalent in stomach, small intestine, and colon. They occur only rarely, if at all, in other species.

Leiomyoma and leiomyosarcoma represent the two extremes of a morphologic continuum, which included, toward the malignant end of the spectrum, tumors now classified as gastrointestinal stromal tumor. The latter are thought to be derived from interstitial cells of Cajal, or from a stem cell precursor to both those cells and smooth-muscle cells, and they are distinguished by expressing c-KIT (CD117) antigen. Although some may contain smooth-muscle actin, they rarely express desmin. Leiomyomas and leiomyosarcomas, on the other hand, do not express c-KIT, and should express smooth-muscle actin and desmin. *Immunohistochemical reactivity is the definitive means of differentiating these tumors*, but may be adversely affected by autolysis and duration of fixation, which must be considered in such studies. However, leiomyomas can be recognized based on their histology and cytology.

In **dogs,** as a group these tumors occur in older animals, in many of which they may be asymptomatic and incidental. Signs can include weight loss, lethargy, anorexia, anemia resulting from intestinal hemorrhage, abdominal pain, palpable abdominal masses, diarrhea, vomition, and dehydration or other signs of gastrointestinal obstruction. Based on limited studies in which the immunophenotype of stromal tumors of the gut has been determined, leiomyomas are most common and tend to occur in the esophagus and stomach of predominantly male dogs. Gastrointestinal stromal tumors are the next most common, and may occur in the stomach and intestine, with a tendency to predominate in the large bowel; sex distribution is equal. They have a spectrum of behavior from benign to malignant, and include tumors that were diagnosed as leiomyosarcomas before revision of terminology. Leiomyosarcomas are seemingly least common, and tend to occur in the intestine, with no apparent sex predisposition.

Most symptomatic tumors of this type are expansile nodules arising in the muscularis externa and can be cured by surgical excision, as is certainly the case with leiomyoma. However, a minority, perhaps up to 30%, of the other types have metastasized by the time that they are discovered.

Leiomyomas are sharply circumscribed masses of well-differentiated smooth-muscle cells, and generally lie beneath an intact mucosa, although they may deform the serosal or mucosal profile, and ulceration, perhaps related to pressure necrosis, can occur. They are comprised of swirling bundles of uniform fusiform cells, with abundant eosinophilic cytoplasm, and a central nucleus with blunt ends; usually no mitotic

figures are evident. Areas of coagulative necrosis may occur in the tumor mass.

Leiomyosarcomas often resemble leiomyomas grossly, but they are invasive rather than circumscribed, and may ulcerate mucosa. The cells resemble those in leiomyomas in general cytology, but there is usually some degree of anisokaryosis, multiple nucleoli, scattered bizarre nuclei, and obvious mitotic activity. There may be necrosis in the mass and a mild lymphocytic or eosinophilic inflammatory infiltrate.

Gastrointestinal stromal tumors may be demarcated and grow by expansion, sometimes forming exophytic nodules on the serosal surface, or they may be transmural and invasive. Overlying mucosa, although usually intact, may ulcerate. They are usually comprised of spindle cells arranged as interlacing fascicles, or in a storiform (whorling or matted) pattern, with oval nuclei, and a somewhat basophilic cytoplasm with indistinct boundaries. A minority of cases may have somewhat epithelioid tumor cells arranged in trabeculae or solid sheets, perhaps with a somewhat myxoid intercellular matrix, often infiltrating between normal smooth-muscle fascicles. Epithelioid tumors are thought to reflect some degree of neural differentiation, whereas a storiform pattern is considered to reflect a poor degree of differentiation. There may be nuclear pleomorphism in all patterns of tumor, and mitotic figures are usually evident and may be common. Hemorrhage or necrosis may be present within the tumor, and lymphocytic and/or eosinophilic infiltrates can occur.

The difficulty in determining the *prognosis* of these tumors in dogs has not changed with the recognition that the great majority are gastrointestinal stromal tumors rather than leiomyosarcomas. No objective criteria or nomenclature differentiate benign from malignant gastrointestinal stromal tumors. In humans, larger tumor size and high mitotic activity are considered to be poor prognostic indicators, but there are no data substantiating these tendencies in animals.

Invasion into the mucosa causes ulceration and cavitation on the luminal surface (Fig. 1-76), which may lead to perforation of the bowel. Even in the absence of perforation, microorganisms from the gut lumen may cause local abscessation and secondary septic peritonitis in which there is intermingling of suppuration, granulation tissue, and tumor cells. Based on studies carried out before revision of the nomenclature,

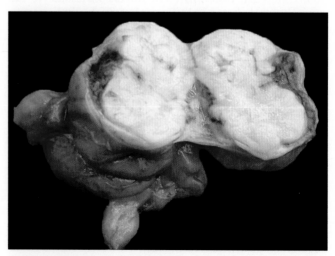

Figure 1-76 **Leiomyosarcoma** in the wall of the cecum obliterating the cecal lumen in a cat. (Courtesy M. Yaeger.)

tumors in cecum and colon, where gastrointestinal stromal tumors predominate, were determined to have a relatively high metastatic risk. They may metastasize to the mesenteric nodes, mesentery, and liver, but in general, these tumors have a more favorable prognosis after complete resection than other malignant neoplasms of the lower gastrointestinal tract.

The large intestinal tumors may also cause *paraneoplastic hypoglycemia,* owing to the production of insulin-like growth factors that may precipitate the search for a neoplasm. Production of erythropoietin, resulting in erythrocytosis, also has been documented.

In old **horses,** tumors of the intestine have been described that in many cases meet morphologic or immunohistochemical criteria for gastrointestinal stromal tumor, as it has been described above. Most are encountered incidentally, at surgery, meat inspection, or autopsy, but tumors of this type, or previously diagnosed as leiomyomas, may cause intermittent bouts of colic that become more frequent with time. They occur in the stomach, small intestine, and most frequently in the cecum and colon, as encapsulated, moderately firm, multinodular, pale tan, or hemorrhagic masses in the muscularis or subserosa, protruding on the serosal surface, or rarely, as somewhat pedunculated tumors projecting from the serosa or into the lumen. They may vary from 1 to >10 cm in diameter, and are usually solitary, but occasionally may be multiple. Malignancy is not described.

Further reading

Del Piero F, et al. Gastrointestinal stromal tumors in equids. Vet Pathol 2001;38:689-697.

Gillespie V, et al. Canine gastrointestinal stromal tumors: immunohistochemical expression of CD34 and examination of prognostic indicators including proliferation markers Ki67 and AgNOR. Vet Pathol 2011;48:283-291.

Hayes S, et al. Classification of canine nonangiogenic, nonlymphogenic, gastrointestinal sarcomas based on microscopic, immunohistochemical, and molecular characteristics. Vet Pathol 2013;50: 779-788.

Maas CP, et al. Reclassification of small intestinal and cecal smooth muscle tumors in 72 dogs: clinical, histologic, and immunohistochemical evaluation. Vet Surg 2007;36:302-313.

Morini M, et al. C-kit gene product (CD117) immunoreactivity in canine and feline paraffin sections. J Histochem Cytochem 2004;52:705-708.

Muravnick KB, et al. An atypical equine gastrointestinal stromal tumor. J Vet Diagn Invest 2009;21:387-390.

Russell KN, et al. Clinical and immunohistochemical differentiation of gastrointestinal stromal tumors from leiomyosarcomas in dogs: 42 cases (1990-2003). J Am Vet Med Assoc 2007;230:1329-1333.

Willard MD. Alimentary neoplasia in geriatric dogs and cats. Vet Clin North Am Small Anim Pract 2012;42:693-706.

APPROACH TO THE DIAGNOSIS OF GASTROINTESTINAL DISEASE

The diagnosis of gastrointestinal disease is facilitated by knowledge of the entities that may be expected in a particular species and age group, and the clinicopathologic syndromes with which they are associated. *In this section, etiologic entities associated with various syndromes in each domestic species are briefly summarized.* The salient diagnostic features of some conditions or the steps required at autopsy to confirm a diagnosis are discussed. The diseases causing gastritis, and those causing typhlocolitis in all species, have been discussed in previous sections. They are only briefly reiterated here; further information on the pathogenesis and diagnosis of most infectious and parasitic conditions is found in the next section.

Diarrhea in neonatal ruminants, swine, and horses

Diarrhea causing dehydration, metabolic acidosis, and electrolyte depletion is an important cause of morbidity and mortality in neonatal piglets, calves, lambs, and kids, and to a lesser extent in foals. Several classes of agents occur in most species of large animals, and mixed infections often occur, such as *Escherichia coli,* coronavirus, rotavirus, and *Cryptosporidium parvum.* These and some other less common agents produce diarrhea in neonatal animals, the etiology of which cannot be readily differentiated on clinical grounds or on the basis of gross postmortem examination.

Undifferentiated diarrhea of neonatal animals requires etiologic diagnosis if appropriate advice is to be rendered regarding prevention and management of the disease. Many of the agents involved are either transiently present or produce lesions such as villus atrophy that is easily obscured by autolysis, which significantly hinders accurate diagnosis. To overcome these obstacles, *one or more live untreated animals in the early phase of clinical disease and representative of the herd problem must be examined.* They should be euthanized and examined immediately using an autopsy procedure modified so that specimens of small intestine are formalin-fixed within a few minutes of death, and so that appropriate samples of tissue and content are quickly collected to facilitate a complete etiologic investigation.

The prevalence of diarrhea and potentially associated agents in neonates is expected to vary considerably on the basis of locality, climate, season, and the management system, as well as by species. The presence of specific microscopic lesions and their distribution within the intestine may suggest an etiology. Bacterial culture or rapid immunologic methods using gut content, formalin-fixed or frozen tissues may identify a bacterial or viral agent. Some agents, such as cryptosporidia and coccidia, may be identified in Giemsa-stained mucosal scrapings or tissue sections. In each species, undifferentiated neonatal diarrhea may be caused by other less common agents; therefore care is required to establish an accurate diagnosis, and to distinguish from other potential diseases that may occur in each species.

In all species, neonates succumbing to the effects of undifferentiated diarrhea are overtly *dehydrated.* The eyes are sunken in the orbits, the skin lacks elasticity, and the subcutis and mucous membranes are tacky. There is usually fecal staining on the perineum, but rare acute cases may display signs of dehydration without significant diarrhea. Animals with diarrhea may continue to suckle during the early phase of their illness; therefore a milk clot or curd may be present in the stomach and internal fat depots may be adequate. Animals that lose interest in feed because of more chronic disease and those taken off nutrients may have serous atrophy of fat and appear cachectic. The small intestine is flaccid and dilated with thin walls, and increased fluid content is present throughout the full intestinal length. The content is usually watery and clear green-yellow and often separates into 2 phases, the more solid of which appears to consist of small masses of

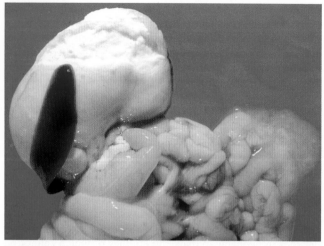

Figure 1-77 The stomach and intestines of a piglet with **undifferentiated neonatal diarrhea**; clotted milk fills the stomach, the small intestine is flaccid, and filled by floccular fluid content, with no gross evidence of inflammation.

clotted milk or mucus (Fig. 1-77). Sometimes the content is more homogeneous and creamy in texture; however, in animals examined sometime after death, this appearance is due to postmortem autolysis of the epithelium. The large intestine also contains fluid, creamy or pasty content, usually white or yellow. The mucosa of the small intestine may appear glistening and mildly congested; that in the large intestine is usually unremarkable. The forestomachs in ruminants that have been tube fed or in which the ruminoreticular groove has apparently failed to close, may contain sour fermented milk or milk replacer and the mucosa may be mildly reddened. The abomasal mucosa of some calves may contain scattered focal stress-associated hemorrhages. In piglets, urates may precipitate in the renal medulla and pelvis as the result of dehydration. The spectrum of agents associated with diarrhea in neonates of each species is considered later in this chapter.

Diarrhea in calves

Several infectious agents have been associated with undifferentiated diarrhea in calves less than ~3 weeks of age, some of which can be distinguished on the basis of gross lesions at postmortem examination. Frequently combinations of these agents occur together, or in sequence; compared with single agent infections, the consequences of combined infections often appear to be more severe. The diagnosis of these infectious problems in a herd can be complex, and examination of more than one untreated animal early in the course of disease is desirable. Causes of noninfectious diarrhea should be considered and eliminated; usually these involve nutritional or management problems.

Enterotoxigenic E. coli *is probably the most common single cause of undifferentiated neonatal diarrhea in neonatal calves.* Little or no morphologic change may be evident in tissue section, although bacteria are seen attached to the surface of enterocytes on villi. The disease usually occurs within the first 4 days of life, and is confirmed using culture along with molecular techniques to identify virulence factors and toxins. Enterotoxigenic colibacillosis is distinct from the less-common **enteropathogenic colibacillosis**, which occurs in older calves and is caused by attaching and effacing *E. coli*, and from **septicemic colibacillosis** or other gram-negative infections seen

in hypogammaglobulinemic neonates. **Enterohemorrhagic colibacillosis**, caused by **Shiga toxin (verotoxin) producing *E. coli***, seen as fibrinohemorrhagic enterocolitis, occurs in calves usually within the first 2 weeks of life.

Rotavirus and **bovine coronavirus** are common, and responsible for a significant proportion of neonatal calf diarrhea, alone, together, or in combination with other agents. Disease caused by these viruses may begin at any time in the first 1 or 2 weeks of life. Both viruses produce villus atrophy by causing lysis or exfoliation of surface enterocytes. Recent prevalence data suggest that bovine rotavirus group A plays a primary role in neonatal calf diarrhea. Bovine coronavirus also commonly causes microscopic and occasionally gross lesions in the colon. Both agents may be confirmed by demonstration of viral antigen or nucleic acids in feces or intestinal epithelial cells.

Cryptosporidium parvum, a minute apicomplexan protist, is very commonly associated with undifferentiated diarrhea and villus atrophy in calves often along with other pathogens, particularly viruses. It is most common in animals ~4-20 days of age. Cryptosporidia organisms can be identified in their intracellular but extracytoplasmic location, along the brush border of epithelium on villi, and in mucosal smears, fecal smears, or flotations.

Beta toxin–producing **Clostridium perfringens** type C infection can occur in calves, and causes acute hemorrhagic and necrotizing enteritis with enterotoxemia. Confirmation is by detection of beta toxin in the intestinal contents or feces by ELISA. **Clostridium perfringens** type B may be a rare cause of hemorrhagic enteritis in neonatal calves. **Clostridium perfringens** type A also has been suggested to cause necrotizing and hemorrhagic enterocolitis in calves; however, it is a common inhabitant in normal calf intestine and its role as a primary pathogen remains unclear.

Salmonellosis, usually caused by *Salmonella enterica* serovar Typhimurium, or *S.* Dublin or *S.* Muenster in enzootic areas, occurs in calves as young as 4 or 5 days of age. Salmonellosis may mimic undifferentiated neonatal diarrhea, particularly in peracute cases; later there is often development of fibrinous and necrotizing enterocolitis, with septicemia in a proportion of cases.

Bovine herpesvirus 1 (infectious bovine rhinotracheitis virus) in calves <2 weeks of age causes multifocal necrotizing lesions throughout the gastrointestinal tract; these are often seen together with lesions in other organs because of systemic infection. **Bovine viral diarrhea virus** can be implicated in enteritis of calves as young as 1 week of age, on the basis of microscopic lesions in the small intestine and colon similar to those found in older animals, with confirmation by virus isolation or detection of viral antigen or nucleic acid.

Bovine torovirus (formerly Breda virus), in genus *Torovirus* and family *Coronaviridae*, has been documented as the sole pathogen from diarrheic calves, usually in calves <3 weeks of age. Although disease is uncommon, serologic surveys suggests that exposure is widespread. The pathogenesis and lesions caused by this virus are similar to other coronavirus infections, although epithelial cells from the lower half of the villi of small intestine and crypt cells of the ileum, colon, and cecum appear to be the first cells infected. **Astrovirus** infections usually appear to be subclinical, and their implication as a cause of diarrhea in calves is rare. Astrovirus infects dome enterocytes overlying the Peyer's patches causing mild transient villus atrophy.

Several **caliciviruses** (family *Caliciviridae*, genus ***Norovirus***; formerly Norwalk-like viruses, and genus ***Nebovirus***) are considered emerging pathogens in calf neonatal diarrhea. Both viruses have been significantly associated with diarrhea in neonatal calves; however, their role in disease remains unclear as they also have been detected in clinically healthy calves. **Enteroviruses** are commonly isolated from the feces of clinically normal animals with highest prevalence on high-density farms. They have been thought to be not associated with significant disease; however, bovine enterovirus 1 has been correlated with enteritis and typhlocolitis in naturally and experimentally infected calves. **Birnavirus** also has been isolated from the feces of diarrheic calves, but with no proof of pathogenicity.

A **bovine enteric group B rotavirus**, or bovine enteric syncytial virus, was identified as a cause of diarrhea in beef calves. Experimentally, this virus causes diarrhea and syncytia of enterocytes on small intestinal villi. **Bovine parvovirus** (family *Parvoviridae*, genus *Bocavirus*) is associated with gastrointestinal, respiratory and reproductive disease in cattle. In neonatal calves, lesions include small intestinal crypt cell necrosis, villus atrophy, and fusion and lymphoid necrosis.

Chlamydophila infection is described as a cause of acute enteritis in young calves; however, current epidemiologic data suggest widespread distribution and a limited role as a primary pathogen. Chlamydiae are more likely significant as causes of economic loss caused by chronic low-grade infections, but the pathogenesis remains poorly understood.

Heavy infestation of ***Strongyloides papillosus*** may result in villus atrophy, diarrhea and sudden death in calves as young as 2-3 weeks of age. Enterotoxigenic ***Bacillus fragilis*** has been suggested as a cause of diarrhea in neonatal calves, but its role is unproved. ***Giardia***, a flagellate protist, has been implicated in diarrhea of calves and other young ruminants; however, its role as a primary etiologic agent of calf diarrhea is controversial. Probably in some circumstances, *Giardia* may cause intestinal lesions and lead to diarrhea.

Diarrhea in neonatal small ruminants

Undifferentiated diarrhea in neonatal lambs and goats is mainly associated with enterotoxigenic **E. coli**, **rotavirus**, and ***Cryptosporidium parvum*. Lamb dysentery** is due to *Clostridium perfringens* type B in lambs and kids <8-10 days of age is usually recognized at autopsy as severe hemorrhagic and necrotizing enteritis. ***Clostridium perfringens*** **type A** has been identified as a significant cause of ovine and caprine enterotoxemia in some parts of the world; however, this type is commonly isolated from the intestine of healthy goats and sheep, so its role as a primary pathogen is unproved. Beta 2 toxin-producing ***Clostridium perfringens*** **type D** has been reported to cause fibrinonecrotic enterocolitis and enterotoxemia in a goat kid. **Coccidiosis** caused by *Eimeria* spp. in lambs and kids may occur in animals as young as 3 weeks of age. Raised white plaques of coccidia-infected *proliferative epithelial cells* are found in the terminal ileum; there may be some degree of hemorrhage in severe cases.

A variety of other pathogens have been associated with diarrhea in neonatal small ruminants. ***Giardia*** is prevalent on some farms and in certain conditions may contribute to clinical disease; its significance is poorly defined. **Salmonellosis** may occur rarely in young lambs. Certain serotypes of **E. coli** or other bacterial species may be the cause of watery mouth disease in lambs, which is characterized by drooling, sepsis,

and possibly diarrhea. Enterotoxin-producing ***Bacteroides fragilis*** has been implicated as a cause of diarrhea in neonatal lambs. **Astrovirus** has been found in lambs and experimentally produces diarrhea. An **adenovirus** antigenically related to ovine adenovirus-2 is reported as a cause of enteritis in goat kids. ***Strongyloides*** may be associated with diarrhea in ruminants only a few weeks old.

Diarrhea in neonatal swine

Agents commonly implicated in undifferentiated diarrhea in piglets <3 weeks of age include enterotoxigenic *E. coli*, coronaviruses, rotavirus, and *Cystoisospora suis*.

Enterotoxigenic *E. coli* is a significant cause of diarrhea in piglets <1 week of age, and the organisms use F4 (formerly K88) fimbriae to adhere to the brush border of enterocytes, but induce no other specific gross or microscopic lesions. **Rotavirus** and **transmissible gastroenteritis virus** (TGEV, coronavirus) infections cause villus atrophy, in contrast with most types of *E. coli*. ***Cystoisospora suis*** tends to occur in piglets >5-6 days of age, and the severity of clinical signs wanes with increasing age. It also causes villus atrophy, and in heavy infections necrotic enteritis in the distal small intestine. Meronts or gamonts may be found in mucosal smears and histologically within epithelium.

A number of other agents are less commonly associated with undifferentiated neonatal diarrhea in pigs. **Porcine epidemic diarrhea virus** (PEDV, family *Coronaviridae*) infection is clinically and pathologically indistinguishable from epidemic transmissible gastroenteritis. PEDV, which is endemic in Europe and China, has emerged recently as a significant cause of diarrhea and mortality of suckling piglets in North America. **Porcine deltacoronavirus** (PDCoV, SDCV) also has emerged as a cause of neonatal piglet diarrhea in North America. **Non–group A rotaviruses** may be more prevalent than once thought in pigs. They may act as primary pathogen or co-pathogen and cause lesions similar to group A rotavirus. **Adenovirus** infection can be seen as intranuclear inclusion bodies in epithelium on the dome over Peyer's patch in tissue sections, and is a rare cause of villus atrophy. **Enteroviruses, astroviruses,** and **calicivirus** have poorly defined significance as pathogens in piglets, though a calici-like virus causes villus atrophy in gnotobiotic pigs. ***Cryptosporidium*** and ***Giardia*** are described in pigs of all ages; these seem to play minor role as enteric pathogens. ***Salmonella*** and ***Klebsiella*, *Bacteroides fragilis***, and some strains of *E. coli* can cause villus atrophy and diarrhea in neonatal pigs, although these are rare. ***Strongyloides ransomi*** is transmitted in the milk and may infect young piglets, causing villus atrophy, malabsorption, protein loss, and diarrhea.

Hemorrhagic and necrotizing enteritis caused by beta toxin–producing ***Clostridium perfringens*** **type C** in piglets in the first week of life is readily recognized at autopsy. ***Clostridium perfringens*** **type A** has been associated with nonhemorrhagic mucoid diarrhea with mucosal necrosis in suckling piglets, although the role of this microorganism in the disease remains controversial. ***C. difficile*** also causes diarrhea in 1-7-day old piglets; lesions include edema of the mesocolon and fibrinonecrotizing colitis.

Diarrhea in foals

In the young foal, nonspecific diarrhea may be associated with **rotavirus**, ***Cryptosporidium***, and ***Strongyloides***. Enterotoxigenic *E. coli* and coronaviruses are not proven pathogens in foals, although their role in diarrhea of foals has not been ruled out yet. *Actinobacillus equuli* may cause severe diarrhea and hemorrhagic enteritis, with lesions of bacteremia evident in other organs at autopsy. **Salmonellosis** in foals may be seen as fatal diarrhea with few gross lesions, or as fibrinous enterocolitis and septicemia, similar to that seen in older horses. *Escherichia coli* and *Klebsiella pneumoniae*, with occasional gram-positive infections, are common causes of neonatal septicemia and possibly diarrhea, predisposed by failure of passive transfer of immunoglobulin. Fibrinonecrotic enterocolitis in foals <1 week of age may be due to *C. perfringens* type C, *C. difficile*, or co-infection by both microorganisms. *C. perfringens* type B infection has been reported rarely in foals; the disease has not been diagnosed in North America. *Rhodococcus equi* may cause chronic diarrhea and wasting in foals. Pyogranulomatous ulcerative lesions of the large bowel, and purulent mesenteric lymphadenitis, often associated with chronic purulent bronchopneumonia, are characteristically found in *R. equi* infection. *Enterococcus (Streptococcus) durans*, an enteroadherent coccus, has been associated with diarrhea in a foal. Moderate atrophy of villi covered with adherent gram-positive cocci was characteristic; the large bowel not being colonized. *Strongyloides westeri* is capable of causing diarrhea in young foals occasionally. **Tyzzer's disease**—caused by *Clostridium piliforme* (formerly *Bacillus piliformis*)—which is restricted to foals less than ~6 weeks of age, may be associated with diarrhea. However, the liver lesion dominates the pathologic picture.

Further reading

Blanchard PC. Diagnostics of dairy and beef cattle diarrhea. Vet Clin North Am Food Anim Pract 2012;28:443-464.

Cho YI, Yoon KJ. An overview of calf diarrhea - infectious etiology, diagnosis, and intervention. J Vet Sci 2014;15:1-17.

Cooper VL. Diagnosis of neonatal pig diarrhea. Vet Clin North Am Food Anim Pract 2000;16:117-133.

Diab SS, et al. Pathology of *Clostridium perfringens* type C enterotoxemia in horses. Vet Pathol 2012;49:255-263.

Diab SS, et al. Pathology and diagnostic criteria of *Clostridium difficile* enteric infection in horses. Vet Pathol 2013;50:1028-1036.

Foster DM, Smith GW. Pathophysiology of diarrhea in calves. Vet Clin North Am Food Anim Pract 2009;25:13-36.

Garcia JP, et al. The pathology of enterotoxemia by *Clostridium perfringens* type C in calves. J Vet Diagn Invest 2013;25:438-442.

Li G, et al. Full-length genome sequence of porcine deltacoronavirus strain USA/IA/2014/8734. Genome Announc 2014;2:pii: e00278-14.

Moeller RB, et al. Systemic bovine herpesvirus 1 infections in neonatal dairy calves. J Vet Diagn Invest 2013;25:136-141.

Mohler VL, et al. *Salmonella* in calves. Vet Clin Norht Am Food Anim Pract 2009;25:37-54.

Reinhold P, et al. *Chlamydiaceae* in cattle: Commensals, trigger organisms or pathogens? Vet J 2011;189:257-267.

Slovis NM, et al. Infectious agents associated with diarrhoea in neonatal foals in central Kentucky: a comprehensive molecular study. Equine Vet J 2014;46:311-316.

Songer JG. The emergence of *Clostridium difficile* as a pathogen of food animals. Anim Health Res Rev 2004;5:321-326.

Songer JG, Uzal FA. Clostridial enteric infections in pigs. J Vet Diagn Invest 2005;17:528-536.

Stevenson GW, et al. Emergence of porcine epidemic diarrhea virus in the United States: clinical signs, lesions, and viral genomic sequences. J Vet Diagn Invest 2013;25:649-654.

Uzal FA, Songer G. Diagnosis of *Clostridium perfringens* intestinal infections in sheep and goats. J Vet Diagn Invest 2008;20:253-265.

Uzal FA, et al. *Clostridium perfringens* type C and *Clostridium difficile* co-infection in foals. Vet Microbiol 2012;156:395-402.

Wyatt CR, et al. Cryptosporidiosis in neonatal calves. Vet Clin North Am Food Anim Pract 2010;26:89-103.

Gastroenteritis in cattle >3 weeks of age

Acute or subacute gastroenteritis associated with systemic disease and, usually, upper alimentary lesions, may be due to **bovine viral diarrhea/mucosal disease** or **malignant catarrhal fever**. In the latter disease, lymphadenopathy occurs, and gross lesions also may be expected in other organ systems. **Acute salmonellosis** occurs as enterocolitis with enlarged mesenteric lymph nodes, but usually without upper alimentary lesions. **Arsenic** poisoning, **oak** poisoning, **oleander** poisoning, and consumption of **mustard seed** or **superphosphate fertilizer** may cause acute hemorrhagic and/or ulcerative gastroenteritis and/or enteritis. Acute diarrhea, hemorrhagic enteritis, and/or enterocolitis may be caused by **adenovirus** infection in calves, feeder cattle, and moose and mule deer of any age. **Winter dysentery**, a hemorrhagic colitis caused by bovine coronavirus infection, is only occasionally fatal. Diarrhea caused by **grain overload** is associated with lesions of chemical rumenitis and usually with a history or evidence of excess carbohydrate intake. **Hemorrhagic bowel syndrome** (jejunal hemorrhage syndrome or jejunal hematoma) with segmental jejunal mucosal necrosis and intramural and intraluminal hemorrhage, and functional or mechanical obstruction of the gut causing severe abdominal discomfort or sudden death, is an entity of unknown etiology that can cause acute diarrhea in cattle.

Gastrointestinal parasitism may be associated with acute or chronic diarrhea and wasting in calves and young cattle at pasture. **Coccidiosis** in calves >3 weeks of age and older cattle usually causes dysentery and fibrinohemorrhagic typhlocolitis. The nematode fauna is usually mixed, but certain genera of helminths may dominate in particular epidemiologic circumstances. Most important is **Ostertagia**, which causes abomasitis with mucous metaplasia and hyperplasia. Intestinal nematodes such as **Strongyloides** and **Nematodirus** may cause diarrhea in calves at pasture or in semiconfinement. **Trichostrongylus** and **Cooperia** in adequate numbers are commonly pathogenic for pastured animals. **Toxocara vitulorum** may have some significance in warm climates.

Enteritis is often not grossly recognized in the small bowel at necropsy of animals with intestinal helminthosis. Therefore the pathologist needs a high index of suspicion to come to a diagnosis in some cases. To make a firm diagnosis of intestinal helminthosis, it is necessary to demonstrate substantial populations of nematodes by worm count in intestinal content or digests, and ideally to observe villus atrophy in tissue sections of infected intestine. These findings should be associated with a compatible syndrome—in the case of *Ostertagia*, *Strongyloides*, and the intestinal trichostrongyles, inefficient weight gain or wasting, and usually diarrhea. The hematophagous genera **Haemonchus** and **Bunostomum** cause anemia and hypoproteinemia, and associated poor growth but without diarrhea. **Oesophagostomum radiatum,** in the colon, may result in anemia, hypoproteinemia, and diarrhea as well as causing nodule formation in the gut wall. ***Trichuris*** may also cause occasional significant hemorrhagic typhlitis, wasting, and diarrhea.

Subacute-to-chronic diarrhea and poor growth or emaciation in cattle also may result from **copper deficiency, chronic bovine viral diarrhea, salmonellosis, yersiniosis, chronic coccidiosis,** and, in cattle >2 years of age, **Johne's disease** (paratuberculosis). **Congestive heart failure** and other causes of portal hypertension may also cause chronic diarrhea associated with alimentary tract congestion in individual animals.

Further reading

Adaska JM. Jejunal hematoma in cattle: A retrospective case analysis. J Vet Diagn Invest 2014;26:96-102.

Elhanafy MM, et al. Understanding jejunal hemorrhage syndrome. J Am Vet Med Assoc 2013;243:353-358.

Saliki JT, Dubovi EJ. Laboratory diagnosis of bovine viral diarrhea virus infections. Vet Clin North Am Food Anim Pract 2004;20:69-83.

Soto-Blanco B, et al. Acute cattle intoxication from *Nerium oleander* pods. Trop Anim Health Prod 2006;38:451-454.

Gastroenteritis in sheep and goats >3 weeks of age

The major causes of diarrhea and ill-thrift in sheep and goats at pasture are parasitic. The main helminth species causing this syndrome are ***Ostertagia, Nematodirus,*** and ***Trichostrongylus.*** The genera and species involved vary with the geographic area and climate, and perhaps seasonally, as well as with the age group and other local epidemiologic factors. Larval **paramphistomes** will also cause enteritis in lambs in enzootic areas. ***Strongyloides*** may affect lambs up to several months of age, even those held in confinement. Where it occurs, ***Nematodirus*** is usually a disease of lambs 1-3 months of age. **Trichostrongylosis** usually affects lambs 3 months to yearling age. ***Oesophagostomum columbianum*** may cause significant disease in sheep, as well as causing nodule formation in the intestinal submucosa. ***Trichuris*** typhlitis is an uncommon problem in sheep, as is ***Chabertia*** infection of the colon. ***Bunostomum*** and especially ***Haemonchus*** cause marked anemia and hypoproteinemia without diarrhea. Hemonchosis is a particular problem in lambs and kids at pasture or held in semiconfinement in warm humid climates. It is also important in ewes and does during the postparturient period, or spring, when retarded larvae emerge synchronously from the abomasal mucosa, and mature.

Coccidiosis is a problem mainly in lambs and kids reared in confinement, on feedlot or heavily stocked on pasture. The disease is most severe between 2 and 8 weeks of age. Villus atrophy caused by mixed-species infections may be responsible for ill-thrift and diarrhea in older animals, whereas *Eimeria arloingi* and *E. christenseni* or *E. ovina* and *E. ahsata* may be responsible for mortality in very young kids and lambs, respectively.

Acute enterocolitis and septicemia caused by ***Salmonella* Arizonae** infection may occur in lambs and sheep. **Yersiniosis** causes fibrinous enterocolitis and caseous mesenteric lymphadenitis in both species. **Grain overload** may cause acute diarrhea in feedlot lambs and in sheep offered supplemental feed. Diarrhea and enterocolitis also may be associated with **C. perfringens** type D enterotoxemia in goats, although animals may die very acutely without the opportunity to show

diarrhea. Intestinal lesions and/or diarrhea are uncommonly observed in type D enterotoxemia of sheep. Where it occurs, ***Peste-des-petits-ruminants* virus** causes acute severe enteritis with upper alimentary lesions in sheep and goats.

Johne's disease causes a syndrome of wasting, usually without diarrhea, in sheep and goats; in goats, caseous mesenteric lymphadenitis may occur. **Schistosomiasis** may cause ill-thrift in sheep in enzootic areas.

Terminal (regional) ileitis of lambs is a syndrome of unknown etiology characterized by reduced weight gain, diarrhea, and apparent abdominal pain, usually in 1-4 month-old animals. It is reported from the United Kingdom, continental Europe, and North America. At autopsy, animals are typically in poor body condition, with evidence of diarrhea. There is marked enlargement of the caudal small intestinal mesenteric lymph node. The terminal small intestine is thickened, with transmural edema, and a corrugated appearance on the serosal aspect. The mucosa is reddened, and thrown into thick transverse nodular folds. There may be superficial erosion and fibrin exudation. The mucosa of the cecum and spiral colon also may be grossly thickened.

Microscopic lesions are always evident in the ileum, and consist of moderate to severe villus atrophy, hypertrophy of crypts, hyperplasia of crypt epithelium, and a heavy mixed inflammatory cell infiltrate in the lamina propria. Microerosions or ulcers may be present, through which neutrophils exude. In the large intestine, the crypt epithelium is hyperplastic, causing thickening of the mucosa, which is infiltrated by a mixed, mainly mononuclear, inflammatory cell population, and is thrown into folds superficially. Peyer's patches and submucosal lymphoid aggregates are hypertrophic, with lymphoid hyperplasia.

Further reading

Chalmers GA, et al. Border disease—a cause of terminal ileitis in lambs? Can Vet J 1990;31:611.

Uzal FA, Songer JG. Diagnosis of *Clostridium perfringens* intestinal infections in sheep and goats. J Vet Diagn Invest 2008;20:253-265.

Van Metre DC, et al. Diagnosis of enteric disease in small ruminants. Vet Clin North Am Food Anim Pract 2000;16:87-115.

Gastroenteritis in swine >3 weeks of age

Rotavirus and **coronaviruses** (transmissible gastroenteritis virus and porcine epidemic diarrhea virus) may be responsible for villus atrophy and diarrhea in susceptible pigs of any age, although significant mortality is generally restricted to neonates and nursing pigs. Considerable morbidity but low mortality occurs in the later suckling, weanling, and feeder age groups. **Postweaning diarrhea** is associated with villus atrophy of uncertain etiology; it is discussed with villus atrophy in the section on epithelial renewal in health and disease. ***Escherichia coli*** causes postweaning enterocolitis, and Shiga toxin–producing strains of *E. coli* produce **gut edema,** as part of edema disease, causing sudden death or nervous signs in weaner and feeder pigs. No mucosal lesions are evident, but edema of the gastric submucosa and mesocolon may be found, among other lesions.

Enterocolitis resulting from ***Salmonella, Lawsonia intracellularis, Brachyspira hyodysenteriae,*** and **intestinal spirochetosis** generally occurs in weaner and feeder swine, although proliferative hemorrhagic enteropathy, swine dysentery, and intestinal spirochetosis occasionally involve suckling animals older than ~3 weeks of age. The differential diagnosis of these conditions and **trichuriasis** was discussed in the section on typhlocolitis in swine. **Coccidiosis,** other than that in neonates caused by *Cystoisospora suis*, is rare in swine. Occasional ileitis or, less commonly, typhlitis is caused by infection with several species of *Eimeria*.

Porcine circovirus 2 (PCV-2) has been associated with watery diarrhea and weight loss, often accompanied by pneumonia, and occasionally inflammatory changes in liver, kidney, pancreas, and/or myocardium in weaned pigs. Grossly, the mucosa of the distal small intestine and colon is thickened and mesocolonic edema may be present. Microscopically, a prominent lymphoplasmacytic/histiocytic infiltrate is evident in the lamina propria and submucosa of these intestinal segments. There is lymphocytolysis and atrophy of follicles in gut-associated lymphoid tissue, and irregular basophilic intracytoplasmic inclusions characteristic of PCV-2 infection are evident in macrophages in lamina propria and lymphoid tissue. Immunohistochemical staining for circoviral antigen stains these inclusions, which are presumably phagocytosed viral inclusions from lytic/infected lymphocytes. Similar inclusions are evident in bronchiolar epithelium and alveolar macrophages in lungs affected with bronchointerstitial pneumonia. Other lesions characteristic of PCV2 infection, including lymphadenopathy, hepatitis, and interstitial nephritis, are also present.

Hemorrhage into the intestine may occur in **proliferative hemorrhagic enteropathy** and **volvulus**, and should be differentiated from the melenic content found in animals with **esophagogastric ulcer.**

Ascaris suum may contribute to diarrhea and ill-thrift in weaner and feeder pigs. The thorny-headed worm ***Macracanthorhynchus hirudinaceus*** may, under rare circumstances, cause ill-thrift or intestinal perforation. Submucosal nodules in the intestinal wall may be caused by **Oesophagostomum** infections, which are otherwise usually relatively inconsequential in swine. Thin-sow syndrome has been attributed to **gastric hyostrongylosis.**

Enteritis in horses

Most of the significant gastrointestinal diseases of horses are discussed elsewhere, including salmonellosis, *Lawsonia*-associated proliferative enteropathy, clostridial enterocolitis, antibiotic-associated diarrhea, Potomac horse fever, granulomatous enteritis, and parasitism. The reader should consult portions of the chapter dealing with displacements, obstruction, ischemic disease of the bowel, syndromes associated with malassimilation and protein-losing enteropathy, and typhlocolitis for discussions putting these conditions into a diagnostic context. The capacity of the equine large intestine probably compensates for the additional fluid load posed by diseases of the small intestine that in other species might be expected to produce diarrhea. Horses presented with a syndrome reflecting hypoproteinemia, usually without diarrhea, may have *Lawsonia* infection, chronic salmonellosis, chronic inflammatory bowel disease, granulomatous enteritis, or enteric lymphosarcoma.

Duodenitis-proximal jejunitis, also known as *proximal enteritis* or *ulcerative duodenitis*, is characterized by signs of upper small intestinal ileus, including depression and nasogastric reflux. There is debate about including ulcerative duodenitis of foals, associated with gastric ulcers, in the syndrome.

We do so here, on the grounds of similar lesions in advanced cases.

At surgery or autopsy, there is fibrinous enteritis or ulceration involving the duodenum, and a variable amount of more distal small bowel. The lesions may be segmental and circumferential, only a few centimeters long, or more diffuse, involving much of the small intestine, but sparing the ileum. The affected segment of bowel may be thickened, congested, or hemorrhagic on the serosal aspect, and there may be fibrinous peritonitis with adhesions, and pancreatitis. Perforation may occur. If the lesion is of some standing, there may be significant stricture at the site. Affected animals often have a distended stomach, with abnormally fluid content, and gastric ulcers, particularly of the pars esophagea. Perforation or rupture of the stomach may occur. Duodenal lesions always should be sought in foals with gastroesophageal ulceration.

Microscopically, there is edema and congestion, with progressive necrosis from the tips of villi in early lesions, advancing to mucosal or transmural acute fibrinonecrotic enteritis, grading to the development of granulation tissue and fibrosis in the bed of more chronic ulcerative lesions.

The etiology is undetermined. *Clostridium difficile, Salmonella*, mycotoxicosis, and ischemia associated with the use of NSAIDs have been proposed, but not firmly implicated. The segmental, often circumferential, nature of the lesions is compatible with ischemia, perhaps complicated by secondary bacteria.

Fibrinous enteritis in the small bowel may also occur in *blister beetle* intoxication. Enterocolitis associated with use of NSAIDs is discussed in the section Intestinal ischemia and infarction.

Further reading

Arroyo LG, et al. Potential role of *Clostridium difficile* as a cause of duodenitis-proximal jejunitis in horses. J Med Microbiol 2006;55:605-608.

Segalés J, Domingo M. Postweaning multisystemic wasting syndrome (PMWS) in pigs. A review. Vet Q 2002;24:109-124.

Stevenson GW, et al. Emergence of porcine epidemic diarrhea virus in the United States: clinical signs, lesions, and viral genomic sequences. J Vet Diagn Invest 2013;25:649-654.

Enteritis in dogs

Rotavirus and **canine coronavirus** infection appear to be causes of uncommon, generally nonfatal, diarrhea in young dogs. Various other viral agents have been associated with diarrhea in dogs, usually on the basis of electron microscopic observations or virus isolation from feces. These include **astroviruses, adenovirus,** and **paramyxovirus,** as well as **calicivirus** and **herpesvirus** antigenically related to feline calicivirus and feline herpesvirus. The pathogenic significance of these agents is unclear. **Circoviruses** have been incriminated recently as being involved in canine gastroenteritis, and may be a co-factor with other etiologies.

Canine parvovirus 2 is by far the most significant cause of gastroenteritis in the dog. It is distinguished by severe fibrino-hemorrhagic enteritis usually evident at autopsy, and the radiomimetic microscopic lesions in the gastrointestinal mucosa, lymphoid, and hematopoietic tissues. Dogs with **canine distemper** often develop diarrhea; canine distemper virus apparently does infect the intestinal cryptal epithelium.

However, the enteric lesions of canine distemper have not been well described.

Salmonella infection occurs, especially in dogs that eat raw food diets. However, salmonellosis and enteritis caused by other gram-negative bacteria such as *Yersinia* is rare in dogs. Likewise, *Campylobacter* infection has been detected in both healthy dogs and those with diarrheal disease, and the role of *Campylobacter* in causing disease remains to be established. Histiocytic colitis in Boxer dogs and French bulldogs may have a bacterial etiology, with *E. coli* suspected. These dogs have been shown to improve with appropriate antimicrobial therapy, which supports an underlying infectious cause. *Enterococcus durans* has been associated with diarrhea in dogs. "**Salmon poisoning**" in the Pacific Northwest of the United States is due to *Neorickettsia helminthoeca* infection transmitted by the fluke *Nanophyetus*.

Hemorrhagic enteritis is associated with **clostridial overgrowth**, and also may be due to **reduced perfusion**, and **coagulation defects**, which may be congenital, part of disseminated intravascular coagulation, or caused by anticoagulant rodenticide intoxication. **Castor beans** (*Ricinus communis*) contain ricin, a glycoprotein known to cause gastroenteritis, vomiting, diarrhea, and occasionally death.

Ascarid infection in puppies may be associated with illthrift, diarrhea, and, in heavy infestations, occasionally with death. **Hookworms** may cause anemia, hypoproteinemia, and ill-thrift, or, in neonatal puppies, occasional acutely fatal infection. *Isospora* infection may cause diarrhea in puppies, and occasional mortality. **Giardiasis** is associated with chronic diarrhea in some dogs.

Syndromes of malabsorption and protein loss associated with granulomatous or eosinophilic enteritis, "filled villi," and lymphangiectasia have been discussed elsewhere. The differential diagnosis of colitis, including idiopathic colitis, parasitic colitis, protothecosis, histoplasmosis, *Campylobacter*, and spirochetal colitis, is discussed in the section on typhlocolitis in dogs. Ulcerating or widely infiltrating **colonic neoplasms** may be associated with diarrhea.

Further reading

Castro TX, et al. Clinical, hematological, and biochemical findings in puppies with coronavirus and parvovirus enteritis. Can Vet J 2013;54:885-888.

Decaro N, et al. Canine distemper and related diseases: report of a severe outbreak in a kennel. New Microbiol 2004;27:177-181.

Marks SL, et al. Enteropathogenic bacteria in dogs and cats: diagnosis, epidemiology, treatment, and control. J Vet Intern Med 2011;25:1195-1208.

Naylor MJ, et al. Canine coronavirus in Australian dogs. Aust Vet J 2001;79:116-119.

Pratelli A, et al. Severe enteric disease in an animal shelter associated with dual infections by canine adenovirus type 1 and canine coronavirus. J Vet Med B Infect Dis Vet Public Health 2001;48:385-392.

Sykes JE, et al. Salmon poisoning disease in dogs: 29 cases. J Vet Intern Med 2010;24:504-513.

Enteritis in cats

Feline panleukopenia virus causes necrotizing enteritis in the small intestine with features similar to canine parvovirus. **Feline leukemia virus** has been associated with a syndrome of cryptal necrosis in the intestine, resembling panleukopenia, but without lymphoid or bone marrow depletion. **Astrovirus**, enteric **coronavirus, calicivirus, rotavirus,** and other viruses are reported from the feces of cats, but are only rarely associated with diarrhea, and even less frequently associated with mortality. A **torovirus** has a questionable association with a syndrome of diarrhea and bilateral protrusion of the nictitating membranes. Diarrhea is a common sign in cats with **feline immunodeficiency virus** infection, and may occur in cats with feline leukemia virus infection. Bacterial infections such as **salmonellosis, shigellosis, yersiniosis, helicobacteriosis,** and **Tyzzer's disease** are unusual, as is significant parasitic enteritis resulting from **helminths, Cystoisospora, Toxoplasma, Giardia,** or **Cryptosporidium.** Chronic inflammatory small bowel disease and the forms of colitis occasionally encountered in cats are considered in previous sections.

Further reading

Hoskins JD. Coronavirus infection in cats. Vet Clin North Am Small Anim Pract 1993;23:1-16.

Kipar A, et al. Comparative examination of cats with feline leukemia virus-associated enteritis and other relevant forms of feline enteritis. Vet Pathol 2001;38:359-371.

Kipar A, et al. Fatal gastrointestinal infection with 'Flexispira rappini'-like organisms in a cat. J Vet Med B Infect Dis Vet Public Health 2001;48:357-365.

Marks SL, et al. Enteropathogenic bacteria in dogs and cats: diagnosis, epidemiology, treatment, and control. J Vet Intern Med 2011;25:1195-1208.

INFECTIOUS AND PARASITIC DISEASES OF THE ALIMENTARY TRACT

Viral diseases of the alimentary tract

Foot-and-mouth disease

Foot-and-mouth disease (FMD) *is a highly contagious viral infection of all cloven-hoofed animals.* It is a problem of worldwide concern, being enzootic in large areas of Africa, Asia, and parts of Europe and South America. The presence of the virus imposes serious trade restrictions that effectively thwart the development of a healthy agricultural economy.

FMD is an acute febrile condition characterized by the formation of vesicles in and around the mouth, on the feet, teats, and mammary glands. The disease is not notable for high mortality, except in sucklings, but morbidity is very high, with a concomitant loss of productive efficiency.

Species **FMD virus** (FMDV) belongs to genus *Aphthovirus* (aphtha = ulcer) in family *Picornaviridae*. The virus is highly resistant under many circumstances, but is inactivated by direct sunlight, because of drying and increase in temperature, and by moderate acidity (pH <5.0). The acid production that accompanies rigor mortis in carcasses and meat inactivates the virus. However, the alteration in pH is not dependable and the virus survives in viscera, lymph nodes, and bone marrow for an indefinite period under refrigeration. Next to the movement of infected animals, contaminated animal products are likely the most common mechanism of spread. FMDV may survive on hay and other fomites for several weeks.

The resistance of FMDV is of epidemiologic significance, especially where control policies involve slaughter rather than vaccination. The importance of a carrier state in the epidemiology of FMD is uncertain. The carrier state has been observed in cattle, sheep, goats, and African buffalo (*Syncerus caffer*), but not in pigs, although the latter play a significant role in transmission because of the high number of viral particles that they produce. The carrier state may persist for up to 2 years post infection in cattle, even in animals with a significant level of serum-neutralizing antibody. Sheep and goats are considered to be a frequent inapparent source of dissemination of the virus because disease can be mild and lesions difficult to identify. Infection in wild ruminants is an obstacle to control. African buffalo can carry FMDV for at least 5 years. Field outbreaks have been associated with buffalo-cattle contact in Africa, but these appear to be rare. Although Asian water buffaloes (*Bubalus arnee*) may be affected in FMD outbreaks, it is not known whether they remain carriers.

Of equal importance to the persistence of the virus is its *antigenic heterogeneity and instability*. There are 7 principal antigenic serotypes, namely, the classical A, O, and C types, and SAT-1, SAT-2, SAT-3, and Asia-1. These can be distinguished by serologic tests. Six of the 7 serotypes (O, A, C, SAT-1, SAT-2, SAT-3) are known to occur in Africa, 4 (O, A, C, Asia 1) in Asia, and 3 (O, A, C) in Europe and South America, although recent pandemics are blurring these geographic distinctions. These serotypes are sufficiently different immunologically that *infection with one type does not confer resistance to the other six*. Within these 7 major types there are antigenic subtypes, each different, to variable degrees, from the parent type. Generally, the subtypes cross-immunize to a useful degree, but exceptions do arise and become recognizable, especially when vaccination fails. *Antigenic drift* also can be demonstrated experimentally; new subtypes can be produced by passing the virus in immune or partially immune animals, or by growing the virus in vitro in the presence of immune serum. There are presently >70 distinct antigenic strains of the virus of natural origin.

As well as differences and variability in antigenic characters, strains of the virus differ in virulence, and a given strain is probably able to vary in virulence. Certainly, comparing different outbreaks, there is considerable variation in the severity of the disease produced in a given host species. Virulence also varies among species. Although the vast majority of strains affect a wide range of species, there have been occasional viruses that show a distinct predilection for one species. An example is the porcinophilic strain that originated in China in the late 1990s and spread to Taiwan, destroying the swine industry there.

The main portal of entry and primary site of viral multiplication are the epithelia of the pharynx and lung. In the pharynx, this is often associated with mucosal-associated lymphoid tissue. Subsequent to the first round of replication, there is widespread viremic dissemination to surface epithelium, with subsequent development of lesions in sites of mechanical or physiologic stress, such as oral and pedal epithelium, or teats in lactating animals. FMDV probably gains entry to these areas via Langerhans cells, with replication in a contiguous group of cells in the stratum spinosum. The resulting cellular degeneration and lysis result in an **epidermal vesicle**, *which is the hallmark of the disease.*

Virus is present at high titer in the vesicular fluid, and is present in large amounts in expired air from acutely infected animals, which is the main source of spread—pigs in particular liberate large quantities of airborne virus. Virus persists in lesions for 3-8 days after the appearance of significant neutralizing titers in serum, but seldom beyond day 11 of clinical illness. It is believed that FMDV is localized in epithelial cells of the oropharynx during persistent infection of ruminants, so that virus may be found in esophagopharyngeal fluid for a considerable period of time.

Within a week of development of neutralizing antibody, the titer of virus in circulation declines. Ordinarily, serum antibody titers decline progressively and fairly rapidly. The duration of persistence of antibody is correlated with the initial titer. In general, animals are resistant to reinfection with homologous strains by natural exposure for ~2-4 years; susceptibility increases as the antibody titer declines.

The characteristic **lesions** of FMD are only seen in those animals that are examined at the height of disease. As the infection progresses lesions heal or are obscured by secondary bacterial infection. Lesions develop mainly in areas subject to trauma: the *oral mucosa*, especially the *tongue*; the *interdigital cleft*; and the *teats* in lactating animals. In cattle, there is appreciable loss of weight and the buccal cavity may contain much saliva. In the living animal, there is diffuse buccal hyperemia and mild catarrhal stomatitis, but the hyperemia disappears at death. Vesicles form on the inner aspects of the lips and cheeks, the gums, hard palate, dental pad, and especially on the sides and rostral portion of the dorsum of the tongue. Sometimes they form on the muzzle and exterior nares. The primary vesicles are small, but coalesce to produce *bullae* which may be 5-6 cm across; these bullae rupture in 12-14 hours, leaving an intensely red, raw, and moist base to which shreds of epithelium may still adhere (Fig. 1-78). The eroded to ulcerated area may be replaced by regenerated epithelium in <2 weeks. Secondary infection may complicate this course.

Foot lesions occur in the majority of cases. There is inflammatory swelling with blanching of skin of the interdigital space in ruminants, coronet in swine, and heels in all species a day or so before vesicles form. The swellings persist until the vesicles rupture and the resultant erosions heal; healing may be considerably delayed on the feet. Vesicles may also occur in the other sites, but much less frequently.

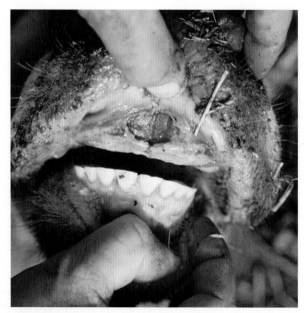

Figure 1-78 Foot-and-mouth disease. Ruptured vesicle on the gingiva of a cow. (Courtesy Noah's Arkives.)

A *malignant form of the disease*, without vesiculation, does occur in young animals and occasionally in adults. In these, death is common, as a result of *myocarditis*. Poorly defined pale foci of variable size are seen anywhere within the ventricular muscle. Although historically referred to as "tiger-heart," these gross lesions are no different from those generated in any other syndrome of severe, acute myocardial damage, but necrosis of fibers may be striking. Animals that survive the acute phase of FMDV infection (or are not slaughtered during depopulation) can progress to develop a set of chronic lesions. Chronic lesions include myocardial necrosis and scarring, heat intolerance, pancreatitis with acinar necrosis, and regeneration. Diabetes mellitus occurs in experimental cases, as does hypophysitis, leading to a constellation of endocrinopathies because of a range of expressions of pituitary dysfunction.

In **sheep**, the infection runs a milder course, although there may be exceptions. Lesions may be subtle or not develop. When lesions do develop, the *dental pad* is the preferred site in the oral cavity. Lingual lesions tend to occur on the caudal dorsal portion as under-running necrotic erosions rather than vesicles. These are small and easily missed, and they heal within a few days. *Lameness* may be prominent in acute outbreaks. Typical vesicles develop in the interdigital cleft, on the coronet and bulb of the heel. Occasionally they may involve the entire coronet and lead to eventual shedding of the hoof. Vesicles also occasionally occur on the teats, vulva, prepuce, and on the pillars of the rumen. The peracute form with myocardial necrosis may occur in lambs.

The disease in **goats** is similar to that described for sheep. Both species may be inapparent carriers, and many outbreaks worldwide have been due to transport of inapparently infected small ruminants.

In **pigs**, lesions occur in the usual sites, although more commonly on the feet than in the mouth. Sloughing of the hooves leads to severe lameness. Lesions also may be present on the snout and behind its rim (Fig. 1-79), and on the teats of lactating sows. Abortion and stillbirth of infected piglets are recorded. The peracute form, with high mortality caused by myocarditis, occurs in sucklings, often before vesicle formation is noticed in sows.

FMD must be differentiated from other viral vesicular diseases such as vesicular stomatitis, vesicular exanthema, and swine vesicular disease in susceptible species, and in the latter stages, from diseases producing erosive/ulcerative lesions of the oral cavity. *Gross lesions alone cannot differentiate these entities.* The disease must be considered in the differential diagnosis in cases of vesicular lesions in the oral cavity, teats, and feet, and sudden death among cloven-footed animals, especially the young. Definitive **diagnosis** requires virus isolation and characterization, demonstration of viral antigen by enzyme-linked immunosorbent assay, or detection of viral genome by polymerase chain reaction in lesional material. The regulatory status of FMD dictates that this must be carried out in accredited laboratories. In areas where vaccination is performed, vaccinated animals need to be differentiated from infected animals.

Further reading

Alexandersen S, et al. The pathogenesis and diagnosis of foot-and-mouth disease. J Comp Pathol 2003;129:1-36.

Arzt J, et al. The pathogenesis of foot-and-mouth disease I: viral pathways in cattle. Transbound Emerg Dis 2011;58:291-304.

Arzt J, et al. The pathogenesis of foot-and-mouth disease II: viral pathways in swine, small ruminants, and wildlife; myotropism, chronic syndromes, and molecular virus-host interactions. Transbound Emerg Dis 2011;58:305-326.

Saraiva V. Foot-and-mouth disease in the Americas: epidemiology and ecologic changes affecting distribution. Ann NY Acad Sci 2004;1026;73-78.

Thomson GR, et al. Foot and mouth disease in wildlife. Virus Res 2003;91:145-161.

Zhang ZD, Kitching PR. The localization of persistent foot and mouth disease virus in the epithelial cells of the soft palate and pharynx. J Comp Pathol 2001;124:89-94.

Vesicular stomatitis

Vesicular stomatitis (VS) affects horses, cattle, and pigs, and may also affect wildlife species such as white-tailed deer, raccoons, feral swine, and some rodents. Experimentally, various rodent species are susceptible and persistence has been demonstrated in hamsters. Also, persistence of viral RNA has been shown in both experimentally and naturally infected cattle, but the reservoir of the virus is unknown. *The disease is important because it causes a loss in production, especially in dairy herds, and it must be differentiated from foot-and-mouth disease in cattle and pigs.* VS is the only vesicular disease naturally occurring in horses (Fig. 1-80). Sheep and goats do not appear to be susceptible to the disease, but a severe, although nonfatal, influenza-like syndrome may occur in infected humans.

Species **Vesicular stomatitis virus** (VSV) belongs to family *Rhabdoviridae*, genus *Vesiculovirus* (type species: *VS Indiana virus* (VSIV)). It is an enveloped single-stranded RNA virus, bullet-shaped and ~80 × 120 nm. Apart from being inactivated by pasteurization temperatures, it shares qualities of resistance with the aphthoviruses. There are several serologically and immunologically distinct types of virus based on epitopes of the surface glycoproteins, including New Jersey, Indiana, Piry, Isfahan, and Chandipura. The 2 most common serotypes of VSV infecting domestic animals in the Americas are New Jersey and Indiana.

VS is enzootic in Central and South America and occurs sporadically elsewhere in the rest of the Americas. It has a seasonal occurrence; outbreaks occur in the warmer seasons

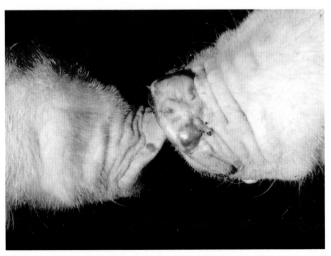

Figure 1-79 Foot-and-mouth disease. Vesicles on the snouts of two pigs. (Courtesy Noah's Arkives.)

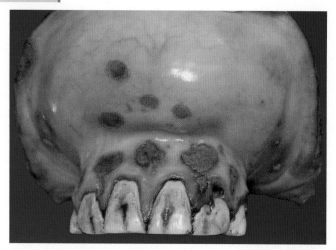

Figure 1-80 Vesicular stomatitis. Ulceration of vesicular lesions in the oral mucosa of a horse.

and usually cease with the onset of cold weather. The seasonal nature of the disease suggests that it is transmitted by *insects*; however, insect transmission is not essential and *contact transmission* has been proved experimentally. VSV has been isolated from both biting and nonbiting insects and black flies have transmitted the virus to pigs. Biting insects most likely become infected from feeding on lesions rather than blood, because viremia is transient, if present. Nonbiting insects act as mechanical carriers of the virus. It is not known how the virus spreads from one geographic area to another. There is some indication that VSVs adapt to specific regions, developing distinct genotypes based on specific vectors or reservoirs in an ecologic area. The intact mucosa is resistant to infection, but abrasions in a susceptible site readily result in infection when contaminated with saliva or exudate from a lesion. Environmental factors that increase the chance of causing abrasions to the skin, teats, or oral mucosa may predispose to infection.

Morbidity in lactating dairy cows may be as high as 100%, although only ~60% of the affected animals drool or froth around the mouth. The lesions of VS occur mainly on the *oral mucosa*; occasionally they do occur elsewhere, including on the *feet*, and in swine, foot lesions are common. This is by no means a dependable feature, and outbreaks of the disease in cattle have been described in which the lesions were predominantly on the *teats*.

The incubation period following exposure by abrasion is 24-72 hours. Experimentally, VS New Jersey virus inoculation in cattle led to viral replication at the inoculation site from 24-48 hours and in the draining lymph nodes within the first 24 hours. In horses, experimental inoculation in the oral cavity and lips also led to local viral infection of the inoculation site, tonsil, and retropharyngeal lymph nodes. The viremic phase seems to be short-lived, because the virus cannot be cultured from blood. Secondary lesions are rare. In cattle, intramuscular injections will not initiate the disease, a distinguishing feature from foot-and-mouth disease. After experimental infection of swine, infectious viral particles can be recovered from a wide variety of tissues within 6 hours postinfection, including salivary gland, tonsils, snout, skin, and lymph nodes. However, infective virus, viral antigens, and nucleic acids cannot be demonstrated 6 days postinfection.

Specific serum neutralizing antibodies persist for months in swine and years in cattle. There is no evidence that animals with persistent antibodies may act as a source of infection to herd mates. Animals are immune against the homologous but not the heterologous strains of the virus.

The lesions of VS are indistinguishable from those of foot-and-mouth disease. Initially, in cattle, there is a raised flattened pale pink to blanched papule a few millimeters in diameter in or near the mouth. These papules rapidly become inflamed and hyperemic. In the course of a day or so they develop into vesicles 2-3 cm in diameter and by coalescence may involve large areas. The shallow erosions that follow rupture of vesicles heal within 1-2 weeks unless secondary infections occur; in the mouth, the latter are common. Oral lesions heal rapidly in swine, but coronary band lesions often become secondarily infected to the point where the claw may separate and slough. Serous rhinitis, with the development of tags of necrotic mucosa, has been described in experimentally infected swine.

The first microscopic changes are seen in the deeper layers of the stratum spinosum, where the virus replicates. Increasing prominence of the intercellular spaces and stretching of the desmosomes are accompanied by a reduction in volume of the cell cytoplasm. This dissociation of cells proceeds to distinct intercellular edema (*spongiosis*) followed by further cytoplasmic retraction until the affected epithelial cells float freely in enlarging vacuoles, which in turn are loculated by strands of cytoplasmic debris. There is no hydropic degeneration of the epithelial cells and the nuclei until now remain normal. *There are no inclusion bodies.* With the onset of epithelial cell necrosis, there is a pleocellular inflammatory reaction in the mucosa and underlying lamina propria. Electron microscopic examination of epithelial cells adjacent to the vesicles confirms the intercellular edema and keratinocyte necrosis seen under the light microscope. The microscopic appearance of the lesions is not diagnostic.

In light of the similarity of VS to foot-and-mouth disease, *laboratory confirmation of VS is essential.* Vesicular fluid and mucosa from the tongue are good sources of the virus. *Diagnosis* is accomplished through virus isolation in tissue culture or embryonated eggs, fluorescent antibody techniques, complement fixation to identify viral antigen, polymerase chain reaction, and inoculation of suckling mice.

Further reading

Green SL. Vesicular stomatitis in the horse. Vet Clin North Am Equine Pract 1993;9:349-353.

Hubálek Z, et al. Arboviruses pathogenic for domestic and wild animals. Adv Virus Res 2014;89:201-275.

McCluskey BJ, et al. Vesicular stomatitis outbreak in the southwestern United States, 2012. J Vet Diagn Invest 2013;25:608-613.

Reis JL Jr, et al. Lesion development and replication kinetics during early infection in cattle inoculated with Vesicular stomatitis New Jersey virus via scarification and black fly (*Simulium vittatum*) bite. Vet Pathol 2011;48:547-557.

Vesicular exanthema of swine

Vesicular exanthema (VE) of swine is an acute, febrile disease of swine that is characterized by formation of vesicles on the snout, mouth, nonhaired skin, and feet. *The lesions are indistinguishable from those of foot-and-mouth disease, vesicular stomatitis, and swine vesicular disease.* VE of swine was first diagnosed in California in the 1930s and eventually spread to most swine-producing states in the United States. An eradication campaign was undertaken and the last reported outbreak of VE was in New Jersey in 1956.

Species ***Vesicular exanthema of swine virus*** (VESV) is the type species of the genus *Vesivirus*, family *Caliciviridae*. It has a single-stranded RNA genome and has only one major polypeptide. It is 35-40 nm in diameter and characteristic cup-shaped structures (calyces) are evident in electron microscopic preparations. There are 13 immunologically distinct serotypes, which vary in virulence.

In 1973, a virus that is biophysically and morphologically similar to VESV was recovered from sea lions (*Zalophus californianus*) with vesicles on their flippers, off the coast of California near San Miguel Island. Several strains of this virus, called **San Miguel sea lion virus** (SMSV), produce milder but otherwise identical lesions to those of vesicular exanthema when inoculated into swine, and SMSV is classified as a serotype of VESV. The host range of SMSV is very broad. One serotype, SMSV-7, has been isolated from opaleye fish (*Girella nigricans*) and it produces lesions identical to VE when inoculated into swine, with horizontal transmission to contact swine. Evidence of SMSV infection continues to be identified in fish and marine mammals. It is thought that VE of swine arose through the feeding of ocean fish to swine, with some adaptation of the virus allowing for very efficient spread through swine.

Most outbreaks of VE were associated with feeding of raw garbage containing pork waste, indicating that the disease was transmitted by direct contact and fomites. VESV now exists only as viral stocks archived in freezers and should be considered a *disease of historical significance only*. The possibility of a recurrence remains, however, if swine are fed uncooked tissues from ocean-origin fish or marine mammals.

Further reading

Calle P, et al. Viral and bacterial serology of six free-ranging bearded seals *Erignathus barbatus*. Dis Aquat Organ 2008;81:77-80.

Gelberg HB, Lewis RM. The pathogenesis of vesicular exanthema of swine virus and San Miguel sea lion virus in swine. Vet Pathol 1982;19:424-443.

Thiel HJ, Konig M. Caliciviruses: an overview. Vet Microbiol 1999;69:55-62.

Van Bonn W, et al. Epizootic vesicular disease in captive California sea lions. J Wildl Dis 2000;36:500-507.

Swine vesicular disease

Swine vesicular disease (SVD) is a highly contagious viral disease of pigs that is characterized by formation of vesicles around the coronary bands and heels of the feet, and, to a lesser extent, on the mouth, lips, tongue, and teats. *Clinically, the disease is indistinguishable from the other vesicular diseases of swine*, including foot-and-mouth disease, vesicular stomatitis, and vesicular exanthema of swine.

The disease was first recognized in Italy in 1966 and it has since been reported from Hong Kong, the United Kingdom, continental Europe, and Asia. The economic importance of SVD is related less to the rather limited losses in production and more to the fact that it is difficult to differentiate from other vesicular diseases and hence restricts trade.

Species ***Swine vesicular disease virus*** (SVDV) is a small RNA virus in the family *Picornaviridae*, genus *Enterovirus*. It is a porcine variant of human coxsackievirus B5, which is a serotype of human enterovirus B. SVDV is highly resistant to environmental factors. Unlike FMDV, it is not inactivated at the low pH in muscle commonly associated with rigor mortis.

Many outbreaks of SVD appear to originate by feeding raw garbage containing pork products. Transmission within and among affected herds is by direct contact, especially during the early stages of the disease, or by exposure to the virus in the environment, where it is very persistent. The portal of entry is most likely oral or by exposure of excoriated skin. Following contact with infected pigs, vesicles develop within 2 days and consistent virus isolation from tonsil is possible for 1-7 days. Viremia lasts for 2-3 days. SVDV has a strong affinity for the epithelial cells of the coronary band, tongue, snout, lips, lymphoid follicles of the tonsils, myocardial cells, and brain. Virus titers in tissue decrease with the appearance of circulating antibodies, which peak after 2-3 weeks and apparently persist for years. Secretions and excretions have high viral titers for a period of 12-14 days. Feces may contain virus for up to 3 months. There is some evidence that pigs may become carriers, with stress reactivating viral shedding several months postinfection.

Clinically, *vesicles are most common on the feet*. Oral lesions occur in only ~10% of affected pigs. The foot lesions appear first at the junction between the heel and the coronary band. Initially, there is a 5-mm wide, pale, swollen area that encircles the digit. In later stages a 1-cm wide band of necrotic skin is located along the coronet. Vesicles on the mouth, lips, and tongue occur in clusters and they are small, ~2 mm in diameter, white, and opaque. They coalesce and rupture within 36 hours and may be covered by a pseudodiphtheritic membrane resulting from secondary bacterial infections. Affected pigs usually recover in 2-3 weeks.

The development of vesicles tends to follow a similar course as that reported for FMD. The virus infects individual epithelial cells in the stratum spinosum, which leads to focal areas of keratinocyte degeneration and vesicle formation. There is an intense leukocytic reaction in the necrotic areas, which is mainly neutrophilic. As with the other vesicular diseases, after 1 week there are indications of epithelial regeneration.

Nervous signs and lesions of *nonsuppurative meningoencephalomyelitis* have been reported in field outbreaks and reproduced experimentally in SVD. Lesions involve most areas in the brain and sometimes spinal cord, and are centered on ganglia and spinal nerve roots. Clinically, the severe lameness tends to overshadow any nervous signs that might be present.

Laboratory diagnosis depends on demonstration of the agent by virus isolation, antigen capture enzyme-linked immunosorbent assay, or polymerase chain reaction, in accredited laboratories, on account of its regulatory status.

Further reading

Dekker A. Swine vesicular disease, studies on pathogenesis, diagnosis, and epizootiology: a review. Vet Q 2000;22:189-192.

Lin F, Kitching RP. Swine vesicular disease: an overview. Vet J 2000;160:192-201.

Martín-Acebes MA, et al. Subcellular distribution of swine vesicular disease virus proteins and alterations induced in infected cells: a comparative study with foot-and-mouth disease virus and vesicular stomatitis virus. Virol 2008;374:432-443.

Bovine viral diarrhea

Species **Bovine viral diarrhea virus** (BVDV) is an RNA virus in genus *Pestivirus*, family *Flaviviridae*. **Pestivirus** is composed of 4 recognized species, **BVDV-1** and **BVDV-2** (previously referred to as genotypes 1 and 2), **Classical swine fever virus**, and **Border disease virus.** It is widespread in cattle populations and this or closely related viruses can infect most even-toed ungulates, including swine. Although evidence for BVDV infection has been found in farmed and free-ranging wildlife in North America, the risk of transmission of the disease from wildlife to cattle remains unknown. As an RNA virus, BVDV is highly mutable because of the error-prone nature of the RNA polymerases responsible for replication of viral RNA. As a result, "swarms" of viral mutants form "quasispecies" that circulate within an infected individual and among individuals in a population. Although most quasispecies lack a selective advantage, or suffer deleterious point mutations, preventing them from becoming dominant, the ability to generate mutants enables BVDV to adapt to host responses, and to establish chronic or persistent infections in some circumstances. Although low virulence would seem to promote prolonged viral shedding, there may be advantages in high virulence that favor the emergence of quasispecies capable of causing severe disease and high virus shedding.

Viral genotype may be linked to specific manifestations of BVDV infection; noncytopathic (NCP) BVDV-2 has been associated with thrombocytopenia, for instance. However, there is a range of virulence among both BVDV-1 and BVDV-2 isolates, varying from subclinical infections or mild clinical disease to severe fatal syndromes.

Recombination of RNA from homologous (BVDV) or heterologous (other viral or host) sources, usually involving the region encoding the nonstructural protein NS2-3 of noncytopathic virus, results in a shift in biotype of either genotype of virus, from the more common **NCP biotype,** in which inapparent persistent infection is produced in cultured cells, to a **cytopathic (CP) biotype,** capable of inducing cytoplasmic vacuolation and apoptotic death of cells in tissue culture. Recombination splits NS2-3, resulting in a small NS3 protein, which induces apoptosis, and is a marker for CP BVD viruses. Reversion of CP viruses to an NCP biotype also occurs, less commonly. *Cytopathogenicity in vitro is not directly related to virulence in vivo.*

A new pestivirus species, tentatively called **HoBi-like, BVDV-3,** or **atypical pestivirus,** was recently identified in fetal bovine serum imported from Brazil into Europe. These viruses are genetically and antigenically related to BVDV and cause disease similar to that traditionally associated with BVDV infection. HoBi-like viruses may not be detected by conventional BVDV diagnostic techniques. Current BVDV vaccines confer limited protection cross-protection against HoBi-like viruses. These viruses have been identified in Brazil, Southeast Asia, and Europe.

BVDV gains access to the oropharyngeal mucosa by ingestion or inhalation, and primary replication is in oropharyngeal lymphoid tissues, including tonsils. The outcome of the ensuing viremia is a product of the genotype and virulence of the virus, the immune status of the host, whether or not the animal is pregnant, and if so, the stage of pregnancy.

Infection of immunocompetent, seronegative, nonpregnant animals usually results in subclinical infection or mild clinical disease. Affected animals develop slight fever, leukopenia, and specific neutralizing antibodies, the outcome in 70-90% of

BVDV infections. In a few situations, animals, mainly those >6 months of age, develop a more obvious clinical syndrome, with a high morbidity and low mortality—classical **bovine viral diarrhea (BVD).** The infecting agent is usually an NCP BVDV. After an incubation period of 5-7 days, the affected animals develop fever, leukopenia, and viremia that may persist up to 15 days. The virus is present in leukocytes (buffy coat), especially lymphocytes and monocytes, and in plasma. There is a transient decrease in the number of B and T lymphocytes and a decline in responsiveness to mitogen stimulation. Clinically, the disease is characterized by lethargy, anorexia, mild oculonasal discharge, and occasional mild oral erosions and shallow ulcers. Diarrhea may occur. In dairy herds there is a transient drop in milk production. Affected animals develop neutralizing antibodies that peak in 10-12 weeks, and probably are immune for life.

A syndrome of **severe acute BVD,** characterized by high morbidity and mortality in all age groups of susceptible animals, has been recognized since the early 1990s. Sometimes termed BVD type 2, because it is caused mainly, although not exclusively, by primary infections with BVDV-2, this syndrome usually has a peracute to acute course, with fever, sudden death, diarrhea, or pneumonia. It should be noted that not all BVDV-2 isolates are highly virulent. In some cases a **thrombocytopenic syndrome,** characterized clinically by epistaxis, hyphema, mucosal hemorrhages, bleeding at injection sites, and bloody diarrhea, is superimposed on the alimentary syndrome caused by BVDV-2, or occurs independently. The pathogenesis of BVD type 2 is most frequently linked to increased strain virulence. However, production of inflammatory cytokines, in response to widespread infection of mononuclear phagocytes, has also been postulated as a cause for the severe disease seen clinically. The mechanism of thrombocytopenia is not completely defined, although infected megakaryocytes in the bone marrow undergo necrosis.

Fetal infections may occur in pregnant immunocompetent seronegative acutely infected females, and in persistently infected counterparts. The outcome of fetal infection is primarily dependent on the stage of gestation. The most serious consequences occur if an NCP BVDV crosses the placental barrier during the first 4 months of gestation. It may result in fetal resorption, mummification, abortion, congenital anomalies, or, if the calf survives, a **persistently infected (PI)** calf. PI calves remain viremic for life, and are immunotolerant to homologous NCP BVD viruses because of failure of the immature fetal immune system to recognize the infecting viral antigens as foreign.

PI calves may be clinically normal, weak, or undersized at birth. They may appear normal, but are often unthrifty, and may have a rough or curly hair coat. The prevalence of these calves in a herd is usually <2%, but may be as high as 25-30% in herds in which a large number of naïve cows, early in pregnancy, have been exposed to NCP BVDV. *Most PI calves succumb to mucosal disease* (see later), usually between the ages of 6 months and 2 years. The offspring of the few animals that reach sexual maturity and become pregnant are also persistently infected, which can result in families of animals persistently infected with BVDV. PI animals are viremic, and lack antibody to the infecting virus (are antigen-positive but seronegative), which they shed constantly, acting as the *most important source of infection in the population.*

In PI animals, virus is present in a wide variety of tissues, and antigen can be demonstrated by immunohistochemistry in skin biopsies—in keratinocytes, hair follicle epithelium, hair matrix cells of the hair bulb, and dermal papillae. Use of skin biopsies for diagnosis of persistent infections by immunohistochemistry or enzyme-linked immunosorbent assay has been exploited diagnostically, but it should be recognized that acutely infected animals may have virus in skin biopsies as well, and detection of BVDV antigen in skin is therefore not specific for PI animals. Lesions in PI animals are minimal and subclinical, in spite of the widespread infection of virtually all tissues.

Mucosal disease is a clinicopathologic syndrome occurring in PI animals that subsequently become infected with a closely related CP strain, or probably more commonly, when the virus causing persistent congenital infection spontaneously develops a recombination encoding NS3. The result is an overwhelming infection that destroys cells, and to which the animal is incapable of responding. Characterized by *low morbidity but very high mortality*, mucosal disease most commonly occurs in cattle that are 6 months to 2 years of age. Although deaths may occur within a few days of illness, and almost always within 2 weeks, some cases may survive for months. The incubation period after experimental infection with a CP strain in an animal persistently infected with an NCP BVDV is usually 7-14 days, but may be considerably longer. Mucosal disease occurred in yearling steers shortly after vaccination with a multivalent vaccine containing modified-live BVDV. Genetic studies of the BVDV isolate obtained from the affected animals, combined with the epidemiologic evidence, was considered as strong evidence that the BVDV vaccine was the cause of mucosal disease.

Basically, there are *2 forms of clinically severe BVDV infection:* mucosal disease in persistently infected animals, and the more recently recognized severe acute form of BVD caused by primary infections with very virulent strains of virus. At autopsy, one cannot confidently differentiate spontaneous cases of severe acute BVD caused by BVDV-1 or BVDV-2 from each other, or from cases of mucosal disease, other than by the more hemorrhagic character of some cases of severe acute BVD caused by BVDV-2 isolates. Tentative differentiation of mucosal disease from severe acute BVD rests on the epidemiologic picture; antigenic or molecular characterization of the involved viruses is required for definitive diagnosis of the various syndromes.

Fulminant severe acute BVD or mucosal disease closely resembles rinderpest clinically and grossly. At the onset the animal is febrile, with serous to mucoid nasal discharge. Discrete oral lesions are preceded by acute stomatitis and pharyngitis, the mucosae being hyperemic and pink and covered by a thin gray film of catarrhal exudate. There is severe diarrhea and tenesmus with feces containing little or no blood or mucus. Affected animals become lethargic, anorexic, and dehydrated; they have ptyalism, polypnea, and tachycardia, and may die quickly.

In more chronic cases, the development of the oral lesions is like that found in acute cases; however, by the time they die there is usually some evidence of healing. The watery diarrhea of the early phase gradually gives way to feces that are passed frequently, are scant in volume, and contain a large proportion of mucus flecked with blood. Late in the clinical course, there is lethargy, emaciation, ruminal stasis, and frequent attempts at defecation accompanied by severe tenesmus. Interdigital dermatitis, dermatitis of pastern (Fig. 1-81A), coronitis, and laminitis affecting all 4 feet may be present in

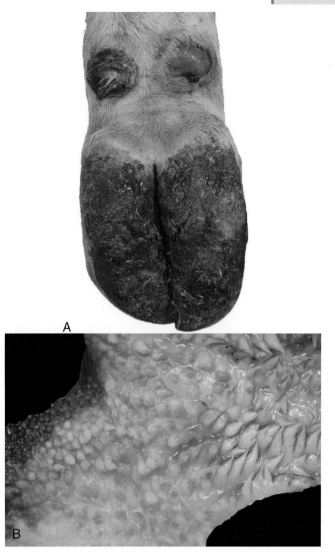

Figure 1-81 Bovine viral diarrhea. A. Erosive-ulcerative dermatitis of pastern in BVD. (Courtesy D. O'Toole.) **B.** Blunting and hemorrhage of papillae on the buccal mucosa as a result of necrosis induced by BVDV infection. A few remaining normal papillae are long with sharp points. (Courtesy R. Moeller.)

chronically affected animals, resulting in lameness. In these too, the skin is dry and scurfy, especially over the neck, withers, back, perineal and preputial areas, and vulva, whereas that on the medial aspect of the thighs and forelegs becomes moist and dirty yellow.

At autopsy, the **gross lesions** vary considerably, especially in acute cases, in which either upper alimentary or intestinal lesions rarely may be absent, and less so in the chronic disease, in which a broader pathologic picture often is present, perhaps partially obscured by healing or evolution of lesions.

Crusts, erosions, and shallow ulcers are present on the muzzle and nares of many affected cattle. There is loss of epithelium from much of the oral cavity. The most conspicuous oral erosions are on the palate, the tips of the buccal papillae (Fig. 1-81B), and the gingiva. Many, especially on the papillae, the hard palate, and in the pharynx, are sharp punched-out ulcers, and expose a denuded, intensely hyperemic lamina propria. In more chronic cases, ulcers may have a margin of thickened proliferative epithelium. The tongue is

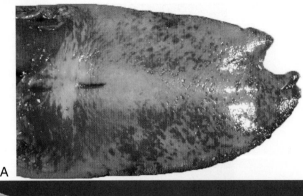

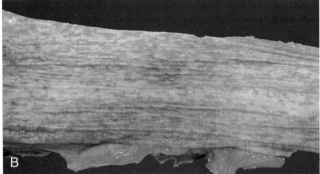

Figure 1-82 **Bovine viral diarrhea.** **A.** Ventral surface of tongue showing multiple confluent ulcers. **B.** Longitudinal erosions and ulcers on the esophageal mucosa. (Courtesy R. Moeller.)

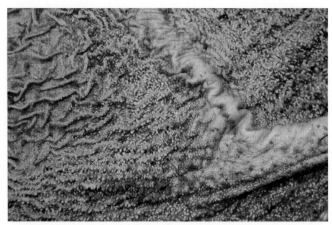

Figure 1-83 Focal and confluent ulcerative lesions on mucosa of dorsal sac of rumen in **bovine viral diarrhea**. (Courtesy D. O'Toole.)

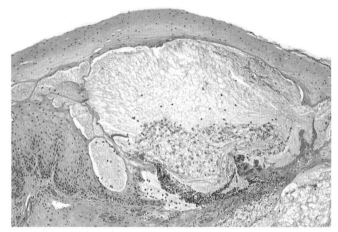

Figure 1-84 Histologic appearance of acute esophageal lesion in **bovine viral diarrhea**. (Courtesy J.P. Garcia.)

not always affected; when present, lesions may be evident on all surfaces (Fig. 1-82A).

Esophageal lesions are usually present, most commonly in the upper third. In some acute cases, the lesions are shallow erosions, rather than ulcers. The erosions are more or less linear but otherwise irregular, have a dirty brown base, and little or no hyperemia, and may be covered by shreds of necrotic epithelium in animals that have not been swallowing (Fig. 1-82B). In more advanced cases, discrete ulcerations occur. In many chronically affected animals the ulcers are beginning to heal and have yellow-white slightly elevated plaques of proliferative epithelium at the periphery of the mucosal defect.

Lesions are found in the *reticulorumen and omasum*, but usually not in the esophageal groove. The ruminal content in chronically affected animals with prolonged anorexia is usually scant and dry. In most acute cases, the ruminal content is unusually liquid and putrid. The lesions on the wall of the rumen resemble those present elsewhere in the upper alimentary tract and, although they occur anywhere, they are best seen on the pillars and other smooth or nonvillus portions of the mucosa (Fig. 1-83). The omasal lesions are most numerous along the edges of the leaves, sometimes causing a scalloped margin or perforation.

The morphogenesis of the lesions in the squamous mucosa of the upper alimentary tract begins with necrosis of the epithelium (Fig. 1-84). Individual cells and groups of cells deep in the epithelium are eosinophilic and swollen, with pyknotic nuclei. These foci enlarge progressively and form areas of necrosis that extend to, and may involve, the basal layer. In the early stages there is little or no inflammation of the lamina propria, but leukocytes infiltrate the necrotic epithelium. These necrotic foci enlarge progressively tending to coalesce, and may form small cleavage vesicles along the

proprial-epithelial junction (Fig. 1-85A), leading to erosions or ulcers as necrotic epithelium is abraded away. The ulcerations of the squamous epithelium of the upper alimentary tract are accompanied by inflammation in the lamina propria, especially where this forms papillae (Fig. 1-85B).

Changes are regularly present in the *abomasum*. The sides of the rugae bear ulcers that may be punctate to 1 cm or more in diameter (Fig. 1-86). The histologic changes in the glandular epithelium of the abomasum are characterized by epithelial necrosis, mainly in the depths of the glands, and accompanying interstitial inflammation.

The mucosa of the *small intestine* often appears normal over much of its length. However, in some cases the mucosa of the small intestine may have patchy or diffuse congestion. In rare cases, fibrin casts may be in the lumen of the small bowel.

In acute cases, it is usual to find *coagulated blood and fibrin overlying and outlining Peyer's patches*, the covering of which is eroded. This, when present, is a very distinctive lesion that is only paralleled in rinderpest. Severely affected Peyer's patches are often obvious through the serosa as red-black oval areas up to 10-12 cm long on the antimesenteric border of the gut (Fig. 1-87A). Less acutely affected Peyer's patches may be overlain by a diphtheritic membrane, whereas in milder or more chronic cases the patches may be depressed and covered

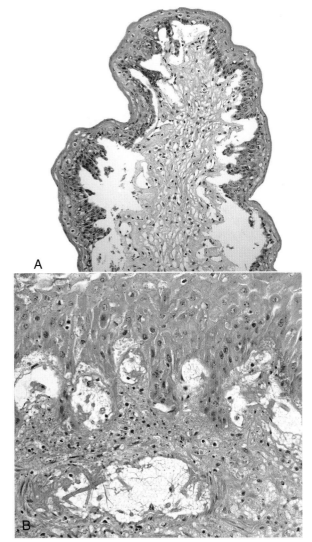

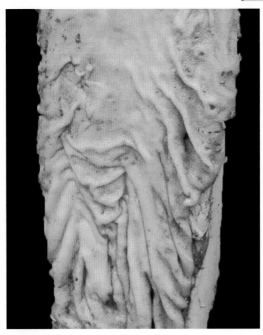

Figure 1-86 Bovine viral diarrhea. Hemorrhage and ulceration of the abomasal mucosa. (Courtesy E. Odriozola.)

Figure 1-85 Bovine viral diarrhea. A. Subepithelial cleavage vesicles in rumen papilla. **B.** Edema and acute focal inflammation of papilla and propria. There is necrosis of scattered cells deep in the epithelium.

by tenacious mucus. Mesenteric lymph nodes may or may not be enlarged.

Lesions in the *large bowel* are highly variable. The mucosa may be congested, often in a "tiger-stripe" pattern following the colonic folds, a reflection of tenesmus. In acute cases there may be fibrinohemorrhagic typhlocolitis (Fig. 1-87B). In more chronic cases, fibrinous or fibrinonecrotic lesions and focal or extensive ulceration may be present at any level of the large bowel, but particularly in the cecum and rectum.

The characteristic **microscopic lesion** in the intestinal mucosa is *destruction of the epithelial lining of the crypts of Lieberkühn*. In the duodenum, only a few crypts are affected, but more crypts are affected more severely in the lower reaches of the small intestine and in the cecum and colon. Affected crypts are dilated and filled with mucus, epithelial debris, and leukocytes. Remaining crypt-lining cells are attenuated in an attempt to cover the basement membrane. Reparative hyperplasia of crypt lining is rarely encountered. Crypt drop-out may be evident microscopically. In the cecum and colon, extensive damage to crypts and associated collapse of

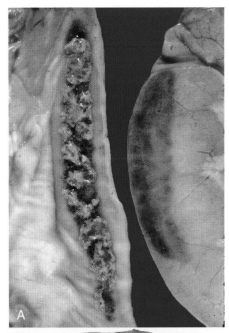

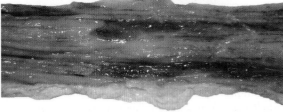

Figure 1-87 Bovine viral diarrhea. A. Fibrinohemorrhagic exudate over Peyer's patch in the ileum (left). Deep red Peyer's patch visible through serosa of small intestine (right). **B.** Fibrinohemorrhagic colitis. (Courtesy D. O'Toole.)

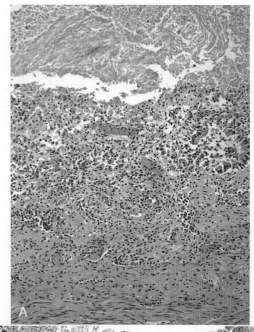

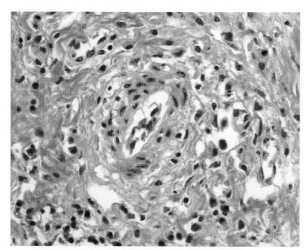

Figure 1-89 Bovine viral diarrhea. Fibrinoid necrosis and mild periarteritis of a mesenteric arteriole in the colon.

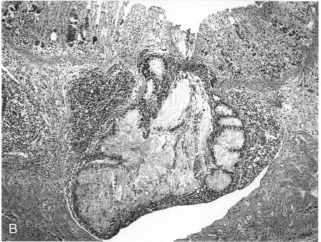

Figure 1-88 Bovine viral diarrhea. A. Colon, with dilated and denuded glands, collapse of lamina propria, and pseudomembrane formation. **B.** Herniation of crypts of Lieberkühn into the submucosa replacing necrotic lymphoid follicles in Peyer's patch. Mucus and inflammatory exudate are in the cystic glands.

the lamina propria are the probable cause of ulceration seen grossly (Fig. 1-88A). Congestion of mucosal capillaries, and in acute or ulcerated cases, effusion of fibrin and neutrophils from the mucosal surface may be evident.

The microscopic lesions of Peyer's patches are distinctive in BVD, comparable lesions being caused only by rinderpest. In the acute phase of the disease, severe acute inflammation in the mucosa over Peyer's patches accompanies almost complete destruction of the underlying glands, collapse of the lamina propria, and lysis of the follicular lymphoid tissues (Fig. 1-88B). Later in the course of the disease, dilated crypts, lined at least in part by cuboidal epithelium and filled with necrotic epithelial cells, mucus, and inflammatory cells, appear to *herniate* into the submucosal space previously occupied by involuted lymphoid follicles. Peyer's patches should be sought assiduously at autopsy because their gross and microscopic appearance may provide useful evidence for diagnosis.

Microscopically, the mesenteric and sometimes other lymph nodes show a diminished population of lymphocytes and necrosis of germinal centers. By immunohistochemistry, there is a marked decrease in most lymphocyte subpopulations.

An important microscopic lesion is *hyaline degeneration and fibrinoid necrosis of submucosal and mesenteric arterioles* (Fig. 1-89). A mild-to-moderate mononuclear inflammatory cell reaction is frequently present in the walls of the vessels and in perivascular areas. The vascular lesions also may be present in a variety of other organs, such as the heart, brain, and adrenal cortices, which may make it difficult to differentiate the disease from malignant catarrhal fever. The vascular lesions in acute mucosal disease are less consistently present and are usually milder, and there is *involution of lymphoid tissue in BVD,* in contrast with the lymphoproliferation characteristic of malignant catarrhal fever.

Coronitis may extend completely around the coronary band, with some separation of the skin–horn junction causing disturbance and overgrowth of the horn. Dermatitis may extend from the coronet up the back of the pastern. Milder dermatitis is generalized, with scurfiness, especially from the ears to the withers. In sections of the skin of animals with chronic mucosal disease, there is hyperkeratosis and parakeratosis with focal accumulations of necrotic epithelium with intense hyperemia of the adjacent superficial dermis. The epithelial lesions are basically similar to those in the squamous mucosa of the upper alimentary tract. Necrosis often extends deeply to or through the basal layers; it results in minute erosions or ulcerations. There is massive infiltration of macrophages and some lymphocytes in the underlying dermis. These deeper lesions occur in the inner aspects of the legs and the perineum, and there is exudation of serum in these areas. The overlying degenerate epithelium becomes disorderly and eventually is lifted off.

Some animals with chronic disease develop *mycotic infections* secondary to lesions in the forestomachs, abomasum, and Peyer's patches. The lesions are areas of hemorrhagic necrosis involving the mucosa, submucosa, and sometimes deeper layers of the wall. Fungal hyphae are found invading the stroma and causing thrombosis in venules.

Infection of oocytes and cumulus cells in the ovaries has been well-documented, causing speculation concerning ovarian dysfunction and reduced fertility in animals surviving BVDV infection.

After *experimental inoculation with virulent BVDV-2,* animals are febrile by 7 days post infection. Prominent clinical signs are anorexia, depression, and episodes of profuse watery and bloody diarrhea that persist until the animal is moribund at 13-14 days post infection. Pregnant animals may abort. Leukopenia and thrombocytopenia are often marked. In cases with severe thrombocytopenia, hemorrhage may be evident clinically.

Lesions are found in the digestive and respiratory systems. There is mild tracheitis, bronchitis, and bronchiolitis, which can progress to secondary bacterial pneumonia. Strains may vary in their ability to infect the pulmonary tree and result in disease. Intestinal lesions strongly resemble those seen in mucosal disease, with severe lymphoid depletion and necrosis of epithelial cells. However, with these BVDV-2 infections, there is often also a significant amount of hemorrhage evident externally, as described previously, and there may be extensive subserosal hemorrhages in the thoracic and abdominal cavities (Fig. 1-90). Similarly, edema may be more noteworthy in this form than in mucosal disease. Severe necrotizing vasculitis, especially arteritis, is noted in multiple organs but is most readily identifiable in lymphoid tissue. Meningoencephalitis associated with neuronal infection by BVDV-2 has been reported.

By immunohistochemistry, there is widespread viral antigen within epithelial cells (including oral and esophageal epithelium), smooth-muscle cells, and mononuclear phagocytes in multiple organs, although lesions often do not correspond to sites of antigen staining.

Bovine viral diarrhea virus and secondary infections. BVDV infection suppresses interferon production and impairs lymphocyte function, monocyte proliferation and chemotaxis, humoral antibody production, neutrophil function, and bacterial clearance. These changes are fairly persistent in chronically infected animals and in those with mucosal disease. The failure of immunogenic response may be associated with immunotolerance, or destruction of immunocompetent cells, which is reflected in lymphopenia. In addition to a lack of humoral antibody response, there is also depression of cell-mediated immunity, as indicated by a poor response of cultured peripheral lymphocytes to various mitogens. The impairment of neutrophil function in cattle infected with BVDV may explain in part the apparent susceptibility of such cattle to *secondary bacterial infections.*

Fetal infection with bovine viral diarrhea virus. In addition to the early embryonic death and abortions that can be ascribed to BVDV, infections of seronegative immunocompetent dams, usually between 90 and 120 days of gestation, may result in a wide spectrum of *teratogenic lesions,* including microencephaly, hypomyelinogenesis, cerebellar hypoplasia and dysgenesis, hydranencephaly, hydrocephalus, and defective myelination of the spinal cord. Ocular lesions, such as microphthalmia, cataracts, retinal degeneration, atrophy and dysplasia, and optic neuritis, have all been associated with fetal infections by BVDV (see Vol. 1, Nervous system; Vol.1, Special senses; Vol. 3, Female genital system). Infections of the immunocompetent fetus, usually after 135 days of gestation, result in antibody production that is detectable in precolostral serum samples of the newborn calf.

Fetal infection later in gestation may produce lesions unrelated to teratogenesis in the fetus, including alimentary tract lesions. Punctate hemorrhages with ulcers 1-3 mm in diameter may be profuse in the oral cavity, excepting the dorsum of the tongue, and in the esophagus, larynx, trachea, conjunctiva, and abomasum. The fetal lesions of squamous epithelium evolve in somewhat the same manner as those described earlier, with focal hemorrhages in the lamina propria and epithelial necrosis beginning in the basal layer.

Further reading

Bauermann FV, et al. HoBi-like viruses: an emerging group of pestiviruses. J Vet Diagn Invest 2013;25:6-15.

Bell CR, et al. Idiopathic bovine neonatal pancytopenia in a Scottish beef herd. Vet Rec 2010;167:938-940.

Euler KN, et al. Bovine neonatal pancytopenia—Comparative proteomic characterization of two BVD vaccines and the producer cell surface proteome (MDBK). BMC Vet Res 2013;9:18.

Fulton RW, et al. Lung pathology and infectious agents in fatal feedlot pneumonias and relationship with mortality, disease onset, and treatments. J Vet Diagn Invest 2009;21:464-477.

Hansen TR, et al. Maternal and fetal response to fetal persistent infection with bovine viral diarrhea virus. Am J Reprod Immunol 2010;64:295-306.

Lindberg ALE. Bovine virus diarrhoea virus infections and its control: a review. Vet Q 2003;25:1-16.

Miller MM, et al. Vaccine associated mucosal disease case study: demonstrating the importance of subsequent herd PI testing. Bov Practit 2013;47:84-93.

Ridpath JF, et al. Change in predominance of bovine viral diarrhea virus subgenotypes among samples submitted to a diagnostic laboratory over a 20-year time span. J Vet Diagn Invest 2011;23:185-193.

Strong R, et al. Increased phylogenetic diversity of bovine viral diarrhoea virus type 1 isolates in England and Wales since 2001. Vet Microbiol 2013;162:315-320.

Van Campen H. Epidemiology and control of BVD in the U.S. Vet Microbiol 2010;142:94-98.

Weber MN, et al. Clinical presentation resembling mucosal disease associated with 'HoBi'-like pestivirus in a field outbreak. Transbound Emerg Dis 2014. doi: 10.1111/tbed.12223.

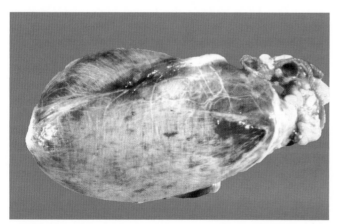

Figure 1-90 Hemorrhages on the serosal aspect of the urinary bladder in the **thrombocytopenic form of bovine viral diarrhea.**

Bovine viral diarrhea virus infection in pigs. The prevalence of naturally occurring antibodies to BVDV in swine has increased dramatically in the last several years with seroconversion in different countries varying between 2% and 43%.

The presence of antibodies to BVDV may complicate the diagnosis of classical swine fever, especially in those countries considered to be free of this disease. Cattle, and modified live virus vaccines containing contaminated fetal bovine serum, are considered to be common sources of infection for swine. Infection of pigs with BVDV usually occurs without clinical signs, allowing an opportunity for the virus to spread without detection. There are sporadic reports of disease in pigs associated with BVDV infection, including stillbirth, and poorly viable piglets, some showing tremors. A few 2-4-week-old pigs in infected herds are anemic, have a rough hair coat, growth retardation, wasting, and diarrhea. Affected pigs fail to develop neutralizing antibodies to the infecting homologous BVDV. Littermates that remain normal develop neutralizing antibodies. The suggestion is that the infections are congenital. In pigs infected postnatally with BVDV, usually no lesions, or very mild lesions, are observed. Experimental in utero BVDV infection of sows may result in prenatal and perinatal deaths, persistently infected immunotolerant or normal pigs. Many of these conditions resemble the effects of in utero infection with NCP BVDV in cattle.

Further reading

Tao J, et al. Bovine viral diarrhea virus (BVDV) infections in pigs. Vet Microbiol 2013;165:185-189.

Walz PH, et al. Experimental inoculation of pregnant swine with type 1 bovine viral diarrhoea virus. J Vet Med B Infect Dis Vet Public Health 2004;51:191-193.

Border disease. Border disease is a congenital infection of sheep and goats, usually with one of several NCP genotypes of **border disease virus** (BDV), a pestivirus antigenically related to BVDV and classical swine fever virus, but apparently also with some BVDV-2 strains. The disease was first reported in lambs from border areas between England and Wales. It is characterized by embryonic and fetal death, abortion, mummification, and birth of weak lambs or kids. The affected animals have an abnormal body conformation, long hairy fleece, clonic rhythmic tremors ("hairy shakers"), unthriftiness, and poor viability (see Vol. 1, Nervous system; Vol. 1, Integumentary system; Vol. 3, Female genital system).

A syndrome resembling mucosal disease has been reported in lambs that survived the initial border disease; they were persistently infected with an NCP BVDV. Immunohistochemical examination of tissues from persistently infected sheep reveals viral antigen in smooth muscle cells of hollow organs and blood vessels, epithelial cells in the gastrointestinal tract, lymphocytes, neurons, and glial cells. When cytopathic BDV is superimposed on persistent infection, affected sheep develop chronic diarrhea, wasting, nasal discharge, and polypnea. Macroscopic lesions are particularly present in the cecum and colon and in a few sheep also the terminal ileum. There is marked thickening of the gut wall caused by subserosal and mucosal edema and diffuse polypoid hyperplasia of the mucosa, which is hemorrhagic and focally ulcerated.

The *microscopic lesions* in the gut are similar to those described for mucosal disease in cattle. Lymphoid cell reactions are evident in the choroid plexus, portal triads of the liver, kidney, myocardium, thyroids, lungs, spleen, and lymph nodes. In addition, some lambs have marked hypertrophy and edema of the muscularis of the terminal ileum. The lesions in the terminal ileum resemble "terminal ileitis," and BDV and

BVDV should be considered as possible causes of that syndrome.

The pathogenesis of fetal infections, resultant border disease, and related enteric lesions in sheep appear to be similar to the multitude of conditions associated with NCP BVDV prenatal infections in cattle. Seronegative ewes infected before 80 days of gestation may produce persistently infected, immunotolerant, chronically viremic lambs.

Further reading

Braun U, et al. Sheep persistently infected with Border disease readily transmit virus to calves seronegative to BVD virus. Vet Microbiol 2014;168:98-104.

Cabezón O, et al. Experimental infection of lambs with Border disease virus isolated from a Pyrenean chamois. Vet Rec 2010;167:619-621.

Monies RJ, et al. Mucosal disease-like lesions in sheep infected with border disease virus. Vet Rec 2004;155:765-769.

Nettleton PF, et al. Border disease of sheep and goats. Vet Res 1998;29:327-340.

Rinderpest

Otherwise known as "cattle plague," rinderpest was an *acute or subacute highly contagious disease of cattle, domestic buffalo, and some other species of even-toed ungulates, including buffaloes, large antelopes, deer, giraffes, wildebeests, and warthogs, characterized by erosive or hemorrhagic lesions of all mucous membranes.* After a global eradication campaign, including limitations on animal movement and the use of highly efficacious vaccine, *the disease was eradicated from the planet,* with the virus last detected in 2001 in wild buffaloes in Meru National Park in Kenya, located on the edge of the Somali ecosystem, the last known remaining reservoir. For several years after that, studies in the region detected antibodies to the rinderpest virus in cattle, but it is thought that they came from old vaccinations. More recent surveillance confirmed the absence of the virus in the region. Vaccination against rinderpest is no longer used anywhere in the world. Before eradication, pandemics of rinderpest occurred in the Middle East and sub-Saharan and equatorial Africa.

Species **Rinderpest virus** (RPV) is in the family *Paramyxoviridae*, genus *Morbillivirus*. It is a highly pleomorphic single-stranded RNA virus with a core diameter of 120-300 nm and a spiked envelope. The virus is highly fragile under ordinary environmental conditions; it is incapable of surviving more than a few hours outside the animal body under normal circumstances.

Probably all cloven-hoofed animals are naturally susceptible to infection, but the expression of infection varies considerably. Goats and sheep do respond, but inconsistently, to experimental inoculations of RPV. Infection in Asiatic pigs may be severe but it tends to be mild in European breeds, which are considered dead end hosts for rinderpest. Rinderpest strains that are responsible for mild disease in cattle might cause severe disease in susceptible wildlife species. Although different strains of RPV vary considerably in their pathogenicity, they are grouped in a single serotype and, when suitably modified, make effective vaccines. The infection impacted heavily on wildlife populations in close contact with cattle, and wildlife was important in virus spread.

The disease in cattle could be mild, especially in endemic areas, but it was acute or peracute and severe in new foci. The different degrees of severity were due in part to real differences in virulence of strains, and largely because of differences in susceptibility of breeds or races of cattle. Rinderpest could also persist for prolonged periods as a very mild disease in endemically infected cattle and wild ungulate herds and it was thought to remain stable for years before the emergence of more pathogenic strains that induced the characteristic disease.

The *nasopharyngeal mucosa* appears to be the main portal of entry in rinderpest. The virus uses glycoproteins expressed on activate lymphocytes and monocytes and on dendritic cells as receptors, and destruction of such cells may be a means by which it causes immunocompromise. It localizes and replicates initially in the palatine tonsils and regional lymph nodes. This is followed after an 8-11 day incubation by a 2-3 day period of viremia that coincides with the fever seen clinically. In circulation, the virus is associated with mononuclear cells. After the viremic stage, the virus replicates in all lymphoid tissues, the bone marrow, and the mucosa of the upper respiratory tract and gastrointestinal tract. Nasal, oral, and ocular secretions, as well as feces, contain high titers of the virus. In general, excretion of virus ceases by about day 9 of the clinical disease, with the onset of neutralizing antibodies. Recovered animals do not appear to be carriers, although there are reports to the contrary.

Fever and its attendant signs usher in the **clinical syndrome**, with early leukopenia. Fever reaches its peak in ~3 days and falls with the onset of diarrhea, which may be bloody. There is severe abdominal pain, anorexia, ocular and nasal discharge, tachypnea, fetid breath, occasional cough, lethargy, severe dehydration and emaciation, and prostration. Death occurs in 5-8 days. Explosive outbreaks with high morbidity and mortality were more likely to occur in naïve populations. Vaccinated or recovered animals usually had lifelong immunity. Secondary bacterial, viral, protozoal, and rickettsial infections were common.

The **gross changes** in rinderpest are characteristic but not pathognomonic. They are similar to bovine viral diarrhea and mucosal disease (Fig. 1-91), and they also bear some similarities with malignant catarrhal fever. The lesions in the upper alimentary tract are *necrotizing and erosive-ulcerative.*

RPV has an affinity for the alimentary epithelium. Most severely affected areas in the oral cavity are those contiguous with lymphoid aggregates. Consequently, the caudal part of the oral cavity is affected preferentially. There is some strain variation with respect to presence of oral lesions. In nonfatal cases there is rapid regeneration of the oral mucosal lesions. Esophageal erosions are usually mild and affect the proximal portion. The forestomachs rarely exhibit any lesions.

The **histologic lesions** of stratified squamous epithelium originate in the stratum spinosum. Entrance into the epithelium may be via infected Langerhans cells that then pass virus along to adjacent cells. Irregularly shaped rafts of acanthocytes are infected with virus as evidenced by immunohistochemistry. These same cells then undergo degeneration and necrosis. Multinucleated syncytia form in the epithelium (Fig. 1-92) and these may have *cytoplasmic and nuclear inclusions.* Abrasion causes the necrotic tissue to lift off and produce shallow erosions or ulcers. This occurs so readily that they are usually the first lesions observed. Their margins are sharp, and the bases are reddened by the underlying congested capillaries. The initial minute erosions enlarge and coalesce to form extensive defects.

The abomasum is often severely reddened, which may just be a reflection of generalized stress for, although immunohistochemically abomasal epithelium is infected with virus, the extent of infection and resulting necrosis is far less than that seen in intestinal mucosa.

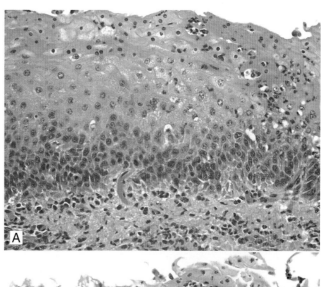

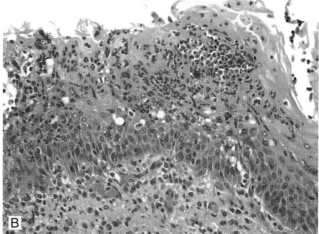

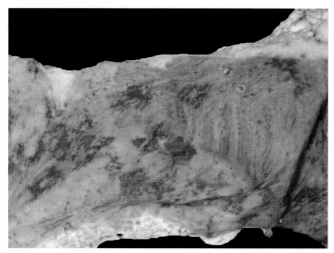

Figure 1-91 Rinderpest in a cow. Multifocal to coalescing fibrinohemorrhagic colitis. (Courtesy Elizabeth Clark, U.S. Department of Agriculture, Animal and Plant Health Inspection Service, Plum Island, NY.)

Figure 1-92 Rinderpest lesions in the tongue of an ox. A. Early stage of oral lesion showing disorganization of epithelium above the basal layer and formation of syncytial cells. **B.** Slightly later stage of (**A**).

Lesions in the intestine are severe and severity correlates with amount of lymphoid tissue in subjacent areas. Consequently, greatest mucosal damage is seen in ileum and the proximal colonic patch. Peyer's patches are almost universally involved. These areas become hemorrhagic and necrotic (Fig. 1-93A), and are associated with necrosis of the overlying mucosa, leaving deep ulcers.

There is replication of virus at all levels of intestine, with both crypt and villus epithelium involved. Replication is associated with formation of inclusion bodies, both nuclear and cytoplasmic, degeneration, necrosis, denuding of epithelium, formation of crypt abscesses and, if prolonged enough, villus atrophy. The formation of syncytia within gut epithelium is a rare event, in contrast with the oral cavity lesions, where it is seen with some regularity.

Receptor affinity dictates that *RPV is trophic for lymphoid tissues.* Infection and replication have been documented in both lymphocytes and macrophages. Necrosis of follicular lymphocytes is extreme (Fig. 1-93B), and gross inspection, which reveals little abnormality of nodes, is misleading.

Multinucleated cells, similar to those in the oral mucosa, occasionally form in the lymph and hemolymph nodes. All or only some follicles may be involved and there is often an increase of other leukocytes in the sinuses. Similar lesions occur in the spleen, tonsils, and, as already noted, in the Peyer's patches.

Acute congestion and edema of the conjunctiva may be followed by purulent conjunctivitis and corneal ulceration. Petechiae are common in the mucosa of the upper respiratory tract, which is usually covered with mucopurulent exudate.

Although the gross lesions of rinderpest resemble those of severe acute bovine viral diarrhea, mucosal disease, and malignant catarrhal fever, *rinderpest is distinguished microscopically most readily by the presence of syncytia and inclusion bodies.*

Further reading

Normile D. Rinderpest. Driven to extinction. Science 2008;319:1606-1609.

Roeder PL, Taylor WP. Rinderpest. Vet Clin North Am Food Anim Pract 2002;18:515-547.

Wohlsein P, et al. Viral-antigen distribution in organs of cattle experimentally infected with rinderpest virus. Vet Pathol 1993;30:544-554.

Peste des petits ruminants

Peste des petits ruminants is an acute viral disease of sheep and goats that closely resembles rinderpest and is also known as kata, *stomatitis-pneumoenteritis complex*, goat plague, ovine rinderpest, and pseudorinderpest. The disease was first recognized in West Africa, and is now distributed in north and sub-Saharan Africa, the Arabian Peninsula, Anatolia, the Indian subcontinent, including Nepal and Bangladesh, and China. Species **Peste-des-petits-ruminants virus** (PPRV), genus *Morbillivirus*, family *Paramyxoviridae*, is closely related to species *Rinderpest virus*, with which it shares common antigenic determinants. The virus cross-reacts with RPV in immunodiffusion and complement fixation tests. It may be differentiated from RPV using monoclonal antibody techniques and cDNA probes. Peste des petits ruminants is currently being considered for global eradication.

The clinical signs, pathogenesis, and lesions of the disease in sheep and goats in general are similar to those of rinderpest (Figs. 1-94 and 1-95), except that the disease is more acute in onset, especially in goats, and follows a more rapid course. Goats have been reported to be more susceptible than sheep in some outbreaks. West African goats appear to be more susceptible than European varieties, and, among the former, the dwarf varieties are most susceptible. Another difference is the marked involvement of the respiratory tract; affected animals have dyspnea, hyperpnea, and cough. There is also a marked serous to mucopurulent nasal and ocular discharge. Erosion/ulceration of the oral and pharyngeal epithelium may be diffuse and pseudomembranes are characteristically observed in the oral cavity (see Fig. 1-95A). The erosions can spread into the pharynx.

The pulmonary lesions of peste des petits ruminants are similar to pneumonia caused by canine distemper virus in dogs and measles virus infections in humans. The gross respiratory tract lesions include fibrinonecrotic tracheitis, and consolidation, atelectasis, and dark-red discoloration of the cranioventral lobes of the lungs. Some animals have fibrinous pleuritis

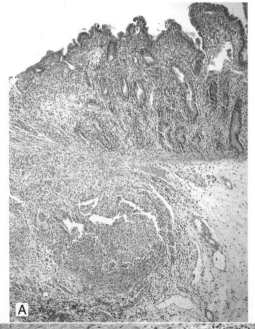

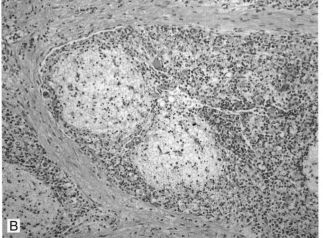

Figure 1-93 Rinderpest in an ox. A. Necrosis of Peyer's patch in ileum. **B.** Necrosis of germinal centers in a lymph node.

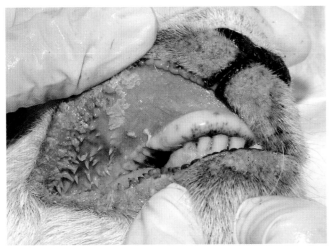

Figure 1-94 Peste-des-petits-ruminants. Oral ulceration and fibrinonecrotic inflammation in a sheep. (Courtesy Plum Island Animal Disease Center.)

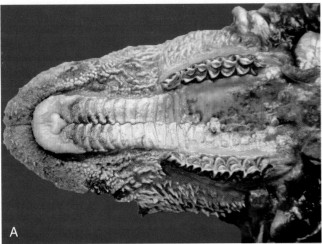

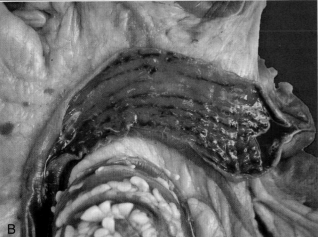

Figure 1-95 Peste-des-petits-ruminants. A. Ulceration and fibrinonecrotic pseudomembrane on the oral mucosa of a sheep. **B.** Hemorrhagic colitis in a goat. (Courtesy S. Perl.)

(see Vol. 2, Respiratory system). Hemorrhagic colitis is almost always present (see Fig. 1-95B). Microscopically, there is mild to severe tracheitis, bronchitis and necrotizing bronchiolitis, and diffuse proliferative *interstitial pneumonia*, with formation of alveolar syncytial cells. Other microscopic lesions

include diffuse colitis, multifocal hepatic necrosis, and severe lymphocytolysis in lymphoid tissues. Syncytial cells are conspicuous, particularly in the oral mucosa, pulmonary alveoli, liver, and lymphoid tissues.

Eosinophilic cytoplasmic and nuclear inclusions are present in the epithelial cells of the renal pelvis, abomasal mucosa, air passages, type II pneumocytes, and syncytial cells. Viral antigen may be demonstrated in the same cells and in brain, rumen, abomasum, heart, and myocytes of the tongue with appropriate immunohistochemical techniques. The primary viral lesions often are complicated by secondary bacterial infections.

Concurrent infection with PPRV and pestivirus was diagnosed in stillborn twin lambs that grossly showed several anomalies typical of border disease, including scoliosis, brachygnathism, prognathism, arthrogryposis, hydranencephaly, cerebellar hypoplasia, and hairy fleece. Microscopically these lambs had epidermal syncytial cells and necrotizing bronchitis/bronchiolitis with PPRV detected by immunohistochemistry in the skin, lungs, kidneys, rumen, and thymus.

Experimental inoculation of PPRV into cattle or pigs does not produce clinical disease, but these animals will resist subsequent challenge with rinderpest virus. These species are considered to be dead end hosts because they do not seem to spread the infection to other species. Natural infection or vaccination of sheep and goats with rinderpest virus protects them against PPRV.

A zoo outbreak of peste-des-petits-ruminants that involved several species of wild ungulates has been reported and Indian buffalo are also susceptible. The distribution of the virus in free-ranging wild ungulates has not been investigated.

Further reading

Baron MD, et al. Peste des petits ruminants: a suitable candidate for eradication? Vet Rec 2011;169:16-21.

Dhar P, et al. Recent epidemiology of peste des petits ruminants virus (PPRV). Vet Microbiol 2002;88:153-159.

Kul O, et al. Concurrent peste des petits ruminants virus and pestivirus infection in stillborn twin lambs. Vet Pathol 2008;45:191-196.

Truong T, et al. Peste des petits ruminants virus tissue tropism and pathogenesis in sheep and goats following experimental infection. PLoS One 2014;9:e87145.

Malignant catarrhal fever

Malignant catarrhal fever (MCF) is an infectious disease primarily of ungulate species in the order *Artiodactyla*, principally in the families *Bovidae*, *Cervidae*, and *Giraffidae*. MCF is also known as malignant head catarrh, and snotsiekte. The disease is characterized by *lymphoproliferation, vasculitis, and erosive-ulcerative mucosal and cutaneous lesions*.

MCF is distributed worldwide. It is generally sporadic, although severe herd outbreaks have been reported in feedlot, dairy, and range cattle, in farmed bison and deer, and in zoos. Among cervids, all species except fallow deer are probably susceptible. Other susceptible species of ruminants include banteng, Cape buffalo, and greater kudu. *Lethality in susceptible species approaches 100%*, although there are rare recorded cases of chronic infection and also of recovery from the disease, especially in infected goats, bison, cattle, and pigs. Although the agent is transmissible, the disease is apparently not contagious among cattle or bison by direct contact.

MCF is caused by cross-species infections with members of the MCF virus group of ruminant gammaherpesviruses (genus *Macavirus*, subfamily *Gammaherpesvirinae*, family *Herpesviridae*). At least 10 members of the MCF virus group have been identified, 6 of which are associated with clinical MCF under natural conditions: (1) ***Alcelaphine herpesvirus 1*** (AlHV-1), carried by wildebeest (*Connochaetes* sp.); (2) ***Ovine herpesvirus 2*** (OvHV-2), endemic in domestic sheep; (3) ***Caprine herpesvirus 2*** (CpHV-2), endemic in domestic goats; (4) ***Caprine herpesvirus 3*** (CpHV-3) causing MCF in white-tailed deer and red brocket deer; (5) ***Alcelaphine herpesvirus 2*** (AlHV-2), carried by hartebeest (*Alcelaphus* sp.) and topi (*Damaliscus* sp.) and causing MCF in Barbary red deer and bison; and (6) ***Ibex MCF virus*** (Ibex-MCFV), carried by the Nubian ibex and producing MCF in bongo and anoa.

Related gammaherpesviruses, as yet unassociated with MCF, have been detected in a number of bovids. Gammaherpesviruses of ruminants are highly cell-associated lymphotropic herpesviruses, difficult or impossible to isolate, which are typically transmitted from adults to offspring within the first 2-3 months of life, probably via free virus shed in nasal secretions. In the natural host, infection is latent or inapparent, with intermittent virus shedding, although disease has been incited in sheep by experimental aerosol inoculation of a large dose of OvHV-2.

Most natural outbreaks of MCF are due to 2 agents originally incriminated in MCF outbreaks: AlHV-1 and OvHV-2. **AlHV-1** is responsible for the "African" or **wildebeest-associated (WA-MCF)** form. **OvHV-2** causes **sheep-associated (SA-MCF)**. Each member of the MCFV group has an asymptomatic reservoir host species and, for those known to be pathogenic, one or more clinically susceptible host species that develop clinical disease. The division is not absolute and lesions and/or disease can be induced in some reservoir species when the challenge dose is sufficiently high. Nevertheless, as a general rule, reservoir species are well adapted to subclinical infection and efficiently shed cell-free virus, whereas MCF-susceptible species are poorly adapted and shed little or more commonly no cell-free virus. This absence of viral shedding accounts for end-stage hosts.

The classical form of MCF resulting from AlHV-1 and OvHV-2 are identical in clinical and pathological terms. However, the epidemiology of the 2 agents has important differences. The blue, brindled, or white-bearded wildebeest (*Connochaetes taurinus*) carries AlHV-1. Wildebeest calves become infected during the first 2-3 months of life, when they are also viremic and shed cell-free AlHV-1 in nasal and ocular secretions. Most wildebeest older than 7 months are serologically positive for AlHV-1. In utero infections have also been reported. Wildebeest are infected for life and transmit AlHV-1 to their calves without showing clinical signs. *Wildebeest calves are considered to be the main source of infection for cattle in East Africa.* They may shed virus in nasal and ocular secretions until they are 3-4 months old. Transmission to cattle may occur even without intimate contact, suggesting aerosol spread.

Viremia apparently ceases with the development of active neutralizing antibodies in animals >6 months old. It may be reactivated during late pregnancy or periods of stress, such as transportation. Although AlHV-1 produces MCF in many captive exotic species of ruminants, apparently most species that are exposed in their native habitat do not develop disease. AlHV-1 has been transmitted and adapted to domestic rabbits,

hamsters, rats, and guinea pigs, in which it produces MCF-like lesions.

The etiologic agent of SA-MCF has never been isolated from sheep; however, polymerase chain reaction probes have permitted its differentiation. *Most sheep have polymerase chain reaction-detectable specific OHV-2 sequences in cells*, and identical sequences are detectable in spontaneous cases of SA-MCF. Experimental transmission of OHV-2 between sheep has been accomplished using an aerosol of virus-infected nasal secretions, and natural transmission from adults to offspring probably takes that route, producing very high rates of infection in the sheep population, where it can be considered ubiquitous. The other 2 gammaherpesviruses associated with MCF have also been identified and implicated by molecular diagnostic techniques.

MCF has been reproduced by infecting bison via intranasal nebulization with sheep nasal secretions containing OvHV-2. MCF-like disease can be induced in rabbits, hamsters, and guinea pigs by transfer of lymphocytes or T lymphoblast cell lines derived from MCF-affected cattle and deer. The domestic rabbit is the most commonly used model to study the pathogenesis of both forms of MCF. MCF caused by OHV-2 occurs spontaneously and experimentally in pigs, and the relative rarity of the disease in swine may be due to lack of exposure to ruminant gammaherpesviruses under most conditions of husbandry. Most sheep are presumed to be carriers of OHV-2 virus. However, spontaneous disease does not appear to occur in this species, although clinical signs and lesions resembling MCF were produced in sheep experimentally exposed to a high dose of aerosolized OvHV-2.

SA-MCF occurs where bovids and deer come in contact with sheep. There is considerable variation in the susceptibility of various ruminant species to SA-MCF. Domestic cattle (*Bos taurus* and *B. indicus*) appear to require high levels of exposure to induce disease. Bali cattle or banteng (*B. javanicus*), the domestic water buffalo (*Bubalus bubalis*), American bison (*Bison bison*) and most species of deer, with the exception of fallow deer (*Dama dama*), seem to be highly susceptible. MCF is one of the most serious diseases of farmed deer in New Zealand, Australia, and the United Kingdom. Multiple case outbreaks have also been reported in captive North American cervids.

The *mucosa of the upper respiratory tract and/or the tonsil* is the most likely natural route of entry for the agents of MCF. Both WA-MCF and SA-MCF can be transmitted to susceptible hosts with large volumes of whole blood or lymphoid tissues administered intravenously, but not by cell-free filtrates, indicating that the agents are cell-associated, probably with lymphocytes. The incubation period of MCF is usually 2-10 weeks, but may, on occasion, be very much longer than this.

Antibodies against the gammaherpesvirus involved can be detected in animals with MCF, and often in herdmates, implying subclinical infection. Development of antibodies does not prevent a fatal outcome.

The **pathogenesis**, clinical signs, and lesions are similar, whatever the agent inducing MCF. Viremia in WA-MCF usually starts ~7 days before the onset of fever, and persists throughout the course of the disease. MCF is characterized by *marked T-lymphocyte hyperplasia*. A population of large granular lymphocytes appears to be infected and transformed by gammaherpesviral infection, and OHV-2 genome has been detected in CD8+ T cells, the predominant cell infiltrating around vessels in the brains studied. These cells are probably cytotoxic T lymphocytes or T-suppressor cells, but the mechanism by which they mediate the lesions of MCF is unclear. Dysfunction of this cell population may result in de-repression of T-lymphocyte replication, permitting lymphoproliferation. Deranged cytotoxic T-cell activity may then create the epithelial and vascular lesions, through a type of graft-versus-host response, attacking epithelium of the respiratory and gastrointestinal systems, as well as medium-sized arteries throughout the body. This is a unifying, but unproved, hypothesis explaining the lymphadenopathy, mucosal epithelial lesions, and vasculitis characteristic of MCF. Vascular lesions may mediate infarction of some affected tissue fields, as well.

There is wide variation in the presenting **clinical syndromes**, which are potentially pansystemic. Quite consistently, affected animals have enlarged lymph nodes, although this may be less the case in bison, and there is usually some degree of ocular and oral disease, and exudative dermatitis. There is edema of the eyelids and palpebral conjunctivae and congestion of the nasal and buccal mucosae. Photophobia is accompanied by copious lacrimation. There is conjunctivitis and an increasing rim of corneal opacity, starting at the limbus and progressing centripetally. Corneal ulceration occurs in some cases, but in those that die quickly, the infiltration of the filtration angle may be all that is seen, and this is easily overlooked. Hypopyon may be seen. In some cases there are nervous signs, such as hyperesthesia, head pressing, trembling, nystagmus, incoordination, and behavioral changes. Other animals may have gastroenteritis with diarrhea, which may be bloody in acute cases. This is most commonly seen in deer. The disease may take an acute course of ~1-3 days, particularly in animals with hemorrhagic enteritis. Those with less severe gastroenteritis, central nervous signs, or generalized disease may linger for as long as 9-10 days. Mortality in MCF has been considered to approach 100% of clinical cases, but recovery may occur, although chronic ocular lesions and vasculitis persist. Clinical signs in bison are more subtle than in cattle, with a high percentage of animals dying without clinical signs being observed or with animals dying very soon after onset of clinical disease.

Gross changes involve multiple organs and are the consequence of 3 basic microscopic lesions: widespread arteritis-phlebitis of medium caliber vessels, lymphoid proliferation and production of atypical lymphoblastoid cells, and mucosal ulceration in digestive, urinary, and respiratory tracts. Gross changes may not be present in occasional animals that die of peracute MCF, and in these the diagnosis must rest on the detection of the characteristic histologic changes, and demonstration of the genome of an implicated gammaherpesvirus in tissue. The carcass is dehydrated, and may be emaciated if the course has been prolonged. Conjunctivitis may be evident. The muzzle and nares are heavily encrusted and, if wiped, often reveal irregular eroded or ulcerated surfaces, although in some cases there may be only a slight serous discharge. Cutaneous lesions, especially in SA-MCF, are common, but often overlooked. Affected areas include the thorax, abdomen, inguinal regions, perineum, udder, and occasionally the head. There may be, acutely, more or less generalized exanthema with sufficient exudation to wet and mat the hair, and to form detachable crusts; in unpigmented skin there is obvious hyperemia. The crusts may become several millimeters thick, and there is patchy loss of hair. Sometimes these cutaneous changes begin locally about the base of the hooves and horns, the loin, and perineum; they may remain localized or become

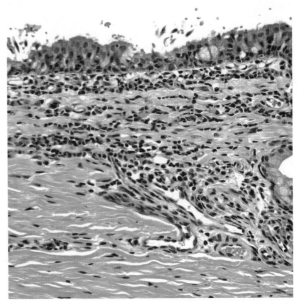

Figure 1-96 Erosive tracheitis in **malignant catarrhal fever.** (Courtesy D. O'Toole.)

generalized. In severe cases, the horns and hooves may slough. Caprine herpesvirus-2 has been associated with syndromes in deer that include dermatitis and alopecia, alone, or in combination with gastrointestinal or neurological disease.

The respiratory system may have minor or severe lesions (Fig. 1-96). When the course is short, the nasal mucosa may only have congestion and slight serous exudation. Later, there is a copious discharge. Lesions are most severe in the rostral third of the nasal cavity, corresponding to the zone of stratified squamous epithelium. In some cases, fibrinous tracheobronchitis may occur (see Fig. 1-96).

The lower alimentary mucosae may have no significant lesions in the peracute disease, although *oral lesions are present in most cases* of MCF (Fig. 1-97). Minor erosions are first observed on the lips adjacent to the mucocutaneous junction. Sometimes apparently normal epithelium on the surface of the tongue peels off in sheets. Later, erosive and ulcerative lesions may involve a large area of oral mucosa, frequently occurring on all surfaces of the tongue, the dental pad, the tips of the buccal papillae, gingivae, both areas of the palate, and the cheeks. In some areas the cheesy or tattered necrotic epithelium may not be sloughed at the time of inspection. Esophageal erosions or ulcers, similar to those that occur in the other diseases causing ulcerative stomatitis, occur in MCF, and, as in rinderpest, are most consistent in the cranial portion. Lesions of the same sort may be present in the forestomachs. Focal ulceration or generalized hyperemia may be evident in the abomasal mucosa. In deer, especially, hemorrhagic or fibrinohemorrhagic typhlocolitis may be a prominent finding.

The *liver* may be slightly enlarged. Close inspection will reveal, in some cases, diffuse mottling with white foci, which are periportal accumulations of mononuclear cells (Fig. 1-98). There may be numerous petechiae and a few erosions of the mucous membrane of the gallbladder.

Characteristic lesions may occur in the *urinary system*. Renal changes are not always present. They are infarcts or 2-4 mm foci of nonsuppurative interstitial nephritis (Fig. 1-99). They may be numerous enough to produce a mottled

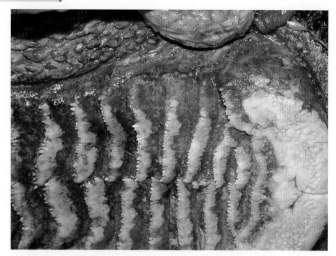

Figure 1-97 Ulcerative lesions in the hard palate of a bison with **malignant catarrhal fever**.

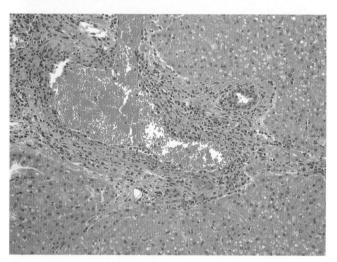

Figure 1-98 Accumulations of lymphocytes in portal triads in **malignant catarrhal fever**.

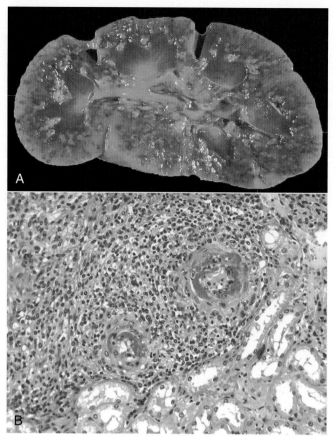

Figure 1-99 Malignant catarrhal fever. A. Focal nonsuppurative interstitial nephritis. **B.** Extensive cuff of mononuclear cells, and fibrinoid necrosis in the wall of a small arteriole in the kidney. (Courtesy D. O'Toole.)

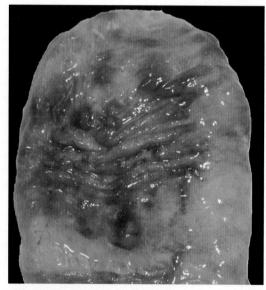

Figure 1-100 Hemorrhages in the mucosa of urinary bladder in **malignant catarrhal fever**. (Courtesy D. O'Toole.)

appearance, and may form slight rounded projections from the capsular surfaces. The pelvic and ureteral mucosa frequently has petechial and ecchymotic hemorrhages. Similar lesions are present on the mucosa of the urinary bladder, or there may be more severe hemorrhage associated with erosion and ulceration of the epithelium, and hematuria (Fig. 1-100). Superficial lesions may occur in the vagina and vulva, similar to those of the oral cavity and skin.

Enlargement of lymph nodes is a characteristic lesion of MCF in most species, perhaps except in bison, where lymphadenopathy has been found, in one large study, in only 62% of cases. This lesion is almost invariably present in cattle. All nodes may be involved, or some may appear grossly normal. Affected nodes may be many times the normal size, and some, including hemolymph nodes, which are usually too small to recognize, may become quite obvious. There is edema of the affected nodes and the pericapsular connective tissue. On microscopic examination it is apparent that the increase in size is due to *lymphocytic hyperplasia*. Some of the nodes are congested or hemorrhagic. The spleen is slightly enlarged, and the lymphoid follicles are prominent.

Most animals may have *meningoencephalitis* as a result of *vasculitis* that may be accompanied by meningeal edema

and is one of the most consistent histologic lesions of the disease.

The **histologic changes** usually must be relied on for the diagnosis of MCF, and its differentiation from similar diseases, although access to molecular diagnosis of specific gammaherpesvirus infections is increasing. The characteristic histologic changes are found in lymphoid tissues and in the adventitia and walls of medium-sized vessels, especially arteries in any organ, and these will be described before other lesions. They are characterized by *perivascular accumulation of mainly mononuclear cells, and fibrinoid necrotizing vasculitis* (see Fig. 1-99B). These changes may be focal or segmental, and may involve the full thickness of the wall, or be confined more or less to one of the layers. When the intima is involved, there is often endothelial swelling. Thrombi are difficult to demonstrate in damaged vessels. The media may be selectively affected, or occasionally, the adventitia alone. Severely affected segments of vessel are replaced by a coagulum of homogeneous, eosinophilic material, in which fragmented nuclear remnants are seen. The perivascular accumulation of cells is particularly characteristic. They are mainly lymphoid cells with large open nuclei and prominent nucleoli; small lymphocytes and plasma cells may be present occasionally. The vascular lesions may be more subtle in other species (especially bison, deer and elk) than in cattle, and in bison this lesion tends to be less widely disseminated than that in cattle.

Cattle that recover from SA-MCF also have distinctive vascular lesions 90 days after clinical onset. Concentric fibrointimal plaques, disrupted inner elastic lamina, focally atrophic tunica media, and vasculitis of variable severity are evident in many organ systems.

In *lymph nodes*, there is active proliferation of lymphoblasts, which form extensive homogeneous populations of cells in the T-cell–dependent areas of the interfollicular cortical and paracortical zones. In bison, lymphoid hyperplasia is either absent or subtle in paracortical areas of lymph nodes. Focal areas of hemorrhage and necrosis associated with arteritis may be seen in all areas of the nodes. The lymphoid reaction in the spleen varies from marked lymphoid cell hyperplasia, in the periarteriolar sheaths, to atrophy and depletion of lymphocytes. In addition, there is marked proliferation and infiltration of lymphocytic and lymphoblastic cells, mainly perivascular in distribution, in a variety of organs. The lymphoreticular proliferation may become so severe in some organs that it is difficult to determine whether it is hyperplastic or neoplastic.

Microscopic arteritis similar to that present in other organs occurs in the nervous system of many cases. Necrotizing arteritis, plasma exudation into the meninges or Virchow-Robin space, and the predominantly adventitial lymphocytic response are, in the brain of cattle, *unique to MCF*, and allow it to be differentiated from other nonsuppurative encephalitides. Degenerative changes in nervous parenchyma can be explained on the basis of the vascular changes.

The lesions in *skin and squamous mucosae* of the alimentary tract consist of a lichenoid infiltrate, as the altered and proliferating lymphoid population moves into the upper dermis and then the epidermis (Fig. 1-101). Often typical arteritis, involving small- and medium-sized vessels, is present in underlying tissue. Groups of epithelial cells become necrotic, with swollen, strongly acidophilic cytoplasm; ultimately the full thickness of epithelium in affected areas undergoes necrosis and ulcerates. Granulomatous mural folliculitis was the prominent microscopic finding in alopecic sika deer infected with CpHV-2.

The mucosa of the abomasum may be infiltrated by lymphocytes, and undergo mucous metaplasia or focal ulceration. The mucosa of the lower alimentary tract, especially the

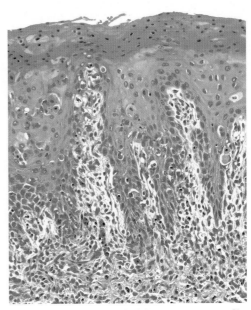

Figure 1-101 **Malignant catarrhal fever** in an ox. Infiltration of lamina propria by lymphocytic cells with developing ulcer over papilla in the tongue. (Courtesy D. O'Toole.)

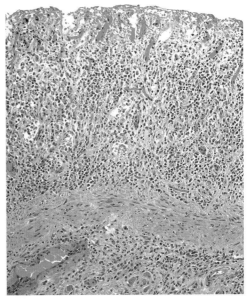

Figure 1-102 Colitis with collapse of glands in **malignant catarrhal fever.**

cecum and colon in deer, may similarly be heavily infiltrated by lymphocytes, often with fibrin and blood exuding into the lumen where surface and glandular epithelium has undergone necrosis and collapsed, sometimes over wide areas (Fig. 1-102). Submucosal arterioles in affected areas of abomasum and intestine are affected by the characteristic arteritis.

The *mottling of liver and the focal nephritis* seen grossly are due to the perivascular accumulation of mononuclear cells in the portal triads of the liver (see Fig. 1-98) and in the cortices of the kidney. In the liver, these cuffs may be very large and invest the branches of the hepatic artery, which may undergo fibrinoid necrosis. Microscopic lesions are frequently present

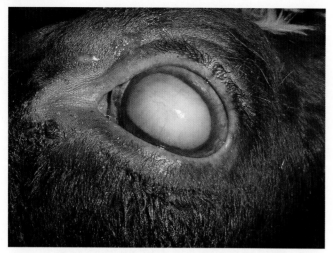

Figure 1-103 Corneal edema in **malignant catarrhal fever.** (Courtesy A. P. Loretti.)

in the kidneys, even though gross lesions are not; they consist of vasculitis involving the smaller arteries and afferent arterioles (see Fig. 1-99B). Extensive diffuse lymphocytic infiltrates disrupt the normal renal cortical architecture, and in some cases, infarcts appear to be associated with vasculitis involving arcuate arteries.

Ophthalmitis often occurs, and its presence is a useful differential criterion from other ulcerative diseases of the alimentary tract. Corneal edema, secondary to vasculitis, is responsible initially for the opacity (Fig. 1-103). Later there may be lymphocytic infiltration of various structures within the globe. There is retinal vasculitis and, in some cases, hemorrhagic or inflammatory detachment of the retina in focal areas. Lymphocytic optic neuritis and meningitis may be seen (see Vol. 1, Eye and ear).

Differentiation of acute severe BVD and mucosal disease from MCF is sometimes difficult, but MCF usually affects one or more organ systems or tissues (liver, kidney, bladder, eye, brain, tracheobronchial tree) not involved in mucosal disease, and typically produces lymphoid hyperplasia in cattle, whereas lymphoid tissue in BVDV infections is expected to be atrophic. Arteritis may be seen in some cases of BVDV infection, mainly in the submucosa in the lower alimentary tract. Fortunately, arteritis is present in more than one tissue in all cases of MCF, whether peracute, acute, or mild with recovery, although it may be necessary to examine many sections to find it. The best organs to examine for vascular lesions are the brain and leptomeninges, carotid rete, kidney (renal arcuate vessels and rete mirabile), liver, adrenal capsule and medulla, salivary gland, and any area of skin or alimentary tract showing gross lesions. In bison, no single tissue can be relied on to establish a morphologic diagnosis of MCF, and a range of tissues should be examined to confirm or rule out the disease. A combination of arteritis, lymphoid hyperplasia, and lymphocytic infiltrates into affected epithelia is very characteristic of MCF.

Bali cattle as well as other species of cattle and buffalo are affected with a disease that closely resembles MCF, and both diseases occur geographically together in Indonesia. **Jembrana disease** is caused by a *lentivirus* distinct from but genetically related to bovine immunodeficiency virus, which initially was described in Bali, where it is endemic, and that has now spread to other islands in Indonesia, including Kalimantan, West Sumatra, and Java. Jembrana disease is characterized by a severe lymphoproliferative response. Gross changes include lymphadenopathy, splenomegaly, and hemorrhages associated with vascular damage. Microscopically, lymphoid tissues of all organs show proliferating lymphoblastic cells. This is particularly marked in the enlarged peripheral lymph nodes and spleen, where proliferating lymphoblastic cells are present throughout the parafollicular T-cell areas; and B-cell follicles are atrophied. Proliferation of T lymphocytes and atrophy of follicles in lymph nodes and spleen, with lymphoid infiltrates in multiple organs in Jembrana disease, appear similar to lesions of MCF.

Further reading

Desport M, Lewis J. Jembrana disease virus: host responses, viral dynamics and disease control. Curr HIV Res 2010;8:53-65.

Dettwiler M, et al. A possible case of caprine-associated malignant catarrhal fever in a domestic water buffalo (*Bubalus bubalis*) in Switzerland. BMC Vet Res 2011;7:78.

Gailbreath KL, et al. Experimental nebulization of American bison (*Bison bison*) with low doses of ovine herpesvirus 2 from sheep nasal secretions. Vet Microbiol 2010;143:389-393.

Li H, et al. Characterization of ovine herpesvirus 2-induced malignant catarrhal fever in rabbits. Vet Microbiol 2011;150:270-277.

Li H, et al. Experimental induction of malignant catarrhal fever in pigs with ovine herpesvirus 2 by intranasal nebulization. Vet Microbiol 2012;159:485-489.

O'Toole D, Li H. The pathology of malignant catarrhal fever, with an emphasis on ovine herpesvirus 2. Vet Pathol 2014;51: 437-452.

O'Toole D, Li H: Malignant catarrhal fever (MCFV). In: Shapshak P, et al., editors. Global Virology I—Identifying and Investigating Viral Diseases. Berlin: Springer-Verlag; 2014.

Schultheiss PC, et al. Epizootic malignant catarrhal fever in three bison herds: differences from cattle and association with ovine herpesvirus-2. J Vet Diagn Invest 2000;12:497-502.

Bluetongue and related diseases

Bluetongue is caused by a reovirus—species ***Bluetongue virus*** (BTV), genus *Orbivirus*, family *Reoviridae*. There are at least 26 recognized serotypes of BTV, distinguished initially by serum neutralization tests and more recently by RT-PCR amplification of the serotype-specific genome segment 2. Immunity to one serotype does not confer resistance against another, and may cause sensitization, with a more severe syndrome following infection by a second type. Apparently not all serotypes are pathogenic.

Epizootic hemorrhagic disease of deer and other ruminants, including cattle, is caused by a virus which represents another serogroup of genus *Orbivirus.* The virus causing Ibaraki disease, recognized in cattle in Japan, is a variant of ***Epizootic hemorrhage disease virus*** (EHDV); seropositive animals also have been found in Taiwan and Indonesia, and an identical virus has been isolated in Australia.

BTV, EHDV, and related viruses are spread by vector-competent *Culicoides* spp., also known as midges or gnats. The virus multiplies by a factor of 10^3-10^4 in the *Culicoides* within a week of the infected blood meal being ingested, and transmission can occur after infection of the salivary glands, 10-15 days after the initial blood meal. Transovarial transmission of virus in *Culicoides* does not occur.

BTV circulates in a broad belt across the tropics and warm temperate areas, from about latitude 49°N to 35°S, with incursions or recrudescence during the *Culicoides* season, annually, or at irregular longer intervals in cooler temperate areas. The condition is enzootic or seasonally epizootic in most of Africa, the Middle East, the eastern Mediterranean basin, the Indian subcontinent, the Caribbean, northern Australia, and the United States. It appears sporadically in the Okanagan valley of western Canada. It also has made persistent incursions into the Iberian peninsula, Corsica and Sardinia, Italy, the Balkans, and northern Europe, including the United Kingdom, perhaps associated with climate change. Seasonality of infection toward the periphery of its distribution probably reflects the unavailability of vectors because the virus may be able to overwinter in latently infected cells in the skin of sheep, which express virus once vector feeding occurs again.

Sheep, goats, and cattle are the primary susceptible domestic species. Severe disease has been described in numerous species of wild and domestic ruminants. South American camelids traditionally have been considered resistant to bluetongue, but serological surveys have identified apparently subclinical infection of alpacas, and lethal cases of bluetongue have been reported in llamas and alpacas. Sheep are the domestic species most highly susceptible to bluetongue, but there is considerable variation in expression of the disease, depending on the breed, age, and immune status of the sheep, the environmental circumstances under which they are held, and the strain of virus. Typically, indigenous breeds seem more resistant to clinical disease than do exotics. Goats, although susceptible to infection, rarely show signs; however, disease has occurred in goats in the Middle East and India. Infection in cattle usually produces only inapparent infection or mild clinical disease. In Africa, a wide variety of nondomestic ungulates and some small mammals may be infected inapparently; mortality has occurred in naturally or experimentally infected topi, Cape buffalo, and kudu. In North America, wildlife species, particularly white-tailed deer, black-tailed or mule deer, elk, bighorn sheep, bison, and pronghorn antelope are also infected. Bluetongue is responsible for significant mortality in all these species except elk, which usually develop mild or inapparent infection, and bison, which are infrequently demonstrated to be serologically positive. Clinical cases of bluetongue have been described only in individual South American camelids. Vaccine inadvertently contaminated with BTV and administered to dogs caused significant mortality, but BTV is not normally considered a pathogen in dogs.

Epizootic hemorrhagic disease occurs in North America, Europe, Africa, and Asia. In North America the white-tailed deer is extremely susceptible, and widespread epizootics have occurred among this species in the United States. The rate of survival is much higher among black-tailed deer and pronghorn antelope; elk are only very mildly affected.

Although sheep are not considered to develop disease when infected with EHDV, occasional mild clinical signs and lesions resembling bluetongue have been reported in sheep inoculated with some Australian isolates. In Japan, the *Ibaraki virus* strain of EHDV produces a clinical syndrome resembling bluetongue in cattle, but not in sheep.

BTV and EHDV circulate together in North America. Both viruses may be involved simultaneously in outbreaks of hemorrhagic disease in wild ruminants, and both have been isolated from *Culicoides* in a single locality at the same time. The role of cattle as reservoirs of BTV is uncertain. Cattle may act as reservoirs in that the virus will be associated with the erythrocytes for the life-span of that cell. Detectable viremia in cattle is thought to be <9 weeks.

The **pathogenesis** of bluetongue, epizootic hemorrhagic disease, and Ibaraki disease is fundamentally similar in all species in which disease is seen. Primary viral replication following insect bite occurs in regional lymph nodes and spleen. Viremia ~4-6 days after inoculation results in secondary infection of endothelium in arterioles, capillaries, and venules throughout the body, but especially in lung microvascular endothelium. Microscopic lesions, fever, and lymphopenia begin a day or so later, about a week after inoculation. BTV in the blood appears to be closely associated with, or in, both leukocytes and erythrocytes, and it may co-circulate with antibody.

Endothelial damage caused by viral infection initiates local *microvascular thrombosis and permeability*. This is reflected microscopically by the presence of swollen endothelium, and fibrin and platelet thrombi in small vessels, with edema and hemorrhage in surrounding tissue. These lesions in turn mediate the full spectrum of gross findings. These are fundamentally *ischemic necrosis* of many tissues; *edema* caused by vascular permeability; and *hemorrhage* resulting from vascular damage compounded (Fig. 1-104A, B), in severe cases, by consumption coagulopathy caused by thrombocytopenia and depletion of soluble clotting factors. Differences in the expression and activity of vasoactive and procoagulant and anticoagulant mediators by infected pulmonary endothelium may explain the greater propensity of sheep to show signs, in comparison with cattle.

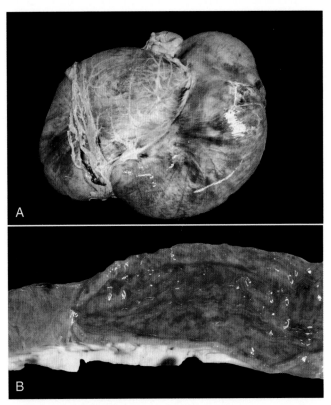

Figure 1-104 Epizootic hemorrhagic disease in a pronghorn antelope. A. Subserosal hemorrhage of the reticulorumen. **B.** Hemorrhage of the small intestine.

Bluetongue in sheep is highly variable; it may cause inapparent infection or acute fulminant disease. Typically, leukopenia and pyrexia occur, even in mild infections, coincident with viremia. The degree and duration of fever do not correlate with the severity of the syndrome otherwise.

In the early phase there is hyperemia of the oral and nasal mucosa, drooling, and nasal discharge within a day or two of the onset of fever. Hyperemia and edema of the eyelids and conjunctiva may occur, and edema of lips, ears, and the intermandibular area becomes apparent. Hyperemia may extend over the muzzle and the skin of much of the body, including the axillary and inguinal areas. Focal hemorrhage may be present on the lips and gums, and *the tongue may become edematous and congested or cyanotic*, giving the disease its name. Infarcted epithelium thickens and becomes excoriated; erosions and ulcerations develop along the margins of the tongue opposite the molars, and the mucosa of much of the tongue may slough.

Excoriation and ulceration also occur on the buccal mucosa, the hard palate, and dental pad. Affected areas of skin also may become encrusted and excoriated with time, and a break in the wool can result in parts or much of the fleece being tender or cast. The coronet, bulbs, and interdigital areas of the foot may become hyperemic. Coronary swelling and streaky hemorrhages in the periople may be evident as a result of lesions in the underlying sensitive laminae. These hemorrhages may persist in the hoof as brown lines that move down the hoof as it grows. A defect parallel to the coronet also may be evident in the growing hoof in recovered cases.

Internally, in acute cases, there is *subcutaneous and intermuscular edema*, which may be serous or suffused with blood. Superficial lymph nodes are enlarged and edematous. Bruise-like gelatinous hemorrhages and contusions, which may be small and easily overlooked if not numerous, often are present in the subcutis and intermuscular fascial planes. Focal or multifocal pallid areas of streaky myodegeneration may be present throughout the carcass, sometimes partly obscured by petechial or ecchymotic hemorrhage. Resolving muscle lesions may be mineralized or fibrous. Stiffness, reluctance to move, and recumbency seen clinically are due to these muscle lesions.

Necrosis may be present deep in the papillary muscle of the left ventricle, and elsewhere in the myocardium. The lesion that is perhaps most consistent and closest to pathognomonic for bluetongue is *focal hemorrhage*, petechial or up to 1 cm wide × 2-3 cm long, in the tunica media at the *base of the pulmonary* artery. These hemorrhages are visible from both the internal and adventitial surfaces and may be present in clinically mild cases with few other lesions. Petechial hemorrhage also may be present at the base of the aorta and in subendocardial and subepicardial locations over the heart.

There also may be edema and petechial or ecchymotic hemorrhage in the pharyngeal and laryngeal area. In severe cases the lungs may assume a purple hue, with marked edematous separation of lobules, and froth in the tracheobronchial tree, probably because of pulmonary microvascular damage and heart failure. Animals with pharyngeal or esophageal myodegeneration suffer from dysphagia, or regurgitate, and may succumb to aspiration pneumonia.

Hyperemia, occasionally marked hemorrhage, or in advanced cases, ulceration of the mucosa may occur on rumen papillae, the pillars of the rumen, and the reticular plicae. In convalescent animals, stellate healing ulcers or scars on the wall of the forestomachs may be apparent.

Microscopically, acute lesions are characterized by microvascular thrombosis, and edema and hemorrhage in affected sites recognized at autopsy. In squamous mucosa and skin, capillaries of the proprial and dermal papillae are involved, resulting in vacuolation and necrosis of overlying epithelium. In acute lesions there is a mild, local neutrophilic infiltrate, and a similarly mild mononuclear reaction in the dermis or propria in uncomplicated chronic lesions, which may granulate if widely or deeply ulcerated. Similar microvascular lesions are associated with necrosis and fragmentation of infarcted muscle. Muscle during the reparative phase follows the usual course of regeneration of fibers or fibrous replacement, depending on whether or not the sarcolemma retains its integrity.

In **cattle,** *clinical bluetongue is rarely apparent;* in endemic areas it may never be evident. Mortality is low and it is often attributed to secondary infection. Clinical disease may be a function of hypersensitivity in previously exposed animals, and disease in experimentally infected animals is poorly defined. Fever, loss of appetite, and leukopenia are usually seen after an incubation period of 6-8 days, and there may be a drop in milk production in dairy cattle. There is reddening of the epithelium of the mucous membranes, and of thin exposed skin, especially notable on the udder and teats. Edema of the lips and conjunctiva may be present. Drooling may become profuse, and as the disease progresses over the next several days, hyperemia and congestion of the mucosae become more intense. Ulcerations of the gingival, lingual, or buccal mucosa occur, most consistently on the dental pad. There may be necrosis of epithelium on the muzzle. Muscle stiffness is a feature of the disease in some animals. Laminitis, characterized by hyperemia and edema of the sensitive laminae at the coronet, may be apparent, and in some cases, hooves on affected feet may eventually slough. Sloughing or cracking of crusts of necrotic epithelium may also occur on affected parts of the skin, but the ulcerative or erosive defects heal readily. Viral antigen and thrombosis are present in small vessels in affected tissues during the acute phase.

Although traditionally *South American camelids* have been considered to be resistant to BTV, individual cases of the disease have been described in alpacas and llamas with lesions including hydrothorax, hydropericardium, pulmonary edema, myocardial hemorrhage, and pericarditis, but no alimentary tract lesions. Experimental inoculation of llamas and alpacas with BTV serotype 8 produced seroconversion, but minimal and mild clinical signs and no significant gross or microscopic lesions.

EHDV can also induce disease in cattle. Clinically and pathologically, EHD in cattle is similar to bluetongue.

Ibaraki disease has been described in Japan and it is produced by a virus that is now considered serotype 2 of EHDV. The signs and lesions of Ibaraki disease are similar to those of bluetongue and EHD in cattle, though more severe in some cases. As well as the signs and lesions described in cattle with bluetongue, there may be difficulty in swallowing in 20-30% of clinically affected animals, and the swollen tongue may protrude from the mouth. At autopsy, in addition to the lesions observable externally, there may be congestion, erosion, or ulceration of the mucosa of the abomasum, and less commonly, the esophagus and forestomachs. Ischemic necrosis and hemorrhage of the striated muscle in the tongue, pharynx, larynx, and esophagus cause the difficulty in swallowing seen clinically, and similar changes are seen in other skeletal muscles. Necrotizing aspiration pneumonia is a sequel to dysphagia in some animals.

The *hemorrhagic diseases* in bighorn sheep, pronghorn antelope, and white-tailed and black-tailed or mule deer in North America resemble bluetongue in sheep. White-tailed deer and pronghorn may develop a particularly severe and fulminant hemorrhagic disease, with high mortality. There may be necrosis of velvet antler, and hooves may slough in survivors. Bluetongue in goats, although usually inapparent, can resemble bluetongue in sheep.

Bluetongue in sheep must be differentiated from foot-and-mouth disease, peste des petits ruminants, contagious ecthyma, and photosensitization in particular. In cattle, the condition must be differentiated from foot-and-mouth disease, vesicular stomatitis, bovine viral diarrhea, rinderpest, malignant catarrhal fever, and photosensitivity. In Japan, Ibaraki disease of cattle in addition must be differentiated clinically from ephemeral fever virus.

In addition to the systemic disease described, *abortion*, perhaps unobserved, and birth of progeny with various *congenital defects* may follow BTV infection of pregnant sheep and cattle. In sheep, BTV infection of ewes early in gestation may result in hydranencephaly. Anomalous calves produced by BTV-infected cattle have excessive gingiva, an enlarged tongue, anomalous maxillae, dwarf-like build, and rotations and contractures of the distal extremities. Porencephaly, hydranencephaly, and arthrogryposis are also reported in calves infected in utero with BTV. Antibody may be sought in neonates that have not sucked, and attempts should be made to isolate virus, because some prenatally infected animals may have immune tolerance, and persistent infection. Anomalies of the brain are considered further in Vol. 1, Nervous system.

Further reading

Breard E, et al. Epizootic hemorrhagic disease virus serotype 6 experimentation on adult cattle. Res Vet Sci 2013;95:794-798.

Maan NS, et al. Identification and differentiation of the twenty six bluetongue virus serotypes by RT-PCR amplification of the serotype-specific genome segment 2. PLoS One 2012;7:e32601.

Ortega J, et al. Fatal bluetongue virus infection in an alpaca (*Vicugna pacos*) in California. J Vet Diagn Invest 2010;22:134-136.

Sailleau C, et al. Cocirculation of bluetongue and epizootic haemorrhagic disease viruses in cattle in Reunion Island. Vet Microbiol 2012;155:191-197.

Savini G, et al. Epizootic haemorrhagic disease. Res Vet Sci 2011;91:1-17.

Schulz, C et al. Experimental infection of South American camelids with bluetongue virus serotype 8. Vet Microbiol 2012;154:257-265.

Parapoxviral infections

Bovine papular stomatitis. Papular stomatitis of cattle occurs worldwide. *It is generally not a clinically significant infection*, but needs to be differentiated from other more serious diseases affecting the oral cavity and skin. Bovine papular stomatitis is usually an indicator of immunity problems associated in many cases with poor colostrum administration. It is caused by species **Bovine papular stomatitis virus** (BPSV),

genus *Parapoxvirus*, family *Poxviridae*, which is closely related to *Pseudocowpox virus* that causes pseudocowpox in cattle and milker's nodules in humans. The disease in humans is usually very mild although severe skin lesions have been reported in at least one case. BPSV is morphologically similar to, and shares antigens with, *Orf virus* of sheep and goats (see Vol. 1, Integumentary system). However, analysis of the genome indicates that these viruses are distinct.

BPSV is relatively host-specific. As with many of the poxviruses, neutralizing antibody is not readily demonstrated. Infection does not confer significant immunity, and successive episodes of lesions and relapses can occur. The disease is more common in calves than in older animals, although the susceptibility of, or recrudescence in, the latter may be increased by intercurrent debility, disease such as bovine viral diarrhea, infectious bovine rhinotracheitis, or other stressors.

The *papular lesions* of this disease occur on the muzzle and in the rostral nares, on the gums, the buccal papillae, the dental pad, the inner aspect of the lips, the hard palate (Fig. 1-105A), the floor of the oral cavity behind the incisors, the ventral and lateral (not dorsal) surfaces of the tongue, occasionally in the esophagus (Fig. 1-105B) and forestomachs.

The initial lesions, which are likely to be detected on the muzzle or lips, are erythematous roughly round macules, ~2 mm-2 cm in diameter. Shortly, the central portion becomes elevated as a low papule, although the elevation is not easy to see, and by the second day a gray central zone of epithelial hyperplasia has developed on which there is superficial scaliness and necrosis. A central necrotic area may slough to form a shallow craterous defect surrounded by a slightly raised red margin. Lesions may coalesce. The course of individual lesions is about a week.

Histologically, there is focal but intense hyperemia and edema in the papillae of the lamina propria, with accumulation of a few mononuclear leukocytes. The epithelium is thickened, sometimes to twice its normal depth, by hyperplasia and ballooning degeneration in the deeper layers (Fig. 1-105C). The cytoplasm of affected cells is clear, and the nucleus may be shrunken. *Dense eosinophilic inclusion bodies lie in the vacuolated cytoplasm*, especially in cells at the active margin of the lesion. These inclusion bodies are present during the initial period of the infection but are difficult to see in the more advanced lesions. In the central, more advanced part of the lesion, a mainly neutrophilic infiltrate into the superficial propria and epithelium is associated with erosion of the upper layers of necrotic cells. The basal layer survives and may be very flattened in eroded areas. Vesicles do not form.

A *chronic form* has been reported, with necrotic and proliferative stomatitis, represented histologically by extensive parakeratotic hyperkeratosis, pseudoepitheliomatous hyperplasia, and occasional intracytoplasmic inclusion bodies.

Papular stomatitis is probably more common and widespread than reports indicate. Variation in the extent and gross appearance of the lesions is to be expected, depending on the usual host-parasite factors and the nature of superimposed infections. They may predispose to the development of necrotic stomatitis, and must be differentiated from the lesions of bovine viral diarrhea, foot-and-mouth disease, alimentary infectious bovine rhinotracheitis, and other causes of ulcers and erosions in the upper alimentary tract. The infection can be transmitted to humans to produce small papules that may persist for several weeks on the skin, usually of the fingers or forearms.

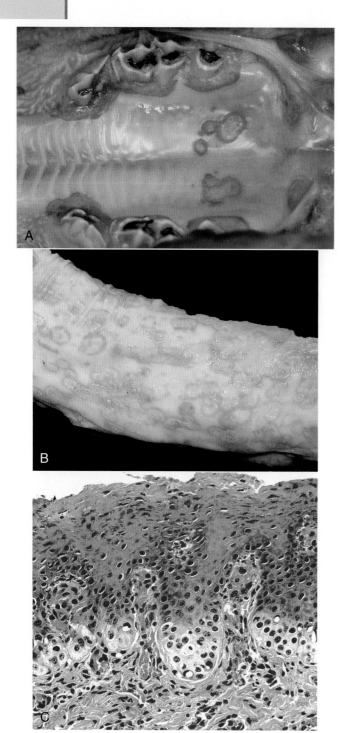

Figure 1-105 Bovine papular stomatitis. A. Lesions at various stages of evolution in palate. **B.** Lesions in esophagus. (Reprinted with permission from Jeckel S, et al. Vet Rec 2011;169:317.) **C.** Thickened epithelium at the margin of a lesion with ballooning degeneration of cells in the deeper layers. (Courtesy P. Loukopoulos.)

Co-infection with vaccinia virus and a parapoxvirus with 85-86% homology with BPSV was described in dairy cattle in Brazil. Affected cows showed gross and histologic lesions similar to those of bovine papular stomatitis in the teats and udder.

Rapid diagnosis is readily accomplished by demonstration of characteristic parapoxvirus particles in negatively stained material from lesions examined under the electron microscope or by PCR. Histology is highly suggestive when the characteristic inclusion bodies are present.

Contagious pustular dermatitis. Contagious pustular dermatitis, also called **orf** or **contagious ecthyma,** is a parapoxviral disease of sheep and goats that is characterized mainly by *proliferative scabby lesions on the lips, face, udder, and feet* (see Vol. 1, Integumentary system). The disease also has been reported in camels and a gazelle. Lesions may extend into the oral cavity, involving the tongue, gingiva, dental pad, and palate. Involvement of the esophagus and forestomachs occurs, but is very unusual. In general the evolution of the alimentary lesions is similar to papular stomatitis of cattle, although they are more exudative and usually much more proliferative. *Intracytoplasmic inclusion bodies* similar to those observed in bovine papular stomatitis also can be observed in the initial stages of the infection. Morbidity may be high, and death can occur in suckling animals. In the upper alimentary tract, lesions may consist of focal red, raised areas, which coalesce to form papules followed by pustules. The latter rupture, and on the muzzle and in the mouth they may become covered by a gray to brown scab, although scab formation may not occur in the mucosa of the upper alimentary tract. As with bovine papular stomatitis, rapid diagnosis is readily accomplished by demonstration of characteristic parapoxvirus particles in negatively stained material from lesions examined under the electron microscope or by PCR. Histology is highly suggestive when the characteristic inclusion bodies are present.

Further reading

de Sant'Ana FJF, et al. Coinfection by Vaccinia virus and an Orf virus–like parapoxvirus in an outbreak of vesicular disease in dairy cows in midwestern Brazil. J Vet Diagn Invest 2013;25:267-272.

Holmes P, et al. Zoonotic transmission of bovine papular stomatitis virus. Vet Rec 2011;169:235-236.

Jeckel S, et al. Severe oesophagitis in an adult bull caused by bovine papular stomatitis virus. Vet Rec 2011;169:317.

Roess AA, et al. Surveillance of parapoxvirus among ruminants in Virginia and Connecticut. Zoon Pub Hlth 2013;60:543-548.

Zhao H, et al. Specific qPCR assays for the detection of orf virus, pseudocowpox virus and bovine papular stomatitis virus. J Virol Methods 2013;194:229-234.

Infectious bovine rhinotracheitis. Species ***Bovine herpesvirus 1*** (Infectious bovine rhinotracheitis virus, BoHV-1), genus *Varicellovirus,* subfamily *Alphaherpesvirinae,* has been associated with a wide range of clinicopathologic syndromes in cattle. These include necrotizing rhinotracheitis, conjunctivitis, infectious pustular vulvovaginitis and balanoposthitis, vesicular lesions of the udder, abortions, systemic infections in neonatal calves and latent infection (see appropriate chapters). Clinical significance of BoHV-1 in other species such as bison that have serological evidence of exposure is not known.

A *systemic form* of the disease, which usually involves the alimentary tract, may occur spontaneously in neonatal calves (in which it may be congenital, or acquired shortly after birth) and in feedlot cattle. It has been reproduced experimentally in young calves.

The pathogenesis of systemic infection with BoHV-1 is poorly understood. Colostrum-deprived calves are especially susceptible, and the disease can be prevented by feeding colostrum from actively immunized dams. The virus probably

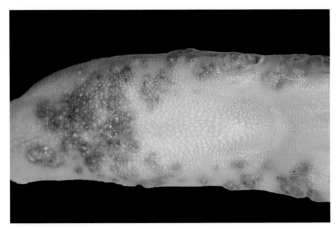

Figure 1-106 Foci of necrosis on mucosa of tongue in a neonatal calf with **infectious bovine rhinotracheitis**. (Courtesy R. Moeller.)

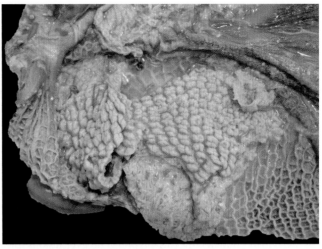

Figure 1-107 Infectious bovine rhinotracheitis in a neonatal calf. Cheesy necrotic debris in rumen and reticulum. (Courtesy V. Psychas.)

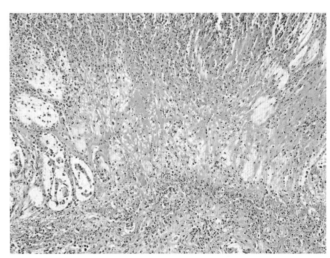

Figure 1-108 Necrosis of epithelium in the crypts of Lieberkühn in the small intestine of a neonatal calf with **infectious bovine rhinotracheitis**. (Courtesy R. Moeller.)

spreads from the mucosa of the upper respiratory tract to other tissues by circulating leukocytes. Peripheral blood mononuclear leukocytes may exhibit apoptosis in response to BoHV-1, but the significance of this is unknown.

Experimental infection of calves with noncytopathic bovine viral diarrhea virus (NCP-BVDV) followed by BoHV-1 inoculation results in dissemination of the latter to a variety of tissues. BVDV impairs cell-mediated immunity, and this may allow BoHV-1 to escape from the respiratory tract and lead to a systemic infection. Dual infections of BVDV and BoHV-1 occur under field conditions, but coinfection of these two viruses is not a prerequisite for the disease to develop.

Clinically affected animals have hyperemic oral and nasal mucosae, and focal areas of necrosis, erosion, and ulceration on the nares, dental pad, gums, buccal mucosa, palate, and the caudal, ventral, and dorsal surfaces of the tongue. Characteristically, the lesions tend to be punctate with a slightly raised margin; the necrotic areas are covered by a gray-white layer of fibrinonecrotic exudate, which leaves a raw red base when removed.

The **lesions** may be present in the oral cavity and extend into the esophagus, usually only the upper third, and the forestomachs. In the oral cavity and esophagus, the erosions and ulcers may be irregular, circular, or linear, and often they have a punched-out appearance and a hyperemic border (Fig. 1-106). The ruminal lesions, which are most commonly located in the dorsal and cranioventral sacs, vary considerably. The earliest lesions consist of foci of necrosis and hemorrhage, a few millimeters in diameter. In some cases the necrosis may involve almost the entire surface of the ruminal mucosa, which becomes covered by a thick, dirty gray layer of exudate, resembling curdled milk, which adheres tightly to the wall (Fig. 1-107). Similar lesions may be evident in the reticulum. Focal areas of necrosis result in the formation of holes, as large as 1.5 cm in diameter, in the leaves of the omasum. In addition, these calves may have focal areas of necrosis in the abomasal mucosal folds, which may coalesce to form areas of necrosis 2-3 cm in diameter. The intestines are red and dilated, and the serosal surface may be covered by a thin layer of fibrinous exudate.

The enteric lesions may be accompanied by changes in the upper respiratory tract. When present the respiratory lesions are similar to those described for older cattle, although they

are milder and generally limited to the nasal mucosa, larynx, and upper third of the trachea (see Vol. 2, Respiratory system). Gray to yellow necrotic foci 2-5 mm diameter may be evident macroscopically on the capsular and cut surfaces of the liver, the adrenal cortices, the spleen, and in Peyer's patches.

Microscopically, the lesions in the squamous mucosa are characterized by *focal areas of necrosis, erosion, and ulceration. Severe* necrosis may involve the entire papilla or mucosa more diffusely. *Nuclear inclusions* may be present in epithelial cells in the periphery of the lesion, although these are an inconsistent finding. They are more likely to be found if tissues are collected in the early stages of the disease and fixed in Bouin's fluid. The abomasal lesions consist of necrosis of glandular epithelial cells. Affected glands are dilated, and filled with necrotic debris. Focal necrotic lesions involving crypts and lamina propria may be present in both the small intestine and large bowel (Fig. 1-108). Abomasal and intestinal lesions may predispose to the development of *secondary mycosis*, which is a common complication.

Foci of coagulative necrosis may occur in the liver, lymph nodes, thymus, Peyer's patches, spleen, and adrenal cortices. Typically there is little inflammation associated with the necrosis. Herpesviral inclusions are inconsistently seen in cells at the periphery of the necrotic foci. In a study of systemic BoHV-1 infection in neonatal calves in California, a large proportion of affected calves had histologic lesions compatible with BoHV-1 only in the adrenal gland. Although most of those animals had enteritis and/or colitis, these lesions were considered to be due to other enteric pathogens (coronavirus, cryptosporidia, rotavirus, and attaching-and-effacing *E. coli*).

The lesions in the upper alimentary tract of cattle associated with BoHV-1 infection must be differentiated from those of calf diphtheria, bovine papular stomatitis, and bovine viral diarrhea. The ruminal lesions must be differentiated from those of bovine adenovirus infection and nonspecific rumenitis, described elsewhere in this chapter. The liver lesions may be confused with focal necrosis associated with septicemias, for example, listeriosis or salmonellosis (see Vol. 2, Liver and biliary system).

Further reading

Moeller RB Jr, et al. Systemic *Bovine herpesvirus 1* infections in neonatal dairy calves. J Vet Diagn Invest 2013;25:136-141.

Nandi S, et al. Bovine herpes virus infections in cattle. Anim Health Res Rev 2009;10:85-98.

Caprine herpesvirus

Species **Caprine herpesvirus 1** (CpHV-1), genus *Varicellovirus*, subfamily *Alphaherpesvirinae*, has been isolated from neonatal goat kids in various parts of the world. CpHV-1 is different from, but shows genomic similarity to, other viruses of this group, such as *Bovine herpesvirus 1*, *Bovine herpesvirus 5*, *Suid herpesvirus 1*, *Cervid herpesvirus 1*, and *Rangiferine herpesvirus 1*. CpHV-1 is associated with 2 different syndromes in goats, depending on the age of the animals at the time of infection. In neonatal kids, CpHV-1 causes an often severe and generalized disease *affecting the digestive tract where it produces erosions and ulcerations*. Infection in adult goats remains inapparent (adult goats may be latent carriers), or may cause respiratory distress, abortion, vulvovaginitis, or balanoposthitis (see Vol. 3, Female genital system). CpHV-1 is able to establish latent infection in trigeminal ganglia and to cause immunosuppression. Although capable of infecting sheep, cattle, and goats, severe disease caused by CpHV-1 is restricted to goats.

The disease in neonatal kids is characterized clinically by fever, conjunctivitis, ocular and nasal discharges, dyspnea, anorexia, abdominal pain, weakness, and death, usually within 1-4 days after onset of clinical signs. Affected kids have leukopenia and hypoproteinemia.

Macroscopic lesions are most obvious throughout the entire alimentary tract. Round or longitudinal erosions, which have a hyperemic border, are evident in the oral mucosa. These are particularly prominent on the gums around the incisor teeth and to a lesser extent in the pharynx and esophagus. Focal red areas of necrosis, which may be slightly elevated above the surrounding mucosa, occur in the rumen. In the abomasum, numerous longitudinal, red erosions are located in the mucosa. The most severe lesions occur in the *cecum and spiral colon*, which are dilated, with a thickened wall, and

contain focal to large areas of mucosal necrosis and ulceration, frequently covered by a diphtheritic membrane. The contents are yellow and mucoid. Hemorrhagic foci may be visible in the bladder mucosa.

Microscopically, the lesions in the upper alimentary tract are typical areas of necrosis and erosion of squamous epithelial cells. The epithelial cells at the periphery of necrotic areas are swollen and vacuolated and these may contain typical *intranuclear herpesviral inclusions*. There is marked inflammatory reaction in the underlying lamina propria. The abomasal lesions consist of acute foci of mucosal necrosis. Inclusions are particularly evident in this area. Lesions in the cecum and colon are more extensive and consist of large areas of mucosal ulceration and necrosis, which may involve the entire thickness of the wall. The submucosa is edematous and markedly infiltrated by inflammatory cells. The mesenteric nodes are edematous and germinal centers are depleted of lymphoid cells. Focal areas of necrosis with a mild inflammatory cell reaction also may be present in liver, urinary bladder, and kidney.

Further reading

Montagnaro S, et al. Modulation of apoptosis by caprine herpesvirus 1 infection in a neuronal cell line. J Cell Biochem 2013;114:2809-2822.

Piper KL, et al. Isolation of caprine herpesvirus 1 from a major outbreak of infectious pustular vulvovaginitis in goats. Aust Vet J 2008;86:136-138.

Thiry J, et al. Isolation and characterisation of a ruminant alphaherpesvirus closely related to bovine herpesvirus 1 in a free-ranging red deer. BMC Vet Res 2007;3:26.

Uzal FA, et al. Abortion and ulcerative posthitis associated with caprine herpesvirus-1 infection in goats in California. J Vet Diagn Invest 2004;16:478-484.

Other herpesviruses

Canid herpesvirus 1 causes systemic disease of neonatal puppies characterized by foci of necrosis and hemorrhage in a wide variety of organs, especially the lungs and renal cortices (see Vol. 3, Female genital system). Focal areas of necrosis may occur in the intestine as part of the systemic syndrome. A similar syndrome also has been described in an adult dog. As with most other herpesvirus, the trigeminal ganglion is an important latency site for canid herpesvirus. However, latency of this virus also occurs in the lumbosacral ganglia and retropharyngeal lymph nodes. Latently infected dogs may or may not shed virus, and shedding may occur continuously or intermittently.

Felid herpesvirus 1 (feline viral rhinotracheitis virus) causes oral lesions (see previous section on Inflammation of the oral cavity). Primary infection by felid herpesvirus 1 may be followed by viremia with the virus distributed to several distant organs. Viruses antigenically related to felid herpesvirus 1 have been isolated from dogs with diarrhea, but descriptions of lesions are not available.

Natural infections with **Suid herpesvirus 1** (SuHV-1; pseudorabies virus, Aujeszky's disease virus) often result in necrotizing tonsillitis. Experimental infection of pigs with SuHV-1 may cause necrotizing enteritis of the distal small intestine. The enteric lesions are characterized by focal areas of necrosis of the cryptal mucosa, muscularis mucosae, and tunica muscularis. Immunohistochemically, antigen is documented in the dome area, the lymphoid follicles of Peyer's patches, and ganglion cells of Meissner's and Auerbach's plexuses.

Necrotizing enterocolitis in adult horses because of **Equid herpesvirus 1** has been reported rarely. A single case with similar intestinal lesions was also reported in a yearling filly. At autopsy there are multiple areas of hemorrhage, necrosis, and ulceration, some several centimeters in diameter, of the mucosa in both small and large intestine. Microscopically, these lesions consist of erosions and ulcerations of the mucosa, and necrosis of cryptal epithelial cells in adjacent areas. Cryptal epithelial cells and some proprial mononuclear cells may have acidophilic and amphophilic nuclear inclusions.

Further reading

Del Piero F, et al. Fatal nonneurological EHV-1 infection in a yearling filly. Vet Pathol 2000;37:672-676.

Evermann JF, et al. Canine reproductive, respiratory, and ocular diseases due to canine herpesvirus. Vet Clin North Am Small Anim Pract 2011;41:1097-1120.

Gadsden BJ, et al. Fatal Canid herpesvirus 1 infection in an adult dog. J Vet Diagn Invest 2012;24:604-607.

Swenson CL, et al. Infectious feline herpesvirus detected in distant bone and tendon following mucosal inoculation of specific pathogen-free cats. Vet Microbiol 2012;160:484-487.

Adenoviral enteritis

The adenoviruses that have been associated with enteric infections in humans, cattle, swine, horses, sheep, cervids, camelids and dogs belong to the family *Adenoviridae*, genera *Mastadenovirus*, and *Atadenovirus*. Serologic surveys show that widely divergent serotypes occur both within and between host species and their distribution is worldwide. All serotypes are morphologically similar; the virus consists of a nonenveloped icosahedral capsid, 70-80 nm in diameter, which has 252 capsomeres. Virus neutralization tests and molecular methods are used to distinguish serotypes. Adenoviral infection of cells causes *intranuclear inclusions*. Adenoviruses are relatively heat-resistant and can survive for several days at room temperature. Most adenoviruses are transmitted by feces, aerosols, or possibly fomites, to susceptible, usually suckling or recently weaned, animals. Infected animals may remain carriers for weeks.

Adenoviruses are highly host-specific. Infections in both humans and animals appear, in general, to be subclinical, and disease seems to occur more commonly in immunologically compromised individuals. Most infections are systemic; certain strains have a tropism for the respiratory tract, and others for the alimentary tract, vascular endothelial cells, or hepatocytes. Their enteric manifestations are considered here.

Further reading

Hartmann NM, et al. Monitoring of adenovirus serotypes in environmental samples by combined PCR and melting point analyses. Virol J 2013;10:190.

Woods LW, et al. Systemic adenovirus infection associated with high mortality in mule deer (*Odocoileus hemionus*) in California. Vet Pathol 1996;33:125-132.

Bovine adenoviruses. Serotypes of bovine adenovirus (BAdV) are in the genera **Mastadenovirus** and **Atadenovirus**,

and are hence being renamed, such as bovine adenovirus serotype 1 (BAdV-1) becomes bovine mastadenovirus A. Infection has been mainly associated with keratoconjunctivitis and respiratory disease. Many strains have been isolated from normal cattle. Serotypes 3, 4, 7, and 10 have been associated with enteric disease. It appears that after an initial viremic stage, the virus localizes in the *endothelial cells* of vessels in a variety of organs, resulting in thrombosis with subsequent focal areas of ischemic necrosis.

Clinically, enteric infections with BAdV occur sporadically in 1-8 week-old calves and in feedlot animals. Affected animals have fever, and diarrhea that may contain blood, and some animals will die peracutely from dysentery. They are dehydrated and the mucous membranes of the muzzle and mouth are congested. Dry, encrusted exudate may cover the muzzle and there may be serous to mucopurulent ocular and nasal discharges.

Macroscopic lesions may be present in the forestomachs, abomasum, and intestine. Those in the forestomachs are characterized by irregular, raised, red-to-gray necrotic areas, 2-4 mm in diameter on the mucosa of both the dorsal and ventral sacs of the rumen. In some cases, the areas of necrosis coalesce to give rise to diffuse necrotizing rumenitis. Ulcers up to 1.5 cm in diameter may be located on the ruminal pillars and these may be visible through the serosa. Similar lesions may be evident in the omasum. The abomasal mucosal folds are edematous and congested, with focal necrosis and ulceration in the mucosa that, like those in the forestomachs, may be visible on the serosal surface.

The intestinal lesions vary from slight dilation and distention with excessive fluid to severe multifocal or diffuse necrosis, which may be covered by a pseudodiphtheritic membrane. In young calves, the lesions are most severe in the jejunum and ileum, especially over the Peyer's patches. In feedlot cattle, the lesions may be most prominent in the colon. The mucosa is dark red (Fig. 1-109) and there is marked edema of the mesocolon. The mesenteric lymph nodes are enlarged and edematous.

Microscopically, foci of ischemic necrosis are evident in the intestinal mucosa, and in more advanced lesions, the necrosis extends across the muscularis mucosae. Fibrinocellular exudate often covers the mucosal surface. Intestinal crypts are dilated, lined by flat epithelial cells, and usually contain necrotic debris (Fig. 1-110A). There is usually marked submucosal edema, congestion, and fibrinous exudation. Foci of necrosis are evident in the lymphoid follicles of the Peyer's patches, which are also depleted of lymphocytes. *Large basophilic to amphophilic inclusions* completely or partially fill the nuclei of endothelium in the vessels of the lamina propria and submucosa of affected areas of the rumen, abomasum, and intestine (Fig. 1-110B). The endothelial cells are swollen and necrotic, and

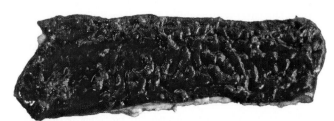

Figure 1-109 Congested and hemorrhagic colon caused by **bovine adenovirus** infection. (Courtesy J.A. Smyth.)

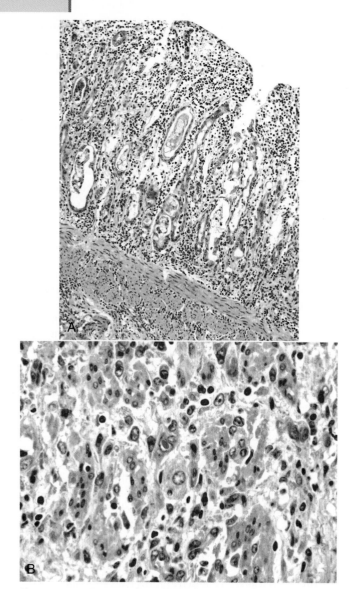

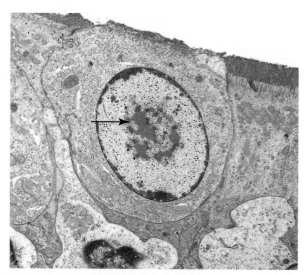

Figure 1-111 Porcine adenovirus–infected cell in epithelium of dome over Peyer's patch. Note inclusion (arrow). (Courtesy D.M. Hoover, S.E. Sanford.)

Lehmkuhl HD, et al. Isolation of a bovine adenovirus serotype 10 from a calf in the United States. J Vet Diagn Invest 1999;11:485-490.

Smyth JA, et al. Bovine adenovirus type 10 identified in fatal cases of adenovirus associated enteric disease in cattle by in situ hybridization. J Clin Microbiol 1996;34:1270-1274.

Porcine adenovirus. According to serological surveys, the 5 serotypes of species *Porcine adenovirus* (PAdV), genus *Mastadenovirus*, are all common. Serotype 4 appears to be the most widely distributed strain of the virus in Europe and North America. Asymptomatic infections are most common in swine, and PAdV may be isolated from feces of normal pigs; PAdVs are actually of more interest as viral vaccine vectors than as pathogens.

The importance of adenoviruses as a cause of enteric disease in the field remains controversial. When disease occurs, the macroscopic lesions in the intestine consist of excessive yellow watery to pasty contents and moderate enlargement of the mesenteric lymph nodes, which cannot be differentiated from other causes of diarrhea in neonatal pigs.

In contrast to the situation in calves, in which inclusions are located mainly in the nuclei of endothelial cells, *inclusions in pigs are in enterocytes* in the distal jejunum and ileum, where primary viral replication likely occurs. The infected nuclei are enlarged, round, and displaced to the apical portion of the cell. The villi may be short and blunt. There may be a moderate mononuclear cell reaction in the lamina propria. Inclusions are also found in the squamous epithelial cells of the tonsils and in endothelial cells of capillary and small blood vessels throughout the body.

Ultrastructurally, infected nuclei of enterocytes are round and swollen and contain numerous typical adenoviral particles (Fig. 1-111). Affected enterocytes are cuboidal and the apical portion protrudes slightly into the lumen. The cell membrane and microvilli are irregular and the terminal web is absent. The rough endoplasmic reticulum shows local distension with formation of large multivesicular bodies. Eventually there is complete loss of microvilli, and the cell membrane ruptures with the release of cell contents and virus particles into the gut lumen.

Figure 1-110 Bovine adenovirus infection. A. Necrosis and hemorrhage of the colon with dilated crypts. **B.** Large basophilic to amphophilic inclusion bodies in the nuclei of endothelium in the vessels of the intestinal lamina propria. (Courtesy C. Buergelt.)

some veins and lymphatics contain thrombi. Similar inclusion bodies may occasionally be seen in nuclei of enterocytes. Typical inclusions also may be found in endothelial cells of vessels and sinusoids of the adrenal glands, mesenteric lymph nodes, liver, spleen, glomeruli, and interstitial capillaries in the kidney, and in the mucosa of the urinary bladder.

Confirmation of enteric BAdV infection depends on the demonstration of the virus in tissue, through electron microscopy, in situ hybridization, PCR or isolation of the virus in cell culture. The latter is often difficult because different serotypes and strains of the virus require specific cell cultures, and several blind passages may be required before cytopathic changes are evident.

Further reading

Adair BM, et al. Bovine adenovirus type 10: properties of viruses isolated from cases of bovine haemorrhagic enterocolitis. Vet Rec 1996;138:250-252.

The significance of adenoviral inclusions in enterocytes must be interpreted with caution. A survey in Canada revealed that 4.4% of 5-day to 24-week-old pigs had adenoviral inclusions in enterocytes, mainly in the ileum. More than 50% of the pigs had diarrhea; however, other enteropathogens were found in most of these animals.

Further reading

Guardado-Calvo P, et al. Crystallographic structure of porcine adenovirus type 4 fiber head and galectin domains. J Virol 2010;84:10558-10568.

Loving CL, et al. Porcine granulocyte-colony stimulating factor (G-CSF) delivered via replication-defective adenovirus induces a sustained increase in circulating peripheral blood neutrophils. Biologicals 2013;41:368-376.

Nagy M, et al. The complete nucleotide sequence of porcine adenovirus serotype 5. J Gen Virol 2001;82:525-529.

Equine adenovirus. Two serotypes of species *Equine adenovirus* (EAdV), genus *Mastadenovirus*, designated EAdV-1 and EAdV-2, have been isolated to date. EAdV-1 has a worldwide distribution and it is mainly responsible for upper respiratory tract infections in foals <3 months of age, whereas EAdV-2 has been isolated mainly from horses with gastrointestinal tract infections.

EAdV-2 has been isolated in Australia from foals with diarrhea. Rotavirus also was identified in the feces of these foals. A serologic survey showed that 77% of adult horses in the area had neutralizing antibodies to this particular serotype.

An unidentified alimentary tract adenoviral infection has been reported in an Arabian foal that did not have lesions of combined immunodeficiency. The foal had diarrhea and progressive weight loss over a 2-month period. The macroscopic lesions consisted of ulcers in the distal esophagus and nonglandular mucosa of the stomach. The intestine contained soft to semifluid ingesta. Histologically, there was necrosis and ulceration of the esophageal and gastric squamous mucosa. Typical adenoviral inclusions were found at all levels of the small intestine. These were most commonly located in the villus epithelial cells, less often in the crypts, and only occasionally in the submucosal glands. There was focal-to-diffuse villus atrophy through the small intestine.

Further reading

Cavanagh HM et al. Genetic characterization of equine adenovirus type 1. Vet Microbiol 2012;155:33-37.

Giles C, et al. Prevalence of equine adenovirus antibodies in horses in New South Wales, Australia. Vet Microbiol 2010;143:401-404.

Adenoviruses in other species. Seven serotypes of *Ovine adenovirus* (OAdV) have been isolated from **sheep**. Serotypes 1-6 belong to the genus **Mastadenovirus**. However, serotype 7 is phylogenetically different from mastadenoviruses, and has been renamed *Ovine adenovirus D*, and subsequently *Ovine atadenovirus D*, the type species in genus **Atadenovirus**. Serotypes 1, 2, and 3 have been recovered from feces of normal sheep, and lambs with enteritis and pneumoenteritis. Experimental inoculation of specific-pathogen-free lambs with OAdV-4 did not cause disease but the virus was re-isolated from feces and nasal secretions for several days post infection. However, occasionally there are reports of enteritis associated

with abundant adenoviral inclusions in lambs and kids. In the former, inclusions were found predominantly in the lamina propria, whereas in the latter they were mostly epithelial.

Goat adenovirus (GAdV) serotypes 1 and 2 can cause enteritis and diarrhea in **goat** kids; GAdV-1 is a serotype of *Ovine adenovirus D*, which also includes serotype 7 and isolate 287.

Two distinct but serologically related adenoviruses have been isolated from **dogs**. *Canine adenovirus 1* (CAdV-1) infection is usually subclinical, but it may cause infectious hepatitis, and diarrhea may be present in these cases. The virus has a particular tropism for hepatocytes and endothelial cells. The serosal hemorrhages in the gastrointestinal tract and possibly the diarrhea may be related to vascular damage in the serosa and mucosa, respectively (see Vol. 2, Liver and biliary system). CAdV-2 is usually associated with upper respiratory infections in dogs (see Vol. 2, Respiratory system). Viruses serologically similar to CAdV-2 have been isolated from feces of diarrheic dogs. DNA fingerprinting of two of these isolates indicated that they are distinct from CAdV-2. It may be that the fecal isolates are due to swallowing of virus originating from upper respiratory tract infections.

A newly recognized cervid *Atadenovirus* known as *Odocoileus adenovirus 1* (OdAdV-1) was the cause of an outbreak of a hemorrhagic disease that caused high mortality in **mule deer** species in California in the 1990s. OdAdV-1 infection has since been diagnosed as a frequent cause of herd mortality in other deer species in other states of the United States and Canada. The OdAdV-1 is phylogenetically most closely related to bovine adenovirus 7, goat adenovirus 1, and ovine adenovirus 7. Experimentally, OdAdV-1 has been demonstrated to be noninfectious to cattle and sheep.

There are 2 manifestations of the disease in deer; systemic and localized. Both forms were experimentally reproduced in black and white-tailed deer. The disease mimics the orbivirus hemorrhagic diseases in that it triggers DIC through endothelial cell necrosis; however, OdAdV-1 targets first endothelial cells of medium and large vessels, whereas bluetongue and epizootic hemorrhagic disease viruses target primarily the microvasculature. With *systemic infection*, gross findings include pulmonary edema and/or gastrointestinal hemorrhage (Fig. 1-112). Microscopically there is widespread vasculitis

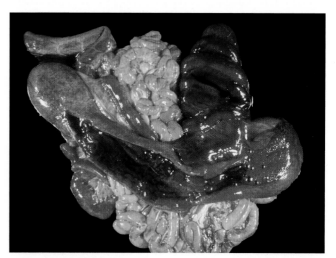

Figure 1-112 Deer adenovirus hemorrhagic disease. Disseminated hemorrhages throughout the gastrointestinal tract. (Courtesy L. Woods.)

characterized by endothelial cell hypertrophy and necrosis, disruption of the tunica intima, leukocytic margination, fibrinoid necrosis, and leukocytic infiltration of the tunica intima and sometimes media. Intranuclear inclusion bodies are seen primarily in the endothelium of large vessels in the lungs and serosa and submucosa of the intestine and less often seen in endothelium of interalveolar septal capillaries in the lungs and lamina propria of the intestines. *Localized infection* is grossly characterized by necrosis and ulceration of the upper alimentary tract. Microscopically there is necrosis of multiple tissues in areas of gross lesions, but vasculitis with intranuclear inclusions is frequently not present.

A novel adenovirus was isolated from an **alpaca** presented with diarrhea and enteritis. Microscopically, multiple intranuclear inclusion bodies were seen in enterocytes throughout the small intestine.

Further reading

Gu Y, et al. Comparative analysis of ovine Adenovirus 287 and human Adenovirus 2 and 5 based on their codon usage. DNA Cell Biol 2012;31:360-366.

Morse BW, et al. Population health of fallow deer (*Dama dama*) on little St. Simons Island. Georgia, USA. J Wild Dis 2009;45: 411-421.

Shilton CM, et al. Adenoviral infection in captive moose (*Alces alces*) in Canada. J Zoo Wildl Med 2002;33:73-79.

Twomey DF, et al. Enteritis in an alpaca (*Vicugna pacos*) associated with a potentially novel adenovirus. J Vet Diagn Invest 2012;24:1000-1003.

Woods LW, et al. Evaluation of the pathogenic potential of cervid adenovirus in calves. J Vet Diagn Invest 2008;20:33-37.

Enteric coronaviral infections

Coronaviruses cause disease affecting a number of organ systems in a variety of species. Among domestic mammals they mainly cause enteric infections, although coronaviruses are implicated in pneumonia in swine and cattle, and in feline infectious peritonitis.

Coronaviruses have a single-stranded RNA genome. They are pleomorphic or roughly spherical and vary in size from ~70-200 nm in diameter, averaging 100-130 nm. They have a phospholipid-bearing envelope, probably derived in part from host cell membrane. They gain their name from the characteristic "corona" of petal- or droplet-shaped radial surface projections ("peplomers") visible under the electron microscope in negatively stained preparations.

The coronaviruses infecting each species of host appear to be distinctive; some species are infected by more than one type of coronavirus. There are antigenic relationships among viruses from various hosts, and experimental cross-infection will occur between some host species, usually without pathologic consequences. Persistent infections can occur.

Coronaviruses are classified as genera *Alphacoronavirus*, *Betacoronavirus*, *Deltacoronavirus*, and *Gammacoronavirus*, in subfamily *Coronavirinae*, family *Coronaviridae*. Species of mammalian veterinary significance include:

- Genus *Alphacoronavirus*
  - Species *Canine coronavirus* (CCoV), *Feline coronavirus* (FCoV), *Porcine epidemic diarrhea virus* (PEDV), *Porcine respiratory coronavirus* (PRCoV), *Transmissible gastroenteritis virus* (TGEV)
- Genus *Betacoronavirus*
  - Species *Bovine coronavirus* (BCoV), *Canine respiratory coronavirus* (CRCoV), *Equine coronavirus* (EqCoV), *Porcine hemagglutinating encephalomyelitis virus* (PHEV)
- Genus *Deltacoronavirus*
  - Species *Porcine deltacoronavirus* (PDCoV, SDCV)

Viral replication in the intestinal epithelium by coronaviruses is similar in all the species studied. Coronavirus infects and replicates in the apical cytoplasm of absorptive enterocytes on the tips and sides of intestinal villi. Virions are probably taken up by the apical border of the cell, by fusion with the plasmalemma. Replication and maturation appear to involve budding of virions from the cytosol through the membrane and into the lumen of vacuoles or cisternae in the smooth endoplasmic reticulum, where they accumulate. Virions are found in tubules of the Golgi apparatus. They may exit via that route from infected cells, by exocytosis at the apical cell membrane, or on the lateral cell surface, because viral particles are often seen lined up between microvilli or in the basolateral intercellular space between infected cells. Virus also may be released by lysis of infected cells. Coronaviruses also infect some mesenchymal cells in villi and probably mesenteric lymph node.

Changes in the infected cell occur by ~12-24 hours after infection. Mitochondria in virus-infected cells swell, cisternae of smooth and rough endoplasmic reticulum dilate, the cytoplasm of infected cells loses its electron density, and cells lose their columnar profile. The terminal web is fragmented; microvilli swell and become irregular, perhaps in association with blebbing of the apical membrane. Damaged epithelium may lyse in situ, releasing virus retained in cytoplasmic vacuoles, or it may exfoliate into the lumen. Profuse diarrhea usually begins about the time that early cytologic changes are becoming apparent, but before there is extensive epithelial exfoliation.

Exfoliation of damaged epithelium may be massive over a relatively short period of time, leading to the development of *villus atrophy*, the severity of which largely reflects the degree of initial viral damage. Villi may appear fused along their sides or tips, and during the exfoliative phase some villi with denuded tips may be present. The enterocytes present on villi shortly after the initial exfoliative episode are mainly poorly differentiated low columnar, cuboidal, or squamous cells, with stubby irregular microvilli. Within 2-3 days, villi begin to regenerate and the epithelium becomes progressively more columnar, although still lacking a well-developed brush border and its complement of enzymes. Defective fat absorption is reflected in the accumulation of lipid droplets in the cytoplasm of enterocytes on villi. This is particularly marked over the period of ~2-5 days after experimental inoculation.

With progressive epithelial regeneration from the crypts, the *villus fusion*, which may be the result of adhesion of temporarily denuded lamina propria of adjacent villi, regresses. Separation begins along the basal margins of the adhesions and progresses toward the tips of the villi. There may be focal acute inflammation in the lamina propria of temporarily denuded villi, and a mild mononuclear infiltrate in the stroma of collapsed villi. Although several cycles of viral replication may occur, poorly differentiated enterocytes appear relatively refractory to infection, and the virus titer falls, presumably as local immune mechanisms also come into play. Hyperplasia of epithelium in crypts usually results in eventual resolution of the villus atrophy, restoring normal function.

The diarrhea that occurs is a result of electrolyte and nutrient malabsorption, with some contribution by secretion by crypt cells, and probably by poorly differentiated surface epithelium in the reparative phase. Mechanisms of diarrhea in villus atrophy are discussed in the section on the Pathophysiology of enteric disease. Remission of signs occurs within ~4-6 days as regeneration of villi occurs, providing the animal survives the dehydration, electrolyte depletion, and acidosis brought about by diarrhea.

Diagnosis is achieved by detection of viral particles by negative-staining electron microscopy or detection of the virus by fluorescent antibodies, immunohistochemistry, PCR, and/or virus isolation.

Further reading

Decaro N, Buonavoglia C. An update on canine coronaviruses: viral evolution and pathobiology. Vet Microbiol 2008;132: 221-234.

Rossen JW, et al. Feline and canine coronaviruses are released from the basolateral side of polarized epithelial LLC-PK1 cells expressing the recombinant feline aminopeptidase-N cDNA. Arch Virol 2001; 146:791-799.

Swine coronaviruses. Four coronaviruses cause gastrointestinal signs in swine. In genus *Alphacoronavirus*, species *Porcine epidemic diarrhea virus* (PEDV), *Transmissible gastroenteritis virus* (TGEV); in genus *Betacoronavirus*, species *Porcine hemagglutinating encephalomyelitis virus* (PHEV); and in genus *Deltacoronavirus*, species *Porcine deltacoronavirus* (PDCoV, SDCV). PEDV, TGEV, and PDCoV cause vomiting and diarrhea in suckling piglets, with high morbidity and mortality caused by severe enteritis. PHEV also causes vomiting and wasting disease in suckling piglets; but mainly mediated by infection of the central and peripheral nervous system (see Vol. 1, Nervous system).

Transmissible gastroenteritis (TGE) may affect swine of any age, causing vomiting, severe diarrhea, and, in piglets, high mortality. The disease is recognized throughout most of the world. The epidemiology of TGE depends on the overall immune status of the herd and of the various age groups within the herd. Introduction of TGEV into a naive herd results in rapid spread of disease with high morbidity affecting all age groups. Sows and older pigs show transient inappetence, and possibly diarrhea and vomiting. Signs may be more severe in sows exposed to high virus challenge from infected baby pigs. Agalactia may occur in recently farrowed sows, perhaps related to TGEV infection of the mammary gland. *Suckling piglets develop severe diarrhea*, and mortality may approach 100% in piglets <10-14 days old. Older pigs usually develop less severe signs and have lower mortality. In herds with enzootic infection, high piglet mortality may occur in the offspring of recently introduced naive sows, and diarrhea with lower mortality may occur in piglets greater than ~2-3 weeks of age as milk intake and concomitant lactogenic immunity wane. Infected pigs in the late suckling or weanling age group may runt. TGE is more prevalent in the winter, perhaps because the virus is not resistant to summer environmental conditions of warmth and sunlight. Baby pigs that are chilled also seem less able to survive the effects of infection.

The severity of disease in baby pigs is partly related to their inability to withstand dehydration because of their small size, and to their susceptibility to hypoglycemia. Probably as significant is the differentiation, and low rate of turnover, of small intestinal epithelium in the neonate. The surface epithelium is mature and has an extensive vesicular network in the apical cytoplasm associated with uptake of macromolecules and colostrum during the first day or two after birth. Crypts are short and relatively inactive. Therefore the population of epithelium susceptible to infection on each villus is large, and the capacity to regenerate new enterocytes is small. By ~3 weeks of age, epithelium is actively proliferative. Virus production by infected enterocytes in older pigs seems less efficient, and replacement of cells lost to infection is more rapid, contributing to the relative resistance seen in swine greater than ~3 weeks of age.

Piglets with TGE have the nonspecific gross appearance at autopsy of undifferentiated neonatal diarrhea. The stomach may contain a milk curd or bile-stained fluid. The small bowel is flaccid and contains yellow frothy fluid with flecks of mucus; chyle is not usually evident in mesenteric lymphatics because there is fat malabsorption.

The microscopic lesions are those of villus atrophy resulting from exfoliation of surface enterocytes (Fig. 1-113), the severity of which is a function of the age of the pig and the stage of the disease. In young piglets, the lesions are most severe about the time of the onset of diarrhea. In later phases or in older pigs there may be subtotal to moderate atrophy, and the mucosa may be lined by cuboidal to low columnar epithelium, with irregular nuclear polarity and an indistinct brush border. Severe atrophy is readily recognized at necropsy of neonatal piglets by examination of the mucosa under a dissecting microscope. Lesions are most common in the middle and lower small intestine, and villi in the duodenum are usually tall and cylindrical. Lesions may be patchy, and several areas of lower small intestine must be examined before atrophy is considered not to be present. In animals beyond the neonatal age group, atrophy may not be so severe and readily recognized under the dissecting microscope, and the contrast with the normally shorter villi in the duodenum of older pigs is not as marked. Histologic assessment of the gut is essential.

Porcine respiratory coronavirus (PRCoV) is genetically and antigenically extremely close to TGEV. It cross-reacts serologically, and vaccinated sows successfully induce passive immunity against enteric infections. PRCoV is spread by inhalation, and infects lining cells of the upper respiratory tract. Mild bronchointerstitial pneumonia results from experimental infection, and the agent has been associated with outbreaks of respiratory disease.

Porcine epidemic diarrhea virus (PEDV), an *Alphacoronavirus* antigenically distinct from TGEV, has been reported for many years from Europe and Asia. In 2013 a diagnosis of this condition was made in Iowa, from where it spread quickly to several other states of the United States and Canada. Traditionally the disease was considered to be essentially similar to TGE in epidemiology, pathogenesis, and lesions, but milder. However, the recent US epidemic occurred as explosive epidemics of diarrhea and vomiting affecting all ages, with 90-95% mortality in suckling pigs. Clinically, grossly, and histologically, disease produced by PEDV cannot be differentiated from TGE. The diagnosis should be confirmed by PCR or immunohistochemistry. Although PEDV is related to TGEV, diagnostic tests for TGEV will not detect PEDV.

Porcine deltacoronavirus (PDCoV), a deltacoronavirus first detected in Hong Kong in 2012 and now present in North

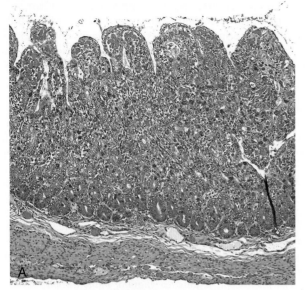

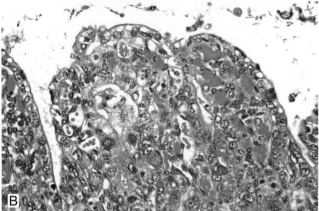

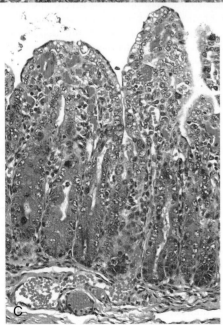

Figure 1-113 Transmissible gastroenteritis in a pig. **A.** Atrophy of villi in small intestine. **B.** Severely attenuated enterocytes on surface of an atrophic villus. **C.** Atrophy of villi, with compensatory hypertrophy of crypts of Lieberkühn. Surface epithelium is cuboidal or flattened.

America, causes infection that is clinically similar to, but distinct from, PED and TGE. It causes diarrhea and vomiting in all age groups and mortality in nursing pigs. Mortality rates appear to be lower than in cases of PED.

Further reading

Chen Q, et al. Isolation and characterization of porcine epidemic diarrhea viruses associated with the 2013 disease outbreak among swine in the United States. J Clin Microbiol 2014;52:234-243.

Huang YW, et al. Origin, evolution, and genotyping of emergent porcine epidemic diarrhea virus strains in the United States. MBio 2013;4:e00737-13.

Li G, et al. Full-length genome sequence of porcine deltacoronavirus strain USA/IA/2014/8734. Genome Announc 2014;2:e00278-14.

Stevenson GW, et al. Emergence of *Porcine epidemic diarrhea virus* in the United States: clinical signs, lesions, and viral genomic sequences. J Vet Diagn Invest 2013;25:649-654.

Bovine coronavirus. In **neonatal calves,** *Bovine coronavirus* (BCoV) infection is a common cause of diarrhea, either alone or in combination with other agents, particularly *Rotavirus* and *Cryptosporidium*. The disease may be severe in combination with BVDV infection. BCoV is capable of infecting absorptive epithelium in the full length of the small intestine, and in the large bowel. Viral antigen is also found in macrophages in the lamina propria of villi and in mesenteric lymph nodes. In field infections, microscopic lesions are found most consistently in the lower small intestine and colon. Calves with BCoV infection usually develop mild depression, but continue to drink milk despite developing profuse diarrhea. With progressive dehydration, acidosis, and hyperkalemia, the animals become weak and lethargic; death can ensue as a result of hypovolemia, hypoglycemia, and potassium cardiotoxicosis. Diarrhea in survivors resolves in 5-6 days.

At autopsy, affected animals have the nonspecific lesions of undifferentiated neonatal calf diarrhea. Rarely, mild fibrinonecrotic typhlocolitis is recognized in calves with coronaviral infection. Mesenteric lymph nodes may be somewhat enlarged and wet.

Virus replication is cytocidal and initially occurs throughout the length of the villi in all levels of the small intestine, eventually spreading throughout the large intestine up to the end of the large colon and rectum, causing a malabsorptive diarrhea. Large concentration of BCoV can be typically found in the spiral colon. Infected epithelial cells die, slough off, and are replaced by immature cells. The microscopic lesions of coronaviral infection in calves vary with the severity and duration of the infection; *villus atrophy in combination with mild colitis is typical* (Fig. 1-114). In the calf *small intestine,* villus atrophy is rarely as severe as that seen in neonatal swine with TGE. Rather, villi are moderately shortened, or have subtotal atrophy with stumpy, club-shaped, or pointed tips, and villus fusion may be common. In the early phase of the clinical disease, villi are often pointed and covered by cuboidal to squamous epithelium. Exfoliation of epithelium and microerosion may be evident. Later, the epithelium is cuboidal to low columnar, basophilic, with irregular nuclear polarity and an indistinct brush border. Cryptal epithelium is hyperplastic. The lamina propria may contain a moderate infiltrate of mainly mononuclear inflammatory cells, some of which may have pyknotic or karyorrhectic nuclei. In the early stages of infection, necrosis of cells in mesenteric lymph nodes is

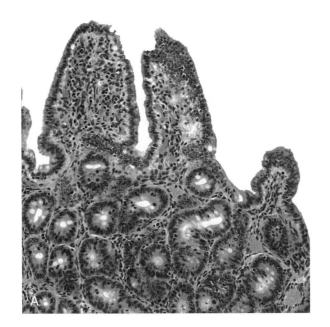

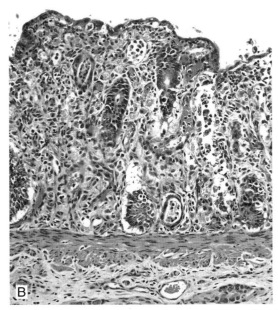

Figure 1-114 Bovine coronavirus infection. **A.** Blunt, fused villi with cuboidal surface epithelium in small intestine. **B.** Attenuation of surface epithelium and necrosis of gland epithelium in colon.

associated with viral replication. Peyer's patches in animals examined after 4-5 days of clinical illness often appear involuted, and are dominated by histiocytic cells. Whether this is the result of viral activity or the effect of endogenous glucocorticoids is unclear.

In the *colon* during the early phase of infection, surface epithelium may be exfoliating, flattened, and squamous or eroded in patchy areas. Some colonic glands may be dilated, lined by flattened epithelium and contain exfoliated cells and necrotic debris. A moderate mixed inflammatory reaction is present in the lamina propria, and neutrophils may be in damaged glands or effusing into the lumen through superficial microerosions. Later in infection, some dilated debris-filled colonic glands will remain, but other glands will be lined by hyperplastic epithelium, and the surface epithelium will be restored to a cuboidal or low columnar cell type. Goblet cells are usually relatively uncommon. Colonic lesions may be recognizable in tissues from animals submitted dead, even though postmortem change has obscured changes in the small intestine.

Live calves in the early stages of clinical disease are the best subjects for confirmation of an etiologic diagnosis. In calves becoming ill <7 days of age, enterotoxigenic *Escherichia coli* is the main alternative diagnosis. *Rotavirus, Cryptosporidium,* and combined infections must be considered in calves 5-15 days of age. Infectious bovine rhinotracheitis, salmonellosis, and bovine viral diarrhea must also be considered. Both salmonellosis and bovine viral diarrhea may be associated with depletion of Peyer's patches and colitis that can be confused with that of coronaviral infection; neither is common in the strictly neonatal age group (<7-14 days of age).

Respiratory tract infection also occurs in calves and feeders infected with BCoV. The virus replicates in the epithelium of the nasal turbinates and tracheobronchial tree, and *respiratory infection may precede, be concurrent with, or follow enteric infection.* Calf pneumonia caused by BRCoV can be observed in calves 6-9 months of age. Affected animals may develop fever, serous to mucopurulent nasal discharge, coughing, tachypnea, and dyspnea. Respiratory infections may play a role in maintaining the virus within a herd, and significant, but poorly characterized, pneumonia has been reported in some experimentally infected calves. In addition, coronaviral infection may predispose to subsequent respiratory bacterial infections or contribute to more severe respiratory disease as part of the shipping fever syndrome. Virus may be identified in tissue or nasal secretions by immunofluorescence or immunohistochemistry.

Winter dysentery is a syndrome in adult cattle that has been associated with BCoV in a number of areas around the world. Animals develop blood-tinged diarrhea, nasolacrimal discharge or cough, anorexia, and drop in milk production. Mortality is rare, but may occur. The disease is characterized by a high morbidity rate ranging from 50-100%, but usually low mortality rate, typically <2%. Winter dysentery outbreaks are predominantly seen in young postpartum dairy cows, which then experience a drop of 25-95% in milk production. Occasional cases are also observed in adult dairy and beef cattle. Despite its name, cases of winter dysentery can be observed, albeit infrequently, during the warmer season. The pathophysiologic characteristics of winter dysentery are mostly attributed to lesions of the colonic mucosa. *Grossly,* the colon of affected animals has linear congestion and hemorrhage along the crests of mucosal folds and there may be a large amount of blood mixed with colonic contents (Fig. 1-115). The *histologic lesions* are similar to those seen in calves with classical BCoV diarrhea, although they are mostly restricted to the colon with only occasional lesions seen in the terminal small intestine. Large amount of BCoV can be detected in colonic epithelium by immunohistochemistry. Coronaviruses are commonly demonstrated in the feces of cattle with winter dysentery; seroconversions occur, and seroprevalence increases in affected herds. Coronavirus antigen is found in the colonic glands of affected animals, in which there is necrosis and exfoliation of epithelial cells. Certain management practices, notably housing animals in stanchions and use of equipment that handles both manure and feed, have been associated with the development of winter dysentery.

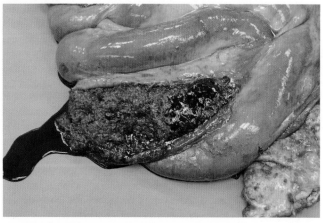

Figure 1-115 Winter dysentery in a cow. A large amount of blood mixed with intestinal content is present in the lumen of the spiral colon.

Further reading

Blanchard PC. Diagnostics of dairy and beef cattle diarrhea. Vet Clin North Am Food Anim Pract 2012;28:443-464.

Boileau MJ, et al. Bovine coronavirus associated syndromes. Vet Clin North Am Food Anim Pract 2010;26:123-146.

Kanno T. Bovine coronavirus infection: pathology and interspecies transmission. J Disast Res 2012;7:293-302.

Natsuaki S, et al. Fatal winter dysentery with severe anemia in an adult cow. J Vet Med Sci 2007;69:957-960.

Park SJ, et al. Dual enteric and respiratory tropisms of winter dysentery bovine coronavirus in calves. Arch Virol 2007;152:1885-1900.

Canine coronavirus. *Canine coronavirus* (CCoV) is widely prevalent in the dog population. Although dogs of all ages appear to be susceptible to infection by CCoV, the condition is probably most important as an *uncommon, transient, generally nonfatal diarrhea in puppies.* Fatal infections have been reported in pups previously infected with parvovirus. Infection with a pantropic canine coronavirus characterized by deadly acute systemic disease was diagnosed recently in several European countries. This was concurrent in most cases with *Canine parvovirus 2c.*

Viral replication occurs in the enterocytes of the small intestine, and in experimental infections in neonatal puppies, the lesion resembles the *villus atrophy* associated with coronaviral infection in other species. Diarrhea begins as early as 1 day after inoculation and in most animals by 4 days. Onset of signs coincides with the development of moderate villus atrophy and fusion. Enterocytes on villi become cuboidal, contain lipid vacuoles, and have an indistinct brush border. Lesions are most consistent and severe in the ileum. Resolution of villus atrophy within 7-10 days is associated with remission of signs.

Colonic infection by CCoV was not demonstrated by immunofluorescence in experimental animals, although mild colonic lesions were described, including loss of sulfomucins from goblet cells and some epithelial shedding. However, in a report of lesions caused by spontaneous CCoV infection, colonic infection and lesions were demonstrated. There was watery content in the lumen of the small and large intestine, and fibrin mixed with blood was evident in the cecum and colon. Mesenteric lymph nodes were enlarged and edematous.

Villus atrophy in the jejunum was inconsistent, but there was necrotic debris in many glands in the cecum and colon. Virus-infected cells were exfoliating into the lumen.

In the recently observed infections with pantropic coronavirus, gross lesions were mostly confined to the small intestine and included pink to red intestinal mucosa that occasionally had a slightly dry and rough surface with rare petechiae. Regional mesenteric lymph nodes and spleen were enlarged and congested. Microscopic lesions included villus atrophy and fusion together with dilated crypts containing degenerated and necrotic cells.

Further reading

Decaro N et al. European surveillance for pantropic canine coronavirus. J Clin Microbiol 2013;51:83-88.

Naylor MJ, et al. Molecular characterization confirms the presence of a divergent strain of canine coronavirus (UWSMN-1) in Australia. J Clin Microbiol 2002;40:3518-3522.

Zicola A. Fatal outbreaks in dogs associated with pantropic canine coronavirus in France and Belgium. J Small Anim Pract 2012;53:297-300.

Feline and other enteric coronaviruses. Our understanding of the enteric implications of coronaviral infections of **cats** is still incomplete. It appears that *Feline enteric coronavirus* (FECV) can establish persistent infection in the intestine, which in rare cases may be clinically apparent. Infection is very common. When it occurs, diarrhea is usually mild or moderate, perhaps with some blood, and kittens are most susceptible. Viral antigen is in cells on the tips of villi, and mild villus atrophy has been illustrated. Approximately 13% of all infected cats are not able to clear the virus, which persists for long periods of time in the colonic epithelium. During replication, mutations may occur in the viral genome giving rise to feline infectious peritonitis virus, which causes the highly lethal feline infectious peritonitis, a disease of far greater clinical significance.

Coronaviruses have been recovered from the feces of **sheep** with transient diarrhea, and they have been associated with severe villus atrophy in several spontaneous outbreaks of diarrhea. No experimental confirmation of the pathogenicity of coronavirus in sheep is available.

Equine coronavirus (EqCoV) is a betacoronavirus that has been associated with enteric and neurologic disease in **horses** in the United States and Japan. Necrotizing enteritis associated with EqCoV has been diagnosed in a horse in California and a donkey in Idaho. EqCoV infection of adult horses can occur in outbreaks, but is usually limited to individual cases of anorexia, lethargy, and fever.

Epizootic catarrhal enteritis of ferrets (ECE) is a highly contagious, diarrheal disease with close to 100% morbidity, but low overall mortality rate (<5%). ECE is produced by *Ferret enteric coronavirus*, genus *Alphacoronavirus*. The disease is clinically characterized by lethargy, hyporexia or anorexia, vomiting, diarrhea with a high mucus content, and dehydration. Feces of chronically affected animals frequently contain gritty material that has been described as resembling birdseed. *Grossly*, the affected small intestinal mucosa is hyperemic and the intestinal wall is thin. *Microscopically*, ECE is characterized by diffuse lymphocytic enteritis, with villus atrophy, fusion, and blunting; vacuolar degeneration and necrosis of the apical epithelium; or a combination of these lesions. Large numbers of coronavirus-infected epithelial cells can be detected by immunohistochemistry using a monoclonal antibody against group 1c coronavirus antigen. Coronavirus-like particles can be seen in cytoplasmic vacuoles of apical enterocytes and at the cell surface by transmission electron microscopy.

Further reading

Kipar A, et al. Sites of feline coronavirus persistence in healthy cats. J Gen Virol 2010;91:1698-1707.

Lowiese MB, et al. Establishment of feline intestinal epithelial cell cultures for the propagation and study of feline enteric coronaviruses. Vet Res 2013;44:71.

Murray J et al. Ferret coronavirus-associated diseases. Vet Clin North Am Exot Anim Pract 2010;13:543-560.

Oue Y, et al. Isolation of an equine coronavirus from adult horses with pyrogenic and enteric disease and its antigenic and genomic characterization in comparison with the NC99 strain. Vet Microbiol 2011;150:41-48.

Pusterla N, et al. Emerging outbreaks associated with equine coronavirus in adult horses. Vet Microbiol 2013;162:228-231.

Rotaviral infections

Members of the genus **Rotavirus,** in the family *Reoviridae*, infect the gastrointestinal tract of most mammals and birds. Rotaviruses are classified according to antigenic properties with group, subgroup, and serotype categories. Segment 6 of the *Rotavirus* genome codes for the VP6 intermediate capsid protein, which is used to classify the virus into seven serogroups, A-G. *Group A rotaviruses (RV-A) are the most diverse and common*, and infect all species of domestic animals, as well as humans, laboratory animals, and wildlife. RV-A can be subdivided into G and P serotypes based on VP7 and VP4 external capsid proteins, respectively; there are 14 G serotypes and 20 P serotypes. The serotypes isolated most commonly from piglets with diarrhea are P[7],G5, P[6],G4, P[7],G3, and P[7],G11. Individual rotavirus serotypes have a surprisingly wide range of host susceptibility. Non–group A rotaviruses infect pigs and ruminants, among domestic animals.

The ability to infect cells, and the serotype specificity of rotaviruses, are conferred by elements of the outer capsid layer. The viruses are probably generally host-specific, with little significant zoonotic potential. However, if epidemiologic circumstances are favorable, cross-species transmission may occur.

Rotaviruses infect the absorptive enterocytes and occasionally goblet cells on the tips and sides of the distal half or two thirds of villi in the small intestine. Rotaviruses infect cells on the apical half (ruminants) or the entire villus (pigs), mainly in the jejunum and ileum. Virus production and the pathogenesis of infection are similar in all species studied. Rotaviruses adhere to cell receptors (e.g., integrins, sialic acid), and inner capsid components are internalized into the cell. Granular "viroplasm" containing incomplete virions is seen in the apical cytoplasm of infected cells, and virions acquire their complete capsid after budding into dilated cisternae of endoplasmic reticulum, where they accumulate. Elongate tubular structures are found in the nuclei and rough endoplasmic reticulum of some infected cells.

Virus-infected cells are most prevalent 18-24 hours after experimental infection, and they tend to diminish in number rapidly, so that by 3-4 days after infection few cells containing viral antigen are present. Infected enterocytes lose cytoplasmic electron density, and mitochondria swell, as does the cell generally. Swollen rarified cells and syncytia may occur in the enterocytes at the villus tips, but cells are fragile and shed readily, particularly if autolysis intervenes. Syncytial cell formation has been recognized in porcine, bovine, and laboratory animal infections with rotavirus. Microvilli become irregular and somewhat stunted, and there may be some blebbing of membranes. Infected cells exfoliate into the intestinal lumen, and virus is released by lysis of damaged epithelium prior to or after exfoliation.

The *pathogenesis of diarrhea with rotavirus* involves 3 mechanisms. First, malabsorption occurs secondary to destruction of enterocytes. Second, a vasoactive agent is released from infected epithelial cells and causes villus ischemia and activation of the enteric nervous system. Third, rotaviruses are capable of producing a nonstructural protein, NSP4, which acts as a *secretory enterotoxin*. This is the first viral pathogen known to produce a toxin.

Exfoliation of infected epithelium over a relatively short period of time results in villus atrophy. The mucosal surface is covered by cuboidal, poorly differentiated epithelium that has an ill-defined microvillus border and that may contain lipid droplets in the cytoplasm. Diarrhea is probably mediated by electrolyte and nutrient malabsorption, perhaps exacerbated by the effect of cryptal secretion. It begins about the time of early viral cytopathology 20-24 hours after infection, and may persist for a variable period, from a few hours to a week or more. Regeneration of the mucosa by epithelium emerging from crypts, and differentiating on reformed villi, is associated with remission of signs in animals surviving the effects of diarrhea.

Rotaviruses are widespread, if not ubiquitous, among populations of most species, and they are relatively resistant to the external environment. Protection against infection in neonates is apparently largely conferred by the presence of *lactogenic immunity*. Many individuals in a population probably undergo inapparent infection. Disease is seen in the various species when viral contamination of the environment is heavy, perhaps as a result of intensive husbandry practices, and lactogenic immunity is waning or absent. Although rotaviral infection is usually associated with younger age groups, and viral receptors on cells diminish with age in some species, naïve older animals may become infected, sometimes with the development of diarrhea.

Bovine rotaviral infection. Rotaviral infection is mainly implicated in *diarrhea of neonatal beef and dairy calves*, both suckled and artificially reared, although there are reports of its association with diarrhea in adult cattle. Combinations of agents, including *Rotavirus*, are frequently involved in outbreaks of diarrhea in neonatal calves. Diarrhea may be produced in calves by rotaviral infection alone, but the condition is usually considered to be relatively mild or transient in comparison with that induced by enterotoxigenic *Escherichia coli* or *Bovine coronavirus*. *Rotavirus* may be implicated in animals developing signs at any time over the period up to ~2-3 weeks of age, and it is more commonly encountered in animals >4-5 days of age. Rotaviral diarrhea is most severe in calves that have slower enterocyte regeneration times. Rotavirus has a prepatent period of 1-3 days, and diarrhea lasts 2-5 days if uncomplicated.

The gross lesions of rotaviral infection are the nonspecific findings of undifferentiated neonatal diarrhea in calves,

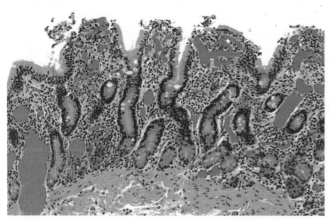

Figure 1-116 Bovine rotavirus infection. Blunted villi with severely attenuated surface epithelium. (Courtesy J. Edwards.)

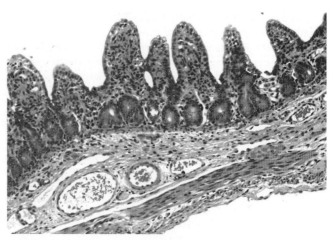

Figure 1-117 Villus atrophy and fusion caused by **rotavirus** infection in the small intestine of a piglet.

described previously. *Microscopic lesions in the small intestine cannot be differentiated from those of coronaviral infection.* They may vary somewhat depending on the severity of the initial viral damage and the stage of evolution of the sequelae. Blunt club-shaped villi, mild or moderate villus atrophy, and perhaps villus fusion may be present (Fig. 1-116). Villi are covered by low columnar, cuboidal, or flattened surface epithelium with a poorly defined brush border. There is usually a moderate proprial infiltrate of mononuclear cells and eosinophils or neutrophils, and hypertrophic crypts may be evident. The distribution of lesions may vary between animals and perhaps with time after infection within an individual animal because the onset of maximal viral damage may not occur synchronously throughout the full length of the intestine. Lesions and viral antigen always should be sought in the distal small intestine, and preferably at several sites along its length. *Rotavirus* does not cause gross or microscopic lesions in the colon, in contrast to coronavirus.

Swine rotaviral infection. *Rotavirus* infection is widespread and enzootic in most swine herds, and subclinical infection of piglets is common. It assumes particular importance as a cause of diarrhea in pigs with reduced lactogenic immunity, either as a result of early weaning or after normal weaning. High environmental levels of virus may result in disease in piglets suckling the sow, but in these circumstances the signs are usually relatively mild. *Rotavirus* may be a cause of "3-week," "white," or postweaning scours in piglets 2-8 weeks of age.

The signs may resemble those of transmissible gastroenteritis (TGE), although *Rotavirus* infection is considered to be less severe. Vomition is less commonly encountered than with TGE, but depression, diarrhea, and dehydration are usual. The character of the feces varies with the diet. Steatorrhea occurs in white scours of suckling piglets. *Rotavirus* infection in swine is frequently associated with other causes of diarrhea, including *E. coli*, coccidiosis, adenoviral infection, and *Strongyloides*.

The gross and microscopic lesions and pathogenesis of rotavirus infection in pigs resemble those of TGE (Fig. 1-117). As in TGE, severity of lesions seems inversely related to age.

Rotaviral infection in other species. Neonatal lambs have proved a useful model for the demonstration of the importance of lactogenic immunity in preventing disease caused by *Rotavirus*. *Rotavirus* may cause diarrhea in neonatal lambs

alone or in combination with enterotoxigenic *E. coli* and/or *Cryptosporidium*. In older, weaned lambs, an outbreak of diarrhea with 17% mortality was reported, produced by a novel ovine rotavirus group A G8 P strain and no other intestinal pathogens associated. The pathogenesis and lesions of *Rotavirus* infection in lambs are like those caused in other species, with the exception that viral infection of the colon may occur.

In **foals** <3-4 months of age, *Rotavirus* infection is considered a major cause of diarrhea, although mortality is rare. Outbreaks have been reported in many areas of the world. Equine rotaviruses are ubiquitous in horse populations and dual infections with more than one strain of rotavirus, including viruses of different G types, have been reported, but the clinical significance of this is poorly understood. Co-infections with other pathogens, including *Salmonella* spp., *Cryptosporidium* spp., and equine coronavirus have also been observed. The natural and experimental disease resembles that seen in other species, with significant viral infection limited to enterocytes in the small intestine, where villus atrophy occurs.

In young **puppies**, especially those <1-2 weeks of age, diarrhea, occasionally fatal, may be caused by *Rotavirus* infection. In experimentally infected pups, green fluid content filled the lower small bowel and colon, and moderate villus atrophy was induced by exfoliation of epithelium from the distal half of villi.

Rotavirus has also been associated with diarrhea in **kittens**, although rotavirus also can be isolated from asymptomatically infected kittens.

Rotavirus infection should be sought in cases of diarrhea in young animals of any species and it should be particularly suspected in animals with villus atrophy in the small intestine. Rotavirus is part of the syndrome of undifferentiated neonatal diarrhea in any species.

Further reading

Bailey KE, et al. Equine rotaviruses—Current understanding and continuing challenges. Vet Microbiol 2013;167:135-144.

Blanchard PC. Diagnostics of dairy and beef cattle diarrhea. Vet Clin North Am Food Anim Pract 2012;28:443-464.

Galindo-Cardiel I, et al. Novel group A rotavirus G8 P[1] as primary cause of an ovine diarrheic syndrome outbreak in weaned lambs. Vet Microbiol 2011;149:467-471.

Kang BK, et al. Genetic characterization of canine rotavirus isolated from a puppy in Korea and experimental reproduction of disease. J Vet Diagn Invest 2007;19:78-83.

Papp H, et al. Review of group A rotavirus strains reported in swine and cattle. Vet Microbiol 2013;165:190-199.

Papp H, et al. Global distribution of group A rotavirus strains in horses: A systematic review. Vaccine 2013;31:5627-5633.

Tupler T, et al. Enteropathogens identified in dogs entering a Florida animal shelter with normal feces or diarrhea. J Am Vet Med Assoc 2012;241:338-343.

Parvoviral enteritis

The *Parvoviridae* are small nonenveloped viral particles ~18-26 nm in diameter, with icosahedral symmetry and a short single-stranded DNA genome. They replicate and produce inclusion bodies in the nucleus of infected cells. Members of the genus *Parvovirus* infect many species of laboratory and domestic animals. Among syndromes associated with parvovirus infection are: disease in cats, dogs, and mink (distinct from *Aleutian mink disease virus*) dominated clinically by enteritis; diarrhea in neonatal calves; and reproductive wastage in swine.

Feline panleukopenia virus (FPV), Mink enteritis virus (MEV), and Canine parvovirus 2 (CPV-2) are considered host range variants or strains of the species *Feline panleukopenia virus* within the genus *Parvovirus*. Based on the nucleotide sequence in the gene for capsid proteins, VP1/VP2, FPV, and MEV are very closely related to each other, and somewhat less related to CPV-2. These viruses are nonetheless biologically distinct, varying in their hemagglutination characteristics, in vitro host cell ranges, and virulence in experimentally inoculated hosts. CPV has been shown to evolve very rapidly in comparison to FPV. Antigenic differences can be detected by monoclonal antibodies and there are differences in host specificity conferred by variations in only very small segments of the viral genome. However, host range is overlapping. Although the originally identified cause of canine parvoviral enteritis (CPV-2) was unable to infect cats, two new antigenic types have evolved from CPV-2, namely, CPV-2a and CPV-2b, which are able to replicate and cause disease in cats. Another variant, CPV-2c, has a more diverse carnivore host range, including skunks, raccoons, foxes, dogs, and cats. Although it is controversial whether CPV-2c is more virulent than other types, CPV-2c is shed at high concentration in feces and it is extremely stable.

The host ranges of FPV and CPV are determined by receptor binding, particularly to the transferrin receptor TfR. Canine parvovirus 2 is distinct from canine minute virus (CMV, or canine parvovirus 1) that also has enteric lesions associated with infection.

Although autonomous parvoviruses may infect cells at any phase of the cell cycle, replication is dependent on cellular mechanisms only functional during nucleoprotein synthesis before mitosis. Hence *the effects of parvoviral infection are greatest in tissues with a high mitotic rate*. These may include a variety of tissues during organogenesis in the fetus and neonate. In older animals, the proliferative elements of the enteric epithelium, hematopoietic and lymphoid tissue are particularly susceptible. At the time of virus assembly, *large basophilic or amphophilic Feulgen-positive nuclear inclusions* may be found in infected cells, especially in Bouin's fixed tissues. Parvovirus is demonstrated in these inclusions by electron microscopy. The chromatin in inclusion-bearing nuclei is usually clumped at the nuclear membrane. Inclusions are most prevalent late in the incubation period, before extensive exfoliation or lysis of infected cells. Hence they are not commonly encountered in animals submitted for autopsy after a period of clinical illness culminating in death. Large nucleoli, seen in proliferative cells encountered in the intestine of parvovirus-infected animals, should not be confused with intranuclear viral inclusions.

The *pathogenesis* of FPV and of CPV-2 infection is sufficiently similar for them to be considered together here, followed by separate discussions of the specific diseases. Oronasal exposure results in uptake of virus by epithelium over tonsils and Peyer's patches. Infection of draining lymphoid tissue is indicated by isolation of virus from mesenteric lymph nodes 1-2 days after experimental inoculation. Release of virus into lymph, and dissemination of infected lymphoblasts from these sites, may result in infection of other central and peripheral lymphoid tissues, including thymus, spleen, lymph nodes, and Peyer's patches, 3-4 days after infection. Lymphocytolysis in these tissues releases virus, reinforcing cell-free viremia. Viremia is terminated when neutralizing antibody appears in circulation ~5-7 days after infection. Moderate pyrexia occurs at about this time.

Cell invasion is mediated via capsid-mediated attachment to one or more receptors on cell membranes and receptor-mediated endocytosis. In the dog, capsid proteins bind to transferrin receptors, whereas in the cat capsid proteins bind to neuraminic acid and transferrin receptors. These receptors confer cell and animal-species specificity to each parvovirus strain. After the replication cycle is completed, parvovirus particles are released from infected crypt enterocytes, killing the cells. Infection of the gastrointestinal epithelium is a secondary event, following dissemination of virus by circulating lymphocytes and cell-free viremia. Peyer's patches are consistently infected at all levels of the intestine, and epithelium in crypts of Lieberkühn over or adjacent to Peyer's patches usually becomes infected a day or so later. Infection of gastrointestinal epithelium at other sites in the gut is less consistent, but is usually more severe in the lower small intestine. It may be the result of virus free in circulation, or carried by infected lymphocytes homing to the mucosa. Maximal infection of cryptal epithelium occurs during the period ~5-9 days after infection.

The occurrence and severity of enteric signs are determined by the degree and extent of damage to epithelium in intestinal crypts. This seems to be a function of two main factors. The first is the availability of virus, which is influenced by the rate of proliferation of lymphocytes, and therefore their susceptibility to virus replication and lysis. The second factor influencing the degree of epithelial damage is the rate of proliferation in the progenitor compartment in crypts of Lieberkühn. If many cells are entering mitosis, large numbers will support virus replication and subsequently lyse. Destruction of cells in the crypts of Lieberkühn, if severe enough, ultimately results in focal or widespread villus atrophy and perhaps mucosal erosion or ulceration. The recognition, evolution, and sequelae of radiomimetic insult to the intestine, such as that caused by parvovirus, are described elsewhere (see previous section on Epithelial renewal in health and disease).

Regeneration of cryptal epithelium and partial or complete restoration of mucosal architecture will occur, if undamaged stem cells persist in most affected crypts, and the animal survives the acute phase of clinical illness. In some survivors, focal villus atrophy is associated with persistent dilated crypts containing cellular debris, and with local "drop-out" of crypts completely destroyed by infection. In rare animals that have recovered from acute disease, chronic malabsorption and protein-losing enteropathy are associated with persistent areas of ulceration caused by more extensive loss of crypts and collapse of the mucosa.

The low rate of replication of intestinal epithelium in germ-free cats explains failure to produce significant intestinal lesions and clinical panleukopenia in experimentally infected animals. In spontaneous cases, the lower prevalence of parvoviral lesions in the colon and stomach, in comparison with the small intestine, reflects the relatively lower rate of epithelial proliferation in those tissues. The consistency of epithelial lesions in the mucosa over Peyer's patches probably results from high local concentrations of virus derived from infected lymphocytes in the dome and follicle. This may be coupled with local stimulation of epithelial turnover by cytokines released by T lymphocytes in the vicinity. Variations in the rate of epithelial proliferation related to age, starvation, and refeeding, or concomitant parasitic, bacterial, or viral infections, may also influence the susceptibility of crypt epithelium to infection, and therefore affect the extent and severity of intestinal lesions and signs.

Diarrhea in parvoviral infections is mainly the result of reduced functional absorptive surface in the small intestine. Effusion of tissue fluids and blood from a mucosa at least focally denuded of epithelium probably also contributes to diarrhea. Dehydration and electrolyte depletion are the result of reduced fluid intake, enteric malabsorption, effusion of tissue fluid, and, in some animals, vomition. Hypoproteinemia is common, and anemia may occur because of enteric blood loss; both are exacerbated by rehydration. Anemia reflects hemorrhage into the gut.

Proliferating cells in the *bone marrow* also are infected during viremia. Lysis of many infected cells is reflected in hypocellularity of the marrow caused by depletion of myeloid and erythroid elements, particularly the former. Megakaryocytes also may be lost, but seem the least sensitive cell population in the marrow. The number of neutrophils in circulation drops quickly in severely affected animals. This is due to failure of recruitment from the damaged marrow, and peripheral consumption, especially in the intestine. Transient neutropenia, of ~2-3 days' duration, occurs consistently in cats, and less commonly in dogs. In surviving animals, regeneration of depleted myeloid elements from remaining stem cells restores the circulating population of granulocytes within a few days. Neutrophilia with left shift may occur during recovery.

Lymphopenia, relative or absolute, results from *viral lymphocytolysis* in all infected lymphoid tissue. Relative lymphopenia is more consistently observed in dogs than neutropenia. When lymphopenia and neutropenia occur together, *the combined leukopenia may be profound in both dogs and cats.* In dogs surviving the lymphopenic phase, circulating lymphocytes return to normal numbers within 2-5 days, as regenerative hyperplasia occurs in lymphoid tissue throughout the body. Lymphocyte numbers increase rapidly, sometimes producing lymphocytosis in recovering dogs. However, there may be transient immunosuppression in gnotobiotic pups subclinically infected with CPV-2. Transient depression of T-cell response to mitogens occurs in cats a week after experimental infection with FPV. But immunosuppression by these agents appears to be of little clinical significance.

Most infected cats and dogs do not develop clinical disease. When it occurs, signs usually begin during the late viremic phase, ~5-7 days after infection. Severe enteric damage is the major cause of mortality. Shedding of infective virus in feces begins ~3-5 days after infection, when Peyer's patches and cryptal epithelium first become infected. Virus shedding persists until coproantibody appears to neutralize virus entering the gut, ~6-9 days after infection. Virus-infected cells may still be detected in crypts and Peyer's patches at this time, and virus complexed with antibody may be found in feces or intestinal content by direct electron microscopy. However, attempts to demonstrate virus in tissues or feces after several days of clinical disease, or at death, are often thwarted by the fact that virus is neutralized by antibody present in tissue fluids. Persistent or sporadic shedding of virus by recovered animals may be the result of virus replication in cells entering mitosis days or weeks after they were infected during the viremic phase.

Infection of the fetus during late prenatal life by FPV causes *anomalies of the central nervous system*, mainly hypoplasia of the cerebellum; anomalies of the central nervous system have not been reported in puppies with CPV-2, although there is mounting evidence from polymerase chain reaction studies that central nervous system lesions in puppies can be induced by fetal CPV-2 infections. Infection of proliferating cardiac myocytes in young puppies with CPV-2 results in nonsuppurative myocarditis and sequelae of acute or chronic heart failure (see Vol. 3, Cardiovascular system), but this is rarely seen in populations with a high prevalence of maternal immunity. A tentative association has been made between infection of kittens with FPV and myocarditis, as well as subsequent cardiomyopathy.

Further reading

Goddard A, Leisewitz AL. Canine parvovirus. Vet Clin North Am Small Anim Pract 2010;40:1041-1053.

Hueffer K, Parrish CR. Parvovirus host range, cell tropism and evolution. Curr Opin Microbiol 2003;6:392-398.

Ikeda Y, et al. Feline host range of canine parvovirus: recent emergence of new antigenic types in cats. Emerg Infect Dis 2002;8:341-346.

Miranda C, et al. Canine parvovirus 2c infection in a cat with severe clinical disease. J Vet Diagn Invest 2014;26:462-464.

Parrish CR. Pathogenesis of feline panleukopenia and canine parvovirus. Baillieres Clin Haematol 1995;8:57-71.

Schoeman JP, et al. Biomarkers in canine parvovirus enteritis. N Z Vet J 2013;61:217-222.

Feline panleukopenia. Feline panleukopenia virus (FPV) infects all members of the *Felidae*, as well as mink, raccoons, and some other members of the *Procyonidae*. FPV is ubiquitous in environments frequented by cats, and infection is common, although generally subclinical. The disease panleukopenia (infectious feline enteritis, feline distemper) usually occurs in young animals exposed after decay of passively acquired maternal antibody, but it may occur in naïve cats of any age. Clinical signs of several days' duration, including pyrexia, depression, inappetence, vomition, diarrhea, dehydration, and perhaps anemia may be evident in the history. However, many cases, particularly poorly observed animals or those prone to wander, may be presented as "sudden death." The pathogenesis of panleukopenia has been considered

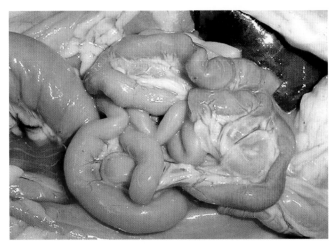

Figure 1-118 Dilated and hemorrhagic small intestine in **feline panleukopenia**. (Courtesy J. Caswell.)

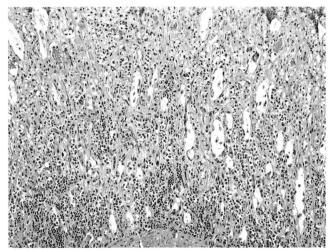

Figure 1-119 Necrosis and dilation of crypts of Lieberkühn, caused by **feline panleukopenia virus** infection in a cat.

above. Lesions of the central nervous system in kittens are considered in Vol. 1, Nervous system.

At **autopsy**, external evidence of diarrhea may be present, the eyes may be sunken, and the skin is usually inelastic, with a tacky subcutis reflecting dehydration. Rehydrated animals may have edema, hydrothorax, and ascites resulting from hypoproteinemia. There is pallor of mucous membranes and internal tissues in anemic animals. Gross lesions of internal organs most consistently involve the thymus and the intestine. The thymus is markedly involuted and reduced in mass in young kittens. Enteric lesions may be subtle and easily overlooked. Hence *it is mandatory that intestine be examined microscopically despite the apparent absence of gross change.*

The intestinal serosa may appear dry and nonreflective, with an opaque ground-glass appearance. Uncommonly in cats, there may be petechiae or more extensive hemorrhage in the subserosa, muscularis, or submucosa of the intestinal wall. The small bowel may be segmentally dilated and can acquire a hose-like turgidity in places, perhaps because of submucosal edema (Fig. 1-118). However, turgidity is difficult to assess in the intestine of the cat. The content is usually foul-smelling, scant, and watery, and yellow-gray at all levels of the intestine. The mucosa may be glistening gray or pink, with petechiae, perhaps covered by fine strands of fibrin. Patchy diphtheritic lesions may be present, especially over Peyer's patches in the ileum. Flecks of fibrin and sometimes casts may be in the content in the lumen. Formed feces are not evident in the colon. Lymph nodes may be prominent at the root of the mesentery. Gross lesions elsewhere in the carcass are usually restricted to pulmonary congestion and edema in some animals, and pale gelatinous marrow in normally active hematopoietic sites.

Microscopic lesions are consistently found in the intestinal tract in fatal cases, and are usual in lymphoid organs and bone marrow. The *intestinal lesions* vary with the severity and duration of the disease. Lesions may be patchy, and several levels of gut should be examined, preferably including ileum and, if possible, Peyer's patch. During the late incubation period and early phase of clinical disease, crypt-lining epithelium is infected. Intranuclear inclusions may be found, and damaged epithelium containing inclusions exfoliates into the lumen of crypts. Crypts are dilated and lined by cuboidal or more

severely attenuated cells. The lamina propria between crypts contains numerous neutrophils and eosinophils at this time, and some emigrate into the lumen of crypts, where they join the epithelial debris.

Subsequently severely damaged crypts may be lined by extremely flattened cells, and by scattered large bizarre cells with swollen nuclei and prominent nucleoli (Fig. 1-119). Enterocytes covering villi are not affected. But as they progress off the villus, they are replaced by a few cuboidal, squamous, or bizarre epithelial cells, so that villi in affected areas undergo progressive collapse. If cryptal damage is severe and widespread, the mucosa becomes thin and eroded or ulcerated, with effusion of tissue fluids, fibrin, and erythrocytes. Inflammatory cells are usually sparse in the gut of such animals, and superficial masses of bacteria may be present, occasionally accompanied by locally invasive fungal hyphae. In less severely affected animals with disease of longer duration, corresponding to ~8-10 days after infection, scattered focal drop-out of crypts, or focal mucosal collapse and erosion or ulceration, may be evident. In these animals, remaining crypts recovering from milder viral damage show regenerative epithelial hyperplasia. Mucosal lesions are often most marked in the vicinity of Peyer's patches.

Lesions in the *colon* generally resemble those found in the small bowel, although they are often less severe or more patchy in distribution. Colonic lesions are present in about half of fatal cases of panleukopenia. Gastric lesions resulting from damage to mitotic epithelium are relatively uncommon in cats. They are recognized by flattening of basophilic cells lining the narrowed isthmus of gastric fundic glands, with some reduction in number of parietal cells in the upper portion of the neck of glands.

Lesions of *lymphoid organs* during the early phase of the disease consist of lymphocytolysis in follicles and paracortical tissue in lymph nodes, thymic cortex and splenic white pulp, and gut-associated lymphoid tissue. Lymphoid necrosis has been associated with induced apoptosis of virus-infected lymphocytes. Lymphocytes are markedly depleted in affected tissue and large histiocytes are prominent, often containing the fragmented remnants of nuclear debris. Follicular hyalinosis, the presence of amorphous eosinophilic material in the center of depleted follicles, may be seen. Erythrophagocytosis by sinus histiocytes may occur in lymph nodes, especially those draining the gut. Severely depleted Peyer's patches may be difficult to recognize microscopically. Later in the course of clinical disease, corresponding to the period beyond ~7-8 days after infection, prominent regenerative lymphoid hyperplasia may be found.

In severely affected animals at the nadir of the leukopenia, virtually all proliferating elements in the *bone marrow* may be depleted. The extremely hypocellular, moderately congested marrow is only populated by scattered stem cells. Milder lesions mainly affect the neutrophil series, generally sparing megakaryocytes and the committed erythroid elements. During the later phases of the disease, marked hyperplasia of stem cells, and eventually of amplifier populations in the various cell lines, is evident.

In the *liver*, dissociation and rounding up of hepatocytes, and perhaps some periacinar atrophy and congestion, may be evident. This is probably associated with dehydration and anemia. Pancreatic acinar atrophy also is common, reflecting inappetence. The lung may be congested and edematous. In leukopenic animals, few leukocytes are seen in circulation in any organ.

A **diagnosis** of feline panleukopenia may be made on the basis of the characteristic microscopic intestinal lesions, in association with evidence of involution or regenerative hyperplasia of lymphoid and hematopoietic tissues. *Inclusion bodies* may be sought in these tissues, but are usually present in significant numbers only during the late incubation and early clinical period. Cryptal necrosis is also reported in the intestines of some cats with FeLV infection, which must be differentiated from feline panleukopenia. Application of immunohistochemical techniques may identify viral antigen in tissue as late as 8-10 days after infection. Viral antigen also may be identified in intestinal content or feces by ELISA or PCR testing.

Further reading

Streck AF, et al. An updated TaqMan real-time PCR for canine and feline parvoviruses. J Virol Methods 2013;193:6-8.

Truyen U, Parrish CR. Feline panleukopenia virus: Its interesting evolution and current problems in immunoprophylaxis against a serious pathogen. Vet Microbiol 2013;65:29-32.

Canine parvovirus 2 infection. Canine parvovirus 2 (CPV-2) resulted from mutation of a closely related virus, likely an FPV-like virus from wild carnivores, such as foxes. It appeared spontaneously and virtually simultaneously in populations of dogs on several continents in 1978, and rapidly spread worldwide. Retrospective serologic studies suggest that it was circulating unnoticed in western Europe by 1976. In addition to domestic dogs, several species of wild canids, including coyotes, gray wolves, and raccoon dogs, are susceptible to infection.

Enteric disease caused by this virus was epizootic for several years in naive populations of dogs, affecting animals of all ages. As the prevalence of antibody caused by natural infection and vaccination increased, the problem subsided to one of an enzootic disease. It now affects those animals with reduced levels of passively acquired maternal immunity, or scattered naive individuals.

During the epizootic period, nonsuppurative viral myocarditis caused by CPV-2 was prevalent in the offspring of naive bitches unable to protect pups with maternal antibody during the first 15 days of life, when replicating myocardial cells are susceptible to parvoviral damage. Myocardial disease in pups caused by CPV-2 is now fairly uncommon, as most bitches have antibody. Enteric and myocardial diseases rarely occur together in the same individual or cohort of animals. Occasional cases of generalized parvoviral infection have been reported in susceptible neonates. Necrosis and inclusion bodies are found in organs such as kidney, liver, lung, heart, gut, and vascular endothelium. They are presumably related to mitotic activity during organogenesis.

Dogs with typical disease caused by CPV-2 become anorectic and lethargic and may vomit and develop diarrhea, perhaps in association with transient moderate pyrexia. Relative or absolute lymphopenia or leukopenia of 1-2 days' duration may occur. Diarrhea may be mucoid or liquid, sometimes bloody, and is malodorous. After a period of 2-3 days, dogs either succumb to the effects of dehydration, hypoproteinemia, and anemia, or begin to recover.

Gross findings at autopsy of fatal cases are those of dehydration, accompanied by enteric lesions characteristic of the disease. There is often segmental or widespread subserosal intestinal hemorrhage, which may extend into the muscularis and submucosa. The serosa frequently appears hemorrhagic and granular because of superficial fibrinous effusion (Fig. 1-120). Peyer's patches may be evident from the serosal and mucosal aspects as deep red oval areas several centimeters long. The intestinal contents may be mucoid or fluid; sometimes they look like tomato soup because of hemorrhage. The mucosa is usually deeply congested and glistening, or covered by patchy fibrinous exudate. Severe mucosal lesions may be widespread or segmental, and their distribution is irregular; thus tissues from several levels of the small intestine should be selected for microscopic examination. Gross changes in the colon are similar but less common. The stomach may have a congested mucosa and contain scant bloody or bile-stained fluid. Mesenteric lymph nodes may be enlarged, congested, and wet, or be reduced in size. Thymic atrophy is consistently

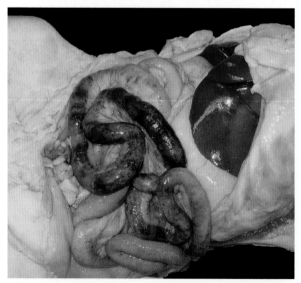

Figure 1-120 Segmental subserosal hemorrhage and mild fibrinous exudation on intestinal serosa in **canine parvovirus 2** infection. (Courtesy J. Ortega-Porcel.)

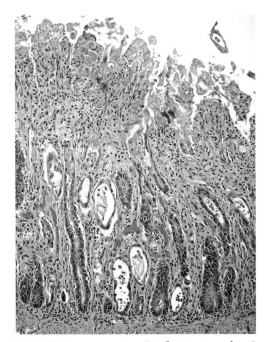

Figure 1-121 Canine parvovirus 2 infection in a dog. Loss and dilation of crypts of Lieberkühn and collapse of proprial stroma in small intestine. Remnants of crypt lining epithelium persist deep in lamina propria.

present in young animals, and the organ may be so reduced in size as to be difficult to find. The lungs often appear congested and have a rubbery texture.

The **microscopic lesions** in stomach, small intestine (Fig. 1-121), colon, lymphoid tissue, and bone marrow caused by CPV-2 infection do not differ significantly from those described earlier in cats with panleukopenia. Gastric lesions are perhaps more frequently encountered in dogs with parvoviral infection. Small intestinal lesions are invariably severe in fatal cases. The colon is involved in a minority of animals. Pulmonary lesions such as alveolar septal thickening by mononuclear cells, congestion, and effusion of edema fluid and fibrin into the lumina of alveoli may be related to terminal gram-negative sepsis and endotoxemia, which is common in fatal cases. Periacinar atrophy and congestion in the liver are attributable to anemia, hypovolemia, and shock, and prominent Kupffer cells probably reflect endotoxemia. Some studies have shown that viral inclusions may occur in tongue epithelium cells as well. Although these inclusions are nuclear, they often appear to be in the cytoplasm (pseudocytoplasmic). A case of erythema multiforme as a result of CPV-2 infection of keratinocytes has been described in a dog with concurrent parvoviral enteritis; viral inclusions were present in oral and skin epithelial cells.

The **diagnosis** of parvoviral enteritis in dogs follows the principles described for that of panleukopenia in cats. The disease must be differentiated from *Canine coronavirus* infection, which is very rarely fatal, and from canine intestinal hemorrhage syndrome, shock gut, intoxication with heavy metals or warfarin, infectious canine hepatitis, and other causes of hemorrhagic diathesis. Involution of gut-associated lymphoid tissue and cryptal necrosis caused by parvovirus must be differentiated from similar lesions occasionally seen in canine distemper.

Further reading

Goddard A, Leisewitz AL. Canine parvovirus. Vet Clin North Am Small Anim Pract 2010;40:1041-1053.

Hoelzer K, Parrish CR. The emergence of parvoviruses of carnivores. Vet Res 2010;41:39.

Streck AF, et al. An updated TaqMan real-time PCR for canine and feline parvoviruses. J Virol Methods 2013;193:6-8.

Canine minute virus. Species *Canine minute virus* (CMV, Minute virus of canines, *Canine parvovirus 1*) is most closely related to *Bovine parvovirus*, and is distinct from members of the feline panleukopenia parvovirus subgroup. Serologic prevalence in the United States is ~50% in adult dogs. The virus is capable of transplacental transmission to the fetus, and exposure of pregnant bitches was associated with fetal resorption, or birth of dead or weak pups. CMV causes enteric or respiratory symptoms in puppies <3 weeks of age. Enterocyte hyperplasia in the duodenum and jejunum with large intranuclear viral inclusion bodies is evident, but the crypt necrosis characteristic of infection by canine parvovirus type 2 does not occur. Interstitial pneumonia and myocarditis are variably present in naturally infected puppies, with death occurring sporadically.

Further reading

Ohshima T, et al. Sequence analysis of an Asian isolate of minute virus of canines (canine parvovirus type 1). Virus Genes 2004;29:291-296.

Schwartz D, et al. The canine minute virus (minute virus of canines) is a distinct parvovirus that is most similar to bovine parvovirus. Virology 2002;302:219-223.

Truyen U, Parrish CR. Feline panleukopenia virus: Its interesting evolution and current problems in immunoprophylaxis against a serious pathogen. Vet Microbiol 2013;65:29-32.

Bovine parvovirus infection. The antigenically distinct species *Bovine parvovirus* (BPV) also known as hemadsorbing enteric virus, is the type species of genus *Bocavirus*, with 3 significant subspecies: BPV1, 2, and 3. BPV has been recognized for many years and occurs widely in cattle populations on all continents. It has been isolated from the feces of normal and recently diarrheic calves as well as from conjunctiva and aborted fetuses. *The status of BPV as an enteric pathogen is unclear*, although it is believed to cause diarrhea in neonatal calves and respiratory and reproductive disease in adult cattle. Virus shedding is not always associated with diarrhea, and it may be part of a mixed infection in diarrheic animals. Serologic prevalence of antibodies to BPV is high, with 83% of cattle and 100% of herds being positive over 2 years of testing in one study. It is rarely diagnosed as a cause of death, and unless sought specifically by culture, direct electron microscopy, or molecular probe, would be missed as a cause of clinical diarrhea. Its significance may be greatest in neonatal calves and animals exposed while passive maternal antibody levels are waning, or in animals in the postweaning period.

The pathogenesis of infection with BPV resembles that in carnivores. Initial viral replication following oral inoculation is in tonsils and gut, with spread to systemic lymphoid tissues, resulting in transient lymphopenia. Viral antigen has been identified in the nuclei of epithelium in intestinal crypts and in cells in thymus, lymph nodes, adrenal glands, and heart muscle. Transient lymphocytolysis in infected tissues, and exfoliation of epithelium in crypts of the small and large intestine, with moderate villus atrophy, depletion of colonic goblets, and mixed inflammatory cell infiltration of the mucosa, have been seen experimentally. Intranuclear inclusions are present at the time when lesions are prevalent. Gross lesions other than abnormally fluid content in the gut are subtle or absent. Intravenous inoculation of BPV into young calves causes severe watery diarrhea and prostration. Milder diarrhea occurs in calves infected orally. The severity of the disease may be potentiated by concurrent infection with other enteric pathogens, or other factors that may increase intestinal epithelial proliferation.

Further reading

Allander T, et al. A virus discovery method incorporating DNase treatment and its application to the identification of two bovine parvovirus species. Proc Natl Acad Sci USA 2001;98:11609-11614.

Dudleenamjil E, et al. Bovine parvovirus uses clathrin-mediated endocytosis for cell entry. J Gen Virol 2010;91:3032-3041.

Manteufel J, Truyen U. Animal bocaviruses: a brief review. Intervirol 2008;51:328-334.

Bacterial diseases of the alimentary tract

Virulence of bacterial pathogens

Evolutionary processes for bacterial survival, persistence, and proliferation are controlled by virulence genes and are subject to complex mechanisms of regulation of expression. Similarly, evolutionary processes for resisting the effects of bacteria on the host are determined by genetic factors and equally complex regulatory processes in the host. *Bacterial virulence can be resolved into 5 components:* (1) attachment; (2) colonization or entry into the host; (3) evasion of host defense; (4) multiplication and/or spread within the host, and damage to the host, by direct virulence attributes, or by stimulation of an immunoinflammatory response; and (5) transmission to other susceptible animals. The interplay between host and pathogen has been extensively studied for a number of important enteric bacterial pathogens, including *Salmonella* and *Escherichia coli.* Genes encoding a range of virulence characteristics in pathogenic bacteria, including adhesion factors, toxins, proteolytic enzymes, and other agents that promote tissue invasion, are often clustered in discrete regions of the genome known as *pathogenicity islands.* These appear to be sites of relative instability, and are thought to facilitate the horizontal transfer of virulence factors between bacteria, and their continued evolution. Similarities in the regulatory mechanisms for pathogenicity islands of important enteric pathogens, including *Salmonella, Shigella, Vibrio, Yersinia,* and *E. coli,* are providing new insights into the reasons why strains of many genera of bacteria vary greatly in their host range and ability to cause disease. Among the factors in the mucosal barrier that resist pathogen virulence there is growing interest in the role of the luminal microbiota and their metabolites. Disruption of the intestinal microbiota may facilitate virulence factors of invading pathogens listed earlier.

Further reading

Ashida H, et al. Bacteria and host interactions in the gut epithelial barrier. Nat Chem Biol 2011;8:36-45.

Cotter PA, DiRita VJ. Bacterial virulence gene regulation: an evolutionary perspective. Annu Rev Microbiol 2000;54:519-565.

Gyles CL, Prescott JF. Themes in bacterial pathogenic mechanisms. In: Gyles CL, et al., editors. Pathogenesis of Bacterial Infections in Animals. 3rd ed. Ames, Iowa: Blackwell; 2004. p. 3-12.

Hacker J, Kaper JB. Pathogenicity islands and the evolution of microbes. Annu Rev Microbiol 2000;54:641-679.

Escherichia coli

Escherichia coli have several virulence attributes that result in disease in animals. Principally, these promote *colonization or adhesion* to the mucosa; they cause *metabolic dysfunction or death of enterocytes*; they affect the *local or systemic vasculature*; or they promote *invasion and septicemia.* Disease syndromes caused by *E. coli* in domestic animals can be related to the combinations of virulence attributes expressed. Many terms have been applied to the mechanisms of action of *E. coli*, with some becoming obsolete and others applying mainly to *E. coli* infections of laboratory animals and humans, rather than to domestic animals.

"**Enterotoxigenic**" *E. coli* (**ETEC**) cause secretory small-bowel diarrhea stimulated by enterotoxins produced by *E. coli* colonizing the mucosa of the small intestine. This condition is an important, common cause of diarrhea in neonatal animals of many species, and in postweaning pigs.

"**Enteropathogenic**" *E. coli* (**EPEC**) in humans and animals may colonize the mucosa of the intestine by a mechanism involving adhesion-effacement ("**enteroadherent**" *E. coli* [**EAEC**] or "**attaching-effacing**" *E. coli* [**AEEC**]). Some do not produce recognized toxins, but are associated with villus atrophy; they are an uncommon cause of disease in domestic animals.

Other strains of *E. coli*, many of which are attaching-effacing, in addition secrete *cytotoxins* (Shiga toxins = verotoxins) that have an effect locally or systemically. Depending on the manifestation of this effect, such *E. coli* have been categorized as "**Shiga toxin-producing**" (**STEC**) = "**verotoxin-producing**" (**VTEC**), or "**enterohemorrhagic**" (**EHEC**). EHEC are a serious cause of foodborne illness in humans and have been incriminated as a cause of hemorrhagic enterocolitis in calves <1 month of age. The reservoir for EHEC that cause human disease is thought to be ruminants.

Shigatoxigenic infections in swine that are not attaching-effacing are associated with some outbreaks of postweaning *E. coli* enteritis and also cause edema disease of weaned pigs, which is a systemic toxemia.

"**Enteroinvasive**" *E. coli* (**EIEC**) can be internalized by surface enterocytes and subsequently disseminate through the body to become septicemic. Although EIEC are poorly documented in domestic animals, **septicemic colibacillosis** is a common manifestation of *E. coli* infection caused by strains adapted to avoid specific or innate systemic defense mechanisms, often in compromised hosts. The intestine is not necessarily the portal of entry and there may not be alimentary disease. The signs of *E. coli* septicemia are mainly referable to bacteremia, endotoxemia, and the effect of bacterial localization in a variety of tissue spaces throughout the body.

Further reading

Dubreuil JD. The whole Shebang: the gastrointestinal tract, *Escherichia coli* enterotoxins and secretion. Curr Issues Mol Biol 2012;14:71-82.

Gyles CL, Fairbrother JM. *Escherichia coli.* In: Gyles CL, et al., editors. Pathogenesis of Bacterial Infections in Animals. 4th ed. Ames, Iowa: Blackwell; 2010. p. 267-308.

Moxley RA, Smith DR. Attaching-effacing *Escherichia coli* infections in cattle. Vet Clin North Am Food Anim Pract 2010;26:29-56.

Smith JL, et al. Shiga toxin-producing *Escherichia coli.* Adv Appl Microbiol 2014;86:145-197.

Enterotoxigenic colibacillosis. Enterotoxigenic colibacillosis caused by enterotoxigenic *E. coli* (ETEC) is one of the major forms of diarrhea in neonatal pigs, calves, and lambs, as well as in humans.

Two major attributes confer virulence on these strains of *E. coli.* These are the ability to colonize the intestine, and the capacity to produce toxins that stimulate secretion of electrolyte and water by the intestinal mucosa. *Colonization and enterotoxin production must occur together for disease to ensue.* The diarrhea produced by ETEC is accompanied by relatively minor microscopic evidence of inflammation, and by little or no architectural change in the mucosa. As a result, overt enteritis is usually not evident at autopsy, and the disease is part of the syndrome of undifferentiated diarrhea of neonatal animals.

Intestinal colonization results from the adhesion of *E. coli* to the surface of enterocytes on villi in the small intestine, and proliferation there (Fig. 1-122A). By adhering to the mucosa, bacteria are able to resist the normal peristaltic clearance mechanisms. Large numbers of organisms, of the order of $>10^7$ per gram of mucosa, or 20-30 per enterocyte, cover the surface of villi. The ability to attach to enterocytes is conferred on ETEC by pili, and may be enhanced by the presence of a capsule.

Fimbriae or **pili** (also known as *colonization factor antigens [CFA]*, with specific names in transition to a system of "F" numbers) are rod-like or filamentous projections from the cell wall of *E. coli* that attach to specific glycoconjugate receptors on the surface of enterocytes (Fig. 1-122B). They are distinct from type 1 fimbriae, which do not promote colonization of the gut. Fimbriae are polymers of protein (pilin) subunits, which are coded by plasmid (F4 [K88], F5 [K99], F18; some F6 [987P]) or chromosomal (F6 [987P], F17, F41) DNA. They are antigenically distinct, permitting recognition by specific antibody.

Fimbrial adhesins include **F5** (K99) and **F41** in strains affecting calves, lambs, and pigs; **F42, F165, F17, F18** in calves and pigs; and **F4** (K88), **F6** (987P), **F18** in pigs. Combinations of adhesins may be expressed by the same strain of ETEC; typically, F41 is expressed by strains also expressing F5, and seems to be of minor importance. Bacteria possessing F4 colonize the entire small bowel, whereas those with F5, F6, and F41 mainly adhere in the jejunum and ileum.

Susceptibility to bacterial fimbrial adhesins, especially F5 and F6, appears to be somewhat age-related; the ability of fimbria-bearing *E. coli* to colonize the small intestine is greatest in animals only a few days old. F5 receptors on enterocytes decline in availability with age, whereas receptors for F6 are shed into the lumen in older pigs, facilitating clearance of bacteria from the mucosa, and interfering with colonization. F18 receptors are not found in neonatal pigs, but are produced with increasing age to weaning. Stimulation of maternal immunity to fimbrial antigens causes secretion of lactogenic antibody, which combines with adhesins in the gut lumen, preventing colonization of the gut of suckling animals.

A nonfimbrial plasmid-encoded *adhesin involved in diffuse adherence* (**AIDA**) of *E. coli* to enterocytes in humans also occurs in strains from pigs associated with edema disease and postweaning diarrhea, often in combination with F18.

Enterotoxigenic strains of *E. coli* produce 2 classes of plasmid-encoded proteins—heat-labile toxin (LT) and heat-stable toxin (ST)—which act locally in the intestine to alter secretion and absorption of electrolyte and water by enterocytes. However, these toxins usually do not alter enterocyte morphology.

Heat-labile toxin is a large immunogenic plasmid-encoded molecule, with two subgroups (LTI and LTII) and comprised

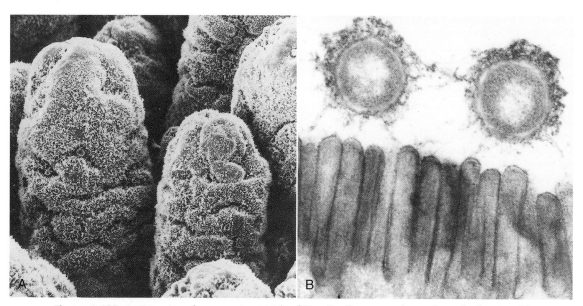

Figure 1-122 A. Scanning electron micrograph of *E. coli* adherent to the surface of villi in a calf. **B.** Transmission electron micrograph of **fimbriate** *E. coli* adherent to microvilli in the small intestine of a calf. (Courtesy J.J. Hadad, C.L. Gyles.)

of a small A subunit with two fragments (A1 and A2), which links A1 to a large pentamer of five B subunits. LTI is antigenically similar to cholera toxin, whereas LTII toxins have B subunits that differ from LTI. The B subunits bind to ganglioside receptors (GM1 gangliosides) on the enterocyte surface; the toxin complex then dissociates, and the A1 subunit is internalized into the cell. It operates via an adenylate cyclase pathway to cause chloride secretion by enterocytes, sodium, and water following osmotically from the mucosa. Co-transport of sodium chloride by enterocytes, and associated water uptake, is probably also shut down at the same time. LT may also promote mucosal secretion by stimulation of local prostaglandin production, the enteric nervous system, and cytokine activation. LT has been shown to decrease host defenses through interference with antimicrobial peptide production by human enterocytes. LT has a latent period before the development of secretion, but the effects on the cell are irreversible.

Heat-stable toxin is classified as STa and STb based on biological properties, and is plasmid-encoded. STa causes an increase in cyclic guanosine monophosphate, which inhibits Na/Cl co-transport and therefore water absorption by surface enterocytes, whereas in crypt epithelium it promotes Cl⁻ and water secretion. STb acts through a different mechanism than STa and is mainly produced by ETEC associated with pigs. STb causes increased intracellular calcium, chloride secretion, and may cause secretion by stimulation of prostaglandin E_2 and 5-hydroxytryptamine production. In pigs, STb can cause exfoliation of surface enterocytes, resulting in mild atrophy of villi.

Enteroaggregative *E. coli* heat stabile toxin (EAST1) has also been reported in ETEC isolated from pigs and cattle. This toxin has been associated with *E. coli*–induced diarrhea in children. However, the role of EAST1 in *E. coli* disease in pigs and cattle is not certain.

Enterotoxigenic colibacillosis is among the commonest causes of diarrhea in **neonatal pigs**, from a few hours to ~1 week of age. ETEC are present in the environment and are ingested. Commonly, serogroups O8, O45, O138, O141, O147, O149, and O157, expressing F4, are involved in enterotoxigenic colibacillosis in piglets, though the prevalence of F4-bearing strains may be declining because of vaccination of sows. Less commonly, F5, F6, and F41 pilus adhesins are involved. STb is the most common toxin produced by porcine ETEC; when LT is found, it is in association with STb, which may be encoded on the same plasmid. STa also occurs in strains of ETEC in swine, alone or in combination with other enterotoxins.

At autopsy, enterotoxigenic colibacillosis cannot be readily separated from the other common causes of undifferentiated neonatal diarrhea without laboratory assistance. Generally there is dehydration, usually with evidence of diarrhea, or a history of its occurrence in the herd. Lipopolysaccharide (LPS) from the bacterial cell membrane may promote inflammatory cascades and contribute to shock. Other than the presence of characteristic fluid content in the flaccid small and large bowel, usually with clotted milk still in the stomach, the internal findings are unremarkable.

In contrast to the viruses and *Cystoisospora*, *ETEC usually does not cause significant villus atrophy* (Fig. 1-123A). Small clumps, or a continuous layer, of bacteria may be found on the surface of enterocytes on villi in mucosal tissue sections, most consistently in ileum (Fig. 1-123B). Some neutrophils

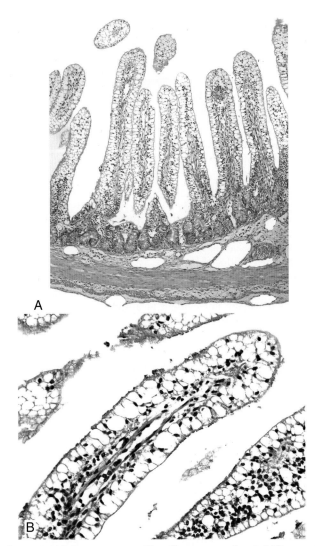

Figure 1-123 Enterotoxic colibacillosis in a piglet. **A.** Villi are tall and crypts are short, as is expected in a 2-3 day old animal. **B.** Bacteria are present on surface of enterocytes. Cytoplasmic vacuoles are normal in the ileal mucosa of young piglets.

may be present in the proprial core of villi, and transmigrating the epithelium into the lumen.

The involvement of ETEC expressing F4 in postweaning diarrhea of pigs >3 weeks of age, and distinct from postweaning colibacillosis caused by VTEC, discussed later, may be related to colonization of intestine in weaned pigs in which *Rotavirus* infection, changes in diet, or villus atrophy associated with hypersensitivity to dietary protein constituents, provide adhesin-bearing *E. coli* with a competitive advantage. It causes diarrhea for up to a week or so, with ill-thrift, but is uncommonly fatal, although a syndrome probably caused by endotoxic shock, similar to that associated with shigatoxigenic stains associated with postweaning colibacillosis, described later, may occur.

In **calves**, many cases of undifferentiated neonatal diarrhea are accounted for by enterotoxigenic colibacillosis, usually involving strains of serogroups O8, O9, O20, O64, O101 with fimbrial adhesins F5 and F41, and producing STa. Infection is typically restricted to the first 2-3 days of life, probably because of the loss of receptors for F5 in older calves.

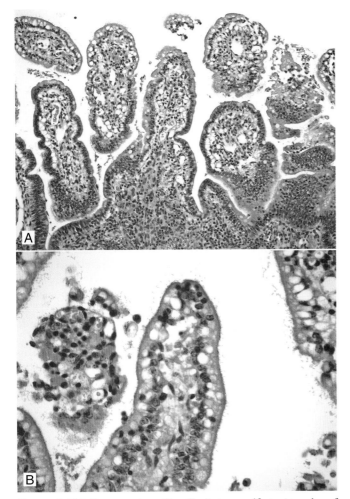

Figure 1-124 Enterotoxic colibacillosis in a calf. **A.** Atrophy of villi is not evident and surface epithelium is normal. **B.** Higher magnification of (**A**); numerous bacteria are attached to the epithelial surface.

ETEC must be differentiated from the other major causes of undifferentiated diarrhea in neonatal calves—*Bovine coronavirus* (BCoV), *Coronavirus*, *Rotavirus*, and *Cryptosporidium*—which typically dominate in calves older than a few days of age. However, ETEC is commonly found in combination with BCoV or *Rotavirus* infection.

The gross findings in calves with enterotoxigenic colibacillosis are the nonspecific appearance of diarrhea and dehydration. The infection is differentiated in tissue sections from the other infectious causes of this syndrome by the *absence of severe villus atrophy* (Fig. 1-124A) and by the presence of *bacteria on the surfaces of villi* in the distal small intestine (Fig. 1-124B). As in piglets, application of a variety of presumptive or specific tests for the presence of ETEC in the intestine confirms the diagnosis.

Enterotoxigenic colibacillosis is a significant problem in **lambs** in some areas. The serotypes involved, pathogenesis, and diagnosis of the condition are similar to those in calves. Synergism with *Rotavirus* infection may occur.

There are several reports of ETEC isolated from **foals** with diarrhea. The organisms have pili, probably F41, and secrete LT or STa. However, their capacity to produce disease in foals is unproved. Diarrhea has not ensued in foals inoculated with

F4-bearing *E. coli*, despite the presence of F4 receptors on enterocytes, and it seems that ETEC has little significance in this species.

Strains of *E. coli* have been associated with diarrhea in neonates of **other species** of animals, especially young dogs, where they mainly produce STa. Generally the enterotoxigenicity and other attributes of virulence have not been well described in strains from other species.

Further reading

Beutin L. *Escherichia coli* as a pathogen in dogs and cats. Vet Res 1999;30:285-298.

Dean EA, et al. Age-specific colonization of porcine intestinal epithelium by 987P-piliated enterotoxigenic *Escherichia coli*. Infect Immun 1989;57:82-87.

Fleckenstein JM, et al. Molecular mechanisms of enterotoxigenic *Escherichia coli* infection. Microbes Infect 2010;12:89-98.

Gyles CL, Fairbrother JM. *Escherichia coli*. In: Gyles CL, et al., editors. Pathogenesis of Bacterial Infections in Animals. 4th ed. Ames, Iowa: Blackwell; 2010. p. 267-308.

Jin LZ, Zhao X. Intestinal receptors for adhesive fimbriae of enterotoxigenic *Escherichia coli* (ETEC) K88 in swine – a review. Appl Microbiol Biotechnol 2000;54:311-318.

Nagy B, Fekete PZ. Enterotoxigenic *Escherichia coli* (ETEC) in farm animals. Vet Res 1999;30:259-284.

Tang Y, et al. Enterotoxigenic *Escherichia coli* infection induces intestinal epithelial cell autophagy. Vet Microbiol 2014;171:160-164.

Wieler LH, et al. Longitudinal prevalence study of diarrheagenic *Escherichia coli* in dairy calves. Berl Munch Tierarztl Wochenschr 2007;120:296-306.

Enteropathogenic colibacillosis. Enteropathogenic *E. coli* (EPEC) are those that cause direct damage to the mucosa, through a *characteristic mechanism of attachment to, and effacement of, epithelium. These* **attaching-effacing *E. coli* (AEEC)** are more common in humans than in animals, where they are most important in pigs, dogs, and rabbits, although they also have been isolated from cats. Control of attaching-effacing activity resides in the *locus for enterocyte effacement* (LEE), a chromosomal pathogenicity island. EPEC have a complicated and sequential relationship with host cells. Long polar fimbriae may mediate initial bacterial interaction with the enterocyte. Secretion of bacterial proteins ensues, including *intimin*, which is an adhesin. A second protein, the *translocated intimin receptor*, is transported via a type III secretion system into the enterocyte cytoplasm, emerging on the cell membrane as the intimin receptor. In response to translocated EPEC proteins, the cell's cytoskeleton is reorganized, resulting in formation of cupped *pedestal-like structures* beneath the attached bacteria, and the subsequent loss of microvilli (Figs. 1-125 and 1-126). Paracellular permeability increases as tight junctions between enterocytes loosen, and neutrophils migrate between cells into the lumen.

In animals and humans, some strains of AEEC are pathogenic despite failure to secrete enterotoxins or cytotoxins. A heavy layer of plump coccobacilli may be found over the luminal aspect of enterocytes on villi throughout the small intestine, and on the surface of the large intestine. *The degree of diarrhea seems related to the extent of bacterial colonization, which is most consistent in lower small intestine and large bowel.* Enterocytes to which bacteria are adherent round up or contract, and exfoliate from the mucosa singly or in clumps,

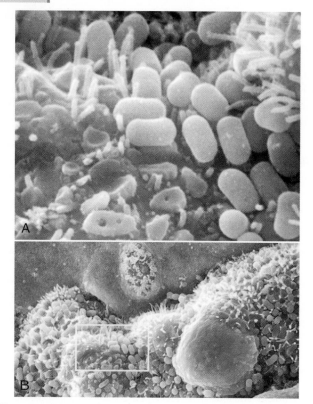

Figure 1-125 A, B. Scanning electron micrograph of the colon of a calf with **enterohemorrhagic *Escherichia coli* infection. B.** Note irregularity of microvilli on cells infected by attaching-effacing *E. coli*, in comparison with microvilli on uninfected cells in background. Outline indicates field illustrated in (**A**). Adherent bacteria are on pedestals projecting from the surface of enterocytes. Occasional bacteria have been lost artifactually, exposing underlying "mushroom-like" pedestals. (Courtesy M. Schoonderwoerd, R. Clarke.)

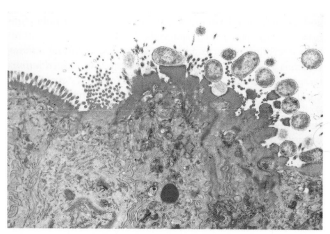

Figure 1-126 Transmission electron micrograph of enterocytes in the colon of a calf infected with enterohemorrhagic *E. coli*. **Enterocyte attaching-effacing *E. coli*** are on pedestals projecting from surface of infected cells. Microvilli are irregular and effaced on infected cells. Normal cell (left). (Reprinted with permission from Schoonderwoerd M, et al. Can J Vet Res 1988;52: 484-487.)

resulting in mild to severe atrophy of villi in the small bowel, and attenuation of surface cells, or microerosions, in the large intestine. Fusion of villi may occur in small intestine, and goblet cell numbers are depleted in both large and small bowel. There is moderate mucosal congestion and local infiltration by neutrophils.

Diarrhea is presumably related to maldigestion and malabsorption of nutrients and electrolytes in small intestine, perhaps with the additive effect of increased mucosal permeability, overloading the colon, the absorptive ability of which is also compromised by damage to surface cells. *Microscopic diagnosis is based on recognition of bacteria on the mucosal surface.*

In **pigs,** EPEC belonging to serogroups O45 and O103, infecting small and large intestine, are responsible for some cases of postweaning diarrhea. In young **dogs,** and occasionally in cats, EPEC have been associated with diarrhea, often as a component of co-infections with viral or protozoal agents. Microscopic lesions characteristic of AEEC are typically found in the jejunum and ileum, less commonly in the colon, and in dogs, sometimes in the stomach.

A distinct subset of EPEC is the **Shiga toxin-producing *E. coli*** (STEC), also known as **enterohemorrhagic *E. coli*** (EHEC). In addition to their ability to attach and efface, these strains produce cytotoxic Shiga toxins (Stx1 and its homologue Stx2 with its variants, c, d, e, f). Shigatoxin 1 is structurally identical to the Shiga toxin produced by *Shigella dysenteriae*, which has a profound cytopathic effect. Because of their effect on Vero cells in culture, these *E. coli* are also referred to as **verotoxin-producing *E. coli*** (VTEC). Shiga toxins, encoded in the genome of bacteriophages, are composed of an A subunit that has enzymatic activity and a B subunit that binds the toxin to the glycolipid receptor globotriaosylceramide (Gb3) on the cell surface. Once endocytosed and transferred via the Golgi apparatus to the rough endoplasmic reticulum, the toxin inhibits protein synthesis, which may be lethal to the target cell, and via separate mechanisms may induce apoptosis. The presence or absence of Gb3 on cell surfaces is a major determinant of the distribution of tissue susceptibility to Shiga toxins, which mainly affect intestinal epithelium and vascular endothelium. Some EHEC also produce hemolysins, which may assist survival in the gut by increasing iron availability. Acid tolerance may also promote colonization efficiency by enhancing survival in the stomach.

The EHEC strains produce disease predominantly in humans, although involvement of domestic animals has been highlighted in the public health arena because of the tendency for cattle and some other species to carry the organism asymptomatically, adherent to epithelium over lymphoid follicles in the rectal mucosa. Different variants of the Stx encoded by phage have been associated with clinical disease and carrier states in cattle. The most widely recognized EHEC serotype is **O157:H7**, a major pathogen in humans, although >200 other STEC serotypes have been identified. In addition to Shiga toxin production, virulence is attributable to attaching and effacing capability, encoded on the LEE.

In **calves <4 weeks of age** (generally >3 days of age, and most commonly in the second week of life), strains of EHEC (O5:NM, O8:H9, O26:H11, O103:H2, O111:NM, O111:H8, and O111:H11) have been associated with a syndrome of *erosive fibrinohemorrhagic enterocolitis*, with the development of dysentery. Fever is not characteristic, and animals may remain bright until the effects of dehydration and blood loss supervene. Death may occur within several days of onset of illness, but some cases will recover in 7-10 days.

At autopsy, gross lesions are usually confined to the spiral colon and rectum, although the ileum and cecum are occasionally involved with mild fibrinous or fibrinohemorrhagic enteritis/typhlitis. In the colon, changes vary from mild patchy congestion of the mucosa to marked mucosal reddening, with adherent mucus, necrotic debris, and blood; colonic contents are fluid and frequently blood-tinged (Fig. 1-127). There may be congestion of the margins of mucosal folds in the rectum, or overt fibrinohemorrhagic proctitis. Mesenteric lymph nodes are often enlarged, especially along the ileum, and occasionally there are lesions (arthritis, serositis) suggesting septicemia.

Microscopically, in affected small intestine the profile of villi is ragged or markedly scalloped, and they are blunted, moderately atrophic, or fused. Epithelial cells on villi in small bowel, and on the colonic surface, where lesions are most severe, are short, rounded up, and in some cases exfoliating singly or in small clumps, causing focal microerosions. Cells in some areas may be markedly attenuated. The microvillus border is indistinct, and covered by a heavy layer of prominent gram-negative coccobacilli (Fig. 1-128). Lesions in large bowel may extend down into glands, which may be dilated, lined by

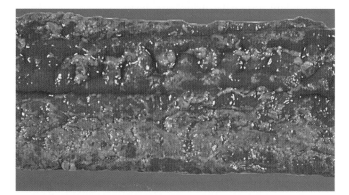

Figure 1-127 Fibrinohemorrhagic enteritis in the ileum of a calf. (Courtesy Noah's Arkives.)

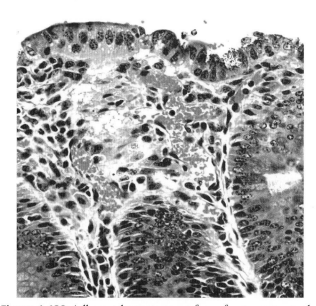

Figure 1-128 Adherent bacteria on surface of enterocytes in the colon of a calf with **enterohemorrhagic *E. coli* infection.**

flattened epithelium, and filled with sloughed epithelium and leukocytes. In the small intestine, foci of bacterial adhesion may be patchy, on the sides of the upper third of villi, with extensive surrounding areas of normal epithelium. Crypts in areas of atrophic small intestine may be elongate, with numerous mitotic figures. In severely affected bowel, the mucosa and submucosa are congested, edematous, and occasional microvascular thrombi may be present. Sloughed enterocytes, erythrocytes, neutrophils, fibrin, and bacteria are in the lumen.

In **dogs,** STEC have been associated with dysentery, and in some dogs, hemolytic uremic syndrome and cutaneous edema and ulceration. In Greyhounds, the syndrome involving this triad has been termed *cutaneous and renal glomerular vasculopathy,* and has been attributed to consumption of beef contaminated with O157:H7 *E. coli,* and other STEC. Renal and cutaneous lesions are attributable to vascular damage caused by Shiga toxin (see Vol. 2, Urinary system; Vol. 1, Integumentary system).

Further reading

Beautin L. *Escherichia coli* as a pathogen in dogs and cats. Vet Res 1999;30:285-298.

DebRoy C, Maddox CW. Identification of virulence attributes of gastrointestinal *Escherichia coli* isolates of veterinary significance. Anim Health Res Rev 2001;2:129-140.

Fröhlicher E, et al. Characterization of attaching and effacing *Escherichia coli* (AEEC) isolated from pigs and sheep. BMC Microbiol 2008;8:144.

Goffaux FB, et al. Genotypic characterization of enteropathogenic *Escherichia coli* (EPEC) isolated from dogs and cats. Res Microbiol 2000;151:865-871.

Harmon BG, et al. Enterohemorrhagic *Escherichia coli* in ruminant hosts. In: Brown CC, Bolin CA, editors. Emerging Diseases of Animals. Washington, DC: ASM Press; 2000. p. 201-216.

Janke BH, et al. Attaching and effacing *Escherichia coli* infections in calves, pigs, lambs, and dogs. J Vet Diagn Invest 1989;1:6-11.

Moxley RA. Escherichia coli 0157:H7: an update on intestinal colonization and virulence mechanisms. Anim Health Res Rev 2004;5:15-33.

Moxley RA, Smith DR. Attaching-effacing *Escherichia coli* infections in cattle. Vet Clin North Am Food Anim Pract 2010;26:29-56.

Shringi S, et al. Carriage of stx2a differentiates clinical and bovine-biased strains of *Escherichia coli* O157. PLoS One 2012;7:e51572.

Edema disease and postweaning *E. coli* enteritis. Edema disease is a distinct syndrome in pigs, characterized by sudden death, or the development of nervous signs associated with enteric colonization by STEC, especially serotypes O138, O139, and O141. The disease occurs most commonly in pigs within a few weeks after weaning, or after other change in feeding or management. Colonization may be related to transient enterocyte malabsorption soon after weaning, which allows for increased dietary protein accumulation in the gut lumen. It often occurs in association with outbreaks of postweaning *E. coli* enteritis. Rare reports exist of edema disease in suckling and mature animals. The disease may be sporadic or occur as an outbreak, usually affecting the best animals in a group, and mortality often approaches 100% of affected animals. Edema disease and postweaning *E. coli* enteritis have apparently declined in prevalence in parts of North America, perhaps with the use of concentrate rations based largely on soybeans and corn, rather than other grains.

Bacterial colonization of the gut is mediated by F18ab fimbriae. Susceptibility of pigs is genetic and related to the presence of receptors for the fimbriae. A Shiga toxin (Stx2e) producing vascular injury and edema has been incriminated in the pathogenesis of edema disease, and vaccination with Stx2e toxoid almost entirely prevents edema disease.

Some strains of *E. coli* that cause edema disease also produce secretory enterotoxin. Diarrhea is not a usual concomitant of edema disease in individual animals. Significant gross or microscopic lesions in the intestinal mucosa do not occur in edema disease, which appears to be a *classical enterotoxemia*, the active principle being absorbed from the gut and acting at a distant site. However, the means by which the toxin enters the circulation is unknown. Stx2e can bind to erythrocytes which may promote its dissemination from the intestine.

Experimentally, the target of Stx2e, like other Shiga toxins, is *vascular endothelium*, particularly of small arteries and arterioles. Preferentially affected organs include spinal cord, cerebellum, eyelid, and colon. However, a study to determine preferential binding sites for Stx2e found receptors on a variety of tissues, not just the aforementioned. Stx2e causes *angiopathy*, which, in its early stages in experimental intoxication, is recognized by swelling of endothelial cells and mild intramural and perivascular hemorrhage. Pyknosis and karyorrhexis of smooth-muscle nuclei, often accompanied by fibrinoid degeneration or hyaline change in the tunica media, may be seen in subacute spontaneous cases. Proliferative mesenchymal elements are found in the tunica media and tunica adventitia in more advanced cases. However, inflammation is not at any stage a prominent component of the angiopathy, nor of the associated edema in most sites, and thrombosis of vessels is rarely encountered. Edema is probably caused by vessel damage during the early stages of the angiopathy. The lesions are distinct from those expected with endotoxemia.

Swine with **edema disease** may die without premonitory signs. Others may have anorexia, or, more characteristically, show nervous signs, usually of <1 day's duration. An unsteady staggering gait, knuckling, ataxia, prostration and tremors, convulsions, and paddling occur. A hoarse squeal, the hoarseness attributed to laryngeal edema and dyspnea, also may be noted clinically.

At autopsy, **gross lesions** in acute deaths may be subtle or absent. Typically, *edema is variably present in one or more sites.* However, it may be mild and must be carefully sought, especially by "slipping" the suspected area over subjacent tissue. Subcutaneous edema may be present in the frontal area and over the snout, in the eyelids, and in the submandibular, ventral abdominal, and inguinal areas. Internally, there may be some hydropericardium, and serous pleural and peritoneal effusion, perhaps accompanied by mild or moderate pulmonary edema. More commonly, the serous surfaces merely appear glistening and wet. Edema of the mesocolon, of the submucosa of the cardiac glandular area of the stomach over the greater curvature, and of mesenteric lymph nodes is most consistently found. The gastric submucosal edema should be sought by carefully cutting through the muscularis to the submucosa. The edema fluid is clear and slightly gelatinous (Fig. 1-129). It is rarely blood-tinged, and overt hemorrhage is usually not present in uncomplicated edema disease. The stomach is often full of feed, but the small intestine is

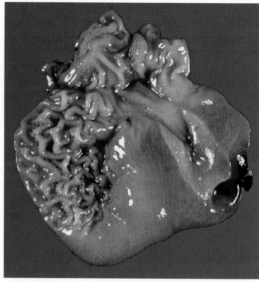

Figure 1-129 Edema of stomach wall in **edema disease** in a pig. (Courtesy Noah's Arkives and A. Doster.)

relatively empty and the mucosa is grossly normal. The colon may contain somewhat inspissated feces.

In swine dying after a more prolonged clinical course, gross edema is often not present, although enlargement of mesenteric lymph nodes is present in a large proportion of cases. A few pigs may show foci of yellow malacia, usually bilaterally symmetrical, in the brainstem at various levels from basal ganglia to medulla.

Microscopically edema in the sites of predilection mentioned earlier is the main lesion in swine dying acutely. It is generally devoid of much protein and contains few erythrocytes and inflammatory cells. A proportion of animals also will have meningeal edema and distended Virchow-Robin spaces in the brain. Vascular lesions may not be well-developed in pigs dying suddenly. When present they usually consist of edema, hemorrhage, myocyte necrosis, and hyaline degeneration in the tunica media. Angiopathy is more consistently found in cases of longer standing. Affected vessels may be found in any tissue in the carcass. Brain edema and focal encephalomalacia in the brainstem are associated with the presence of lesions in cerebral vessels; necrosis may be a sequel to edema and ischemia. *Cerebrospinal angiopathy of swine* is probably a manifestation of edema disease.

A **diagnosis** of edema disease is based on nervous signs or sudden death in growing pigs, in association with typical gross and microscopic lesions, when they are present. In acute cases, heavy growth of hemolytic *E. coli* of one of the serotypes known to produce Stx2e is essential.

Edema disease must be differentiated from enteritis and endotoxemia resulting from *E. coli* in postweaning pigs; from mulberry heart disease in animals dying suddenly; and from salt poisoning, *Salmonella* meningoencephalitis, and other infectious encephalitides, in animals with nervous signs.

Postweaning *E. coli* enteritis (coliform enteritis of weaned pigs) typically occurs during the first week or two following weaning, or after some other change in feed or management. Postweaning diarrhea may be caused by classical enterotoxigenic F4 (K88) *E. coli*, but it is often associated with hemolytic *E. coli* of the same serotypes primarily implicated in edema disease, as well as serotype O149. The two diseases often

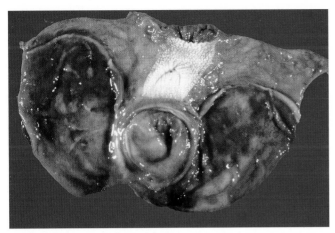

Figure 1-130 Deep red areas of venous infarction in the gastric mucosa in **postweaning colibacillosis** in a pig.

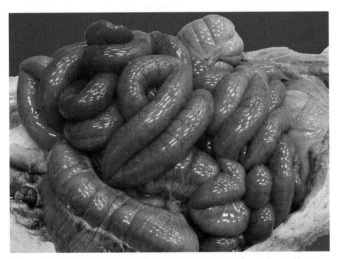

Figure 1-131 Acute enteritis, with congested, flaccid small intestine in **postweaning colibacillosis** in a pig. (Courtesy Iowa State University Veterinary Diagnostic Laboratory.)

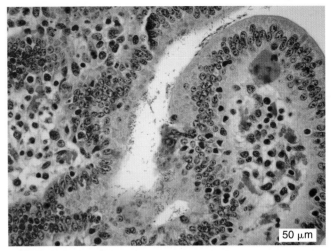

Figure 1-132 *E. coli* attached to the epithelial surface of the villus in **postweaning colibacillosis** in a pig. (Courtesy Iowa State University Veterinary Diagnostic Laboratory.)

occur in the same population of pigs, although usually affecting different animals. Typically, postweaning colibacillosis is a disease of high morbidity and variable mortality, with loss of condition in pigs suffering prolonged illness. Diarrhea is usually yellow and fluid, and stains the perineum. Deaths that occur may or may not follow a prior episode of diarrhea, and often appear to be related to endotoxemia.

In fatal cases there may be blue-red discoloration of the skin and evidence of dehydration. Deep red *gastric venous infarcts* are present in almost all cases (Fig. 1-130). The small intestine is flaccid. The mucosa may be normal in color and the content creamy. In other animals the mucosa of the distal small intestine is congested and the contents watery and perhaps blood-tinged or brown with flecks of yellow mucus or fibrin (Fig. 1-131). Cecal and colonic lesions are usually mild, but there may be some congestion and fibrinous exudate in the proximal large bowel. Mesenteric lymph nodes may be somewhat enlarged, congested, and juicy. Other organs are usually unremarkable grossly.

The **pathogenesis** of postweaning *E. coli* enteritis caused by non-F4 *E. coli* is poorly understood, and the microscopic pathology is not well described. In swine with diarrhea, *E. coli* may be attached to the surface of villi by F18ac fimbriae (Fig.

1-132). Experimentally, stress and decreased mucosal immune functions associated with early weaning have been associated with ETEC and postweaning diarrhea. Like edema disease, high protein levels in the intestinal lumen at weaning may play a role in colonization and disease development. Atrophy of villi does not seem to be evident, and diarrhea is presumed to be mediated by enterotoxins. Mortality may be ascribed to dehydration in animals with prolonged diarrhea and few gross intestinal or extraintestinal lesions. In animals dying of more acute disease, there is local microvascular thrombosis in sections of congested mucosa, and the gross and microscopic lesions in other organs, especially those related to gastric mucosal and submucosal thrombosis and venous infarction, are suggestive of endotoxemia. Hemolytic *E. coli* of the implicated strains are consistently isolated in virtually pure culture from the lower small intestine and colon. However, they are present in the spleen and liver in only a few cases, suggesting terminal bacteremia.

The factors predisposing to the massive colonization of hemolytic *E. coli* are unclear. Loss of lactogenic immunity, a favorable environment for proliferation of bacterial strains with specific nutrient requirements, and promotion of epithelial colonization by the effects of antecedent *Rotavirus* infection have been variously implicated.

A **diagnosis** of postweaning colibacillosis is suggested by the gross lesions in animals dying acutely or subacutely, and it is confirmed by culture and serotyping of associated strains of *E. coli*. The fatal disease must be differentiated from edema disease, proliferative hemorrhagic enteropathy, salmonellosis, and swine dysentery. Postweaning diarrhea caused by uncomplicated *Rotavirus* infection, transmissible gastroenteritis virus, or associated with attaching-effacing O45:K "E65" *E. coli*, is usually nonfatal.

Further reading

Fairbrother JM, et al. *Escherichia coli* in postweaning diarrhea in pigs: an update on bacterial types, pathogenesis, and prevention strategies. Anim Health Res Rev 2005;6:17-39.

Matise I, et al. Binding of shiga toxin 2e to porcine erythrocytes in vivo and in vitro. Infect Immun 2003;71:5194-201.

McLamb BL, et al. Early weaning stress in pigs impairs innate mucosal immune responses to enterotoxigenic *E. coli* challenge and exacerbates intestinal injury and clinical disease. PLoS One 2013;8:e59838.

Moxley RA. Edema disease. Vet Clin North Am Food Anim Pract 2000;16:175-185.

Opapeju FO, et al. Effect of dietary protein level on growth performance, indicators of enteric health, and gastrointestinal microbial ecology of weaned pigs induced with postweaning colibacillosis. J Anim Sci 2009;87:2635-2643.

Paton JC, Paton AW. Pathogenesis and diagnosis of Shiga toxin-producing *Escherichia coli* infections. Clin Microbiol Rev 1998;11:450-479.

Enteroinvasive *E. coli*. Strains of *E. coli* are recognized, infecting humans and certain other species, which have the capacity to invade or to be internalized by surface enterocytes of the small and large intestine, in which they multiply. In this sense they resemble *Shigella* in primates, and *Salmonella*. The enteroinvasiveness of *Shigella* and some strains of *E. coli* appears to be correlated with the presence of a high-molecular-weight plasmid coding for outer-membrane proteins involved in invasion. Multiplication of the organism within epithelial cells results in *local erosion and ulceration*, associated with acute inflammation in the mucosa.

Among domestic animals, *enteroinvasive colibacillosis has only been confirmed experimentally in neonatal swine*, using a strain of O101 *E. coli*. Spontaneous enteritis that appears to be due to enteroinvasive *E. coli* is rarely encountered in piglets up to weaning and in calves <2 weeks of age. Diarrhea in experimentally infected piglets is described as gray-yellow, watery, and containing small clots. The gross findings may not be remarkable, or the intestine may appear congested in comparison with that in most diarrheic piglets. In spontaneous cases suspected of being due to enteroinvasive *E. coli*, the gastric fundus also may be congested, and this correlates with the presence of venous infarction visible microscopically. Experimental enteroinvasive colibacillosis in piglets causes villus atrophy that is comparable in severity to that induced by the common viruses of neonates. Enterocytes appear cuboidal or flattened and some are seen lysing. The lamina propria is edematous; capillaries are congested and infiltrated by neutrophils and other inflammatory cells. In spontaneous cases, thrombi may be evident in proprial capillaries and submucosal lymphatics. Neutrophils and tissue fluid effuse into the lumen between villi through epithelial discontinuities. Similar microthrombosis, proprial inflammation, enterocyte destruction, and effusion may be found in the cecum and colon. Intracellular organisms of O serogroup 101 were demonstrated by immunoperoxidase staining in the experimental study, but are not generally recognized in spontaneous cases suspected to be due to enteroinvasive *E. coli*. Edema and neutrophil accumulation in sinusoids of mesenteric lymph nodes are present. Experimental enteroinvasive colibacillosis in piglets has been associated with malabsorption and protein loss into the gut, presumably a result of villus atrophy and effusive enteritis, respectively.

There is growing evidence that an invasive *E. coli* is involved in the histiocytic and ulcerative colitis of Boxers and French Bulldogs. In these dogs, *E. coli* are noted within lamina propria macrophages and mesenteric lymph nodes. A role for this agent in disease development is supported by improvement of clinical signs and mucosal inflammation after its removal from the mucosa by antimicrobial therapy. It is hypothesized that a genetic predisposition to this invasive *E. coli* exists in these breeds. There are similarities between this *E. coli* and adherent and invasive *E. coli* (AIEC) described as playing a role in human inflammatory bowel disease.

Further reading

Craven M, et al. Granulomatous colitis of boxer dogs. Vet Clin North Am Small Anim Pract 2011;41:433-45.

DebRoy C, Maddox CW. Identification of virulence attributes of gastrointestinal *Escherichia coli* isolates of veterinary significance. Anim Health Res Rev 2001;2:129-140.

Mansfield CS, et al. Remission of histiocytic ulcerative colitis in Boxer dogs correlates with eradication of invasive intramucosal *Escherichia coli*. J Vet Intern Med 2009;23:964-969.

Okerman L. Enteric infections caused by non-enterotoxigenic *Escherichia coli* in animals: occurrence and pathogenicity mechanisms. A review. Vet Microbiol 1987;14:33-46.

Septicemic colibacillosis. Generalized systemic infection with *E. coli* occurs commonly in *calves*, and less commonly or sporadically, especially among young animals of the other domestic species. Predisposition to infection is a prerequisite for *E. coli* septicemia. This usually results from reduced transfer or absorption of maternal colostral immunoglobulin, or from intercurrent disease or debilitation. But certain strains of *E. coli*, especially O8, O9, O15, O26, O35, O45, O78, O86, O101, O117, and O137 in calves and lambs, and O115 in pigs and calves, are particularly associated with septicemia, and may possess characteristics that enhance their ability to invade and proliferate systemically in compromised animals.

Among factors conferring virulence upon these strains are plasmids coding for colicin V (Col V). Col V plasmids carry genes coding for aerobactin, a bacterial hydroxamate siderophore permitting survival in low-iron extracellular environments; outer-membrane proteins resisting bactericidal effects of serum, such as complement activation; and hydrophobic properties that impede phagocytosis, conferred by a capsule. Some produce cytolethal distending toxin, or fimbriae that impede phagocytosis. Endotoxin released by dying bacteria causes the vascular damage and shock associated with *E. coli* septicemia.

The portal of entry of *E. coli* causing septicemia probably varies somewhat. The navel in the neonate, the upper respiratory tract and possibly the tonsil, and the intestine are likely sites. In calves, adhesins such as P, F17, AfaE-VIII, and CS31A may promote enteric colonization and invasion. Enteritis is not a necessary, or even common, concomitant of colisepticemia in animals.

Colisepticemia is most commonly a disease of neonates, and may vary from peracute septicemia and endotoxemia resulting in sudden death, to subacute or chronic disease in which signs are related to sites of bacterial localization, especially in the meninges, joints, and eyes.

The lesions associated with colisepticemia in young animals of any species, especially calves, lambs, and foals, may vary from subtle to obvious. Mortality in hypogammaglobulinemic neonates may occur acutely with little in the way of abnormal gross findings. These may be limited to mildly congested or blue-red, slightly rubbery lungs, and a firm spleen, perhaps with evidence of omphalitis. *Microscopic changes* in the lungs include thickening of alveolar septa by mononuclear cells and neutrophils, and effusion of lightly fibrinous exudate and a few neutrophils into alveoli. There may be a corona of neutrophils around white pulp in the spleen, and neutrophils may be present in abnormal numbers in circulation in many organs, including lung and hepatic sinusoids. Kupffer cells also may be prominent in sinusoids in the liver. Fibrin thrombi may be evident in pulmonary capillaries, glomeruli, and hepatic sinusoids. Some calves develop acute interstitial nephritis with foci of neutrophil accumulation, which with time evolve into "white-spotted kidney" in surviving animals.

More severe acute cases show evidence of serosal hemorrhage, with perhaps some serosanguineous pericardial fluid. The lungs may be deep red-blue, rubbery, and fail to collapse. Interlobular septa may be slightly separated by edema, and froth or fluid may be present in the major airways. Meningeal vessels may be congested, and the meninges wet. The abomasum or stomach may have focal superficial ulcers, or more extensive deep red areas of venous infarction. There may be evidence of diarrhea and dehydration, with congestion of the small intestine. Microscopic lesions resemble those previously described, with more severe congestion, thrombosis, and edema in lungs, and perhaps other tissues. In cases not examined for some time after death, clumps of small bacilli may be seen in vessels throughout the body. The vascular permeability, thrombosis, and hemorrhage reflect endotoxemia and its sequelae.

Subacute cases may develop localized infection on serous surfaces, in the joints and meninges. Fibrinous peritonitis, pleuritis, and pericarditis, fibrinopurulent arthritis and meningitis, and hypopyon are commonly found, alone or in various combinations. Affected animals may have a history of lameness ascribable to arthritis, nervous signs caused by meningitis, or general debilitation. Microscopic examination reveals the lesions already described in animals with active systemic disease, with the addition of extensive congestion and edema of inflamed serous surfaces, associated with an acute fibrinous inflammatory exudate.

In *lambs*, congestion and edema of the mucosa of turbinates and sinuses, perhaps with mucopurulent to hemorrhagic sinusitis, have been described. Fibrinous polyserositis and arthritis are sporadic manifestations of *E. coli* septicemia in growing or adult swine, and must be differentiated from the more significant *Haemophilus*, *Mycoplasma*, and streptococcal infections causing these lesions. Colisepticemia is a sporadic cause of mortality in litters of young puppies.

Diagnosis of colisepticemia is based on the isolation of *E. coli* in large numbers from more than one parenchymatous organ or other internal site, other than mesenteric lymph node (preferably liver, spleen, lung, or kidney), or from a site of serosal localization, in conjunction with compatible gross and/or microscopic lesions.

"Watery mouth," a syndrome characterized by drooling, depression, loss of appetite, and abomasal and abdominal distention, is associated with *E. coli* infection/bacteremia in lambs <3 days of age in the United Kingdom. At autopsy affected lambs are in poor condition. They may have unclotted milk and mucinous fluid in the distended abomasum; there is gas in the abomasum and intestine, and meconium retention is common. It is hypothesized that *E. coli* colonize the bowel, and in some manner cause loss of motility and functional obstruction. Fluid and gas accumulate in the abomasum. Bacteremia/septicemia is terminal.

Further reading

Dezfulian H, et al. Presence and characterization of extraintestinal pathogenic *Escherichia coli* virulence genes in F165-positive *E. coli* strains isolated from diseased calves and pigs. J Clin Microbiol 2003;41:1375-1385.

Fecteau G, et al. Virulence factors in *Escherichia coli* isolated from the blood of bacteremic neonatal calves. Vet Microbiol 2001;78:241-249.

Gay CC, Besser TE. *Escherichia coli* septicaemia in calves. In: Gyles CL, editor. *Escherichia coli* in Domestic Animals and Humans. Oxford: CAB International; 1994. p. 75-90.

Kireçci E, et al. Isolation of pathogenic aerobic bacteria from the blood of septicaemic neonatal calves and the susceptibility of isolates to various antibiotics. J S Afr Vet Assoc 2010;81:110-113.

Salmonellosis

The **taxonomy of Salmonella** is currently based on molecular genetic analysis. The genus *Salmonella* is considered to be comprised of 2 species, **S. bongori** and **S. enterica.** There are 6 subspecies of *S. enterica* (*enterica, salamae, arizonae, diarizonae, indica,* and *houtenae*) and many (>2,400) antigenically distinct serotypes or serovars. About 60% of *Salmonella* serotypes belong to *S. enterica* subsp. *enterica*, and occur in birds and mammals. Members of *S. e. enterica* are the predominant cause of salmonellosis in humans and domestic animals, but <50 of these serotypes have been isolated from mammals or birds with any frequency worldwide. The remainder of *S. enterica* and *S. bongori* serotypes are found in ectothermic animals or the environment. In conventional terminology, the serotypes have been treated as species, but in the new terminology the names of serotypes are capitalized, but not italicized (e.g., *S. enterica* Typhimurium when first used, followed later by *S.* Typhimurium). They are usually named on the basis of the locality in which the serotype was first isolated or identified, or on their host association and the clinical syndrome they may produce. Identification of isolates at the subserotype level, by phage typing, plasmid profile analysis, or other molecular techniques, is desirable when there is evidence of zoonotic transmission, or when epidemiologic tracing is necessary.

The **clinical and pathologic syndromes of salmonellosis** typically vary from localized enterocolitis to septicemia; abortion may also occur, with or without obvious systemic disease. Although some serotypes are strongly host-adapted, others have a very wide host range. Highly host-adapted serotypes, such as *S.* Typhi (humans), *S.* Dublin (cattle), and *S.* Choleraesuis (swine), tend to produce severe systemic disease in adult, as well as juvenile animals, whereas serotypes with a broad host range, e.g., *S.* Typhimurium, tend to affect predominantly young animals in most species, and mainly cause enterocolitis, though septicemia may occur. There may be overlap between the two forms of disease, and if the animal survives, a carrier state of variable duration usually follows.

Asymptomatic carriage of Salmonella may be common, depending on the species, and transmission can occur directly, or indirectly, by contamination of feed, water, or the environment from which the organism is ingested or inhaled. Stressors that compromise immune competence or disrupt the enteric bacterial ecosystem are often implicated in salmonellosis, and disease is usually more common and severe in young animals. The more common *stressors* associated with salmonellosis in domestic animals include transportation, starvation, changes in the ration, overcrowding, pregnancy, parturition, exertion, anesthesia, surgery, intercurrent disease, immunosuppressive drugs, and oral treatment with antibiotics and anthelmintics. Consequent changes in the anaerobic bacterial ecosystem that alter the volatile fatty acid composition of the enteric environment are permissive of *Salmonella* colonization.

There are many examples of enhanced susceptibility to salmonellosis associated with intercurrent disease. The best known is that between the *Classical swine fever virus* and *S.* Choleraesuis, an association so close as to have caused early pathologists to disregard the bacterium as a significant pathogen. The disease in adult cattle is usually sporadic, and often there are predisposing conditions, such as parturient paresis, ketosis, mastitis, and parasitic infestations. The stress of anesthesia and surgery may account in part for the serious outbreaks of salmonellosis that occur in hospitalized animals, especially horses, at veterinary schools.

The **pathogenesis of salmonellosis** may be divided into several stages: *entry* of the bacteria into the host and attainment of the primary site of infection, usually the enterocyte; attachment to the surface (*colonization*); and *invasion* of enterocytes.

For infection to take place, *Salmonella* must be present in sufficient numbers; generally a minimal infective oral dose of 10^7-10^9 organisms is needed to infect large domestic animals. After ingestion, the *Salmonella* must overcome nonspecific resistance factors, including the bactericidal effects of salivary enzymes, and the acid pH of the gastric environment. Mucus and lysozymes in the glycocalyx, peristalsis, commensal luminal microbial population, and constant sloughing of enterocytes may interfere with attachment. Those organisms that survive the nonspecific resistance factors may colonize and invade enterocytes.

Invading *Salmonella* in some species enter the mucosa through M cells in the Peyer's patches, and host specificity of some *Salmonella* serotypes may be associated in part with specific receptor sites on these cells. *Salmonella* have been demonstrated in the Peyer's patches as early as 6 hours postinoculation. When bacteria invade through M cells, smaller numbers of *Salmonella* may enter through enterocytes in other areas of the small intestine. However, the M cell is not the main site of attachment in some circumstances, for instance in *S.* Typhimurium infections of calves and pigs.

In salmonellosis characterized primarily by enterocolitis, the organisms do not usually disseminate beyond the mucosa and the mesenteric lymph nodes, and the ensuing inflammation remains confined to the intestine. In those cases where bacteremia ensues, the organisms must be able to survive and replicate in macrophages and disseminate to other systemic sites, such as liver, lung, joints, meninges, or placenta and fetus. In *S.* Dublin infection, the bacteria are present within macrophages in the intestinal mucosa, but are free in lymph in the draining lymphatics and dissemination is likely via lymphatics.

The ability to attach, invade, and penetrate enterocytes is crucial to virulence, and the first step in the development of salmonellosis. A number of known virulence factors contribute to the pathogenesis of salmonellosis, including motility, pili, or fimbriae, effector proteins modifying the metabolism or causing death of host cells, and lipopolysaccharides. The information for such virulence attributes is often encoded in chromosomes in clusters of genes known as *Salmonella* pathogenicity islands (SPI).

Invasion of enterocytes, especially those in the ileum, occurs within 12 hours of oral infection. Ability to invade cells is dependent on a type III protein secretion system encoded in SPI-1. Protein targets of the secretion system are translocated into host cells, where they facilitate bacterial invasion by causing changes in the cytosol and ruffling of the cell membrane. Outer membrane vesicles are secreted from the surface of the bacterium and are internalized by the host cells. These vesicles also carry bacterial proteins into the cell that are important for internalization.

Motility, associated with the presence of flagella, is characteristic of many *Salmonella* serovars. Bacterial motility is generally not considered to be an important virulence determinant. However, it may enhance the movement of bacteria through the glycocalyx and facilitate attachment to specific receptor sites on enterocytes.

Fimbriae (pilus adhesins) encoded in chromosomes and on virulence plasmids are present on salmonellae, and they may play a role in colonization of the gut. Adherence of *Salmonella* to intestinal epithelial cells takes place in 2 stages. The first step is reversible because the organisms can be easily washed off. Weak ionic and nonionic interactions between bacterial and host cell membrane surfaces are thought to be the binding forces responsible for this attachment. The second stage, referred to as *receptor-mediated endocytosis*, is irreversible. It occurs after a lag period and it is characterized by degeneration of the microvilli on the epithelial cells, "ruffling" of the cell membrane, and macropinocytosis, resulting in internalization into membrane-bound vacuoles (endosomes) containing *Salmonella*.

The ultrastructural changes of *Salmonella* infection in the intestine were first described in experimental infections of guinea pigs. Large numbers of organisms are present in the lumen, on the surface of the brush border, and in enterocytes. There is an increase in the number of neutrophils in the gut lumen and within intercellular spaces, and some of these contain bacteria. Degeneration of microvilli, characterized by loss of filamentous cores, is associated with close adherence of bacteria. Other changes consist of elongation, swelling, budding and fusion of microvilli, and loss of the terminal web.

The organisms usually invade the cells through the brush border; however, they may also enter the mucosa through the intercellular junctional complex. In the cytoplasm, the bacteria are located within membrane-bound vacuoles, which may also contain remnants of microvilli and cytoplasmic debris. Most organisms remain intact and multiply during their transcellular migration in endosomes. Often, many bacteria are present in a single enterocyte during the early stages of infection, but cellular damage is mild and transient. The *Salmonella*-receptor complex dissociates as a result of the acidification of the endosomal content, allowing the receptor site to return to the apical plasma membrane and repeat the processes of endocytosis. After 24 hours, most bacteria are located within membrane-bound vacuoles in macrophages in the lamina propria. Many organisms are evident in the lumina of crypts, but invasion of cryptal epithelial cells evidently does not take place.

The **lipopolysaccharide** (LPS) moiety of *Salmonella* with smooth cell walls consists of an *O-specific side chain, a core portion, and a lipid A portion.* Most *Salmonella* isolated from animals have smooth cell walls, which influences virulence in several ways. These strains are more invasive, and are more successful at avoiding phagocytosis, and lysis in phagolysosomes after invasion, than are "rough" counterparts with incomplete LPS. LPSs reduce the susceptibility of the organisms to the host's cationic proteins; they stimulate local prostaglandin synthesis; and they prevent the activation and deposition of complement on the bacterial surface.

The main function of LPS may be to facilitate survival in the intestinal mucosa and eventual entry into deeper tissues. The involvement of LPS in invasion apparently varies among *Salmonella* serotypes because some strains of *S.* Typhimurium do not require intact LPS to invade epithelial cells in vitro. On the other hand, more host-specific *Salmonella* serotypes, such as *S.* Typhi and *S.* Choleraesuis, require intact LPS or O-side chains. The lipid A portion of LPS is responsible for the endotoxin-mediated effects of *Salmonella* infection that are seen in systemic disease. Septicemia (endotoxemia) typically causes fever, leukopenia, hemoconcentration, lactic acidosis, coagulopathies, hypotension, and death.

Diarrhea in salmonellosis is not mediated by enterotoxins such as those involved in cholera and *E. coli* infections. Rather, *effector proteins* associated with SPI-1 induce secretory diarrhea by blocking chloride channel closure, whereas others attract neutrophils and induce apoptosis of enterocytes. Proteins encoded in SPI-5 also promote neutrophil recruitment and electrolyte secretion. Mucosal inflammation leads to the accumulation of a number of mediators, including prostaglandin E_2, capable of causing hypersecretion of chloride by enterocytes, and consequent passive osmotic movement of water into the lumen. Loss of enterocytes, dying as a sequel to *Salmonella* invasion and neutrophil-induced tissue injury, results in a reduction in absorptive surface area, and causes defects in mucosal integrity, through which the protein- and neutrophil-rich exudate leaking from permeable vessels effuses.

Thus diarrhea is an outcome of active secretion of electrolyte, malabsorption resulting from reduced mucosal surface area and enterocyte competence, and inflammatory exudation, which may contain sufficient fibrinogen to form a pseudomembrane over the affected surface. The volume of fluid originating in lesions in the small intestine may overwhelm the capacity of the colon to compensate; as often as not in salmonellosis, the large intestinal mucosa is also involved, further compounding the compromise to electrolyte and water homeostasis in the gut.

Thrombosis of mucosal venules is common in *Salmonella* enteritis, and may contribute to loss of mucosal viability. Such lesions may be due in part to the large amounts of **endotoxin** absorbed through the damaged mucosa, or released locally.

Enteritis in salmonellosis is thus characterized by fibrinous or fibrinohemorrhagic exudates over denuded small and large intestinal mucosae, directly mediated by the apoptosis and necrosis induced by invading bacteria, and by the necrotizing effects of local neutrophil activity and microvascular thrombosis.

The **systemic outcome of an infection with *Salmonella*** is determined by the genetic virulence determinants of the invading organism and the ensuing innate, humoral, and cell-mediated immune response of the host. *Salmonella* are considered to be *facultative intracellular pathogens*, and invading strains must have the ability to survive and replicate within macrophages to cause bacteremia or septicemia. This capacity is conferred by components coded in SPI-2, perhaps largely through inhibition of NADPH oxidase-mediated oxidative

killing of *Salmonella* in cytoplasmic vacuoles, and in some species by factors encoded in SPI-2 and SPI-3. The virulence of several serotypes commonly associated with systemic infections in animals, including *S.* Typhimurium, *S.* Dublin, and *S.* Choleraesuis, is enhanced by intracellular survival in macrophages mediated by attributes encoded on virulence plasmids.

Salmonella taken up by resident macrophages elicit a *major immune response* in the host. Initiation of the innate immune response commences with pattern recognition receptors, such as toll-like receptors (TLR), which recognize conserved bacterial motifs. Ligation of these receptors promotes proinflammatory cytokine production and recruitment of neutrophils. There is considerable controversy about the roles played by cell-mediated and humoral immunity in the pathogenesis of salmonellosis, but *Salmonella* infection results in the release of cytokines by specifically stimulated T lymphocytes. They activate macrophages that phagocytose the organisms, and in such a circumstance, cell-mediated immunity is of paramount importance.

Once *Salmonella* bacteria have crossed the mucosa, they may enter the bloodstream via the lymphatics, perhaps carried in macrophages, and cause septicemia or transient bacteremia. Or they may remain indefinitely in the gut-associated lymphoid tissues and mesenteric lymph nodes. Increased susceptibility to salmonellosis in animals with intercurrent disease, or subjected to stress, may be related to relaxation of cell-mediated immunity to the organism. Septicemia may be of variable duration and severity but, as a rule, it is rapidly fatal in young animals. If, however, there is transient bacteremia, the organisms are removed by fixed macrophages, especially those of the spleen, liver, and bone marrow. They may continue to proliferate in such extravascular locations and subsequently may cause another bacteremic phase that may result in fatal septicemia or secondary localization in other tissues.

The carrier state is important in the epidemiology of the disease. Whether *Salmonella* can maintain themselves in the intestinal lumen is not clear; to some extent fecal shedding is likely to depend on intermittent seeding from the bile, or from macrophages in the lamina propria and gut-associated lymphoid tissue. The duration of the carrier state may be prolonged, or animals may rid themselves of the infection, probably by means of cell-mediated immunity. The carrier state is an unstable one, for it appears that if the carrier is subjected to some stress or debilitating disease it may succumb to disease; this often seems to occur in adult cattle. The carrier animal is a potential threat to any other animal that it contacts, either directly or through the medium of its excreta, or by-products such as bone or meat meal.

Further reading

Darwin KH, et al. Molecular basis of the interaction of *Salmonella* with the intestinal mucosa. Clin Microbiol Rev 1999;12:405-428.

de Jong HK, et al. Host-pathogen interaction in invasive salmonellosis. PLoS Pathog 2012;8(10):e1002933.

Jepson MA, Clark MA. The role of M cells in *Salmonella* infection. Microbes Infect 2001;3:1183-1190.

Libby SJ, et al. *Salmonella*. In: Gyles CL, et al., editors. Pathogenesis of Bacterial Infections in Animals. 3rd ed. Ames, Iowa: Blackwell; 2004. p. 143-167.

Monack DM. *Salmonella* persistence and transmission strategies. Curr Opin Microbiol 2012;15:100-107.

Ohl ME, Miller SI. *Salmonella*: a model for bacterial pathogenesis. Annu Rev Med 2001;52:259-274.

Santos RL. Pathobiology of *Salmonella*, intestinal microbiota, and the host innate immune response. Front Immunol 2014;5:252.

Yoon H, et al. Discovery of *Salmonella* virulence factors translocated via outer membrane vesicles to murine macrophages. Infect Immun 2011;79:2182-92.

Zhang S, et al. Molecular pathogenesis of *Salmonella enterica* serotype typhimurium-induced diarrhea. Infect Immun 2003;71:1-12.

Salmonellosis in swine. Many serotypes of *Salmonella* have been isolated from swine, and with poultry and cattle they form an *important reservoir of the organism*. The bacteria are carried in the lamina propria of the intestine, but also in the regional lymph nodes of the alimentary tract, so that carrier animals may not excrete the organism in the feces.

Three syndromes are associated with *Salmonella* infections in swine. (1) *Septicemic salmonellosis* is usually associated with the host-adapted *S.* Choleraesuis var. kunzendorf, although enteric lesions may be present with this serovar. Sporadic infections with *S.* Dublin have also been associated with septicemia in nursing pigs. (2) *S.* Typhimurium most commonly causes *acute or chronic enterocolitis*, including necrotizing proctitis which may lead to rectal stricture. (3) *S.* Typhisuis infection is characterized by *ulcerative enterocolitis*, as well as caseous tonsillitis and lymphadenitis. *S.* Choleraesuis and *S.* Typhimurium are the most common serovars that cause disease in pigs. However, *S.* Derby is also frequently detected in pigs.

Salmonella Choleraesuis was once thought to be the cause of classical swine fever (formerly hog cholera) because gross lesions of septicemic salmonellosis and acute classical swine fever are similar. The latter disease is often complicated by *S.* Choleraesuis, the bacterium being recovered from 10-50% of pigs with classical swine fever.

The major clinical manifestations of *S.* Choleraesuis infection are *septicemia and enteritis*; they usually occur separately and septicemia is more common. *S.* Choleraesuis can cause disease in both young and adult pigs. Oral inoculation of *S.* Choleraesuis initially results in septicemia and acute enterocolitis, followed in some cases by large necrotic and ulcerative lesions (*button ulcers*) in the colonic mucosa. Enteritis is not necessarily chronic, or even clinically evident. Interstitial pneumonia and multifocal hepatic necrosis are the most consistent systemic lesions. In Europe, infection has also been associated with the development of fulminant fibrinous pneumonia. Immunohistochemical techniques reveal the preferential location of *S.* Choleraesuis in the colon and surface of ileal M cells in Peyer's patches. The invasive capability of this serovar is indicated by the presence of large numbers of organisms in proprial macrophages and regional lymph nodes.

Salmonellosis that is clinically septicemic is usually fatal. Death may occur quickly without observed illness, or after a course of a week or more. There is a high fever; characteristic but not pathognomonic blue discoloration of the skin, especially of the tail, snout, and ears (Fig. 1-133); caudal weakness; dyspnea that often leads to misdiagnosis of primary pneumonia; and sometimes terminal convulsions. Sows may abort during the septicemic phase of infection. Pigs that have recovered from this phase may have dry gangrene of the ears and tail, caudal paralysis, blindness, and diphtheritic enteritis. The *chronic or enteric form* may develop from the acute, but is usually insidious from the onset. It is characterized by loose

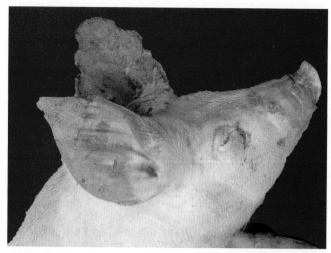

Figure 1-133 Note congestion of skin of ears and snout owing to microvascular thrombosis caused by endotoxemia in **septicemic salmonellosis** in a pig. (Courtesy D. Driemeier.)

yellow feces containing flakes of fibrin, progressive emaciation and debility, and eventual death. Some recover but fail to thrive, often partly owing to chronic bronchopneumonia.

At **autopsy,** there is blue or purple discoloration of the *skin*, which may be very intense about the head and ears. There may be superficial ischemic necrosis of the ears. Typically there are petechial hemorrhages in many organs and tissues. The lymph nodes are almost invariably hemorrhagic. The visceral nodes are more frequently and obviously involved than the peripheral ones, with the exception of those of the throat, which are usually hemorrhagic. The mesenteric lymph nodes are greatly enlarged, and they may be speckled with hemorrhages.

There may be hemorrhages, petechial or as small discrete ecchymoses, on the *laryngeal mucosa*. The *lungs* do not collapse because there is frothy fluid in the respiratory passages. They may be pale blue or purple. Beneath the visceral pleura there are small dark foci of hemorrhage. The lungs are wet and there is fluid in the interlobular tissue. The changes are best appreciated in the caudal lobes because the cranial lobes are often the seat of acute lobular pneumonia. These pulmonary changes, attributable in part to endotoxin, account for the respiratory signs observed clinically. The *pneumonia* is interstitial because of endotoxemia and embolic organisms. The lobar cranioventral pneumonia may be due to ascending *Salmonella* alveolitis and bronchiolitis. Occasionally, the injury to the alveolar septa by *Salmonella* results in extensive fibrinous pneumonia of the caudal lobes. The cardiac serosae often bear petechiae, and in some more virulent infections there is fibrinohemorrhagic pericarditis with scant fluid exudation.

The *spleen is enlarged*, deep blue, firm with sharp edges; little blood oozes from the cut surface. There may be petechiae on the capsule, but the marginal infarcts of classical swine fever are not present. Other causes of splenomegaly, such as erysipelas, other septicemias, and African swine fever, must be differentiated.

The *liver* is usually congested, and focal hemorrhages may be visible in the capsule. In some cases the hemorrhages are very large, involving up to half of the central area in a lobule. They may be scattered at random throughout the liver or grouped, often at the edge of a lobe. In some, there are tiny

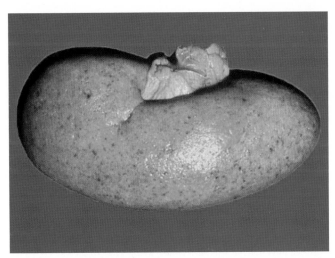

Figure 1-134 *Salmonella* septicemia in a pig. Petechiae in the kidney. (Courtesy Joint Pathology Center.)

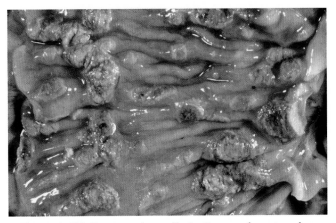

Figure 1-135 Porcine salmonellosis. Button ulcers in colon.

yellow foci of necrosis, referred to as *paratyphoid nodules*. Pinpoint hemorrhages are consistently present in the renal cortex (Fig. 1-134). There may be only a few in each kidney or they may be so numerous as to cause the "turkey egg" appearance.

The *stomach* shows the intense red-black color of the severe congestion and venous infarction common to endotoxemia in pigs. If the animal survives a week or more, the superficial necrotic layer of the affected gastric mucosa sloughs. There may be no lesions in the *intestine*. There may be catarrhal enteritis or, more frequently, the enteritis is hemorrhagic, increasing in severity lower in the tract and terminating in a hemorrhagic ileitis. The mucosae of the colon and cecum may be normal but, if the course is prolonged, there is hyperemia, fibrinohemorrhagic inflammation, or button ulcers (Fig. 1-135).

Petechial hemorrhages may occur in the *meninges and brain*, but there is no gross inflammation. Localization sometimes occurs in *synovial membranes*, producing polysynovitis and sometimes *polyarthritis*. It is more usual to have an increase in the volume of fluid with red velvety hypertrophy of the synovial villi. The gross features described are usually not all present in any one case.

The **histologic changes** that occur in internal organs in acute disease are mainly associated with *endothelial damage*

resulting from endotoxin, and *focal localization of bacteria*. The discoloration of the skin is initially caused by intense dilation, congestion, and thrombosis of capillaries and venules in the dermal papillae. There is activation and necrosis of the endothelial cells in affected vessels. The renal lesions vary but principally affect the glomeruli. In some there is diffuse glomerulitis, and this is associated with mild nephrosis and hyaline casts. In others the glomerulitis is exudative and hemorrhagic and in these a great many capillary loops contain hyaline thrombi. Embolic bacterial colonies are occasionally seen in the glomerular and intertubular capillaries. Fibrin thrombi also may be found in the afferent arterioles and interlobular arteries.

The pulmonary lesions are also characterized by thrombosis and vasculitis and a largely mononuclear cellular response in alveolar septa. There is flooding of the alveoli by edema fluid and moderate numbers of alveolar macrophages. This is the usual histologic picture; the extremes are acute fibrinous inflammation or a few scattered parenchymal hemorrhages.

In the liver the *paratyphoid nodules* may be found in all transitional stages from foci of nonspecific necrosis to reactive granulomas. Typically there are few neutrophils, and whether the nodules are necrotic or reactive depends on their duration. The initial change is focal coagulative necrosis. Macrophages accumulate about the margin, expanding and displacing the surrounding parenchymal cords.

In the spleen there are scattered hemorrhages, but the overall histologic impression is of increased histiocytes with a scattering of neutrophils. The follicles are small and rather inactive. Very small foci of necrosis, containing many bacteria, may be sparse or relatively numerous, and these develop a reactive macrophage response and form the typical paratyphoid nodules.

Meningoencephalomyelitis occurs in a proportion of cases of septicemic salmonellosis. The lesion is fundamentally a vasculitis. There may be petechiae in the meninges but, microscopically, there is infiltration of large mononuclear cells in the pia-arachnoid and concentrated about the veins. The organism is relatively fastidious and cultures from postmortem samples may not be uniformly positive.

***Salmonella* Typhimurium** infection in swine produces a syndrome that differs from *S.* Choleraesuis in a number of ways. Clinically, the disease occurs in *feeder pigs* and is characterized by fever, inanition, and yellow watery diarrhea that may contain blood and mucus, especially in the later stages. The diarrhea may be chronic and intermittent. There is high morbidity but low mortality. Most pigs recover but may remain *carriers* for variable periods of time; some may develop rectal stricture. The organism persists in tonsils, lower intestinal tract, and submandibular and ileocolic lymph nodes.

The pathogenesis and morphology of the enteric lesions differ from those described for *S.* Choleraesuis enteritis. The lesions with *S.* Typhimurium infection are mainly confined to the colon, cecum, and rectum, with minor involvement of the distal small intestine. There is acute enterocolitis with formation of a diphtheritic membrane on the mucosal surface (Fig. 1-136). Button ulcers are not associated with this or other non–host-adapted serovars. Systemic dissemination and septicemia are rare.

Rectal stricture is thought to be a *sequel in most cases to ulcerative proctitis of ischemic origin*, caused by *S.* Typhimurium. It is characterized clinically by marked progressive distention of the abdomen, loss of appetite, emaciation, and soft feces.

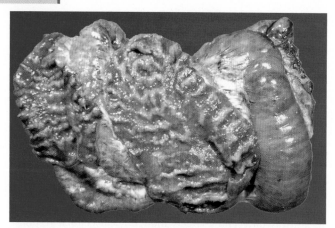

Figure 1-136 Fibrinous colitis in a pig infected with *Salmonella* Typhimurium.

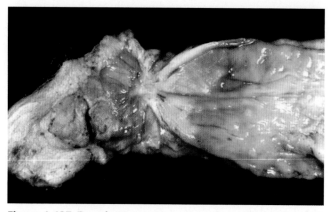

Figure 1-137 Rectal stricture in porcine salmonellosis. (Courtesy Noah's Arkives.)

At autopsy, there is marked dilation of the colon, which is caused by narrowing of the rectum, 1-10 cm cranial to the anus (Fig. 1-137). The stricture is usually <1.0 cm in diameter and varies in length from 0.5 to 20 cm. There is marked fibrous thickening of the rectal wall, which may contain microabscesses. The dilation of the colon, proximal to the stricture, may consist of a well-demarcated widened area several centimeters long and wide. The colonic mucosa in this area is usually ulcerated and may be covered by fibrinous exudate. In some cases there is more gradual but sometimes massive dilation of the entire colon and cecum, which are full of digesta, with ulceration of the mucosa just proximal to the stricture. The mucosa is always excessively corrugated; this is mainly the result of marked thickening of the internal muscularis. Anastomoses of the small intestine and/or colon to the dilated portion of the descending colon may occur. Localized chronic peritonitis is often associated with the dilated segments of the colon.

The stricture is located in an area of rectum that has a relatively poor blood supply, namely, the junction of the circulatory fields of the caudal mesenteric and pudendal arteries. Ulcerative proctitis is consistently found in swine with typhlocolitis caused by *S.* Typhimurium infection. Granulation of such lesions probably leads to cicatrization and stricture. The location, the persistent nature of this lesion in some pigs, and its limited capacity to heal are probably related to the restricted blood supply of the affected area.

***Salmonella* Typhisuis** infection is an *uncommon* condition in pigs. The disease, called *paratyphoid* in Europe, is now known to cause disease in pigs in the Americas and Asia. It is a progressive disease of 2-4 month-old pigs that is clinically characterized by intermittent diarrhea, emaciation, and frequently, massive enlargement of the neck region, the latter associated with caseous palatine tonsillitis, cervical lymphadenitis, and parotid sialoadenitis. There is also circular or button-like to confluent ulceration of the mucosa of the ileum, cecum, colon, and rectum. Other less frequent findings are caseous lymphadenitis of the mesenteric lymph nodes, interstitial pneumonia, hepatitis, and pericarditis.

Further reading

Barrow PA, et al. *Salmonella*. In: Gyles C, editor. Pathogenesis of Bacterial Infections in Animals. Ames, Iowa: Wiley-Blackwell; 2010. p. 231-265.

Clothier KA, et al. Comparison of *Salmonella* serovar isolation and antimicrobial resistance patterns from porcine samples between 2003 and 2008. J Vet Diagn Invest 2010;22:578-82.

Horter DC, et al. A review of porcine tonsils in immunity and disease. Anim Health Res Rev 2003;4:143-155.

Moxley RA, Duhamel GE. Comparative pathology of bacterial enteric diseases of swine. Adv Exp Med Biol 1999;473:83-101.

Wood RL, et al. Distribution of persistent *Salmonella typhimurium* infection in internal organs of swine. Am J Vet Res 1989;50: 1015-1021.

Salmonellosis in horses. The most common serovar in horses in most areas is **S. Typhimurium**, and its prevalence is increasing, especially that of multidrug-resistant definitive phage type 104 (DT104). Other serovars are usually associated with sporadic cases of disease. *Many horses are* Salmonella *carriers, and when they are stressed, diarrhea follows.* Abortion of pregnant mares has been associated with S. Abortusequi. *Salmonella* Infantum has been associated with disseminated infection localizing in a variety of tissues, including muscle, in a horse.

Treatment with antibiotics, especially orally, increases the risk of salmonellosis. Resistance to certain antibiotics is associated with the presence of *resistance (R) plasmids* that may be transferred to other bacteria, of the same or different species, by conjugation or transduction. Antibiotic-resistant *Salmonella* may not respond to treatment, and antimicrobial therapy may increase the potential for infection and disease because of the suppression of the normal intestinal microbiota. Antibiotic-resistant strains have been associated with outbreaks of salmonellosis at veterinary teaching hospitals.

Salmonellosis in horses may be manifested clinically as *peracute* (usually septicemic), *acute*, and *chronic* forms, and as an *asymptomatic carrier state*.

The septicemic form occurs most commonly in foals 1-6 months of age. These animals are usually with their dams at pasture and predisposing factors are unclear. The infection in foals tends to be fatal. Affected animals are lethargic and develop severe diarrhea, often with characteristic green color, which may contain casts and blood. They are febrile and waste rapidly, to die in 2-3 days. Some survive for a week or more and these may develop signs of pneumonia, osteitis, polyarthritis, and meningoencephalitis.

The primarily enteric forms of the disease are more likely to occur in older horses. Most of the predisposing factors mentioned earlier apply to horses. *Salmonellosis is an occupational hazard of horses,* since many are exposed to long periods of transport, and to exertion owing to overwork or excessive training.

Clinically, the acute disease is characterized by diarrhea and fever for a period of 1-2 weeks, followed by recovery or death. The chronic form persists for weeks or months. Affected horses pass soft, unformed manure that resembles cow feces. They lose their appetite, with subsequent progressive loss of weight and condition. In later stages they become dehydrated and emaciated.

The gross lesions are those of enteritis and/or septicemia; the former are most consistently found at autopsy. As a rule, the longer the course, the lower in the intestine does one find the most severe lesions.

Acute septicemic cases have small hemorrhages on the serous or mucosal membranes. The visceral lymph nodes are always enlarged, juicy, and often hemorrhagic. Marked pulmonary congestion and edema, and renal cortical pallor and medullary congestion may occur. The main lesions are in the stomach and intestines. In **peracute or septicemic cases** there is intense hyperemia of the gastric mucosa, probably venous infarction, with some edema and scattered hemorrhage. The small intestine may be congested with a mucous or hemorrhagic exudate. In **acute cases** there is diffuse and intense fibrinohemorrhagic inflammation of the cecum and colon overshadowing any lesions in the upper intestine, and leading rapidly to superficial necrosis of the mucosa and a gray-red pseudomembrane (Fig. 1-138A). In **chronic salmonellosis,** enteric lesions may be few or subtle. Some animals have extensive or patchy fibrinous or ulcerative lesions of the cecum and colon. In others, raised circumscribed lesions ~2-3 cm in diameter may be evident, with a gelatinous submucosa and ulcerated mucosa. Some such lesions are more fibrinous, and resemble button ulcers (Fig. 1-138B).

Histologic alterations of significance are usually limited to the intestine. However, in septicemic animals lesions typical of endotoxemia are present in lung, liver, kidney, spleen, and adrenal. There may be acute ileocecocolic lymphadenitis, and inflammation in sites of localization, such as growth plates in long bones and the meninges. Depending on the duration of the enteritis, hemorrhage, necrosis, or diphtheresis may predominate, but the infiltrating leukocytes are largely mononuclear. The superficial coagulative necrosis of the mucosa may extend over large areas. A layer of fibrinocellular exudate may cover the necrotic mucosa. Fibrin thrombi are frequently present in the capillaries or venules of the lamina propria (Fig. 1-138C). There is usually marked congestion of submucosal vessels, which is accompanied by considerable edema.

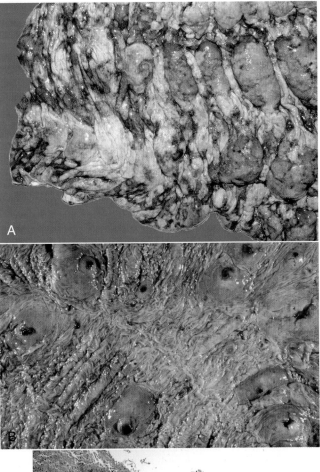
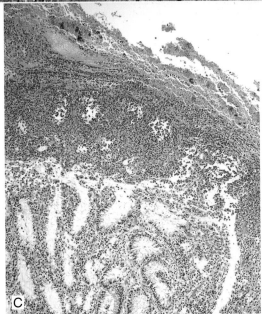

Figure 1-138 Salmonellosis in a foal, *Salmonella* Typhimurium. A. Fibrinonecrotic membrane over the mucosal surface of the colon. **B.** Nodular ulcerative lesions in colon in chronic salmonellosis. **C.** Full-thickness necrosis and effusion from colonic mucosa; several thrombosed vessels are in the lamina propria.

Further reading

Alinovi CA, et al. Risk factors for fecal shedding of *Salmonella* from horses in a veterinary teaching hospital. Prev Vet Med 2003;60:307-317.

Barr BS, et al. Antimicrobial-associated diarrhoea in three equine referral practices. Equine Vet J 2013;45:154-158.

Ernst NS, et al. Risk factors associated with fecal *Salmonella* shedding among hospitalized horses with signs of gastrointestinal tract disease. J Am Vet Med Assoc 2004;225:275-281.

McCain CS, Powell KC. Asymptomatic salmonellosis in healthy adult horses. J Vet Diagn Invest 1990;2:236-237.

Raisis AL, et al. Equine neonatal septicaemia: 24 cases. Aust Vet J 1996;73:137-140.

Weese JS, et al. Emergence of *Salmonella typhimurium* definitive type 104 (DT104) as an important cause of salmonellosis in horses in Ontario. Can Vet J 2001;42:788-792.

Salmonellosis in cattle. The serotypes usually incriminated are **S. Typhimurium** and **S. Dublin**; both are distributed worldwide. Wherever *S.* Dublin is found, it tends to be adapted to cattle and to occur in epizootics, whereas other serotypes usually cause more sporadic disease. **S. Newport** has been identified as an emerging pathogen in cattle.

It is unusual to find salmonellosis in **calves** <1 week of age, in contrast to enteric and septicemic colibacillosis, which usually affect very young animals. *In calves, salmonellosis is a febrile disease typified by dejection, dehydration, and usually diarrhea.* Diarrhea is not always present, but when it is, the feces are yellow or gray, and have a very unpleasant odor. In older calves, there may be blood and mucus in the feces. In less acute cases there may be delayed evidence of localization in the lung and synovial structures. Morbidity and mortality may be considerable, especially in calves that are confined, such as in vealer operations. Experimental infections in calves indicate that survival is inversely related to the numbers of *Salmonella* in the inoculum, and directly to the age of the calves.

The general appearance at **autopsy** of a calf with salmonellosis may resemble one with septicemic colibacillosis. However, *enlargement of mesenteric lymph nodes and gross enteric lesions* are generally observed in salmonellosis. There is moderately severe gastrointestinal inflammation, acute swelling, and hemorrhage of the visceral lymph nodes, and some petechiation of serous membranes. The enteritis may be catarrhal, but sometimes it is hemorrhagic or more commonly causes exudation of yellow fibrin (Fig. 1-139). The mucosa overlying the lymphoid tissues may become necrotic and slough. In animals with fibrinous enteritis, the bowel wall is somewhat turgid and the serosa may have a ground-glass appearance. There is often diffuse, but perhaps mild, fibrinous peritonitis.

The intestinal lesions are usually most severe in the ileum, especially during the early stages of the disease. With time the jejunum and colon become involved but the duodenum remains relatively normal. The regional distribution of the lesions may, in part, be related to differences in the level of bacterial colonization of the mucosa. Twelve hours after oral infection of calves with *S.* Typhimurium, the numbers of bacteria are generally lower in the abomasum and duodenum than in the lower intestinal tract, whereas they are relatively constant from the jejunum through to the rectum.

The early **microscopic lesions** in the small intestine consist of a thin layer of fibrinocellular exudate on the surface of short and blunt villi. This is followed by extensive necrosis and ulceration of the mucosa, with fibrin and neutrophils exuding from the ulcerated areas into the lumen. The lamina propria may be moderately infiltrated by mononuclear inflammatory cells. Fibrin thrombi are often evident in proprial capillaries and venules. There is also marked submucosal edema and the centers of lymphoid follicles in the Peyer's patches are completely involuted. Similar erosion, ulceration, and fibrinous effusion occur in the proximal large bowel (Fig. 1-140).

Scanning electron microscopy of small intestine shows large numbers of bacteria on a tattered mucosal surface. Clusters of enterocytes slough off short villi (Fig. 1-141). Strands of fibrin emerge from the mucosal defects and cover the mucosa. Ultrastructurally, the lesions are similar to those described originally in guinea pigs, except that there is more damage to epithelium in calves experimentally infected with *S.* Typhimurium.

Characteristic changes usually occur in the *liver and spleen,* but may be absent in peracute septicemic cases. There is often fibrinous cholecystitis. In acute cases the spleen is enlarged and pulpy as a result of congestion, but this is soon replaced by acute splenitis, present as miliary, tiny foci of necrosis or as reactive nodules. The liver is often pale with many minute *paratyphoid nodules.* In the spleen, macrophage reaction is sometimes diffuse. Paratyphoid granulomas also may be found microscopically in the kidney, lymph nodes, and bone marrow. These probably represent a cell-mediated immune response to embolic bacteria. In those animals that survive the acute phase of the disease, the inflammatory changes in lymphoid tissues progress to an immunologic response, characterized by a diffuse reaction of medium-sized and large lymphocytes in the follicles, and plasma cells in the sinusoids. There may be marked cortical atrophy of the thymus. In calves with acute septicemia, pulmonary congestion and edema are visible at

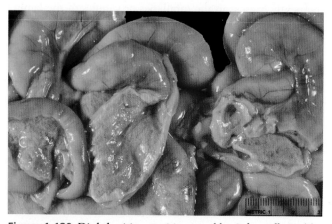

Figure 1-139 Diphtheritic enteritis caused by *Salmonella* Dublin infection in a calf. (Courtesy M. Miller, J. Ramos Vara.)

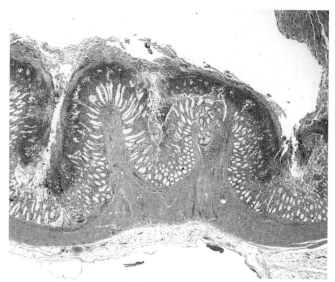

Figure 1-140 Necrosis of lamina propria, effusion of neutrophils, and fibrin and pseudomembrane formation in colon of a calf infected with **S.** Dublin.

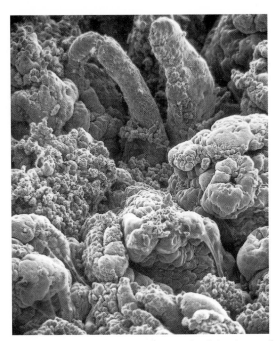

Figure 1-141 Scanning electron micrograph of the ileum of a calf 12 hours postinoculation with **S. Typhimurium.** Villi are atrophic, and rounded cells are exfoliated from surface. (Courtesy R. Clarke, C.L. Gyles.)

autopsy, with interstitial thickening of pulmonary alveolar septa by mononuclear cells in tissue section. There may be thrombosis of septal capillaries, and some effusion of edema fluid and macrophages into alveolar spaces.

In subacute salmonellosis of calves, there may be cranial bronchopneumonia, usually with adhesions and abscessation. Purulent exudate is in synovial cavities, and the organism is recoverable in pure culture from such affected joints and tendon sheaths. It may be mixed with *Trueperella pyogenes* and *Pasteurella* in the lungs.

Salmonellosis in **adult cattle** may occur in *outbreaks* as it does in calves, but more often it is sporadic, and it may cause *chronic diarrhea and loss of condition.* The source of infection is usually the carrier animal. Other sources, such as feed containing protein of animal origin, or bone meal, should be considered when the disease is caused by an uncommon serovar. *Abortions* are most common with S. Dublin, but may occur with any serovar. In some herds, this may be the only clinical evidence of infection, although other animals often excrete the offending serovar in the feces. The *carrier state* of S. Dublin infection in adult cattle may persist for years, sometimes for life, in contrast to infections with other serovars, which rarely persist >18 months. Dairy cows may persistently shed *Salmonella*, especially S. Dublin, in milk and cause infections in humans who drink raw milk. In cattle admitted to a teaching hospital a higher risk for shedding was identified in those that were admitted to the hospital in the fall, suggesting a seasonality to shedding. The morbid changes in adult cattle correspond to those in calves except that there is more pleural hemorrhage and the enteritis may be more hemorrhagic and fibrinous. The histologic changes in the liver and other organs are the same as those seen in calves.

The multidrug-resistant strain *Salmonella* Typhimurium definitive phage type 104 (DT104), first seen in the UK in the late 1980s, has now spread worldwide and in some parts of the United States is the leading cause of bovine salmonellosis. The potential for this strain to emerge as a major foodborne pathogen has caused great consternation among both agricultural and public health communities. Multidrug-resistant strains of S. Newport have also been identified.

Further reading

Brichta-Harhay DM, et al. Diversity of multidrug-resistant *Salmonella enterica* strains associated with cattle at harvest in the United States. Appl Environ Microbiol 2011;77:1783-1796.

Cummings KJ, et al. Fecal shedding of *Salmonella* spp among cattle admitted to a veterinary medical teaching hospital. J Am Vet Med Assoc 2009;234:1578-1585.

Hancock D, et al. The global epidemiology of multiresistant *Salmonella enterica* serovar typhimurium DT104. In: Brown CC, Bolin CA, editors. Emerging Infectious Diseases of Animals. Washington, DC: ASM Press; 2000. p. 217-244.

Mohler VL, et al. *Salmonella* in calves. Vet Clin North Am Food Anim Pract 2009;25:37-54.

Nielsen LR. Review of pathogenesis and diagnostic methods of immediate relevance for epidemiology and control of *Salmonella* Dublin in cattle. Vet Microbiol 2013;162:1-9.

Pender AB. Salmonellosis in a herd of beef cows. Can Vet J 2003;44:319-320.

Toth JD, et al. Survival characteristics of *Salmonella enterica* serovar Newport in the dairy farm environment. J Dairy Sci 2011;94:5238-5246.

Salmonellosis in sheep. As well as abortion caused by S. Abortus-ovis, abortion and neonatal death may follow infection of pregnant ewes by any species of *Salmonella*. Although the prevalence of S. Abortus-ovis in the United Kingdom seems to be waning, S. Montevideo, on the other hand, has been associated with abortions in several flocks in the British Isles. S. Brandenburg has been reported in sheep in New Zealand.

Salmonellosis is not a common disease in sheep, but outbreaks are always severe and may cause very heavy losses. Predisposing influences are necessary, and these are usually provided by circumstances that enforce congregation. Deprivation of food and water for 2-3 days may be sufficient and, coupled with fatigue, is the usual predisposing factor when sheep are transported or confined in holding yards. Deaths usually continue for 7-10 days after debilitating circumstances have been remedied.

The serovars usually found in sheep are **S. Typhimurium, S. Arizonae,** and **S. Enteritidis.** *Salmonella* Dublin is increasing in prevalence in the United Kingdom and the midwestern states of the United States. Experimental inoculation of sheep with S. Arizonae produces infection but rarely disease. Under natural conditions this host-adapted organism is frequently considered to be an infection secondary to some other disease, or an incidental finding in apparently healthy animals. Most serovars produce the same sort of disease, which closely resembles that seen in cattle both clinically and at autopsy. The major findings are fibrinohemorrhagic enteritis and septicemia.

Further reading

Hjartardottir S, et al. *Salmonella* in sheep in Iceland. Acta Vet Scand 2002;43:43-48.

Kerslake JI, Perkins NR. *Salmonella* Brandenburg: case-control survey in sheep in New Zealand. N Z Vet J 2006;54:125-131.

Van Metre DC, et al. Diagnosis of enteric disease in small ruminants. Vet Clin North Am Food Anim Pract 2000;16:87-115.

Salmonellosis in carnivores. *Salmonella can often be recovered from apparently healthy dogs and cats.* However, primary disease rarely occurs. *Salmonella* has been recovered in high frequency from normal sled dogs lacking clinical disease. Raw meat fed to dogs has been shown to have a high incidence of *Salmonella* contamination. In dogs and cats, nosocomial infections are sometimes associated with hospitalization and antibiotic therapy. In dogs, salmonellosis may be secondary to canine distemper. It can cause bronchopneumonia, acute hemorrhagic gastroenteritis, swelling of the spleen and mesenteric lymph nodes, serosal hemorrhages, and foci of necrosis in the liver and other organs. Septicemia in puppies has been associated with *S.* Dublin infection. Salmonellosis has been reported in dogs with lymphosarcoma, shortly after the initiation of chemotherapy. The immunosuppressive effect of the treatment, or depressed cell-mediated immunity, probably predisposes to the development of disease.

Various serovars have been isolated from cats and most of these appear to cause subclinical infections. However, salmonellosis may be a problem in catteries and hospitals, affecting animals that are subjected to stressful conditions. Spillover of *Salmonella* spp. from wildlife populations to cats through predator/prey relationships has been documented. Immunosuppression associated with feline leukemia virus, feline immunodeficiency virus, *Salmonella*-contaminated panleukopenia vaccine, or other intercurrent diseases is thought to predispose to salmonellosis in cats. *S.* Typhimurium is most commonly associated with such outbreaks. The disease is characterized by gastroenteritis and septicemia or a more chronic, nonspecific febrile illness, with neutrophilia and left shift. Conjunctivitis and abortions have also been associated with *Salmonella* infection in cats.

Because of their close association with humans, especially children and the aged, dogs and cats that are carriers are a potential source of zoonotic infection.

Further reading

Cantor GH, et al. *Salmonella* shedding in racing sled dogs. J Vet Diagn Invest 1997;9:447-448.

Giovannini S, et al. Epidemic of salmonellosis in passerine birds in Switzerland with spillover to domestic cats. Vet Pathol 2013;50:597-606.

Marks SL, et al. Enteropathogenic bacteria in dogs and cats: diagnosis, epidemiology, treatment, and control. J Vet Intern Med 2011;25:1195-1208.

Stiver SL, et al. Septicemic salmonellosis in two cats fed a raw-meat diet. J Am Anim Hosp Assoc 2003;39:538-542.

Weese JS. Bacterial enteritis in dogs and cats: diagnosis, therapy, and zoonotic potential. Vet Clin North Am Small Anim Pract 2011;41:287-309.

Yersiniosis

Yersinia enterocolitica and **Y. *pseudotuberculosis*** are gram-negative organisms that, in domestic animals, cause *enterocolitis, mesenteric lymphadenitis, septicemia* and, less commonly, conjunctivitis, hepatitis, abortion, neonatal death, epididymitis-orchitis, mastitis and pneumonia. *Y. pestis*, the cause of plague in animals and humans, is not considered here.

The *epidemiology* of yersiniosis is complex and poorly understood. These organisms may be shed in the feces by asymptomatic animals in the herd or flock, and by other species, such as rodents and birds, in the environment. The organisms can survive and grow in the environment at low temperatures, and in cool weather environmental contamination by *Yersinia* spp. may be considerable, resulting in significant oral challenge. Disease may in part be due to compromise of cell-mediated immunity, permitting establishment of invading organisms, or recrudescence of latent infection. Often, outbreaks occur under stressful circumstances, such as poor weather, flooding, after transport, during the breeding season, or in animals on a poor plane of nutrition.

Subsequent to ingestion, *the organisms invade through the intestinal epithelium or M cells* overlying Peyer's patches and reach the lamina propria or submucosal lymphoid follicles. Enormous recruitment of neutrophils and ensuing destruction of cytoarchitecture of the Peyer's patch and overlying epithelium result in formation of suppurative foci in place of follicles in Peyer's patches, and microabscesses in the lamina propria of the small or large intestine if invasion occurs elsewhere. *Yersinia* spp. disseminates via lymphatics and hepatic portal venous drainage to mesenteric lymph nodes or to liver and the systemic circulation.

Pathogenicity in the main *Yersinia* species is associated primarily with the 70-kb virulence plasmid, pYV, and with other proteins that are chromosomally encoded. After bacteria are ingested and they reach the terminal ileum, they present on their surface the outer membrane protein invasin; this protein is expressed in stationary phase at low temperatures. Invasin facilitates translocation of the bacteria across the intestinal epithelium, after which invasin binds to $\beta 1$ integrins in the host tissue, which induces production of chemokines such as IL-8. In the Peyer's patches, bacteria replicate and express another adhesin, YadA. The latter down-regulates expression of invasin and protects bacteria against phagocytosis. YadA and another protein, Ail, protect bacteria against the host immune system enabling bacterial propagation to mesenteric lymph nodes and, occasionally, other tissues.

Although *Yersinia* reside extracellularly as microcolonies in suppurative foci in the lamina propria of the intestine and lymph nodes, at least some appear to reside intracellularly, since a T-cell–mediated immune response is required to clear infection. Giant cells wall off foci of infection in subacute to chronic lesions, hence the specific name *pseudotuberculosis*.

Disease may be gradual in onset, subtle and chronic, producing a syndrome of diarrhea and ill-thrift in cattle, sheep, and goats. Mild diarrhea and enteritis with low mortality has been reported in Australia in weaned pigs with *Y. pseudotuberculosis*. More fulminant disease, characterized by severe, sometimes hemorrhagic, diarrhea, systemic infection, and prostration, may occur in cattle, some species of deer, especially chital and red deer, water buffalo, and exotic ungulates. Yersiniosis is an apparently uncommon cause of diarrhea, and occasionally fatal enterocolitis, mesenteric lymphadenitis, and systemic infection in carnivores. *Yersinia* also causes sporadic pneumonia and septicemia in foals.

Yersiniosis has been described worldwide, as a cause of disease in sheep, cattle, goats, deer, and pigs. The lesions of *Y. pseudotuberculosis* and *Y. enterocolitica* cannot be differentiated reliably grossly or microscopically.

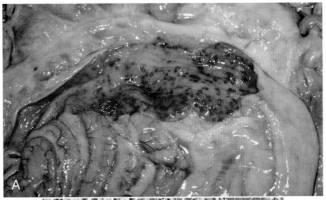

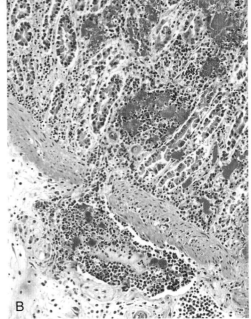

Figure 1-142 Yersinia pseudotuberculosis infection in a goat.
A. Ulcerative colitis. (Reprinted with permission from Giannitti
F, et al. J Vet Diagn Invest 2014;26:1-8.) **B.** Mucosal and submu-
cosal colonies of coccobacilli are observed.

In all species, **gross lesions** in clinically subacute to chronic
yersiniosis may be mild. They are usually limited to abnormally fluid intestinal content, with congestion, edema, roughening, and perhaps small foci of pallor, focal hemorrhages,
erosion, or mild ulceration and fibrin effusion. Raised nodules
up to 5 mm in diameter, with depressed centers, or ulcers may
be evident in affected large bowel (Fig. 1-142A). Mesenteric
lymph nodes are enlarged, congested, and edematous, perhaps
with foci of necrosis. There may be mild fibrinous cholecystitis, and pale foci of necrosis scattered in the liver.

The infection is characterized **histologically** by *masses of
gram-negative coccobacilli forming microcolonies*, in the lamina
propria of villi and around the necks of crypts in the distal
half of the small intestine, in Peyer's patches, and in the superficial mucosa of the large intestine. Intense local infiltrates of
inflammatory cells, predominantly neutrophils, accumulate to
form *microabscesses* up to about 300 μm in diameter around
the bacteria, and effuse into the lumen through microerosions
on the mucosal surface or in crypts. Small crypt abscesses may
be present. In small intestine, there may be moderate atrophy
of villi and hyperplasia of crypts, associated with increased
infiltrates of chronic inflammatory cells. Microabscesses, or

pyogranulomas surrounded by macrophages or giant cells, and
sometimes containing bacterial microcolonies, may be present
in the subcapsular and medullary sinuses of mesenteric lymph
nodes.

In fulminant *Yersinia* infection in all species, there is *fibrinous or fibrinohemorrhagic enterocolitis*, with heavy local mucosal
colonization by masses of coccobacilli, and marked neutrophil
infiltration (Fig. 1-142B). Peyer's patches may be particularly
involved, with grossly visible foci or confluent masses of
caseous necrotic debris, as may be found in draining mesenteric lymph nodes, which are enlarged. There may be serosal
hemorrhages on the gut, fibrinous peritonitis and pleuritis, and
foci of necrosis also may be present in the liver, lungs, and
occasionally other parenchymatous organs; the characteristic
microcolonies of coccobacilli are usually evident in them.

Caseous mesenteric lymphadenitis, with mature pyogranulomas containing microcolonies of bacteria, surrounded by neutrophils and giant cells, may occasionally be found as an
incidental lesion, or in animals with *Yersinia* abscesses in other
organs.

Yersiniosis is **diagnosed** in tissue section by finding characteristic microcolonies of coccobacilli in microabscesses (see
Fig. 1-142B), and is confirmed by bacterial isolation. Microscopic lesions may not be detected in the intestinal mucosa
of some clinically affected animals from which isolates are
made, perhaps because lesions are patchy. Because *Yersinia*
spp. are psychrophiles, cold enrichment and culture at temperatures <37°C are used in their isolation.

Further reading

Dube PH, et al. Protective role of interleukin-6 during *Yersinia enterocolitica* infection is mediated through the modulation of inflammatory cytokines. Infect Immun 2004;72:3561-3570.

Fallman M, et al. Resistance to phagocytosis by *Yersinia*. Int J Med
Microbiol 2002;292:501-509.

Giannitti F, et al. *Yersinia pseudotuberculosis* infections in goats and
other animals diagnosed at the California Animal Health and Food
Safety Laboratory System: 1990-2012. J Vet Diagn Invest 2014;26:
1-8.

Mecsas J, Chafel R. *Yersinia*. In: Gyles CL, et al. editors. Pathogenesis
of Bacterial Infections in Animals. 3rd ed. Ames, Iowa: Blackwell;
2004. p. 295-307.

Mikula KM, et al. *Yersinia* infection tools: characterization of structure
and function of adhesins. Front Cell Infect Microbiol 2013;2:169.

Stamm I, et al. *Yersinia enterocolitica* in diagnostic fecal samples from
European dogs and cats: identification by fourier transform infrared
spectroscopy and matrix-assisted laser desorption ionization-time
of flight mass spectrometry. J Clin Microbiol 2013;51:887-893.

Lawsonia intracellularis infection

Lawsonia intracellularis infects a variety of species including
swine, horses, donkeys, deer, rodents, rabbits, foxes, dogs,
ferrets, and nonhuman primates. It causes a *characteristic proliferative lesion of cryptal epithelium in distal small and/or large
intestine* that is associated with diarrhea and ill thrift. *L. intracellularis* is a microaerophilic nonflagellated gram-negative,
curved or S-shaped rod bacterium. Because it is an obligate
intracellular organism, cultivation requires use of tissue
culture. Formerly referred to as *intestinal adenomatosis complex*,
the conditions in swine now known to be caused by *L. intracellularis* including *porcine intestinal adenomatosis, necrotic*

enteritis, and *proliferative hemorrhagic enteropathy* are collectively known as **porcine proliferative enteropathy** (PPE). Identification of the etiologic agent was elusive for decades. The intracellular bacterium was initially thought to be *Campylobacter* spp., then putatively identified as *ileal symbiont intracellularis*, until the taxonomy was formalized as *Lawsonia intracellularis* in 1995.

PPE is a prevalent and important infection in swine worldwide. The syndrome occurs mostly in postweaned pigs; however, pigs from 3 weeks of age to adults may be affected. Severity of clinical effects varies from mild subclinical disease with reduced growth rate to persistent diarrhea and severe weight loss. Once infected, pigs shed the organism for weeks. Death may follow a period of diarrhea and progressive cachexia, or it may occasionally occur as a result of perforation of an ulcerated intestine, or through peracute hemorrhage. Mortality may be very high.

Development of disease is dependent on undefined interactions with other bacteria in the gut, because gnotobiotic pigs inoculated with *L. intracellularis* fail to develop disease, whereas conventional pigs are quite susceptible. Experimental studies and mild spontaneous cases suggest that infection occurs first in glandular epithelial cells near lymphoid aggregates of the ileocecocolic region, whereas the cecal and colonic cryptal epithelial cells are infected later in the course of disease. The **pathogenesis of PPE** is related to active uptake of *L. intracellularis* by epithelial cells, although specific receptors remain unknown. Once endocytosed by the host cell, the entry vacuole breaks down and the bacteria persist and replicate freely within the apical cytoplasm, causing hyperplasia and propagation of the bacteria throughout the epithelium. Cell division is required for bacterial replication, which may explain its tissue tropism. Bacteria are passed on to daughter epithelial cells and exit via extrusion from the cytoplasm of enterocytes on villi or between crypt openings. Disruption of intestinal cell differentiation by the pathogen is theorized to be a central event; however, specific virulence factors of *L. intracellularis* and molecular details of the host cell-pathogen interaction remain undescribed.

Infected epithelium is thus transformed into a population of mitotically active and poorly differentiated cells. Glands are lined by dysplastic pseudostratified columnar epithelial cells with basophilic cytoplasm; goblet cells often are reduced in number. Mucosal glands are elongated, dilated, and branched, resulting in a thickened mucosal layer (Fig. 1-143A). Hyperplastic glands may protrude multifocally into the underlying submucosal lymphoid tissue or epithelial cells may form elevated plaques above the mucosal surface; use of the term *adenomatosis* to describe such a change is obvious. Occasionally, microscopic foci of adenomatous epithelium may be found in submucosal lymphatics or the regional lymph node. Small intestinal villi in infected animals undergo progressive atrophy, and they may be absent in well-established lesions. The proliferative lesion in the crypts is considered a primary lesion, and not a secondary hyperplastic response to increased epithelial exfoliation. *L. intracellularis* organisms are readily recognized as *curved rods* within the *apical cytoplasm of glandular epithelial cells* in silver-stained tissue sections (Fig. 1-143B) or by immunohistochemistry (Fig. 1-143C). *L. intracellularis* also have been identified ultrastructurally in degenerate cells and macrophages in the lamina propria. Inflammation in areas of uncomplicated adenomatosis is usually not a prominent feature.

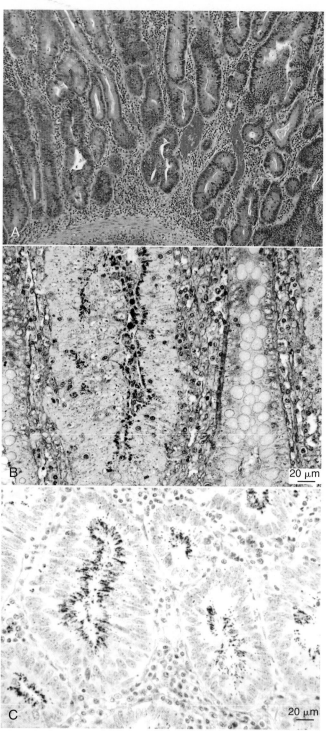

Figure 1-143 Porcine proliferative enteropathy. **A. Adenomatous change** in glands in the lamina propria. **B.** Masses of silver-stained *Lawsonia* organisms in the apical cytoplasm of hyperplastic epithelium lining intestinal glands. **C.** *Lawsonia* organisms in the apical cytoplasm of hyperplastic epithelium lining intestinal glands by immunohistochemistry. (Courtesy E.R. Burrough.)

In the least complicated forms of the disease, **lesions** *are always found in the terminal portion of the ileum*, extending proximally for a variable distance, usually <1 meter. In a significant proportion of cases, lesions occur in the cecum and proximal spiral colon primarily, or in addition to the ileum. In mild cases, only a few ridges or plaque-like thickened areas

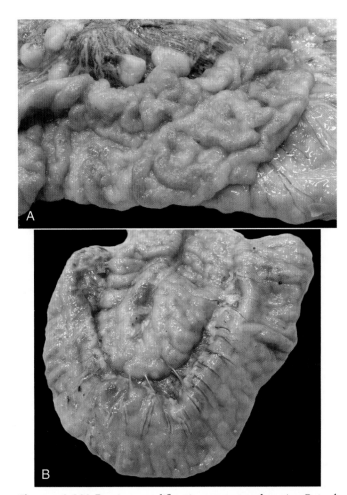

Figure 1-144 Porcine proliferative enteropathy. A. Raised nodular or **ridge-like areas of thickened mucosa** in the colon, resulting from hypertrophy of glands. **B.** Exaggerated **reticular pattern of folds** on serosal aspect of the proximal colon. (Courtesy E.R. Burrough.)

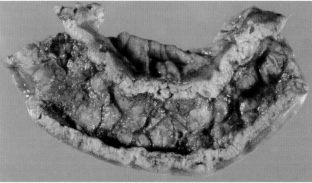

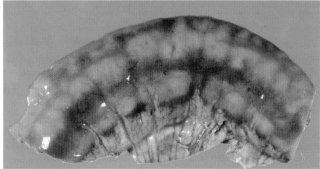

Figure 1-145 Necrotic enteritis, thick ileal wall in **porcine proliferative enteropathy.**

project above the normal mucosa; however, there are typically more widespread lesions with thickened mucosa and irregular longitudinal or transverse folds or ridges (Fig. 1-144A). The mucosal surface in proliferative lesions of the small or large intestine may be intact, but small foci of necrosis or fibrin exudation may be evident. In affected small or large intestine, hyperplastic mucosal epithelium and some degree of submucosal edema is reflected in the *cerebriform pattern of projections and depressions on the serosal aspect of the intestine, which is virtually pathognomonic for this condition* (Fig. 1-144B). The ileocolic lymph nodes are enlarged and hyperplastic.

Coagulative necrosis of adenomatous mucosa commonly occurs and when extensive areas are affected, this form of the disease is referred to as **necrotic enteritis**. It may be partly the result of pathogenic anaerobic large-bowel flora colonizing the affected terminal ileum and large intestine. Necrotic epithelial cells, neutrophils, and fibrin exudation from superficial lesions contribute to formation of diphtheritic membranes or luminal fibrin casts, which can be found in the small or large intestine (Fig. 1-145). The cerebriform pattern of serosal folding is evident in necrotic enteritis. Necrotic enteritis may be a sequel to other enterocolitides in swine, *PPE caused by L intracellularis infection is the most common primary lesion.*

Microscopically, coagulative necrosis of the mucosal epithelium may be focal and superficial but can involve the full thickness of the mucosa or even extend into the submucosa. A few islands of viable hyperplastic crypts or glands may remain, and masses of bacteria, presumably fecal anaerobes, are observed among the necrotic debris. With time, granulation tissue develops in ulcerated areas. Proximal ileum along the margin of the zone of mucosal necrosis should be examined for hyperplastic epithelium because, in severe cases of necrotic enteritis, few remnants of mucosa persist. Repeated bouts of epithelial proliferation, necrosis, ulceration, and granulation may result in progressive stricture of the lumen that may be accompanied by hypertrophy of the external muscle layer. This should be differentiated from idiopathic ileal muscular hypertrophy of swine, which is known to occur independent of antecedent PPE.

Acute or subacute intestinal hemorrhage and anemia also occur in PPE, and is generally considered as a distinct syndrome referred to as **proliferative hemorrhagic enteropathy**. Some animals exsanguinate and die quickly without hematochezia, whereas others display melena or hematochezia for several days. This syndrome is more common in young adults than in growing pigs. It is usually sporadic and of relatively low morbidity, but up to half of clinically recognized cases may die. Animals that die of *massive intestinal hemorrhage* are pale, and the perianal area may be smeared with blood. The typical cerebriform pattern is evident on the serosal surface of the distal ileum, which is thickened and turgid. The ileum may contain variable combinations of free blood, fibrin or clotted blood, and the cecum and colon may contain dark bloody digesta (Fig. 1-146). The ileal mucosa usually resembles that in uncomplicated PPE. Overt regions of hemorrhage or ulceration are rarely discernible grossly, and there appears to be widespread mucosal diapedesis. **Microscopically,** there is extensive proliferation, erosion, and necrosis of superficial

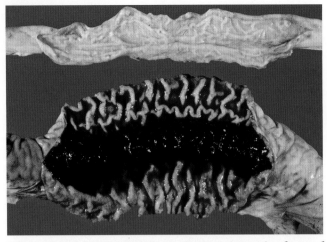

Figure 1-146 Proliferative hemorrhagic enteropathy form of porcine proliferative enteropathy. Hemorrhage in the lumen of the terminal ileum. Normal ileum (top).

epithelium. An acute inflammatory infiltrate is present in the superficial lamina propria. Small blood vessels are frequently thrombosed and there is effusion of neutrophils, fibrin and extensive hemorrhage into intestinal glands, and onto the mucosal surface and intestinal lumen.

In **horses,** the lesions and pathogenesis of **equine proliferative enteritis (EPE)** are similar to those in PPE. This disease affects mostly weanling foals, and causes fever, lethargy, diarrhea, hypoproteinemia, edema, and weight loss. Thickening of the mucosa is most commonly observed in the distal small intestine near the ileal-cecal junction; however, gross lesions are not always evident, or they are subtle and can be easily overlooked. In severe or long-standing cases, there can be marked irregular hyperplasia and thickening of the mucosa with fibrinonecrotic membrane and variable edema of the submucosa. As for PPE, EPE is definitively diagnosed by documenting adenomatous proliferation of epithelial cells in the crypts of the small intestine and by demonstrating the intracellular curved bacteria in the apical cytoplasm of enterocytes using silver stains or by immunohistochemistry. The **epidemiology** of EPE remains incompletely understood and the source of infection for horses remains unconfirmed, although rodents and rabbits have been proposed as reservoir hosts. Pigs have been suggested as a potential source of infection for horses; however, in most equine cases no evidence of exposure to pig feces has been documented.

In all species, including swine, diarrhea is probably related to loss of functional mucosal surface area in distal small intestine and large bowel, whereas ill-thrift or wasting syndromes are attributable to protein-losing enteropathy. A presumptive **diagnosis** of proliferative enteritis in any species can be based on typical gross and histologic lesions, and supported by Warthin-Starry staining to visualize the intracellular bacteria. Confirmation can be obtained by immunohistochemistry using a specific antibody for *L. intracellularis* or by polymerase chain reaction.

Further reading

Boutrup TS, et al. Early pathogenesis in porcine proliferative enteropathy caused by *Lawsonia intracellularis*. J Comp Pathol 2010;143:101-109.

Gebhart CJ, Guedes RMC. *Lawsonia intracellularis*. In: Gyles CL, et al., editors. Pathogenesis of Bacterial Infections in Animals. 3rd ed. Ames, Iowa: Blackwell; 2004. p. 363-372.

Kroll JJ, et al. Proliferative enteropathy: a global enteric disease of pigs caused by *Lawsonia intracellularis*. Anim Health Res Rev 2005;6:173-197.

Pusterla N, Gebhart C. Equine proliferative enteropathy caused by *Lawsonia intracellularis*. Eq Vet Educ 2009;21:415-419.

Pusterla N, Gebhart CJ. Equine proliferative enteropathy-a review of recent developments. Eq Vet J 2013;45:403-409.

Vannucci FA, Gebhart CJ. Recent advances in understanding the pathogenesis of *Lawsonia intracellularis* infections. Vet Pathol 2014;51:465-477.

Enteritis associated with Campylobacter *spp.*

Campylobacter spp. are common causes of gastrointestinal disease in humans, and some species also may be capable of causing enteritis in animals. **Campylobacter jejuni** and **C. coli** are the most studied, but recent work has implicated other fastidious *Campylobacter* species as pathogens in humans and animals. Pathogenic strains penetrate the surface mucus layer, then adhere to and invade the epithelial cells where they avoid delivery to lysosomal compartments and thus prolong their intracellular survival. Central to the pathogenesis of *Campylobacter*-associated disease are type IV and VI secretion systems and the production of toxins, most notably the cytolethal distending toxin. Many human infections are acquired by ingestion of contaminated milk products, water, meat, or other animal products, making this an important potential zoonosis. *Chickens* are common asymptomatic shedders of C. *jejuni*, and C. *coli* can be frequently isolated from the feces of diarrheic or asymptomatic swine.

C. *jejuni* has been associated with diarrhea characterized by the presence of blood and mucus in some dogs, despite the fact that it can often be isolated from asymptomatic animals. It has also been isolated from dogs with parvoviral enteritis or other viral infections; pre-existing infections may predispose to the development of pathologic effects of C. *jejuni*. C. *jejuni* has been implicated as the primary pathogen in some canine cases of mild to moderate lymphoplasmacytic enterocolitis by associating large numbers of the organism with the lesions and by ruling out other known etiologies. In experimentally infected gnotobiotic and conventional dogs, lesions are limited to mild mucosal colitis. Mild to moderate inflammatory lesions limited to the colon has been documented in some pigs where *Campylobacter* sp. was the only potential pathogen isolated. Erosive colitis has been associated with C. *jejuni* infection in mink, and was reproduced experimentally. Young cats are probably asymptomatic carriers of C. *jejuni*. Several *Campylobacter* spp., including C. *jejuni*, C. *coli*, and C. *fetus* subsp. fetus, rarely have been associated with diarrhea and enterocolitis in young foals; the pathogenesis is not clear and infection may be more common in immunocompromised individuals.

Weaner colitis of sheep is described in Australia as a diarrheal syndrome of high morbidity and low mortality, and is associated with an unidentified *Campylobacter* sp., not C. *jejuni*. Affected sheep have watery colonic content; chronically affected animals may have edema and loss of body condition suggestive of enteric protein loss. Histologically there is mild erosive to ulcerative typhlocolitis with a layer of bacteria adherent to surface epithelial cells and in crypts. The disease has been reproduced by inoculation of the thermophilic catalase-negative *Campylobacter*-like organism previously isolated from spontaneous cases.

Further reading

Backert S, et al. Transmigration route of *Campylobacter jejuni* across polarized intestinal epithelial cells: paracellular, transcellular or both? Cell Commun Signal 2013;11:72.

Burrough E, et al. Prevalence of *Campylobacter* spp. relative to other enteric pathogens in grow-finish pigs with diarrhea. Anerobe 2013;22:111-114.

Joens LA. *Campylobacter* and *Helicobacter*. In: Gyles CL, et al., editors. Pathogenesis of Bacterial Infections in Animals. 3rd ed. Ames, Iowa: Blackwell; 2004. p. 353-361.

Kaakoush NO, Mitchell HM. *Campylobacter concisus*-a new player in intestinal disease. Front Cell Infect Microbiol 2012;2:4.

Marks SL, et al. Enteropathogenic bacteria in dogs and cats: diagnosis, epidemiology, treatment, and control. J Vet Intern Med 2011;25:1195-1208.

Spirochetal colitis in swine

Swine dysentery caused by ***Brachyspira*** (formerly *Serpulina, Treponema*) ***hyodysenteriae,*** family *Spirochaetaceae,* is a historically well-recognized and now re-emergent production-limiting disease of swine worldwide, characterized by moderate to severe *mucohemorrhagic to fibrinous colitis.* **Porcine spirochetal colitis** refers to a less severe nonhemorrhagic colitis caused by *B. pilosicoli,* which is discussed later. Additional *Brachyspira* species, such as ***B. murdochii, B. intermedia,*** and ***B. innocens,*** have been associated with variably severe disease. Strains have traditionally been distinguished by morphologic and phenotypic features, including biochemical properties and strength of beta-hemolysis. Recent work in Canada and the United States has documented mucohemorrhagic diarrhea in pigs, indistinguishable from classic swine dysentery caused by *B. hyodysenteriae,* that is caused by emergent, strongly beta-hemolytic but phylogenetically distinct strains of the proposed novel species ***"B. hampsonii."*** The virulence of these novel species has been experimentally confirmed in both mice and pigs.

Since 1921, **classical swine dysentery** has been recognized as a highly infectious disease, mainly of weaned pigs. *B. hyodysenteriae* is a gram-negative, anaerobic, oxygen-tolerant, strongly beta-hemolytic *spirochete.* The loosely coiled motile organism has 7-13 periplasmic flagella. Although the bacterial genus *Brachyspira* includes several species capable of colonizing a wide spectrum of hosts, *B. hyodysenteriae* is predominantly a pathogen of pigs, although the bacterium has been associated with necrotizing typhlocolitis in rheas. Experimental reproduction of swine dysentery in gnotobiotic pigs requires the presence of anaerobic bacteria indigenous to the normal colon, along with *B. hyodysenteriae;* there is apparently a *synergistic action between B. hyodysenteriae and the intestinal microbiota,* mainly *Bacteroides* and *Fusobacterium.* Several studies have implicated dietary factors, specifically an elevated protein:carbohydrate ratio in the hindgut, as a predisposing factor for enhanced pathogenicity of *B. hyodysenteriae* in pigs. The mechanisms remain poorly understood; however, alterations in fermentation activity and altered microbiota in the hindgut likely are important.

The **pathogenesis** of swine dysentery is still incompletely understood, but gene studies have identified virulence traits for *Brachyspira* that include hemolysins, cytotoxins, outer membrane proteins, motility factors such as flagella, and NADH oxidase that is thought to be required for the bacterium to successfully colonize the colonic epithelium. *B. hyodysenteriae* first colonizes mucus on the luminal surface of the large bowel before invading the cytoplasm of enterocytes and goblet cells; spirochetes can be observed by electron microscopy or in situ hybridization. This process is likely mediated by flagella and outer membrane proteins that enable the pathogen to successfully colonize the host. Following invasion by the pathogen, there is enhanced and altered mucin secretion, degeneration, and necrosis of epithelial cells and hemorrhage, which are thought to be mediated by cytotoxins and endotoxin. Exfoliation of surface epithelial cells has been associated with large numbers of spirochetes and other anaerobic bacteria on the mucosa. *Brachyspira* do not usually invade beyond the epithelial cells, and the result is *mucosal colitis* characterized by superficial erosion with hyperplasia of cells in colonic glands, hypersecretion of mucus, and a mixed inflammatory infiltrate in the lamina propria. Thrombosis of capillaries and venules in the superficial areas of the colonic mucosa is probably due to absorption of endotoxin through the damaged mucosal epithelium. Diarrhea is due to *malabsorption of fluids and electrolytes in the colon;* this presumably results from damage to the superficial epithelium of the colon, which in the pig normally has tremendous absorptive capacity. Active fluid secretion by the colon, associated with bacterial enterotoxins, probably does not play a major role in swine dysentery.

Transmission occurs by ingestion of feces, and introduction of *asymptomatic carrier* pigs into a herd usually precedes an outbreak; the involvement of vectors including rodents is also considered a risk factor. Once established in a herd, the infection tends to remain *enzootic,* and although treatment can effect a rapid clinical amelioration, relapses often occur cyclically in individuals or groups. The morbidity and mortality may reach 90% and 30%, respectively. Immunity is variable following bouts of dysentery, and recovered pigs are apparently protected against subsequent challenge for several months though some animals remain susceptible.

The disease occurs in pigs of all ages >2 or 3 weeks old, but particularly in pigs 8-14 weeks of age. Once initiated, it spreads rapidly by pen contact. The disease is initially febrile, and the initial diarrheic feces are thin, semisolid, and lack blood or mucus. After 1-2 days, blood and copious mucus appear in the feces and this progresses to watery feces with blood, mucus, and fibrin. Some pigs die peracutely without showing diarrhea, but most pigs recover slowly, although their rate of growth is reduced. Experimentally, the severity of disease depends on overall stress on the animals, diet, body weight, group size, and the quantity and growth phase of the inoculum.

Early intestinal lesions can be subtle and include hyperemia and edema of the colonic walls and mesentery with mucosal exudate containing small amounts of fibrin or blood (Fig. 1-147). Mucosal lesions become more severe as the disease progresses, and there is increased mucus, fibrin, hemorrhage, and perhaps a fibrinonecrotic membrane forming along the mucosal surfaces of the large intestine and cecum. Lesions can be multifocal, patchy, or involve the entire large intestine. The colonic content in these cases is usually scant, and

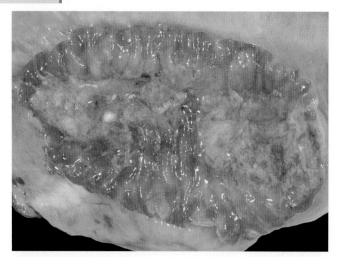

Figure 1-147 Swine dysentery. Fibrinocatarrhal exudate on the hemorrhagic colonic mucosa. (Courtesy E.R. Burrough.)

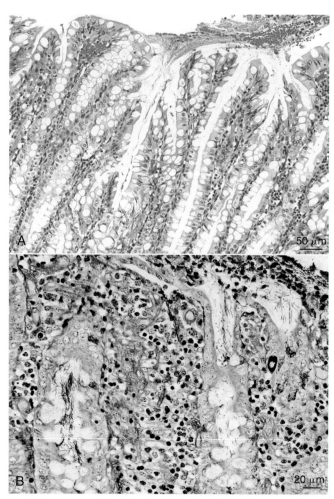

Figure 1-148 Swine dysentery. A. Mucus, fibrin, and hemorrhage covering the mucosa of the colon. There is also goblet cell hyperplasia, increased mucus in the crypts, and lymphoplasmacytic infiltration of the lamina propria. **B.** Warthin-Starry stain of colonic mucosa showing numerous delicate spirochetes. (Courtesy E.R. Burrough.)

porridge-like dirty gray to red-brown and greasy in appearance. The most severe lesions can appear similar to those of salmonellosis in extent and severity. The production of mucus in swine dysentery becomes copious in many chronic cases because of *remarkable goblet cell hyperplasia.*

The earliest **microscopic lesions** are also limited to the colon and cecum. Lesions are characterized by discrete areas of epithelial erosion and necrosis of the superficial mucosa. Thin layers of exudate composed of mucus, fibrin, neutrophils, and erythrocytes cover the areas of damaged epithelium (Fig. 1-148A). In more advanced cases these areas become more diffuse and exudation is more copious; however, deep ulceration is not common. There may be minor bleeding or small fibrin thrombi in the superficial vessels of the lamina propria underlying eroded mucosa. There is usually some edema of the lamina propria, submucosa, and serosa. Initially mucus is expelled from the basilar portions of the crypts. In concert with the increased turnover of epithelial cells associated with the superficial erosion, there is hyperplasia of goblet cells as well as epithelial cells deeper in the glands. The crypts are elongated and lined by proliferative basophilic epithelial cells with large hyperchromatic nuclei, and few differentiated goblet cells. Crypts often subsequently become dilated and contain necrotic debris; some have marked goblet cell hyperplasia, and copious mucus production.. Large delicate spirochetes can be observed within dilated crypts and goblet cells using Warthin-Starry staining (Fig. 1-148B).

Porcine intestinal spirochetosis is caused by ***Brachyspira pilosicoli*** (formerly *Anguillina coli*), which differs from *B. hyodysenteriae* in that it is weakly beta-hemolytic. *B. pilosicoli* has a wide host range and has been isolated from a number of other animal species with lesions of intestinal spirochetosis, and it may be zoonotic.

Porcine intestinal spirochetosis has been seen in most major swine-producing areas of the world. The disease is characterized by *generally transient watery to mucoid diarrhea without blood.* Reduced weight gain is a significant clinical finding. As for *B. hyodysenteriae,* gross lesions are limited to the colon and cecum and may be subtle. Mesocolonic edema, swollen lymph nodes, variable mucosal erosion, and abundant watery large intestinal contents are early gross lesions. Later, the mucosa becomes thickened and in severe cases there is

exudation of fibrin, which intermixes with necrotic debris and hemorrhage on the mucosal surface forming a diphtheritic membrane.

Virulence factors of *B. pilosicoli* are also still poorly defined, but motility and chemotaxis for mucus may be important. The organism is capable of polar attachment by one end of the bacterium to the apical membrane of colonic or rectal epithelial cells, resulting in a palisade of upright bacteria perpendicular to the epithelial cells and displacement or effacement of microvilli. Thus spirochetes can often be observed histologically as a *false brush border* on the luminal surface early in infection; visualization of the bacteria is enhanced by Warthin-Starry silver stains or fluorescence in-situ hybridization. Although the molecular receptors for attachment have not been identified, the organism can invade paracellularly, especially at the extrusion zone between colonic crypt units. *B. pilosicoli* can be observed within colonic crypts, goblet cells, or invading tight junctions into the lamina propria, but is not disseminated systemically in pigs. In chronic infections, there are large numbers of inflammatory cells in the lamina propria, including lymphocytes, plasma cells, and monocytes. There is also goblet cell hyperplasia and crypt hyperplasia so that crypts are lined by immature basophilic mitotically active cells. The diarrhea and ill-thrift characteristic of infection may be related to loss of absorptive function, secondary to disruption of the brush border of enterocytes, and increased exfoliation of poorly differentiated cells and perhaps enteric loss of plasma protein. Given the existence of long-term colonization by *B. pilosicoli* in pigs, it is unlikely that protective immunity develops after infection; however, the immune responses against this organism are poorly understood.

In **dogs, colonic spirochetosis** with mucosal colitis has also been described, in association with *B. pilosicoli* and perhaps with other *Brachyspira* spp., but a causal relationship has not been established experimentally.

Further reading

Burrough ER, et al. Comparative virulence of clinical *Brachyspira* spp. isolates in inoculated pigs. J Vet Lab Diagn Invest 2012;24:1025-1034.

Burrough ER, et al. Comparison of atypical *Brachyspira* spp. clinical isolates and classic strains in a mouse model of swine dysentery. Vet Microbiol 2012;160:387-394.

Chander Y, et al. Phenotypic and molecular characterization of a novel strongly hemolytic *Brachyspira* species provisionally designated "*Brachyspira hampsonii.*" J Vet Lab Diagn Invest 2012;24:903-910.

Hampson DJ. Brachyspiral colitis. In: Zimmerman JJ, et al., editors. Diseases of Swine. 10th ed. Ames, Iowa: Blackwell; 2012. p. 680-699.

Rubin JE, et al. Reproduction of mucohaemorrhagic diarrhea and colitis indistinguishable from swine dysentery following experimental inoculation with "*Brachyspira hampsonii*" strain 30446. PLOS One 2013;8:e57146.

Wilberts BL, et al. Comparison of lesion severity, distribution and colonic mucin expression in pigs with acute swine dysentery following oral inoculation with "*Brachyspira hampsonii*" or *Brachyspira hyodysenteriae*. Vet Pathol 2014; in press.

Diseases associated with enteric clostridial infections

Most of the important enteric clostridial diseases occur in herbivores and are caused by 1 of the 5 toxigenic types of **Clostridium perfringens** or by **Clostridium difficile**. Enteritis in dogs is associated with C. *perfringens* and C. *difficile*. **Clostridium piliforme** (formerly *Bacillus piliformis*) causes Tyzzer's disease, characterized by multifocal necrotic hepatitis and occasionally enteritis, colitis and myocarditis, in many animal species. **C. *chauvoei*** may affect the tongue causing blackleglike glossitis (see Vol. 1, Muscle and tendon). Enteritis produced by C. *chauvoei* has also been described in an outbreak in heifers. **C. *septicum*** causes clostridial abomasitis (braxy) in sheep and calves, discussed in the earlier section, Stomach and abomasum. **C. *botulinum*** causes botulism in horses, cattle, and several other species by ingestion of preformed toxins (see Vol. 1, Nervous system).

The virulence of C. *perfringens* is mostly attributable to its capacity to produce up to 16 toxins, including 4 so-called *major (typing) toxins* (i.e., alpha, beta, epsilon, and iota), which are used to classify this microorganism into 5 toxinotypes, designated A-E (Table 1-2). However, no single strain produces this entire toxin set. Besides producing 1 or more of the 4 typing toxins (see Table 1-2), some C. *perfringens* strains produce additional toxins, such as enterotoxin, beta 2, necrotic enteritis B-like toxin (NetB), kappa, and lambda, some of

Table • 1-2

Classification of Clostridium perfringens *into five toxinotypes based on the presence of genes for four major exotoxins (alpha, beta, epsilon, and iota)*

C. Perfringens type	Toxin gene			
	Alpha	Beta	Epsilon	Iota
A	+	−	−	−
B	+	+	+	−
C	+	+	−	−
D	+	−	+	−
E	+	−	−	+

+, toxin gene present; −, toxin gene not present.

which are also critical for virulence of a given strain. There is not always a clear distinction between the different types of C. *perfringens*. Some strains lose their ability to produce one or more of their toxins when stored or cultured, and this complicates the identification of isolates and the assessment of their significance in disease outbreaks. Additionally, plasmid conjugation occurs both in vitro and in vivo and it is now thought that previously avirulent strains may become virulent by acquiring toxin genes.

The 4 major typing toxins are produced during active growth.

- The **alpha toxin** is a lecithinase that acts on cell membranes, producing hemolysis and necrosis of cells. The role of alpha toxin in intestinal disease of mammals is controversial, although most evidence indicates that this toxin on its own does not produce significant intestinal damage.

- The **beta toxin** is a pore-forming toxin that induces intestinal necrosis and occasionally a variety of neurologic effects through a yet unknown mechanism. This toxin is exquisitely sensitive to the action of trypsin, which inactivates it in a few minutes; this property is very important for the pathogenesis of beta toxin–related diseases as explained later in this chapter.

- The **epsilon toxin** is produced as a relatively inactive prototoxin that is activated by enzymatic digestion. Intestinal trypsin and chymotrypsin, and lambda toxin produced by C. *perfringens* itself are the main enzymes responsible for activation of epsilon prototoxin. Epsilon toxin is also a pore-forming toxin that induces mainly neurologic and respiratory effects, which are mostly the result of increased vascular permeability, although there is evidence that this toxin can also produce a direct effect on neurons in the brain.

- The **iota toxin** is a binary toxin with 2 components, iota a and iota b, which is also elaborated as a prototoxin and activated by proteolytic enzymes.

- **Beta2 toxin**, which despite its name is not related to beta toxin, has been associated with enteric disease in swine and horses caused by C. *perfringens* type A, although its pathogenicity is uncertain.

- Some strains of C. *perfringens*, especially type A, produce **enterotoxin**, which is a specific toxin; the name *enterotoxin* should therefore not be used to refer to all C. *perfringens* toxins produced in the intestine. The enterotoxin is only elaborated during sporulation and is released upon lysis of vegetative cells. It may be produced by most strains, but most cases of disease are associated with type A. Enterotoxin-producing *C. perfringens* type A is the second and third most important cause of human food poisoning in humans in the United States over the past decades. Enterotoxigenic type A strains are also associated with antibiotic treatment–related diarrhea in humans. The significance of enterotoxin in animal disease is limited. It is also a pore-forming toxin.

Clostridial diseases originating in the intestine are often called **enterotoxemias,** which by definition are diseases produced by toxins generated in the intestine and absorbed into the circulation and that act on distant organs such as the brain and lungs. However, although several clostridial diseases of the intestine are true enterotoxemias, some of them are not. For instance, disease produced in sheep by *C. perfringens* type D, whose epsilon exotoxin is elaborated in the intestine but in this species exerts its important effects on distant organs such as brain and lungs, is a true enterotoxemia. The same toxinotype can produce an enterocolitis in goats with, in the chronic cases, no systemic absorption of epsilon toxin, in which case, no enterotoxemia occurs.

The **pathogenesis** of enteric infection with *C. perfringens* and *C. difficile* requires: (1) the presence of these microorganisms in the intestine (sometimes they can be normal inhabitants of the gut), and (2) *a change in the enteric microenvironment* favorable to massive expansion of luminal populations of clostridia and/or production of their toxins. Such changes may include a change in feed, abnormally nutrient-rich digesta, antimicrobial therapy, altered pancreatic exocrine function or trypsin inhibitors, reduced motility, and/or primary infections with agents such as coccidia.

C. perfringens bacteria alone are most likely nonpathogenic; exotoxins are required to induce disease, as it has been recently demonstrated in several animal experiments using so-called reverse genetics, in which bacterial strains genetically engineered to remove one or more toxin genes were inoculated into animals. The absence of a particular toxin gene eliminated the virulence, which was, however, restored when that gene was reintroduced into the genome.

C. difficile produces 2 exotoxins: A, which is an enterotoxin, and B, which is a cytotoxin but also an enterotoxin. Tissue damage is probably due to the effects one or of both toxins, which glycosylate and inactivate Ras GTPases, disabling signaling pathways in the cell. As well, they glycosylate Rho and interfere with its ability to regulate cytoskeletal actin. Under the influence of these toxins, the cytoskeleton condenses, tight junctions open, cells round up and undergo apoptosis. They also cause release of proinflammatory mediators, attracting neutrophils, and activate secretion stimulated by the enteric nervous system. Hence, disease is characterized by fluid intestinal content, with focal or diffuse small intestinal or colonic epithelial necrosis, through which neutrophils may exude into the lumen, producing a so-called "volcano" lesion. Not all isolates of *C. difficile* are toxigenic; 34 toxinotypes, based on sequence variations in the genes for the A and B toxin molecules, have now been described. Molecular epidemiologic investigation may permit associations of toxinotype with virulence.

C. piliforme, the cause of Tyzzer's disease and the only gram-negative clostridia, is an obligate intracellular pathogen

that in the alimentary tract infects small intestinal or colonic epithelial cells causing necrosis and inflammation. The pathogenesis of Tyzzer's disease is not clearly dependent on toxin production, although some strains do produce cytotoxic proteins.

Diagnosis of disease because of the toxin-producing clostridia is mostly dependent on demonstration of toxin in gut content or feces of affected animals, by the most specific test available. Although the presence of large numbers of a particular type of *C. perfringens* suggests causation of the disease, some types of this organism are commonly present in the gut in a variety of circumstances, where they cannot be implicated as etiologic agents. *C. perfringens* type A is by far the most ubiquitous toxinotype in the intestine of animals, and isolation of this type alone is the least significant from a diagnostic standpoint. However, other types (e.g., type B and C) are less frequently found in the intestine of healthy animals, which makes isolation of these types more diagnostically significant.

Further reading

Li J, et al. Toxin plasmids of *Clostridium perfringens*. Microbiol Mol Biol Rev 2013;77:208-233.

Marks SL. Bacterial-associated diarrhea in the dog: a critical appraisal. Vet Clin North Am Small Anim Pract 2003;33:1029-1060.

McClane BA. An overview of *Clostridium perfringens* enterotoxin. Toxicon 1996;34:1335-1343.

Uzal FA, Songer JG. Diagnosis of *Clostridium perfringens* intestinal infections in sheep and goats. J Vet Diagn Invest 2008;20:253-265.

Uzal FA, et al. Towards an understanding of the role of *Clostridium perfringens* toxins in human and animal disease. Future Microbiol 2014;9:361-377.

***Clostridium perfringens* type A.** *C. perfringens* type A is the toxinotype *most commonly found in the environment and in the intestine of clinically healthy animals.* Its major toxin is the *alpha toxin*; and some strains may also produce $beta_2$ toxin and enterotoxin in addition to a variable number of other toxins.

This is one of several clostridia that produce *gas gangrene* in humans and animals. The production of gas gangrene in wound and puerperal infections is mostly mediated by alpha toxin with assistance by perfringolysin O. *C. perfringens type A is responsible for necrotic enteritis in chickens,* and it has been associated with *several alimentary syndromes in mammals,* including enteritis in foals; enterocolitis in horses; necrotizing enterocolitis in neonatal piglets; enterotoxemia and hemorrhagic enteritis in lambs and neonatal calves and older cattle; and diarrhea and hemorrhagic enteritis in dogs. However, absolute proof of involvement of *C. perfringens* type A in these alimentary syndromes of mammals is lacking.

Many strains of *C. perfringens* type A produce $beta2$ (CPB2) toxin and recent information suggests a role for this toxin in porcine clostridial enteritis, as nearly all type A strains isolated from pigs with enteric disease carried the *cpb2* gene for CPB2 toxin. Involvement of CPB2 toxin-producing *C. perfringens* in enterocolitis of horses also has been suggested.

A very rare disease of **lambs** characterized by *acute intravascular hemolysis,* known as *yellow lamb disease,* has also been associated with type A infections and, at least in one occasion, with type D infection. Affected animals may be found dead or moribund, and jaundice and hemoglobinuria may be evident clinically. At autopsy, icterus, anemia, hemoglobinuric nephrosis, and other changes of severe, acute, intravascular hemolysis are prominent. Microscopically the most prominent changes are centrilobular hepatic necrosis and hemoglobinuric nephrosis, both presumably associated with acute intravascular hemolysis and anemia. This hemolytic disease must be distinguished from other causes of acute intravascular hemolysis such as leptospirosis, necrotic hepatitis, and bacillary hemoglobinuria caused by C. novyi type B and D, respectively, and chronic copper poisoning. Presumably, the hemolytic effect of alpha toxin is responsible for the intravascular hemolysis. Given that type A strains and alpha toxin are commonly found in the intestines of ruminants, diagnosis of this condition cannot be confirmed by detection of either of these and it has to be established presumptively based on clinical, gross, and microscopic findings coupled with ruling out other possible causes of intravascular hemolysis. It has been suggested that the disease is associated with unusually high alpha toxin type A strains, although this has not been confirmed.

Strains of C. perfringens type A, some determined to be enterotoxin producers, have been associated with diarrhea, sometimes bloody, in dogs. **Hemorrhagic canine gastroenteritis** (canine gastrointestinal hemorrhage syndrome) is a sporadic, peracute, hemorrhagic gastroenteritis, associated in some cases with C. perfringens type A, although in other cases the etiology has not been identified. Dogs with the peracute hemorrhagic disease are often found dead lying in a pool of bloody excreta; sometimes hemorrhagic diarrhea is noted before death. Autopsy reveals hemorrhagic enteritis and colitis, and sometimes hemorrhagic gastritis is present. Colonic lesions tend to be more severe. Microscopically there is hemorrhagic necrosis of the gastrointestinal mucosa, which extends from the luminal surface into the mucosa. Numerous clostridia may line the necrotic intestinal structures or be distributed through the detritus, but they do not invade the intact tissue. Recurrent diarrhea, sometimes bloody, has been associated with enterotoxin-secreting type A strains. Multiple serotypes of clostridia have been associated with nosocomial, usually nonfatal, cases of diarrhea in dogs. C. perfringens enterotoxin has been demonstrated twice as frequently in hospitalized dogs with diarrhea compared with controls without diarrhea.

Further reading

Giannitti F, et al., Diagnostic exercise: hemolysis and sudden death in lambs. Vet Pathol 2014;51:624-627.

Marks SL, et al. Enteropathogenic bacteria in dogs and cats: diagnosis, epidemiology, treatment, and control. J Vet Intern Med 2011;25:1195-1208.

Songer JG. Clostridial enteric diseases of domestic animals. Clin Microbiol Rev 1996;9:216-234.

Valgaeren BR, et al. Intestinal clostridial counts have no diagnostic value in the diagnosis of enterotoxaemia in veal calves. Vet Rec 2013;172:237.

Valgaeren BR, et al. Lesion development in a new intestinal loop model indicates the involvement of a shared Clostridium perfringens virulence factor in haemorrhagic enteritis in calves. J Comp Pathol 2013;149:103-112.

***Clostridium perfringens* type B.** *Clostridium perfringens* type B has been reported from Europe, South Africa, and the Middle East, but not from the Americas and Australasia. It

causes "*lamb dysentery*," usually in lambs up to 10-14 days of age, dysentery in calves of approximately the same age, and rarely dysentery in foals within the first few days of life.

In **lambs,** death may occur without premonitory signs, but there is usually abdominal pain, especially when animals are forced to rise, and passage of semifluid dark feces mixed or coated with blood. The abdomen is often tympanitic. A more chronic form in older lambs, which among other diseases is known as "pine" in England, is characterized by unthriftiness and depression, reluctance to suckle, and a peculiar stretching when the animal rises; such cases are reputed to respond well to specific antiserum.

Typical **gross lesions** are usually present, although in exceptional peracute cases they may be absent. The characteristic lesion is *extensive necrohemorrhagic enteritis.* The peritoneal cavity often contains a small amount of serous or blood-stained fluid. In cases with more severe and deeply penetrating mucosal ulcerations, there may be overlying peritonitis with red fibrin strands on the local mesentery and intestinal adhesions. On the mucosal surface, the ulcers are irregular but are well defined by a sharp margin and rim of intense hyperemia, and they contain a yellow necrotic deposit; they may coalesce to form extensive areas of necrosis. Usually the intestinal contents are blood stained and may appear to be composed of pure blood, but in lambs that live for 3-4 days, there may be little or no hemorrhage evident. **Histologically,** the wall of the intestine is hemorrhagic, and the areas of necrosis extend deeply into the mucous membrane, in some cases penetrating to the external muscle layers and serosa. There are large numbers of typical bacilli in the necrotic tissue, but few inflammatory cells.

The lesions present in other organs are those of *severe toxemia.* The liver is usually pale and friable, but may be congested. The spleen is normal or slightly enlarged and pulpy. The kidneys may be enlarged, edematous, pale, and soft from toxic degeneration. The pericardial sac contains abundant clear gelatinous fluid, the myocardium is pale and soft, and epicardial and endocardial hemorrhages are almost constant. The lungs are often slightly congested and very edematous. Occasionally foci of symmetrical encephalomalacia similar to those observed in cases of type D enterotoxemia are observed in chronic cases.

The disease in **calves** caused by type B C. perfringens closely resembles that in lambs, usually affecting sucklings <10 days of age, with a course of 2-4 days characterized by prostration and dysentery. Older calves up to 10 weeks of age are sometimes affected. It appears that calves are more likely to recover, albeit slowly, than are lambs. The intestinal lesion is acute hemorrhagic enteritis with extensive mucosal necrosis and patchy diphtheritic membrane formations, especially in the ileum. Information on the disease in **foals** is very scant as only a few cases in this species have been reported.

Further reading

Songer JG. Clostridial enteric diseases of domestic animals. Clin Microbiol Rev 1996;9:216-234.

Uzal FA, et al. Diagnosis of Clostridium perfringens intestinal infections in sheep and goats. J Vet Diagn Invest 2008;20:253-265.

***Clostridium perfringens* type C.** *Clostridium perfringens* type C is present worldwide, and causes disease mostly in neonatal individuals of several species, including particularly sheep, cattle, horses, and pigs. Occasionally, type C disease occurs in adult individuals of these species. The main virulence factor of *C. perfringens* type C is beta toxin as demonstrated in animal experiments using toxin mutants of this microorganism in rabbits, mice, and goats. Beta toxin is trypsin-labile, and circumstances such as low trypsin levels in neonatal animals, trypsin inhibitors in the diet and/or very high levels of toxin are critical in the pathogenesis of type C disease. The high susceptibility of neonatal animals to type C disease is considered to be a consequence of the trypsin inhibitor effect of colostrum, a mechanism apparently aimed to protect immunoglobulins present in the colostrum. "Pig-bel," also known as "enteritis necroticans," is a necrotizing enteritis of humans caused by *C. perfringens* type C, which was the most important cause of human deaths in the 1960s in Papua New Guinea and still occurs sporadically in that island and other countries of the region. The disease has been associated with consumption of trypsin inhibitors in sweet potatoes, a significant component of the diet in Papua New Guinea. This, coupled with the low level of protein in the diet, results in low trypsin in the intestine, which allows persistence of beta toxin in the intestinal lumen. Intraduodenal inoculation of *C. perfringens* type C in combination with trypsin inhibitor produces acute necrohemorrhagic enteritis and/or enterotoxemia in guinea pigs, rabbits, lambs, and goats.

The diseases caused by type C in **lambs, calves, piglets, goat kids,** and **foals** are very similar. Affected animals are usually neonates, which contract the disease within the first few days of life, often within the first few hours.

Sick **lambs** may shiver, show abdominal pain, abdominal distention, diarrhea, and prostration, and die in 12 hours or less. Frequently, lambs with type C disease are found dead without clinical signs having been observed. In lambs, the **gross** intestinal changes are characterized by *acute necrohemorrhagic enteritis* that may be segmental and can sometimes be confused with intestinal strangulation. *The most prominent changes occur in the jejunum and ileum*, the lumen of which may contain *free blood*, which forms a clotted cast in fresh cadavers. Sometimes there is merely acute hyperemia of a segment of jejunum with edema of the wall, scant creamy intestinal content, and a few small ulcerations of the mucosa. A fibrinous pseudomembrane may be observed over the mucosa of the small intestine. The peritoneal cavity contains a small quantity of serous blood-stained fluid, and the local mesentery and peritoneum are often mildly to severely hyperemic, and bear red strands of fibrin. The mesenteric nodes are enlarged, edematous, and congested. There is usually excess pericardial fluid and pulmonary interstitial edema. Ecchymoses on the serous membranes are nearly constant, and in a few cadavers all tissues, but especially the meninges and brain, are liberally sprinkled with small hemorrhages. There might be terminal bacteremia by *C. perfringens* with bacterial embolism in multiple organs.

Histopathologic changes in lambs with type C disease are not specific, but can be highly suggestive of this infection. The changes consist of acute necrosis that involves mostly the intestinal mucosa, although it can progress to be transmural in severe cases. In most cases this is coagulative necrosis, but in animals that survive longer, the mucosa is completely replaced by a fibrinous pseudomembrane. Thrombosis of mucosal and submucosal vessels is a common finding, and inflammation is usually not a striking component, although it might be more marked in subacute cases. Diffuse or multifocal

distribution of gram-positive bacilli free in the intestinal lumen is common. Although they may be in close contact with the mucosa and attachment has been suggested, no definitive evidence of attachment has been demonstrated in *C. perfringens* infections in ruminants.

In adult **sheep,** *C. perfringens* type C causes *"struck,"* a disease of pastured animals that has a mortality rate of 5-15% in some areas. Death usually occurs suddenly with terminal convulsive episodes, but less acute cases may adopt a straining position that probably indicates acute abdominal pain. In adult sheep, diarrhea or convulsions rarely occur. Gross and microscopic lesions are similar to those described in lambs except that small intestinal ulceration may be prominent and the mucosal necrosis is deeper, with a peripheral leukocytic rim separating the more or less normal deeper layers of the intestine.

Calves with type C disease show abdominal pain, some show diarrhea of sudden onset, and death may be preceded by spasmodic convulsions. Occasionally, sudden death occurs without premonitory clinical signs. Gross and microscopic lesions in calves are similar to those described in lambs.

Type C disease can apparently also occur, albeit rarely, in **feedlot cattle.** The condition is similar to "struck." Animals are found either dead or moribund, and congestion and hemorrhage of the gastrointestinal tract are prominent. The jejunal and ileal content are bloody with fibrin clots and necrotic debris. Excessive straw-colored pleural and pericardial fluid and petechiation of epicardium and endocardium are present. Autolysis and postmortem bloat occur rapidly, and differentiation from ruminal tympany and other clostridial diseases is necessary.

C. perfringens type C also causes *necrohemorrhagic enteritis* mostly in neonatal **piglets.** Rarely, epizootics occur in 2-4 week-old and weaned pigs. The disease occurs as epizootics in affected herds and regions, and may then remain enzootic. Poor hygienic conditions, overcrowding, and antibiotic treatment are thought to be predisposing factors in some outbreaks. Clinical disease can be peracute, acute, or chronic, with signs of the acute and peracute condition including intense abdominal pain, depression, and bloody diarrhea, which begins 8-22 hours after exposure to *C. perfringens* type C. Sow feces contain small numbers of type C organisms, and these multiply rapidly in the small intestine of piglets, outcompeting other bacteria and becoming the dominant organisms in the population. The course of the disease is usually 24 hours or less in 1- to 2-day-old piglets, but chronic disease (usually in older animals) can persist for 1 or 2 weeks and is characterized by persistent diarrhea without blood and dehydration. Marked anal hyperemia can be observed just before death in both acute and chronic forms.

Beta toxin has been shown to bind to small intestinal mucosa endothelial cells of piglets with type C infection. It was therefore suggested that beta toxin–induced endothelial cell damage plays an important role in the early lesion development of *C. perfringens* type C enteritis in pigs. The predominant lesions occur in the small intestine, especially the jejunum, but the cecum and spiral colon are often involved, and occasionally lesions are confined to the large intestine. **Gross lesions** are similar in all areas of the intestine, and in acute cases consist of *intestinal and mesenteric hyperemia, extensive necrosis of the intestinal mucosa, which may be covered by a pseudomembrane* (Fig. 1-149A), *and blood-staining of the contents.* There may be emphysema of the intestinal wall, which

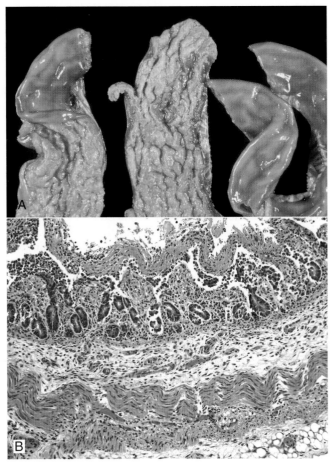

Figure 1-149 Necrotizing enteritis in a piglet, caused by *Clostridium perfringens* type C. A. Fibrinonecrotic membrane covers the mucosal surface. (Courtesy P Blanchard.) B. Necrosis of the superficial mucosa, which is covered by a pseudomembrane.

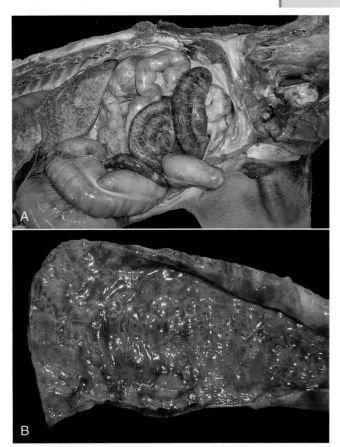

Figure 1-150 Hemorrhagic and necrotizing enteritis caused by *Clostridium perfringens* type C in a newborn foal. A. Serosal view. B. Mucosal view. (Reprinted with permission from Diab SS, et al. Vet Pathol 2012;49:255-263.)

becomes fragile. Mesenteric lymph nodes are red, and sanguineous peritoneal and pleural fluid is present. Fibrinous intestinal adhesions may develop.

Histologically, the hallmark of acute disease in young piglets is hemorrhagic necrosis of the intestinal wall, which starts in the mucosa but usually progresses to affect all layers of the intestine. Lesions are morphologically similar in all segments of intestine; the luminal surface is covered by a pseudomembrane composed of degenerate and necrotic desquamated epithelial cells, cell debris, inflammatory cells including neutrophils, lymphocytes, plasma cells, and macrophages, fibrin (Fig. 1-149B), and a variable number of large, thick bacilli with square ends with occasional subterminal spores. These bacteria occur singly or in clusters, free in the lumen, or lining the margin of the denuded mucosal surface. Although the bacterial population is usually greater in the central intestinal lumen, a few bacilli also can be seen in crypts and glands and invading necrotic lamina propria. Superficial epithelium and superficial layers of lamina propria are necrotic, showing a homogeneous acidophilic appearance with scattered pyknotic or karyorrhectic nuclei and an inflammatory cell infiltrate composed of neutrophils and mononuclear cells. Fibrin thrombi occluding superficial arteries and veins of the lamina propria and submucosa are characteristic of this condition. Fibrin also can be seen in mucosal and submucosal lymphatics and in the interstitium. Diffuse edema with variable amounts of protein and inflammatory cell exudate can be seen throughout all intestinal layers, including serosa. The mucosa is severely thickened by edema and inflammatory exudate. As the infection progresses, necrosis becomes deeper, including epithelium of crypts and glands and, later, all intestinal layers. Severe congestion of subserosal vessels is observed throughout the course of the infection. Lesions are usually diffuse, although they can be multifocal. Mucosal necrosis without hemorrhage may be observed in older pigs with chronic disease.

The disease caused by *C. perfringens* type C in **foals** has been reported from the United States, Canada, Australia, and several European countries. It usually occurs in foals <4 days of age, although occasional cases in older foals and adult horses may also occur. Typical clinical signs include weakness, yellow to brown watery diarrhea, colic, and dehydration. Affected foals usually die in <24 hours. Sudden death without clinical signs being observed may also occasionally occur. **Gross lesions** are those of *acute hemorrhagic necrotizing enteritis*, usually in the distal two thirds of the small intestine (Fig. 1-150A, B), although in some cases most of the small and large intestine may be affected. The **microscopic lesions** are similar to those described previously for *C. perfringens* type C infection in other species (Fig. 1-151) and in foals, histologically the lesions are very similar to those caused by *C. difficile* and *Salmonella* sp. In a series of cases of combined infection with *C. perfringens*

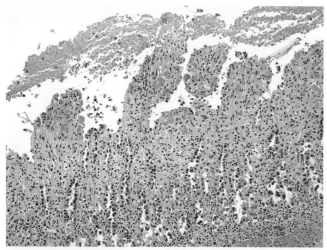

Figure 1-151 Hemorrhagic and necrotizing enteritis caused by *Clostridium perfringens* **type C in a newborn foal.** A fibrinous pseudomembrane covers the mucosa, and numerous fibrin thrombi occlude mucosal vessels. (Reprinted with permission from Diab SS, et al. Vet Pathol 2012;49:255-263.)

type C and *C. difficile* in foals, both the gross and microscopic pathology were indistinguishable from those in foals infected with either of these two microorganisms individually.

A disease clinically and pathologically identical to that described in sheep has been experimentally produced in **goats** inoculated intraduodenally with *C. perfringens* type C.

A presumptive **diagnosis** of type C disease can be established based on clinical and pathologic findings, but confirmation of the disease relies on detection of beta toxin in intestinal contents and/or feces. However, because this toxin is so sensitive to trypsin, failure to detect this toxin in intestinal content does not preclude a diagnosis of *C. perfringens* type C infection. Because this microorganism is infrequently found in the intestine of normal animals, isolation is considered to be diagnostically significant.

Further reading

Diab SS, et al. Pathology of *Clostridium perfringens* type C enterotoxemia in horses. Vet Pathol 2012;49:255-263.

Garcia JP, et al. The effect of *Clostridium perfringens* type C strain CN3685 and its beta toxin mutant in goats. Vet Microbiol 2012;15:412-419.

Songer JG, Uzal FA. Clostridial enteric infections in pigs. J Vet Diagn Invest 2005;17:528-536.

Uzal FA, et al. *Clostridium perfringens* type C and *Clostridium difficile* co-infection in foals. Vet Microbiol 2012;156:395-402.

Uzal FA, et al. Recent progress in understanding the pathogenesis of *Clostridium perfringens* type C infections.Vet Microbiol 2011;153: 37-43.

***Clostridium perfringens* type D.** Enterotoxemia ("*pulpy kidney*" *disease*, "*overeating*" *disease*) caused by *Clostridium perfringens* type D is an important disease of *sheep and goats* with a worldwide distribution. It occurs occasionally in cattle. The rarely observed subacute and chronic forms of the disease in sheep have been called *focal symmetrical encephalomalacia* (FSE), because for many years they were thought to be a different disease, but FSE is only one of pathologic manifestations of the subacute and chronic forms of type D enterotoxemia.

By definition, type D isolates must produce both alpha and epsilon toxins, although some type D isolates can express several other toxins. However, it has been demonstrated by the use of reverse genetic experiments in animal models that epsilon toxin is sufficient to cause all the clinical signs and lesions of type D enterotoxemia in sheep and goats. Epsilon toxin is the third most potent clostridial toxin (after botulinum and tetanus toxins) and, until recently it was considered a class B select agent by the USDA and CDC in the United States. Activated epsilon toxin apparently facilitates its own absorption through the intestinal mucosa and it is then transported to several target organs, including the brain, lungs, and kidneys. In the brain and possibly also in other organs, epsilon toxin affects endothelial cells, producing the lesions described later. It also has been suggested that epsilon toxin acts directly on neurons within the brain.

Lambs and goats suddenly fed large amounts of grain or concentrate are highly susceptible; thus the synonym *overeating disease*. The manner in which overeating leads to clostridial enterotoxemia is complex and not fully understood. Cultures of *C. perfringens* type D given orally are largely destroyed in the rumen and abomasum. However, when the intestinal environment is favorable, the few organisms that reach the intestine proliferate rapidly and produce toxin.

It was accepted traditionally that the critical factor for type D enterotoxemia to occur is the *presence of undigested starch in the small intestine*, providing a suitable substrate for these saccharolytic bacteria, which allows them to proliferate to immense numbers—perhaps $>10^9$ organisms per gram of intestinal contents—and produce correspondingly large amounts of toxin. However, it has been demonstrated in vitro that the absence of glucose in a culture medium stimulates epsilon toxin production. Therefore it is possible that the presence of starch in the intestine stimulates the growth of *C. perfringens* type D, whereas the absence of glucose stimulates epsilon toxin production. When the animal is suddenly provided with excessive quantities of food, particularly starch-rich food, there is a delay before the ruminal flora can adapt. In this period, undigested or partially digested starch may escape into the intestine, and *C. perfringens* type D is likely to take advantage of it. The lack of digestion of starch also would be responsible for the absence of glucose in the small intestine. The epsilon prototoxin is produced as a relatively inactive prototoxin, which is fully activated by digestive enzymes, especially the combination of trypsin and chymotrypsin, but also by some proteases produced by *C. perfringens* itself.

Epsilon toxin facilitates its own absorption from the intestine, probably in part by increasing the permeability of the mucosa. No damage to the intestinal mucosa, except for occasional congestion and mild hemorrhage, is observed in sheep, as opposed to goats, in which severe necrotizing colitis and/or enterocolitis is frequently observed.

The acute disease in *goats* likely has a similar pathogenesis as in sheep, but the chronic disease, with lesions confined to the intestine, appears to be caused by local effects of type D toxins. Although very little information is available in *cattle*, probably the disease develops in the same way in cattle as in sheep.

Type D enterotoxemia may occur in **lambs >2 weeks or adult sheep**. In most lambs with type D enterotoxemia, the course is acute and the animal is found dead without clinical signs being observed or after a short period of acute neurological and respiratory signs, including convulsions and tachypnea, and often bawling as from severe pain. Animals that survive longer may show drooling, rapid breathing, hyperesthesia, wide stance, blindness, opisthotonos, and terminal coma or convulsions. In older sheep or younger but vaccinated sheep, subacute or chronic cases are most frequently seen. Neurologic clinical signs are characteristic of the subacute and chronic forms of type D disease and include blindness, ataxia, head pressing, and paraparesis. Diarrhea occasionally may be observed, although this is not a common clinical sign in sheep type D disease.

In **goats**, type D produces acute, subacute, or chronic disease as well. The acute form occurs more frequently in young, unvaccinated animals and is clinically similar to the acute disease in sheep and characterized by sudden death or acute neurologic signs. The subacute form is more frequently seen in adult goats, vaccinated or not, and is characterized by hemorrhagic diarrhea, abdominal discomfort, tachypnea, opisthotonos, and convulsions. The disease may result in death 2-4 days after onset, but some animals recover. Adult animals, often vaccinated, can also exhibit chronic disease, which is characterized by profuse, watery diarrhea (often containing blood and mucus), abdominal discomfort, weakness, anorexia, and agalactia in milking does. This chronic form may last for days or weeks and may culminate in either death or recovery.

Grossly, in sheep dead of acute enterotoxemia, the carcass is usually well nourished. In those with a course of 1-2 days, there may be occasional evidence of scours about the rump, although diarrhea is rarely observed. Often there is excessive straw-colored pericardial, thoracic, and abdominal fluid with strands of fibrin (Fig. 1-152) that clots on exposure to air, and congestion and edema of the lungs that may be severe enough to produce froth in all the respiratory passages; and hemorrhage beneath the endocardium of the left and occasionally right ventricles of the heart. There may be hemorrhages beneath other serous membranes such as the epicardium, and blotchy hemorrhages beneath the parietal peritoneum are characteristic. Sometimes the liver is congested and the spleen enlarged and pulpy. There is no gastrointestinal inflammation visible at autopsy, although the content of the small and large intestine may be moderately fluid and short lengths of the small intestine occasionally may be distended with gas and be hyperemic.

The so-called "pulpy kidney" (softening of the renal parenchyma) may be present in a small proportion of cases, but it is of little diagnostic significance because its occurrence is so inconsistent. It is best regarded as a poorly understood example of accelerated autolysis because it is not seen in freshly dead carcasses. Glucosuria is present in a relatively small percentage of animals with type D enterotoxemia and it is a useful, though nonspecific, diagnostic indicator when detected. The absence of glucosuria does not preclude a diagnosis of type D enterotoxemia.

In adult sheep, the gross lesions are the same as those in lambs, but are more consistent and more advanced. *Brain gross lesions* may occur in lambs and older sheep with subacute or chronic enterotoxemia and these are sufficiently unique to be of diagnostic significance. They include herniation of the cerebellar vermis (Fig. 1-153) and/or **focal symmetrical encephalomalacia** (FSE) (Fig. 1-154). The commonest distribution of FSE involves the corpus striatum, thalamus, and cerebellar peduncles; there are some minor variations of the pattern, but

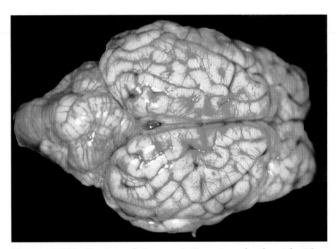

Figure 1-153 Coning of the cerebellum in a lamb with *Clostridium perfringens* type D enterotoxemia. (Courtesy B. Barr.)

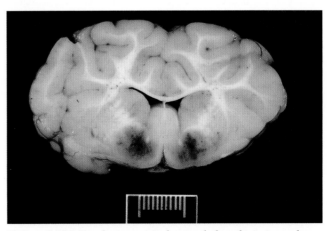

Figure 1-154 Focal symmetrical encephalomalacia in a sheep. Hemorrhage and softening in internal capsules and cerebellar white matter in a sheep with *Clostridium perfringens* type D enterotoxemia. (Courtesy University of California-Davis Anatomic Pathology.)

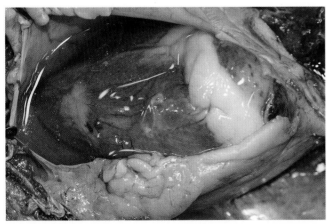

Figure 1-152 Hydropericardium with presence of fibrin strands in a **sheep with *Clostridium perfringens* type D enterotoxemia.**

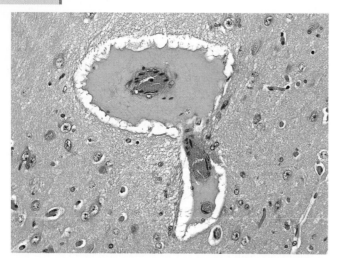

Figure 1-155 Perivascular proteinaceous edema in the corpus striatum of a sheep with *Clostridium perfringens* type D enterotoxemia. (Courtesy J.P. García.)

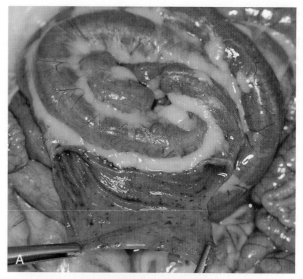

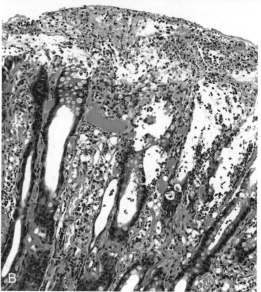

Figure 1-156 Colitis in a goat with *Clostridium perfringens* type D enterotoxemia. **A.** Mucosal hemorrhage and ulceration. **B.** Mucosal necrosis, neutrophilic exudation, and incipient pseudomembrane formation.

the lesions are always of the same type. Less frequently FSE can be seen also in substantia nigra, white matter of the frontal gyri, rostral cerebral peduncles and other areas. The white matter is preferentially affected in all of these areas.

The **histologic changes** in the brains of sheep with type D enterotoxemia are unique and pathognomonic, and although they are present in the vast majority of cases, occasionally they may be absent. The most consistent change, observed in ~90% of acute and subacute cases, is *perivascular proteinaceous edema*, also known as microangiopathy, which is seen mostly as homogeneous acidophilic accumulations of protein surrounding small- and medium-sized arteries and veins (Fig. 1-155). Occasionally, accumulation of protein hyaline droplets around small vessels is also seen. These lesions are first evident a few hours after onset of clinical signs. Apparently, no other conditions of sheep produce this highly proteinaceous perivascular edema in brain, and *this change therefore should be considered diagnostic for type D enterotoxemia in this species*. In subacute and chronic disease, FSE can be observed. This lesion is usually multifocal and characterized by degeneration of white matter, hemorrhage, and astrocyte and axonal swelling. Perivascular edema and FSE in the brain are always bilateral and roughly symmetrical, and they have been described most frequently in corpus striatum, thalamus, midbrain, cerebellar peduncles, and cerebellar white matter. These areas are not exclusively affected, and lesions sometimes can be seen in other parts of the brain, such as cortex and hippocampus. Usually, no significant histologic changes are found in intestines of sheep dying from enterotoxemia. Histologic changes were not observed in kidneys of experimentally inoculated lambs autopsied immediately after death, supporting suggestions that these lesions are due to postmortem change. Thus microscopic lesions in kidney should not be considered a diagnostic indicator of ovine enterotoxemia.

Ultrastructurally, *severe damage to vascular endothelium* is apparent and there is swelling of protoplasmic astrocytes. The foot processes around blood vessels and the processes around neurons are most severely swollen.

Immunohistochemistry has revealed that Alzheimer precursor protein 1 (APP1) is very early upregulated in axons surrounding areas of vasculopathy, suggesting that neuronal stress is an early event in ovine enterotoxemia.

Type D enterotoxemia may be seen in both adult **goats** and kids. As in sheep, 3 forms of the disease are recognized in goats: *acute*, *subacute*, and *chronic*. The acute disease is similar to that seen in lambs, and usually manifests as sudden death. The subacute form is characterized by diarrhea and severe abdominal discomfort with or without neurologic signs. Affected animals usually die within 1-2 days of the onset of clinical signs. The chronic form of the disease may last for a few days or weeks. Weight loss and diarrhea are its main clinical features. The principal **gross lesions** in the acute form of the disease are similar to those seen in sheep, except that gross brain lesions are absent. In the subacute and chronic disease, there is mild to severe mesocolonic edema, hyperemia, and ulceration of the mucosa (Fig. 1-156A), especially of the distal small intestine, cecum, and spiral colon. The affected areas may be covered by a layer of fibrin that reveals multifocal to diffuse ulceration when peeled off. The intestinal contents are olive-green to red and mucoid and frequently contain strands of fibrin. The mesenteric lymph nodes are enlarged and edematous. Hydropericardium, ascites, and pulmonary edema can be seen in the subacute form but not in the chronic form of the disease. FSE similar to that describe in sheep has been described in one case of subacute enterotoxemia in goats.

Microscopic changes are usually absent in acute cases, but perivascular edema similar to that described in sheep occasionally may be observed. The main microscopic lesions in subacute and chronic forms are seen in the colon and, occasionally in the caudal segments of the small intestine. These lesions vary from a mild pleocellular leukocytic reaction in the lamina propria to a suppurative and fibrinonecrotizing enteritis, colitis, and/or enterocolitis (Fig. 1-156B). Changes in the lungs may be similar to, but are less consistent than, those seen in lambs. Only rarely has FSE been described in subacute type D enterotoxemia of goats. The reasons for the different manifestations of enterotoxemia in sheep and goats are unknown.

Information on type D enterotoxemia in **cattle** is sparse and the disease seems to occur very rarely in this species. A spontaneous disease with gross brain lesions similar to those observed in FSE of sheep occasionally is seen in cattle. However, a causal relationship between the lesions and C. *perfringens* type D or its epsilon toxin has not been established in any of these cases, and the etiology of these lesions in cattle remains undetermined.

Experimentally, a disease very similar to the acute form of type D enterotoxemia in sheep was observed in calves inoculated intravenously with epsilon toxin. These animals developed severe respiratory and neurologic clinical signs very shortly after inoculation. Gross findings included severe pulmonary edema and hydropericardium. Histologic changes were proteinaceous perivascular edema of the brain and lungs. Intraduodenal inoculation of calves with C. *perfringens* type D also resulted in a disease similar to the acute form of type D enterotoxemia in sheep, with clinical and pathologic findings similar to those seen in epsilon toxin inoculated calves in most animals; one animal developing chronic neurologic disease with gross and microscopic lesions of FSE as described in the subacute and chronic ovine form of the disease.

These experimental results indicate that cattle are susceptible to C. *perfringens* type D infection and its epsilon toxin. However, natural type D disease in this species seems to be a rare occurrence. Microangiopathy similar to that described in in sheep and goat enterotoxemia was described in the brain of two 1-day-old calves and in a heifer, in which epsilon toxin was detected in the intestinal content.

A **diagnosis** of type D disease in sheep can be established based on the presence of FSE and/or perivascular edema in the brain. The same applies for goats in the rare cases in which these lesions are present. Absence of these lesions in either species does not preclude a diagnosis of enterotoxemia. Although it has been suggested that epsilon toxin may be produced in the intestine after death, this has never been proved, and demonstration of epsilon toxin in intestinal content is therefore considered diagnostic for the disease in both animal species. It is likely that the same diagnostic criteria apply for enterotoxemia in cattle, although much less information is available about the disease in this species and diagnostic criteria have not been established in cattle.

Further reading

Filho EJ, et al. Clinicopathologic features of experimental *Clostridium perfringens* type D enterotoxemia in cattle. Vet Pathol 2009;46:1213-1220.
Finnie JW. Pathogenesis of brain damage produced in sheep by *Clostridium perfringens* type D epsilon toxin: a review. Aust Vet J 2003;81:219-221.
Oliveira DM, et al. Focal symmetrical encephalomalacia in a goat. J Vet Diagn Invest 2010;22:793-796.
Uzal FA. Diagnosis of *Clostridium perfringens* intestinal infections in sheep and goats. Anaerobe 2004;10:135-143.
Uzal FA, et al. The pathology of peracute experimental *Clostridium perfringens* type D enterotoxemia in sheep. J Vet Diagn Invest 2004;16:403-411.
Uzal FA, Songer JG. Diagnosis of *Clostridium perfringens* intestinal infections in sheep and goats. J Vet Diagn Invest 2008;20:253-265.

***Clostridium perfringens* type E.** *Clostridium perfringens* type E has been blamed for enterotoxemia of lambs, calves, and rabbits. Pathogenesis of type E infections is not very well understood, although it is assumed that iota toxin plays an important role.

In the few reported cases of this condition in **calves**, the animals died acutely and had a congested ulcerated abomasum and hemorrhagic enteritis that occurred segmentally along the small intestine. Mesenteric nodes were enlarged and red, and pericardial effusion and serosal hemorrhages may be present.

No comprehensive descriptions of clinical disease, gross and microscopic lesions of type E enterotoxemia in **other ruminants**.

The few diagnoses of type E enteritis that have been reported were based on isolation of C. *perfringens* type E from the intestinal content of sick animals. This procedure, however, is not universally accepted as a diagnostic criterion for C. *perfringens* intestinal diseases because this organism is present in many healthy animals.

Although C. *perfringens* type E also has been suspected as a cause of enterotoxemia in **rabbits**, cross-reactivity of the iota toxin with the toxins of C. *spiroforme*, has created doubt regarding the role of C. *perfringens* type E in disease in rabbits.

Further reading

Songer JG, Miskimmins DW. *Clostridium perfringens* type E enteritis in calves: two cases and a brief review of the literature. Anaerobe 2004;10:239-242.
Uzal FA, Songer JG. Diagnosis of *Clostridium perfringens* intestinal infections in sheep and goats. J Vet Diagn Invest 2008;20:253-265.

Clostridium difficile. *Clostridium difficile* is a gram-positive rod that may be found in the soil and gut of many animal species. C. *difficile* is the most commonly identified cause of antibiotic-associated and nosocomial diarrhea in humans but, in the past few years, it has also been associated with cases of colitis and diarrhea in people that have not been treated with antibiotics or exposed to hospital environments (community-associated C. *difficile* infections). C. *difficile* disease occurs spontaneously in several animal species including horses, hares, rabbits, pigs, nonhuman primates, dogs, cats, ostriches, and black-tailed prairie dogs. C. *difficile* has been isolated from cattle with enteritis but also infected by other pathogens, and although it is very likely that this microorganism plays a role in enteritis of cattle, final evidence to support this assertion is lacking.

C. difficile disease has been reproduced experimentally in several animal species that are used as models for human disease, including Syrian hamsters, guinea pigs, mice, rats, and rabbits. Lesions in most nonhuman mammals are similar to those in humans, but vary extensively in severity and distribution within the gastrointestinal tract. Differences in distribution of lesions within the gastrointestinal tract also exist between different age groups of the same animal species. Over the past few years, highly virulent ribotypes responsible for severe human outbreaks (i.e., 027 and 078) have been associated with disease in several animal species, prompting speculation that animal-to-human transmission and/or vice versa occurs.

Pathogenesis of *C. difficile* disease in domestic animals is likely mediated by toxins A (an enterotoxin) and B (a cytotoxin and also an enterotoxin). Much controversy exists about the relative importance of each of these toxins in the pathogenesis of *C. difficile* infection. However, animal experiments using toxin mutant strains of *C. difficile* (i.e., strains that do not produce toxin A or B or both), have shown that both toxins are able to cause lesions and disease.

The major predisposing factors for *C. difficile* disease in most species are antibiotic therapy and, at least for humans and horses, hospitalization. Although clindamycin and vancomycin therapy pose a higher risk than other antibiotics for many animal species, disturbance of normal flora with development of *C. difficile* disease can occur after administration of almost any antibiotic, including antibiotics that are effective against *C. difficile* itself. However, in horses the disease has been most frequently associated with administration of β-lactam antibiotics, probably because of the prevalence of their use.

Confirmation of a diagnosis of *C. difficile* disease should be based on identification of toxins A, B, or both in gut content or feces by tests with high sensitivity and specificity, mostly ELISAs. However, because of the lower carrier rate of this microorganism in some animal species (e.g., horses), isolation of toxigenic strains of this microorganism from intestinal content and/or feces is considered diagnostically significant for *C. difficile* infection by some authors. Typing of isolates is necessary because nontoxic strains can occur and isolation of those is of no diagnostic significance.

In **horses**, *C. difficile* causes enteritis, enterocolitis, and/or colitis. Diarrhea and colic have been reproduced in foals using inocula of *C. difficile* spores and vegetative cells. Horses of any age can be affected and although there are exceptions, it is generally accepted that the distribution of lesions throughout the intestinal tract seems to be dependent on the age of the horse. In foals <1 month old, the small intestine is invariably affected, whereas colon and cecum may or may not have lesions. In older foals and adult horses, the disease has a more caudal distribution, affecting the colon and sometimes the cecum, and generally sparing the small intestine. Although this age-related distribution of lesions within the gastrointestinal tract is seen in the majority of cases, exceptions do occur and lesion distribution should not be used to confirm/rule out *C. difficile* infection in horses.

The clinical signs of *C. difficile* disease in horses are highly variable, not specific and may occur with highly variable

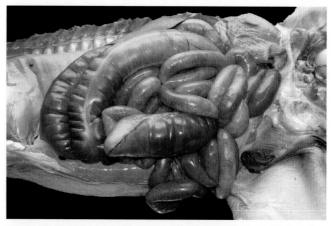

Figure 1-157 Enterocolitis caused by *Clostridium difficile* infection in a foal. Marked congestion and hemorrhage of the small and large intestine serosal surfaces. (Reprinted with permission from Diab SS, et al. Vet Microbiol 2013;167:42-49.)

severity. The main clinical sign is diarrhea, which may be accompanied by hyperemic mucous membranes, prolonged capillary refill time, pyrexia, tachycardia, tachypnea, dehydration, abdominal distention, and colic. The mortality rate in foals and adults varies from 0 to 42%. A syndrome known as *duodenitis-proximal jejunitis*, characterized clinically by large volumes of enterogastric reflux, has been known since the early 1980s. Although an association has been suggested between *C. difficile* and duodenitis-proximal jejunitis, a conclusive relationship has been neither proved nor ruled out.

C. difficile gross and microscopic lesions may be characteristic but are not pathognomonic, as other infectious (*C. perfringens* type C, *Salmonella* sp., and *Neorickettsia risticii*) and noninfectious (NSAIDs) causes of intestinal disease can produce very similar lesions.

Grossly, the serosa of the small and large intestine is multifocally red or blue as the result of intense hyperemia and/or hemorrhage (Fig. 1-157). The wall of the small intestine can be slightly thickened; the mucosa is often diffusely reddened and may have an overlying, multifocal, tan to orange pseudomembrane. The wall of the colon and cecum is typically diffusely and severely thickened by clear to hemorrhagic, gelatinous submucosal and mucosal edema; the mucosa is multifocally or diffusely dull green or red and may be multifocally covered by a tan or light green pseudomembrane (Fig. 1-158). The intestinal content in young foals is often hemorrhagic but may be yellow and pasty or green/brown and watery. In older foals and adult horses, the colon and cecum are characteristically filled with large amounts of green or light brown, watery contents, and occasionally dark brown or red, hemorrhagic, watery contents (Fig. 1-159). Bloody content may be present caudally to the small colon and rectum. When present, gross lesions outside the gastrointestinal tract are those of endotoxic shock and/or disseminated intravascular coagulation, including serous or serosanguineous pericardial effusion, pulmonary edema and congestion, and multifocal subendocardial and subserosal petechiae and ecchymoses.

Microscopic lesions in horses are mostly restricted to the gastrointestinal tract and they can be present in the small and/or large intestine. They are almost identical to those seen in horses with *C. perfringens* type C infection and consist mainly of multifocal to diffuse, often hemorrhagic, coagulative

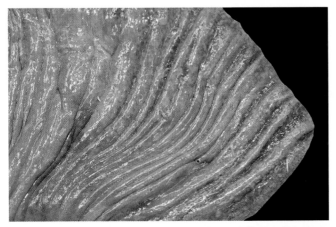

Figure 1-158 Colitis caused by *Clostridium difficile* infection in an adult horse. Mucosal necrosis and edema of mucosal folds. (Reprinted with permission from Diab SS, et al. Vet Microbiol 2013;167:42-49.)

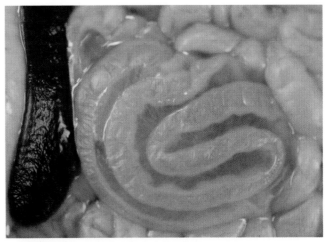

Figure 1-160 Marked edema of the mesocolon in a neonatal piglet infected with *Clostridium difficile*.

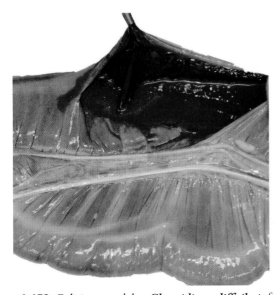

Figure 1-159 Colitis caused by *Clostridium difficile* infection in an adult horse. Dark red content in the large colon. (Courtesy S.S. Diab.)

necrosis of the mucosa, which may be covered by a pseudo-membrane, frequently accompanied by submucosal edema and congestion. Thrombosis of small to mid-size blood vessels in the mucosa and/or submucosa is a very frequent, although not constant, finding, and it is especially useful in those cases in which autolysis has partially masked the mucosal necrosis. Mild to moderate mucosal and submucosal fibrino-neutrophilic infiltration with fewer plasma cells, lymphocytes, and macrophages is frequently observed. The so-called "volcano" lesions, as described in the human disease and characterized by patchy focal erosions on the small intestinal or colonic mucosa through which fibrin and neutrophils exude, are not very frequently seen in horses and it has been speculated that the reason is that, at the time of autopsy and sample collection, the lesions are usually too advanced to show the delicate volcano-like lesions. Few to numerous clusters of short and thick, gram-positive rods can be observed in the intestinal lumen and/or on the surface or within the necrotic mucosa.

Co-infection of foals with *C. difficile* and *C. perfringens* type C can also occur. The clinical signs, gross and microscopic lesions are almost identical to those produced by either of these microorganisms alone.

C. difficile is increasingly being recognized as a cause of diarrhea resulting from *fibrinous colitis* in **neonatal pigs** under about a week of age, and the disease has been reproduced experimentally using pure cultures of the organism. Piglets have diarrhea, dyspnea, scrotal edema, and mild abdominal distention. Affected litters experience lost productivity (mainly shown as decreased weaning weight).

Grossly, hydrothorax and characteristic although not pathognomonic, *edema of the mesocolon* (Fig. 1-160) are evident grossly, usually in association with patchy to extensive fibrinous typhlocolitis (Fig. 1-161A), with yellow pasty to fluid content and feces. Microscopically, fibrinous colitis similar to that described in horses is a common lesion, with colonic serosal and mesenteric edema and infiltration of mononuclear inflammatory cells and neutrophils in the lamina propria. Segmental erosion and ulceration of colonic mucosal epithelium is common, and volcano lesions may be seen in acute cases of the disease (Fig. 1-161B). Occasionally deeper necrosis of the mucosa and colonic wall may occur.

Information on *C. difficile* infection in domestic **dogs and cats** is scant and the role of this microorganism in canine and feline enteric disease is currently unclear. Although a possible association between the detection of *C. difficile* toxins in feces of dogs and disease has been reported in multiple studies, diagnostic criteria for *C. difficile* infection in these species have not been defined. This is complicated by the fact that prevalence of *C. difficile* in normal dogs and cats may be up to 50% and *C. difficile* toxins also have been detected in a small percentage of asymptomatic dogs. Descriptions of lesions of *C. difficile* infections in dogs or cats are not available.

The role of *C. difficile* in enteric disease of **cattle** has been proposed in several studies, but no conclusive evidence has been provided to confirm or rule out this possibility. This microorganism, including the highly virulent ribotypes 027 and 078, and its toxins, has been detected in the intestine of healthy and diarrheic calves. Ribotype 078 has been found to be predominant strain in cattle in North America. The fact that several of the highly virulent ribotypes of *C. difficile* for humans have been found in cattle suggests that zoonotic transmission (and/or vice versa) may occur. There is growing concern that some *C. difficile* infections may be acquired from

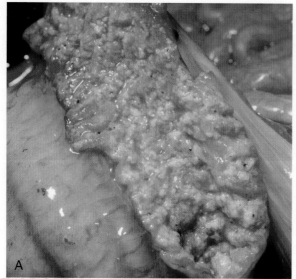

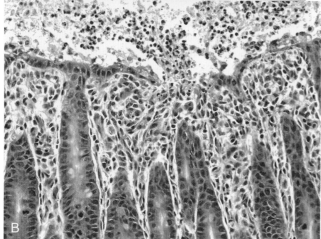

Figure 1-161 Fibrinonecrotic colitis in a neonatal piglet infected with _Clostridium difficile_. A. The colonic mucosa is covered by a pseudomembrane. (Courtesy W.R. Kelly.) **B.** Effusion of neutrophils through the superficial epithelium **(volcano lesion)**.

ingestion of C. _difficile_ spores in contaminated foods of animal origin. Although a correlation between the presence of fecal C. _difficile_ and its toxins and calf diarrhea was found, frequently this microorganism is detected in diarrheic calves together with other enteropathogens (e.g., bovine coronavirus, bovine rotavirus, _Cryptosporidium_ spp.), and ascribing the enteropathogenic effects to one of these pathogens alone is difficult. One study failed in the attempt to provoke diarrhea in calves by oral administration of virulent C. _difficile_ strains.

Tyzzer's disease is caused by the obligate intracellular bacterium **_Clostridium piliforme,_** the only gram-negative organism among the pathogenic clostridia. It is a disease of many species of mammals, among them horses, cats, dogs, rabbits, hamsters, and cattle, although there seem to be bacterial strain differences that determine host susceptibility. Affected animals are often very young or appear to be immunocompromised in some way.

The classical triad of lesions in most animal species include changes in the heart, intestinal tract, and liver. However, frequently lesions are observed only in the liver, which is the organ most frequently affected in the majority of animal species. Animals become infected initially through the

epithelium of the ileum, cecum, and colon, where, when present, inflammation may vary from subtle catarrhal to fibrinohemorrhagic. Bacilli can be observed faintly in hematoxylin and eosin preparations but are better demonstrated using silver stains, often forming characteristic "pick-up-sticks" arrays, in the cytoplasm of enterocytes. Ultimately, in most cases they disseminate elsewhere in the body, especially to liver and myocardium, where they cause acute to subacute necrotic lesions. The organism cannot be cultured in conventional media and diagnosis is usually based on histologic examination by demonstration of the classical intracellular bacilli. The disease is discussed more fully in Vol. 2, Liver and biliary system.

Further reading

Arroyo LG, et al. Experimental _Clostridium difficile_ enterocolitis in foals. J Vet Intern Med 2004;18:734-738.

Diab SS, et al. Pathology and diagnostic criteria of _Clostridium difficile_ enteric infection in horses. Vet Pathol 2013;50:1028-1036.

Hammit MC, et al. A possible role for _Clostridium difficile_ in the etiology of calf enteritis. Vet Microbiol 2008;127:343-352.

Hoover DG, Rodriguez-Palacios A. Transmission of _Clostridium difficile_ in foods. Infect Dis Clin North Am 2013;27:675-685.

Keel MK, Songer JG. The comparative pathology of _Clostridium difficile_–associated disease. Vet Pathol 2006;43:225-240.

Rodriguez-Palacios A, et al. Natural and experimental infection of neonatal calves with _Clostridium difficile._ Vet Microbiol 2007;124:166-172.

Uzal FA, et al. _Clostridium perfringens_ type C and _Clostridium difficile_ co-infection in foals. Vet Microbiol 2012;156:395-402.

Paratuberculosis (Johne's disease)

Johne's disease is caused by **_Mycobacterium avium_ subsp. _paratuberculosis_** (MAP) infection. The etiologic agent of Johne's disease is classified as a subspecies within the _M. avium_ complex based on DNA hybridization studies and other genotypic and phenotypic tests. MAP in culture is slow growing, and its dependence on the iron chelator mycobactin classically has been the key distinguishing phenotypic characteristic. Genetically, the IS900 insertion sequence element seems unique to MAP, and has been used broadly as a diagnostic tool in animals and humans. Highly homologous but not identical IS900-like sequences have been detected in other mycobacteria. At least 2 distinct MAP strains are known to cause paratuberculosis in various hosts, and these are generally referred to as type I, or S strain first isolated from sheep, and type II, or C strain first isolated from cattle. Type I strains have been isolated mostly from sheep, particularly in Australia; there are rare reports of cattle infected with type I strains. Type II strains, on the other hand, are the most common; they have a broad host range and have been isolated from domestic and wildlife species as well as nonruminants. The strains have distinct phenotypic, genotypic, host preference, virulence, and pathogenic traits that continue to be clarified.

Paratuberculosis is most common in _domestic ruminants_, but spontaneous disease also occurs rarely in a number of free-ranging and captive nondomestic ruminants, camelids and rabbits, equids, swine, and captive primates. Wild mammals including lagomorphs, rodents, and carnivores, and several species of wild birds are naturally infected with MAP, but do not necessarily develop disease. MAP has been recovered from tissue and blood samples of human patients inflicted with *Crohn's disease*, a chronic granulomatous enteritis of importance in humans that shares several pathologic and immunologic features with Johne's disease. These findings are suggestive of a causal relationship; however, Koch's postulates have not yet been fulfilled, so it seems more likely that MAP is coincidental, or plays a potentially opportunistic role in these cases.

The **epidemiology and pathogenesis** of Johne's disease are best understood in cattle, and are assumed to be similar in other species. MAP is transmitted predominantly by the fecal-oral route, either directly by ingestion in feces or indirectly via MAP-contaminated milk, colostrum, or water. Organisms may be present in semen or urine, and may cross the placenta, particularly during advanced disease. A distinct age-dependent susceptibility to MAP infection is observed; the infectious dose for adults is considerable higher than for neonates. The basis for this is unknown, and control programs aimed at blocking transmission are almost exclusively focused on neonates. Johne's disease is often categorized into 3 (or 4) stages: silent infection, subclinical infection, clinical disease (and advanced clinical disease), based on severity of clinical signs, potential for shedding of MAP organisms into the environment, and ease of diagnosis. Of particular importance is the subclinical period, which can last 2-5 years before infected animals develop clinical signs. Because shedding of MAP into the environment by subclinical cows is variable and progressive, this period represents a significant risk for spread of the infection to susceptible herdmates. This long and unpredictable incubation period has given rise to the concept of *the iceberg effect* because in any infected herd, although few animals may be showing clinical signs of Johne's disease, a much greater number of animals are likely MAP infected. Sheep, goats, and cervids are considered to be more susceptible to MAP infection compared with cattle, and have a shorter incubation period before development of clinical signs. Survivability of MAP in the environment is proposed to have a significant effect on the epidemiology of MAP infection in animals; however, the biologic relevance of these factors for transmission of infection is still unclear.

MAP gains access to the small intestinal mucosa and subepithelial dome via microfold (M cells) or epithelial cells overlying submucosal Peyer's patches. Macrophages are the preferred host cell for MAP, and the ability of pathogenic mycobacteria including MAP to inhibit phagosome-lysosome fusion is fundamental to its survival and persistence within the host. Experimental in vitro and in vivo work indicates that MAP-infected cattle develop a proinflammatory immune response early after intestinal infection, which is probably driven by innate intestinal T lymphocytes including gamma-delta T cells and natural killer cells. However, in animals that fail to clear the infection, the early proinflammatory response eventually gives way to an apparently ineffective but robust MAP-specific antibody response. This transition correlates with the progression from subclinical to clinical disease in affected adults, but the mechanisms for this remain largely unknown. The rate of disease progression and the length of the subclinical period of Johne's disease are irregular and can be protracted; clinical cows are rarely <2 years of age. The reasons for this remain unclear, although there is likely a complex interplay of factors, including age of initial exposure, dose, re-exposure over time, environment, nutrition, production stage, and genetics. As an animal progresses toward clinical disease, the population of MAP within the intestinal mucosa increases and live MAP are shed in the feces more frequently and in greater numbers. Appetite often remains normal, and intermittent to progressive diarrhea may persist for weeks before eventual development of hypoproteinemia, cachexia, emaciation, and death.

The major lesions of Johne's disease are usually confined to the ileum, large intestine, and draining lymph nodes; however, the infection is generalized and the organism is widely distributed in lymph nodes, and can be cultured from a variety of parenchymatous organs or even blood in fulminating infections. Diarrhea during Johne's disease is related to the *granulomatous inflammatory response in the lamina propria of the small intestine,* and the associated villus atrophy that develops. Malabsorption and filtration secretion caused by the inflamed small intestinal mucosa overloads the capacity of the colon to resorb electrolytes and fluid. The function of the colon itself may be compromised by MAP infection, especially in severe or advanced cases. There is malabsorption of amino acids, enteric loss of plasma protein, and hypoproteinemia causing reduced productive efficiency, and when negative nitrogen balance occurs, a decline in body condition, and ultimate emaciation.

The **gross lesions** of Johne's disease include small intestinal mucosal lesions that may be segmental or continuous, and can be distributed from the duodenum to the rectum. Lesions are usually best developed in the *lower ileum and upper large intestine.* The ileocecal valve is considered by some to be the site that is earliest and most consistently affected; however, lesions in the ileocecal valve can be variable. The classic intestinal change is *diffuse thickening of the mucosa,* which is folded into transverse rugae, the crests of which may be congested (Fig. 1-162). Mucosal thickening is due to accumulation of predominantly macrophages, as well as edema fluid, in the mucosa and submucosa. The mucosa and/or serosa may have a slightly granular appearance because of increased cellularity and edema. *The ileocecal and mesenteric lymph nodes are enlarged, pale, and edematous. Lymphangitis is common,* and the lymphatic vessels can often be traced as thickened cords from

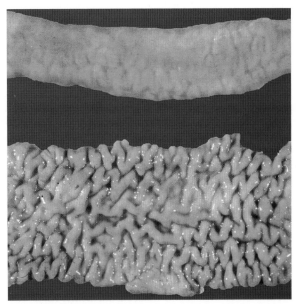

Figure 1-162 Thickened mucosal folds that can also be seen from the serosal surface in the jejunum of a cow with **Johne's disease.**

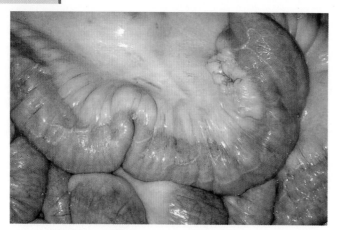

Figure 1-163 Serosal edema and **lymphangitis** in a goat with Johne's disease. (Courtesy J. Caswell.)

the intestinal serosa through the mesentery to the mesenteric nodes (Fig. 1-163). In some cases mucosal lesions are subtle and lymphangitis is the only readily recognizable gross lesion, which is specific enough to justify a presumptive diagnosis of Johne's disease at gross postmortem examination. Additionally, there is marked loss of muscle mass and serous atrophy of fat depots, intermandibular edema, and fluid effusion in various body cavities. Plaques of intimal fibrosis and mineralization may be evident in the thoracic aorta.

When gross lesions are well developed, the **characteristic microscopic lesions** of *transmural granulomatous enteritis and lymphangitis* are obvious (Figs. 1-164 and 1-165), although in cattle with minimal gross lesion, microscopic abnormalities can be more subtle. Depending on the severity and stage of the infection, villi are moderately to markedly atrophic; macrophages are increased in number and are focally or diffusely distributed in the lamina propria, submucosa, muscular layers or the serosa of the intestine. Epithelioid macrophages and Langhans-type multinucleated giant cells are often present in aggregates or diffuse sheets. The inflammatory infiltrate may abnormally separate and displace crypts, which are elongate and lined by hyperplastic epithelial cells. Crypts may be distended with mucus and exfoliated cells, probably because of compression and obstruction of their mouths by inflammatory cells and edema. Foci of necrosis may occur within these aggregates of macrophages, but in cattle formation of classic tuberculoid granulomas with caseation and mineralization are extremely rare.

Granulomatous lymphangitis is one of the most consistent changes, and inflammatory cells can be observed along the lacteal vessels of villi, or in the submucosa (see Fig. 1-165). Initially the lymphatics are surrounded by lymphocytes and plasma cells and many contain plugs of epithelioid cells in the lumen. Granulomas may form in the wall and project into the lumen. These nodules may undergo some central necrosis. *Granulomatous lymphadenitis* occurs in ileocecal or mesenteric lymph nodes in advanced cases. In the early stages, there are increased numbers of macrophages within the subcapsular sinuses; with time, these progress to nodular or diffuse infiltrates of epithelioid macrophages and giant cells that replace much of the lymph node cortex and infiltrate the medullary sinusoids.

Of the other organs and tissues from which MAP can be isolated in cattle, *focal granulomas* attributable to MAP have only been described in the liver, hepatic lymph nodes, and very

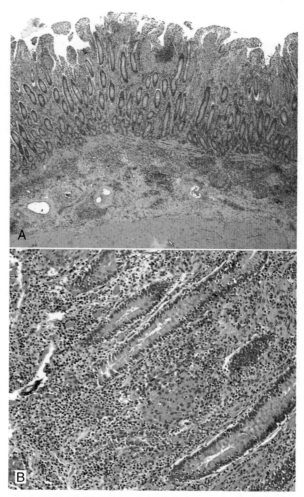

Figure 1-164 Johne's disease in a cow. A. Blunt **atrophic ileal villi,** and hyperplastic crypts. Note heavy **inflammatory infiltrate** in lamina propria and submucosa. **B.** Aggregate of **macrophages** in hypercellular lamina propria.

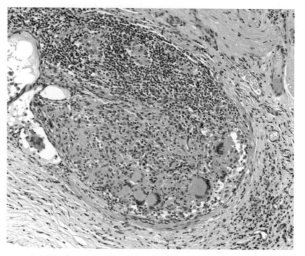

Figure 1-165 Ileal subserosal granulomatous lymphangitis with prominent giant cells in a cow with Johne's disease.

rarely, the kidney and lungs. Granulomas are most common in the liver, and are found in portal triads or scattered throughout the hepatic parenchyma. Acid-fast bacilli are usually demonstrable in these lesions.

In sheep and goats, Johne's disease mainly occurs in adults and is characterized by *chronic wasting*; there may be breaks in the wool in sheep, and submandibular edema resulting from hypoproteinemia. Feces are often normal and may be soft and unpelleted, but overt diarrhea is unusual except intermittently in the terminal stages of disease. The reason for this is unknown, but may relate to the innately greater efficiency of electrolyte and fluid absorption in the colon of these species. In **farmed deer**, Johne's disease is clinically similar, but there are reports of disease in animals well under a year old.

In sheep, goats, and deer, a distinct age and dose susceptibility pattern has been described such that animals exposed to higher doses of MAP at earlier ages probably progress faster and develop more severe disease. Goats are thought to be more susceptible to MAP infection compared with sheep or cattle. Enteric **gross lesions** in sheep and goats tend to be more sporadic and subtle compared with cattle. Lesions appear to occur most commonly in the distal jejunum, and can range from focal or multifocal subtle lesions that are easily missed at postmortem examination, to diffuse and severe intestinal thickening with prominent transverse ridges and mesenteric adhesions. There may be lymphadenomegaly and lymphangitis as seen in cattle. **Microscopically**, there can be focal or multifocal accumulations of epithelioid cells and lymphocytes, with relatively few organisms; this is the paucibacillary form. Others may have a dense transmural intestinal inflammatory infiltrate with abundant organisms; this is the multibacillary form. Microscopic lesions also tend to be most severe in the distal jejunum and/or the ileocecal valve. Goats and sometimes sheep develop foci of tubercle-like caseation necrosis, often with mineralization and fibrosis in the mucosa, submucosa, serosa, and lymphatics of the intestine or in the lymph nodes. These nodules may be grossly visible as white foci 1-4 mm in diameter. Scattered lymph nodes elsewhere in the body, and liver, lung, spleen, and other organs, may contain focal granulomatous lesions in sheep and goats. Pigmented strains of MAP have been described in sheep, and in these cases the mucosa and lymph nodes may be discolored orange.

The organism is usually readily demonstrable by acid-fast staining within macrophages and giant cells in the lesions, especially in diffuse multibacillary forms of the disease (Fig. 1-166). However, some clinical cases may have multifocal paucibacillary lesions in sheep, so an extensive search must be made for individual macrophages or giant cells bearing low numbers of acid-fast bacilli. Antibodies with well-defined specificity for MAP have allowed the development of immunohistochemical tests, but these are typically not helpful when there are very few organisms. Polymerase chain reaction techniques are useful for confirming the diagnosis in individual cases. Culture can be reliable to detect MAP in goats, because they tend to be infected with the cattle strain; however, culture of MAP from sheep is difficult because of its fastidious growth requirements.

Further reading

Coussens PM, et al. Host-pathogen interactions and intracellular survival of *Mycobacterium avium* subsp. *paratuberculosis*. In: Berhs MA, Collins DM, editors. Paratuberculosis: Organism, Disease, Control. Cambridge: CAB International; 2010.

Fecteau M, Whitlock RH. Paratuberculosis in cattle. In: Berhs MA, Collins DM, editors. Paratuberculosis: Organism, Disease, Control. Cambridge: CAB International; 2010.

MacKintosh CG, Griffin JF. Paratuberculosis in deer, camelids and other ruminants. In: Berhs MA, Collins DM, editors. Paratuberculosis: Organisms, Disease, Control. Cambridge: CAB International; 2010.

Manning EJ, Collins MT. Epidemiology of paratuberculosis. In: Berhs MA, Collins DM, editors. Paratuberculosis: Organism, Disease, Control. Cambridge: CAB International; 2010.

Plattner BL, Hostetter JM. Comparative gamma delta T cell immunology: a focus on mycobacterial disease in cattle. Vet Med Int 2011;2011:214-384.

Stevenson K. Comparative differences between strains of *Mycobacterium avium* subsp. *paratuberculosis*. In: Berhs MA, Collins DM, editors. Paratuberculosis: Organism, Disease, Control. Cambridge: CAB International; 2010.

Sweeney RW. Pathogenesis of paratuberculosis. Vet Clin North Am Food Anim Pract 2011;27:537-549.

Rhodococcus equi *enterocolitis of foals*

Rhodococcus equi is an intracellular pathogen found in soil and as part of the normal intestinal flora of horses and other animals. This microorganism is a major pathogen of horses, and it also causes disease in pigs and cattle. In the past few years, *R. equi* pneumonia in HIV-infected or otherwise immunocompromised humans has become common.

R. equi isolated from foals and many recovered from humans carry an approximately 81-kb plasmid named pVAPA1037. This plasmid is essential for disease in horses; removal of this plasmid results in loss of the capacity of *R. equi* to replicate in macrophages. The genes on the virulence plasmid are divided into 4 groups, but only the genes within 1 of those groups, the PAI region, have been evaluated and reported to play significant roles in virulence. In particular, the

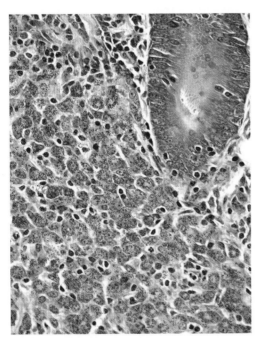

Figure 1-166 Large number of acid fast bacteria in the cytoplasm of macrophages and giant cells of a cow with Johne's disease. (Modified Ziehl Neelsen stain.)

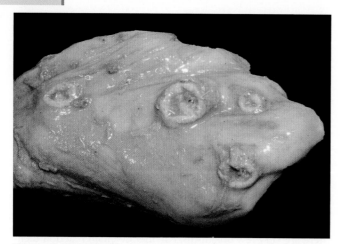

Figure 1-167 *Rhodococcus equi* infection in a foal. Craterous ulcerated lesions on colonic mucosa. (Courtesy L. Minatel.)

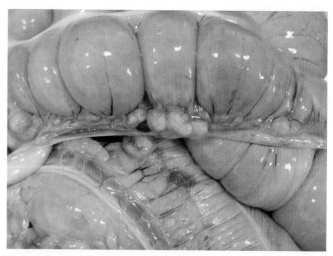

Figure 1-168 *Rhodococcus equi* infection in a foal. Enlarged suppurative cecal and colic lymph nodes. (Courtesy L. Minatel.)

PAI-encoded, virulence-associated protein A (*vapA*) and its positive regulators (*virR* and *ORF8*) are critical for resistance to macrophage attack and for bacterial multiplication in vivo. A *R. equi vapA* knockout mutant is incapable of intracellular replication and unable to establish a persistent infection in severe combined immunodeficient mice. There are both virulent and avirulent strains in nature, and on farms where disease caused by *R. equi* is endemic, there is a much higher proportion of virulent forms. Virulence factors may not be necessary for production of disease in an immunocompromised host. *R. equi* is usually associated with *suppurative bronchopneumonia of foals*. Abdominal lesions are identified in ~50% of foals with *R. equi* pneumonia that are presented for autopsy, and include any of the following, alone or in combination(s): pyogranulomatous enterotyphylocolitis, pyogranulomatous lymphadenitis of the mesenteric or colonic lymph nodes, large intra-abdominal abscesses, and peritonitis.

The development of intestinal lesions appears to be dose-related, in that experimental reproduction of the disease requires repeated oral infection. In natural disease, continual exposure to bacteria in swallowed respiratory exudate is probably an important source of infection in those animals with pneumonia.

Gross lesions may occur throughout the small and large intestines, but are usually most severe over Peyer's patches in small intestine, and in the cecum, large colon, and related lymph nodes (Figs. 1-167, 1-168). Mucosal lesions consist of multifocal irregular, elevated, and crateriform lesions with central ulcers up to 1-2 cm in diameter, often covered by purulent or necrotic debris (see Fig. 1-167). Edema of the wall of the gut may be severe. Mesenteric or colonic lymph nodes often are massively enlarged by edema and caseous or purulent foci that may obliterate the structure of the node. Occasionally, massively enlarged abscessed lymph nodes (see Fig. 1-168) are found without evidence of concurrent enteritis or colitis.

Microscopically, infection seems to occur by penetration of the specialized epithelium over Peyer's patches or intestinal lymphoid follicles. An initial neutrophilic response occurs and erosions of the epithelium develop subsequently. Macrophages and neutrophils accumulate in the lamina propria. The macrophages contain aggregates of *R. equi* but do not destroy them. Later necrosis of lymphoid follicles occurs, and deep ulcers develop that contain masses of neutrophils, macrophages, and multinucleated giant cells. Pyogranulomatous lymphangitis and mesenteric lymphadenitis characterize the chronic enteric disease.

Further reading

Giguère S, et al. *Rhodococcus equi*: clinical manifestations, virulence, and Immunity. J Vet Intern Med 2011;25:1221-1230.

Reuss SM, et al. Extrapulmonary disorders associated with *Rhodococcus equi* infection in foals: 150 cases (1987–2007). J Am Vet Med Assoc 2009;235:855-863.

Tripathi NV, et al. Conjugal transfer of a virulence plasmid in the opportunistic intracellular actinomycete *Rhodococcus equi*. J Bacteriol 2012;194:6790-6801.

Enterococcus *spp. enteritis*

Enterococcus spp. are gram-positive cocci, which are common inhabitants of the environment and gastrointestinal tract of clinically healthy humans and several animal species. However, some enterococci, mainly *Enterococcus hirae* and *Enterococcus durans*, may colonize extensively the mucosal surface of the small intestine in piglets, puppies, foals, calves, and suckling rats, in a manner similar to that of enteropathogenic *E. coli* and produce diarrhea. These bacteria adhere to the microvillus surface of enterocytes by fine filamentous pili. In tissue section they form a layer of small cocci crowded on the entire surface of epithelial cells, from the tips to the base of villi. There may be mild to moderate villus atrophy and some desquamating enterocytes.

The organisms from rats have been described, on genetic grounds, as *E. ratti*, whereas those from piglets have been described as *E. villorum* or *E. porcini*, which may be synonyms. *E. faecalis* that had numerous virulence traits and was resistant to multiple antimicrobials was isolated from young kittens with enteritis, diarrhea and up to 15% mortality. These kittens had been given probiotics that contained enterococci.

Malabsorption associated with reduced brush border enzyme activity may explain diarrhea in all animal species. Although in spontaneous cases in piglets, *Enterococcus* is frequently associated with other pathogens, the organism isolated from foals produced diarrhea when inoculated alone into gnotobiotic pigs.

Further reading

Arias CA, Murray BE. The rise of the *Enterococcus*: beyond vancomycin resistance. Nat Rev Microbiol 2012;10:266-278.

Ghosh A, et al. Mortality in kittens is associated with a shift in ileum mucosa-associated enterococci from *Enterococcus hirae* to biofilm-forming *Enterococcus faecalis* and adherent *Escherichia coli*. J Clin Microbiol 2013;51:3567-3578.

Nicklas JL, et al. *In situ* molecular diagnosis and histopathological characterization of enteroadherent *Enterococcus hirae* infection in pre-weaning-age kittens. J Clin Microbiol 2010;48:2814-2820.

Vancanneyt M, et al. *Enterococcus villorum* sp. nov., an enteroadherent bacterium associated with diarrhoea in piglets. Int J Syst Evol Microbiol 2001;51:393-400.

Bacteroides fragilis–associated diarrhea

Bacteroides fragilis is a non–spore-forming obligate anaerobe that is part of the normal enteric flora. Some enterotoxin-secreting strains have been associated with diarrhea in piglets, calves, lambs, foals, and humans. This enterotoxin is a *protease*, and probably damages the zonula adherens at the tight junction between enterocytes. Enterotoxigenic strains or cell-free culture filtrates cause secretion in ligated lamb or calf intestinal loops, and bacterial inocula cause diarrhea when administered orally to gnotobiotic piglets.

Bacteria do not adhere to the surface. Enterocytes round up and exfoliate, with villus attenuation and crypt elongation and hyperplasia. Infiltration of neutrophils is common. Damage may be seen in both small and large intestines. Ultrastructurally, affected cells lose their intercellular interdigitations, microvilli are shortened or absent, and the terminal web is disrupted.

Further reading

Almeida FS, et al. Occurrence of enterotoxigenic and nonenterotoxigenic *Bacteroides fragilis* in calves and evaluation of their antimicrobial susceptibility. FEMS Microbiol Lett 2007;272:15-21.

Sears CL. The toxins of *Bacteroides fragilis*. Toxicon 2001;39:1737-1746.

Anaerobiospirillum *ileocolitis*

The genus *Anaerobiospirillum*, small spiral gram-negative bacteria, comprises 2 species, *A. succiniciproducens* and *A. thomasii*, which have been isolated from dogs and cats, although only a few studies have related them to diarrhea. In **cats,** ileocolitis has been associated with *Anaerobiospirillum*. Cats may be asymptomatic, lethargic, and anorexic, or have vomiting and diarrhea. Microscopically, exfoliated epithelial cells and neutrophils are in dilated crypts in the ileum and colon, and bacteria stained with silver can be found in the lumen of crypts, in goblet cells, and sometimes in the lamina propria. Septicemia may occur, and renal failure has been associated.

Further reading

Rossi M, et al. Occurrence and species level diagnostics of *Campylobacter spp.*, enteric *Helicobacter spp.* and *Anaerobiospirillum spp.* in healthy and diarrheic dogs and cats. Vet Microbiol 2008;129:304-314.

Enteritis caused by Chlamydiaceae

Members of the family *Chlamydiaceae* are *obligate intracellular parasites*. The order Chlamydiales has been re-classified several times over the last decades. The latest revision led to the separation of the family *Chlamydiaceae* into the genera *Chlamydophila* and *Chlamydia*, with a total of 9 species, namely, *Chlamydophila abortus*, *Chlamydophila pecorum*, *Chlamydophila psittaci*, *Chlamydophila pneumoniae*, *Chlamydophila felis*, *Chlamydophila caviae*, *Chlamydia trachomatis*, *Chlamydia suis*, and *Chlamydia muridarum*. However, this division into 2 *Chlamydiaceae* genera has been widely criticized, and it was recently proposed that all *Chlamydiaceae* species should be grouped into a single *Chlamydia* genus.

Among all the *Chlamydiaceae* species, only **Chlamydia pecorum** and **C. suis** are associated with enteritis, in cattle and pigs, respectively. Other syndromes associated with *Chlamydiaceae* in domestic animals include respiratory disease, polyarthritis, orchitis, hepatitis, conjunctivitis, abortion, and encephalomyelitis, discussed in appropriate chapters elsewhere in these volumes.

The intestinal tract is the natural habitat for C. *pecorum*. Most infections are probably inapparent, but the intestine may be an important portal of entry in the development of systemic infections leading to hepatitis, arthritis, encephalitis, and pneumonia in ruminants. Enteritis may accompany or presage these diseases, and occasionally C. *pecorum* causes severe enteric disease in calves. Also, asymptomatic calves with C. *pecorum* intestinal infections may suffer up to 48% reduction in growth rates. This is associated with increased conjunctival reddening, increased serum globulin, and decreased plasma albumin and insulin-like growth factor-1. Based on these results, it was suggested that suppression of chlamydial asymptomatic infections may be a major contributor to the growth promoting effect of feed-additive antibiotics.

Following oral infection, C. *pecorum* infects mainly the enterocytes on the tips of ileal villi. These cells are in the G_1 phase of the cell cycle, which is required by *Chlamydia* for multiplication. C. *pecorum* also infects other cells, including goblet cells, enterochromaffin cells, and macrophages, and the latter cells may transport the organisms systemically before being destroyed by them.

C. *pecorum* adsorbs to the brush border of enterocytes and enters the cell by pinocytosis. Following multiplication of organisms in the supranuclear region, the cells degenerate. C. *pecorum* is released into the gut lumen and the lamina propria, where it infects endothelial cells of lacteals, whence they are released and become systemic.

Gastrointestinal disease caused by C. *pecorum* is usually a problem of **calves** <10 days old, but it may affect older calves, and can produce recurrent diarrhea. Watery diarrhea, dehydration, and death are often accompanied by lesions, although not necessarily signs, of hepatitis, interstitial pneumonia, and arthritis. Gross lesions may occur in the abomasum and throughout the intestinal tract but are most consistent and severe in the *terminal ileum*. Mucosal edema, congestion, and petechiae, sometimes with ulceration, are usually observed. Serosal hemorrhages and focal peritonitis may occur. Histologically, chlamydial inclusions may be demonstrable with Giemsa, Jimenez, Macchiavello, or immunoperoxidase staining. Central lacteals and capillaries are dilated, and neutrophils and monocytes infiltrate the lamina propria. Occasionally, granulomatous inflammation occurs in the intestinal submucosa and extends into the mesentery and to the serosa, producing the peritonitis observed grossly. Crypts in the small and large intestine may be dilated, lined by flattened epithelium, and contain inflammatory exudate. The centers of lymphoid follicles in Peyer's patches are necrotic.

C. suis in **swine** has been associated with conjunctivitis, rhinitis, pneumonia, enteritis, reproductive disorders, and asymptomatic infections. *C. suis* has been recognized in the intestinal mucosa of swine, with approximately equal frequency in diarrheic and nondiarrheic animals. Enteric chlamydial infections of pigs with *C. suis* are frequent and often subclinical. After experimental inoculation of *C. suis* into gnotobiotic piglets, there was moderate diarrhea, anorexia, weakness, and body weight loss. Microscopic changes consisted of necrosis and exfoliation of enterocytes on the apical half of villi, resulting in mild to severe villus atrophy in the distal jejunum and ileum. Lymphangitis and perilymphangitis were also evident in affected gut. Chlamydial replication was particularly marked at 2-4 days postinoculation and primarily located in the small intestinal villus enterocytes. Further sites of replication included large intestinal enterocytes, lamina propria, submucosa, and the mesenteric lymph nodes. In weanling pigs, similar lesions, but no diarrhea, were induced.

Further reading

Greub G. International Committee on Systematics of Prokaryotes. Subcommittee on the taxonomy of the Chlamydiae: minutes of the closed meeting, 21 June 2010, Hof bei Salzburg, Austria. Int J Syst Evol Microbiol 2010;60:2694.

Guscetti F, et al. Experimental enteric infection of gnotobiotic piglets with *Chlamydia suis* strain S45. Vet Microbiol 2009;135:157-168.

Poudel A, et al. Asymptomatic endemic *Chlamydia pecorum* infections reduce growth rates in calves by up to 48 percent. PLoS ONE 2012;7:e44961.

Schautteet K, et al. Chlamydiaceae infections in pig. Vet Res 2011;42:29.

Yousef K, et al. Recent advances in the understanding of *Chlamydophila pecorum* infections, sixteen years after it was named as the fourth species of the Chlamydiaceae family. Vet Res 2010;41:27-37.

Potomac horse fever (equine neorickettsiosis)

This condition, also described as *equine monocytic ehrlichiosis*, *equine ehrlichial colitis*, and *equine neorickettsiosis*, was first defined clinically in 1979, and is characterized by fever, leukopenia, depression, loss of appetite, colic, diarrhea, and lameness. It is caused by **Neorickettsia** (formerly *Ehrlichia*) **risticii**, a member of the order Rickettsiales, which are *obligate intracellular bacterial pathogens*. Potomac horse fever typically occurs in the summer. It was first described in the Potomac river valley of Maryland, Virginia, and Pennsylvania but it is now found in most areas of the United States and Canada, with cases also reported in Brazil and Uruguay, where it has been known for many years as *churrido*. Considering the current distribution of the disease, the name *Potomac horse fever* is probably no longer appropriate, and the term **equine neorickettsiosis** has been proposed.

Neorickettsia spp. replicate within the phagosome in the host cell, and use trematodes as hosts. The life cycle of the fluke includes freshwater snails from where it goes back into water, where it is ingested by the larval stages of several aquatic insects, including caddis flies and mayflies. The main mode of infection is most likely by accidental ingestion of infected adult insects that may accumulate in water containers. Insectivorous birds and bats are definitive hosts, which themselves become infected with *N. risticii*. Experimental infection has been produced with oral administration of infected insects and subcutaneous inoculation of *N. risticii*. All attempts to transmit the disease using ticks have failed.

The disease may be highly variable. Many infected horses seem not to get sick. Others develop severe colic, subcutaneous edema, laminitis, and shock: mortality can be up to 30% in untreated cases. Abortions of pregnant mares have been attributed to *N. risticii* infection.

The incubation period in experimental infections is ~9-14 days, and diarrhea begins 1-3 days after the onset of fever. Not all experimentally infected animals develop disease.

At **autopsy** of spontaneous cases, small vesicles are reported in the oral cavity, and epicardial hemorrhages and pulmonary congestion and hemorrhage, compatible with endotoxemia, are described. These are not reported in experimental cases, nor is laminitis. The lesions of the gastrointestinal tract are the most significant, in both spontaneous and experimental cases. In some animals there may be focal or more extensive erosions in the gastric mucosa, sometimes with overlying fibrinous exudate. Lesions in the small intestine are generally limited to segmental areas of mucosal congestion or hyperemia, with occasional focal ulcers or hemorrhage, and are much less consistent and severe than those in the *cecum and colon*. The content of the large bowel is abnormally fluid, and may have a brown or red-brown color, and foul odor. In the cecum and colon, there may be patches of hyperemia 5-10 cm in diameter, aggregates of small ulcers a few millimeters in diameter, and petechial hemorrhages. Sometimes the mucosa of the entire cecum is widely hyperemic. Ulcers and petechial hemorrhage are more severe and consistent in the right dorsal colon. The small colon is usually unaffected grossly.

Microscopic lesions are most consistent in the large intestine; similar changes may be evident in the small bowel. In areas of gross hyperemia, there is marked congestion and superficial hemorrhage in the mucosa. Associated with these lesions are superficial epithelial necrosis, erosion, and fibrin effusion. The mucosal surface is denuded, or perhaps covered by fibrinocellular exudate, and epithelium in the upper half of crypts is attenuated. Deeper parts of crypts are dilated and may contain necrotic epithelium and inflammatory cells. An abnormally intense mixed inflammatory cell population is in the lamina propria, and sometimes, the submucosa. Lymphoid tissue in the gut, mesenteric lymph nodes, and spleen is moderately involuted, compatible with the effects of the stress of systemic illness.

Organisms are not evident in hematoxylin and eosin–stained tissue. They are visible in large colon, and less consistently, in cecum, small colon, and small intestine, with *modified Steiner silver stain*. They appear as small clusters of 10-15 fine brown dots, <1 μm in diameter, in the apical cytoplasm of epithelial cells deep in crypts, or as more numerous, smaller black structures distributed in the cytoplasm of macrophages in the periglandular lamina propria, or in a few glandular epithelial cells. Ultrastructurally, small dense elementary bodies may be found, alone or in small clusters in vacuoles in the cytoplasm of macrophages, mast cells, and crypt epithelium, or as morulae—aggregates of larger, more open organisms, in the same locations. *N. risticii* can be identified in feces or peripheral blood buffy coat by polymerase chain reaction, providing a more sensitive and specific means of diagnosis.

Further reading

Baird JD, Arroyo LG. Historical aspects of Potomac horse fever in Ontario (1924-2010). Can Vet J 2013;54:565-572.

Bertin FR, et al. Clinical and clinicopathological factors associated with survival in 44 horses with equine neorickettsiosis (Potomac horse fever). Vet Intern Med 2013;27:977-981.

Coffman EA, et al. Abortion in a horse following *Neorickettsia risticii* infection. J Vet Diagn Invest 2008;20:827-830.

Dutra F, et al. Equine monocytic ehrlichiosis (Potomac horse fever) in horses in Uruguay and southern Brazil. J Vet Diagn Invest 2001;13:433-437.

Mycotic diseases of the gastrointestinal tract
Intestinal zygomycosis and aspergillosis

Formerly referred to as *phycomycosis*, the term *zygomycosis* denotes infections caused by one of several genera of fungi in the class Zygomycetes, which is divided into the orders of Mucorales and Entomophthorales. The gastrointestinal mucosa is the main portal of entry; *fungal invasion is a common sequel to many mucosal diseases and lesions*, and it may be the precursor to systemic infection. Heavy fungal challenge, disruption of the normal flora, a primary local lesion, and/or lowered host resistance are probably required for establishment of mycotic disease in the gut. Spores are probably normally carried across the mucosa by macrophages, and only if host immunity is compromised in some way will they establish in the deeper tissues or become disseminated.

The most common organisms associated with alimentary tract mycoses are zygomycetes of the family *Mucoraceae* (*Lichtheimia*, *Mortierella*, *Mucor*, *Rhizomucor*, and *Rhizopus*); other organisms that also may be involved include family *Entomophthoraceae* (*Basidiobolus* and *Conidiobolus*) and rarely *Aspergillus* sp., *Candida* spp., and *Histoplasma capsulatum* also may invade the wall of the alimentary canal; these are considered separately later in this chapter. *Mucoraceae* are characterized in their invasive mycelial form by broad (6-25 μm), coarse irregular hyphae, with infrequent septation and random branching, sometimes surrounded by an eosinophilic sleeve in tissue sections. *Entomophthoraceae* hyphae vary from 5 to 25 μm in diameter, with thin irregularly parallel walls, infrequent septa, and rare random branching. They are characteristically surrounded by a wide sheath or sleeve of eosinophilic material in tissue section. *Aspergillus* has relatively uniform narrow (3-6 μm) septate hyphae; it typically displays acute angled dichotomous branching.

Lesions occur anywhere in the gastrointestinal tract, including the forestomachs of ruminants, and in the mesenteric lymph nodes. Clinical signs may be related to the location of lesions (vomition, bloody diarrhea), nonspecific (malaise, weight loss), or entirely absent. Two primary types of lesion are produced: (1) *necrosis and hemorrhage*; or (2) *granulomatous inflammation*.

Mucorales fungi and **Aspergillus** typically cause *hemorrhage and infarction*. Cases in cattle are mostly seen following rumen acidosis caused by grain overload, mastitis, downer cow syndrome, parturition, or subsequent to immunosuppression or prolonged antimicrobial usage. Fungi have been reported in cattle secondary to erosive viral diseases including infectious bovine rhinotracheitis and bovine viral diarrhea, and can cause mycotic abomasitis in calves with bacterial septicemia. These fungi can be found at any level of the gastrointestinal tract; however, the rumen and omasum are the most common sites. *Aspergillus* tends to be most common in the abomasum. These organisms have a propensity to invade mucosal and submucosal veins, producing *thrombosis and venous infarction*. Characteristic gross lesions are focal or multifocal areas of edema and red-black discoloration caused by venous stasis and hemorrhage. Histologic lesions include mucosal to transmural necrosis of the gastrointestinal wall, and there may be a relatively mild inflammatory response to the fungi. Dissemination to the liver and more distant organs via the portal and systemic circulations is not uncommon.

Mycotic ileitis and colitis in cats (*Aspergillus* spp.) has been described, and may be associated with feline parvovirus infection or antibiotic therapy. Intestinal lesions can be subtle, particularly in the face of concurrent intestinal pathogens, but are hemorrhagic and necrotizing with a cellular immune response; dissemination to other organs can also occur and the lung appears to be the favored site in cats. Mycotic enteritis with dissemination is a rare sequel to canine parvovirus-2 enteritis in dogs.

The gastrointestinal tract is probably a common portal of entry for many sporadic, disseminated zygomycoses and aspergillosis in animals. Fungi may produce a localized granulomatous lesion in the Peyer's patches or be carried to the regional mesenteric lymph node while the mucosal lesion heals. The presence of zygomycete fungal hyphae in mesenteric lymph node granulomas of clinically normal feedlot cattle is recognized, and indicates that *invasion by these agents across the intestinal mucosa does not lead invariably to systemic disease*. Grossly, affected lymph nodes are variably enlarged with areas of necrosis and fibrosis evident on the cut surface. Histologically, there is granulomatous inflammation with numerous foreign body and Langhans-type giant cells. The lesions also contain areas of mineralization, variable degrees of fibrosis and PAS and/or GMS-positive fungal hyphae free or within the cytoplasm of giant cells. Asteroid bodies may form around *Aspergillus* spp. or zygomycetes.

Entomophthoromycosis involving the gastrointestinal tract is far less common and sporadic, but has been rarely reported in dogs. *Basidiobolus ranarum* has been associated with subcutaneous, respiratory, or intestinal infections involving the stomach and small intestine, whereas *Condiobolus* sp. has been more commonly associated with cutaneous or rhinofacial and nasopharyngeal lesions in humans, horses, dogs, and sheep. Histologically, there is granulomatous inflammation with thin-walled non- or poorly septate hyphal organisms.

Definitive **diagnosis** of mycotic lesions requires culture, which may be difficult, and molecular genetic identification of the isolate. Granulomatous lesions of the gut should be cultured for fungi as well as bacteria, to increase the frequency of an etiologic diagnosis. Mycotic lymphadenitis must be differentiated from a mycobacterial, actinomycotic, or nocardial lesion. A presumptive diagnosis may be based on morphologic characteristics of organisms in tissue sections. Immunochemical procedures using specific antibody may add to the confidence of a morphologic diagnosis.

Further reading

Njaa BL, et al. Gross lesions of alimentary disease in adult cattle. Vet Clin North Am Food Anim Pract 2012;28:483-513.

Ortega J, et al. Zygomycotic lymphadenitis in slaughtered feedlot cattle. Vet Pathol 2010;47:108.

Candidiasis

Candida spp. are commensal inhabitants of the alimentary and biliary tract of animals, existing as *budding yeasts* in association with mucosal surfaces. With changes in the mucosal surface itself, particularly squamous mucosae, or in the mucosal flora, these yeasts may become opportunistic pathogens and invade as *branching, filamentous pseudohyphae and hyphae that replace the yeast forms. Candida* spp. are occasionally opportunistic invaders of nonsquamous mucosal lesions in the alimentary tract, but other opportunistic fungi are more likely to be associated with nonsquamous lesions, particularly in older animals. *Candidiasis is mainly a disease of keratinized epithelium in young animals, especially pigs, calves, and foals.*

Only a few of the almost 200 *Candida* species cause candidiasis; in animals the most important are **C. albicans** and **C. tropicalis.** Changes in the mucosal flora usually result from systemic antimicrobial therapy that reduces the numbers of anaerobic bacteria and allows proliferation of *Candida* spp. Immunosuppression, environmental and social stress, and treatment with chemotherapeutic, anti-cancer, or anti-inflammatory agents may also predispose to candidiasis. An important factor in the virulence of *Candida* spp., especially C. *albicans*, is the ability to adhere to, colonize, and invade the epithelium. Adherence to the epithelium is mediated by a family of *adhesins* produced by the yeast. *Candida* spp. is a polymorphic fungus that can grow as an ovoid 3-6 μm yeast (with budding), elongated ellipsoid pseudohyphae (chains of tubular yeast) or true hyphae, and binding to the epithelium induces the well-known yeast-to-hypha switch. Epithelial damage may be induced by yeast-produced enzymes, including proteinases and catalases, or by host cell–produced enzymes such as neutrophil myeloperoxidase. These enzymes contribute to local damage, which permits deeper penetration into squamous epithelium and perhaps promote systemic dissemination. Accumulation of keratin caused by anorexia may also contribute to the extensiveness of lesions in all species by increasing the substrate available to the fungus.

In **pigs,** *Candida* spp. often invade the parakeratotic material that accumulates on the *gastric squamous mucosa;* apparently these infections are innocuous. *Thrush* is the term for candidiasis of the oral cavity, which is seen occasionally in young pigs, especially those raised on artificial diets, or in pigs with concurrent disease. Lesions may be confined to the tongue, hard palate, or pharynx, but often involve the esophagus and gastric squamous mucosa as well. Grossly the lesions are yellow-white, smooth, or wrinkled plaques loosely adherent to the mucosa. Histologically, there is vacuolar degeneration of the epithelium, which contains many yeasts, pseudohyphae, hyphae, and pockets of neutrophils and bacteria within and beneath the stratum corneum. Vascular congestion, mild inflammation, and erosion and ulceration of the epithelium may be evident.

In **calves,** candidiasis occurs following prolonged antimicrobial therapy and in association with rumen putrefaction. Lesions are most often seen in the *ventral sac of the rumen*, but may involve the omasum and reticulum and occasionally the abomasum. Grossly the lesions resemble those of *thrush* in pigs, but the keratin layer tends to be thicker, less diffuse, and light gray. Omasal leaves may be adhered together by the mass of fungus-riddled keratin. C. *glabrata* in the abomasum has been implicated as a cause of diarrhea in calves, especially during winter months. Disseminated candidiasis occurs more often in calves than in pigs, probably because of the relatively prolonged survival of calves with alimentary lesions. Candidiasis in calves with prominent ulcers should be differentiated from alimentary herpesviral infections.

Gastroesophageal candidiasis in **foals** also involves the squamous epithelium, and lesions are typically *adjacent to the margo plicatus.* Colic and anorexia can be observed, and are probably related to the development of the ulcers, which may perforate, causing peritonitis.

In **dogs,** *Candida* spp. have been described as the cause of mycotic stomatitis (thrush), peritonitis, and rarely systemic disease or sepsis; these cases have occurred mostly in immunocompromised patients.

In tissues, identification of appropriate lesions composed of foci of necrosis, neutrophilic inflammation, and the presence of one or more of the yeast's polymorphic forms permits a provisional identification of *Candida* spp. Silver or periodic acid-Schiff stain enhances the organisms in section.

Further reading

Bradford K, et al. *Candida* peritonitis in dogs: report of 5 cases. Vet Clin Pathol 2013;42:227-233.

Calderone RA, Fonzi WA. Virulence factors of *Candida albicans*. Trends Microbiol 2001;9:327-335.

Mayer FL, et al. *Candida albicans* pathogenicity mechanisms. Virulence 2013;15:119-128.

Williams DW, et al. Interactions of *Candida albicans* with host epithelial surfaces. J Oral Microbiol 2013;5:10.3402.

Intestinal histoplasmosis

Histoplasma capsulatum is a *dimorphic soil-borne fungus* existing in the environment as a mycelial form and in the host as a yeast. Although the fungus has worldwide distribution, histoplasmosis is endemic in certain areas such as the Mississippi, Ohio, and Missouri river valleys of the United States. In Canada, it is thought to be limited to south central Canada, along the Ottawa and St. Lawrence River valleys with only sporadic cases reported elsewhere. It is an important disease of humans and dogs, and occasionally occurs in other species. Infection generally occurs via *inhalation of spores*, and possibly *by ingestion* of microconidia or macroconidia in the mycelial phase that transition to yeast forms within host macrophages in which they resist host defense mechanisms. Immunocompetent individuals probably have self-limiting infections, but animals that are immunocompromised or receive large doses of organism have greater risk of developing disease.

Given the routes of exposure, infection in **dogs** is usually confined to the lungs, but dissemination can occur to the gastrointestinal tract, and less commonly to the skin, bone, liver, spleen, or brain. Rare cases of histoplasmosis confined to the gastrointestinal tract suggest exposure by ingestion, potentially of infected sputum. *Disseminated histoplasmosis* is predominantly a disease of young dogs that are usually presented with weight loss, generalized lymphadenopathy, hemorrhagic diarrhea, and tenesmus. In **cats,** disseminated disease is most common and may involve lungs, lymph nodes, liver, spleen, kidney, adrenal glands, bone marrow, and the gastrointestinal tract; primary *intestinal histoplasmosis* is probably rare in cats. **Horses** appear to be relatively resistant to histoplasmosis, although sporadic cases have been reported in a variety of organs, including the intestine; a single report of disseminated disease has been reported.

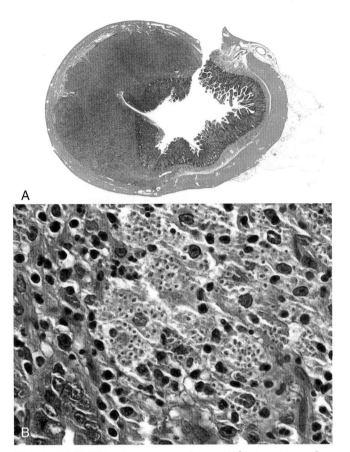

Figure 1-169 Histoplasma capsulatum infection in a dog. A. Marked expansion of the mucosa and submucosa by macrophages containing *H. capsulatum* organisms. **B.** Higher magnification of (**A**) showing *H. capsulatum* organisms within macrophages. (Courtesy J. Caswell.)

Gross intestinal lesions may be absent, or there may be hemorrhagic enteritis of small and/or large intestine, or the lesions mimic neoplasia as they cause granulomatous nodular thickening of the intestinal wall with mucosal ulceration. Mesenteric lymph nodes are often markedly enlarged. Characteristic histologic lesions are *multifocal and coalescing transmural granulomatous inflammation* of the stomach, or small and/or large intestine (Fig. 1-169A). Nonulcerated areas of the mucosa and draining lymph nodes contain multifocal to diffuse infiltrations of macrophages laden with *H. capsulatum* organisms within cytoplasmic vacuoles. Oval to round 2-5 μm diameter yeasts with a characteristic central spherical basophilic body surrounded by a clear halo (Fig. 1-169B) usually can be readily observed with hematoxylin and eosin stain; however, periodic acid-Schiff stain highlights the organisms in tissues. Microscopic diagnosis of gastrointestinal histoplasmosis is not difficult, but grossly the disease must be distinguished from intestinal lymphoma and in the colon, and from colitis of other types. Histoplasmosis is discussed in detail in Vol. 3, Hematopoietic system.

Further reading

Aulakh HK, et al. Feline histoplasmosis: a retrospective study of 22 cases (1986-2009). J Am Anim Hosp Assoc 2012;48:182-187.

Bromel C, et al. Histoplasmosis in dogs and cats. Clin Tech Small Anim Pract 2005;20:227-232.

Schumacher LL, et al. Canine intestinal histoplasmosis containing hyphal forms. J Vet Diagn Invest 2013;25:304-307.

Pythiosis

Although it develops mycelium as do fungi, *Pythium insidiosum* is a fungus-like aquatic oomycete more closely related to diatomeae and algae, and not a true fungus. It has relatively narrow (up to 9-10 μm), thick-walled hyphae, with almost parallel walls, near right-angle branching, and occasional septa. Pythiosis (oomycosis) occurs most commonly in apparently immunocompetent individuals in tropical and subtropical areas, but on occasion can be found in more temperate climates. *P. insidiosum* zoospores display chemotaxis toward animal hair, intestinal mucosa, and wounds, including those caused by insect bites. Therefore lesions commonly involve body parts with direct contact with water containing zoospores.

Best recognized as a cause of *cutaneous lesions in horses* (see Vol. 1, Integumentary system), *P. insidiosum* can cause distinct disease forms including vascular, ocular, gastrointestinal, and rarely systemic disease mostly in dogs and horses but sporadically in calves and sheep. In contrast to horses, the gastrointestinal form is the most common form in dogs, likely acquired by drinking contaminated water. Concurrent cutaneous and gastrointestinal lesions in the same animal are rare. There is segmental thickening and ulceration of the stomach, small intestine, and/or colon, and mesenteric lymph nodes are enlarged and frequently embedded in a granulomatous mass. Small firm white or yellow necrotic coagula, known as *leeches* or *kunkers*, may be embedded in the firm fibrotic reactive tissue.

Histologically, there is multifocal to transmural pyogranulomatous inflammation that may cause obstruction, lymphangitis, lymphadenitis, and sometimes peritonitis with omental adhesions. Granulomas and a local mixed inflammatory infiltrate, including eosinophils, are prominent in some cases. In contrast to zygomycetes, characteristic hyphae are difficult to see with hematoxylin and eosin stain; 3-7 μm-wide hyphae with nondichotomous irregular branching and rarely septate filaments are best exposed, in the areas of necrosis or centers of granulomas, using *silver stains*. Similar lesions are reported in horses, sheep, and cats. A diagnosis of pythiosis should be confirmed by identifying the agent using culture, serology, or PCR.

Further reading

Gaastra W, et al. *Pythium insidiosum*: An overview. Vet Microbiol 2010;146:1-16.

Grooters AM. Pythiosis, lagenidiosis, and zygomycosis in small animals. Vet Clin North Am Small Anim Pract 2003;33:695-720.

Pessoa CRM, et al. Pythiosis of the digestive tract in sheep. J Vet Diagn Invest 2012;24:1133-1136.

Protothecal enterocolitis

Prototheca spp. are *colorless unicellular opportunistic algae* that in some scenarios can be pathogenic for humans and animals. They are ubiquitous in some environmental niches including raw and treated sewage, water, feces, plant sap, and tree slime; they also can be contaminants of various substrates including cow's milk. Two species, **P. zopfii** and **P. wickerhamii**, cause disease in animals with both occurring occasionally in the same animal.

Lesions caused by *Prototheca* spp. are predominantly *cutaneous* infections of cats and human, *mastitis* in cows, and *gastrointestinal* or *disseminated* infections in dogs. The **pathogenesis** of prototothecosis is not completely understood. Traumatic inoculation is thought to lead to cutaneous infection in humans and cats. An environmental pathogen in dairy cows, *P. zopfii* probably gains access to the mammary gland by invasion of the teat canal. In dogs, the colon has been proposed as a primary site of infection, with dissemination to other organs, including eyes, brain, liver, kidneys, bone marrow, and skin. The prognosis following dissemination in dogs is usually considered poor.

Factors predisposing to the development of intestinal protothecosis are poorly understood. Immunosuppression may account for the sporadic incidence of disease in dogs; Collies and Boxer dogs have been overrepresented in some reports, suggesting breed-related susceptibility. Perhaps *Prototheca* spp. is an opportunistic invader of existing mucosal lesions. Cattle, horses, and wild pigs pass *Prototheca* spp. in the feces without apparent clinical disease.

Clinical signs in dogs often include chronic, episodic, and intractable, hemorrhagic large-bowel diarrhea, with progressive weight loss. *Hemorrhagic and ulcerative colitis* is the first and most consistent enteric lesion. In dogs with disseminated disease intestinal lesions may be subtle; dissemination via the hematogenous or lymphatic route most commonly affects the eyes, central nervous system, kidneys, and heart. Mesenteric lymph nodes may be enlarged. **Histologically,** the cellular host inflammatory response to infection can vary; granulomatous to pyogranulomatous ulcerative colitis is typical. Intracellular and extracellular algal organisms are observed in variable numbers, depending on the severity of disease in affected tissue. In cases of disseminated disease, granulomas containing organisms can be found in various organs.

Prototheca in tissue sections stained with hematoxylin and eosin can be difficult to visualize; periodic acid-Schiff or silver stains are helpful. The algae are unicellular, nonbudding, round to oval spherules with a refractile capsule, and range in size from 5-12 μm (*P. wickerhamii*) to 10-25 μm (*P. zopfii*). The presence of multiple wedge-shaped endospores within a single sporangium characterizes *Prototheca* spp. Other potentially pathogenic algal organisms that also undergo endosporulation such as *Chlorella* contain periodic acid-Schiff–positive cytoplasmic starch granules that are PAS-negative after diastase digestion; this test can be helpful for differentiation of these organisms. Culture, cytology, and fluorescent antibody tests are also helpful ancillary diagnostic techniques.

Further reading

Hollingsworth SR. Canine protothecosis. Vet Clin North Am Small Anim Pract 2000;30:1091-1101.

Osterstock JB, et al. Prototothecal enteritis as a cause of protein-losing enteropathy in a bull. J Am Vet Med Assoc 2005;227:1476-1479.

Stenner VJ, et al. Protothecosis in 17 Australian dogs and a review of the canine literature. Med Mycol 2007;45:249-266.

Gastrointestinal helminthosis

Helminths are parasitic organisms that cause a wide variety of diseases in animals. They can be classified into nematodes (roundworms), trematodes (flukes), and cestodes (tapeworms). The diagnosis of disease resulting from gastrointestinal helminths must be made with knowledge of their pathogenic potential and the mechanisms by which it is expressed. *Parasites are much more common than the diseases they cause*, and "helminthiasis," *the state of infection*, must be clearly differentiated from "helminthosis," *the state of disease.*

According to their action on the host and pathogenesis of disease, gastrointestinal helminths fall into 5 *categories*:

1. The first group, including some nematodes and cestodes, **resides free in the lumen of the intestine**, competing with the host for nutrients in the gut content. They are generally of low pathogenicity, except for rare massive infections, and are not likely to be lethal, except by obstruction. Some of these worms, in sufficient numbers, may cause subclinical disease such as inefficient growth, or clinical disease in the form of ill-thrift; others are essentially nonpathogenic. The ascarids, adult small strongyles (cyathostomes) of horses, and tapeworms such as *Moniezia* and *Taenia* spp., fall into this group, as may *Physaloptera* in the stomach of carnivores.

2. A second group of helminths, all nematodes, primarily cause **blood loss**. These worms feed on the mucosa causing bleeding, or they actively suck blood. Anemia, hypoproteinemia, and their sequelae cause production loss, clinical disease, and death. *Haemonchus* in the abomasum, and in the intestine the hookworms of carnivores and ruminants, the large strongyles of horses, and *Oesophagostomum radiatum* in cattle are the main examples.

3. The third group, composed of nematodes and some flukes, mainly causes **protein-losing gastroenteropathy**, usually associated with inappetence and diarrhea. In the abomasum, *Ostertagia* and *Trichostrongylus axei* cause mucous metaplasia and hyperplasia of gastric glands, achlorhydria, and diarrhea. In the small intestine, *Cooperia*, *Nematodirus*, *Strongyloides*, *Trichostrongylus*, and larval paramphistomes in sheep and cattle cause villus atrophy. This may cause malabsorption of nutrients, electrolytes, and water. But probably more important is the loss of endogenous protein into the gut, mainly related to chronic mucosal inflammation. In heavy infestations with *Trichuris* spp., erosion results in loss of absorptive function, and effusion of tissue fluids, or in severe cases, hemorrhagic exudate.

4. The fourth group, composed of nematodes and trematodes, causes **physical trauma to the intestinal wall** by burrowing into or inciting inflammatory foci in the submucosa or deeper layers. In the stomach, various species of spirurids embed in the mucosa, or establish in cystic spaces in the submucosa. In the intestine, acanthocephala cause local ulceration by their thorny hold-fast organ; larval stages of equine cyathostomes and *Oesophagostomum* spp. become encapsulated in the submucosa. Protein loss may occur from ulcerated areas, or when larvae emerge from the submucosa. The potential exists for perforation of the stomach or bowel, or for complications caused by sepsis of submucosal nodules. Adhesion of inflamed serosal surfaces associated with nodules or perforations may impair motility.

5. Finally, some intestinal helminths, among them a few in the categories above, have **effects at sites distant from the gut**. This is usually the result of migrating larval stages of the worm, either in definitive or intermediate hosts. Larval *Habronema*, ascarids, hookworms, and equine strongyles

may cause lesions in a variety of extraintestinal sites in the definitive host. Larval ascarids and taeniid metacestodes may cause lesions or signs because of migration in nonenteric locations in accidental or intermediate hosts.

A **diagnosis of helminthosis** should be reserved for cases in which, ideally, 3 criteria are met: (1) the helminth is present, in numbers consistent with disease; (2) the lesions (if any) typically caused by the agent, are evident; and (3) there is a syndrome compatible with the pathogenic mechanisms known to be associated with the worm.

Further reading

Anderson RC. Nematode Parasites of Vertebrates – Their Development and Transmission. 2nd ed. Wallingford, Oxon, UK: CAB International; 2000.

Ashford RW. Current usage of nomenclature for parasitic diseases, with special reference to those involving arthropods. Med Vet Entomol 2001;15:121-125.

Charlier J, et al. Gastrointestinal nematode infections in adult dairy cattle: impact on production, diagnosis and control. Vet Parasitol 2009;164:70-79.

Gardiner CH, Poynton SL. An Atlas of Metazoan Parasites in Animal Tissue. Washington, DC: Armed Forces Institute of Pathology; 1999.

Garijo Toledo M, et al. Atlas de patología parasitaria en rumiantes. Barcelona: Merial Laboratorios S.A.; 2012. p. 232-264.

Taylor MA. Emerging parasitic diseases of sheep. Vet Parasitol 2012; 189:2-7.

Abomasal and gastric helminthosis

Ostertagiosis. A complex of related genera and species of trichostrongylid nematodes, including *Ostertagia*, parasitize the *abomasum of ruminants*. The nomenclature of these worms is in a state of flux; for the sake of simplicity, the disease that they cause will be termed ostertagiosis. *Ostertagiosis is probably the most important parasitism in grazing sheep and cattle in temperate climatic zones throughout the world.* It causes subclinical loss in production, and clinical disease characterized by diarrhea, wasting, and in many cases, death. **Ostertagia ostertagi** and the associated O. *lyrata* infect cattle. Sheep and goats are infected by **Teladorsagia circumcincta** (formerly *Ostertagia circumcincta*). Some cross-infection by these genera occurs between sheep and cattle, but is of minor significance. Other species of *Ostertagia* and related genera, including *Marshallagia*, *Spiculopteragia*, and *Camelostrongylus*, infect wild ruminants, including farmed deer; some may also parasitize the abomasum of cattle, sheep, and goats. Their behavior in general resembles that of *Ostertagia* and *Teladorsagia*.

The life cycle is direct. Third-stage larvae ex-sheath in the rumen and enter glands in the abomasum, where they undergo two molts. Normally early fifth-stage larvae emerge to mature on the mucosal surface, beginning 8-12 days after infection in *T. circumcincta* infections in sheep, and ~17-21 days after O. *ostertagi* infection in cattle. However, a proportion of larvae ingested may persist in glands in a hypobiotic state at the early fourth stage, only to resume development and emerge at a future time, perhaps many months hence. The prepatent period is ~3 weeks.

During the course of larval development, the normal architecture of the gastric mucosa is altered by *interstitial inflammation*, and *mucous metaplasia and hyperplasia of the epithelium*

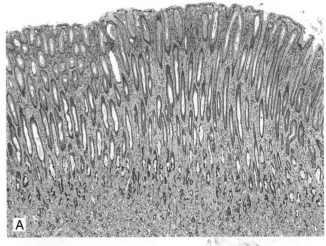

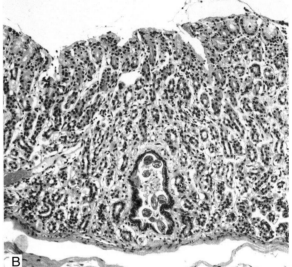

Figure 1-170 **Ostertagiosis in the bovine abomasum. A.** Mucous metaplasia and hyperplasia of fundic mucosa on abomasal fold. **B.** Multiple larval sections in abomasal gland. (Courtesy J. Ortega-Porcel.)

lining glands. In sheep infected with *T. circumcincta*, mucous metaplasia and hyperplasia occur in infected and surrounding glands early in infection, reaching a peak about the time of emergence of larvae on to the mucosal surface. In cattle with O. *ostertagi*, only glands infected with larvae undergo significant mucous change until about the time larvae leave the glands for the surface of the mucosa (Fig. 1-170A, B). Mucosal change then becomes more widespread, involving uninfected glands in the vicinity of those that contained larvae.

Affected areas of mucosa thicken. In infected glands, in many cases the lining is flattened adjacent to worms, but is composed of tall columnar mucous cells elsewhere in the gland. The undifferentiated mucous cells lining uninfected glands also eventually differentiate into tall columnar mucous cells. If infection is not heavy, lesions are limited to a radius of a few millimeters around infected or previously infected glands. These form raised nodular pale areas in the mucosa, often with a slightly depressed center. Confluence of these lesions in heavily infected animals leads to the development of *widespread areas of irregularly thickened mucosa with a*

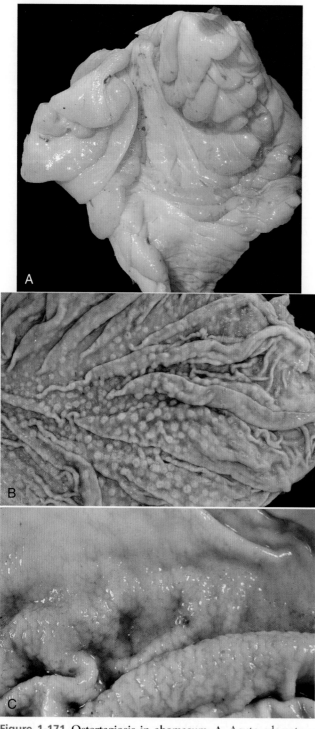

Figure 1-171 Ostertagiosis in abomasum. A. Acute edematous abomasitis in a cow. (Courtesy E. Odriozola.) **B.** Multifocal to coalescent nodules in a sheep. (Courtesy J. Corpa-Arenas.) **C.** Confluent thickening of hyperplastic glandular mucosa in a sheep.

convoluted surface pattern, likened to *Morocco leather* (Fig. 1-171A-C).

Mucous metaplasia and hyperplasia are accompanied by a mixed population of inflammatory cells in the lamina propria. Lymphocytes, plasma cells, eosinophils, and a few neutrophils are present between glands in the infected abomasum, and globule leukocytes are common in gland epithelium. There

may be edema of the lamina propria associated with permeability of proprial vessels. Lymphoid response in local lymph nodes has been characterized as primarily B-cell–oriented, which is a surprising reaction to a nematode parasite.

Mucosal lesions lead to achlorhydria, elevation of plasma pepsinogen levels, and local vascular permeability with loss of plasma protein. Widespread replacement of parietal cells by mucous neck cells results in progressive and massive decline in hydrogen ion secretion, with severe cases having a pH of up to 7 or more. This increased abomasal pH results in elevated levels of gastrin in the circulation. The permeability of the mucosa is also increased, which is reflected in back-diffusion of pepsinogen from the lumen of glands to the propria, and ultimately to the circulation. Intercellular junctions between poorly differentiated mucous neck cells are also permeable to plasma protein in tissue fluids, emanating from the leaky small vessels in the inflamed lamina propria. Significant loss of protein occurs into the lumen of the abomasum.

The cardinal signs of ostertagiosis in sheep and cattle are *loss of appetite, diarrhea, and wasting.* Plasma protein loss into the gastrointestinal tract, in combination with reduced feed intake, seems largely responsible for the weight loss and hypoproteinemia that occur in clinical ostertagiosis, and for loss in productive efficiency that occurs in subclinical disease.

Clinical ostertagiosis occurs under 2 sets of circumstances. The first, **"type I" disease,** is seen in lambs or calves at pasture during or shortly after a period of high availability of *infective larvae.* It is due to the direct development, from ingested larvae, of large numbers of adult worms, over a relatively short period of time and it is characterized by chronic gastritis. In contrast, **"type II" disease** is characterized by acute gastritis due to the synchronous maturation and emergence of large numbers of *hypobiotic larvae* from the mucosa, and it occurs when intake of larvae is likely low or nonexistent. It may occur in yearlings during the winter in the northern hemisphere, or during the dry summer period in Mediterranean climates. Heifers about the time of parturition may succumb, and this syndrome also is seen occasionally in animals experiencing environmental stress of any type.

The **diagnosis** of ostertagiosis is indicated at autopsy by an *abnormally elevated abomasal pH* (>4.5) in association with *typical gross lesions* on the mucosa. The adult worms are brown and thread-like, up to 1.5 cm long, but very difficult to see on the mucosa with the unaided eye. *Abomasal contents and washings* should be quantitatively examined for the presence of emergent or adult *Ostertagia* and other nematodes. A *portion of the mucosa should be digested* to permit recovery and quantitation of pre-emergent stages. Significant worm burdens in sheep are in the range of 10,000-50,000 or more. In cattle >40,000-50,000 adult worms may be present, and in outbreaks of type II disease, hundreds of thousands of hypobiotic larvae are often detected in the abomasal mucosa. Typically there is widespread mucous metaplasia and hyperplasia in dilated glands in sections of abomasum. *Ostertagia* are recognized in sections, on the mucosal surface or in glands, by the presence of prominent longitudinal cuticular ridges (synlophe) that project from the surface of worms cut transversely. In some cases the worm burden may have been lost through attrition or recent treatment, and the diagnosis must be presumptive, based on the characteristic mucosal lesions.

A positive association between *O. ostertagi* antibodies and the presence of abomasal lesions was found in cattle and it has been suggested that measurement of *O. ostertagi* serum antibodies may be a useful indicator of parasite-associated abomasal lesions. Abomasal lesions produced by *Ostertagia* are accompanied by a marked hypergastrinemia and increased level of plasma pepsinogen, both of which are occasionally used as diagnostic tools for ostertagiosis.

Further reading

Forbes AB, et al. Associations between blood gastrin, ghrelin, leptin, pepsinogen and *Ostertagia ostertagi* antibody concentrations and voluntary feed intake in calves exposed to a trickle infection with *O. ostertagi*. Vet Parasitol 2009;162:295-305.

Garijo Toledo M, et al. Atlas de patología parasitaria en rumiantes. Barcelona: Merial Laboratorios S.A.; 2012. p. 232-264.

Larraillet L, et al. Abattoir survey of abomasal lesions associated with ostertagiosis in adult cattle. Vet Rec 2012;171:299-300.

Simpson HV, et al. Effects of *Teladorsagia (Ostertagia) circumcincta* infection on lambs selected for high fleece weight. Vet Parasitol 2009;165:256-264.

Szyszka O, et al. Do the changes in the behaviours of cattle during parasitism with *Ostertagia ostertagi* have a potential diagnostic value? Vet Parasitol 2013;193:214-222.

Hemonchosis. Hemonchosis is a common and severe disease in some parts of the world. *Haemonchus* species require a period of minimum warmth and moisture for larval development on pasture. As a result, they tend to be *most important in tropical or temperate climates with hot wet summers*. **Haemonchus contortus** infects mainly sheep and goats, whereas **H. placei** occurs mainly in cattle. Although *H. contortus* and *H. placei* will infect the heterologous host, the host-parasite relationship appears to be less well adapted, and the species do appear to be genetically distinct. Other species of *Haemonchus* can infect several ruminant species but they are of less clinical significance. **Mecistocirrus digitatus** causes disease very similar to hemonchosis in cattle, buffalo, and sheep in Southeast Asia and Central America.

By exploitation of hypobiosis or retardation of larvae, populations of *H. contortus* are able to persist in the abomasum of the host through periods of climatic adversity, such as excessive cold or dryness. Disease can be expected in animals, especially females, experiencing the synchronous *"spring rise"* or periparturient development and maturation of previously hypobiotic larvae, and in young animals heavily stocked at pasture during periods of optimal larval development and availability.

Haemonchus, commonly called the *large stomach worm, or barber pole worm*, is ~2 cm long. Females give the species its common name by their red color, against which the white ovaries and uterus stand out. The male is a little shorter and uniform deep red. These worms are equipped with a buccal tooth or lancet, and *fourth-stage and adult worms suck blood*. Ingested third-stage larvae enter glands in the abomasum, where they molt to the fourth stage and persist as hypobiotic larvae, or from which they emerge as late fourth-stage larvae to continue development in the lumen. The prepatent period for *H. contortus* in sheep is ~15 days; for *H. placei* in cattle is ~26-28 days; and for *M. digitatus* is ~61-79 days.

Hemonchosis may occur as *peracute or acute disease*, resulting from the maturation or intake of large numbers of larvae. It may cause more insidious *chronic disease* if worm burdens are lower. The pathogenicity of *Haemonchus* infection, whatever its manifestation, is the result of blood-sucking activity, which causes anemia and hypoproteinemia.

Individual *Haemonchus* worms in sheep cause the loss of ~0.05 mL of blood per day. Of the order of one tenth to one fourth of the erythrocyte volume may be lost per day by heavily infected lambs; the plasma loss is concomitant and may be several hundreds of milliliters. The potential for the *rapid onset of profound anemia and hypoproteinemia* in heavily infected animals is obvious. Such animals succumb quickly, some even before the maturation of the worm burden. Less heavily infected animals may be able to withstand the anemia and hypoproteinemia for a period of time. They compensate by expanding erythropoiesis 2-fold to 3-fold, and increasing hepatic synthesis of plasma protein. However, they are unable to compensate adequately for the enteric iron loss, despite intestinal reabsorption of a proportion of the excess, and they ultimately succumb some weeks later to *iron-loss anemia*, when iron reserves are depleted. Low-level infections may contribute to subclinical loss of production or ill-thrift through chronic enteric protein and iron loss. Low protein rations compound the effect of infection.

The clinical syndrome may vary somewhat. Some animals are found dead, without the owner observing illness. Others lack exercise tolerance, fall when driven, or are reluctant to stand or move, so weak are they from anemia. Edema of dependent portions, especially the submandibular area or head in grazing animals, is often observed (Fig. 1-172). In primary hemonchosis there is no diarrhea; diarrhea may occur if intercurrent infection with large numbers of other gastrointestinal helminths occurs.

The **postmortem** appearance of animals with hemonchosis is dominated by the extreme pallor of anemia, apparent on the conjunctiva and throughout the internal tissues. The liver is pale and friable. There is usually edema of subcutaneous tissues and mesenteries, with hydrothorax, hydropericardium, and ascites reflecting the severe hypoproteinemia. The abomasal content is usually fluid, and dark red-brown because of the presence of blood. The abomasal rugae may be edematous because of hypoproteinemia, and focal areas of hemorrhage are evident over the surface. In animals that are not decomposing, the worms will be evident to the naked eye (Fig. 1-173): if alive, writhing on the mucosal surface; if dead, less obvious and free in the content. Lymph nodes draining

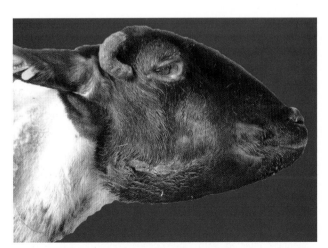

Figure 1-172 Severe **submandibular edema** (bottle-jaw) in **Haemonchus contortus** infection in a sheep. (Courtesy V. Psychas.)

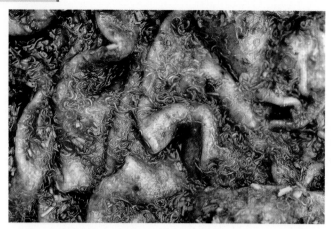

Figure 1-173 *Haemonchus contortus* in abomasal content in a sheep. (Courtesy V. Psychas.)

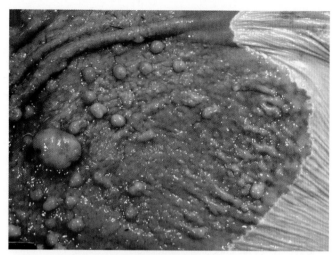

Figure 1-174 Hypertrophic gastritis in the glandular mucosa of a horse with trichostrongylosis. (Courtesy P. Stromberg.)

the abomasum may double in weight within 5 days of infection.

Microscopically, there is abomasitis with increased numbers of mucosal and submucosal lymphocytes, eosinophils and mast cells. Leukocyte levels in the abomasal mucosa peak 5 days after infection, and then may decrease; however, mast cell numbers remain high. Sheep that are resistant to *H. contortus* may have more numerous mucosal mast cells. Abomasal lymph nodes undergo rapid lymphocyte (CD4+ T cell) proliferation. Edema in many organs and centrilobular hepatic necrosis owing to anemia and resultant hypoxia can be seen.

In clinically affected sheep and goats, usually 1,000-12,000 worms are found. The severity of the disease is a function of the number of worms and to some extent, the size of the animal In lambs, 2,000-3,000 worms is a heavy burden, whereas in adult sheep and goats, 8,000-10,000 are associated with fatal infection.

A high egg count is usually found on fecal flotation because *Haemonchus* is a prolific egg-layer. However, in peracute prepatent infections, no eggs will be present in feces. In recently treated animals, no worms may be present, and the diagnosis may have to be presumptive. On the other hand, treated animals returned to contaminated pasture may succumb to reinfection within 2-3 weeks. A serologic test targeting a somatic antigen has been developed.

Further reading

Alba-Hurtado F, Muñoz-Guzmán MA. Immune responses associated with resistance to haemonchosis in sheep. Biomed Res Int 2013;2013:162158.

Garijo Toledo M, et al. Atlas de patología parasitaria en rumiantes. Barcelona: Merial Laboratorios S.A.; 2012. p. 232-264.

MacKinnon KM, et al. Effects of *Haemonchus contortus* on the humoral and cellular immune response of parasite-resistant hair sheep. Vet Immunol Immunopathol 2009;128:288-289.

Rowe JB, et al. The effect of haemonchosis and blood loss into the abomasum on digestion in sheep. Br J Nutr 1988;59:125-139.

Subhadra S, et al. Development and validation of real-time PCR for rapid detection of *Mecistocirrus digitatus*. PLoS ONE 2013;8:e63019.

Yacob HT, et al. Parasitological and clinical responses of lambs experimentally infected with *Haemonchus contortus* (L3) with and without ivermectin treatment. Vet Parasitol 2009;166:119-123.

Trichostrongylus axei infection. *Trichostrongylus axei* infects the *abomasum of cattle, sheep, and goats*, and the *stomach of horses*. It has a direct life cycle: Third-stage infective larvae enter tunnels in the epithelium of the foveolae and neck of gastric glands in both fundic and pyloric areas. The worms live throughout their life *partly embedded in intraepithelial tunnels* at about this level of the mucosa. They molt to the fourth stage about a week after being ingested and to the fifth stage by ~2 weeks after infection. The prepatent period is ~3 weeks in calves and sheep, and ~25 days in horses.

Infections with *T. axei* are usually part of a *mixed gastrointestinal helminthosis*, mostly with *Ostertagia* spp. in ruminants. However, in all hosts this species alone is capable of inducing disease, if present in sufficient numbers. After a period of several weeks, *mucous metaplasia and hyperplasia are seen in glands in infected areas of the mucosa*. In severely affected animals, flattening of surface epithelium with desquamation, or erosion of the mucosa, develops, accompanied by effusion of neutrophils, eosinophils, and tissue fluid. Fibroplasia may occur in the superficial propria in eroded areas.

In light infestations, there may be no changes visible in the abomasum other than congestion of the mucosa. The gross lesions present in heavy *T. axei* infections reflect the hypertrophy of glands, and superficial erosion. *Circular or irregular raised white plaques or nodules of thickened infected mucosa* are present, often with a thick layer of mucus. Erosions or shallow ulcers may be present. In severe infections, the entire mucosa appears edematous and congested.

Infection in horses is uncommon and is usually related to sharing pasture with sheep or cattle. In chronically infected horses, white raised plaques or nodular areas of mucosa are present, covered by tenacious mucus and surrounded by a zone of congestion (Fig. 1-174). Mucosal lesions may be confluent in heavily infected animals, and erosions and superficial ulceration may be encountered. Infection may extend into the proximal duodenum, where polypoid masses of hypertrophic glandular mucosa are occasionally observed. Plasma pepsinogen levels may be elevated.

Achlorhydria develops in heavily infected sheep and cattle, associated with *diarrhea*, particularly in the latter species. Dehydration may prove severe in scouring calves. Plasma pepsinogen and gastrin levels increase, and hypoproteinemia and *wasting* occur. This suggests that the mucous metaplasia in the glands is associated with increased permeability and that plasma protein loss occurs into the gastrointestinal tract.

Although *T. axei* is not commonly seen as a primary cause of disease in any species, it should be sought at autopsy of animals with signs of wasting and perhaps diarrhea. The typical gross lesions in the stomach are distinctive in horses. In ruminants, they must be differentiated from those caused by *Ostertagia*, with which animals may be infected intercurrently. The worms are very fine, and gastric washes or digestion are required to recover them quantitatively. The *distinctive intraepithelial location of T. axei* in section differentiates it from other nematodes inhabiting the abomasum of ruminants and the stomach of horses.

Further reading

Herd RP. Serum pepsinogen concentrations of ponies naturally infected with *Trichostrongylus axei*. Equine Vet J 1986;18:490-491.

Rehbein S, et al. Prevalence, intensity and seasonality of gastrointestinal parasites in abattoir horses in Germany. Parasitol Res 2013;112:407-413.

Torina A, et al. Study of gastrointestinal nematodes in Sicilian sheep and goats. Ann NY Acad Sci 2004;1026:187-194.

Gastric parasitism in horses. The most common parasites of the equine stomach are *larvae of botflies* of the genus **Gasterophilus**. Although they are not helminths, it is convenient to consider them here. There are 6 species of the genus, the most common ones being **G. intestinalis, G. nasalis,** and **G. haemorrhoidalis,** and the uncommon ones being G. pecorum, G. nigricornis, and G. inermis. The flies deposit the ova on the ends of the coat hairs in the face, intermandibular region, or on the lower body and legs. The eggs hatch spontaneously, or when stimulated by licking. The first-stage larvae penetrate the oral mucosa, molt, emerge, and migrate down the alimentary canal.

Gasterophilus intestinalis usually wander about in tunnels in the superficial mucosa of the cheeks, tongue, or gums for 3-4 weeks before moving to periodontal pockets containing purulent exudate in the gingival sulcus on the lingual aspect of molars, especially in the upper arcade. Here they molt before moving on to the base of the tongue, and to the stomach. This is the most common species, and in the stomach it attaches itself to the squamous mucosa of the cardia to complete its subsequent molts. **G. nasalis** first invade the gums, where they may be associated with pockets of purulent exudate in the interdental spaces, then pass to the stomach and settle on the pyloric mucosa and in the first ampulla of the duodenum. Members of any of these species occasionally may be found attached to the pharynx and esophagus but, except for G. pecorum, which congregates in the pharynx and causes pharyngitis, these preliminary migrations are uneventful for the host. In the summer after the deposition of the ova, the larvae leave the stomach and pass out in the feces to pupate. Those of G. pecorum and G. haemorrhoidalis may attach themselves for a short while to the wall of the rectum.

It is generally assumed that the larvae of *Gasterophilus* have little effect on their host. The larvae fasten themselves to the mucosa by chitinous oral hooks and they bore into the mucosa (Fig. 1-175). They apparently subsist on blood, exudate, and detritus, producing focal erosions and ulcerations at the point of contact. These defects in the cardia are surrounded by a

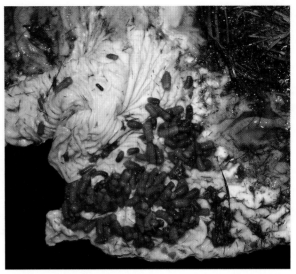

Figure 1-175 *Gasterophilus* **larvae** on gastric mucosa of a horse. (Courtesy A. Barragán.)

narrow rim of hyperplastic squamous epithelium. Usually the number of epithelial defects exceeds the number of larvae, suggesting that they move about on the mucosa.

Severe infestations produce a dense pock-marked appearance of the pars esophagea, with chronic inflammatory thickening. Ulcers may occur in the glandular mucosa and, rarely, a large proportion of the affected pyloric mucosa may be lost. Healing occurs when the larvae migrate on, but may be complicated by secondary bacterial infection. Histologically, the ulcers penetrate the submucosa, which is chronically inflamed. The deep layers of eroded epithelium and the epithelial margins of ulcers in the squamous mucosa become hyperplastic and develop rete pegs. There seems to be no relationship between bot infestations and the development of gastric ulcers in the pars esophagea.

The **spirurid nematodes *Draschia megastoma, Habronema majus,*** and ***H. muscae*** are also parasitic in the stomach of horses. The adult worms are 1-2 cm in length. The latter two species lie on the mucosal surface and are probably insignificant except possibly for a few erosions and mild gastritis. *D. megastoma* burrows into the submucosa to produce large tumor-like nodules (Fig. 1-176).

H. majus mainly uses *Stomoxys calcitrans* as its intermediate host and the other two species use various muscid flies, including the common fly (*Musca domestica*). The *Habronema* larvae in the feces are swallowed by maggots of the appropriate intermediate host and persist through pupation and maturation of the fly. They leave the host fly via the proboscis when it seeks moisture, for instance, on the lips. Larvae deposited on or in cutaneous wounds, or in the eye, invade the skin or conjunctiva and provoke an intense local reaction, which becomes granulomatous and densely infiltrated with eosinophils (see Vol. 1, Integumentary system). Occasionally *Draschia* and *Habronema* larvae may be found in the brain, or in the lungs, where they may become encapsulated and mineralize.

The only one of concern in the stomach is *D. megastoma*, which burrows into the submucosa of the fundus, usually within a few centimeters of the margo plicatus. Within the submucosa, the worms provoke a surrounding granulomatous reaction that contains them in a central core of necrotic and

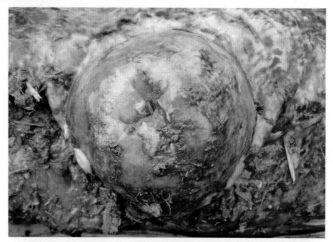

Figure 1-176 Nodules containing *Draschia megastoma* in the glandular region near margo plicatus of the stomach in a horse. (Courtesy L. Minatel.)

cellular detritus, with abundant eosinophils. These lesions form protrusions up to ~5 cm in diameter, with a small fistulous opening to the lumen (see Fig. 1-176). The nodules generally produce no clinical disturbance, though they have been considered to lead rarely to abscessation, adhesions of the stomach to the spleen, or perforation when infected with pyogenic bacteria.

Further reading

Lapointe JM, et al. Septic peritonitis due to colonic perforation associated with aberrant migration of a *Gasterophilus intestinalis* larva in a horse. Vet Pathol 2003;40:338-339.

Schuster RK, et al. Cutaneous and pulmonal habronemosis transmitted by *Musca domestica* in a stable in the United Arab Emirates. Vet Parasitol 2010;174:170-174.

Sequeira JL, et al. Prevalence and macro- and microscopic lesions produced by *Gasterophilus nasalis* (Diptera: Oestridae) in the Botucatu Region, SP, Brazil. Vet Parasitol 2001;102:261-266.

Gastric parasitism in swine. Gastric parasitism is not of great clinical or pathologic importance in swine and is rare in pigs reared in modern total confinement systems. *Ascaris suum*, normally inhabiting the small intestine, may migrate or reflux to the stomach after death. *Hyostrongylus rubidus* is probably the most significant parasite of the stomach of swine; this and the various spirurids are more common in pigs allowed to forage. *Ollulanus tricuspis* is reported in pigs. It is more commonly encountered in cats, and is discussed with gastric parasitism in dogs and cats.

Hyostrongylus rubidus is a trichostrongylid nematode with a typical life cycle. Third-stage larvae enter glands in the stomach, especially in the fundic region, where they develop and molt twice. Pre-adult and adult worms emerge on to the gastric mucosa ~18-20 days after ingestion. The lesions produced by *Hyostrongylus* resemble those caused by *Ostertagia* in ruminants. There is *mucous metaplasia and hyperplasia of the lining of infected and neighboring glands*, and dilation of infected glands. The lamina propria in infected mucosa is edematous and infiltrated by lymphocytes, plasma cells, and eosinophils, and lymphoid follicles develop deep in the mucosa. Neutrophils and eosinophils may transmigrate the

epithelium into dilated glands, the lining of which may become quite attenuated. There may be extensive erosions.

During the course of development of the worms, the mucous metaplasia and hyperplasia cause the formation of pale nodules in the vicinity of infected glands. In heavy infections these may become confluent, causing the development of an irregularly thickened convoluted mucosa, most notable in the fundic area and along the lesser curvature. Adult worms are fine, red, and thread-like in the gastric mucus; they are difficult to see with the naked eye.

Experimental infections of moderate degree do not produce obvious clinical signs or loss of production. However, loss of plasma protein has been documented in heavy *Hyostrongylus* infections. Inappetence, diarrhea, and reduced weight gains and feed efficiency also occur in these circumstances. In the field, hyostrongylosis is mainly associated with the "thin-sow syndrome," in which it seems probable that it may interact with nutritional and metabolic factors.

Spirurid nematodes parasitizing the porcine stomach include *Physocephalus sexalatus*, *Ascarops strongylina*, *A. dentate*, and *Simondsia paradoxa*. *Physocephalus* and *Ascarops* use dung beetles as intermediate hosts. **Ascarops** and **Physocephalus** are common in many parts of the world in swine with access to grazing. Large numbers of worms are required to cause ill-thrift. Worms in affected pigs may be free in the lumen or partly embedded in the mucosa, which may be congested and edematous, or eroded and ulcerated with fibrinous exudate on the surface. There may be chronic interstitial inflammation and fibrosis in the mucosa. **Simondsia** is found in swine in Europe, Asia, and Australia. The caudal portion of the female worm is globular, and is embedded in palpable nodules up to 6-8 mm in diameter in the gastric mucosa. *Gnathostoma doloresi* causes gastric ulcers and granulomas in pigs in eastern Asia. *G. hispidum* may cause lesions in the liver, and submucosal nodules in the gastric wall of pigs, similar to those produced by *G. spinigerum* in carnivores.

Further reading

Chowdhury N, et al. Development of some larval nematodes in experimental and natural animal hosts: an insight into development of pathological lesions vis-a-vis host-parasite interactions. Sci World J 2013;2013:162538.

Fernandez-de-Mera IG, et al. Wild boar helminths: risks in animal translocations. Vet Parasitol 2003;115:335-341.

Stewart TB, et al. Experimental infections with *Hyostrongylus rubidus* and the effects on performance of growing pigs. Vet Parasitol 1985;17:219-227.

Gastric parasitism in dogs and cats. Parasites are uncommonly encountered in the stomach of dogs and cats at autopsy and most are incidental findings, or postmortem migrants from the intestine.

Gnathostoma spinigerum, G. binucleatum, and G. procyonis occur in the stomach of dogs and cats, and of a variety of nondomestic carnivores. It is more common in areas with warm climates. The life cycle of this spirurid nematode involves copepods as an aquatic invertebrate intermediate host, and a variety of fish, amphibian, or reptiles as second intermediate or paratenic hosts. Ingested third-stage larvae may migrate in the liver, leaving tracks of necrotic debris, which eventually heal by fibrosis. In heavy infections, lesions associated with larval migration may be found elsewhere in the abdominal and pleural cavities, and in the skin. Adults are found in groups of up to 10 in nodules in the gastric submucosa. Nodules are up to ~5 cm in diameter, and open into the gastric lumen. Portions of nematodes may protrude through this opening. The worms lie in a pool of blood-tinged purulent exudate in the lumen of the nodule, the wall of which is comprised of granulation tissue and reactive fibrous stroma. Focal granulomas may center on nematode ova trapped in the connective tissue. Infection with *Gnathostoma* is usually subclinical; however, illness and death may be associated with disturbance of motility, chronic vomition, and occasional rupture of verminous nodules on to the gastric serosa, leading to peritonitis.

A number of species of **Physaloptera,** including *P. praeputialis* (cat), *P. rara* (dogs and wild canids and felids), and *P. canis* (dog) are found in the stomach of dogs and cats. These spirurid nematodes use arthropod intermediate hosts and probably some vertebrate transport hosts. The adult worms, which may be mistaken for small ascarids, are found in the stomach, where they may be free in the lumen. More commonly they are attached as individuals or in small clusters to the gastric mucosa. Ulcers may be formed, and the cranial end of the worm may be embedded in the submucosa. Hyaline periodic acid-Schiff–positive material surrounds the cranial end of some worms, perhaps anchoring them in the tissue. These nematodes are not highly pathogenic, although heavy burdens may have the potential to cause significant gastric damage and chronic vomition.

Cylicospirura felineus and members of the genus **Cyathospirura** may be found in the stomach of domestic and wild felids. *Cylicospirura* are usually found in the submucosal nodules, similar to those formed by *Gnathostoma*, whereas *Cyathospirura* is usually found free in the lumen, or sometimes associated with *Cylicospirura* in gastric nodules. The life cycle is unknown; the pathogenicity of these species is poorly defined, but is likely low.

Ollulanus tricuspis is a small trichostrongyle, ~1 mm long, which inhabits the stomach of cats and swine. It is viviparous, and third-stage larvae developing in the uterus of the female are transmitted in vomitus. As a result, infection is usually not detected by fecal examination, and infection with this species may go unnoticed. In some parts of the world it is common, particularly in cat colonies and cats that roam. Clinical signs and gross lesions caused by O. *tricuspis* are uncommon. *Vomition, anorexia,* and *weight loss* are the signs most frequently associated with infection. The worms lie beneath the mucus on the surface of the stomach, or partly in gastric glands. Infection is associated with increased numbers of lymphoid follicles deep in the gastric mucosa, increased interstitial connective tissue in the mucosa, and numerous globule leukocytes in the gastric epithelium. Heavy infection results in mucous metaplasia and hyperplasia of gastric glands, causing the surface of the stomach to be thrown into thickened convoluted folds, grossly resembling idiopathic hypertrophic gastritis of dogs. Gastric glands are often separated by the heavy reactive fibrous stroma in the mucosa. In gastric biopsies, this suite of microscopic changes in the mucosa should be recognized as characteristic of *Ollulanus* infection, even if worms are not present. *Ollulanus* are characterized in section by the numerous longitudinal cuticular ridges (synlophe) recognized as projections on the surface of sectioned worms.

Further reading

Alvarez-Guerrero C, et al. *Gnathostoma binucleatum*: Pathological and parasitological aspects in experimentally infected dogs. Exp Parasitol 2011;127:84-89.

Cecchi R, et al. Demonstration of *Ollulanus tricuspis* in the stomach of domestic cats by biopsy. J Comp Pathol 2006;134:374-377.

Eckstrand CD, et al. Nematode-associated intramural alimentary nodules in pumas are histologically similar to gastrointestinal eosinophilic sclerosing fibroplasia of domestic cats. J Comp Pathol 2013;148:405-409.

Ibba F, et al. Gastric cylicospirurosis in a domestic cat from Italy. J Fel Med Surg 2013;16:522-526.

Naem S, Asadi R. Ultrastructural characterization of male and female *Physaloptera rare* (Spirurida: Physalopteridae): feline stomach worms. Parasitol Res 2013;112:1983-1990.

Intestinal helminth infections

Strongyloides infection. *Strongyloides* spp. parasitize all species of domestic animals considered here. Ruminants are infected by *S. papillosus;* horses by *S. westeri;* swine mainly by *S. ransomi;* dogs by *S. stercoralis;* and cats by *S. felis, S. planiceps* (= *S. catti*), and *S. stercoralis* in the small intestine, and by *S. tumefaciens* in the colon.

The parasitic worms are parthenogenetic females, which produce larvae capable of direct infection of the host, or of uniquely developing into a facultative free-living generation of males and females. Infection by free-living filariform third-stage larvae takes place by skin penetration, or to a lesser extent by ingestion and probably subsequent penetration of the gastrointestinal mucosa. Larval migration occurs primarily through the naso-frontal region and the lungs, during which larvae are carried up the mucociliary escalator and swallowed before establishing as parasitic adults in the small intestine.

Typically infecting the proximal small intestine of all species, *Strongyloides* larvae *establish and persist within tunnels in the epithelium at the base of villi or in upper crypts* (Fig. 1-177). The nematodes are usually found in the surface epithelium, not beneath the basal lamina. Adult worms are small, only 2-6 mm long, depending on species. In sufficient numbers they cause villus atrophy, often associated with hyperplastic

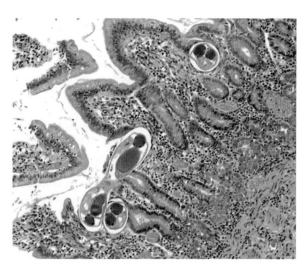

Figure 1-177 Strongyloides westeri in tunnels at base of a moderately atrophic villus in the intestine of a foal with diarrhea.

cryptal epithelium and mixed eosinophilic to lymphocytic inflammation of the lamina propria. Surface epithelial cells are usually low columnar to cuboidal, with an indistinct brush border; there may be squamous metaplasia, or erosions. Embryonated or larvating ova may be retained in epithelial tunnels, and help to distinguish this nematode in tissue section from *Trichostrongylus* in hosts in which both species occur.

Strongyloides ransomi is responsible for *diarrhea in suckling piglets* in some parts of the world. Larvae migrate through the lungs, which may cause minor local hemorrhage, alveolar septal damage, scattered aggregates of lymphocytes and plasma cells and impaired respiration. In the duodenum, villus atrophy results in malabsorption, luminal protein loss, diarrhea, and eventually debilitation of affected piglets. Specific gross lesions other than those associated with diarrhea may be absent. Heavy infestations result in moderate to severe clinical disease in young piglets; adult nematodes are evident in mucosal scrapings at autopsy.

S. westeri infects *foals*, and is associated with diarrhea that can be fatal in heavily infested individuals. It has been hypothesized that skin penetration by third-stage larvae permits entry of *Rhodococcus equi*, an important bacterial pathogen of foals; however, this remains unproven and millions of larvae are necessary to cause fatal infections experimentally.

S. papillosus may cause diarrhea and occasionally death if there is overwhelming infection of *suckling ruminants*. A syndrome of sudden death caused by cardiac failure associated with heavy infections of *S. papillosus* has been described; however, the pathogenesis remains unclear.

S. stercoralis primarily infects dogs. *S. stercoralis* can undergo *autoinfection* in which repeated parasitic generations develop in the same host individual, which can result in rapid expansion of parasitic populations in a host with multi-organ involvement, but this probably only occurs in the face of severe immunosuppression. Infection is most commonly fatal in *puppies* up to 2-3 months old from kennel environments. Affected dogs are dehydrated and emaciated with blood-tinged diarrhea, but the intestine may be grossly unremarkable. *Histologically* there is villus atrophy and mononuclear interstitial infiltrates in the duodenum of affected dogs. Adult nematodes are embedded within the superficial mucosa, and larvae may be observed in granulomas in the intestinal lamina propria and submucosa. Multifocal interstitial pneumonia may be due to pulmonary migration of larvae. *S. stercoralis* also infects humans, and there are rare reports of natural zoonotic transfer from dogs to humans; immunocompromised humans appear to be more susceptible.

S. felis may cause mild focal granulomatous or eosinophilic interstitial pneumonia in **cats**, because of migration of larvae through the lungs. There may be hyperplasia of the crypts of Lieberkühn in the vicinity of worms in the small intestine, but diarrhea is uncommon. *S. tumefaciens* in cats has rarely been associated with chronic diarrhea. It differs from the other species discussed previously, because it causes proliferation of colonic submucosal glands and results in formation of nodules in which the worms are found. It is uncertain whether this lesion is specifically induced by *S. tumefaciens* infection.

Further reading

Dillard KJ, et al. *Strongyloides stercoralis* infection in a Finnish kennel. Acta Vet Scand 2007;49:37-42.

Greaves D, et al. *Strongyloides stercoralis* infection. Brit Med J 2013;347:f4610.

Viney ME. The biology and genomics of *Strongyloides*. Med Microbiol Immunol 2006;195:49-54.

Viney ME, Lok JB. *Strongyloides* spp. (May 23, 2007), WormBook, ed. The *C. elegans* Research Community, WormBook, doi/10.1895/wormbook.1.141.1.

Intestinal trichostrongylosis. Members of the genus *Trichostrongylus* parasitize the *proximal small intestine of ruminants* worldwide. They cause significant subclinical inefficiency in production, or clinical disease characterized by *diarrhea, ill-thrift, and in some cases, death*. The most important species infecting sheep and goats are **T. colubriformis, T. vitrinus,** and **T. rugatus;** others include *T. longispicularis, T. falculatus, T. capricola,* and *T. probolurus. T. colubriformis* and *T. longispicularis* also parasitize cattle. Although some *T. axei* may be found in the duodenum of cattle and sheep, this species is primarily parasitic in the abomasum. Experimental infection studies indicate that the lesions and pathogenesis of disease caused by *Trichostrongylus* species are similar, although some evidence suggests that T. *vitrinus* is more pathogenic than *T. colubriformis* and *T. rugatus.*

Trichostrongylosis is most important in zones with a cool climate at some time of the year, but without extreme winters. It is a significant problem in sheep-grazing areas of New Zealand, Australia, South Africa, South America, and the United Kingdom. The life cycle is direct, and ingested third-stage larvae ex-sheath in the acidic abomasal environment and establish preferentially in the proximal 5-6 meters of the small intestine of sheep. A small proportion of the population colonize the abomasal antral mucosa near the pylorus. The larvae enter tunnels in the superficial intestinal mucosa above the basal lamina at the base of villi, and they persist throughout their life at least partially embedded in the epithelium. Larvae develop over a 2-week period into adults with a prepatent period of 16-18 days.

The disease is marked clinically by variable depression, inappetence, diarrhea, and wasting. Although some local malabsorption of water, electrolytes, and nutrients occurs in the duodenum, it seems unlikely that the absorptive capacity of the remaining small intestine and large bowel would be overwhelmed. Reduced feed consumption and increased loss of endogenous nitrogen into the gut because of considerable effusion of plasma protein into the lumen and exfoliation of the intestinal epithelium, likely play some role in the development of diarrhea. In severe trichostrongylosis, compensation for increased catabolism of plasma protein and mucosal epithelial protein is at the expense of anabolic processes elsewhere in the body; wool and muscle growth are hindered and secondary osteoporosis has been described.

Gross lesions observed in animals succumbing to trichostrongylosis are nonspecific and may include cachexia, dehydration, dark-green diarrhea, serous atrophy of internal fat depots, and atrophy of skeletal muscle. Mesenteric edema and serous effusion into body cavities because of hypoproteinemia is observed, if dehydration is not severe. Mesenteric lymph nodes are enlarged. The intestines are flaccid and the small bowel as well as the large bowel may contain thin watery green foul-smelling feces. The duodenal mucosa may be glistening and pink; however, superimposed postmortem autolysis may rapidly conceal these changes. The proximal third of the small intestine (5-7 meters) contains the bulk of the population of the parasites, and a worm count in the small bowel may reveal 15,000-80,000 *Trichostrongylus* in severe clinical infections; subclinical or mild disease is associated with fewer worms.

The severity of the *histologic lesions* within an individual animal correlates with the local density of worms. The histologic lesion is characterized by *villus atrophy* that may vary considerably in severity. The cause of villus atrophy is unclear, although its likely related to the host mucosal immune response against the parasites. Crypts are hyperplastic, dilated, and elongated; there is goblet cell hyperplasia. The lamina propria is populated by a moderately heavy mixed inflammatory cell population, including lymphocytes, plasma cells, eosinophils, and globule leukocytes, the latter of which are thought to indicate strength of the immune response or repeated infection. The *diagnosis* is based on recovery of substantial populations of *Trichostrongylus* spp. in association with the clinicopathologic syndrome. Mixed infections with other parasitic genera are common.

Further reading

Cardia DFF, et al. Immune response and performance of growing Santa Ines lambs with artificial *Trichostrongylus colubriformis* infections. Vet Parasitol 2011;182:248-258.

Roy EA, et al. The effects of concurrent experimental infections of sheep with *Trichostrongylus colubriformis* and *T. vitrinus* on nematode distributions, numbers and on pathological changes. Parasite 2004;11:293-300.

Trapani F, et al. Histopathological histochemical and immunohistochemical findings of the small intestine in goats naturally infectd by *Trichostrongylus colubriformis*. Vet Parasitol 2013;191:390-393.

Nematodirus and **Cooperia** infection. *Nematodirus* species infect the *proximal third of the small intestine of ruminants*. The most important species are *N. helvetianus*, which infects cattle; *N. spathiger*, *N. filicollis*, and *N. abnormalis*, which infect sheep, goats, and cattle; and *N. battus*, a parasite mainly of sheep, which causes disease in calves.

The life cycle is direct, although infective larvae within eggs of *N. battus* and *N. filicollis* require a period of conditioning by cold (overwintering) before hatching. The epidemiologic pattern is thus one of infection of susceptible lambs during a year because of larvae produced by the previous year's lambs. This has led to devastating outbreaks of spring disease in mostly temperate areas of the world. The larvae of *N. spathiger* and *N. helvetinus* are not delayed in hatching, and their epidemiologic pattern resembles that of *Trichostrongylus* spp. in grazing animals. *Nematodirus* spp. often form part of a mixed population of worms in parasitic gastroenteritis of grazing lambs and calves, although the disease may also occur in confined nonpastured calves. Ingested infective third-stage larvae enter the deeper layers of the mucosa, and perhaps intestinal crypts. Larvae emerge at the fourth or fifth stage to take up residence coiled among the villi, with their caudal ends protruding toward the lumen and do not normally penetrate the epithelium.

Lambs and calves with nematodirosis develop *severe dark-green diarrhea*, anorexia, and wasting that may persist for several weeks before recovering, or they may die acutely. Disease is presumably mainly related to malabsorption and loss of appetite. At autopsy, other than the changes associated with dehydration and cachexia, findings are limited to watery mucoid intestinal contents. The mucosa of the duodenum is usually unremarkable or perhaps hyperemic with excess mucus on the surface. Clinical disease is associated with populations of 10,000-50,000 or more *Nematodirus* adults.

Histologic lesions in the intestine are observed in heavy infections, but are usually milder in comparison with those induced by *Strongyloides* or *Trichostrongylus*. Villus atrophy is characterized by short, stumpy, and perhaps fused or ridge-like surface alterations that may replace the normal villus structures. Crypts are hyperplastic, and appear elongate and dilated. Overlying surface enterocytes may be domed, with loss of the brush border, and irregular nuclear polarity. Biochemically there are reduced levels of mucosal alkaline phosphatase and disaccharidases, and this correlates with the severity of diarrhea in affected sheep. The pathogenesis of villus atrophy is not clear, but as for other strongylids it may be related to the development of a cell-mediated immune response against the nematodes. A moderate mixed inflammatory response with lymphocytes, plasma cells, and eosinophils is evident in the lamina propria.

Cooperia infect the *upper small intestine of ruminants*. The important species include *C. curticei*, mainly in sheep and goats, and *C. pectinata*, *C. punctata*, and *C. oncophora*, mainly in cattle. The latter is regarded as the least pathogenic of the three. Although both sheep and cattle may host mixed burdens of helminths containing or dominated by populations of *Cooperia*, this species seems to be more significant in cattle, especially in cool temperate regions.

Cooperia has a typical trichostrongylid life cycle, but larvae have the capacity to undergo hypobiosis to carry the population through periods of regular climatic adversity. The normal prepatent period is 16-20 days. Like *Nematodirus*, *Cooperia* do not tunnel in the epithelium, but rather brace or coil themselves among villi to maintain their place in the intestine. In light infections, the worms are concentrated in the proximal third of the small intestine. Heavier infections are more evenly distributed along the intestine; this may be because more nematodes cause villus atrophy, and therefore loss of the substrate against which to brace.

Heavy burdens of *Cooperia* in calves, 70,000-80,000 or more nematodes, may be associated with *inappetence, reduced weight gain*, or *weight loss and diarrhea*, with protein-losing enteropathy in experimental infections. Villus atrophy and inflammation are variable; atrophy is concomitant with reductions in the brush-border enzymes, typical of helminthosis. The diagnosis is confirmed by finding large numbers of the fine, coiled *Cooperia* in the small intestine.

Further reading

McCoy MA, et al. Outbreak of *Nematodirus battus* infection in calves. Vet Rec 2004;154:370-371.

Rodrigues RR, et al. Histopathological changes during experimental infections of calves with *Cooperia punctata*. J Helminthol 2004;78:167-171.

Stromberg BE, et al. *Cooperia punctata*: Effect on cattle productivity? Vet Parasitol 2012;183:284-291.

Van Dijk J, Morgan ER. Hatching behavior of *Nematodirus filicollis* in a flock co-infected with *Nematodirus battus*. Parasitol 2009;136:805-811.

Hookworm infection. Members of the family *Ancylostomatidae* infect dogs, cats, ruminants, and swine. Hookworms of the genus *Globocephalus* appear to be of little significance in swine. In dogs, *Ancylostoma caninum*, *A. braziliense*, and *A. ceylanicum* occur. The former is most common in tropical, subtropical, and warm temperate zones of Africa, Australia, Asia, and North America, where adequate humidity for larval development occurs. *A. braziliense* occurs in dogs and cats in the tropics and subtropics, whereas *A. ceylanicum* is found in both species in Sri Lanka and Southeast Asia. *Uncinaria stenocephala* occurs in dogs in cool temperate regions of Europe and North America. *A. tubaeformae* only occurs in the cat.

Ancylostoma spp. are capable of infecting the host by 4 routes: (1) *orally*, with direct development to adult worms in the intestine; (2) by *skin penetration*, resulting in movement through the bloodstream to the lungs, and then by tracheal migration to the pharynx and the intestine; (3) by the *lactogenic* transmission of third-stage larvae mobilized from dormancy in the skeletal muscle of parturient bitches; and (4) occasionally by prenatal *transplacental* transmission of mobilized larvae. The latter route of transmission does not apparently occur in *A. braziliense* infection. Some larvae of *A. caninum* may become arrested at the third stage in the intestine, to resume development at a later time.

Ancylostomosis is the result of persistent blood loss, resulting in anemia and hypoproteinemia in affected individuals. *Ancylostoma* spp. usually inhabit the small intestine, where they move about the surface, intermittently attaching several times a day to feed. They penetrate deeply into the mucosa, sometimes to the muscularis mucosae, as they take a plug of host tissue into their large buccal capsule. Host tissue is lacerated by large teeth and parasite-produced anticoagulant is released locally, which permits persistent blood flow. Blood loss is maximal while worms are attaining maturity between 12 and 16 days after infection, and then again during the peak period of egg production after 3-4 weeks of infection. The prepatent period for *A. caninum* is ~15 days.

There is considerable variation in the blood-sucking activity, and therefore the pathogenicity, of members of the genus. *A. caninum* consumes in the range of 0.01-0.2 mL of blood per worm per day, which in young puppies and kittens can represent a significant percentage of their blood volume. Experimentally, 200 *A. tubaeformae* worms cause anemia, weight loss, and mortality in 1.5-kg cats. Anemia in ancylostomosis is at first normochromic and normocytic; however, suckling pups with ancylostomosis are susceptible to rapid development of microcytic hypochromic anemia because of their poor iron reserves and the low iron levels in the dam's milk.

Acute fatal ancylostomosis occurs most commonly in 2-3 week-old pups infected via the lactogenic route. Heavy infections acquired by this route may result in death from acute anemia and hypoproteinemia before eggs are present in the feces. Chronic anemia may also lead to mortality of pups after a longer course. Percutaneous infection occurs in older dogs housed in suboptimal conditions in which moisture and temperature are conducive to larval development. Dermatitis caused by larval penetration may be observed between the toes or on ventral contact surfaces of the body. Ancylostomosis in older dogs is usually characterized by anemia, exercise intolerance, weakness, and emaciation. Watery feces may contain mucus or blood; however, the major effect of ancylostomosis is due to increased loss of erythrocytes, iron, and plasma protein.

Animals that succumb to ancylostomosis are characteristically *extremely pale*. There is often edema of subcutaneous tissue and mesentery, and serous effusion into body cavities, attributable to hypoproteinemia. In chronic infections, cachexia may be evident. If recent exposure to heavy percutaneous infection has occurred, there may be dermatitis, and multifocal hemorrhages throughout the pulmonary parenchyma because of larval migration. The intestinal mucosa is often diffusely red or has pinpoint red foci where adults have previously fed. Parasites are 1-1.5 cm long, translucent, gray or red depending on when they last consumed blood, and dispersed over the mucosa of the small intestine and less commonly into the large intestine. In a young pup, as few as 20-50 worms may cause fatal infection, and they may be easily overlooked.

Uncinaria stenocephala mainly infects by the oral route. Percutaneous infection is not efficient, although dermatitis may occur; prenatal and lactogenic transmission appear not to occur. This species sucks little blood and is less pathogenic than *A. caninum*; however, heavy infections with this species (burdens of >1,000 worms) may cause clinical disease and occasional mortality in pups. *Nonspecific signs of infection include lethargy, inappetence,* and *ill-thrift* and perhaps diarrhea; hypoproteinemia may be observed, but anemia does not occur.

The lesions are similar to those found in ancylostomosis. Grossly, the intestinal mucosa appears thickened, with scattered focal hemorrhages at sites of attachment. Histologic lesions may include moderate atrophy and thickening of villi and irregularity of the surface epithelium. There are aggregates of inflammatory cells, including neutrophils, secondary to the damage induced by deep attachment of adult worms. Disease caused by *U. stenocephala* is the result of protein loss and malabsorption. A similar syndrome may be associated with heavy infections of *A. braziliense*, in which hypoproteinemia also occurs.

All of these hookworms are zoonotic. In humans, *A. braziliense* is most commonly associated with cutaneous larva migrans; other hookworm species larvae less commonly cause eosinophilic pneumonitis, myositis, or ocular lesions. *A. caninum* has been shown to mature to adulthood and cause eosinophilic enteritis in humans.

The **hookworms of ruminants** include the following: in cattle, *Bunostomum phlebotomum*, and in India and Indonesia, *Agriostomum vryburgi*; in sheep, *B. trigonocephalum* and, in India and Southeast Asia, Africa, and South America, *Gaigeria pachyscelis*. The life cycle of these nematodes is typical of hookworms. *Bunostomum* third-stage larvae infect by the oral or percutaneous routes, whereas *Gaigeria* only infect across the skin. Eggs and larval stages on the ground are extremely susceptible to desiccation, and hookworm disease in ruminants is most common in tropical or subtropical areas during wet seasons. Stabled animals in cooler temperate areas may be affected by larvae invading the skin from contaminated bedding. Following skin penetration, the usual pattern is seen, with migration of larvae to the lungs, where they molt to the fourth stage, and subsequently pass up the trachea to the digestive tract. Larvae taken in by ingestion spend some time in the deep mucosa of the intestine before emerging to mature in the lumen of the small intestine. The prepatent period of *Bunostomum* is long, approximately 7-8 weeks. *Gaigeria* larvae migrate via the lungs, and worms begin to lay eggs 10 weeks after infection.

Both *Bunostomum* and *Gaigeria* cause *hemorrhagic anemia and hypoproteinemia*, especially in animals <1 year of age. These species often occur with mixed gastrointestinal helminth burdens, and their effects are at least additive to those of the other worms. As few as 20-30 *Gaigeria* will cause anemia and hypoproteinemia in lambs and kids, although several times that number may be more usual in fatal cases. The size of the animal, the status of its iron reserves, and the plane of nutrition, especially the level of protein, likely influence the pathogenicity of these species.

Gross lesions are nonspecific, secondary to anemia and hypoproteinemia. *Bunostomum* are often found in the distal half of the small intestine, whereas *Gaigeria* tend to be concentrated in the duodenum. Hemorrhage and bite marks may be evident on the mucosa in the infected areas of intestine. Given that relatively low numbers of worms can cause disease, and their unique distribution, the gut should be examined carefully and thoroughly in suspect cases.

Further reading

Bowman DD, et al. Hookworms of dogs and cats as agents of cutaneous larva migrans. Trends Parasitol 2010;26:162-167.

Epe C. Intestinal nematodes: biology and control. Vet Clin North Am Small Anim Pract 2009;39:1091-1107.

Periago MV, Bethony JM. Hookworm virulence factors: making the most of the host. Microbes Infect 2012;14:1451-1464.

Traversa D. Pet roundworms and hookworms: a continuing need for global worming. Parasit Vectors 2012;5:91-110.

Oesophagostomum* and *Chabertia* infection.** Members of the genus ***Oesophagostomum infect *sheep, cattle,* and *swine.* Two species in **sheep,** O. *columbianum* and O. *venulosum,* are most significant; the former is considerably more pathogenic and is particularly important in warm temperate to tropical areas. After ingestion, infective third-stage larvae penetrate the intestinal wall and encyst deep in the mucosa, inciting the formation of *inflammatory nodules in the wall of the intestine.* After ~1 week, they molt, emerge, and mature into adults in the colon. A proportion of fourth-stage larvae encyst within nodules in the colonic submucosa. Adult worms in the colon may be pathogenic for lambs, and burdens of only a few hundred O. *columbianum* are associated with anorexia, mucoid feces or diarrhea, and ill-thrift.

Gross lesions associated with clinical oesophagostomosis are nonspecific and include emaciation, enlarged mesenteric lymph nodes, and thickened and congested colonic mucosa with a layer of mucus in which the adult worms are scattered. Histologically there is hyperplasia of goblet cells, and the lamina propria contains a heavy mixed inflammatory infiltrate with many eosinophils. Globule leukocytes are in the epithelium of glands. Nodules caused by fourth-stage larvae are found mainly in the large intestine. These nodules are ~0.5-1 cm in diameter and comprised of a central caseous or mineralized core, eosinophils, giant cells, and macrophages often centered on the nematode (or its remnant), and surrounded by a thin fibrous capsule. Similar nodules may be found in liver, lungs, mesentery, and mesenteric lymph nodes. Those in the deeper layers of the gut project from the serosal surface and give rise to the name *pimply gut.* They may cause adhesion to adjacent abdominal viscera, intussusception, or

peritonitis; however, in most cases, nodules are incidental lesions. O. *venulosum* is a much less significant parasite. It seldom causes significant nodule formation; when it does, the nodules are small and mainly in the cecum and colon.

Two species also occur in **cattle,** O. *radiatum* and O. *venulosum,* and the former is the most significant parasite. The life cycle is similar to that of O. *columbianum.* Clinical disease caused by O. *radiatum* is characterized by *loss of appetite, reduced productive efficiency, anemia, hypoproteinemia,* and *diarrhea.* Anemia results from hemorrhage at sites of mucosal damage owing to larval emergence or the presence of adult worms. Considerable exudation of tissue fluids and plasma protein from colonic lesions along with hemorrhage contributes to protein loss and hypoproteinemia. Reduced growth efficiency is the product of significant protein loss and inappetence, whereas diarrhea presumably results from loss of colonic absorptive capacity.

Pathogenic worm burdens in calves are in the range of 1,000-10,000 O. *radiatum;* oesophagostomosis may be fatal in calves. Nonspecific gross lesions include pallor, edema, and cachexia, and are attributable to anemia and hypoproteinemia. Colonic lymph nodes are enlarged. The mucosa of the colon is grossly thickened and folded because of edema and mixed inflammation in the lamina propria. Colonic submucosal lymphoid follicles are large and active. Repeated exposure to infective larvae may result in the accumulation of large numbers of fourth-stage larvae within inflammatory nodules in the colon; this has little pathogenic significance in cattle.

In **swine,** several species occur in the large intestine; however, O. *dentatum* and O. *quadrispinulatum* are most widespread. Oesophagostomosis in swine is a *mild, usually subclinical disease.* Occasional diarrhea, depression in weight gain, and inefficiency of feed conversion may occur, especially during the period of emergence of larvae and maturation of worms in the lumen of the large intestine. Burdens of 3,000-20,000 adult worms are associated with subclinical disease experimentally. The nematodes are 1-2 cm long, white, and are present in mucus on the surface of the gut, or in luminal content. Massive repeated challenge cause severe typhlocolitis, but this seems to be purely an experimental phenomenon. The life cycle, gross and histologic lesions are typical of the genus. Lesions resolve following emergence of larvae.

Chabertia ovina is a robust 1-2 cm long worm that inhabits the *colon of sheep, goats,* and *cattle.* It is mainly a problem for sheep in cooler climatic zones. Phylogenetic analysis based on ribosomal DNA sequence data indicate that C. *ovina* is clustered within the subfamily *Oesophagostominae.* The life cycle of *Chabertia* resembles that of *Oesophagostomum;* third-stage larvae encyst in the wall of the small intestine, then emerge to mature in the cecum and colon. Adults penetrate to the muscularis mucosae and take a plug of mucosa into the buccal capsule, so minor hemorrhage may be related to physical trauma to the mucosa. Significant loss of plasma protein from the mucosa at numerous focal sites of trauma occurs. Disease in sheep is associated with the presence of mature worms in the colon, and nonspecific clinical signs include ill-thrift and soft feces with mucus, and perhaps blood. Grossly the lesions are characterized by edema of all layers of the wall of infected parts of the colon, and enlargement of colonic lymph nodes. Worms generally are concentrated in the proximal portion of the spiral colon, and the area that they inhabit may have numerous hemorrhagic foci corresponding to sites of former attachment. Pathogenic burdens may be as few as 150 worms and the species must be sought in its usual site of predilection or be missed. Histologically, there is often widespread mononuclear infiltration in the mucosa and submucosa and hyperplasia of goblet cells.

Further reading

Makovcová K, et al. Linear distribution of nematodes in the gastrointestinal tract of tracer lambs. Parasitol Res 2008;104:123-126.

Petersen HH, et al. Parasite population dynamics in pigs infected with *Trichuris suis* and *Oesophagostomum dentatum*. Vet Parasit 2014;199:73-80.

Stewart TB, Gasbarre LC. The veterinary importance of nodular worms (*Oesophagostomum* spp. Parasitol Today 1989;5:209-213.

Sweeny JP, et al. Impacts of naturally acquired protozoa and strongylid nematode infections on growth and faecal attributes in lambs. Vet Parasitol 2012;184:298-308.

Equine strongylosis. Members of the family *Strongylidae* are common nematode parasites of the cecum and colon in horses, and are usually present as mixed infections.

- The subfamily *Strongylinae*, or **large strongyles**, includes the important genus *Strongylus* and the less significant genera *Triodontophorus*, *Oesophagodontus*, and *Craterostomum*. Members of this group are *plug feeders or blood suckers*, and *Strongylus* spp. undergo extensive extraintestinal migrations.
- The subfamily *Cyathostominae*, or **small strongyles**, includes 8 genera of nematodes. Adults of this group *feed mainly on intestinal contents*, and are of little pathogenic significance. However, simultaneous emergence of large numbers of *larvae* from the gut wall may cause disease.

Large strongyles. *Strongylus vulgaris* is relatively common, and has been considered the *most significant nematode parasite in horses*. However, infection levels have considerably decreased with the advent of improved anthelmintics. Larval forms cause *endoarteritis* in the mesenteric circulation, resulting in *arterial infarction* of the large bowel and colic, whereas the adults cause *anemia* and *ill-thrift*. Infective third-stage larvae are ingested from pasture and ex-sheath in the small intestine to penetrate the intestinal mucosa and molt to the fourth stage. They enter small arterioles, where they migrate along the endothelium to reach the cranial mesenteric artery within 3 weeks. Following a 3-4 month maturation period, immature adults, or fifth-stage larvae, return to the wall of the cecum or colon via the arterial lumen, where they encapsulate in the subserosa forming 5-8 mm nodules. The nodules eventually rupture into the lumen of the large bowel, especially cecum and right ventral colon, where the parasites mature in another 1-2 months, ~6-7 months after initial infection. Some larvae may become trapped and encapsulated in arterioles in the mesentery on their way back to the gut, and remain there to die eventually.

Endoarteritis associated with migration and establishment of larvae in the cranial mesenteric artery and its branches is discussed in Vol. 3, Cardiovascular system, as are the consequences of aberrant migration in the aorta and other arteries. Syndromes associated with aberrant migration include *cerebrospinal nematodiasis* and *aortic-iliac thrombosis*. Lesions of the cranial mesenteric, cecal, and colic arteries may lead to *colic* as a result of reduced perfusion and thromboembolism, or perhaps owing to impingement upon autonomic ganglia in the

vicinity of the arterial root at the aorta. Although many older horses are infected with adult worms or have arterial lesions, the complications of colic and infarction caused by this parasite are most common in young horses. An *acute syndrome*, characterized by pyrexia, anorexia, depression and weight loss, diarrhea or constipation, colic, and infarction of intestine occurs in foals infected with large numbers of larvae; this is not often observed in animals previously exposed to infection.

S. edentatus now rarely causes infection. It has a life cycle characterized by extensive larval migration. Third-stage larvae enter the intestinal wall and pass in the portal system to the liver, where they incite inflammatory foci. Here they molt to the fourth stage and, ~30 days after infection, begin migrating through the hepatic parenchyma. Inflammatory reaction in the liver consists of necrotic debris, eosinophils, neutrophils, and mononuclear cells with variable amounts of fibrous connective tissue and hemorrhage. By 8-10 weeks after infection, larvae migrate from the liver via the hepatic ligaments. *Parenchymal scars and tags of fibrous tissue on the hepatic capsule*, especially the diaphragmatic surface, are commonly found during postmortem examination of horses, and are thought to be a legacy of migrating *S. edentatus*; however, the prevalence of these lesions has not decreased along with the reduction in incidence of infection, and final association of these lesions with migrating strongyles has not been established. Larvae may be encountered in the retroperitoneal tissue, often associated with local hemorrhage, or they can be observed in aberrant locations, including the omentum, hepatic ligaments, and diaphragm, where they induce formation of eosinophilic granulomas. Omental adhesions also may be a sequel to aberrant larval migration. In the flank, larvae persist for several months, molting to the fifth stage before returning from the right flank via the cecal ligament to the cecum and colon. Here they form nodules and edematous or hemorrhagic plaques in the intestinal wall, eventually perforating to the lumen, where they mature and begin to lay eggs ~10-12 months after infection. Lesions associated with the larval migration of *S. edentatus* are usually incidental findings at autopsy.

S. equinus is very rare today. Ex-sheathed third-stage larvae penetrate to the deeper layers of the wall of the ileum, cecum, and colon, molt to the fourth stage, and produce hemorrhagic subserosal nodules, before moving to the liver through the peritoneal cavity. They migrate in the hepatic parenchyma for 6-7 weeks, then leave the liver, probably via the hepatic ligaments, to the pancreas and peritoneal cavity, where they molt to the fifth stage ~4 months after infection. They regain the lumen of the cecum and right ventral colon by an unknown route, probably by direct penetration from the peritoneal cavity or pancreas. Pancreatic damage is usually mild and is mainly manifested by slight periductal infiltration of eosinophils.

Hemomelasma ilei is the term applied to slightly elevated *subserosal hemorrhagic plaques*, up to 1-2 × 3-4 cm in size, usually found along the antimesenteric border of the distal small intestine, or rarely on the large bowel (Fig. 1-178). The lesion is considered incidental, and has long been associated with trauma by migrating larvae of *S. edentatus* in particular, but may be caused by larvae of any of the *Strongylus* spp. As with the hepatic lesions historically associated with migration of large strongyles, *the incidence of hemomelasma ilei has not apparently declined with the reduction in incidence of large strongyle infections over the last 25 years*. Histologically, there is

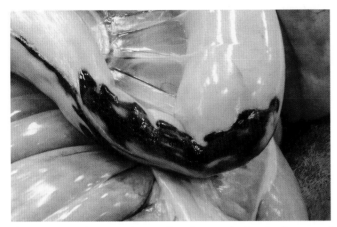

Figure 1-178 Hemomelasma ilei, large subserosal plaques of resolving hemorrhage on the small intestine of a horse. (Courtesy C. Schott.)

edema, hemorrhage, a mixed population of leukocytes and variably mature fibrous tissue; depending on the stage of the lesions, erythrophagocytosis by macrophages can be prominent.

Adults of all species in the *Strongylinae* are plug feeders and blood suckers. In sufficient numbers they may cause ill-thrift and anemia, as the result of active erythrophagia and blood loss from sites of recent feeding activity. Increased albumin catabolism causing accelerated turnover of the plasma pool, and reduced red cell survival, have been demonstrated in horses with relatively low numbers (<100) of adult *S. vulgaris.*

Triodontophorus spp. are also large strongyles found in horses and appear to be less pathogenic compared with *Strongylus* spp. The most important species is *T. tenuicollis,* which can be associated with significant blood loss; these parasites attach to the mucosa of the colon in clusters, causing local congestion and ulceration.

The **small strongyles,** or **cyathostomins** (cyathostomes), a group containing >50 distinct species; these parasites are highly prevalent worldwide. They are *essentially nonpathogenic as adults,* despite the fact that tens or many hundreds of thousands may be in the content of the large bowel. Cyathostominosis is a disease of horses >1 year of age, and little resistance is apparent to repeated infection.

The clinical syndrome *larval cyathostominosis* occurs as a result of simultaneous emergence of inhibited third-stage larvae from the intestinal mucosa, and *is a significant cause of morbidity and mortality in horses.* The cyathostomins have a direct life cycle. Infective third-stage larval cyathostomins are ingested, and they migrate into the deep mucosa or submucosa of the cecum and large colon to encyst and molt, before emerging to the lumen to molt again and mature into adults. Encysted third- or fourth-stage larvae may undergo hypobiosis or developmental inhibition, persisting in nodules in the colonic wall for as long as 2 years. The timing during which inhibition occurs is dependent on the climate: Inhibition occurs during cooler months of the year in temperate climates, and during the hot summer in tropical climates. The most devastating damage occurs when large numbers of encysted inhibited larvae emerge *en masse* to continue their development in the intestinal lumen. This occurs in the late winter, spring, and early summer in northern temperate climates.

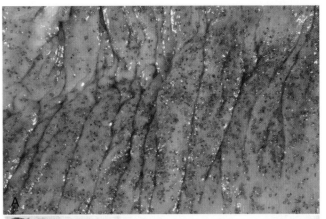

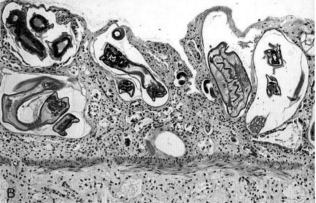

Figure 1-179 Equine cyathostominosis. A. Equine colonic mucosa studded with 2-5 mm diameter nodules formed by **larval cyathostomins.** (Courtesy R. Foster.) **B.** Encysted larvae in the lamina propria surrounded by mixed inflammatory infiltrate. (Courtesy A. Peregrine.)

Development of widespread anthelmintic resistance by cyathostomins, particularly encysted larval stages, is well documented.

Affected horses may be of any age; clinical signs are non-specific and include diarrhea, edema, anorexia, and weight loss. **Grossly,** mucosal nodules formed by encysted larvae are only a few millimeters in diameter, slightly raised red or black (Fig. 1-179A); visualization of the nodules is enhanced by transillumination of the intestine. Incision reveals a small translucent gray or red larval nematode. There will be edema and congestion of the mucosa and submucosa. **Histologically,** a mixed inflammatory response is observed either centered on encysted larvae in the submucosa or more diffusely throughout the lamina propria (Fig. 1-179B).

Further reading

Corning S. Equine cyathostomins: a review of biology, clinical significance and therapy. Parasit Vectors 2009;2:S1-S13.

Matthews JB, et al. Recent developments in research into the Cyathostominae and *Anoplocephala perfoliata.* Vet Res 2004;35:371-381.

Reinemeyer CR, Nielsen MK. Parasitism and colic. Vet Clin North Am Equine Pract 2009;25:233-245.

Stratford CH, et al. An update on cyathostomin: anthelmintic resistance and diagnostic tools. Eq Vet J Suppl 2011;39:133-139.

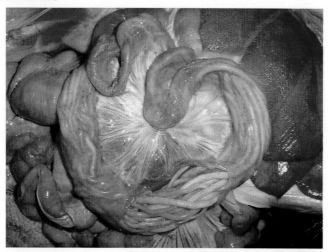

Figure 1-180 A heavy burden of ***Ascaris suum*** impacted in and obstructing the small intestine in a pig. (Courtesy A. Peregrine.)

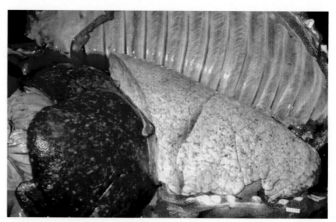

Figure 1-181 Effects of migrating ***Ascaris suum*** larvae in a pig: multifocal hepatitis and scarring in the liver and multifocal hemorrhage in the lung. (Courtesy A. Peregrine.)

Ascarid infection. Members of the family *Ascarididae* are *common and important parasites of swine, horses, dogs, cats, water buffalo, and to a lesser extent, cattle.* They do not normally occur in sheep and goats. Their importance is related to incidental and sometimes significant lesions caused by *larval migration* in the tissues of definitive and accidental hosts, and to the effects of *adult worms* in the small intestine of the definitive host.

Ascaris suum is a large parasite, usually found in the *upper half of the small intestine of swine;* females measure up to 40 cm long. The life cycle is direct. After ingestion, eggs hatch and release third-stage larvae in the intestine. The larvae penetrate the cecal or colonic mucosa to be carried in the portal blood to the liver, then pass to the lungs, where they break out of capillaries into alveoli, as early as 3-5 days after infection. Larvae move up the respiratory tree to the pharynx, where they are swallowed, and arrive in the intestine to mature. After returning to the intestine, most larvae gradually move to the distal small intestine and are expelled between 14 and 21 days post infection, a phenomenon likely mediated by parasite-specific immunoglobulin A–producing plasma cells, eosinophils, and intraepithelial T lymphocytes. The pathogenicity of adult ascarids in the intestine is poorly defined. Heavy infections may be evident as rope-like masses within the intestinal lumen and can potentially result in obstruction or rarely perforation (Fig. 1-180). The presence of ~80-100 worms in young swine may depress feed intake and the efficiency of feed conversion; however, most pigs harboring patent infections are clinically normal. *A. lumbricoides* in humans interferes with carbohydrate, fat, and protein absorption, and *A. suum* probably has a similar influence.

Larval migration induces lesions in the liver and lungs (Fig. 1-181), and respiratory signs characterized by dyspnea (common term, thumps) may occur in piglets if large numbers of larvae migrate through the lungs. Gross lesions in pigs associated with pulmonary migration of ascarids are largely limited to numerous focal hemorrhages scattered over and through the pulmonary parenchyma. In the liver, migrating *A. suum* do not causing clinical disease but do result in considerable economic loss from liver condemnation at slaughter inspection. The lesions are related to mechanical damage caused by the worms, subsequent repair, and hypersensitivity

reactions to excretory and secretory products of the larvae. Initially, hemorrhagic tracks are present near portal areas and throughout lobules. They are visible through the capsule as pinpoint red areas, perhaps slightly depressed and surrounded by a narrow pale zone. These lesions collapse and heal by fibrosis, causing scarring that involves most intensely the adjacent portal tracts. However, fibrosis extends diffusely through more distant tracts, emphasizing lobular outlines.

Microscopically *in the lung* there is eosinophilic bronchiolitis, and in some cases secondary bronchopneumonia. Bronchioles are surrounded by macrophages and eosinophils, and the bronchiolar epithelium is hyperplastic, disorganized, or perhaps eroded. The bronchiolar wall is infiltrated by eosinophils that are also present in the lumen intermixed with necrotic debris. There also may be an eosinophilic and granulomatous vasculitis. *In the liver* there is a heavy eosinophil infiltrate in fibrotic septa, which becomes most obvious beginning ~10-14 days after infection. Inflammatory foci containing giant cells, macrophages, and eosinophils may center on larval remnants trapped and destroyed in the liver. The inflammatory infiltrates in livers of animals exposed to larval ascarids may become severe and generalized; this is reflected in the gross appearance of the liver, which has extensive white "*milk spots,*" and prominent definition of lobules. The liver is firm, and heavy scars may become confluent, obliterating some lobules and extending out to exaggerate interlobular septa throughout the liver. Where pigs are raised intensively, it is now rare to encounter extreme fibrosis of the liver associated with ascarid migration. *Larvae or their remnants are usually readily found in sections of lung.* They may be present in alveoli, alveolar ducts, bronchioles, or bronchi, perhaps surrounded by eosinophils. In more chronic cases, larvae are within eosinophilic granulomas. Like all larval ascarids of mammals, *A. suum* in the lungs have *lateral alae visible in section.*

A. suum also infects animals other than swine. In sheep, and occasionally cattle, immature ascarids may be found in the intestine. Dyspnea and coughing associated with eosinophilic pneumonia, and focal eosinophilic hepatitis, may occur in lambs exposed to *A. suis;* mortality rarely occurs. Liver lesions in lambs are usually too small to be significant at slaughter inspection.

In **calves** exposed to yards contaminated by pig feces containing *A. suum* eggs, *severe acute interstitial pneumonia* may occur. Signs of dyspnea, tachypnea, coughing, and increased expiratory effort are usually first seen ~7-10 days after exposure, when large numbers of larvae are present in the lungs. Deaths may ensue over the following few days, and the lungs are moderately consolidated, light pink to deep red, with alveolar and interstitial emphysema and interlobular edema. Microscopically there is thickening of alveolar septa, and effusion of fibrin, proteinaceous edema fluid, and macrophages into alveoli. Hemorrhage into alveoli may also occur. Larvae are present in alveoli and bronchioles and provoke acute bronchiolitis. Neutrophils are found around larvae in bronchioles; eosinophils may be present but are not prominent in animals dying acutely. In addition to being usually observed readily in tissue sections, larvae may be recovered from the airways by washing with saline, or from minced lung in saline or digestion fluid, by use of a Baermann apparatus. Tens of thousands to millions of larvae may be present in the lungs of fatal cases.

Further reading

Dold C, Holland CV. Ascaris and ascariasis. Microbes Infect 2011;13:632-637.

Masure D, et al. The intestinal expulsion of the roundworm *Ascaris suum* is associated with eosinophils, intra-epithelial T cells and decreased intestinal transit time. PLOS Neg Trop Dis 2013;7:e2588.

Miquel N, et al. Host immune reactions and worm kinetics during the expulsion of *Ascaris suum* in pigs. Parasite Immunol 2005;27:79-88.

Roepstorff A, et al. Helminth parasites in pigs: New challenges in pig production and current research highlights. Vet Parasitol 2011;180:72-81.

Parascaris equorum. *Parascaris equorum* is the *ascarid of horses.* It is widespread and common in young horses; it may contribute to ill-thrift and occasionally causes death by obstruction. *P. equorum* is a large nematode, females being up to 50 cm long. The life cycle resembles that of *A. suum*. Similarly, *hepatic and pulmonary lesions are associated with larval migration*, and coughing may occur at the time larvae are in the lungs, particularly if infections are heavy. The prepatent period is ~10-15 weeks. The lesions in the lungs of foals with migrating *P. equorum* larvae 2 weeks after infection are similar to those described in swine with *A. suum*. Resolving pulmonary lesions may be observed as subpleural nodular accumulations of lymphocytes up to 1 cm in diameter, and there may be residual lymphocytic cuffing of pulmonary vessels.

It is possible to establish heavy infections of *P. equorum* in the intestines of foals a few months old, but not in yearlings wherein larvae appear to be killed during hepatopulmonary migration. In heavily infected foals, many worms are lost from the intestine before patency, suggesting the possibility of an effect of crowding on the population of growing worms. A heavy burden of ascarids in the intestine may reduce weight gains in growing foals. Inappetence occurs but increased plasma protein catabolism or loss into the gut does not. Reduced weight gain may be due to decreased protein intake. Ascarid infection may reduce rate of intestinal transit, and heavy burdens can be associated with obstruction, intussusception or, rarely, perforation of the intestine.

Further reading

Anderson UV, et al. Recent advances in diagnosing pathogenic equine gastrointestinal helminths: the challenge of prepatent detection. Vet Parasitol 2013;192:1-9.

Tatz AJ, et al. Surgical treatment for acute small intestinal obstruction caused by *Parascaris equorum* infection in 15 horses (2002-2011). Equine Vet J Suppl 2012;43:111-114.

Toxascaris leonina. The **ascarids of small animals** are *Toxascaris leonina*, infecting both cats and dogs, and *Toxocara canis* and *T. cati*, infecting the dog and cat, respectively. All occur in the *small intestine*, mainly in young animals.

Toxascaris leonina has a life cycle that may be direct, but can involve a paratenic host. In the definitive host, larvae ingested in infective ova enter the wall of the gut, where they remain for several weeks, molting to the fourth stage and emerging to the intestinal lumen to molt again and mature. The prepatent period is 10-11 weeks.

Toxocara canis has a complex life cycle, and dogs can be infected by ingestion of embryonated eggs from the environment or larvae from paratenic hosts including rodents and rabbits, or by vertical transmission including either intrauterine or transmammary routes. After ingestion of embryonated ova, larvae penetrate the intestinal mucosa, and migrate via the liver to arrive in the lungs 24-36 hours post infection. From the lung, *larvae follow one of two pathways*. Depending on the age and immune status of the host, larvae may penetrate alveoli, and migrate via bronchioles and trachea, where they are swallowed and mature into adults in the intestine. In the second pathway, larvae penetrate alveoli but are distributed by the circulatory system throughout the body where they encyst (*larva migrans*), rather than undergoing development and tracheal migration; this is more common in older animals. Most migrating larvae end up in kidneys, skeletal muscle, liver and central nervous system. Probably *the most important route in young dogs is transplacental transmission*. In the pregnant bitch encysted larvae in tissues are mobilized and cross the placenta to infect the fetus after day 42 of gestation; mechanisms for mobilization of larvae is not clearly understood. In the fetus, they remain in the liver, passing to the lungs within 2-3 days after birth. Mobilized larvae may also result in transmammary transmission.

In some abnormal hosts, including humans, the syndrome *visceral larva migrans* can be caused by ingestion of embryonated *T. canis* or *T. cati* eggs from soil or infective larvae from under-cooked meat. A broad spectrum of pathologic and clinical sequelae are associated with this syndrome, and the severity and range of symptoms depends on the tissue involved (eye, liver, lungs, central nervous system), the number of larvae migrating, and the age of the host.

Baylisascaris procyonis, the raccoon roundworm, is known for the ability of its larvae to cause *visceral larva migrans* in many accidental or "dead-end" hosts, including humans who ingest eggs or infective larvae. Dogs can serve as alternative definitive hosts for *B. procyonis*, and this can lead to patent intestinal infections. This is of significant zoonotic risk for humans because the eggs of *B. procyonis* easily can be mistaken for *T. canis*. Furthermore, dogs have an indiscriminate defecation pattern compared with raccoons, and *B. procyonis* eggs are extremely hardy in the environment.

T. cati may infect cats directly by the transmammary route, ingestion of larvated eggs, or ingestion of an infected paratenic

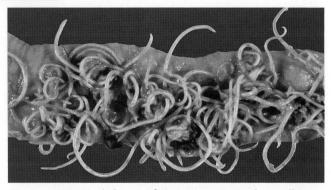

Figure 1-182 Tangled mass of ***Toxocara canis*** in the small intestine of a pup.

host; the latter two routes are most important in cats. Prenatal infection apparently does not occur. Larvae hatching from ingested eggs migrate via the liver, lungs and trachea, whereas those ingested from milk or via a paratenic host exhibit direct development, often involving the gastric mucosa but without tracheal or extraintestinal migration.

Lesions associated with ascariasis in dogs and cats are mostly secondary to larval migration, though in massive infections, adult parasites can cause obstruction or intestinal rupture (Fig. 1-182). Heavy infections of ascarids in puppies and kittens, usually those reared in unhygienic communal environments, may result in *ill-thrift*. The most significant effects are those caused in the stomach and intestine by maturing *T. canis* in young puppies infected prenatally. The animals may develop weakness, lethargy, and vomition that can be fatal. Gross lesions indicate poor growth relative to age, pot-belly, cachexia, and masses of maturing worms in the intestine and perhaps stomach. Up to 20% of the body weight of young puppies may be accounted for by the worm burden. *T. cati* may be associated with clinical disease, but usually not death, in kittens up to several months of age. Disease is rarely attributed to *T. leonina*.

Mature *T. cati* are up to 10 cm long; *T. canis* are up to 18 cm long. In freshly dead animals, adult worms are often coiled; this may help maintain their place in the intestine by bracing against the gut wall. The mechanism by which adults of these ascarids in the intestinal lumen impair growth has not been investigated. Ascarids occasionally enter the bile or pancreatic ducts, and many perforate those structures or the intestine.

Migrating *T. canis* larvae can cause focal hemorrhages in the lungs of puppies; inflammatory foci are commonly seen grossly in the liver or kidney, as white elevated spots 1-2 mm in diameter in the cortex beneath the capsule. Ocular larva migrans has been described in dogs but not cats infected with *T. canis*. Histologic lesions are characterized by aggregates of mixed inflammatory cells, including eosinophils and macrophages in a variety of tissues, most commonly liver, kidney, and lung; some nodules may contain larvae of *T. canis*. Focal scarring may be observed in tissue in which larvae are destroyed. Considering the large numbers of larvae that migrate through tissues of dogs, relatively few are encountered. *T. cati* developing in the mucosa of the stomach and intestine may provoke a mild granulomatous response comprised of lymphocytes and a few macrophages about the coiled larva. Larvae free of such a response are also found in the mucosa and submucosa.

Further reading

Bauer C. Baylisascariosis - Infections of animals and humans with 'unusual' roundworms. Vet Parasitol 2013;193:404-412.

Despommier D. Toxocariasis: clinical aspects, epidemiology, medical ecology, and molecular aspects. Clin Microbiol Rev 2003;16:265-272.

Overgaauw PAM, vanKnapen F. Veterinary and public health aspects of *Toxocara* spp. Vet Parasitol 2013;193:398-403.

Schnieder T, et al. Larval development of Toxocara canis in dogs. Vet Parasitol 2011;175:193-206.

Strube C, et al. *Toxocara* spp. infections in paratenic hosts. Vet Parasitol 2013;193:375-389.

Yee ACY, et al. Epidemiologic and zoonotic aspect of ascarid infections in dogs and cats. Trends Parasit 2010;26:155-161.

Toxocara vitulorum. *Toxocara (Neoascaris) vitulorum* infects the *small intestine of young calves of domestic cattle*, mainly in the tropics and subtropics and rarely in North America; it is especially significant in water buffalo.

The life cycle involves transmammary transmission of third-stage larvae mobilized from the tissues of the dam within a few days of parturition. The larvae reach the liver of the calf and undergo tracheal migration. Patency occurs within the calf ~1 month of age, but worms are expelled within a short time, and by 2-3 months of age, none are present.

Signs of infection include foul-smelling *diarrhea* and *ill-thrift*. Immature and mature worms both contribute to the signs. Heavily infected calves may die in an emaciated state, with burdens of up to 400-500 worms as much as 30 cm long in the intestine. Occasionally, migration up the bile duct or perforation of the gut may occur.

Further reading

Davila G, et al. *Toxocara vitulorum* in beef calves in North Central Florida. Vet Parasitol 2010;168:261-263.

Roberts JA. The life cycle of *Toxocara vitulorum* in Asian buffalo (Bubalus bubalis). Int J Parasitol 1990;20:833-840.

Trichuris **infection.** *Trichuris* species, the **whipworms**, are so called because of their long thin cephalic end and shorter stouter caudal portion. They inhabit the *cecum*, and occasionally the *colon*, of all the domestic animals considered here, except the horse. The host-parasite relationships include: in dogs, *T. vulpis*; in cats, *T. campanula* and *T. serrata*; in swine, *T. suis*; in sheep and goats, *T. ovis*, *T. globulosa*, *T. skrjabini*; and in cattle, *T. discolor* and, less commonly, *T. ovis* and *T. globulosa*.

The life cycle is direct. Larvated ova may remain viable and infective for years in the environment. Ingestion of larvated eggs leads to release of third-stage larvae, which enter the mucosal glands of the proximal small intestine for up to 7-10 days, before returning to the lumen and passing on to the cecum, where they establish their adult existence. The prepatent period varies from 6-7 weeks for *T. suis* to 11-12 weeks for *T. vulpis*. In rare instances disease may occur during the prepatent period, in which case ova will not be in the feces.

In all species, the filamentous cranial end of the worm is embedded at least partially in tunnels within the superficial mucosa of the cecum and colon, while the caudal end lies freely within the intestinal lumen (Fig. 1-183). *Trichuris* ingest

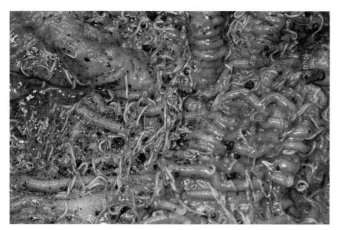

Figure 1-183 Hemorrhagic typhlocolitis in a pig caused by *Trichuris suis*.

blood, yet disease associated with these parasites is not usually related to this activity. A protease produced by *T. globulosa* has been shown to promote degradation of mucosal tissue. Light infections cause little morphologic alteration in the mucosa and no disease; however, heavy infection with *Trichuris* is associated with *severe and often hemorrhagic typhlitis or typhlocolitis in all species*. In the **dog**, large populations of worms overflow their normal habitat and infect the mucosa of the ascending colon, sometimes extending to the rectum. Clinical signs may include chronic diarrhea or dysentery, perhaps with some weight loss. The blood and foul odor of the feces are due to hemorrhage and effusion of tissue fluid from the mucosal surface damaged by the embedded worms. Grossly the mucosa is thickened, red, and edematous. The colonic content is often watery, and contains blood or mucus. Masses of tangled worms are visible on the mucosa. Microscopically the mucosal surface is widely eroded or mildly ulcerated, and effusion of proteinaceous fluid, inflammatory exudate, and blood is evident. The glandular epithelium is hyperplastic. Occasionally, *T. vulpis* infection may be associated with more severe localized or regional lesions characterized by granulomatous inflammation and fibroplasia in deeper layers of the mucosa; rarely ova or worms can be identified in such lesions.

In **swine**, if enough *T. suis* worms are present, they may cause *mucohemorrhagic typhlocolitis* that is associated clinically with anorexia, diarrhea, dysentery, dehydration, ill-thrift, and in some cases death. The disease is most common in animals exposed to dirt yards contaminated with infective *Trichuris* ova. Clinical signs of the disease appear to be referable to loss of colonic absorptive function, and probably are partly due to effusion of protein into the lumen. Erythrocyte loss is a minor component of the pathogenesis.

Typical gross lesions are similar to those described in dogs and the mucosa is thickened, edematous, reddened, and may be eroded with increased mucus secretion. The gross appearance may resemble that of swine dysentery; however, close examination reveals nematodes on the mucosa, and particularly the thicker caudal end of the worms is readily observed. They may resemble *Oesophagostomum* at first glance, and only on more careful observation is the distinct elongate thread-like cephalic end noted.

Histologic lesions include hypertrophy of glandular epithelium, mucosal erosions, and surface effusion of proteinaceous fluid, inflammatory cells, and blood. Lesions are more severe in swine with conventional gut flora than those reared germ-free, or free of known enteric pathogens. *T. suis* may suppress mucosal immunity to resident bacteria.

Trichurosis in **sheep** and **cattle** resembles that described in swine. The disease usually occurs in animals that are concentrated in areas contaminated by ova, and immunocompromise has been suggested to increase susceptibility. Heavily infected animals develop chronic diarrhea, dysentery, and/or loss of condition. The gross lesions are nonspecific, and may include cachexia and hypoproteinemia associated with mucohemorrhagic typhlitis or typhlocolitis.

A **diagnosis** of trichurosis in all species is usually readily made during postmortem examination by identifying adult worms. The worms have a characteristic morphology that can be readily observed on the inflamed mucosal surface. Histologically, the filamentous cephalic end of the adults is embedded in tunnels in the surface epithelium, and contains the stichosome esophagus typical of members of the *Trichuroidea*, and a single bacillary band. The characteristic barrel-shaped ova have thick walls and plugs at each pole, and may be seen in the body of worms, in the gut lumen, or occasionally in tissue. *Capillaria* spp. and their ova may be similar in tissue section, but are not expected in the cecum and colon.

Further reading

Hendrix CM, et al. Whipworms and intestinal threadworms. Vet Clin North Am: Small Anim Pract 1987;17:1355-1375.

Mansfield LS, et al. Enhancement of disease and pathology by synergy of *Trichuris suis* and *Campylobacter jejuni* in the colon of immunologically naive swine. Am J Trop Med Hyg 2003;68:70-80.

Roepstorff A, et al. Helminth parasites in pigs: new challenges in pig production and current research highlights. Vet Parasitol 2011;180:72-81.

Traversa D, et al. Environmental contamination by canine geohelminths. Parasit Vectors 2014;7:67.

Cestode infection. Within the class Cestoda, 2 orders are of importance to veterinarians. Pseudophyllidea include the genera *Diphyllobothrium* and *Spirometra* and are associated with aquatic food chains and require 2 intermediate hosts: The first is a copepod and the second may be a fish, amphibian, or reptile. The order Cyclophyllidae contains several families of interest such as *Taeniidae, Mesocestoididae, Anoplocephalidae, Dipylidiidae,* and *Hymenolepididae*. Most cyclophyllideans require only one intermediate host, which may be a mammal or an arthropod.

Adult tapeworms inhabit the gastrointestinal tract or the ducts of the liver and pancreas, where they are generally of minor significance. They are flattened, segmented organisms with sequentially maturing hermaphroditic reproductive units, or *proglottids*, forming an elongate strobila a few millimeters to many meters long. Cestodes attach to the host by a specialized hold-fast organ, or scolex, which usually has 4 suckers, and perhaps a rostellum, sometimes armed with hooks. Cestodes lack an alimentary tract and absorb nutrients through the specialized absorptive surface or tegument of the proglottids.

The life cycle of tapeworms is complex and often specific to a particular species. The definitive host is infected by ingestion of the intermediate or paratenic host containing infective larvae. Carnivores tend be infected by tapeworms that use prey species as intermediate hosts. Larval cestodes use some species of domestic animals as intermediate hosts, and humans can serve as accidental hosts. Metacestodes, or larval cestodes within their intermediate or paratenic hosts, in domestic animals may cause disease, result in economic loss because of condemnation of tissues or organs at slaughter inspection, or can have zoonotic significance.

Histologically, adult cestodes have flattened solid parenchymatous bodies segmented into proglottids. Internal organs are embedded within the parenchymatous matrix, and contain male and female reproductive organs but lack a digestive tract. Other features that may be observed include anterior muscular suckers and hooks. *Calcareous corpuscles* are basophilic round to oval structures that may have concentric rings, and are embedded within the parenchyma of the outer region; corpuscles are more numerous in the head and neck region of adult and larval cestodes.

Further reading

Bowman DD. Class Cestoda, Helminths. In: Georgis' Parasitology for Veterinarians. 9th ed. Elsevier Inc; 2009. p. 131-152.

Raether W, Hanel H. Epidemiology, clinical manifestations and diagnosis of zoonotic cestode infections: an update. Parasitol Res 2003;91:412-438.

Intestinal tapeworms. In **ruminants**, the more common and widely distributed intestinal tapeworms are *Moniezia expansa*, *M. benedeni*, and *Thysaniezia* (*Helictometra*) *giardi*. *Stilesia globipunctata* is found in the small intestine of sheep and goats in Europe, Asia, and Africa, whereas *S. hepatica* occurs in the bile ducts of ruminants in Africa and Asia. *Thysanosoma actinioides* occurs in the small intestine, and pancreatic and bile ducts of ruminants in North and South America. *Avitellina* spp. occur in the small intestine of sheep and other ruminants in parts of Europe and Asia. The intermediate hosts of these tapeworms are oribatid mites or psocids (book lice).

Heavy infestations of the small intestine by *Moniezia*, *Thysaniezia*, and *Avitellina* have been associated with diarrhea and ill-thrift in young lambs and calves; however, the pathogenicity of *Moniezia* is considered very low.

The scolex of *Stilesia globipunctata* may be embedded in 6-10 mm diameter mucosal nodules in the upper small intestine, with their thread-like strobila streaming into the intestinal lumen. There is a chronic inflammatory reaction around the embedded scolex; glands in the vicinity are also hyperplastic, and together with the inflammatory cells cause nodule formation. The presence of many adults is associated with edema, diarrhea, and wasting in small ruminants.

Stilesia hepatica and *Thysanosoma actinioides* may cause mild fibrosis and ectasia of the bile ducts, and worms are often concentrated in the segmented saccular dilations of bile ducts. In areas where infection is common, these worms cause significant economic loss through condemnation of infected livers at slaughter inspection.

Further reading

Denegri G, et al. Anoplocephalid cestodes of veterinary and medical significance: a review. Folia Parasitol (Praha) 1998;45:1-8.

Irie T, et al. Continuous *Moniezia benedini* infection in confined cattle possibly maintained by an intermediate host on the farm. J Vet Med Sci 2013;75:1585-1589.

Moazeni M, Nili M. Mixed infection with intestinal tape worms in sheep. Trop Biomed 2004;21:23-26.

Anoplocephala perfoliata. The cestodes found in **horses** are *Anoplocephala perfoliata*, which attaches to the intestinal mucosa in the region of the ileocecal junction, and *A. magna* and *Paranoplocephala mamillana*, which colonize the small intestine and occasionally the stomach. *P. mamillana* is small, <5 cm in length, and is rarely associated with disease or lesions. *A. magna* tends to live in the lower small intestine, where it can reach a length of up to 80 cm, and a width of 2.5 cm. All use oribatid mites as intermediate hosts.

Anoplocephala perfoliata is the most common cestode in horses and has a worldwide distribution. *A. perfoliata* does not invade the mucosa of the intestine, its attachment via 4 suckers on its scolex causes a localized inflammatory response. In heavy infections, *A. perfoliata* attach in clusters of up to several hundred along the ileocecal junction (Fig. 1-184), and there may be erosion and ulceration of the mucosal epithelium. The depressed surface is often covered by fibrin, perhaps with some hemorrhage, or a local verrucous granulating mass may project into the lumen. Histologic lesions include large numbers of eosinophils and lymphocytes with edema, mucosal ulceration, and fibrosis. Villous atrophy of ileal mucosa, hypertrophy of the cecal epithelium, goblet cell hyperplasia, and hypertrophy of the muscular layers of the cecum occur with heavy infections. Changes in the myenteric ganglia, including loss and degeneration of neurons, edema, and inflammation, have been described. The risk of *spasmodic colic* also increases with parasite burden, which may be at least partially explained by the histologic lesions described. *Ileal muscular hypertrophy, impaction and partial obstruction* of the ileocecal orifice, and *ileocecal and cecocecal intussusception* are also associated with large numbers of *A. perfoliata*. Although histologic lesions correlate well with the parasite burden, whether the development of colic, obstruction, muscular hypertrophy, or intussusception is the result of altered peristaltic waves or mucosal and submucosal lesions remains unclear.

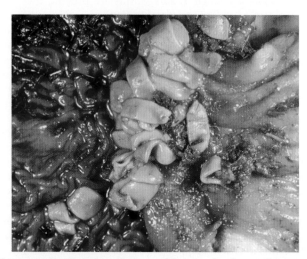

Figure 1-184 *Anoplocephala perfoliata* at the ileocecal junction of a horse.

Further reading

Back H, et al. The association between *Anoplocephala perfoliata* and colic in Swedish horses-a case control study. Vet Parasitol 2013;197:580-585.

Matthews JB, et al. Recent developments in research into the Cyathostominae and *Anoplocephala perfoliata*. Vet Res 2004;35:371-381.

Pavone S, et al. Pathological changes caused by *Anoplocephala perfoliata* in the mucosa/submucosa and in the enteric nervous system of equine ileocecal junction. Vet Parasitol 2011;176:43-52.

Trotz-Williams L, et al. Occurrence of *Anoplocephala perfoliata* infection in horses in Ontario, Canada and associations with colic and management practices. Vet Parasitol 2008;153:73-84.

***Diphyllobothrium* spp. Dogs** may be parasitized by *Diphyllobothrium* spp., as may be humans, **cats**, **swine**, and other fish-eating mammals. The adults can be large, reaching lengths of up to 12-15 meters in humans, though in animals they tend to be shorter. The worm is ~2 cm in width, and characterized by a central uterus containing dark operculate eggs. Intermediate stages occur in copepods and fish, and the adult worm matures in the intestine of piscivorous mammals. Infection by *Diphyllobothrium* spp. is rarely, if ever, associated with clinical disease in animals.

Spirometra species are, like *Diphyllobothrium*, members of the order Pseudophyllidea, and their life cycle is similar. The taxonomy of the genus is difficult, recognized species include *S. mansonoides*, which infects dogs, cats, and raccoons in North and South America; *S. mansoni* infects dogs and cats in East Asia and South America; and *S. erinacei* infects cats and dogs in Australia and the Far East. The definitive host must ingest the third larval form, or plerocercoid, usually via predation of an infected intermediate or paratenic host. Several animal species that are not definitive hosts can serve as paratenic or transport hosts when they ingest the *plerocercoid, or spargana* found in the body cavity, muscle or subcutaneous tissues of the second intermediate host, usually an amphibian or reptile. Spargana are white, ribbon-like, but otherwise structureless worms up to several centimeters long found free or encysted in a thin, fibrous capsule in the peritoneal cavity, muscle, or subcutaneous tissue. A chronic inflammatory reaction may occur around dead spargana, although the adult worms are nonpathogenic. Spargana can also occur in carnivores, swine, or even humans (sparganosis), if the first intermediate host *Cyclops* copepod containing the second larval stage (procercoid) is ingested, usually via contaminated drinking water. Sparganosis is a significant disease in humans, where the plerocercoids migrate mainly in subcutaneous tissues or rarely in other organs.

Mesocestoides spp. occasionally infect dogs, as well as other mammals and some birds, in North America, Europe, Asia, and Africa. These cyclophyllidean tapeworms have a complex life cycle involving an insect or mite, and a vertebrate as second intermediate host. Infective *tetrathyridia* are found in the body cavities, liver, and lung of mammals, reptiles, or birds; ingestion of tetrathyridia causes infection of the definitive host. In the intestine of definitive hosts, *Mesocestoides* adults may also replicate asexually, and heavy infections or continual re-infection may occur as a result of this, or from the consumption of large numbers of tetrathyridia in an intermediate host. Animals infected with intestinal *Mesocestoides* may develop diarrhea. Tetrathyridia replicating in the intestine of the dog may also penetrate the gut wall, and proliferate in the peritoneal cavity, resulting in peritoneal larval cestodosis. Tetrathyridia in the abdominal cavity of dogs and cats may cause peritoneal effusion (*parasitic ascites*), perhaps with the development of pyogranulomatous peritonitis and adhesions. Tetrathyridia 1-2 mm in diameter are scattered in abundant exudate, along with small white cyst-like structures, comprised of necrotic parasite tegument and host cellular debris. Mild infections may be discovered incidentally at autopsy. *Mesocestoides* infection of the abdominal cavity must be differentiated from peritoneal infections by cysticerci of several *Taenia* spp., which occur very rarely in carnivores.

Dipylidium caninum occurs in the dog, cat, fox, and, occasionally, children. It is ubiquitous. The narrow worms, up to 0.5 meters long, have distinctive cucumber-seed–like segments, and are often encountered incidentally in the small intestine at autopsy. They are of no pathologic significance. Cysticercoids develop in fleas and perhaps in the dog louse *Trichodectes canis*. Infection in the normal definitive hosts, or in accidental ones such as humans, is by ingestion of fleas containing cysticercoids.

Further reading

Crosbie PR, et al. Diagnostic procedures and treatment of eleven dogs with peritoneal infections caused by *Mesocestoides* spp. J Am Vet Med Assoc 1998;213:1578-1583.

Gray ML, et al. Sparganosis in feral hogs (*Sus scrofa*) from Florida. J Am Vet Med Assoc 1999;215:204-208.

Patten PK, et al. Cestode infection in 2 dogs: cytologic findings in liver and a mesenteric lymph node. Vet Clin Path 2013;42:103-108.

Toplu N, et al. Massive cystic tetrathyridiosis in a dog. J Small Anim Pract 2004;45:410-412.

Taeniid tapeworms. *Taeniid cestodes are the most important tapeworms in domestic animals*, not because of the effects of the adult worm in the carnivorous definitive host, but rather because of the *metacestodes*, or larval forms, in intermediate or paratenic hosts. Gravid taeniid segments exit from the definitive host and shed their eggs. If ingested by an appropriate intermediate vertebrate host, the egg hatches and the embryo enters the intestinal wall to migrate to the organ of predilection, which is often the liver, peritoneum, or muscle. Here they differentiate into second-stage larvae characterized by a fluid-filled bladder with one or more scolices (bladderworm), which is infective to the definitive host. Once the second-stage larva is ingested by the definitive host, the scolex embeds itself into the small intestinal mucosa, where it begins to bud segments to form strobila. Metacestodes occasionally may be found in organs other than the site of predilection.

Taeniid metacestodes assume 4 basic forms. The **cysticercus** is a fluid-filled, thin-walled muscular cyst into which the scolex and neck of a single larval tapeworm are invaginated. The **strobilocercus** is a modification of this theme: Late in larval development the scolex evaginates, elongates, and segments while still in the intermediate host, so that it resembles a tapeworm up to several centimeters long. The **coenurus** is a single or loculated fluid-filled cyst, in which many scolices are present in clusters on the inner wall. Each scolex is capable of developing into a single adult cestode in the intestine of the definitive host. The **hydatid cyst** is formed by members of the genus *Echinococcus* and is of unilocular or multilocular structure, on the inner germinal membrane of which brood capsules develop. Within the brood capsules, invaginated protoscolices form. Brood capsules may float free in the cyst fluid, where they are termed *hydatid sand*. Release of brood capsules or protoscolices into tissues, as a result of rupture of the hydatid cyst, may lead to development of new cysts. The alveolar hydatid cyst proliferates by budding externally.

Taenia taeniaeformis infects the intestine of domestic cats and some wild felids, and the strobilocercus, *Cysticercus fasciolaris* is found in the liver of small rodents. Formation of hepatic fibrosarcomas has been associated with chronic inflammation resulting from *C. fasciolaris*. The adults are up to 60 cm long, have no neck, and caudal segments are somewhat bell-shaped, so this species is readily differentiated from the other cestodes found in the feline small intestine. Usually only a few worms are present in the cat, and they are of no consequence.

T. pisiformis is common in the small intestine in dogs and some wild canids, which prey on rabbits and hares. *C. pisiformis* migrates in the liver of the intermediate host, causing hemorrhagic tracks that are infiltrated by a mixed inflammatory reaction, and ultimately heal by scarring. The 3-5 mm diameter cysticerci encyst in a thin fibrous capsule on the mesentery, omentum, or on the ligaments of the bladder. Occasionally, cysticerci persist beneath the hepatic capsule. Burdens of up to 20-30 worms, sometimes more, may be present in the intestine of the dog.

T. hydatigena infects the dog, and the metacestode, *C. tenuicollis*, the long-necked bladder worm is found in the peritoneal cavity of sheep, cattle, swine, and occasionally other species. Immature cysticerci in the liver migrate through the parenchyma for several weeks as they develop, before emerging to encyst on the peritoneum anywhere in the abdominal cavity. Immature cysticerci are <1 cm long, ovoid, and translucent. They cause tortuous hemorrhagic tracks similar to those produced by immature liver flukes, and if large numbers are present, they may cause a syndrome of depression and icterus.

Heavily infected livers, with 4,000-5,000 actively migrating cysticerci, are mottled because of the subcapsular and parenchymal hemorrhagic tracks. Cysticerci up to 6-8 mm long may be present beneath or breaching the capsule by ~3 weeks after infection. Rarely, animals may exsanguinate into the abdominal cavity, or the hepatic necrosis may predispose to the development of black disease or bacillary hemoglobinuria. Cysticerci trapped in the liver may persist in a fibrous capsule or be destroyed in a cystic eosinophilic granuloma that may mineralize; this is common on the diaphragmatic surface where the falciform ligament is attached. Usually the intensity of infection is low, and a few, but occasionally scores of cysticerci—delicate translucent fluctuant fluid-filled cysts up to 5 cm or more in diameter—are contained in individual thin, noninflammatory fibrous capsules scattered on the peritoneal serosa. When a cyst degenerates, it is destroyed by a granulomatous reaction and the fibrotic mass may mineralize. Hepatic migration by *C. tenuicollis* may, at any stage, cause condemnation of lamb and swine livers at slaughter inspection.

T. ovis infects the intestine of the dog, whereas the metacestode, *C. ovis* is in the muscle of sheep where it causes cysticercosis or *sheep measles*. Cysticercosis of muscle caused by *C. ovis*; by *C. bovis* in cattle; and by *C. cellulosae* in swine and other species, including dogs, is considered in Vol. 1, Muscle and tendon. The adult stages of the latter two cysticerci, *T. saginata* and *T. solium*, respectively, occur in the small intestine of humans.

T. multiceps occurs in the intestine of dogs and wild canids, but the metacestode **Coenurus cerebralis** develops in the brain and spinal cord of sheep and other ungulates, and rarely in humans. In the goat, coenuri may also occur in other organs, including the subcutaneous space or intramuscularly. Migration of small metacestodes in the central nervous system may cause tortuous red or yellow-gray tracks in the brain because of hemorrhage and malacia, and central nervous signs or death may occur. More commonly, signs of CNS disease termed "sturdy" or "gid," do not develop until coenuri enlarge up to 4-5 cm in diameter and develop more fully, usually 4-8 months after infection. Cysts may be present at any level and depth in the brain and spinal cord, and projecting into the cerebral ventricles, but they are most common near the surface of the parietal cortex in the cerebrum. They cause increased intracranial pressure, hydrocephalus, and necrosis of adjacent brain parenchyma that may extend to the overlying skull. Coenuri developing in the spinal cord may cause paresis or paralysis.

T. serialis infects dogs and foxes throughout the world. The larval coenurus is found in the subcutaneous and intermuscular connective tissue of lagomorphs. Cerebral coenurosis has been reported in cats.

Histologically, cysticerci and coenuri are recognized as cystic structures with an eosinophilic outer layer or tegument, which may appear fibrillar on the outermost surface. Beneath the tegument, a less cellular area, which may contain calcareous corpuscles, gives way to a web-like, lightly cellular matrix, and the central open fluid-filled portion of the cyst. Internal organs are not present in the metacestode. Muscular scolices, with suckers, and hooks on the rostellum (except *C. bovis*), may be encountered extending into the center of the metacestode. The size and shape of hooks may assist in a specific diagnosis if they are fully developed. Immature migrating metacestodes lack organized scolices. Other sources should be consulted for details on the taxonomy and specific identification of adult and larval taeniid tapeworms.

Echinococcus spp. tapeworms occur in the small intestine of a number of species of carnivores, predominantly canids. In enzootic areas, the distinctive metacestodes or *hydatid cysts*, are commonly found in normal or accidental intermediate hosts. Humans may accidentally become infected with the metacestode, and echinococcosis or hydatidosis is a significant public health problem where carnivores shedding *Echinococcus* eggs come in close contact with humans. The important species are *E. granulosus*, *E. multilocularis*, *E. oligarthus*, and *E. vogeli*. The latter two involve sylvatic cycles in Central and South America, with felids and canids as definitive hosts, respectively, and rodents as intermediate hosts in which polycystic hydatidosis occurs; *E. vogeli* may infect humans. The other two species may use domestic animals as definitive hosts, and are considered further here.

E. granulosus uses the dog and some other canids as the definitive host. The most widespread strain or genotype uses a *sheep-dog cycle*, and has been disseminated wherever there is pastoral husbandry of sheep. It is significant as a potential zoonosis in many parts of Eurasia and the Mediterranean region, some parts of the United Kingdom, North America, South America, continental Australia, and Africa. Eradication has been accomplished, or virtually so, in Iceland, New Zealand, and Tasmania. Other cycles affecting domestic animals include horse-; cattle-; camel-; pig-; water buffalo-; goat-; and human-dog. Sylvatic cycles include: in Eurasia and

North America, cervid-wolf; in Argentina, hare-fox; in Sri Lanka, deer-jackal; and in Australia, macropod-dingo. Not all cycles represent different genotypes.

In the small intestine of the definitive host, protoscolices evaginate and establish between villi and in the crypts of Lieberkühn. The scolex distends the crypt and the epithelium is gripped by the suckers and may become eroded, but there is little or no inflammatory response. The worms that develop are short, usually <6-7 mm long; they commonly have only 3-5 proglottids, the caudal gravid one making up almost half the length of the worm. Burdens of *E. granulosus* are often heavy, no doubt because of the large numbers of protoscolices ingested at a meal containing one or more hydatid cysts. The heavily infected intestine is carpeted by the tiny white blunt projections, partially obscured between the villi and resembling lymphangiectasia; enteric signs are not normally observed. Eggs shed from adults are ingested by the intermediate host; oncospheres released from eggs in the intestine of the intermediate host migrate via subepithelial capillaries or lacteals to the liver, lungs, and general circulation. *Hydatid cysts occur most commonly in the liver and lung*, with some strain and host species variation in the relative prevalence in these organs. In sheep they may be more common in lungs, whereas in cattle and horses the liver is the usual site of establishment. Less common sites in domestic animals include the brain, heart, bone, and subcutaneous tissue. A single cyst, or up to several hundreds, may be present, displacing tissue in infected organs. Disease is rarely attributed to hydatidosis in animals, even in those heavily infected. However, strategic location of one or more cysts may lead to heart failure, bloat, or central nervous signs because of space occupation. Condemnation of infected organs at slaughter inspection may cause significant economic loss.

Grossly, hydatid cysts are spherical, turgid, and fluid-filled. They usually measure 5-10 cm in diameter in domestic animals; rarely, cysts in animals may be larger, but in humans hydatid cysts can become huge. In contrast, fertile cysts in equine livers may be as small as 2-3 mm diameter. The lining of fertile cysts is studded with small granular *brood capsules*, which contain protoscolices. "Hydatid sand," comprised of free brood capsules and protoscolices, is typically present within the fluid; smooth lined cysts are sterile. Although the potential exists for development of daughter cysts and exogenous budding by herniated cysts, most hydatid cysts in domestic animals are unilocular. They may be irregular or distorted in shape because of the tissue they are in, and variable resistance of parenchyma and portal tracts or bronchi and by the profiles of bone or other resistant tissues.

Microscopically, immature hydatid cysts are surrounded by an infiltrate of mixed inflammatory cells, including giant cells and eosinophils. As they develop, a layer of granulation tissue surrounds the cyst, and this matures so that in aged lesions the inner portion of the fibrous capsule is comprised of acellular mature collagenous connective tissue. In close apposition is a periodic acid-Schiff–positive staining *acellular lamellar hyaline outer layer* of the hydatid cyst wall, comprised of a polysaccharide-protein complex that may become hundreds of micrometers thick. The cyst is lined by the thin syncytial germinal layer from which the brood capsules form on fine pedicles. If the cyst is ruptured and protoscolices are released into tissue, secondary cysts may form from them. If hydatid cysts degenerate, the inner structures collapse and the mass becomes filled with necrotic debris and may

mineralize; these resemble tuberculous lesions grossly and histologically.

E. multilocularis has a holarctic distribution; adults occur mainly in foxes, and the metacestodes in small rodents, especially voles and lemmings. Dogs and cats may also become infected with adult *E. multilocularis* in enzootic areas. Although the parasite is principally arctic, the cycle is found in the northern prairie area of North America and in eastern and central Europe, and is moving progressively southward. The mature cestodes in the intestine are similar to but smaller than *E. granulosus*. In the intermediate host the metacestode or *multilocular alveolar hydatid* mainly infects the liver by forming a cystic structure with internal brood capsules and many protoscolices. The alveolar hydatid is capable of external budding that continuously proliferates and infiltrates surrounding tissue. They may metastasize via the bloodstream to the lungs or bone, or implant in the peritoneal cavity. The inflammatory reaction to alveolar hydatids is comprised of macrophages, giant cells, lymphocytes, and plasma cells within a fibrous capsular stroma. The metacestodes are rarely found in domestic animals, but may infect humans who ingest eggs shed by infected carnivores.

Further reading

Carmena D, Cardona GA. Canine echinococcosis: Global epidemiology and genotypic diversity. Acta Tropica 2013;128:441-460.

Deplazes P, Eckert J. Veterinary aspects of alveolar echinococcosis—a zoonosis of public health significance. Vet Parasitol 2001;98:65-87.

DeWolf BD, et al. *Taenia ovis* infection and its control: a Canadian perspective. N Z Vet J 2014;62:1-7.

Hoberg EP. *Taenia* tapeworms: their biology, evolution and socioeconomic significance. Microbes Infect 2002;4:859-866.

McManus DP, et al. Echinococcosis. Lancet 2003;362:1295-1304.

Otero-Abad B, Torgerson PR. A systematic review of the epidemiology of echinococcosis in domestic and wild animals. PLOS Negl Trop Dis 2013;7:e2249.

Intestinal fluke infection. Digenetic trematode infections of the intestine of domestic animals are uncommon. Dogs and cats in many parts of the world may be infected with *Alaria* spp., the second intermediate hosts for which are frogs or other amphibia. *Heterophyes heterophyes, Metagonimus yokagawi, Echinochasmus perfoliatus*, and *Phagicola longa* may infect dogs and cats fed fish that contain metacercariae. The former two occur in the Mediterranean area and the Far East; the latter in Eurasia. *Cryptocotyle* spp., most commonly parasitic in piscivorous birds, also may be found in dogs, cats, and mink fed infected marine fish.

Enteritis has been attributed to **Alaria, Echinochasmus, and Cryptocotyle.** The flukes attach to the mucosa by suckers, and perhaps cause their effects by local irritation, erosion, and ulceration when present in large numbers. Excessive intestinal mucus production, hemorrhagic enteritis, vomiting, and illthrift have been associated with intestinal fluke infection in small animals. The flukes involved are small, <4-5 mm long, and must be sought carefully at autopsy.

The digenean trematode **Nanophyetus salmincola**, the vector of *salmon poisoning disease*, occurs in the small intestine of dogs, cats, and humans, and in various fish-eating wild mammals and birds in the northwestern United States; Vancouver Island, Canada; and eastern Siberia. The disease has been thought to be restricted to North America; however, similar organisms have been recognized in dogs with lesions compatible with salmon poisoning disease in southern Brazil. Its distribution is determined by that of the snails that are the first intermediate hosts. The second intermediate hosts are fish, especially members of the family *Salmonidae*. Adult flukes inhabit the small intestine, where they penetrate and attach to the mucosa and release large numbers of ova, which infect the snail. Mature *cercariae*, or free-swimming larvae, are released into water and penetrate the abdominal region of the second intermediate host. Metacercariae locate in the kidneys, liver, and intestine via the circulation of the fish. Adult trematodes attach deeply and develop in the intestine of the definitive host that has ingested metacercariae-infected fish. *N. salmincola* transmits **Neorickettsia helminthoeca**, the etiologic agent of *salmon poisoning disease*, which is released from the trematode and is disseminated via the circulatory and lymphatic system in the definitive host. *N. helminthoeca* is nonpathogenic to either the first or second intermediate host; *N. salmincola* in high numbers can be pathogenic to both intermediate hosts.

Salmon poisoning disease has an incubation period of ~5-7 days, and is characterized clinically by pyrexia, anorexia, depression, weakness, and weight loss. There may be serous nasal discharge, lymphadenopathy, and mucopurulent conjunctivitis. Diarrhea with tenesmus develops; feces are scant yellow and mucoid or watery, often with some blood. The condition is usually fatal; if untreated, only 5-10% of infected dogs survive, but they are immune to reinfection.

Gross lesions are most consistently found in the lymphoid tissues and include *generalized enlargement of lymph nodes*, especially in the abdominal cavity. Enlarged tonsils are everted from their fossae. The thymus is often increased in size in young dogs and the spleen may be swollen and congested. Peyer's patches and other intestinal lymphoid aggregates are elevated above the mucosal surface, and there may be petechial hemorrhages on the mucosa. In some cases there is ulceration and hemorrhage of the intestine near the ileocecocolic valve; intussusception of the small intestine occurs in many cases. There may be hepatomegaly, hepatic rupture, and hemoabdomen. Focal hemorrhages have been described in the pleura, the gallbladder, and the urinary bladder.

Microscopic changes in lymph nodes include *depletion of lymphocytes* and increased numbers of histiocytes in the cortex and medulla. Similar changes may occur in the thymus, and splenic follicles may undergo necrosis. Intracytoplasmic *elementary bodies* of the *Neorickettsia* may be demonstrated in reticuloendothelial cells of lymphoid tissue and other visceral organs, by use of Giemsa or Macchiavello stains or immunohistochemistry. In the small intestine the flukes may be present embedded deep in the mucosa, although usually little reaction to them is present. Additional microscopic lesions may include lymphocytic and histiocytic leptomeningitis or meningitis, which may be most consistent over the cerebellum. Similar inflammatory cells may surround small and medium-sized vessels throughout the neuroparenchyma; focal gliosis is relatively sparsely distributed but seems most common in the brainstem. Elementary bodies are also demonstrable in reticuloendothelial cells of the central nervous system, and the diagnosis is usually made on the basis of this finding in lymphoid tissue and/or brain. The organisms can be isolated and grown on primary canine monocyte cultures and in several other cell culture systems, but this is not a routine procedure.

Paramphistome, or rumen fluke, infections in ruminants may cause significant intestinal disease. Adults of the genera *Paramphistomum*, *Cotylophoron*, *Calicophoron*, *Ceylonocotyle*, *Gastrothylax*, *Fischoederius*, and *Carmyerius* occur in the forestomachs of ruminants in various areas around the world. The species involved vary with the host and geographic area. In cattle, water buffalo, and American bison, the species incriminated in disease include *P. cervi*, *P. microbothrium*, *P. explanatum*, *Calicophoron calicophorum*, and various species of *Cotylophoron*, *Gastrothylax*, and *Fischoederius*. In sheep and goats, *P. microbothrium*, *P. ichikawai*, *P. cervi*, *P. explanatum*, *G. crumenifer*, *Cotylophoron cotylophorum*, and *F. cobboldi* have been associated with disease.

Infection is most common in warm-temperate to tropical areas. In the rumen, the tan to red pear-shaped adult flukes, with their characteristic cranial and caudal suckers, are considered innocuous, although some papillae may become atrophic and slough. When ingested, metacercariae encysted on herbage give rise to immature flukes that inhabit the duodenum, and in heavy infections may cause severe hemorrhagic enteritis. After 3-5 weeks in the small intestine, the worms normally migrate through the abomasum to establish and mature in the reticulorumen (see Fig. 1-34A). However, if massive infection occurs, growth in the small intestine is slowed, and flukes may persist for months in the duodenum, prolonging the course of disease.

Calves and lambs with severe intestinal paramphistomosis are depressed and inappetent. Fetid *diarrhea* usually develops within several weeks of infection, and may contain immature flukes. Hypoproteinemia is reflected in submandibular edema in some animals and anemia is reported to occur occasionally. Morbidity and mortality can be substantial, and survivors may suffer considerable loss in condition. Protein loss into the gut, coupled with loss of appetite, probably accounts for the most important pathophysiologic consequences.

Gross lesions are nonspecific and include cachexia depending on the duration of the disease, edema of subcutaneous tissues, abomasal folds, and mesentery, and multi-cavitary effusion caused by hypoproteinemia. The proximal small intestine appears congested, and the mucosal surface is edematous, thickened, corrugated, and covered with mucus. Myriad immature pink or brown paramphistomes, a few millimeters long, are observed firmly attached and embedded in the proximal intestinal wall and may be visible through the serosa. Occasionally, the organisms perforate the intestinal wall and are found free in the abdominal cavity. In advanced infections, some organisms may be present migrating orally into the abomasum or the forestomachs.

Histologically, larval paramphistomes are found deep in the lamina propria, occasionally in the submucosa, and sometimes in Brunner's glands. Larger immature forms are attached to the surface of the mucosa by a plug of tissue taken into the oral sucker, or acetabulum (see Fig. 1-34B). There is atrophy of villi, elongation of crypts, erosion or ulceration of the mucosa, and potentially fibroplasia in heavily infected areas.

The other fluke occurring in the intestine of ruminants is *Skjrabinotrema ovis*, associated with catarrhal enteritis in sheep in Eurasia.

In **swine,** the paramphistomes *Gastrodiscoides* and *Gastrodiscus* may be found in the colon, where they are of little significance. *Fasciolopsis buski* and *Artyfechinosomum malayanum* may infect the small intestine of swine as well as humans.

They are of little importance in pigs other than as potential reservoirs for human infection.

In **horses** in Africa and India, the paramphistomes *Gastrodiscus aegyptiacus* and *Pseudodiscus colinsi* occur in the large bowel. Larvae of the former species have been associated with severe colitis in horses, but they are generally nonpathogenic.

Intestinal schistosomiasis is due mainly to *Schistosoma* spp. in ruminants and *Heterobilharzia americanum* in dogs. *H. americanum* has been located primarily in the Atlantic or Gulf coast states in North America; however, naturally occurring disease has been reported in the midwestern United States. *H. americanum* has a complex life cycle involving both snail and mammalian hosts such as raccoon and domestic canids. Dogs are infected while swimming or wading in water contaminated with infective free-swimming cercariae, which penetrate the skin. Immature flukes can be found in the liver within several days of infecting the mammalian definitive host; this is where most of their growth and development occurs. Mature adults migrate to mesenteric veins where sexual reproduction occurs; eggs then penetrate the serosal surface of the intestine and migrate through the intestinal wall, which incites a severe inflammatory response. Alternatively, eggs migrate to the liver and are carried by the portal circulation to various other organs, the most common of which include the pancreas and kidneys. Eggs embedded in these organs result in host tissue response and granulomatous inflammatory foci; the number of embedded eggs determines the degree of organic dysfunction in these cases.

Clinical signs include intermittent hemorrhagic diarrhea with excess mucus production, tenesmus, vomiting, anorexia and weight loss; involvement of the gastrointestinal system is common. Gross intestinal lesions are nonspecific, but may include reddened thickened intestinal wall; intestinal intussusception has been associated with this syndrome in a small number of dogs. Histologic lesions in the intestine are typically *multifocal to diffuse granulomatous enterocolitis*; eggs may be present within the mucosa, submucosa, and muscular layers of affected dogs. Other histologic lesions include granulomas surrounding eggs embedded in other organs are also present. For additional information on syndromes caused by *H. americanum*, see Vol. 3, Cardiovascular system.

Adult flukes in tissue section are generally somewhat flattened or globose, with a loose mesenchymal parenchyma in which the internal structures are embedded. The tegument is eosinophilic, and may contain spines. Muscular oral and acetabular suckers and pharynx may be encountered in sections. Ceca are usually present, and elements of the male and female reproductive systems in these typically hermaphroditic adult worms (excepting the schistosomes) may be seen. The uterus may contain ova with a tan-yellow or brown shell, perhaps with an operculum, and ova are often seen in the intestinal lumen or in tissue. The developing miracidium may be present in ova. Schistosomes are recognized by their intravascular location and sexual dimorphism, the leaf-like male perhaps enveloping the slender cylindrical female within the gynecophoric canal.

Further reading

Fabrick C, et al. Clinical features and outcome of *Heterobilharzia americana* infection in dogs. J Vet Intern Med 2010;24:140-144.

Hanzlicek AS, et al. Canine schistosomiasis in Kansas: five cases (2000-2009). J Am Anim Hosp Assoc 2011;47:e95-e102.

Headley SA, et al. *Neorickettsia helminthoeca* and salmon poisoning disease: a review. Vet J 2011;187:165-173.

Mason C, Stevenson H. Disease associated with immature paramphistome infection in sheep. Vet Rec 2012;170:343-344.

Millar M, et al. Disease associated with immature paramphistome infection. Vet Rec 2012;171:509-510.

Sykes JE, et al. Salmon poisoning disease in dogs: 29 cases. J Vet Intern Med 2010;24:504-531.

Acanthocephalan infections. Acanthocephala is a phylum of parasitic worms that have an elongate sac-like body, no internal alimentary canal, and use a spiny protrusible proboscis for attachment to the intestinal wall. The life cycle typically involves obligate development in an intermediate host, usually an arthropod, and perhaps the use of a paratenic host to facilitate transmission. The acanthocephala of concern in domestic animals are in the genera *Macracanthorhynchus* and *Oncicola*.

Macracanthorhynchus hirudinaceus is the *thorny-headed worm* that infects the small intestine of *swine*. The life cycle involves dung beetles or other *Scarabaeidae*, and foraging or rooting swine are prone to infection. Adult males are 10 cm long, and the females up to 30-40 cm long, slightly pink, curved, and taper caudally. The proboscis has ~6 rows of hooks, and is used to penetrate deeply the intestinal wall. Attachment incites a local granulomatous nodule that has been called a *strawberry mark*, which may be visible from the serosal surface as a gray or yellow 1-cm diameter nodule surrounded by a hyperemic rim. The proboscis may penetrate the tunica muscularis and cause peritonitis. Heavily infected pigs may suffer ill-thrift and perhaps anemia, probably related partly to plasma protein loss and hemorrhage from numerous focal ulcerative lesions.

M. catalinum and *M. ingens* are smaller but similar thorny-headed worms that inhabit the intestine of a variety of wild carnivores, and occasionally the dog.

Oncicola canis occurs in the small intestine of wild carnivores, and occasionally the dog and cat. It rarely causes disease. Intermediate hosts are presumably arthropods, with insectivorous vertebrates acting as paratenic hosts. Up to several hundred worms, 0.5-1.5 cm long and dark gray, may infest the small intestine; infections are usually light. The proboscis is embedded to the subserosal level, and a focal nodular lesion develops about it.

Further reading

Zhao B, et al. Light and electron microscopic studies of the histopathogenicity of *Macracanthorhynchus hirudinaceus* (Archiacanthocephala) in experimentally infected domestic swine. Parasitol Res 1990;76:355-359.

Protistan infections

Coccidiosis

The coccidia are members of the protistan phylum Apicomplexa, intracellular parasites characterized at some stage of the life cycle by a typical "apical complex" of organelles at one end of the organism. Members of the subclass Coccidiasina, which are considered together under coccidiosis, all have a similar basic life cycle. It begins with infection of a cell, often, but not always, in the intestinal mucosa, by a **sporozoite** released from a **sporocyst** in the lumen of the gut. One or more cycles of asexual division, termed **schizogony or merogony,** follow, and the **merozoites** produced infect other cells, forming another generation of **meronts,** or transforming to sexual stages, termed **gamonts.** Gamonts subsequently develop into nonmotile female **macrogametes,** and motile male forms or **microgametes.** A nonmotile zygote produced by union of microgametes and macrogametes forms an **oocyst.** Oocysts are released in feces to the environment. **Sporogony,** which is the production of sporocysts containing infectious sporozoites within the oocyst, may occur in the host, or more commonly, after the resistant oocysts are passed in feces.

Members of the genus *Eimeria* and *Isospora* are **homoxenous,** with sexual and asexual development taking place in a single host. *Cystoisospora* (former *Isospora* spp. in carnivores) and the genera *Toxoplasma, Sarcocystis, Hammondia, Besnoitia, Frenkelia, Neospora,* and *Caryospora* are all **heteroxenous,** in which case asexual stages occur in an intermediate host. The heteroxenous genera exploit natural prey-predator relationships. In general, sexual development takes place in the intestinal mucosa of a predator, whereas at least one generation of asexual replication, often several, occurs in the tissues of one or more species of prey.

The *endogenous stages of coccidia are all intracellular,* except, temporarily, the merozoite and microgamete. Mature developmental stages are usually readily recognized; immature forms may not be easily identifiable. **Trophozoites,** small undifferentiated, rounded, basophilic forms with a single nucleus, usually within a parasitophorous vacuole in the host cell, are found at 3 stages of the life cycle. They occur after invasion by the infective sporozoite, before merogony; after invasion by a merozoite, before a subsequent generation of merogony; and after invasion by a merozoite, before differentiation into a recognizable gamont. Developing meronts are multinucleated. Merogony may involve **endopolygeny,** which is multiple fission or apparent "budding" of merozoites from the periphery of the meront or from infoldings of it. A single residual body, surrounded by slightly curved, fusiform, or banana-shaped uninucleate merozoites, or many spherical clusters of merozoites with a central residuum, may be present. A second form of replication, termed **endodyogeny,** occurs in meronts of many of the heteroxenous coccidia. Two daughter organisms develop within a mother organism, which is destroyed when they are released. The location of a meront, and the number of merozoites it contains, vary with the species and the generation of merogony. A very few, or up to tens or hundreds of thousands of merozoites, may be released from a single meront.

Microgamonts mature in 2 steps. The first involves enlargement of the gamont and proliferation of nuclei. During the second phase, the microgametes differentiate about the periphery of the gamont, which may become deeply folded or fissured by invaginations. Immature microgametocytes during these stages may resemble developing schizonts. However, *fully differentiated microgametes* differ from merozoites in being small, densely basophilic, and comma-shaped, with 2-3 flagella. They may be present in swirling masses, perhaps with some residual bodies, in mature microgametocytes. Macrogametes, the female stage, have a large nucleus with a prominent nucleolus, and with time they usually enlarge to contain refractile eosinophilic "plastic granules" or wall-forming bodies, which give rise to the layers of the oocyst

wall. *Mature macrogametes* typically have prominent wall-forming bodies, and contain clear or periodic acid-Schiff–positive amylopectin granules, and a large nucleus and nucleolus.

Fertilization by the microgamete leads to development of the zygote, and subsequent formation of the oocyst wall. The contained *sporont* is spherical, with nucleus and nucleolus, and amylopectin granules in the cytoplasm. Sporulation usually occurs outside the host, but in *Sarcocystis* and *Frenkelia* it occurs in the tissue of the definitive host; in *Caryospora,* sporulated oocysts develop in tissues of the prey host. Sporozoites are enclosed within sporocysts, which in turn are contained by the oocyst wall. Oocysts of most coccidia, or sporocysts of *Sarcocystis* and *Frenkelia,* are passed in the feces.

Coccidia of domestic animals are relatively host-, organ-, and tissue-specific. Asexual stages of *Toxoplasma* and *Neospora* are the obvious exception to this generalization. Species of *Eimeria, Isospora,* and *Cystoisospora* rarely occur in more than one genus of definitive host. Similar coccidia occurring in related genera of hosts, when tested, usually prove incapable of cross-infection.

The economic cost of coccidiosis in the food-animal species is considerable, in terms of mortality, morbidity, subclinical disease, and the cost of prevention and treatment. It is even more so in chickens. In dogs and cats, coccidiosis is a minor problem.

Virulence reflects a number of factors. Among these are the location and type of cell infected by various stages of the organism, the function of infected cells, and the degree of host reaction stimulated by infection. The effects of infection on the host cell are several, and vary somewhat with the infecting species. Infected cells may be functionally compromised. They may hypertrophy; nuclei may enlarge or a considerable amount of cytoplasm may be displaced; and the outer membrane of infected cells may be highly modified, perhaps to facilitate metabolic exchange. The intercellular relationships may be affected. The rate of movement of infected epithelial cells up villi is altered. *E. bovis* also induces apoptosis by interfering with both the receptor-mediated and inner pathways of apoptosis. Necrosis is also likely to occur.

Immune reactions may be incited by coccidial infection. In experimental systems resistance to coccidial infection is thymus-dependent, and is largely mediated by T-cell–driven intracellular killing directed mainly against asexual stages in the life cycle.

In mammals, acute inflammatory reactions in intestinal coccidiosis are most commonly associated with heavy infection and destruction of cells by the sexual stages and oocysts, rather than in response to asexual stages. In toxoplasmosis and neosporosis, necrosis and focal acute or chronic inflammatory reactions may be incited by actively replicating asexual stages in many organs. A syndrome characterized by hemorrhage occurs in some species infected with asexual stages of *Sarcocystis,* about the time that merogony occurs in vascular endothelium.

The effects of *intestinal coccidiosis* in mammals vary with the host-parasite system. They are mainly related to malabsorption induced by *villus atrophy,* or to anemia, hypoproteinemia, and dehydration caused by exudative enteritis and colitis caused by *epithelial erosion and ulceration.* A not yet fully characterized heat-labile *neurotoxin* has been associated with the development of nervous disorders in cattle with coccidiosis. Many species of coccidia appear to have little pathogenic effect under normal circumstances.

Coccidiosis is typically a disease of *intensively managed animals*. It is especially important in naive young animals exposed to a high level of infection. This is predisposed by high contamination rates associated with crowding, yarding, or high stocking rates on pasture. A damp substrate promotes oocyst sporulation and survival, and practices such as feeding on the ground or the natural propensity of young animals to nibble or perhaps indulge in coprophagy may promote infection. Although infections may not proceed to patency, chronic ingestion of oocysts may cause an intestinal immune response, villus atrophy, and in some situations perhaps ill-thrift. Immune reactions may only halt development of, but not kill, endogenous asexual stages. Epidemiologic evidence suggests that under some circumstances there may be relaxation of resistance and resumption of development of the organisms, ultimately expressed in disease. This seems the likely explanation for outbreaks of bovine coccidiosis occurring during midwinter in freezing climates, or in postparturient stabled dairy cattle.

Coccidiosis caused by members of the genera *Eimeria* and *Isospora* in the various species are considered further here. The heteroxenous organisms, including *Cystoisospora*, *Toxoplasma*, *Neospora*, and *Sarcocystis*, are considered subsequently, as are *Cryptosporidium*.

Further reading

Barta JR, et al. The genus *Atoxoplasma* (Garnham 1950) as a junior objective synonym of the genus *Isospora* (Schneider 1881) species infecting birds and resurrection of *Cystoisospora* (Frenkel 1977) as the correct genus for *Isospora* species infecting mammals. J Parasitol 2005;91:726-727.

Hermosilla C, et al. *Eimeria bovis*: an update on parasite-host cell interactions. Int J Med Microbiol 2012;302:210-215.

Samarasinghe B, et al. Phylogenetic analysis of *Cystoisospora* species at the rRNA ITS1 locus and development of a PCR-RFLP assay. Exp Parasitol 2008;118:592-595.

Coccidiosis in cattle. More than a dozen species of *Eimeria* parasitize cattle; of these, **Eimeria zuernii** and **E. bovis** are potentially highly pathogenic, whereas several others, notably *E. ellipsoidalis*, *E. alabamensis*, and *E. auburnensis* may cause diarrhea but probably not death. *Coccidial infection is common, and it usually comprises several species.* Almost half the calves and yearlings in confinement operations shed oocysts, with calves shedding high numbers, whereas a much smaller proportion of cows shed low numbers of oocysts.

Disease occurs mainly in calves or weaned feeder cattle less than ~1 year of age, when one or both of the potentially pathogenic species produce heavy infection. It may occur in animals at pasture or on range, concentrated at water holes, but is most common in animals in feedlots or yards where the level of sanitation is not high. The stress of shipping, cold weather, or intercurrent disease may be associated with outbreaks, which can occur in midwinter when oocyst transmission is expected to be poor. Bovine parvovirus infections have been associated with outbreaks of coccidiosis in a dry environment in northern Australia. Reactivation of latent schizonts in tissue may explain coccidiosis in stressed animals, or at a time when transmission is unlikely.

Coccidiosis is characterized by *diarrhea that may progress to dysentery* with mucus, and tenesmus, perhaps causing rectal prolapse. Animals dehydrate, and become hyponatremic and sometimes anemic. Morbidity may be high, but mortality is usually low. The duration of severe disease is ~3-10 days, after which most cases recover, because infection is essentially self-limiting. Some animals develop concurrent nervous signs, including tremors, nystagmus, opisthotonos, and convulsions, and many of these die within a few days.

The signs in bovine coccidiosis resulting from *E. zuernii* and *E. bovis* occur when the epithelium in the glands of the cecum and colon is infected by second-generation schizonts and gametocytes. In heavily infected animals, disease and sometimes death can occur before many oocysts are passed in the feces. The life cycles of both agents are similar, two schizogonous generations preceding gametogony. The first-generation schizont of **E. bovis** infects hypertrophic endothelial cells in lacteals on the upper part of villi in the *lower small intestine*, several meters proximal to the ileocecal valve. These schizonts may be large, up to ~300 μm in diameter, and are visible to the naked eye as *pinpoint white nodular foci in the mucosa*. They contain tens of thousands of merozoites, but are invested by only a narrow rim of mononuclear inflammatory cells, unless they degenerate, when a marked local mixed reaction develops, including neutrophils and macrophages. Merozoites released from these schizonts ~14-18 days after infection enter cells deep in cecal and colonic glands. In heavy infections, crypts of Lieberkühn in the terminal ileum also may be infected. Here they produce small second-generation schizonts, which in turn release merozoites, infecting other cells in the gland. Gametogony may begin as early as 15 days after infection, and oocyst production peaks ~19-21 days after infection.

The first-generation schizonts of **E. zuernii** may be about the same size as those of *E. bovis*. However, they are most common in the *terminal meter of the ileum* and are located in the lamina propria below the crypt-villus junction, often deep near the muscularis mucosae, rather than in the endothelium of the lacteal. Hence they are not so readily visible grossly as those of *E. bovis*. The second-generation schizonts and gamonts of *E. zuernii* also occur in glands of the cecum and colon, but not the terminal ileum. The merozoites tend to be somewhat longer (up to 15 μm) and schizonts more numerous and of greater diameter (~14 μm) than those of *E. bovis*. The timing of the development of *E. zuernii* infection is similar to that of *E. bovis*. First-generation schizonts of *E. bovis* occasionally reach the mesenteric lymph node, where they may mature, with no significance.

Animals dying of coccidiosis have fecal staining of the hindquarters, and may be somewhat cachectic and anemic. The **gross** enteric lesions in severe cases are those of *hemorrhagic or fibrinohemorrhagic typhlocolitis*, which may extend to the rectum (Fig. 1-185); if *E. bovis* is involved, the terminal ileum also may be affected and sometimes a few schizonts are visible in the ileal villi. The contents of the large bowel are usually abnormally fluid, and may vary from brown to black to overtly red, possibly with flecks of mucus or fibrin. The mucosa is edematous, with exaggerated longitudinal and perhaps transverse folds, which may be congested. Submucosal edema is also marked. Fibrin strands or a patchy diphtheritic membrane may be present on the mucosa, and fibrin casts can form. In milder cases lesions are limited to congestion and edema of the mucosa.

Microscopically, in animals dying at the peak of infection, virtually all cells lining cecal and colonic glands in many areas are infected by small schizonts, gamonts, or developing oocysts. Cells infected by *E. bovis* tend to dissociate and project into

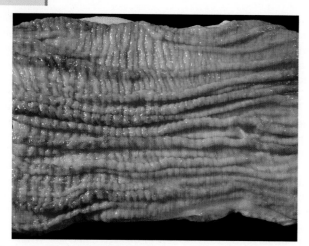

Figure 1-185 Acute colitis, with mucosal hemorrhage and minute ulcerations, in **bovine coccidiosis**. (Courtesy L. Craig.)

the lumen of the gland. As cells are disrupted and oocysts are released into the lumen of glands, the remaining glandular epithelium becomes extremely attenuated, or the gland collapses (Fig. 1-186A, B). Concurrently, the surface epithelium becomes squamous, or the mucosa is eroded, and effusion of fibrin, neutrophils, and hemorrhage occurs from dilated, congested superficial vessels. Oocysts released into the glands and lumen of the colon may be seen in the exudate. At the same time, the mucosa begins to collapse, and the lamina propria is infiltrated by neutrophils, eosinophils, lymphocytes, macrophages, and plasma cells. Oocysts trapped in denuded glands in the collapsed mucosa may be surrounded by small giant cells.

If destruction is widespread, and the animal survives sufficiently long, the *mucosa may ulcerate* to the level of the muscularis mucosae, and begin to granulate. In areas where the lesion is patchy, glands that have been relatively spared may become lined with hyperplastic epithelium, making an attempt to regenerate the mucosa. Flattened epithelial cells spread from these glands across the denuded surface, beneath the diphtheritic exudate. A few crenated oocysts in small giant cells in the stromal remnants of the mucosa may be all the evidence of coccidiosis found in lesions in animals surviving for 7-10 days.

Malabsorption caused by mucosal damage in the cecum and colon, and inflammatory effusion and hemorrhage explain the enteric signs of coccidiosis. The nervous signs in bovine coccidiosis are not associated with recognized lesions in the brain; they have been related to a yet not fully characterized neurotoxin found in the blood of affected animals.

The gross lesions of coccidiosis in cattle must be differentiated from those in salmonellosis, bovine viral diarrhea, rinderpest, malignant catarrhal fever, and bovine adenoviral infection, all of which may cause typhlocolitis. Coccidiosis often can be confirmed simply at autopsy by finding large numbers of developing stages in mucosal scrapings. Oocysts of *E. bovis* are ovoid, smooth, and ~28 × 21 μm; those of *E. zuernii* are subspherical to ovoid, smooth and −18 × 15 μm.

Although other coccidia are unlikely to be the primary cause of diarrhea or death in cattle, several have distinctive endogenous stages that may be recognized in tissue section. ***Eimeria auburnensis*** has a giant first-generation schizont that may be confused with those of *E. bovis* and *E. zuernii*. However, they are present usually 6-12 meters cranial to the ileocecal

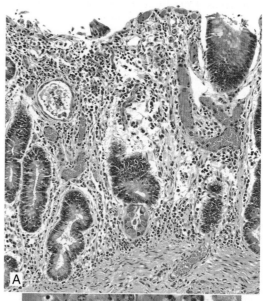

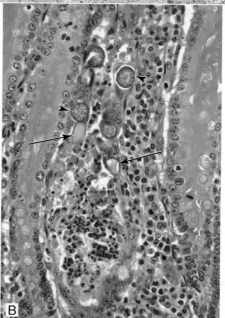

Figure 1-186 **Bovine coccidiosis. A.** Heavy infection and destruction of colonic glands by gamonts. **B.** Destruction of colonic glands by developing gamonts (arrowheads). Oocysts are in the lumen of a necrotic gland (arrows).

valve and form in the epithelium deep in crypts of Lieberkühn, although this may not be apparent because of plane of section, or following their migration into the lamina propria. Second-generation schizonts and gamonts of *E. auburnensis* develop in the lamina propria in the ileum, small schizonts in villi, and gamonts in the deeper lamina propria. Microgametocytes may be several hundred micrometers across. Oocysts are ~38 × 23 μm.

The other bovine coccidium with gamonts apparently developing in the lamina propria is **E. bukidnonensis**. Oocysts of this species are large, ~48 × 35 μm and thick-walled, with a micropyle, and have been found in the lamina propria. **E. alabamensis** develops in vacuoles within the nucleus of epithelial cells in small intestine and, in heavy infections, the large bowel. Both schizonts and gamonts may be found together within the same nucleus. Gamonts of **E. kosti** have been described in the epithelium deep in the abomasal glands. None of these organisms is particularly pathogenic.

Eimeria bareillyi is associated with clinical coccidiosis in water buffalo calves. The serosal vessels in the distal half of the small intestine are congested, and the lumen of the lower small bowel contains creamy or yellow fluid content in which some mucus, fibrin, or blood may be present. Focal to coalescent pale raised plaques or polypoid masses may be present on the mucosa, or the surface may appear granular and necrotic, with petechial hemorrhages. The gross changes are caused by hypertrophy of crypts and villi, upon which virtually every cell is infected with developing gamonts or oocysts. *E. bareillyi* will not cross-transmit to domestic cattle, although *E. ellipsoidalis* and *E. zuernii* of bubaline origin will. *E. zuernii* is pathogenic in water buffalo.

Further reading

Dubey JP, et al. Fatal intestinal coccidiosis in a three week old buffalo calf (*Bubalus bubalus*). J Parasitol 2008;94:1289-1294. (*Eimeria bareillyi*)

Enemark HL, et al. Eimeriosis in Danish dairy calves—correlation between species, oocyst excretion and diarrhoea. Parasitol Res 2013;112(Suppl. 1):169-.

Hermosilla C, et al. *Eimeria bovis*: an update on parasite-host cell interactions. Int J Med Microbiol 2012;302:210-215.

Jolley WR, et al. Ruminant coccidiosis. Vet Clin North Am Food Anim Pract 2006;22:613-621.

Lucas AS, et al. A study of the level and dynamics of *Eimeria* populations in naturally infected, grazing beef cattle at various stages of production in the Mid-Atlantic USA. Vet Parasitol 2014;202: 201-206.

Coccidiosis in sheep and goats. *Coccidial infection is universal in sheep and goats,* and coccidiosis can be a significant problem in the young of both species. The etiology of coccidiosis in these species is complicated by the morphologic similarity of the coccidia infecting sheep and goats. Assumptions on the potential for cross-infection of coccidia between sheep and goats, and of the species found in each host, have been revised as new taxonomic and biologic information has come to light.

About a dozen species of coccidia are found in each of sheep and goats. Of these, three (*Eimeria pallida, E. caprovina, E. punctata*) may occur in both sheep and goats, although the validity of *E. punctata* as a species is questioned. Eight species pairs of *Eimeria* occur, in which the coccidia look and behave similarly in sheep and goats, but do not cross-infect. Listing the sheep-adapted species of each pair first, these are: *E. ahsata–E. christenseni; E. ovinoidalis–E. ninakohlyakimovae; E. bakuensis (=ovina)–E. arloingi; E. granulosa–E. jolchijevi; E. crandallis–E. hirci; E. faurei–E. apsheronica; E. parva–E. alijevi; E. intricata–E. kochrii.* Two species are unique to sheep, *E. weybridgensis* (formerly *E. arloingi* "B"), and *E. marsica;* in goats, one species, *E. caprina,* is unique. In addition, giant schizonts of an unknown coccidian, termed *Eimeria (Globidium) gilruthi,* are seen incidentally as pinpoint white foci in the abomasum of sheep and goats. An individual case of proliferative abomasitis associated with this parasite was described in a sheep. The taxonomic confusion has been carried over into descriptions of the natural or experimental disease, because many infections were of mixed species, resulted from inocula of poorly defined species of coccidia, or occurred under circumstances in which the oocysts associated were not described. However, although the taxonomic picture has changed, the syndromes associated with coccidiosis in sheep and goats have not.

Coccidiosis in sheep and goats is a disease of young animals. Under conditions of intensive pastoral husbandry or confinement, lambs and kids are exposed to oocysts of many species of coccidia within the first few days of life. Weaned lambs, presumably exposed to only light infections while at range, are also prone to coccidiosis when brought into feedlots. In young suckled animals and those in feedlots exposed to large numbers of oocysts, signs may occur before oocysts are passed. Suckling lambs, ~4-8 weeks old, reared at pasture at relatively heavy stocking rates, may also develop signs and occasionally die. Under these conditions, the disease needs to be differentiated from gastrointestinal helminthosis, which may be concurrent.

Outbreaks of coccidiosis in confined lambs and kids are usually acute and characterized by moderate morbidity and low mortality; there is green or yellow watery *diarrhea,* occasionally with blood or mucus. Yarded and grazing animals may also suffer weight loss, or subclinical ill-thrift. Signs are usually associated with lesions in the lower small intestine, caused by *E. ahsata* and *E. bakuensis* in lambs, and their analogues in goats, *E. christenseni,* and *E. arloingi,* or with typhlocolitis, caused by *E. ovinoidalis* in sheep, and *E. ninakohlyakimovae* in goats. Some pathogenicity is also ascribed to *E. faurei, E. intricata, E. parva,* and *E. crandallis* in sheep, and presumably to their analogues in goats. Infections may be mixed, and gross and microscopic lesions may reflect this.

E. ovinoidalis in sheep and *E. ninakohlyakimovae* in goats presumably have similar endogenous development. In the sheep, giant schizonts up to 300 µm in diameter develop in cells deep in the lamina propria, in the terminal ileum. They release merozoites that enter epithelium in the glands of the cecum and colon, and sometimes distal ileum. Here small second-generation schizonts evolve, and other cells in glands in the same area subsequently become infected by the gametocytes. These species are considered highly pathogenic and *E. ovinoidalis* often is associated with disease in feedlot lambs. Lesions other than those related to diarrhea, dehydration, and hypoproteinemia are limited to the terminal ileum, and especially the cecum and proximal colon, and are associated with second-generation schizogony and gametogony. Affected areas of gut are edematous and thickened. The most significant microscopic lesions are those in the cecum and colon, which resemble those in cattle caused by *E. bovis* and *E. zuernii. E. caprina* in goats also seems to have pathogenic potential. Like *E. ninakohlyakimovae,* it causes typhlocolitis; the small intestine is not involved.

E. christenseni and *E. arloingi* in goats and their analogues, *E. ahsata* and *E. bakuensis* in sheep, are also associated with serious disease. They seem to have somewhat similar developmental cycles and lesions, although interpretation of the literature is clouded by confusion among these species. Many cases of coccidiosis in lambs attributed to *E. bakuensis* (as *E. arloingi*) may in fact have been due to *E. ahsata* because the unsporulated oocysts, although of differing sizes, can be confused.

E. christenseni has a developmental cycle that involves giant schizonts up to nearly 300 µm across in the endothelium of the lacteal in villi in the middle small intestine. In heavy

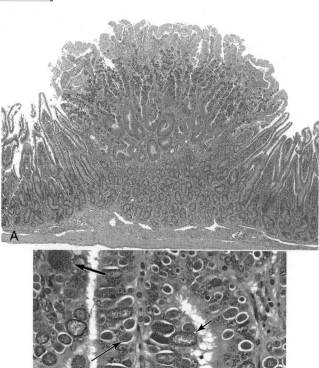

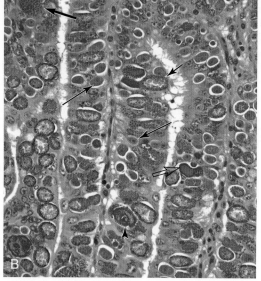

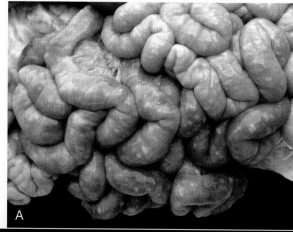

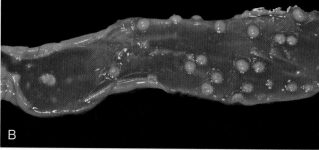

Figure 1-188 Coccidiosis (presumably *Eimeria arloingi*) in a goat. **A.** White nodules can be seen through the serosa. (Courtesy V. Psychas.) **B.** White nodules present in the mucosa. (Courtesy F. Giannitti.)

Figure 1-187 Coccidiosis (presumably *Eimeria arloingi*) in a goat. **A.** Mucosal polyp with coccidial forms within most epithelial cells. **B.** Undifferentiated gamonts (long arrows), macrogametocytes (short arrow), microgametocytes (arrowhead), large schizonts (thick arrow), and developing oocysts (hollow arrow) in epithelium of ileal crypts and villi.

infections, every cell in a number of contiguous crypt-villus units may be infected. Although there may be an acute local reaction around ruptured primary schizonts, clinical disease is associated with the subsequent stages of development, diarrhea occurring during the late prepatent and patent periods. Affected intestine may be congested and edematous. Numerous pale white or yellow foci from a few millimeters to up to a centimeter in diameter, often visible from the serosa, are present as slightly raised plaques on the mucosa of the small bowel. These foci are areas of intense infection of cryptal and villus epithelium by gamonts and developing oocysts, and have been dubbed "*oocyst patches.*" There may be some hemorrhage into the intestine, but the feces are rarely bloody.

E. arloingi undergoes a development similar to that of *E. christenseni* (Fig. 1-187A, B) and causes similar gross and microscopic lesions in goats, with minor differences. First-generation schizonts are most numerous in the lacteals of villi in the lower jejunum, gamonts are mainly above the host cell nucleus. The associated gross lesions consist of nodules in the

mucosa that also can be seen from the serosa (Fig. 1-188A, B); they tend to be more distal in the small intestine, and occasionally involve the large bowel. *E. ahsata* and *E. bakuensis* in sheep are similar.

Nodular polypoid structures, sometimes pedunculate, and ~0.3-1.5 cm in diameter, are encountered in the small intestinal mucosa of sheep and goats, usually as an incidental finding. These masses are comprised of hypertrophic crypt-villus units, in which virtually every epithelial cell is infected by mainly gametocytic stages of coccidia, which, in sheep, are probably *E. bakuensis* and *E. ahsata.*

Adjacent mucosa appears normal and is uninfected. The term "pseudoadenomatous" has been used to describe these polypoid lesions, and the oocyst patches or plaques was discussed earlier in the section on coccidian-infected sheep and goats. The infected epithelial cells appear somewhat hypertrophic, with eosinophilic cytoplasm and prominent brush borders. Often these coccidia-infected cells do not slough rapidly postmortem, in contrast with their uninfected fellows.

Why masses of infected cells apparently persist in chronically infected animals without clinical disease is unclear. However, the plaques and polyps may be the result of mitogenic stimuli from progamonts, the immature stages in crypt epithelium, which appear to divide by binary fission in synchrony with the infected host cell.

Coccidiosis may also cause ill-thrift and diarrhea in suckling or weanling lambs 5-6 weeks old heavily stocked on pasture. In the United Kingdom, *E. crandallis,* which develops largely in the ileum, and *E. ovinoidalis* are mainly associated with this syndrome. *E. weybridgensis* (*E. arloingi* "B"), which infects most of the length of the small intestine, may also contribute. The only gross lesion in affected lambs is congestion and thickening of the mucosa of the lower small intestine.

Under some circumstances, probably sudden exposure to large doses of oocysts, *E. crandallis,* at least, causes *villus atrophy* in infected areas of intestine. Giant first-generation schizonts develop in crypt cells that after infection migrate into the lamina propria. As the infection progresses, villi become stumpy or disappear, and in small bowel and cecum, crypts are straight, hypertrophic, and contain proliferative epithelium. Asexual or, more commonly, sexual stages of coccidia are present in epithelium on the surface of the mucosa. In hyperplastic crypts, epithelial cells are infected by progamonts, which seem to be dividing in synchrony with host cells. Masses of macrophages may invest and invade the base of infected crypts, and apoptosis of infected and uninfected cells may occur, resulting in attenuation of surviving crypt epithelium. In heavy infections, there also may be thickening of the cecal mucosa by hyperplastic coccidia-infected cells. Occasionally, areas of small intestine and cecum, in which there has been severe damage to crypts, may become eroded.

Such lesions, if widespread, may cause malabsorption or perhaps protein-losing enteropathy. It is unclear whether atrophy of villi is the result of excess loss of epithelium directly because of the effects of coccidial infection, or whether it is mediated by an immune response.

E. apsheronica in the goat has minor pathogenic potential. Giant schizonts develop in the lamina propria of villi throughout the small intestine and in the cecum; second-generation schizonts are in the epithelium on villi in the small intestine, and in the cecum, but not the colon. Gametocytes have the same distribution. Pale foci in the mucosa, where gametocytes are concentrated, and focal areas of erosion and hemorrhage may occur in heavily infected animals.

Large schizonts are often encountered incidentally in submucosal lymphatics, or in the subcortical or medullary sinusoids of mesenteric lymph nodes in sheep and goats. Sometimes they may be visible grossly in these locations as pinpoint white foci. Occasionally, coccidial gametocytes or oocysts may also develop in intestinal lymphoid aggregates and mesenteric lymph nodes, where they may provoke a mild granulomatous reaction. Stages in lymph nodes probably result from establishment of sporozoites or primary merozoites swept from the lacteal into the lymphatic drainage early in infection. Development in such sites is not uncommon, but aberrant and likely dead-end. The species involved appear mainly to be those considered in the previous section, with a giant primary schizont developing in the lacteal.

In coccidiosis, *oocysts are usually numerous in feces,* but this is neither constant in, nor necessarily indicative of, disease. Mucosal scrapings or tissue sections of mucosa containing large numbers of asexual and gametogenous coccidial forms, in association with diarrhea, and perhaps some hemorrhage into the intestine, support the diagnosis, in the absence of other syndromes such as gastrointestinal helminthosis.

Further reading

Hashemnia M, et al. Experimental caprine coccidiosis caused by *Eimeria arloingi*: morphopathologic and electron microscopic studies. Vet Res Commun 2012;36:47-55.

Jolley WR, et al. Ruminant coccidiosis. Vet Clin Food Anim 2006;22: 613-621.

Maratea KA, Miller AA. Abomasal coccidiosis associated with proliferative abomasitis in a sheep. J Vet Diagn Invest 2007;19: 118-121.

Razavi SM, et al. *Eimeria arloingi*: further studies on the development of some endogenous stages. Exp Parasitol 2014;140:12-17.

Ruiz A, et al. Isolation of an *Eimeria ninakohlyakimovae* field strain (Canary Islands) and analysis of its infection characteristics in goat kids. Res Vet Sci 2013;94:277-284.

Coccidia in horses. The only coccidium of horses reported with any frequency is *Eimeria leuckarti*, which is found in horses and donkeys the world over. In one survey of foals in Germany, it was found in 100% of animals, but prevalence elsewhere is usually very low. Although the infection by *E. leuckarti* is most common in foals, it also occasionally has been seen in adult animals. Its reputation for pathogenicity rests largely on the *distinctive large gamonts* found in the lamina propria of the small intestine in animals dead of enteric disease of undetermined etiology. However, implication of *E. leuckarti* in the disease process is rarely, if ever, convincing, and this parasite is encountered incidentally in the intestine of horses dead of other clearly defined conditions. Furthermore, heavy experimental inoculations, producing many gamonts in the gut and heavy oocyst passage, have failed to elicit clinical signs.

The stages present in the lamina propria of villi are giant microgametocytes and macrogametes, developing in markedly hypertrophic host cells, probably of epithelial origin (Fig. 1-189). The microgametocytes are up to ~250 μm in diameter, and when mature they contain swirling masses of microgametes. Immature microgametocytes very much resemble some of the giant schizonts of other species of coccidia, and have frequently been referred to as such; this stimulated the application of the term *Globidium* to the organism. However, the only schizont containing merozoites that has been recognized in horses was very small (12.5 μm in diameter), and in the epithelium of the ileum. The macrogametes have distinctive large eosinophilic or Schiff-positive granules that may be individual or confluent. The host cells are markedly hypertrophic with a fibrillar periphery, and the enlarged nucleus forms a crescent along one side of the parasitophorous vacuole. There is no inflammatory response to the gamonts, and only a mild reaction to degenerate stages in the lamina propria.

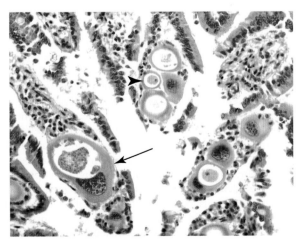

Figure 1-189 Microgametocyte (arrow) and developing oocyst (arrowhead) of *Eimeria leuckarti* in lamina propria, in a horse.

Further reading

De Souza PN, et al. Natural infection by *Cryptosporidium sp.*, *Giardia sp.* and *Eimeria leuckarti* in three groups of equines with different handlings in Rio de Janeiro, Brazil. Vet Parasitol 2009;160:327-333.

Hirayama K, et al. *Eimeria* organisms develop in the epithelial cells of equine small intestine. Vet Pathol 2002;39:505-508.

Lyons ET, Tolliver SC. Prevalence of parasite eggs (*Strongyloides westeri, Parascaris equorum,* and strongyles) and oocysts (*Eimeria leuckarti*) in the feces of thoroughbred foals on 14 farms in central Kentucky in 2003. Parasitol Res 2004;92:400-404.

Coccidiosis in swine. At least 8-10 species of *Eimeria* are thought to occur in swine, along with a single species of *Cystoisospora*. The latter, **Cystoisospora (Isospora) suis**, is the most important; it causes *porcine neonatal coccidiosis*, a disease of piglets from ~5-6 days to ~2-3 weeks of age. This disease is recognized in the United States, Canada, the United Kingdom, and western Europe; it also occurs in Australia, and probably wherever swine are reared intensively. The condition is most severe in herds where continuous farrowing and total confinement are practiced, and some laboratories report a prevalence of 10-50% among scouring baby pigs. Rapid sporulation (12 hours) and short prepatent period (5 days) promote rapid build-up of infection in a farrowing house.

Porcine neonatal coccidiosis has high morbidity, and usually low but variable mortality. It causes yellow watery diarrhea, dehydration, loss of condition, and death, or at least a temporary check in growth. Some animals may runt severely. Illness usually begins at ~7-10 days of age. Piglets continue to nurse, but may vomit clotted milk. At autopsy, many piglets have the typical appearance of undifferentiated neonatal diarrhea, with no specific gross findings in the gastrointestinal tract other than fluid yellow content. However, the intestine in some animals with coccidiosis may look turgid, rather than flaccid, and in a minority of animals a fibrinous or fibrinonecrotic exudate is present in the lower portion of the small intestine. Occasionally, casts form.

C. suis replicates in the epithelium on the *distal third of villi* (Fig. 1-190), mainly in the *jejunum and ileum*, although infected cells may be found in the duodenum and colon in a few animals. Piglets usually become infected within the first day or two of life, perhaps by ingestion of the sow's feces. Merogony occurs in vacuoles in the cytoplasm, usually beneath the nucleus of the host cell. Infection of host cells is maximal 4-5 days after infection, and by 5 days gametogony is evident. Thick- and thin-walled sporulated oocysts have been observed in feces of infected pigs, but either form may cause disease. The onset of lesions and clinical signs corresponds with this period of heavy infection of cells, which undergo lysis. Villi may become markedly atrophic. The lumen contains massive numbers of exfoliated epithelial cells, inflammatory cells, and coccidial stages (Fig. 1-191). The surface epithelium that remains is cuboidal to squamous, and infected epithelial cells may be seen degenerating or exfoliating. Erosions may develop at the tips of villi, through which there is effusion of neutrophils and fibrin. In the remnant of the villus, neutrophil infiltration, a moderate increase in mononuclear leukocytes and eosinophilic proteinaceous material, probably collagen, may be present in the lamina propria. Effusion of neutrophils and fibrin from the eroded tips of villi contributes to the fibrinonecrotic membrane seen in some animals, and ulceration can occur. Gram-positive bacilli are often present in the exudate.

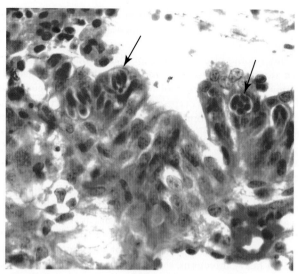

Figure 1-190 Meronts containing merozoites (arrows) in epithelial cells of a pig with **Cystoisospora suis** infection.

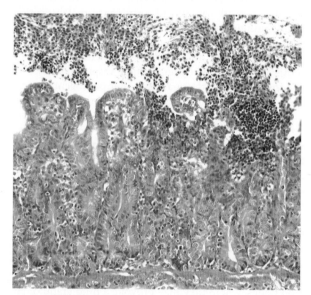

Figure 1-191 Blunting and atrophy of villi in a pig with **Cystoisospora suis** infection. Erosions are present at the tip of villi and there is effusion of neutrophils and fibrin into the lumen.

In animals surviving for a few days, the cryptal epithelium may be markedly hyperplastic.

The severity of the lesions is a function of the size of the inoculum and the age of the pigs. Heavier inocula, within limits, produce more cellular damage and villus atrophy; fibrinonecrotic enteritis indicates ingestion of a large dose of oocysts. However, severe lesions may not be associated with heavy shedding of oocysts because relatively few gamonts are able to develop in the reduced population of epithelial cells remaining on villi. The severity of lesions and signs is much greater in piglets a few days old in comparison with those 2 weeks of age. This partly relates to the lower rate of replication of epithelium in the crypts of young piglets, and therefore the development of more severe villus atrophy. The smaller size of young piglets also makes them more susceptible to the effects of malabsorption and diarrhea. Animals previously exposed to *C. suis* have relatively strong resistance to challenge.

A **diagnosis** of coccidiosis must be considered in scouring neonatal piglets, and is strongly suggested by the presence of *fibrinonecrotic enteritis in the distal small bowel*. Atrophy of villi may be recognized at autopsy using a hand lens or stereomicroscope, or in tissue section. Asexual or sexual stages may be found in smears of mucosal scrapings. The distinctive binucleate type I meronts and pairs of large (12-18 μm in smears, 8-13 μm in sections) type I merozoites may be found in jejunal mucosa in the early phase of diarrheal disease. Multinucleated type II meronts and numerous small type II merozoites are the predominant stage during the clinical phase of disease. In section, these form clusters of 2-16 organisms like bunches of bananas, perhaps with a small residual body, in the parasitophorous vacuole in the enterocyte (see Fig. 1-190).

Macrogamonts and microgamonts are present in moderate numbers by day 5 of infection, and a few oocysts also may be seen. Microgametocytes are ~9-16 μm in diameter, and are multinucleated. Oocysts in tissue sections are oval, ~15 × 12 μm, whereas those in smears are ~18 × 16 μm. Coccidial stages may be difficult to find in animals that have been ill for several days. Oocysts may not be found in feces, because the infection is not yet patent, the patent period has passed, or the lesions are very severe, reducing the number of oocysts produced.

Coccidiosis in older swine caused by several *Eimeria* species is uncommon; speciation can be accomplished. It typically occurs in animals with access to yards or pasture contaminated with oocysts. Weaners and growing pigs are affected. The species considered potentially pathogenic include *E. scabra*, *E. debliecki*, and *E. spinosa*. It is difficult to produce disease in experimentally inoculated pigs; *E. scabra* is probably the most pathogenic. Coccidiosis in older swine is usually sporadic or affects a few pigs in a group. Typically it causes diarrhea of a few days' duration, loss of appetite, and perhaps transient ill-thrift, or, in severe cases, emaciation. Occasionally animals die.

Lesions are usually limited to the lower small intestine, which may be congested or hemorrhagic, although overt blood is rarely found in the feces. Large numbers of schizonts, gamonts, and developing oocysts are in epithelial cells on villi and sometimes in crypts. Atrophy of villi, or erosion and local hemorrhage or inflammatory effusion may be evident, the lamina propria is edematous, and desquamated epithelium and oocysts are in the lumen of the gut. Rarely, heavily infected animals may have lesions in the large intestine. The species involved are diagnosed on the basis of the morphology of oocysts in feces or mucosal scrapings.

Coccidial gamonts and oocysts of a species resembling *E. debliecki* have been found infecting epithelium on the papilliform mucosa of cystic bile ducts in porcine liver. This is probably an aberrant site of development.

Further reading

Barta JR, et al. The genus Atoxoplasma (Garnham 1950) as a junior objective synonym of the genus *Isospora* (Schneider 1881) species infecting birds and resurrection of *Cystoisospora* (Frenkel 1977) as the correct genus for *Isospora* species infecting mammals. J Parasitol 2005;91:726-727.

Mengel H, et al. Necrotic enteritis due to simultaneous infection with *Isospora suis* and clostridia in newborn piglets and its prevention by early treatment with toltrazuril. Parasitol Res 2012;110:1347-1355.

Stuart BP, Lindsay DS. Coccidiosis in swine. Vet Clin North Am Food Anim Pract 1986;2:455-468.

Worliczek HL, et al. Porcine coccidiosis—Investigations on the cellular immune response against *Isospora suis*. Parasitol Res 2009;105: S151-S155.

Heteroxenous apicomplexan protists

Cystoisospora (Isospora), Toxoplasma, Neospora, Hammondia, Sarcocystis, Besnoitia, and **Frenkelia** comprise this group of protists. All of these heteroxenous members of the Apicomplexa are known to *use carnivores as definitive hosts*, and have one or more generations of merogony in the tissues of various species of prey. *Frenkelia*, which some would place in the genus *Sarcocystis*, as far as is known uses only raptorial birds as definitive hosts and small rodents as intermediate hosts. It is not considered further.

Coccidiosis in dogs and cats. Although several species of *Eimeria* have been reported from dogs and cats, their status as genuine parasites of these hosts is in doubt. The significant coccidia of dogs and cats are members of the genus *Cystoisospora*, considered here, and of the genera *Toxoplasma*, *Sarcocystis*, *Hammondia*, *Besnoitia*, and *Neospora*, dealt with subsequently. *Caryospora* spp. may occasionally produce dermal coccidiosis in immunosuppressed dogs.

Cystoisospora spp. are characterized by oocysts that are passed unsporulated in feces, and which, when sporulated, have two sporocysts lacking a Stieda body, each with four sporozoites. Following ingestion of sporulated oocysts of heteroxenous species, transport hosts, usually prey species such as mice and other small rodents, but sometimes other hosts, are infected by large sporozoite-like "hypnozoites" in phagocytic cells in lymph nodes and other tissues. These, when ingested by the predator, resume development in the intestine, and lead to asexual and sexual development in the definitive host. Heteroxenous passage is not obligatory, and sporulated oocysts are also directly infective to the definitive host.

In **dogs,** 4 species of *Cystoisospora* are recognized. Meronts of *C. canis* develop in the subepithelial lamina propria of the villi in the distal small intestine and, to a lesser extent, in large bowel. Gamonts occur beneath and within the epithelium of the ileum and large intestine, and the oocyst is the largest among *Cystoisospora* spp. of dogs, being ~38 × 30 μm. The other three are members of the "*C. ohioensis* complex." *C. ohioensis* develops exclusively in epithelial cells, mainly in the distal portions of villi along the length of the small bowel, especially in the ileum, and occasionally in the large bowel. It may be the most pathogenic species in dogs. The oocysts of *C. burrowsi*, *C. ohioensis*, and *C. neorivolta* are similar. Original literature should be consulted for details that will permit differentiation of these species in tissue. Endogenous stages of *C. burrowsi* occur in epithelial cells, and in the lamina propria of the tips of villi in the distal two thirds of the small intestine. *C. neorivolta* mainly develops in proprial cells beneath the epithelium in the tips of villi in the distal half of the small intestine, and rarely in the cecum and colon. Occasional stages may be in the epithelium. *C. canis* and *C. ohioensis* are known to be heteroxenous. Meronts of an unknown coccidian, probably a *Cystoisospora* sp., have been found in the intrahepatic bile ducts of a dog, associated with severe suppurative cholangiohepatitis.

In **cats,** 2 species of *Cystoisospora* occur. Meronts and gamonts of *C. felis* develop in epithelium of villi in the small intestine, and occasionally in epithelium in the large bowel. The oocyst is large, ~43 × 33 μm. **C. rivolta** also develops in epithelium on villi and in crypts and glands in the small and large intestine. Oocysts are ovoid, ~25 × 23 μm. Subepithelial schizonts and gamonts of an unknown coccidian, possibly a *Cystoisospora* species, have been associated with fatal enteritis in a cat.

Coccidiosis in the dog and cat is largely a clinical entity, *usually nonfatal.* The lesions of coccidiosis in small animals are poorly defined, and care must be taken not to ascribe disease to these organisms simply on the basis of the presence of endogenous stages in the mucosa of animals dead of enteric disease. Rotavirus and coronavirus might be expected to produce similar signs. However, genuine cases of fatal coccidiosis do occur, although few are recorded in the literature. Affected animals are young, and usually from environments such as pet shops, animal shelters, or kennels in which standards of sanitation may not be high. There is a history of diarrhea of several days' duration, and the animal is dehydrated. Other than mild hyperemia of the mucosa and excessively fluid content of the small intestine and colon, gross lesions in the gut may not be evident. Microscopically, there may be moderate atrophy of villi, with attenuation of surface enterocytes, and perhaps effusion of acute inflammatory exudate from the tips of some eroded villi. Asexual and sexual stages of coccidia are evident in moderate to large numbers in the epithelium or lamina propria of villi. In some cases the large bowel may be infected, with exfoliation of surface epithelium, and accumulation of necrotic debris in some dilated glands.

Further reading

Houk AE, et al. Experimentally induced clinical *Cystoisospora canis* coccidiosis in dogs with prior natural patent *Cystoisospora ohioensis*-like or *C. canis* infections. J Parasitol 2013;99:892-895.

Lappin MR. Update on the diagnosis and management of *Isospora* spp infections in dogs and cats. Top Companion Anim Med 2010;25:133-135.

Mitchell SM, et al. *Cystoisospora canis* Neméseri, 1959 (syn. *Isospora canis*), infections in dogs: clinical signs, pathogenesis, and reproducible clinical disease in beagle dogs fed oocysts. J Parasitol 2007;93:345-352.

Toxoplasmosis. *Toxoplasma gondii* uses felids as definitive hosts. It is optionally heteroxenous; cats may be infected directly by ingestion of oocysts, but probably most commonly by ingestion of asexual stages in the tissues of prey species. Cats excrete oocysts 3-10 days after ingesting *bradyzoites*, ~13 days after ingesting tachyzoites, and 18 days after ingesting oocysts. Transmission efficacy varies and cats can become infected after ingestion of one bradyzoite, whereas ingestion of 1,000 oocysts is required to establish infection. Intermediate hosts are infected by oocysts shed in the feces of cats, or by a variety of other routes considered later. Five stages of asexual development are recognized in the intestinal epithelium of cats infected with tissue cysts from intermediate hosts. The gametocytes also develop in epithelium on villi, especially in the *ileum*. Most cats will shed oocytes once, however, in cases of immunosuppression repeated oocyte shedding may occur. In heavy infections, exfoliation of infected epithelium from villi is associated with the development of *villus atrophy*, and occasional spontaneous cases of diarrhea in kittens seem to be caused by *Toxoplasma*-induced atrophy of villi and malabsorption.

In intermediate hosts and in cats, extraintestinal asexual development occurs in a variety of organs and tissues. Rapidly dividing forms (*tachyzoites*) may by endodyogeny proliferate in cells in many sites for an indefinite number of generations, and are the stage associated with acute toxoplasmosis in cats and other species. Eventually, tachyzoites induce the formation of a cyst wall in a host cell, and divide slowly, forming bradyzoites, which reside in quiescent tissue cysts.

T. gondii, with *Neospora caninum*, is unique among protists in its ability to parasitize a wide range of hosts and tissues. *It is one of the most ubiquitous of organisms;* experimentally, essentially all homeothermic animals can be infected, and natural infections occur in birds, nonhuman primates, rodents, insectivores, herbivores, and carnivores, including domestic species and humans. Serologic surveys indicate that infection is widespread in most species of domestic animals; however, except for abortions in sheep and goats, overt disease is sporadic and rare.

Transmission may occur by a number of different routes. The shedding of oocysts in the feces of cats and wild felids has been mentioned earlier. Transplacental infection occurs commonly in sheep and goats and sporadically in swine and humans. Carnivorous animals and humans may become infected by ingesting oocysts from cats, or more commonly from cysts containing bradyzoites in tissues of infected animals, implying that the cycle of infection can be maintained by means of facultative homoxenous transmission, without a definitive host. It has been shown that infected rodents will lose avoidance behaviors to feline odor, and instead become attracted to areas where cats are present. This may favor transmission to the definitive host.

Systemic toxoplasmosis occurs most often in young animals, especially immunologically immature neonates and in immunocompromised hosts. *Toxoplasma gondii* infection leads to alterations of proinflammatory and anti-inflammatory cytokine production, which includes production of IL-10, which is a negative regulator of IL-12 and interferon gamma. Low levels of interferon gamma and the associated inability to activate macrophages are predisposing factors for systemic toxoplasmosis. In dogs, canine distemper, ehrlichiosis, and lymphosarcoma are commonly concomitant with toxoplasmosis. The infection in juveniles may be acquired prenatally or postnatally. After ingestion, *Toxoplasma* organisms penetrate the intestinal mucosa. In cats, the enterointestinal cycle and systemic infection occur almost simultaneously. In other animals the tachyzoites are the first stage of infection, after invasion of the lamina propria by sporozoites released from the oocyst, or by bradyzoites released from the tissue cyst digested from food in the intestine.

Dissemination of *Toxoplasma* occurs in lymphocytes, macrophages, granulocytes, and as free forms in plasma. From the intestine the organism may follow 2 routes. It may spread via the lymphocytes to the regional nodes and from there in the lymph to the bloodstream, or it may pass in the portal circulation to the liver and from there to the systemic circulation. Further dissemination occurs to a wide variety of organs. Tachyzoites actively invade or are phagocytosed by host cells and are surrounded in a parasitophorous vacuole formed of host cell membrane. Tachyzoites proliferate, destroying the host cell, and cell-to-cell transmission may occur within infected organs.

Focal necrosis is common, and appears to be directly related to the rapid replication of tachyzoites. The outcome of infection is determined by a number of factors, including the number and strain of *Toxoplasma* in the infecting dose, and the species, age, and immune status of the host. Lesions in visceral organs are usually evident within 1–2 weeks after oral infection. Variable numbers of tachyzoites are usually found in the vicinity of the necrotic areas.

Specific immunity develops within a few days after infection; the cell-mediated arm is most significant in toxoplasmosis, mediated in large part by interleukin-12 and interferon gamma production. This reduces the severity of infection but usually does not terminate it. Infection by *Toxoplasma* interferes with the cell-mediated immune response, but does not completely inhibit it. The remaining cell-mediated immune capacity may control pathogen proliferation and promote progression to chronic disease. In experimental models lacking cytokines associated with cell-mediated immunity, including γ-interferon, *Toxoplasma* infection is nearly always fatal. The *chronic or dormant form* of *Toxoplasma* infection is characterized by the formation of *cysts* containing bradyzoites. These are mainly located in the brain, skeletal muscle, and myocardium. Cysts may form as early as 1–2 weeks after infection and they may persist for months, possibly years. Intracellular encystment protects the bradyzoites from both cellular and humoral immune mechanisms. *Inflammation is usually not associated with cysts.* When the level of resistance drops below a critical level, for example, because of treatment with immunosuppressive drugs, intercurrent disease, or other factors that depress immunity, particularly decreased levels of γ-interferon, *a chronic infection may become reactivated*. The cysts rupture and cause severe local inflammation. In experimental murine models, bradyzoites have been shown to revert to tachyzoites in the absence of γ-interferon.

The **clinical signs** of toxoplasmosis vary considerably, depending on the organs affected. The most consistent signs reported are fever, lethargy, anorexia, ocular and nasal discharges, and respiratory distress. Neurologic signs include incoordination, circling, tremors, opisthotonos, convulsions, and paresis. Paresis is often associated with radiculitis and myositis. In the dog signs may coexist with those of canine distemper and are not sufficiently distinctive to allow ready differentiation.

Systemic toxoplasmosis has been reported in most species of domestic animals. The hallmarks are *interstitial pneumonia*, *focal hepatic necrosis*, *lymphadenitis*, *myocarditis*, and *nonsuppurative meningoencephalitis*. Pulmonary lesions are probably most consistently found, followed by central nervous system lesions. The lesions in the various organs are morphologically similar in most species, varying mainly in degree.

Macroscopic lesions in the lung vary from irregular gray foci of necrosis on the pleural surface to hemorrhagic pneumonia with confluent involvement of the ventral portions. Careful examination of the liver usually reveals either areas of focal necrosis or irregular mottling, and edema of the gallbladder. The spleen is enlarged, as are lymph nodes, which are wet and often red. Pleural, pericardial, and peritoneal effusions occur irregularly. Pale areas may be evident in the myocardium and skeletal muscle. Occasionally the pancreas is the most severely affected organ, in which case an acute hemorrhagic reaction may involve the entire organ. Yellow, small, superficial intestinal ulcers with a hyperemic border have been reported in piglets. Large pale areas of necrosis

may be present in the renal cortices, mainly in goats and kittens.

Microscopically, the early pulmonary lesions are characterized by *diffuse interstitial pneumonia*; the alveolar septa are thickened by a predominantly mononuclear inflammatory cell reaction with a few neutrophils and eosinophils. Macrophages and fibrinous exudate fill the alveoli. Foci of necrosis involving the alveolar septa, bronchiolar epithelial cells, and blood vessels are scattered throughout the lobules. These lesions are soon followed by regenerative changes that are characterized by hyperplasia and hypertrophy of alveolar lining cells, mainly type II pneumocytes: so-called *epithelialization of alveoli*. In some areas this may be so marked as to give the affected areas an adenomatous appearance. Tachyzoites are usually evident in alveolar macrophages and also may be found in bronchiolar epithelial cells and the walls of blood vessels.

In the *liver*, irregular foci of coagulative necrosis are scattered at random throughout the lobules. There is usually little evidence of inflammation associated with the necrotic areas. Variable numbers of tachyzoites may be present in hepatocytes and Kupffer cells, usually at the periphery of the lesions, but often at some distance. If the pancreas is involved, there is extensive peripancreatic fat necrosis, with areas of coagulative necrosis in parenchyma. Numerous tachyzoites usually are evident in both ductal and acinar cells.

Lesions in *lymph nodes* often are associated with infection in the corresponding organ. They are characterized by irregular areas of coagulative necrosis, mainly in the cortex. A moderate inflammatory reaction may be evident at the periphery of the necrotic areas. There may be necrosis and depletion of lymphocytes in the follicles. In more chronic cases, the changes are those of nonspecific hyperplasia of lymphoid cells in cortical and paracortical areas, with a large macrophage population in the medullary sinusoids. Tachyzoites may be seen in phagocytic cells in sinusoids. Similar lesions may occur in the spleen. Necrotic areas are mainly located in the red pulp in this organ.

In the *heart and skeletal muscle*, foci of necrosis and mononuclear cell inflammation may be part of toxoplasmosis. There is often some difficulty in distinguishing between tachyzoites and mineralization of mitochondria in myocytes but, at some distance from areas of acute reaction, inert cysts usually can be identified in healthy fibers.

Brain lesions may vary in appearance. In the most fulminating cases cerebral lesions may be relatively inconspicuous. They consist of nonsuppurative meningoencephalitis with multifocal areas of necrosis and often malacia. There is swelling of endothelial cells, necrosis of vessel walls, and vasculitis. There may be marked perivascular edema and hyperplasia of perithelial cells. Tachyzoites and occasionally cysts may be found in vessel walls and in necrotic areas in both gray and white matter at all levels of the brain. If survival is prolonged, residual cerebral lesions consist of *microglial nodules* along with more extensive hyperplasia of perithelial cells and perivascular fibrosis that tends to make the vessels very obvious. At this stage tachyzoites are rare, and cysts 30 μm in diameter with a wall of amorphous acidophilic material ~0.5 μm thick, located in areas away from the lesions, may be the only form seen. Spinal cord lesions resemble those seen in the brain.

Systemic toxoplasmosis is reported from *cats*, but is certainly seen less commonly in this species than in some others. Lesions are similar to those described for other species. Chronic granulomatous toxoplasmosis may involve the intestine in older cats and produce annular areas of thickening. The mucosa overlying the granulomas may be ulcerated.

The finding of tachyzoites and/or cysts in association with areas of coagulative necrosis in one or more organs is highly suggestive of toxoplasmosis. Often the *Toxoplasma* organisms are difficult to distinguish within the necrotic foci, and immunohistochemical techniques are very useful in highlighting their presence. Serologic tests are of limited value in the diagnosis of disease associated with *T. gondii* infection.

The placental and fetal lesions associated with *Toxoplasma* infection and abortion are described in Vol. 3, Female genital system, and ocular lesions in Vol. 1, Special senses.

Further reading

Aliberti J, et al. Turning it on and off: regulation of dendritic cell function in *Toxoplasma gondii* infection. Immunol Rev 2004;201:26-34.

Davidson MG. Toxoplasmosis. Vet Clin North Am Small Anim Pract 2000;30:1051-1062.

Dubey JP. History of the discovery of the life cycle of *Toxoplasma gondii*. Int J Parasitol 2009;39:877-882.

Elmore SA, et al. Trends *Toxoplasma gondii*: epidemiology, feline clinical aspects, and prevention. Parasitol 2010;26:190-196.

House PK, et al. Predator cat odors activate sexual arousal pathways in brains of *Toxoplasma gondii* infected rats. PLoS One 2011;6:e23277.

Lang C, et al. Subversion of innate and adaptive immune responses by *Toxoplasma gondii*. Parasitol Res 2007;100:191-203.

Malmasi A, et al. Prevention of shedding and re-shedding of *Toxoplasma gondii* oocysts in experimentally infected cats treated with oral clindamycin: a preliminary study. Zoonoses Public Health 2009;56:102-104.

Skariah S, et al. *Toxoplasma gondii*: determinants of tachyzoite to bradyzoite conversion. Parasitol Res 2010;107:253-260.

Sullivan WJ Jr, et al. Mechanisms of *Toxoplasma gondii* persistence and latency. FEMS Microbiol Rev 2012;36:717-733.

Neosporosis. *Neospora caninum* causes disease in *dogs and ruminants* over much of the world. *Dogs, Australian dingoes, and coyotes are definitive hosts;* cattle, water buffalo, and white-tailed deer can act as intermediate hosts. *Neospora* has been associated with systemic and central nervous system disease in dogs, and with abortion and CNS disease in neonatal ruminants. Tachyzoites undergoing endodyogeny and cysts containing bradyzoites are found in the tissues of affected animals. Transplacental transmission occurs in ruminants and dogs. Infection may be maintained in lines of cattle in this manner, whereas some subclinically infected bitches have given birth to successive litters of pups that became affected within the first few months of life. Transmission may also occur by ingestion of infected tissue, as in toxoplasmosis.

Dogs of all ages may be affected, but disease seems most characteristic as *encephalomyelitis, polyradiculoneuritis,* and *polymyositis* in puppies greater than ~5 weeks of age, and perhaps involving several animals in a litter. Ascending paralysis, muscle contraction causing hyperextension of the limbs, cervical weakness, and dysphagia may progress to death, or animals stabilize with caudal paralysis. In adult dogs there are signs of widespread involvement of the CNS, and disseminated disease may be evident, with polymyositis, myocarditis, and dermatitis associated with parasite infection. Although disease may be precipitated or exacerbated by glucocorticoid administration, *Neospora* is regarded as a *primary pathogen.*

Cell-mediated immunity including production of IL-12 and γ-interferon may be related to immune resistance.

In acute systemic infections, there may be hepatic enlargement with coalescing areas of pallor related to widespread necrosis of hepatocytes; streaky pallor of muscles resulting from myonecrosis, mineralization, and nonsuppurative myositis; and pulmonary congestion and edema resulting from subacute alveolitis. Tachyzoites are common in affected tissues.

Nonsuppurative encephalomyelitis is associated with the presence of tachyzoites and tissue cysts in neurons and neuropil; the degree of necrosis, gliosis, neovascularization, and demyelination presumably depends to some extent on the duration of the lesion. Retinitis is also reported in association with *Neospora*, as is pyogranulomatous ulcerative dermatitis, occasionally.

In **ruminant abortion**, *Neospora* may be associated with *necrotizing placentitis*, and with *myositis* and *nonsuppurative encephalomyelitis* of the fetus after ~90 days' gestation. Gestation may lead to diminished γ-interferon production and this may promote dissemination of parasites to the fetus. Although a well-documented etiologic agent of abortion in cattle, the extent of natural *Neospora*-induced abortions in sheep and goats is unknown. Experimentally, sheep and pigs experience placental infection and necrotizing encephalitis in the fetuses. *N. caninum* also has been reported from a case of equine protozoal myelitis. *Neospora* has been isolated from wildlife including white tailed deer and water buffalo.

Tachyzoites are approximately ovoid, ~5-7 μm long, and are found in small groups or large clusters, free in the cytoplasm or in parasitophorous vacuoles in many types of cells throughout the body. Tissue cysts are found in only the brain and spinal cord. They are spherical or slightly elongate, up to ~110 μm in greatest dimension. The cyst wall is ~1-4 μm thick, usually greater than the width of the bradyzoites, which are slender (1.5 × 7 μm), slightly curved, with an obvious nucleus; they stain weakly periodic acid-Schiff–positive.

Neospora must be distinguished from *Toxoplasma* in all species, and from *Sarcocystis* in aborted fetuses. *Neospora* tachyzoites resemble those of *Toxoplasma* in tissue section. Ultrastructurally, *Neospora* tachyzoites have >11 rhoptries, whereas there are few in *Toxoplasma*. *Toxoplasma* is always found in a membrane-bound vacuole in the cytoplasm; *Neospora* tachyzoites are often not within a parasitophorous vacuole. *Neospora* tissue cysts are relatively uncommonly encountered, especially in acute cases. They are distinguished from *Toxoplasma* by the thicker wall (thinner than 0.5 μm in *Toxoplasma*). Perhaps the most common method of distinction is by immunohistochemistry using specific antibodies; polymerase chain reaction is also useful. *Sarcocystis* meronts divide by endopolygony in endothelium in domestic animals; they are not in a parasitophorous vacuole; and merozoites lack rhoptries. Sarcocysts in muscle cells are within a parasitophorous vacuole; they have a distinct wall; and they are usually subdivided internally by septa.

Further reading

Dubey JP, Lindsay DS. A review of *Neospora caninum* and neosporosis. Vet Parasitol 1996;67:1-59.

Dubey JP, et al. Epidemiology and control of neosporosis and *Neospora caninum*. Clin Microbiol Rev 2007;20:323-367.

Dubey JP, Schares G. Neosporosis in animals—the last five years. Vet Parasitol 2010;180:90-108.

Gondim LF, et al. Transmission of *Neospora caninum* between wild and domestic animals. J Parasitol 2004;90:1361-1365.

Khan IA, et al. *Neospora caninum*: role for immune cytokines in host immunity. Exp Parasitol 1997;85:24-34.

McAllister MM, et al. Dogs are definitive hosts of *Neospora caninum*. Int J Parasitol 1998;28:1473-1478.

***Hammondia* infection.** *Hammondia* spp. are obligatorily heteroxenous organisms, with the cat (**H. hammondi**) and dog (**H. heydorni**) as definitive hosts. They also have been known as *Toxoplasma hammondi* and *Isospora bahien*sis, respectively. *Toxoplasma*-like oocysts are shed in the feces of the definitive host and are infectious to intermediate hosts, mammals and birds (*H. hammondi*), and ruminants (*H. heydorni*). Here, bradyzoites develop in cysts in striated muscle, which are infective when ingested by the carnivore. Disease is not associated with infection of intermediate hosts; diarrhea may occur in heavily infected dogs.

Further reading

Dubey JP, Sreekumar C. Redescription of *Hammondia hammondi* and its differentiation from *Toxoplasma gondii*. Int J Parasitol 2003;33:1437-1453.

Dubey JP, et al. Clinical *Toxoplasma gondii*, *Hammondia heydorni*, and *Sarcocystis* spp. infections in dogs. Parasitologia 2003;45: 141-146.

***Sarcocystis* infection.** *Sarcocystis* is comprised of ~200 obligatorily heteroxenous species. Inconspicuous sexual stages occur in the epithelium at the tips of villi in the small intestine, and oocysts sporulate in the subepithelial lamina propria, producing two sporocysts within a thin oocyst wall. Sporocysts containing four sporozoites are shed in feces. These are infective to intermediate hosts, in which three generations of merogony occur in vascular endothelium, and a final cyst containing first *metrocytes* (mother cells), which produce *merozoites* (bradyzoites), is formed in myocytes and occasionally other cells. Ingestion of tissue cysts containing bradyzoites initiates gametogony in the definitive host. There is apparently no resistance to the development of gamonts, and no disease is associated with them in the definitive host.

Many species of *Sarcocystis* are recognized, based on prey-predator cycles, for instance, between cattle and dogs, and cattle and cats. Sporogony of a given species usually occurs in only one or a few genera of carnivores. The number of species capable of acting as intermediate hosts may be narrow or wide, depending on the species of *Sarcocystis*.

Sarcocystis cysts in ovine and, occasionally, bovine muscle may be grossly visible, causing losses at meat inspection. *Eosinophilic myositis* can result from granulomas caused by *Sarcocystis* infection of muscle. However, studies have shown that unaffected muscle often harbors more of these organisms than the inflamed portions. *Sarcocystis* infection in cattle (**S. cruzi**), sheep (**S. tenella**), and swine (**S. miescheriana**), and, experimentally, in goats (**S. capracanis**), may cause acute fatal disease characterized by anemia and widespread hemorrhage, which is associated with clotting disorders. As the disease progresses, cattle may develop inappetence, weight loss, reduced milk yield, hyperexcitability, hair loss, and in some animals, nervous signs. Ill-thrift associated with *Sarcocystis* infection may also occur in other species. Both syndromes are initiated during the endothelial phase of the infection. As well,

abortion occurs during this phase in some species. Abortion associated with the acute disease is the result of the systemic illness, and the fetus is usually not infected. However, in cattle, some abortions, seen in otherwise clinically normal animals, are associated with meronts of *Sarcocystis* in the placenta and in vascular endothelium of the fetus, especially in the brain, and with nonsuppurative encephalitis. Encephalitis is occasionally associated with *Sarcocystis* infection in sheep, and in horses **S. neurona** is the cause of protozoal myeloencephalitis. Details of these syndromes are discussed in Vol. 1, Muscle and tendon; Vol. 3, Female genital system; Vol. 1, Nervous system.

Sarcocystis spp. have been identified as causing rare incidents of severe myositis in dogs and encephalomyelitis in cats. A *Sarcocystis*-like agent also has been implicated in mortality of Rottweiler dogs with hepatitis, encephalitis, and dermatitis.

Further reading

Bisby TM, et al. *Sarcocystis* sp. encephalomyelitis in a cat. Vet Clin Pathol 2010;39:105-112.

Dubey JP, et al. A review of *Sarcocystis neurona* and equine protozoal myeloencephalitis (EPM). Vet Parasitol 2001;95:89-131.

Fayer R. *Sarcocystis* spp. in human infections. Clin Microbiol Rev 2004;17:894-902.

Sykes JE, et al. Severe myositis associated with *Sarcocystis* spp. infection in 2 dogs. J Vet Intern Med 2011;25:1277-1283.

Tenter AM. Current research on *Sarcocystis* species of domestic animals. Int J Parasitol 1995;25:1311-1330.

***Besnoitia* infection.** *Besnoitia* spp. are also obligatorily heteroxenous, but the definitive host for many species has not been identified. Some stages of merogony and gametogony occur in the intestine of the only definitive host yet known, the cat, where they are not known to be pathogenic. Oocysts are shed unsporulated, and resemble those of *Toxoplasma* and *Hammondia* when sporulated. Meronts in the intermediate host develop in mesenchymal cells, probably fibroblasts, which become massively hypertrophic, forming cysts containing many clusters of merozoites (bradyzoites) in the host cell cytoplasm. Among domestic animals, cysts of *B. besnoiti* may assume some significance in the skin of cattle and goats (Vol. 1, Integumentary system), and *Besnoitia* cysts have been reported in association with laryngeal polyps in a horse.

Further reading

Alvarez-García G, et al. Dynamics of *Besnoitia besnoiti* infection in cattle. Parasitol 2014;29:1-17.

Cortes H, et al. A review on bovine besnoitiosis: a disease with economic impact in herd health management, caused by *Besnoitia besnoiti* (Franco and Borges). Parasitol 2014 Apr 2:1-12.

Cryptosporidiosis

Cryptosporidium is a small apicomplexan protist, found on the surface of epithelium in the gastrointestinal, biliary, and respiratory tracts of mammals, birds, reptiles, and fish. Respiratory infection is most significant in birds, and disease in mammals is generally enteric.

Although its taxonomic position in relation to other apicomplexan protists, and its species nomenclature, are in a state of flux, on molecular genetic grounds ~15 morphologically

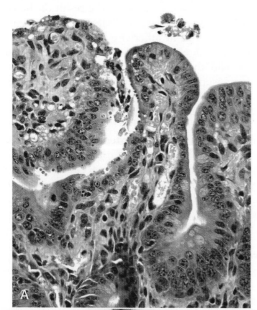

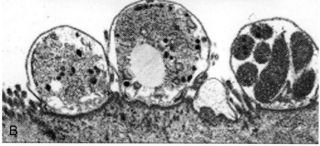

Figure 1-192 Cryptosporidia. A. Appearing as minute basophilic dots on the brush border of enterocytes in the small intestine of a calf. **B.** Attached to apex of enterocytes in small intestine. Two macrogametes and a schizont containing merozoites. (Transmission electron micrograph Courtesy S. Tzipori.)

similar species of *Cryptosporidium* are recognized. Five of these occur in domestic animals: (1) **C. parvum**, small, and initially described in the mouse intestine, but parasitic in cattle, other ruminants, and humans; (2) **C. andersoni** in cattle; (3) **C. suis** in pigs; (4) **C. felis** in cats; and (5) **C. canis** in dogs. C. parvum is zoonotic, as are C. suis, C. felis, and C. canis to a lesser extent, and disease in humans has been associated with contamination of water sources, food and milk products, as well as close contact with infected animals. However, humans also have a primate-adapted species, **C. hominis,** and it is probably responsible for the majority of outbreaks of cryptosporidiosis not associated with direct animal contact.

All 3 stages of the *Cryptosporidium* life cycle—merogony, gametogony, and sporogony—occur extracytoplasmically in a vacuole within the apical region of epithelial cells, protruding above the cell surface (Fig. 1-192A, B). The prepatent period of C. parvum in calves is ~7 days and infections usually persist for weeks or, if the animal is immunocompromised, perhaps months. Type I merozoites recycle in a new host cell to produce another meront generation, whereas type II merozoites differentiate to gamonts. Thin-walled oocysts excyst in the gut of the same host, resulting in autoinfection by the sporozoites released, whereas thick-walled oocysts are excreted to the external environment and are responsible for transmission

to another host. Multiple generations of merogony, and autoinfection by excystment of thin-walled oocysts, result in a large biotic potential and promote heavy colonization of the gut.

The organisms are enclosed within a parasitophorous vacuole formed by apposition of two unit membranes of the host cell, probably caused by inversion of a microvillus by the infecting sporozoite or merozoite. A specialized "feeder" organelle is present at the attachment zone in the base of the vacuole, between the infecting organism and the cytoplasm of the host cell. Developmental stages are small, in most cases ~2-6 μm in diameter. Undifferentiated meronts and gamonts are recognized as small basophilic trophozoites. Mature schizonts contain small falciform merozoites. Macrogamonts are ~5 μm in diameter, and contain small granules. Oocysts in tissue sections are often collapsed into a crescent shape. The various stages may be recognized in wax- or plastic-embedded sections under the light microscope, but are best studied with the electron microscope. Oocysts containing 4 sporozoites may be demonstrated by fecal flotation, or in fecal smears stained with Giemsa, by a modified Ziehl-Neelsen technique, or with Auramine O or fluorescein-labeled antibody and examined with ultraviolet light.

Cryptosporidia are found in many circumstances, and in some species infection appears to be asymptomatic. Neonates are particularly susceptible to intestinal infections, and this is especially so among ruminants (calves, lambs, kids, red deer calves) infected with C. parvum. Diarrhea, anorexia, and depression in calves usually occur between ~1 and 4 weeks of age, and in lambs ~5-14 days old. However, naïve calves up to 3 months of age are susceptible to infection and may develop diarrhea.

Cryptosporidial infections are mainly eliminated by cell-mediated immune responses, including γ-interferon production by CD4 T lymphocytes, but the humoral arm also contributes. Immunosuppression is contributory to, but not essential for, the development of disease. Heavy infections are reported in Arabian foals with combined immunodeficiency, and cryptosporidiosis has occurred in cats with feline leukemia virus infection, and in dogs with canine distemper. In immunocompromised individuals organisms may be present at any level of the gastrointestinal tract, from esophagus to colon. Liver, gallbladder, pancreas, and their ducts also may be involved, as may the respiratory tract. Cryptosporidia frequently occur concurrently with enterotoxigenic *Escherichia coli*, rotaviral, or coronaviral infection in neonatal ruminants, but can be primary pathogens.

In all species, *intestinal cryptosporidiosis is associated with villus atrophy of variable severity*, characterized by blunting and some fusion of villi, and by hypertrophy of crypts of Lieberkühn. Surface epithelium is usually cuboidal, rounded, or low columnar, and sometimes exfoliating or forming irregular projections at tips of villi. *Large numbers of cryptosporidia are usually visible in the microvillus border of cells on the villi* (Fig. 1-193), and not in crypts of Lieberkühn, although occasionally, the reverse is true. Organisms typically are most heavily distributed in the distal half of the small intestine, especially in ileum, although occasionally cryptosporidia may occur in the cecum and colon. Mild proprial infiltrates of neutrophils and mixed mononuclear cells are present, probably attracted by proinflammatory cytokines released from infected epithelium. An increase in intraepithelial T lymphocytes has been documented in the intestine of infected calves.

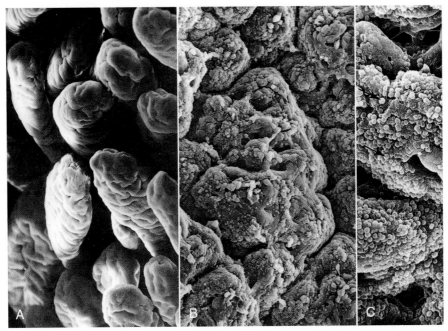

Figure 1-193 Cryptosporidia: scanning electron micrographs. A. Normal villi. **B.** Villus atrophy associated with cryptosporidiosis. Cryptosporidia are visible as minute spheres on mucosal surface. **C.** Detail of (**B**) showing cryptosporidia (arrows). (Courtesy S. Tzipori.)

Diarrhea in cryptosporidiosis is mainly attributable to malabsorption associated with villus atrophy and a population of immature enterocytes; and perhaps to the occupation of a large proportion of the surface area of absorptive cells by the organisms. Release of inflammatory mediators, principally prostaglandins, may stimulate mucosal secretion, and an increase in epithelial cell permeability to macromolecules has been demonstrated in vitro.

Cryptosporidium parvum is most significant in **calves,** as a cause of undifferentiated neonatal diarrhea, in which it must be differentiated particularly from coronaviral and rotaviral infection. Frequently it is concurrent with other agents causing this syndrome; it tends to be most prevalent in animals ~2 weeks old. A similar situation occurs in lambs, although disease does not appear to be as common or well recognized in that species. It is a sporadic or minor cause of sometimes fatal diarrhea in other species of ruminants.

Several species are susceptible to *Cryptosporidium* infection; however, many infections are subclinical. Although cryptosporidiosis can be induced experimentally in **piglets,** it is a very rare cause of spontaneous disease in swine. It is only occasionally associated with disease of carnivores, and then often in probably immunocompromised animals. Although infection of **foals** is not uncommon, *Cryptosporidium* has been associated with disease mainly in animals with combined immunodeficiency, complicated by adenoviral infection. Disease has not occurred in successful experimental infections in foals, and the role of cryptosporidia in the etiology of neonatal diarrhea in foals is poorly defined, although occasional outbreaks attributable to *C. parvum* may occur.

The diagnosis is based on the presence of large numbers of cryptosporidia in sections of freshly fixed lower small intestine, preferably in association with villus atrophy. Examination of smears of ileal mucosa stained with Giemsa may allow a rapid diagnosis, or permit a diagnosis on tissue from an animal dead for some hours.

C. andersoni, in the *abomasum of weaned calves and older cattle,* is not associated with diarrhea, but plasma pepsinogen levels rise, and weight gains of some growing animals may be adversely affected. There is mucous metaplasia/hyperplasia in the fundic glands, which are dilated, with attenuation of the lining epithelium, on which cryptosporidia are numerous. Infections have been associated with decreased milk production.

Rarely, cryptosporidia are seen in gastric biopsies from **cats,** sometimes associated with mild gastritis. There is some indication that concurrent infection with *Helicobacter felis* will precipitate disease because of cryptosporidia. A mixed infection of *C. muris* (stomach) and *C. felis* (small intestine) was identified in an adult cat with diarrhea that was refractory to therapy.

Further reading

Barr F. Cryptosporidiosis. J Small Anim Pract 1997;38:319-320.

Deng M, et al. Host intestinal epithelial response to *Cryptosporidium parvum*. Adv Drug Deliv Rev 2004;56:869-884.

Gookin JL, et al. Host responses to *Cryptosporidium* infection. J Vet Intern Med 2002;16:12-21.

Olson ME, et al. Update on *Cryptosporidium* and *Giardia* infections in cattle. Trends Parasitol 2004;20:185-191.

Petry F, et al. Host immune response to *Cryptosporidium parvum* infection. Exp Parasitol 2010;126:304-309.

Ramirez NE, et al. A review of the biology and epidemiology of cryptosporidiosis in humans and animals. Microbes Infect 2004;6:773-785.

Santín M. Clinical and subclinical infections with *Cryptosporidium* in animals. N Z Vet J 2013;61:1-10.

Amebiasis

Entamoeba histolytica is the cause of amebiasis in humans, nonhuman primates, and, rarely, in other species, including dogs and cattle; cats are susceptible to experimental infection. Infection in dogs is sporadic, probably acquired by exposure to cysts in feces from infected humans. Dogs tend not to pass encysted amebae; hence it has been suggested that they present little public health hazard, and are unlikely to support spread from dog to dog. However, under some circumstances, cysts may be shed, and fecal material containing motile trophozoites has been used to transmit infection orally to other dogs.

Amebae are usually nonpathogenic inhabitants of the lumen of the large bowel, but sometimes they cause colitis. The diet and immune status of the host, and virulence attributes of various strains of the organism, seem to influence pathogenicity. Adhesion to mucus by specific lectins, enzymatic degradation of mucus, and lectin-mediated adherence of amebae to host epithelium are essential steps leading to tissue damage. Cysteine proteinases produced by *E. histolytica* contribute to epithelial cell damage and to induction of inflammation, both of which are involved in initiation of mucosal lesions. Cytolysis is induced by in-contact amebae.

Amebiasis in dogs is associated with diarrheic or mucoid feces, perhaps with some blood, or with dysentery. *Erosive mucosal colitis or ulcerative colitis* occurs in dogs with amebiasis, and disease seems more common or severe in animals with concomitant *Trichuris* or *Ancylostoma* infection.

Early lesions in human amebiasis seem to be diffuse acute mucosal colitis, with focal erosions or ulcerations. Amebae, although scarce, may be found in mucus on the colonic surface, but are most numerous in the fibrinocellular exudate over erosions or superficial ulcers. Ulcers advance as an area of necrosis and predominantly neutrophilic infiltrate, causing loss of glands, and extending for the full depth of the mucosa. Initial lesions consist of tiny erosions of the surface epithelium that evolve to deeper, more extensive ulcers. Established ulcerative amebic colitis classically has a flask-shaped ulcer, the narrow neck through the mucosa, and the broad base in the submucosa. There amebae, and necrosis, expand laterally, apparently less constrained by the architecture of the tissue. Intestinal perforations and intramural abscesses may form.

Amebae may be present, commonly in small clusters, in necrotic debris or in adjacent viable tissue, frequently not involved in an inflammatory reaction. Amebae in tissue, often surrounded by a clear halo, may be spherical or irregular, with extended pseudopodia, and are ~6-50 μm in diameter. The nucleus has a central dense karyosome and peripheral chromatin clumps. The cytoplasm may appear foamy, can contain remnants of erythrocytes in phagolysosomes, and contains glycogen, which makes the cytoplasm periodic acid-Schiff–positive. The lesions of established amebiasis in the colon of dogs resemble those in humans; the early lesions may as well.

Although dissemination of amebae, with abscessation in other organs, especially liver, lung, and brain, is a relatively common complication in humans, it seems rare in dogs. One such case occurred in an animal with canine distemper.

Further reading

Huston CD. Parasite and host contributions to the pathogenesis of amebic colitis. Trends Parasitol 2004;20:23-26.

Wittnich C. *Entamoeba histolytica* infection in a German shepherd dog. Can Vet J 1976;17:259-263.

Yoshida N, et al. Invasion mechanisms among emerging food-borne protozoan parasites. Trends Parasitol 2011;27:459-466.

Giardia *and other flagellates*

Giardia spp. are flagellate protists that inhabit the small intestine of a wide range of vertebrates. The taxonomy of the genus is difficult. It appears that 4 or 5 morphologically distinct "species" exist, each with a relatively wide host range within amphibians, birds, rodents, and other mammals. ***Giardia duodenalis*** (= *G. lamblia*) infection is common in humans, and it also occurs in a wide array of mammals. Although morphologically similar, molecular genetic investigations have identified at least 7 genotypes within *G. duodenalis*, several of which (assemblages A and B) infect humans. Hoofed animals are infected by assemblages A and E, the former being potentially zoonotic, dogs by assemblages C and D, and cats by assemblage F. *Giardia* infection has been associated with disease, with various degrees of credibility, in most of these hosts. In an experimental model, genotypes A and B appear to be more infectious and cause more severe mucosal injury.

Giardia trophozoites are pyriform in outline, ~10-20 μm long by 5-15 μm wide and 2-4 μm thick, and convex on the dorsal surface. The concave ventral surface is modified by the presence of a disk that functions in attachment. Nutrient absorption seems to occur through the dorsal surface. A pair of nuclei, 2 axonemes, 2 medial bodies, and 4 pairs of flagella are present, and the organisms multiply by binary fission in the gut lumen. They apply their ventral aspect to the microvillus surface of enterocytes, usually between villi, in folds on the villus surface, or occasionally in crypts of Lieberkühn. Giardia has been demonstrated in the mucosa, but this is an unusual and probably aberrant location. Relatively resistant oval cysts are passed in the feces, and transmission is by the fecal-oral route.

The significance of *Giardia* as a pathogen in humans and other species has been controversial because *asymptomatic infection is the rule.* However, under some circumstances *Giardia* may cause disease. How the host-parasite relationship is modified, and the pathogenesis of the disease, are still unclear.

In *young dogs and cats,* in which giardiosis is most important, although still uncommon, the main sign is intermittent or chronic *diarrhea,* which may persist for several months. The stool is soft, pale, mucoid, and greasy. Although appetite is not usually impaired, there may be a reduced growth rate or weight loss, suggesting malabsorption. A poor hair coat is attributed to deficiency of fat-soluble vitamins. Among animals other than dogs and cats, *Giardia* seems most convincingly to be associated with *enteric signs in neonatal calves,* which may pass soft mucoid feces, and have a reduced growth rate.

Gastrointestinal dysfunction has not been extensively documented in domestic animals. However, in a variety of experimental systems, deficiencies in microvillus-associated digestive enzymes, electrolyte and glucose malabsorption, and microvillus shortening or injury have been documented, although not consistently. Some humans with *Giardia* infection have malabsorption of D-xylose and vitamin B_{12}, with steatorrhea and hypocarotinemia. Excess fecal fat has been found in infected cats, but was not demonstrated in experimentally infected rats.

Also, D-xylose malabsorption was not demonstrated in a dog with giardiosis.

Selective deficiencies in some brush border enzymes occur in humans with giardiosis, and in *Giardia*-infected calves. Possibly these are related to the direct effects of *Giardia* on microvilli, which may be deformed adjacent to adherent organisms or diffusely shortened. *Giardia* may also inhibit the activity of pancreatic lipase, causing fat malabsorption. However, bacterial overgrowth of the small intestine may occur with *Giardia* infection, and associated bile salt deconjugation could explain steatorrhea in giardiosis.

Several mechanisms have been proposed to explain these findings. Although villus atrophy may occur in humans with giardiosis, this mainly occurs in a subgroup of patients with hypogammaglobulinemia. Marked histologic abnormality is not found in many cases of giardiosis in humans, and this also seems to be true for dogs, cats, and calves. In experimental murine giardiosis, infection is associated with hypertrophy of crypts and increased production of cells, combined with an increased rate of movement of enterocytes along villi, with an increased crypt:villus ratio. Deficiencies in brush border form and function may be attributable to incomplete differentiation of enterocytes in this circumstance, or perhaps to damage mediated by mucosal T cells. Intraepithelial lymphocytes are common in infected intestine, and altered epithelial kinetics may be related to cell-mediated immune reactions in the mucosa. Infection may lead to increased enterocyte apoptosis, and alterations in epithelial barrier function. Infection has been shown in experimental models to interfere with tight junctions in the epithelium. Atrophy of villi has been associated with restoration of cell-mediated immune competence in *Giardia*-infected athymic mice, reinforcing the notion that immune phenomena may be involved in the pathogenesis of giardiosis.

Giardiosis is usually *diagnosed clinically* on the basis of typical cysts in fecal flotations, or trophozoites in intestinal aspirates or fecal smears, coupled with remission of clinical signs following therapy, and an inability to identify other potential causes of the signs. Sometimes a diagnosis is based on findings in biopsies of small intestine or at autopsy.

In all species, morphologic changes in the mucosa are not well defined in spontaneous cases of giardiosis. The mucosa may appear normal but there may be equivocal blunting of villi, perhaps associated with a moderate infiltrate of mononuclear cells into the core of the villus, or a heavy population of intraepithelial lymphocytes. *Giardia* should be sought in animals with malabsorption syndromes. They lie between villi, and are usually evident as crescent shapes, applied by their concave surface to the brush border of epithelial cells. In favorable sections through the level of the nuclei, they may appear to have a pair of "eyes." Trophozoites oriented along the plane of section may look as they do in smears, the paired nuclei giving the organism a "face-like" appearance. An abnormal number of bacteria, suggestive of overgrowth, may be present in the mucus and content in the vicinity in symptomatic animals. A diagnosis of giardiosis always should be reserved for those cases in which no other explanation for the syndrome can be identified. Giardiosis has been associated with colitis in dogs but the association is not clearly causal.

Trichomonads, small flagellate protists that reproduce by binary fission, and are transmitted directly between hosts, are sometimes encountered in the feces of horses, cattle, dogs, and cats with diarrhea. Only in cats is there a causal association with disease. **Tritrichomonas foetus** is associated with *persistent large-bowel diarrhea*, refractory to treatment, in **cats** <1 year of age, and the syndrome has been reproduced experimentally. The microscopic lesions are typical of chronic mucosal colitis, most severe in areas colonized by the organisms. The diagnosis is confirmed in section by detection of pyriform or crescent-shaped organisms, ~5 × 7 μm in size, with a faint nucleus and eosinophilic cytoplasm, applied to the surface epithelium, or in the lumen of colonic glands, usually in large numbers. However, the organisms are present in only a little more than half the sections examined from infected cats, and multiple samples may be necessary to have a high probability of detecting them. In some cases trichomonads appear to disrupt the epithelium, attaining the subepithelial lamina propria around crypts, or they are associated with ulceration and foci of necrosis and pyogranulomatous inflammation that are distributed transmurally in affected areas of colon, and in draining lymph nodes.

Further reading

Foster DM, et al. Outcome of cats with diarrhea and *Tritrichomonas foetus* infection. J Am Vet Med Assoc 2004;225:888-892.

Kirkpatrick CE. Feline giardiasis: a review. J Small Anim Pract 1986; 27:69-80.

Oberhuber G, Stolte M. Giardiasis: analysis of histological changes in biopsy specimens of 80 patients. J Clin Pathol 1990;43: 641-643.

Olson ME, et al. Update on *Cryptosporidium* and *Giardia* infections in cattle. Trends Parasitol 2004;20:185-191.

Scott KG-E, et al. Role of CD8+ and CD4+ T lymphocytes in jejunal mucosal injury during murine giardiasis. Infect Immun 2004;72:3536-3542.

Xenoulis PG, et al. Intestinal *Tritrichomonas foetus* infection in cats: a retrospective study of 104 cases. J Feline Med Surg 2013;15:1098-1103.

Yaeger MJ, Gookin JL. Histologic features associated with *Tritrichomonas foetus*-induced colitis in domestic cats. Vet Pathol 2005; 42:797-804.

Balantidium

Balantidium is a large oval protist ~50-60 μm or more long, and ~25-45 μm wide, with a macronucleus and micronucleus, and covered by many cilia arrayed in rows. **B. coli** occurs in the large bowel of swine, humans, and nonhuman primates. It is very common in pigs, and many infected humans live in close contact with swine. It has been reported from a horse and from several dogs with access to swine yards, as a complication of trichurosis.

Balantidium is normally present as a commensal in the lumen of the cecum and colon, but is capable of opportunistic invasion of tissues injured by other diseases. On rare occasions it may be a primary pathogen. In swine, in which the organisms are most commonly encountered by veterinary pathologists, *Balantidium* may be found at the leading edge of the crateriform necrotizing or ulcerative lesions of the large intestine that develop secondary to intestinal adenomatosis (Fig. 1-194), swine dysentery, or perhaps salmonellosis. *Balantidium* is recognized in tissue by large size, ovoid shape, the dense curved or kidney-shaped macronucleus, and the presence of cilia (which may be accentuated by silver stains) in rows on the surface.

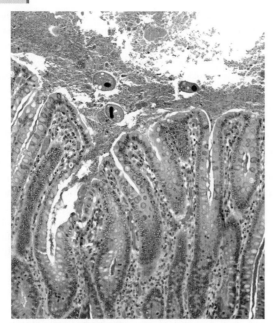

Figure 1-194 *Balantidium coli* in the colon of a pig.

Further reading

Headley SA, et al. *Balantidium coli*-infection in a Finnish horse. Vet Parasitol 2008;158:129-132.

Hindsbo O, et al. Age-dependent occurrence of the intestinal ciliate *Balantidium coli* in pigs at a Danish research farm. Acta Vet Scand 2000;41:79-83.

Nakauchi K. The prevalence of *Balantidium coli* infection in fifty-six mammalian species. J Vet Med Sci 1999;61:63-65.

PERITONEUM AND RETROPERITONEUM
General considerations

Peritoneal diseases are commonly secondary to processes either involving the organs covered by peritoneum or arising in the retroperitoneum. The peritoneum lines the abdominal cavity, which is incompletely divided into compartments by the mesentery, omentum, and ligaments covered by the peritoneum, with a total surface area greater than that of the skin. During organogenesis, the coelomic cavity is partitioned into peritoneal, pleural, and pericardial cavities lined by mesothelial cells that become known as peritoneum, pleura, and pericardium, respectively. *The normal peritoneum is a smooth, shiny membrane that is semipermeable to the movement of water and small solute molecules. There is normally just enough fluid present in the cavity to keep it moist.* Peritoneal fluid is normally clear and watery, but in neonatal pigs and lambs fluid may contain strands of mucinous coagulum lying on the intact serosal surfaces of abdominal viscera. The fluid is in osmotic equilibrium with plasma, but does not contain fibrinogen or other high-molecular-weight proteins, and generally does not clot, except in pigs.

The peritoneum consists of a single serosal lining layer of **mesothelial cells** on a basement membrane supported by submesothelial connective tissue containing a mixture of resident inflammatory cells, fibroblasts, blood vessels, and lymphatics. The submesothelial layer is inapparent in some places such as the liver, and prominent in other places such as the mesenteries. Mesothelial cells vary in appearance from squamous to low cuboidal with single small round nuclei and share characteristics of both epithelial and mesenchymal cells. Surface microvilli play a role in retention of hyaluronate-based secretions, and are more abundant on the visceral than parietal pleural surfaces. Tight junctions and desmosomes are discontinuous in the mesothelial layer, allowing for diffusion of water and small molecules across the membrane. Mesothelial cells are fragile and are readily injured after exposure to such mild insults as air, physiologic saline, intestinal dilation, and transient ischemia. Mesothelial wounds heal rapidly however, and although cell division and migration of adjacent mesothelium is important, a number of studies have suggested other sources of regenerating mesothelial cells, including free-floating serosal progenitor cells, that are capable of mesothelial differentiation.

Traditionally, the *function of the peritoneum* was considered to be providing a protective nonadhesive surface in the abdominal cavity; however, it is now clear that these cells are a dynamic membrane with several physiologic functions, including fluid and solute transport, immune surveillance and production of extracellular matrix, cytokines, growth factors, and other molecules. Both parietal and visceral peritoneum are continuously involved in transport of fluid in both directions. Normal fluid contains only traces of protein and secreted macromolecules that reduce permeability, and the electronegativity of the endothelium relative to mesothelium inhibits transfer of plasma proteins from capillaries into the cavity. Thus the net hydraulic forces favor movement of fluid into the abdominal cavity. *Several pathways contribute to the drainage of peritoneal fluid.* Direct transfer through stomata in the membrane to subserosal lymphatics is the main mechanism, dominated by transfer into lymphatics of the ventral diaphragm, and thence via the sternal lymph nodes to the right lymphatic duct, or via mediastinal lymph nodes to the thoracic duct. Respiratory diaphragmatic movements assist transfer through the diaphragm to ventral mediastinal lymphatics. Less fluid is taken up through the omentum and abdominal viscera, and drains via visceral lymphatics and lymph nodes to the thoracic duct. There is a lesser contribution to drainage by the pelvic serosa. Transfer of peritoneal fluid through and between mesothelial cells occurs but is a minor contributor to overall fluid movement.

Mesothelial cells secrete glycosaminoglycans, proteoglycans and surface lubricants to provide a nonadhesive surface. They also produce many cytokines and growth factors, which regulate inflammatory processes, leukocyte trafficking into and out of serosal cavities, or tissue repair. They produce fibrinolytic mediators, which aid in fibrin clearance and protect against formation of adhesions. Mesothelial cells have been implicated in both the spread and inhibition of tumor growth in serosal cavities.

The basement membrane is absent in minute foci, so-called **peritoneal milky spots,** pale semitransparent *focal nests of macrophages mixed with lesser numbers of lymphocytes and plasma cells* that allow transfer of particulate matter from the peritoneal cavity to lymphatics in the mesentery and omentum. They are also probably preferential sites for leukocyte trafficking and for the migration of neoplastic cells from the peritoneal cavity. Generally recognized as omental structures, milky spots also may be functional on the parietal membranes of peritoneal, pericardial, and pleural cavities and in the mediastinum.

The **retroperitoneum** is the adipose and connective tissue immediately beneath the peritoneal lining of the abdominal cavity. The concept of retroperitoneum properly includes the lymphatics and draining lymph nodes in addition to connective tissues, blood vessels, nerves, and the fixed and migratory mononuclear cell populations, most significant along the dorsum from the diaphragm to the anus. Its volume is small, except when adipose tissue accumulates, commonly around the kidneys, pelvic cavity, omentum, and mesenteries. With emaciation, fat stores of the retroperitoneum undergo *serous atrophy*, as do fat deposits in subcutaneous tissues, the thorax, and bone marrow cavities.

There appear to be no absolute barriers to movement of fluid or exudates within the retroperitoneal space of dogs; it may travel in the fascia around the dorsal and ventral aspects of the sublumbar muscles, to gain access to the fascial planes of the abdominal wall. Suppurative inflammation or exudates in the retroperitoneum of dogs may drain at the flank, by passing along the fascial planes of the abdominal and the iliopsoas muscles, to emerge in the lumbodorsal triangle, cranioventral to the tuber coxae.

Antemortem and postmortem effusions and discoloration in the peritoneal cavity should be distinguished. Fluid accumulates in the peritoneal cavity after death, and this becomes stained with hemoglobin as soon as erythrocytes in the serosal vessels lyse. Such fluid does not clot and similar fluid is often also present in other serous cavities. Diffusion of bile pigments through the wall of the gallbladder, the bile ducts, or the duodenum will also stain adjacent viscera.

Further reading

Mutsaers SE. The mesothelial cell. Int J Biochem Cell Biol 2004;36:9-16.
Rangel-Moreno J, et al. Omental milky spots develop in the absence of lymphoid tissue-inducer cells and support B and T cell responses to peritoneal antigens. Immunity 2009;30:731-743.

Anomalies

Congenital abnormalities affecting the peritoneal membranes are associated most frequently with retention of effete embryonic structures or defective partitioning of the coelomic cavity.

A **persistent vitelline or omphalomesenteric duct** *may form a fibrous ligament between the intestine or Meckel's diverticulum and the umbilicus*. The remnant may be partial and not reach the umbilicus, or it may be attached to the mesentery or to a loop of intestine. These structures may become involved in herniation and obstruction or strangulation of the intestine; persisting ducts may become cystic.

A **mesodiverticular band** is the result of a **persistent vitelline artery**. The band is a fold of mesentery, occasionally carrying a patent vitelline artery in its free edge, which extends from the cranial mesenteric artery, or from a spot partway down the mesenteric veil, to the antimesenteric side of the intestine (the site of Meckel's diverticulum). The pocket formed between this fold and the normal mesentery *may entrap intestine*; defects may develop in it that permit strangulation of intestinal loops. Occasionally, double (left and right) mesodiverticular bands are present. Rarely, fibrous cords of mesenteric tissue may be found that do not appear to be part of embryonic remnants of vitelline structures.

The **falciform ligament**, which in its free margin may contain the remnant of the umbilical vein as the *round ligament*, varies in size among species and individuals; it is typically largest in young animals. There is potential for entrapment or strangulation of bowel if a large persistent falciform ligament is perforated.

Partitioning of the coelom to separate the thoracic cavity from the developing gastrointestinal tract begins with the formation of the *septum transversum* from the ventral body wall, eventually forming the ventral part of the diaphragm. The dorsal part of the diaphragm is provided by downgrowth from the dorsal body wall of the paired *pleuroperitoneal and pleuropericardial folds*. **Congenital pleuroperitoneal diaphragmatic hernias** are most commonly observed in dogs, but occasionally are observed in herd animals. *They usually involve a defect in the left dorsal quadrant of the diaphragm, presumably from failure of the left pleuroperitoneal fold to fuse with the septum transversum;* the reason for the particular susceptibility for the left side is unknown. The lesion in some breeds of dogs may have an autosomal recessive mode of inheritance. Some congenital pleuroperitoneal defects in small animals may be more extensive, to the point that virtually the entire diaphragm is missing. The margins of the diaphragmatic defect are smooth, and a large mass of abdominal viscera may pass into the thoracic cavity through the opening; large defects result in respiratory difficulties, abdominal pain, and bloating if incarceration of herniated viscera occurs. Most small animals born with these defects die at or shortly after birth. In large animals, the lesions may be clinically silent, especially when only a small portion of liver is present in the hernia.

Peritoneopericardial diaphragmatic hernias *are triangular and ventral, and presumably result from abnormal development or fusion of the septum transversum*. They are more common than pleuroperitoneal hernias in small animals, perhaps because the animals live longer. They can be associated with cardiac anomalies, malformations of the sternum and costochondral junctions, or umbilical hernias. Although various portions of the liver, spleen, omentum, and small intestine may herniate into the pericardial sac and cause cardiac tamponade, compromised respiratory function or gastrointestinal tract obstruction, these lesions also can be clinically silent.

External hernias are the result of abnormal openings in the abdominal wall that permit passage of the abdominal contents and may be congenital or acquired. Congenital defects resulting in hernias are of several types and include abnormally increased size of normal opening such as the inguinal canal; persistence of fetal openings as in umbilical hernias; and defects in closure of the abdominal cavity, as in schistosomus reflexus and diaphragmatic hernias.

Reactions of peritoneum to injury

Even minor injuries to peritoneum cause rapid loss of mesothelial cells. The denuded area is rapidly covered by a layer of fibrin, neutrophils and macrophages. If the injury is minor, the mesothelial layer is soon regenerated; however, regeneration may be delayed if the injury is severe or prolonged, and subsurface tissues are damaged. Under normal conditions, the mesothelium is a slowly renewing tissue. Restoration of the mesothelial surface may not be provided solely by proliferation and migration of adjacent mesothelial cells; current experimental evidence favors involvement of multipotent mesenchymal cells either lying in the immediate subserosa or free-floating in the peritoneum. Therefore, unlike other epithelial-like surfaces, in which wounds heal only from the edges, mesothelial healing occurs more rapidly and diffusely across the denuded surface.

Metaplasia of mesothelium is frequently seen in histologic specimens. Simple metaplasia also occurs where alterations to surface contours of organs produce clefts or valleys in which fluid movement slows; for example, in cases of hydroperitoneum. In these cases mesothelial cells become cuboidal, columnar, or if the stimulus persists, nodules of hyperplastic mesothelial cells are generated. Papillary hyperplasia of mesothelium is frequent in some chronic forms of peritonitis, such as those caused by actinomycotic infections in dogs and cats, and in organization of subserosal hemorrhages in spleen and intestine. Proliferative mesothelial cells may mimic neoplasia and in humans they are occasionally observed in lymph nodes where they can be confused with metastatic neoplasia; this phenomenon, known as benign epithelial inclusions in humans, has been described in the lymph nodes of cattle.

Traumatic lesions of the abdomen and peritoneum

Physical trauma to the abdomen is common, and *sequelae* include hemorrhage, peritoneal sepsis, uremia caused by the escape of urine into the abdomen, and dysfunction of traumatized organs.

Blunt trauma to the abdomen may result in contusion of abdominal viscera; avulsion of organs from supporting mesenteries or ligaments, and from their vascular supply; and perhaps laceration of the capsule of solid organs such as the liver, spleen, and kidney. Hollow organs, including the stomach, gallbladder, and urinary bladder, may rupture and release their contents into the abdominal cavity. Sudden increase in intra-abdominal pressure resulting from such trauma may cause acquired hernias by forcing viscera through natural apertures such as the inguinal canal, weak points such as the perineum, or through lacerations in the diaphragm or the abdominal wall, resulting in eventration.

Following abdominal trauma, contusions, lacerations, or perforation may be evident on the underside of the skin or in subcutaneous tissues; these lesions are often in apposition to internal lesions. Lacerations of the liver or spleen may result in internal hemorrhage and diffuse pallor of the animal. Contusion or laceration of the kidney results in subcapsular, retroperitoneal, or peritoneal hemorrhage. The source of hemorrhage may be subtle slits or crevasses in the capsule of the organ involved, or the laceration may be more obvious. In animals that die of exsanguination, the spleen is often contracted. Following splenic rupture, portions of spleen may implant and persist ectopically elsewhere in the abdomen (splenosis), and may be encountered as an incidental finding. Urine in the abdominal cavity may be easily mistaken for ascitic fluid; uroperitoneum should be confirmed by comparing creatinine concentration of the abdominal fluid to that of serum. Lacerations of the urinary bladder may be small and difficult to detect, particularly because the bladder contracts as urine is lost through the laceration or rupture. If the pregnant uterus is ruptured, fetuses may be free in the abdomen. They will die and cause peritonitis if the dam survives and they are not removed.

Endogenous forces may also result in herniation. The additional weight of intestinal contents during pregnancy,

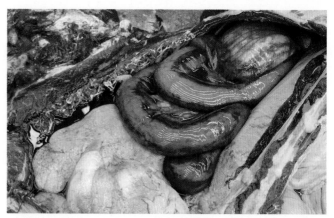

Figure 1-195 Acquired diaphragmatic hernia in a horse. Loops of small intestine and stomach have passed through the diaphragmatic laceration into the thoracic cavity, compressing lung.

especially when complicated by an event such as hydrops amnios, may cause ventral hernia. Straining during defecation or parturition may also cause herniation; the former is associated with perineal hernias in dogs; the latter, with acquired diaphragmatic hernias in horses. Tympany of the large bowel in horses or the forestomachs in ruminants may also cause herniation involving the abdominal wall or diaphragm. Antemortem lesions must be differentiated from postmortem tears resulting from bloating of viscera during postmortem autolysis. *The presence of hemorrhage, fibrin deposits, and acute inflammation in torn muscle, or strangulation of herniated gut, is evidence for an antemortem condition.*

Acquired diaphragmatic hernia can occur secondary to penetrating or blunt trauma; the latter is more common. The diaphragm is weaker than the abdominal wall, so during blunt trauma, a large pressure differential is generated between the abdominal and thoracic sides of the diaphragm, and this is relieved by rupture of the diaphragm and herniation of abdominal contents into the thoracic cavity (Fig. 1-195).

In small animals, the diaphragmatic muscle usually ruptures before the tendinous part; in general the location and orientation of the lesion are the result of the type of trauma and the location or direction of impact. Almost any of the abdominal viscera may herniate into the thoracic cavity through the defect, but liver and small bowel are most commonly involved. The lesion may be clinically silent for a considerable period, but eventually typically causes respiratory difficulty, hydrothorax, ascites, chylothorax, gastric tympany, or intestinal obstruction. At surgery or autopsy, acute diaphragmatic laceration is readily observed. If chronic, the margin of laceration is usually thickened by fibroplasia, and may even be adhered to the viscera. Differentiation from congenital hernias is based on the age, clinical history, and any evidence of scarring or adhesions at the margin of the diaphragmatic defect.

In horses, acquired lesions usually involve the area where the tendinous portion meets the pars costalis, whereas postmortem laceration of the diaphragm in the horse is most common at the ventral midline, near the xiphoid process. Most horses with acquired diaphragmatic hernias develop abdominal pain and signs of colic; respiratory signs are less common.

Further reading

Banz AC, Gottfried SD. Peritoneopericardial diaphragmatic hernia: a retrospective study of 31 cats and 8 dogs. J Am Anim Hosp Assoc 2013;46:398-404.

Gower SB, et al. Major abdominal evisceration injuries in dogs and cats: 12 cases (1998-2008). J Am Vet Med Assoc 2009;12:1566-1572.

Minihan AC, et al. Chronic diaphragmatic hernia in 34 dogs and 16 cats. J Am Anim Hosp Assoc 2004;40:51-63.

Romero AE, Rodgerson DH. Diaphragmatic herniation in the horse: 31 cases from 2001-2006. Can Vet J 2010;51:1247-1250.

Shaw SP, et al. Traumatic body wall herniation in 36 dogs and cats. J Am Anim Hosp Assoc 2003:39:35-46.

Abnormal contents in the peritoneal cavity

Foreign materials within the peritoneal cavity, such as urine, ingesta, blood, or air indicate an abnormality of another organ. **Uroperitoneum** in adults usually results from rupture of the urinary bladder, urethra, or ureters, which most frequently occurs as a consequence of urethral obstruction, particularly in ruminants. Uroperitoneum in neonates is associated with sepsis, and is described as a consequence of inflammation or congenital abnormalities involving the urachus or urethra.

Ingesta in the peritoneal cavity caused by bowel rupture or perforation occurs in horses and cattle, less frequently in swine, sheep, and goats, and rarely in dogs and cats. The site of perforation or rupture is usually easy to find, especially when the animal dies before peritonitis develops; once the intestines and mesenteries become adhered together, the primary site of perforation may be very difficult to discover. Ingesta may leak from any devitalized segment of small or large bowel as a consequence of impaction and pressure necrosis, tympany and rupture, or perforation either from sharp objects or deep mucosal ulceration. Cecal rupture in cattle following overload or impaction is reported; this condition in other species is rare. Rectal perforation can cause contamination of the abdomen with feces, and these lesions may be difficult to discover during postmortem examination. **Rectal perforation** in horses is most commonly secondary to accidental iatrogenic injury during rectal palpation, but can also occur secondary to dystocia; most tears occur 25-30 cm from the anus on the dorsal aspect of the rectum. Deep tears that involve the tunica muscularis have potential for contamination of the peritoneal cavity and secondary peritonitis. If the serosa remains intact, the potential exists for development of subserosal or rectal diverticula, perineal abscessation or fistula, pelvic cellulitis, or other complications. If these lesions progress and eventually perforate the mesorectum, gross fecal contamination of the peritoneum occurs.

Any portion of the bowel may easily rupture as a postmortem artifact; therefore **postmortem rupture of a viscus** must be differentiated from an antemortem lesion. The margin of a postmortem defect lacks hemorrhage and exudate, and the peritoneal surfaces are not inflamed.

Pneumoperitoneum arises from traumatic perforation of the abdominal wall (including surgery), from diaphragmatic tears in horses with concurrent pneumothorax, or from leakage of gas and liquid contents from a gastrointestinal perforation. Rarely, pneumoperitoneum can develop secondary to rupture of the urinary bladder or the female reproductive tract.

Hemoperitoneum *is the presence of blood or hemorrhagic effusion in the peritoneal cavity.* The amount present at death is not necessarily an indication of the volume of bleeding during life, because the blood may be removed quite rapidly via diaphragmatic lymphatics. Blood in the cavity may remain fluid or be partially clotted. Hemoperitoneum can be traumatic or atraumatic (spontaneous), and is seen most commonly in the dog and cat as a result of blunt or penetrating trauma. Spontaneous hemoperitoneum usually is associated with one of many pathologic processes, including hepatic or splenic torsion or rupture, gastric dilation and volvulus, coagulopathies, and neoplastic processes involving the liver, spleen, kidney, or other abdominal organs. When traumatic in origin, the liver and spleen are most commonly involved. Splenic hemangiosarcoma or hematoma, which may bleed into the abdomen, are the most common causes of spontaneous hemoperitoneum in dogs past middle age. Enlargement of liver or spleen because of infiltrating neoplastic cells, fat, or amyloid predisposes to rupture. Fine fissures in the capsule of the liver resulting in hemorrhage have been reported in infectious canine hepatitis.

In several species, acquired coagulopathies following ingestion of *anticoagulant rodenticides* cause hemorrhage that results in unclotted blood in the abdomen. Calves born of cows that have been fed moldy sweet-clover hay hemorrhage from the umbilical vessels into the peritoneal cavity and elsewhere. Manual ablation of a corpus luteum is a source of hemorrhage in cattle. In cattle and horses, laceration of the uterus or rupture of a uterine artery at parturition can result in fatal hemorrhage. In horses, hemoperitoneum may be due to hemorrhage from granulosa-thecal cell tumor of the ovary, and in all species any friable intra-abdominal or retroperitoneal neoplasm may occasionally rupture and hemorrhage if traumatized.

Hemorrhage on or beneath the peritoneal surface without free blood in the cavity may occur in acute bacterial toxemias and in other conditions that interfere with vascular integrity or hemostasis. *Peritoneal hemorrhage must be differentiated from hemorrhagic peritonitis,* which is an important lesion in some diseases. Subserosal hemorrhage and *hemomelasma ilei* occasionally occur on the intestine of the horse; this lesion has long been attributed to migration of strongyles. Rarely, subserosal hematomas may cause intestinal obstruction. Hemorrhage into an omental or mesenteric cyst can cause sudden abdominal enlargement without free blood in the abdomen.

Further reading

Aumann M, et al. Uroperitoneum in cats: 26 cases (1986-1995). J Am Anim Hosp Assoc 1998;34:315-324.

Clas A, et al. Evaluation of risk factors, management, and outcome associated with rectal tears in horses: 99 cases. J Am Vet Med Assoc 2008;233:1605-1609.

Conwell RC, et al. Haemoperitoneum in horses: a retrospective review of 54 cases. Vet Rec 2010;167:514-518.

Lux CN, et al. Perioperative outcome in dogs with hemoperitoneum: 83 cases (2005-2010). J Am Vet Med Assoc 2013;242:1385-1391.

Saunders WB, Tobias KM. Pneumoperitoneum in dogs and cats: 39 cases (1983-2002). J Am Vet Med Assoc 2003;223:462-468.

Ascites

Ascites, or hydroperitoneum, is the presence of excess fluid, usually a modified transudate, in the peritoneal cavity. Ascites occurs because of reduced removal of, or overproduction of, fluid in the abdominal cavity. Ascitic fluid is generally watery and clear or straw-colored, and contains few leukocytes but possibly numerous desquamated mesothelial cells. The serosal lining is normal and glistening but may become slightly opaque as a result of subserosal edema.

Reduced removal of fluid from the peritoneal cavity *is mainly caused by obstruction of lymphatic drainage through the diaphragm.* Limited area for direct-to-lymphatic absorption and the small size of stomata on the diaphragmatic and pelvic serosa explain the ease and rapidity with which peritoneal drainage can be blocked. An example is peritoneal carcinomatosis, in which neoplastic cells implant throughout the abdomen; when they implant on the diaphragm in the region of the lymphatic stomata, obstruction of lymphatic drainage occurs. Ascites may also develop if there is obstruction to sternal lymphatic flow cranial to the diaphragm. This may occur with sclerosing lymphadenitis or space-occupying lesions in the ventral or cranial mediastinum, and is common in lymphosarcoma of adult cattle.

Overproduction of peritoneal lymph *is mainly related to altered hydrostatic pressure gradients in the hepatic and portal circulation,* except for **chylous ascites,** which results when the cisterna chyli leak triglyceride-rich milky fluid into the abdomen. Increased prehepatic portal venous pressure alone does not usually lead to ascites; if present, such fluid is low protein, being derived from intestinal and mesenteric interstitial fluid. Acute portal vein obstruction causes intestinal infarction and death, but not ascites. Slowly developing portal hypertension of prehepatic, hepatic, or hepatic venous origin may cause transient ascites, which resolves with the development of collateral portal-postcaval venous shunts within a few weeks. However, portal hypertension of cardiac origin does not result in portocaval shunts, because the elevation in central venous pressure permits no pressure gradient between the portal and postcaval systems. *The sine qua non of hepatic ascites is increased resistance in the intrahepatic or posthepatic circulation.* The exception is the increase in portal blood flow caused by hepatic arteriovenous fistulas or anastomoses; in this circumstance, hydrostatic pressure at the level of the hepatic sinusoids is elevated by the arterialization of the portal flow.

The usual conditions causing increased hepatic or posthepatic resistance to blood flow are fibrosis of the liver and congestive heart failure, respectively. In diffuse fibrosis, intrahepatic resistance may be compounded by the development of arteriovenous anastomoses in the fibrous septa around nodules; these arterialize the hepatic portal circulation, further elevating hydrostatic pressure. Additional causes of portal hypertension include: primary neoplasms of the liver, especially cholangiocellular carcinomas, which tend to be diffuse and infiltrative; secondary tumors, especially lymphosarcomas, which widely infiltrate the liver; extensive infestation with hydatid cysts; and chronic biliary trematodiasis, or other causes of chronic cholangiohepatitis and portal fibrosis. Tumors or abscesses in or compressing the hepatic vein as it leaves the liver, or obstructions in the caudal vena cava cranial to the entry of the hepatic vein, may also cause posthepatic obstruction.

When the liver is congested, there is increased flow of hepatic lymph, which has a high concentration of protein. The bulk of hepatic lymph comes from the space of Disse, which is separated from the sinusoidal lumen by fenestrated endothelium that is freely permeable to plasma constituents, including large protein molecules. Hence, the formation of hepatic lymph is not regulated by plasma oncotic pressure, but is sensitive to small changes in hydrostatic pressure in the sinusoids. This accounts for the frequency with which ascites is associated with diseases that cause increased central and hepatic venous pressure, or increased intrahepatic resistance to blood flow. If the capacity of the hepatic lymphatics is exceeded, then high-protein lymph oozes from the extensive lymphatic plexus along the hepatic capsule, and it may spill from efferent lymphatics passing from the porta hepatis to the cisterna chyli. In hepatic ascites these efferent lymphatics become very large, numerous, and thick walled.

The fluid that enters the peritoneal cavity is continually in flux. Gross ascites will only develop when the normal high capacity to drain fluid from the abdomen is exceeded by the rate of production, and this requires an increase in renal retention of sodium and water. The initiating factors causing excess of total body salt and water are uncertain, but contributing factors include increase of adrenal medullary hormones, increased sympathetic output leading to reduced natriuresis, and activation of the renin-angiotensin system. Renal factors, including reduced excretion of water and increased reabsorption of sodium, are important in perpetuating the condition. The resultant expansion of plasma volume permits the development of edema and ascites in congestive heart failure, and ascites in hepatic disease. It also further increases hydrostatic pressure in the hepatic sinusoids, driving lymph production to the point that ascites develops. Secondarily, reduced effective vascular volume, associated with sequestration of fluid in ascites, expansion of the splanchnic circulation, and other systemic circulatory events, also causes sodium retention via the renin-angiotensin pathway, with aldosterone secretion, and by parallel mechanisms. In heart failure, activation of the renin-angiotensin system is expected, because of reduced effective vascular volume.

Hypoproteinemia caused by reduced hepatic synthesis may occur in severe liver disease. Normally, oncotic forces are subsidiary to hydrostatic forces at the level of the sinusoid in affecting the formation of lymph. However, in diffuse fibrosis, once advanced capillarization of sinusoids occurs, the free permeability of the hepatic vascular system to the flow of large molecules is reduced. In this circumstance, reduced plasma oncotic pressure caused by hypoalbuminemia promotes continued hepatic lymph formation and ascites; it also promotes fluid flux to the peritoneum across the splanchnic capillary bed.

Hypoproteinemia of nonhepatic origin is most commonly associated with protein-losing enteropathy, such as Johne's disease in ruminants, or with protein-losing nephropathy, such as glomerular amyloidosis. Severe hypoproteinemia reduces plasma oncotic pressure, promoting edema and permitting transudate to accumulate in serous spaces, including the peritoneal cavity.

Vascular injury in the portal circulation allows increased permeability to plasma protein and substantially favors development of ascites. Mild ascites may occur in a variety of systemic illnesses altering vascular permeability, such as the clostridial intoxications, endotoxemia, acute uremic syndromes in ruminants and pigs, and in exudative diathesis of pigs with vitamin E deficiency.

Effusion of fluid into body cavities is part of the postmortem picture in sheep and cattle that die of *urethral obstruction*, and the fluid may have a distinct uriniferous odor. The pathogenesis of this fluid accumulation is uncertain. Although in a few cases there is a rupture of the lower urinary tract that might permit uroperitoneum, in many cases this cannot be demonstrated. Renal uremia, especially that caused by acute toxic nephrosis, also may be accompanied by significant effusions. It is usually the case with ascites of urinary tract disease that the mesenteries and retroperitoneum also become saturated.

Further reading

James FE, et al. Ascites due to pre-sinusoidal portal hypertension in dogs: a retrospective analysis of 17 cases. Aust Vet J 2008;86: 180-186.

Kriedet RT. Peritoneal physiology—impact on solute and fluid clearance. Adv Ren Replace Ther 2000;7:271-279.

Stafford JR, Bartges JW. A clinical review of pathophysiology, diagnosis, and treatment of uroabdomen in the dog and cat. J Vet Emerg Crit Care (San Antonio) 2013;23:216-229.

Uriz J, et al. Pathophysiology, diagnosis and treatment of ascites and cirrhosis. Bailleres Best Pract Clin Gastroenterol 2000;14:927-943.

Wright KN, et al. Peritoneal effusion in cats: 65 cases (1981-1997). J Am Vet Med Assoc 1999;214:375-381.

Abdominal fat necrosis

Necrosis of mesenteric or other abdominal or retroperitoneal fat occurs either as a consequence of pancreatitis in several species, or as a poorly understood condition affecting the abdominal fat predominantly of ruminants.

In **pancreatic necrosis,** enzymatic necrosis of peripancreatic adipose tissue is always seen, and may in fact be the initial morphologic change. In acute pancreatic necrosis, discrete foci or confluent masses of white necrotic adipose tissue are surrounded by a zone of intense hyperemia with fibrin deposited on the surface. Such lesions may be limited to the peripancreatic fat or be distributed throughout the abdominal cavity. Histologically, there is necrosis of adipocytes containing acidophilic, opaque, amorphous, or basophilic fibrillar to granular mineralized material. The necrosis is attributed to release of proteolytic and lipolytic enzymes from damaged pancreatic acini, and to degeneration of neutrophils recruited to the area.

Massive fat necrosis in cattle is reported most frequently in Channel Island breeds and occurs in older animals that may be excessively fat. The disease is characterized by the formation of multifocal masses of necrotic fat of various sizes that may coalesce to involve significant portions of the abdominal cavity. Although it is *often an incidental finding*, it can cause clinical signs and even death if there is compression or obstruction of abdominal viscera. Necrosis may occur in any portion of the omental, mesenteric, and retroperitoneal fat, and has been observed in intermuscular and subcutaneous fat. Initially there is acute inflammation, and the hard necrotic masses are surrounded by a zone of hyperemia; the overlying peritoneum may be necrotic, perhaps with adhesions to adjacent viscera. On cut section these nodular masses are firm, dry, and chalky, or sometimes moist, oily, and deep yellow. Because of the unusual bulk of the necrotic tissue in some cases, and because necrotic fat is sometimes found in abnormal locations, such as under the serosa of the intestine, the condition has been called

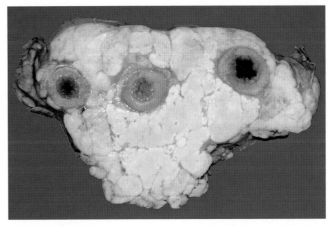

Figure 1-196 Mass of fat enclosing intestinal loops in **abdominal fat necrosis** in a cow.

lipomatosis, but the lesions are not considered to be hyperplastic or neoplastic. The hard lumps of fat may be confused with fetal structures, lymphoid tumors, or other masses on abdominal palpation. Clinical signs, although uncommon, are most often caused by *intestinal obstruction* (Fig. 1-196).

Histologically, the lesions are a mixture of acute and chronic fat necrosis with infiltration of many macrophages and multinucleated giant cells, as well as fewer neutrophils, lymphocytes, and plasma cells. There is variable fibrosis and mineralization. The pathogenesis remains unclear, although it has been linked to alterations in lipid metabolism; there may be a genetic component. Abdominal fat necrosis also is probably related to dietary factors, including ingestion of feeds high in long-chain saturated fatty acids. In several ruminant species, including cattle, sheep, goats, and deer, the condition also has been linked to grazing of endophyte-infested tall fescue pastures.

Massive necrosis of abdominal fat is reported infrequently *in cats*; some cases are subsequent to trauma or pancreatitis, whereas in other cases the cause was not determined. Nodular necrosis of abdominal fat can be an incidental finding in aged dogs and cats.

Steatitis (*yellow-fat disease*) occurs in many species affecting the abdominal and peritoneal fat, along with other adipose tissue. It is associated with diets high in polyunsaturated fat and low in tocopherols, favoring oxidation of fatty acids. Peroxidation of susceptible lipids and membranes creates free radicals that provoke the characteristic inflammatory reaction in response to formation of irritant soaps, cholesterol deposits and ceroid-lipofuscin (see section on Panniculitis in Vol. 1, Integumentary system).

Further reading

Schwarz T, et al. Nodular fat necrosis in the feline and canine abdomen. Vet Radiol Ultrasound 2000;41:335-339.

Tharwat M, Buczinski S. Diagnostic ultrasonography in cattle with abdominal fat necrosis. Can Vet J 2012;53:41-46.

Peritonitis

Inflammation of the serosa of the peritoneal lining, or **peritonitis,** is very common in large domestic animals, and less common in dogs and cats. *Peritonitis may be classified as* *primary or secondary; as acute or chronic; as local or diffuse; as septic or nonseptic; and on the basis of the type of exudate, which may be serofibrinous, fibrinopurulent, purulent, hemorrhagic, or granulomatous.* Differences in distribution, type of exudate, and duration of the lesion can be more or less anticipated from the source and the cause. Most cases of peritonitis in domestic animals are secondary; that is, they arise as complications of other events in the abdomen, but primary serositis in systemic infections is of much importance for agricultural livestock. *The causes of peritonitis are numerous and varied*, so only some of the more common and important of them are considered here.

Chemical peritonitis may be induced by a variety of agents. Intraperitoneal instillation of a number of therapeutic agents causes mild and usually inconsequential peritonitis; however, abdominal lavage has been associated with more severe serosal damage and formation of adhesions. Surgical glove powders, including *talc* or *starch*, provoke granulomatous peritonitis; starch granules have a characteristic Maltese cross appearance in polarized light, and are periodic acid-Schiff–positive. Accidental leakage of *barium sulfate* into the abdomen during contrast studies causes a potentially fatal hemorrhagic peritonitis that progresses over several days to severe granulomatous and fibrosing peritonitis. Leakage of barium is often concurrent with leakage of ingesta, and thus is frequently complicated by intercurrent sepsis.

The most devastating forms of chemical peritonitis are endogenous, and are caused by *bile and pancreatic enzymes.* **Bile peritonitis** is associated with endothelial dysfunction and increased production of proinflammatory cytokines. Bile peritonitis is readily recognized by the typical yellow-green staining of visceral and parietal peritoneal surfaces; the lesions can be intense, and, especially if complicated by sepsis, can be fatal. **Peritonitis associated with pancreatic necrosis** is also common in dogs. The reaction within and adjacent to the pancreas is characterized by acute necrosis and neutrophilic inflammation; there is often adhesion of the lesser omentum to the pancreas, adjacent liver, and other organs. This local peritoneal reaction resolves completely if the animal survives, and only very minor adhesions or slight puckering of the mesentery persist with fibrosis in the pancreas. The peritoneal exudate of mostly neutrophils may be scant, but contains droplets of fats and soaps released from the adipose tissue by the pancreatic enzymes. Rarely, acute accumulation of chyle in the peritoneum occurs secondary to acute pancreatitis, and this causes a peritoneal reaction referred to as **chylous peritonitis.**

Bacterial peritonitis may occur if bacteria reach the peritoneum by direct implantation after perforation of a contaminated external surface. It most commonly originates with peritoneal contamination by ingesta from a perforation or rupture of the gastrointestinal tract; however, bacteria also can be introduced from the skin or in females via the reproductive tract. Endometritis caused by tuberculosis or brucellosis in cows, and brucellosis in sows, may extend to the peritoneum through the uterine tubes. Cystitis and rupture of the urinary bladder may also cause peritonitis. Bacterial peritonitis is also common as an extension from a localized inflammatory reaction in an abdominal viscus or the umbilicus, or as a component of bacteremia or septicemia. For example, acute serofibrinous peritonitis may occur by extension through the wall of an intestine with localized necrosis, or from a uterus just before rupture. Secondary peritonitis occasionally results by extension from retroperitoneal infection, or in ruminants from omental bursitis. When peritonitis develops by direct extension, there is little difficulty in ascertaining its origin, even when the process becomes diffuse.

Consequences of peritonitis

The consequences of peritonitis vary widely from insignificant to catastrophic. Acute generalized peritonitis is a catastrophic sequel of many local diseases of the abdominal cavity, but it may be a relatively insignificant secondary event in generalized infections. Obviously peritonitis does not significantly affect the outcome of *Escherichia coli* septicemia or of clostridial infections such as blackleg or braxy. Within the first few hours of generalized peritonitis, there may be intestinal hypermotility; however, *paralytic ileus*, mediated by autonomic innervation, soon supervenes. Initially ileus may be beneficial as exudates are no longer further distributed by intestinal movement, but development of fibrinous adhesions between loops of intestine can be significant and eventually produce fibrous adhesions and their sequelae.

The systemic effects of generalized peritonitis are largely related to detrimental effects on cardiovascular function, circulatory homeostasis, and acid-base balance. These are partly the result of sequestration of fluid and plasma proteins in the peritoneal exudate; sequestration of fluid and electrolyte in immotile intestinal tract; and loss of intestinal absorptive function. Endotoxin and exotoxins, such as those produced by clostridia, may be absorbed into the circulation, directly through the peritoneum or via the lymphatic drainage, causing increased vascular permeability, shock, and other detrimental cardiovascular effects. Death from toxemia may result before overt peritonitis develops. Bacteria may spread via the lymphatics to the pleura and the sternal or mediastinal nodes, or may reach the general circulation, causing septicemia.

Not all cases of generalized peritonitis are immediately fatal. Depending on the nature, distribution, and severity of the exudate, the lesions may resolve completely, mature into fibrous adhesions, or persist in some localized areas as chronic active peritonitis or abscessation. In uncomplicated situations, peritoneal lesions are debrided by phagocytes; fibroplasia neovascularization and collagen deposition occur within days, and mesothelial restoration is accomplished by 5-8 days after the insult. Because the mesothelium differentiates from mesenchymal elements in the subserosa or from free-floating peritoneal stem cells, reconstitution of the mesothelium is not affected by the size of the defect.

Damage to, or loss of the peritoneal lining may diminish the fibrinolytic activity of mesothelium. Fibrin between damaged serosal surfaces persisting beyond 3-4 days after the original insult becomes progressively organized and mature, resulting in formation of **fibrous adhesions.** Downstream effects vary depending on the location of adhesions, but there may be persistent adhesion of adjacent structures, or stenosis or compression of abdominal viscera resulting in impaired motility, obstruction, or circulatory embarrassment. Fibrous adhesions may remodel and occasionally separate, but often persist as scars on the serosa.

Formation of adhesions seems to be promoted by ischemia, increasing severity of tissue necrosis, foreign material such as sutures on the serosa, and by sepsis; all of these increase and prolong the inflammatory response. Determining the duration of peritonitis may be important in cases such as iatrogenic rectal perforation, and its assessment requires careful gross and microscopic examination of the serosal surface and the adherent exudates. The proliferation and degree of differentiation of fibroblasts and mesothelial cells within and along the margins of any wound will give some indication of the age of the lesion. The thickness of granulation tissue over the old serosa may give an indication of the duration of chronic peritonitis.

Further reading

Dayer T, et al. Septic peritonitis from pyloric and non-pyloric gastrointestinal perforation: prognostic factors in 44 dogs and 11 cats. J Small Anim Pract 2013;54:625-629.

Ko JJ, Mann FA. Barium peritonitis in small animals. J Vet Med Sci 2014;76:621-628.

Tubby KG. Concurrent gall bladder, liver lobe torsion, and bile peritonitis in a German shepherd dog 2 months after gastric dilatation/volvulus gastropexy and splenectomy. Can Vet J 2013;54:784-786.

Wright KN, et al. Peritoneal effusion in cats: 65 cases (1981-1987). J Am Vet Med Assoc 1998;214:375-381.

Peritonitis in horses

Diffuse peritonitis in horses is usually acute and fatal; this is perhaps associated in part with a small omentum, and a poor capacity to heal contaminated areas. In most cases the cause is rupture or perforation of the stomach or intestine with spillage of ingesta into the abdominal cavity. Purulent peritonitis and mesenteric lymphadenitis may be seen in *Rhodococcus equi* infection of foals. Intestinal infection of foals by *Actinobacillus equuli* causes fibrinous mesenteric lymphangitis and peritonitis. *Clostridium perfringens* in foals, and anthrax in older horses, causes acute hemorrhagic enteritis with peritonitis. Peritoneal lavage may cause severe diffuse chemical peritonitis. Seminoperitoneum caused by laceration of the vagina at breeding is an unusual cause of acute diffuse nonseptic peritonitis; sperm are present in the cytoplasm of neutrophils.

Chronic diffuse peritonitis is virtually never recorded in horses, other than rare nocardiosis. Acute or chronic local peritonitis does occasionally occur after castration, and the colon may adhere to the inner inguinal area; from penetrating wounds originating from the skin; and from streptococcal abscesses in the mesentery. It may be secondary to local verminous lesions such as from suppurative gastritis in habronemiasis, or from gastrointestinal perforation associated with *Gasterophilus* or *Anoplocephala* infestation. Migrating *Strongylus equinus* or *S. edentatus* larvae are thought to cause retroperitoneal lesions in the flank, perirenal fat, and diaphragm; fibrous tags on the liver capsule; and chronic diffuse thickening and inflammation in the mesentery, omentum, and hepatorenal ligament. Large strongyles returning to the gut may cause focal peritoneal lesions on the ileum, cecum, and colon, and migration of large strongyles in the wall of the small intestine is thought to be a cause of hemomelasma ilei.

Further reading

Henderson ISF, et al. Study of the short and long-term outcomes of 65 horses with peritonitis. Vet Rec 2008;163:293-297.

Matthews S, et al. Peritonitis associated with *Actinobacillus equuli* in horses: 51 cases. Aust Vet J 2001;79:536-539.

Nógrádi N, et al. Peritonitis in horses: 55 cases (2004-2007). Acta Vet Hung 2011;59:181-193.

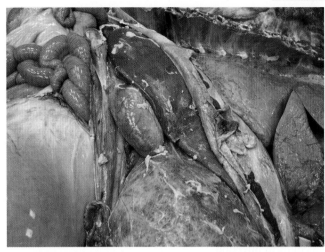

Figure 1-197 Acute diffuse fibrinous peritonitis in a cow.

Peritonitis in cattle

Acute diffuse fibrinopurulent peritonitis is common in cattle, and is usually the result of perforation of a viscus, including the gastrointestinal or reproductive tracts. Perforation initially results in local acute disease, which is typically followed by diffuse chronic peritonitis with adhesions. Diffuse fibrinous **traumatic reticuloperitonitis** (hardware disease) may evolve to include septic **reticulopericarditis** if the offending foreign body migrates as far as the pericardial sac (Fig. 1-197). Disordered motility of the forestomachs, manifest clinically as vagus indigestion, may follow scarring that interferes with esophageal function.

Cattle seem to have a relatively high capacity to localize and wall off septic foci within the peritoneal cavity, and abscesses frequently develop from such foci. Sometimes these may become quite large; mixed bacterial flora is most commonly isolated. Perforation of the abomasum or intestine is more likely to cause diffuse fibrinous or fibrinohemorrhagic peritonitis, but occasionally causes local chronic peritonitis and abscessation.

In neonates, extension of infection from the umbilicus produces fibrinopurulent peritonitis, which tends to be most severe along the ventral abdominal wall, adjacent to associated liver abscesses, or extending along the urachus to the bladder. Fibrinous peritonitis may be an expression of *polyserositis* in neonatal calves with septicemic colibacillosis and neonatal streptococcal infection. Copious serofibrinous peritonitis (with similar lesions on other serous membranes) is typical of sporadic bovine encephalomyelitis. Diffuse fibrinohemorrhagic peritonitis occurs in most cases of clostridial hemoglobinuria, and in some cases of blackleg and septicemic pasteurellosis; a more localized peritonitis of this type occurs in clostridial enteritis of calves caused by *C. perfringens* type B and type C and in braxy.

Tuberculosis, actinobacillosis, and infection with green algae are rarely reported causes of inflammatory lesions in the peritoneum of cattle.

Further reading

Braun U, et al. An unusual cause of traumatic reticulitis/reticuloperitonitis in a herd of Swiss dairy cows nearby an airport. Schweiz Arch Tierheilkd 2009;151:127-131.

Herzog K, et al. Post surgical development of inflammatory adhesions and reticular function in cows suffering from traumatic reticuloperitonitis. Dtsch Tierarztl Wochenschr 2004;111:57-62.

Watts AS, Tulley WJ. Case report: sequelae of traumatic reticuloperitonitis in a Friesian dairy cow. N Z Vet J 2013;61:111-114.

Peritonitis in sheep and goats

Peritonitis of specific cause is uncommon in **sheep**. A local inflammatory reaction accompanies penetration of the intestine by the larvae of *Oesophagostomum columbianum*. Rare cases of peritonitis in sheep with caseous lymphadenitis are described, caused by rupture of caseous lesions in internal organs. The postpartum uterus is probably the most common site in adults from which infection spreads to the peritoneum. Outbreaks of peritonitis in lamb flocks are frequently ascribed to coliform infection.

Mycoplasma mycoides may cause acute fibrinous peritonitis in **goats,** although acute death from septicemia, or arthritis and mastitis are more common. Paratuberculosis caused by *Mycobacterium avium* subspecies *paratuberculosis* frequently produces nodular granulomatous lymphangitis in the mesentery and sometimes caseous or mineralized lymphadenitis.

Further reading

Dennis MM, et al. An outbreak of granulomatous peritonitis caused by injectable selenium in a flock of Merino sheep. Aust Vet J 2011;89:209-212.

Perrin J, et al. Infection with *Mycoplasma mycoides* ssp. *mycoides* LC (large colony type) in bezoar goat kids (*Capra aegagrus cretica*) in the Bern (Switzerland) Zoo. Schweiz Arch Tierheilkd 1994;136: 270-274.

Peritonitis in swine

A few filmy strands of mucin with appearances of fibrin frequently overlie the intestine, mesentery, and liver in many acute infectious diseases of swine, and in conditions that result in vascular damage, such as edema disease and vitamin E/selenium-responsive conditions; this does not qualify as peritonitis (Fig. 1-198). However, peritonitis is well recognized as part of the pathologic picture in several defined infectious syndromes in pigs.

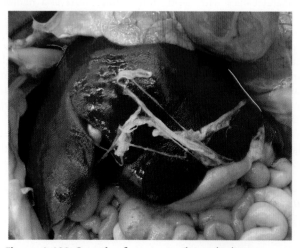

Figure 1-198 Strands of mucin overlying the liver in a pig.

Diffuse fibrinopurulent peritonitis is common in pigs. Acute diffuse serofibrinous peritonitis with fibrinous arthritis and meningitis is characteristic of Glasser's disease, caused by *Haemophilus parasuis*. In chronic infections pigs have reduced growth rate because of severe polyserositis and arthritis. Similar clinical signs and lesions also can be associated with a number of other septicemic bacterial infections, especially *Streptococcus suis* and *Mycoplasma hyorhinis*. Small firm nodules and flattened disks of inspissated fibrin are often found free in the peritoneal cavity in chronic *Mycoplasma* infections. Further diagnostic testing using bacteriology or molecular methods often is required to differentiate these diseases.

A variety of other bacterial organisms can be isolated from cases of peritonitis in pigs, including *Trueperella pyogenes, Escherichia coli*, or several organisms simultaneously. In some cases the cause can be traced to castration or other wounds. Peritonitis may be localized to the inguinal and pelvic regions, or the intestines may be so adhered together with fibrin that they cannot be separated. Occasionally, *T. pyogenes* produces multifocal discrete abscesses on both visceral and parietal peritoneum.

Tuberculosis in swine may cause lymphadenitis or peritonitis and induce adhesions in the peritoneum. In cases of rectal stricture there is marked dilation of the colon and cecum and the serosa may be covered with fibrin tags, similar to that of infectious serositis. Peritonitis also can occur in pigs with perforating gastric ulcers, but many pigs die from acute gastric hemorrhage before perforation.

Stephanurus dentatus larvae cause subserosal focal hepatitis and a mild reaction with edema in the perirenal fat and retroperitoneal tissue, and sometimes in the mesentery and local lymph nodes, as they migrate to the kidney.

Further reading

Kang I, et al. Optimized protocol for multiplex nested polymerase chain reaction to detect and differentiate *Haemophilus parasuis, Streptococcus suis,* and *Mycoplasma hyorhinis* in formalin-fixed, paraffin-embedded tissues from pigs with polyserositis. Can J Vet Res 2012;76:195-200.

Zhang B, et al. Update on the pathogenesis of *Haemophilus parasuis* infection and virulence factors. Vet Microbiol 2014;168:1-7.

Peritonitis in dogs

Septic peritonitis is an inflammatory lesion of the peritoneum that occurs secondary to microbial contamination in a variety of scenarios, including perforation of the gastrointestinal tract, reproductive tract, urinary bladder or other viscera, or bacteremia. Microorganisms associated with septic peritonitis are varied and typically reflect the source of contamination.

Mild *fibrinohemorrhagic peritonitis and serositis* associated with canine parvoviral enteritis, infectious canine hepatitis, and toxoplasmosis can be easily overlooked. There may be edema of the intestinal subserosa and frequent petechiae or larger hemorrhages in these cases.

Suppurative peritonitis is uncommon in dogs; it has been observed in puppies as an extension from umbilical and hepatic streptococcal abscesses. Septic peritonitis involving a variety of agents, including *E. coli* and anaerobes, may follow surgical contamination of the abdomen; a penetrating wound or perforation of the gut; rupture of the urinary bladder; or rupture of pancreatic, hepatic, or prostatic abscesses. Peritonitis also occurs when the uterus ruptures, either as a result of pyometra or septic metritis with fetal putrefaction.

A distinctive pyogranulomatous peritonitis occurs in dogs and cats. Actinomyces spp., most commonly *A. viscosus*, or bacteria of the *Nocardia asteroides* complex, are mainly responsible for the lesions that include copious red-brown exudate. The exudate often contains small yellow sulfur granules free in the exudate or within granulomas adhered to serosal surfaces, including omentum, mesenteries, and mesenteric lymph nodes. The color is from blood derived from proliferation of thin-walled capillaries on serous surfaces that are thickened, red, and edematous.

Chronic pyogranulomatous or granulomatous peritonitis occurs in the rare cases of eumycotic mycetoma and zygomycosis that involve the abdominal cavity. There is usually serosal thickening and fibrosis of affected segments of gut, with formation of adhesions, and the development of firm granulomatous masses on the gut wall, in the mesenteries and omentum. *Mycobacterium microti* (llama-type), the vole bacillus, has been reported as a rare cause of severe diffuse granulomatous peritonitis.

Sclerosing encapsulating peritonitis, a characteristic pathologic syndrome, occurs rarely in the dog. A thick layer of progressively maturing granulation tissue lines parts or all of the abdominal cavity and abdominal visceral organs, which effectively produces one or more thick-walled cystic spaces enclosing some or most of the abdominal cavity and its organs. Within the space is a large volume of clear or serosanguineous fluid, with strands of variably organized fibrin. Involved organs are often atrophic or misshapen because of the thick fibrous capsule on their surface.

Body cavity parasitism by larval stages of some tapeworms, including *Mesocestoides* and *Spirometra*, causes proliferative to granulomatous peritonitis with cysts containing cestode larvae, and occurs mostly in dogs who act as intermediate hosts for these parasites (see later section on Parasitic diseases of the peritoneum).

Further reading

Dayer T, et al. Septic peritonitis from pyloric and non-pyloric gastrointestinal perforation: prognostic factors in 44 dogs and 11 cats. J Small Anim Pract 2013;54:625-629.

Patten PK, et al. Cestode infection in 2 dogs: cytologic findings in liver and a mesenteric lymph node. Vet Clin Pathol 2013;42:103-108.

Ragetly GR, et al. Septic peritonitis: etiology, pathophysiology, and diagnosis. Compend Contin Educ Vet 2011;33:E1-E6.

Peritonitis in cats

Peritonitis occurs when the uterus ruptures because of pyometra or fetal putrefaction. Peritonitis also occurs from penetrating wounds or by extension from retroperitoneal tissues, and occasionally septic peritonitis is caused by anaerobes such as those associated with cat-bite abscesses. Actinomycotic peritonitis similar in appearance to the disease in dogs may complicate feline leukemia virus infection in cats and the other myeloproliferative diseases.

Feline infectious peritonitis. The genus *Alphacoronavirus*, family *Coronaviridae*, includes species *Feline coronavirus* (FCoV), and its two biological pathotypes, feline infectious peritonitis virus (FIPV) and feline enteric coronavirus (FECV). FCoVs can also be divided into two antigenically distinct serotypes (I and II) based on cell culture cytopathic effect and other features; both FIPV and FECV strains are represented among FCoV types I and II, though type I FCoV induce higher antibody titers and are more frequently associated with FIP than type II FCoV. In domestic and wild felids, the various FCoV strains have a spectrum of virulence, from asymptomatic enteric infection and healthy lifelong carrier status, through symptomatic enteric infection (see the section on enteric coronaviral infections) to virulent systemic infection, which is expressed as FIP.

FCoVs are ubiquitous in cats, but the disease FIP is sporadic with a low prevalence that *predominantly affects young, intact male cats.* Purebred cats appear to be more susceptible to FCoV. FECV is transmitted by the fecal-oral route, and the virus initially infects enterocytes but soon becomes restricted to cecum and colon. Some cats become persistently infected and although they remain clinically healthy, continue to shed virus in their feces. FECV is generally regarded as the avirulent pathotype of FCoV, although some cats may develop catarrhal to hemorrhagic enteritis. Enteric infection with FCoV may produce mild, subclinical blunting and fusion of villi.

FIPV was initially thought to have evolved as a deletion mutation of FECV; however, analysis of the viruses has revealed a much more complex picture of several genes and proteins involved in mediating virulence. There is strong evidence that FIPV is not transmitted horizontally, but emerges within each cat that eventually develops FIP. A requirement for development of FIP is likely the capacity of the virus to replicate within monocytes of the host. In comparison to FECV, FIPV strains have less tropism for the gut. *FIPV replicates in macrophages,* and it is thought that macrophages from the intestine acquire virus from the intestinal epithelium and carry it to regional lymph nodes and disseminate the virus to many parts of the body; this is central to their virulence. It has been proposed that mutation and transformation of FECV to FIPV can also take place within these macrophages; however, this has not been definitively demonstrated. Incidence of the disease is apparently not higher in cats infected with feline leukemia virus or feline immunodeficiency virus; however, FCoV replicates 10-100 fold more in macrophages of cats infected with FIV, thus enhancing the probability of spontaneous mutations.

Resistance to FIPV infection is cell mediated, and systemic clinical disease probably only occurs if the cell-mediated response is ineffective; the lack of cell-mediated immunity may allow viral persistence or more pronounced virus production within macrophages. The cytokine response appears to be important in the response to FIPV infection, and immunity against FIPV may be associated with low tumor necrosis factor-α/high interferon-γ responses, whereas high tumor necrosis factor-α/low interferon-γ responses favor disease. There is also evidence that type III and type IV immune reactions play a role in vasculitis and CD4+ cell-heavy granulomatous inflammation of FIPV-infected cats, respectively. Cats that recover from FIP have humoral immune responses and immune complexes that are demonstrable in blood, but although clearance of virus occurs, persistence and fecal shedding may extend for several months.

Cats that do not clear FIPV develop either the dry or wet clinical forms of the disease depending on whether ineffective cell-mediated or humoral immunity dominates the clinical

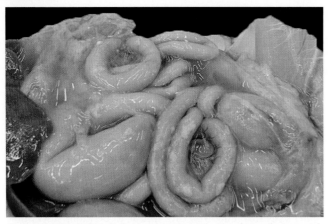

Figure 1-199 Feline infectious peritonitis. Exudative lesion with fibrin on mesentery and viscera, and granulomas in most viscera. (Courtesy M. Yaeger.)

disease. Although often described as distinct entities, *the effusive (wet) and noneffusive (dry) forms of FIP are the extremes of a continuum of syndromes, with* **vasculitis** *and* **pyogranulomatous inflammation** *as the hallmarks.* Effusive disease is more common than the noneffusive form, and mixed forms are probably common.

Cats with the effusive form of FIP often develop severe abdominal distention. Pleural effusion is present in ~25% of cases and may cause dyspnea. Cardiac tamponade caused by pericardial effusion is rare. Ocular and central nervous signs are rare in this form. Up to 1 liter of abdominal exudate may be present in cats with effusive FIP. The fluid is usually viscous, clear, and pale to deep yellow, although it may be flocculent and contain strands of fibrin. The serosal surfaces may be covered with fibrin, giving them a granular appearance; fragile adhesions may be present between viscera. There are foci of necrosis, raised plaques, or nodular cellular infiltrations that vary in size from a few millimeters to a centimeter in diameter on the serosa that extend into the parenchyma of organs. The mesentery is often thickened and opaque; the omentum may be contracted into a mass in the cranial abdomen, and adherent to itself and other abdominal surfaces (Fig. 1-199). Fibrin is usually less prominent in the thoracic cavity, but firm white nodules may be present under the pleura, and the lungs may be dark and rubbery. Abdominal and thoracic lymph nodes may be enlarged. Some cats with FIP are lame because of generalized synovitis caused by migration of macrophages into the synovium. The cats are hypergammaglobulinemic and may have leukocytosis and neutrophilia. The clinical course for effusive FIP is rapid; most cats die within a few weeks and very few recover after passing through a phase of noneffusive disease.

Cats with noneffusive FIP have a chronic disease of insidious onset and frequently develop signs specific to organs severely affected by vascular lesions. These may include ocular disease; central nervous disorders such as ataxia, paraparesis, head tilt; specific nerve palsies, nystagmus, and behavioral changes; renal failure; hepatic or pancreatic insufficiency; and diarrhea caused by ulcerative colitis.

Peritonitis is present in most animals, although marked effusion is not found in those with the noneffusive form of FIP. In cats with *noneffusive FIP*, there may be inflammatory foci in the abdominal or thoracic organs as described previously, or lesions may be restricted to the eyes and nervous system. Diffuse uveitis, chorioretinitis, and sometimes pan-ophthalmitis are present; fibrin is often present in the anterior chamber. Lesions in the central nervous system can involve the leptomeninges, spinal cord, or brain, but usually are subtle grossly and easily overlooked. Occasionally, hydrocephalus, hydromyelia, and syringomyelia may result from ependymitis and obstruction of cerebrospinal fluid flow. The kidneys may be enlarged and nodular with multifocal random variably sized white firm nodules protruding from the cortex. Hepatitis and pancreatitis of variable degree also may be present, characterized by small, white foci of inflammation. The tunica vaginalis may be affected, resulting in periorchitis in intact males. In the intestine, there may be marked thickening of the cecum and colon by nodular, firm, white inflammatory exudate extending through the wall of the affected gut; there is often adhesion to the adjacent enlarged lymph nodes.

The characteristic microscopic lesion is generalized vasculitis and perivasculitis, especially of small to medium-sized venules of the leptomeninges, renal cortex, eyes, and less frequently the lungs and liver. Macrophages predominate and probably mediate lesion development; however, variable numbers of neutrophils, lymphocytes, and plasma cells also accumulate in and around affected veins. The endothelium swells, and medial vascular necrosis may be evident in some cases; narrowed vascular lumina may predispose to thrombosis and infarction in these cats. The proportion of neutrophils in the reaction varies, and some lesions may be comprised mainly of a mixture of macrophages and lymphoid cells. Fibroplasia is variable; occasionally, adventitial fibrosis occurs with little cellular infiltrate. The vascular lesion results in the serofibrinous and cellular exudate on the serosal surfaces, and the nodules visible on the surfaces and deeper in solid organs.

The microscopic changes in the *omentum, mesentery,* and *serosal tissues* vary in severity. Mild changes include proliferation of mesothelial cells, fibrin accumulation, fibroblast proliferation, and scattered neutrophils and mononuclear cells. Severe changes include dense fibrin accumulation on serosal surfaces, with necrosis and/or mesothelial hyperplasia. Large numbers of neutrophils, mononuclear cells, and necrotic debris may be embedded in the fibrin. Vasculitis may extend from the serosa into the intestine, affecting the muscularis, myenteric ganglia, the submucosa, and the mucosa, which may be segmentally infarcted.

Lesions in various organs, including kidney, liver, lung, and pancreas, are largely caused by the vascular damage that occurs because of inflammatory cellular infiltrates in the capsule and stromal connective tissue. Severe multifocal lymphoplasmacytic interstitial nephritis may develop; in addition to focal lung lesions, there may be diffuse interstitial pneumonia, sometimes most severe close to the visceral pleura. Degenerative and necrotic lesions in the parenchyma of the central nervous system, including the meninges, choroid plexus, and ependyma, also appear to be related to vasculitis. The ependyma may be visibly roughened and develop reactive syncytia of lining cells. Ocular lesions are common, but usually subclinical (see Vol. 1, Special senses). *Effusive FIP must be differentiated from bacterial peritonitis. Noneffusive forms may appear grossly similar to lymphosarcoma, steatitis, mycotic infections, and toxoplasmosis.* With thorough postmortem examination, the constellation of lesions is usually sufficiently distinctive to allow a gross diagnosis with a high degree of accuracy.

Serologic tests such as enzyme-linked immunosorbent assay or immunofluorescence may be useful in supporting a diagnosis of FIP or managing the disease in cat populations; however, histopathology with identification of viral antigen in lesions using immunohistochemistry or real-time RT-PCR remains the most conclusive means of diagnosis of FIP.

Further reading

Benetka V, et al. Prevalence of feline coronavirus types I and II in cats with histopathologically verified feline infectious peritonitis. Vet Microbiol 2004;99:31-42.

Kipar A, et al. Feline infectious peritonitis, still an enigma? Vet Pathol 2014;51:505-526.

Malik R, et al. *Nocardia* infections in cats: a retrospective multi-institutional study of 17 cases. Aust Vet J 2006;84:235-245.

Pedersen NC. An update on feline infectious peritonitis: Diagnostics and therapeutics. Vet J 2014;pii:S1090-0233(14)00177-4.

Pedersen NC. An update on feline infectious peritonitis: virology and immunopathogenesis. Vet J 2014;pii:S1090-0233(14)00178-6.

Parasitic diseases of the peritoneum

Most parasites found in the peritoneal cavity are in the normal course of migration to another site, or as an accident. Only a few larval and adult helminths use the abdominal cavity as their normal habitat.

Cysticerci (*Cysticercus tenuicollis* in ruminants; *C. pisiformis* in lagomorphs) may be found on the peritoneum during their normal development; they are nonpathogenic, and excite virtually no tissue response beyond their thin bland fibrous capsule. Rarely, cysticerci have been encountered in the abdomen of carnivores, which are abnormal hosts. **Spargana**, elongate larval forms of *Spirometra* spp., may encyst in a bland fibrous capsule in the peritoneal cavity of carnivores and swine. **Tetrathyridia**, the larvae of the tapeworm *Mesocestoides*, may proliferate extensively in the abdominal cavity of carnivores, where they cause a characteristic pyogranulomatous and proliferative peritonitis known as parasitic ascites.

Fasciola hepatica larvae can cause acute and chronic peritonitis in cattle and sheep; inflammation involves the parietal peritoneum and sometimes the visceral peritoneum, especially that of liver, spleen, and omentum. The lesions may consist of many fibrin tags, or more diffuse thickening of the peritoneum; young flukes may be found in the inflammatory lesions both on and beneath the peritoneum.

Dioctophyma renale seems to be better adapted to dogs compared with cats. In most cases in dogs, worms are located in the kidney; however, they have been observed in the abdominal cavity, suggesting that they did not complete their normal migration pathway from the small intestine to the kidney. Migration of the worm or its ova may initiate chronic perihepatitis or peritonitis.

Stephanurus dentatus, in the course of its migrations through the liver and peritoneal cavity to the kidneys in pigs, may cause local hemorrhage, peritonitis, and perihepatitis. *Strongylus edentatus* and *S. equinus* normally migrate through the liver, as well as the ligaments and lumen of the peritoneal cavity. Fibrous tags on the liver, particularly the diaphragmatic aspect, are thought to be sequelae of *S. edentatus* migration. The larvae of both species may be found in the retroperitoneal tissues of the dorsal abdomen in horses, and in the mesenteries and omentum, where they may incite eosinophilic inflammatory response.

Ascarids of all species may occasionally cause obstruction and rupture of the small intestine or bile duct, such that they may be found in the abdomen as a terminal event.

Some parasites use the peritoneal cavity as their final habitat. *Setaria* spp. are onchocercid filarioid nematodes that inhabit the peritoneal cavity of many wild and domestic ungulates, including horses, cattle, sheep, goats, and swine. They are commonly found during postmortem examination or during surgery of cattle and horses in endemic areas. Some species of *Setaria* have a cosmopolitan distribution and may be found in several species of wild and domestic ungulates (*S. equina* in equids; *S. labiatopapillosa* in cattle, buffalo, and perhaps deer and antelope), whereas others are restricted geographically (*S. digitata*, Asia; *S. marshalli*, Asia) perhaps by the distribution of intermediate hosts.

Adult *Setaria* do not usually cause significant peritoneal lesions in their normal host. There are rare reports of occlusion of the uterine tube by *S. labiatopapillosa* in cattle. Adult *S. labiatopapillosa* in the peritoneal cavity, or in the tunica vaginalis around the testis, may incite granulomatous peritonitis or periorchitis if they die; remnants of the dead nematode may be detected in sections of the granulomatous reaction. Adult *S. digitata* rarely may be found in abnormal locations, such as the heart, lungs, and mesenteric lymph nodes, where they incite eosinophilic granulomatous inflammation. The larval form of *S. digitata* can produce mild peritonitis and granulomas in the retroperitoneum and bladder of cattle. The larvae of *S. equina*, *S. digitata*, and perhaps others that normally spend part of their time in the central nervous system, may occasionally penetrate the neural parenchyma and cause lesions. The sheathed microfilariae deposited by adult females in the peritoneal cavity are found in the blood. The intermediate host may be a mosquito, or for some *Setaria* spp., biting flies (*Haematobia* and *Stomoxys* spp). The microfilariae develop into infective larvae in 2-3 weeks. They are released from the feeding arthropod and enter the final host.

Setaria digitata is normally found as an adult in the peritoneal cavity of cattle and buffalo in Asia, but its larvae can cause *cerebrospinal nematodiasis* in aberrant hosts (see Vol. 1, Nervous system). *Setaria* species that may occur normally in cervids have been reported to cause central nervous system lesions in deer; however, *Elaphostrongylus* larvae produce similar signs and lesions, and differentiation may be difficult.

S. digitata larvae may invade the eye of horses, via the optic nerve to cause endo-ophthalmitis, as do the microfilariae of *S. equina*.

Further reading

Mohanty MC, et al. *Setaria digitata* infections in cattle: parasite load, microfilaraemia status and relationship to immune response. J Helminthol 2000;74:343-347.

Nakagawa TL, et al. Giant kidney worm (*Dioctophyma renale*) infections in dogs from Northern Parana, Brazil. Vet Parasitol 2007; 145:366-370.

Patten PK, et al. Cestode infection in 2 dogs: cytologic findings in liver and a mesenteric lymph node. Vet Clin Pathol 2013;42:103-108.

Tung KC, et al. Cerebrospinal setariosis with *Setaria marshalli* and *Setaria digitata* infection in cattle. J Vet Med Sci 2003;65: 977-983.

Miscellaneous lesions of the peritoneum

Cysts of the peritoneum are rather common but insignificant. Those associated with genital adnexa are described with those systems. Cysticerci were previously discussed; *Echinococcus granulosus* may develop cysts on the peritoneum following the rupture of a mature hydatid into the abdomen. Multiple small fluid-filled cysts are occasionally observed in the omentum; these inconsequential lesions are inclusion cysts or sites of localized lymphatic ectasia.

The normal squamous mesothelial cells of the serosa may undergo **metaplasia** to a cuboidal or columnar epithelium. Such metaplasia is probably the mildest response of the peritoneum to irritation but also may be a response to estrogen. Inflammatory metaplasia leading to ossification may occur in peritoneal scars, especially in swine. It also may be found in the mesenteries and the dorsal retroperitoneum without obvious cause, although ossification may occur following fat necrosis as well. Ossified areas are discoid, of variable size and shape, and are usually found in adipose tissue.

Neoplastic diseases of the peritoneum

Primary tumors of the peritoneum may arise from the serosa itself, from the subserous connective tissues, and from various differentiated tissues such as nerve sheaths. Tumors arising from the serosa are called **mesotheliomas**. The qualification term malignant is applied to mesothelioma; however, this term is without meaning because virtually all mesotheliomas can readily spread by implantation and less commonly by metastasis.

Mesotheliomas are rare. They occur with greatest frequency in cattle and dogs but are occasionally reported in horses, cats, pigs, and other species. Interest in mesotheliomas has increased following the discovery of the association between asbestos fiber and mesothelioma in humans. This association has not been confirmed in animals, although ferruginous bodies, which are suggestive of asbestos exposure, have been found in the lungs of some urban dogs with mesothelioma, and an association has been made between mesothelioma in dogs and exposure of owners to asbestos. *Many fiber types other than asbestos are capable of causing mesotheliomas, and this ability seems to be related mostly to fiber size and solubility.* In domestic animals, mesothelioma is notable because it occurs most frequently as a *congenital neoplasm* in fetal or young cattle.

Mesotheliomas arise from the cells of the serous linings of pericardial, pleural, and peritoneal cavities, and they may involve all 3 locations simultaneously. They are typically pleural in pigs. They usually appear as *multiple firm sessile or pedunculated nodules, from* a few millimeters to 6-10 cm in diameter (Fig. 1-200); *as villus projections* on a thickened mesentery or serosal surface; or as plaque-like *fibrous or sclerosing forms.* In sclerosing tumors in which adhesions more often occur, mesothelioma might resemble chronic granulomatous peritonitis. The tumor is frequently associated with ascites or a milky to blood-tinged effusion as the result of blocked lymphatics.

Mesotheliomas of the pleura, pericardium, or peritoneum may assume a variety of histologic patterns. They appear as *papillary arrangements of epithelial cells* resembling carcinoma, as *spindle cells* resembling fibrosarcoma, or most commonly as biphasic in pattern. The epithelial form is composed of single layers of dark plump cuboidal, columnar, or rounded, epithelioid cells with a distinct border and abundant pink cytoplasm

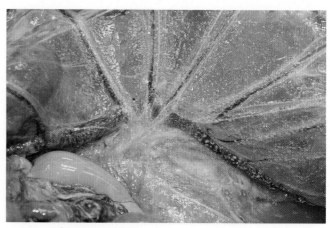

Figure 1-200 Mesothelioma in a horse. Multiple tumor nodules in the mesentery.

supported by thin fibrovascular stroma. Mitotic figures are typically not numerous. Some tumors have atypical cells with marked anisokaryosis and prominent nucleoli, or large multinucleated cells. Mesothelial cells form clusters and whorls, or they line cystic spaces forming tubular structures with mucinous matrix. Mesotheliomas resembling carcinoma can mimic implantation and metastasis via subserosal lymphatics so completely that adequate differentiation from a true carcinoma may rest on very careful examination for, and exclusion of, a primary malignant neoplasm. *Mesothelioma must be differentiated from activated or hyperplastic mesothelium,* which can be extremely challenging. No single feature can be used reliably to distinguish between hyperplastic and neoplastic mesothelium. Histochemistry and immunohistochemistry have not been particularly successful in uniquely identifying malignant mesothelial cells in domestic animals.

Lipomas are the most frequently encountered tumors of the peritoneal interstitium. These benign tumors are well known in horses, in which they usually originate in the mesenteries. They may reach enormous size, but their greatest significance is when they become pedunculated and cause acute strangulation obstruction when the pedicle wraps around a loop of intestine. The core of many lipomas is friable and necrotic, probably from ischemia; in many lipomas, only the superficial centimeter or so remains viable, perhaps nourished by diffusion from the peritoneal environment (Fig. 1-201). In the dog, lipomas arise in the omentum, rather than the mesenteries, and settle on the abdominal floor. They may become very large, but tend not to become pedunculated and therefore do not cause acute distress. Lipomas are benign lesions that do not metastasize.

Other tumors of the subserosal connective tissues, including myxomas, fibromas, and their malignant counterparts, are rare, although fibrosarcomas are observed in dogs, and an omental fibrosarcoma has been reported in a horse. Neurofibromatosis of cattle may involve the abdominal nerves and plexuses, and ganglioneuromas are also observed in this species.

Secondary tumors of the peritoneum are not common, but may occur in any abdominal neoplasia. These mainly arise by direct implantation, rather than by lymphatic or hematogenous metastasis. Carcinomas occur much more commonly than sarcomas. They may induce a robust scirrhous response, and when accompanied by ascites may resemble chronic

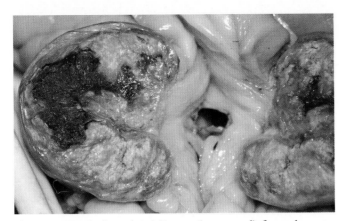

Figure 1-201 Pedunculated lipoma (transected) from the mesentery of a horse. Note necrotic core and thin capsule of viable tissue.

peritonitis. The relative or complete absence of adhesions can be a helpful distinguishing feature grossly. There are obviously many possibilities for the origin of secondary tumors; several common types are listed later.

Ovarian carcinomas are a cause of ascites, and may be difficult to differentiate from mesothelioma; implants of ovarian carcinoma tend to be papillary. Bile duct carcinomas and pancreatic adenocarcinomas tend to be scirrhous, as do intestinal adenocarcinomas in cattle and sheep. Prostatic carcinomas may form discrete firm white nodules on the peritoneum and resemble other carcinomas. Squamous cell carcinomas of the equine stomach form rather discrete implants that may resemble nodules of mesothelioma or granulomas; they may be differentiated enough to be recognizably keratinized on gross inspection. Transitional cell tumors developing in cattle with enzootic hematuria implant locally on the pelvic surfaces; implants from rectal adenocarcinoma in dogs also tend to be confined to the pelvic peritoneum. Malignant melanomas of perineal origin in horses produce pigmented plaques on the peritoneum or in the mesenteries, as may occasional metastatic melanomas in dogs.

Further reading

Bacci B, et al. Ten cases of feline mesothelioma: an immunohistochemical and ultrastructural study. J Comp Pathol 2006;134:347-354.

Churg A., et al. The separation of benign and malignant mesothelial proliferations. Am J Surg Pathol 2000;24:1183-1200.

Gumber S, et al. Disseminated sclerosing peritoneal mesothelioma in a dog. J Vet Diagn Invest 2011;23:1046-1050.

Hammar SP. Macroscopic, histologic, histochemical, immunohistochemical and ultrastructural features of mesothelioma. Ultrastruct Pathol 2006;30:3-17.

Misdorp W. Tumours in calves: comparative aspects. J Comp Pathol 2002;127:96-105.

Diseases of the retroperitoneum

Diseases in the retroperitoneum may originate in the stroma of the space itself, from organs in this space, or as an extension from lesions in adjacent organs.

Retroperitonitis may arise from sepsis involving the pelvic or abdominal urogenital tract, or the mesenteric root; from penetrating wounds; from rectal tears in horses; and from migrating grass awns or other foreign bodies. Frequently it evolves to form a fluctuant abscess or draining fistula in the flank, based on the path of least resistance in the soft tissue of the region. The lesion is usually a poorly encapsulated sinus or abscess, with a wall of granulation tissue and containing purulent exudate. It may extend to involve adjacent vertebrae as periostitis or osteomyelitis. A foreign body may be encountered on exploration, or the lesion may be traced back to a primary septic focus in the abdomen, perhaps a renal or perirenal abscess; an ovarian stump with a remnant of unresorbed suture; or an abscess or pyogranuloma in the root of the mesentery. Mixed bacterial flora are usually isolated, and if *Actinomyces* spp. are present, there may be sulfur granules surrounded by granulomatous inflammation.

Nonneoplastic retroperitoneal masses include hematomas or accumulations of urine, following trauma to the caudal abdominal or pelvic area. Hemorrhage may dissect widely in this area, and the origin may be difficult to detect. Rupture of retroperitoneal hematomas may be fatal. Retroperitoneal hemorrhage in newborn calves is often an indication of fracture of the spinal column caused by inappropriate rotation during assisted calving. Sublumbar hemorrhage is frequent in male lambs castrated by traction of the testis. Renal and perirenal cysts, and pseudocysts or capsular cysts, also may be encountered, and are usually incidental.

Neoplasms of the retroperitoneal space include lipomas, fibrosarcomas, lymphosarcomas, osteosarcomas, and nonchromaffin paragangliomas, as well as primary renal (or other) carcinomas and adrenal tumors.

Metastatic tumors to the region include those commonly involving the sublumbar lymph nodes, such as lymphosarcoma, transitional cell, prostatic, colonic, perianal gland, and anal gland malignancies. Metastatic involvement of the sublumbar lymph nodes may stimulate periosteal reaction on the ventral aspect of adjacent vertebral bodies. Occasionally, tumors metastatic to the region lyse vertebral bodies or transverse processes, and they may occasionally invade the spinal canal. Lytic and osteophytic reactions must be distinguished from the effects of osteomyelitis.

Further reading

Holloway A, O'Brien R. Perirenal effusion in dogs and cats with acute renal failure. Vet Radiol Ultrasound 2007;48:574-579.

Liptak JM, et al. Retroperitoneal sarcomas in dogs: 14 cases (1992-2002). J Am Vet Med Assoc 2004;224:1471-1477.

Marvel SJ, MacPhail CM. Retroperitoneal abscesses in seven dogs. J Am Anim Hosp Assoc 2013;49:378-384.

Roush JK, et al. Diseases of the retroperitoneal space in the dog and cat. J Am Anim Hosp Assoc 1990;26:47-54.

 For more information, please visit the companion site: PathologyofDomesticAnimals.com

CHAPTER 2

Liver and Biliary System

John M. Cullen • Margaret J. Stalker

ACKNOWLEDGMENTS

The authors acknowledge the major contributions of Dr. W. Roger Kelly and Dr. M.A. (Tony) Hayes as previous authors of this section. In addition, the authors thank Drs. W. Roger Kelly and Jeremy Allen for critical review, discussions, and provision of images.

GENERAL CONSIDERATIONS

From a contemporary perspective, the liver is a marvel of biology. It is the guardian of homeostasis, the epicenter of the body's metabolic capability, a massive filter detoxifying the portal blood releasing cleansed blood to the systemic circulation, and a lymphoid organ protecting against infection. However high our regard for the liver, it is dwarfed by the perspective of ancient civilizations that regarded the liver as the seat of life and window to the future. In ancient Mesopotamia and Babylonia, the liver was used to divine the future using a technique termed hepatoscopy. This interest is captured in a Biblical quote from Ezekiel 21:21, *"For the king of Babylon stands at the parting of the way, at the head of the two ways, to use divination; he shakes the arrows, he consults the household idols, he looks at the liver."* Hepatoscopy was continued by the Greeks, Etruscans, and the Romans. The practice is continued in a fashion today. Liver injury or neoplasia foretells a poor future for many pharmaceuticals in development.

The liver plays a central role in processing dietary carbohydrates, lipids, amino acids, and vitamins; in the synthesis and turnover of most plasma proteins; and in the detoxification and biliary excretion of endogenous wastes and xenobiotic compounds. The liver also functions as an important organ of the innate immune system, integrated into the complex system of defense against foreign macromolecules. As such, hepatic disorders have far-reaching consequences, given the dependence of other organs on the metabolic function of the liver.

Origin, structure, and function

The embryonic origin of the liver is an out-pouching of the embryonic endoderm forming the duodenum termed the hepatic diverticulum or the *liver bud*. Primitive epithelial cells of the hepatic diverticulum extend into the adjacent mesenchymal stroma of the septum transversum, a sheet of cells that incompletely separates the pericardial and peritoneal cavity and that will develop into the connective tissue of the liver. The primitive epithelial cells are arranged in close approximation with the vessels that form the vitelline venous plexus, a complex of vessels that drain the yolk sac. Thus the essential sinusoidal arrangement of the liver is established very early in development. The gallbladder and the cystic duct arise from the caudal part of the hepatic diverticulum.

The hepatic diverticulum is also the origin of the biliary epithelium. Development of the biliary tree begins at the hilus and spreads outward to reach the subcapsular zone over time. Intrahepatic bile ducts develop from the **ductal plate,** a structure that is composed initially of a single row of hepatoblasts that surround the portal vein branches and ensheath the mesenchyme of the primitive portal tract. The development of the hepatoblasts adjacent to the portal tract mesenchyme is altered by interactions with the mesenchyme. Initially, these cells form the ductal plate, a single row of cells surrounding the portal tract. The cells of the ductal plate can be identified by expression of cytokeratin 7, differentiating them from the hepatoblasts (Fig. 2-1). A second discontinuous outer layer of cells forms subsequently, and the 2-cell–thick regions remodel into tubules. Most undergo apoptosis, but 1 or 2 ducts become incorporated in the developing portal tract. At about the time the bile ducts are forming, the hepatic artery branches appear in the developing portal tract. Nerves and lymphatics eventually invest the portal tracts as well, completing the mature portal tract. The wave of development from the hilus to the subcapsular region is imperfect, as the veins, arteries, and bile ducts reach their terminal ends separately. Consequently, in human liver, up to 30% of subcapsular portal tracts are "dyads" containing only bile duct and artery profiles. Sinusoidal lining cells other than the endothelium likely arise in the bone marrow and populate the liver via a hematogenous route.

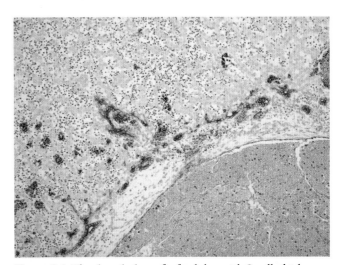

Figure 2-1 The **ductal plate** of a fetal dog with 2-cell–thick rows of cytokeratin 7–positive cells formed at the edge of the developing portal tract.

The liver is the largest internal organ in the body. In adult carnivores, the liver constitutes ~3% of body weight. In adult omnivores, it is ~2% of body weight and ~1% of body weight in adult herbivores. In neonates of all species, the liver is a larger percentage of body weight than in the adult. The liver has a smooth capsular surface, and the parenchyma consists of friable red-brown tissue that is divided into lobes. The number and shape of the liver lobes of the major domestic mammals vary among species. In monogastric animals, the liver abuts the diaphragm and occupies the central area of the cranial abdomen. In ruminants, and to a lesser extent in horses, the liver is displaced to the right side of the cranial abdominal cavity. A series of ligaments maintains the liver in its position. The *coronary ligament* attaches the liver to the diaphragm near the esophagus. The *falciform ligament* attaches the midline of the liver to the ventral midline of the abdomen. The *round ligament*, a remnant of the umbilical vein, is embedded within the falciform ligament.

The liver receives ~25% of the cardiac output, but is also supplied by the **portal vein.** The valveless portal vein drains the digestive tract, forestomachs, glandular stomach, and intestines, as well as the spleen and pancreas. Portal vein flow provides 70-80% of the total afferent hepatic blood flow and ~50% of the oxygen supply. The **hepatic artery** provides the remainder of hepatic blood flow. Portal blood flow is not regulated, but hepatic arterial flow is regulated, primarily by adenosine, and responds to changes in portal flow. When portal blood flow is reduced, less adenosine is washed out of the hepatic circulation, and this increased concentration drives hepatic arterial dilation, creating a **hepatic arterial buffer effect** whereby a consistent hepatic blood flow is maintained. Portal blood flow is important for the rapid clearance of nutrients, xenobiotics, microorganisms, and potentially immunogenic materials that enter the circulation from the gastrointestinal tract. Hepatic arterioles disperse into a peribiliary capillary plexus, a perivenous plexus surrounding the portal vein, or join terminal hepatic arterioles before entering the sinusoids, lowering pressure and preventing reversal of portal venous inflow. Portal and arterial blood eventually mix in the low-pressure hepatic sinusoids. Both terminal portal venules and hepatic arterioles flow into the sinusoids, but flow is closely regulated by a series of inlet sphincters formed by endothelial cells for the venules and smooth muscle for the arterioles. Thus, at any particular time, sinusoidal blood could be entirely venous, mixed arterial and venous, or arterial. This blood flow pattern may account for the interlobular and intralobular heterogeneity of lesions following various toxicities. Blood leaves the liver via the **hepatic vein,** which is very short, and enters the caudal vena cava.

Hepatic sinusoids have an average diameter of 10 μm, but can expand up to 30 μm. The periportal sinusoids are more tortuous than those in the centrilobular region. Hepatic sinusoids are lined by specialized endothelial cells. Hepatic sinusoids differ from vascular structures elsewhere in that they lack a typical basement membrane, and are supported by a specialized, discontinuous or loose extracellular matrix (ECM). Hepatic **sinusoidal endothelial cells** are fenestrated, and these 100-nm diameter sieve-like pores control fluid, solute, and particulate interchange between blood and the perisinusoidal space, regulated by the action of the cellular cytoskeleton. Sinusoidal endothelial cells are actively pinocytotic and internalize and degrade various endogenous glycoproteins, glycosaminoglycans, and immune complexes. **Kupffer**

cells are fixed macrophages attached to the inner sinusoidal wall in direct contact with blood moving at a relatively low velocity. This arrangement facilitates phagocytic removal of particulates, especially bacteria that enter the portal blood via the lower alimentary tract. Kupffer cells also participate in the regulation of inflammatory and repair responses by secretion of various cytokines into the circulation and perisinusoidal space. **Natural killer cells** (formerly referred to as pit cells) are large granular lymphocytes with natural killer activity that adhere to the sinusoidal endothelium, where they are also well situated to participate in various innate immune defenses, for example, targeting infected cells that enter the liver via the blood.

The sinusoids are separated from the adjacent hepatocellular plates by an extracellular space, known as the **space of Disse,** that contains **hepatic stellate cells** (also termed *lipocytes* or *Ito cells*), reticulin fibers, and nerves. The space of Disse is not readily visible by light microscopy unless there is fluid retention, such as can occur with impediment to venous outflow. Although hepatic sinusoids in the normal liver lack a conventional basement membrane, the perisinusoidal space contains a low-density ECM consisting of collagen type IV; laminin; fibronectin; minor amounts of collagen types I, III, V, and VI; nonfibrillar collagen XVIII; tenascin; and various proteoglycans. A conventional ECM composed of fibrillar collagen types I, III, V, and fibronectin is found in the external capsule **(Glisson's capsule),** septa, and around portal triads and central veins. "Reticulin fibers" are the components of the ECM that are stainable by silver impregnation techniques, consisting mainly of collagen type III with attached fibronectin and other glycoproteins. The fenestrated sinusoidal endothelium, coupled with the loose subendothelial matrix, allows for exchange of various macromolecules between hepatocytes and the sinusoidal blood. After hepatic injury, a denser, less permeable matrix resembling a true basement membrane may form, and sinusoidal endothelial cells may lose their fenestrae (so-called **"capillarization" of sinusoids),** reducing uptake and secretion of plasma proteins and other metabolically important substances.

The **terminal hepatic venules** *("central veins")* collect the outflow blood from the sinusoids. These venules converge into the larger **hepatic veins** that empty into the caudal vena cava. In most species, increased pressure in the vena cava during right-sided heart failure or hepatic vein thrombosis causes passive congestion and distension of the hepatic veins and sinusoids. However, the large and small hepatic veins in dogs have a prominent spiral circumferential smooth muscle that can also affect the central venous pressure on the sinusoids. Fluids from the perisinusoidal space drain into **lymphatics** in the extracellular connective-tissue spaces of the liver capsule, the portal tracts, and the connective tissue of the terminal veins. These flow out the portal hilus to the hepatic lymph nodes and eventually enter the thoracic duct. In some species, such as the dog, there are also lymphatics around the larger hepatic veins; these cross the diaphragm into the mediastinum. The liver is the largest lymph producer in the body, contributing 20-50% of the thoracic duct flow. Hepatic lymph is high in protein, containing 85-95% of the protein of plasma and a high cell count composed of lymphocytes and macrophages. In sheep, more lymphocytes pass through the liver than any typical lymphoid organ, and ~2 × 10^8 macrophages leave the liver in lymph daily. **Hepatic nerves** contain both sympathetic and parasympathetic fibers. The fibers invest major blood vessels and also extend along the sinusoids. These may modulate function of hepatocytes, endothelial cells, and hepatic stellate cells.

The vasculature of the liver parenchyma defines its functional microanatomy, but *debate continues as to what best represents the hepatic structural-functional unit*. Mammalian hepatocytes are organized in plate-like monolayer arrays among the sinusoids and in 3 dimensions; *plates, sinusoids, and tracts anastomose in a complex pattern*. Currently, a somewhat baffling array of models exists, each with their own adherents. These include the well-known lobular and acinar patterns (discussed later) and several others. Matsumoto's primary lobule is based on detailed reconstructions of human liver sections, and considers the penetrating venule extending from the portal tract as a "vascular septum" and the origin of the primary lobule's blood flow as it is a starting place for the radially arranged sinusoids flowing to the terminal hepatic vein. In this model, there is a series of branches formed by the portal vein. The first branches provide a conducting portal flow, and the next level of branches drain directly into the sinusoids forming the distributing portal flow. The **choleohepaton,** related to the concept of the nephron, is composed of an isosceles triangle of hepatocytes with its apex in contact with the terminal hepatic venule and drained by a single bile ductule/canal of Hering at the base of the triangle. More detail is available in the cited references.

Arrangements of hepatocytes in the most commonly used nomenclature systems are referred to as either **acini** or **lobules.**

- The **classic hepatic lobule** is a 6-sided anatomic arrangement of hepatocytes centered on the **terminal hepatic venule,** also termed the "central vein" in this context. Peripherally, lobules are outlined by fibrovascular septa extending from the portal tracts. In the pig liver, septa form obvious lobular perimeters, but in most mammalian species, the lobules are less pronounced because connective tissue is more restricted to portal tracts. The terms **periportal** and **centrilobular** are mainly used for pathologic conditions that are centered on the hepatocytes surrounding the *portal tracts* or the *central veins* of the classic lobule.
- The **hepatic acinus** of Rappaport is a functional diamond-shaped subunit divided into *zones* in relation to blood supply:
  - **Zone 1** hepatocytes are arranged around an axis formed by the portal tract and the distributing vascular branches that leave the portal tract and are closest to the oxygen- and nutrient-rich arterial and portal inflow.
  - **Zone 2** is the transitional midzone.
  - **Zone 3 (periacinar)** hepatocytes form the apex of the diamond-shaped acinus, are nearest the outflow (terminal hepatic venule), and are exposed to reduced oxygen and nutrients.

The functional activity of hepatocytes is heterogeneous, and virtually all liver functions have a zonal gradient. Periportal hepatocytes, exposed to the blood with the highest concentration of oxygen, insulin, glucagon, and amino acids, are the principal site of gluconeogenesis, protein synthesis, aerobic metabolism, urea cycle, and lipid and cholesterol metabolism. In the centrilobular region, glycolysis, lipogenesis, and the major biotransformation functions are more active, including the expression of most cytochromes P450, glucuronyl transferases, glutathione S–transferases, and other biotransformation/detoxification enzymes. *Centrilobular hepatocytes are therefore more susceptible to hypoxic injury as well as injury by toxic*

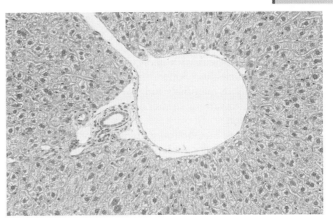

Figure 2-2 The **normal portal tract** contains a branch of the portal vein and hepatic artery, as well as a bile duct. The first row of hepatocytes adjacent to the portal tract connective tissue is termed the **limiting plate.**

substances that are metabolically activated by cytochromes P450. By comparison, *hepatocytes in periportal hepatocytes are more susceptible to direct-acting toxicants,* such as ingested metal salts, given their proximity to the vascular inflow. Under the influences of various inducers, the patterns of enzyme expression can extend beyond the resting limits. Lobular variation is not restricted to parenchymal cells, but is also apparent in the structure and function of sinusoidal endothelial cells, Kupffer cells, perisinusoidal stellate cells, and the composition of the matrix in the space of Disse.

The **portal tract,** or *portal triad,* is a well-defined structure *containing at least one small arterial branch, a portal vein branch, and a bile duct,* surrounded by connective tissue composed primarily of type I collagen (Fig. 2-2). Because of the pattern of progressive branching of the portal tract system, individual tracts exhibit a range of sizes and shapes, from round to triangular or branching. In larger portal tracts, lymphatic channels and autonomic nerve fibers may be seen. The **bile duct** system is a branching outflow that ultimately enters the proximal duodenum. Most species, with the exception of the horse and rat, have a bile storage diverticulum (**gallbladder**). Cats occasionally have divided or bipartite gallbladders. The bile duct joins the pancreatic duct before entry into the duodenum in some species and has a separate entry in others. Intrahepatic bile ducts range in size from the larger septal or trabecular ducts (internal diameter of >100 µm in humans) to the smaller interlobular ducts, and tend to be adjacent to a hepatic artery branch of approximately the same size. Bile ducts are lined by cuboidal to low columnar **bile duct epithelial cells,** subtended by a periodic acid–Schiff (PAS)-positive basement membrane. **Bile ductules** are smaller yet (lumen size of <20 µm) and are located at the periphery of portal tracts.

Cells of the liver

Hepatocytes (referred to as **parenchymal cells**) constitute ~70-80% of the liver mass. However, >50% of liver DNA is found in smaller **nonparenchymal cells** (bile duct epithelium, hepatic stellate cells, sinusoidal endothelium, Kupffer cells) and itinerant cells (such as leukocytes). The hepatocyte is a polygonal epithelial cell, ~30-40 µm in diameter, arranged in single-cell–thick anastomosing plates, separated by hepatic sinusoids. Each hepatocyte is therefore exposed to sinusoidal blood on 2 sides. A discontinuous line of hepatocytes, termed the **limiting plate,** is found at the interface with the collagenous ECM of the portal tract. Normal hepatocytes have abundant eosinophilic cytoplasm, and most have a single, round, centrally placed nucleus with finely dispersed chromatin and at least one nucleolus. Some binucleate hepatocytes are present normally in mammals and can become more numerous in response to various stimuli and injuries that induce or affect regeneration.

Hepatocytes are metabolically highly active cells, containing an array of organelles, including smooth and rough endoplasmic reticulum, mitochondria, lysosomes, peroxisomes, Golgi complexes, and transport vesicles. These organelles support a variety of hepatocellular functions, including the synthesis and secretion of plasma proteins, coagulation factors, and acute-phase proteins. Hepatocytes store nutrients in times of adequate energy and release glucose when needed. They are key modulators of lipid metabolism, and they synthesize and secrete lipoproteins. In addition, they are the only cells capable of bile acid synthesis, and they can absorb and secrete them into bile. Finally, hepatocytes detoxify the large majority of xenobiotics and secrete them into the bile. Because of this central role in metabolism, the liver is subjected to a variety of nutritionally based insults as well as toxin-related damage. A greater proportion of the genome is expressed in the normal liver than has been observed in any other tissue, an indication that brief surveys of liver functions are necessarily oversimplified. However, those constituents that are most abundant have most influence on the microscopic appearance of the liver. The normal hepatocyte contains abundant glycogen, which varies depending on food intake, and which can be demonstrated by PAS staining, as well as variable amounts of stored triglycerides and various proteins, such as ferritin, an iron-binding protein. The cytoplasm of the centrilobular hepatocytes may also contain uniform, golden-brown granules of **lipofuscin,** particularly in older cats. This so-called "wear-and-tear" pigment becomes more prominent with age, and progressively accumulates in midzonal and periportal hepatocytes. Hepatocytes have a cytoskeleton composed of microtubules, microfilaments, and intermediate filaments. Microtubules are found throughout the cytoplasm, and are involved in the movement of secreted proteins into the extracellular perisinusoidal space; accordingly, microtubule inhibitors such as colchicine and *Vinca* alkaloids may reduce hepatic protein secretion. Microfilaments, composed of actin and myosin, are concentrated around the bile canaliculus, where they are involved in canalicular peristalsis and bile secretion; microfilament inhibitors result in cholestasis. Intermediate filaments (predominantly cytokeratins 8 and 18) form an irregular meshwork extending from the plasma membrane to the perinuclear zone, and are responsible for spatial organization of the hepatocyte.

There are 3 morphologically and functionally distinct surfaces of the hepatocyte plasma membrane.

1. The **sinusoidal domain** faces the space of Disse and has numerous irregular microvilli, increasing hepatocyte surface area by ~6-fold (considerably less that that seen in enterocytes). This specialized membrane is modified to facilitate an exchange of substances with the blood. There are ultrastructurally evident pits between the villi, some of which represent secretory vacuoles in the process of exocytosis, sending various products into the plasma, and others are clathrin-coated pits involved in selective receptor-mediated endocytosis. Numerous membrane receptors for glycoproteins, asialoglycoproteins, peptides, hormones, growth factors, immunoglobulin A, and other endocytotic or signaling ligands are found at the sinusoidal pole. In addition, transmembrane proteins involved in plasma exchange of small ionic substances with the sinusoidal plasma, and transmembrane proteins responsible for matrix recognition, are concentrated on the sinusoidal surface.

2. The **lateral domain** extends from the sinusoidal surface to the edge of the canaliculus. This portion of the cell membrane is specialized for adhesion via junctional complexes, including desmosomes, tight junctions, and intermediate junctions, as well as for intercellular communication via gap junctions.

3. The **canalicular domain** is the beginning of the bile drainage system of the liver. *The canaliculus is an intercellular space between 2 adjacent hepatocytes, isolated by junctional complexes.* The canalicular surface is covered with an irregular array of microvilli. Canalicular diameter increases as it approaches the periportal region, enlarging from ~0.5-2.5 µm. Bile is propelled along the canaliculi by a web of contractile microfilaments. This specialized membrane contains various adenosine triphosphate (ATP)-dependent carriers that export many products, including leukotrienes, bile salts, xenobiotics, and their metabolites into the bile.

The **canal of Hering** is partly lined by biliary epithelium and partly by hepatocytes and connects the bile canaliculus to the cholangioles and eventually the interlobular bile ducts.

Cholangiocytes (biliary epithelium) account for ~3-5% of the liver cell population. Although derived from common embryologic progenitor cells, cholangiocytes differ from hepatocytes in both phenotype and function. They contain a strongly developed network of intermediate filaments, including cytokeratins 7 and 19. They also express marked heterogeneity along the anatomic course of the biliary system. Functionally, bile duct epithelial cells actively modify the composition of bile. Secretion is primarily under the control of secretin and somatostatin. Secretin released from the duodenum triggers secretion of bicarbonate-rich fluids that buffer acids released from the stomach. Cholangiocytes secrete immunoglobulin A (IgA) and IgM, but not IgG. Absorption involves the sodium-dependent glucose transporter and aquaporins responsible for glucose and water uptake, as in the renal proximal tubule. They express γ-glutamyltranspeptidase, which removes glutamic acid from glutathione conjugates.

Hepatic progenitor cells (HPCs), formerly known as oval cells in rodents, reside in the region of the canal of Hering. These cells are bipotential and can mature into either biliary epithelium or hepatocytes. They can proliferate and form a type of **ductular reaction.** In cases of massive hepatic necrosis in which the animal survives for a few days after the initial injury, HPCs can proliferate dramatically, forming cords or small caliber ducts lined by cuboidal basophilic cells with abundant mitochondria. These cells can mature and replace lost hepatocytes and bile ducts. HPCs in humans and rats contain both markers of hepatocyte phenotype (i.e., albumin) and biliary phenotype (i.e., cytokeratin 7). Similar markers have been described in dogs and cats as well. Bone marrow–derived pluripotential stem cells also appear to have the ability to differentiate into hepatocytes. Other types of ductular reaction are discussed in the section on Responses of the liver to injury.

Hepatic endothelial cells are specialized, perforated by numerous fenestrations, ~175 nm in diameter, and often clustered together forming sieve plates. Larger, but less frequent, fenestrations are more common at the periportal end of the sinusoid, but opening size is dynamic, responding to endogenous mediators and toxins. The endothelial cells rest on a very thin and discontinuous ECM. The fenestrations allow direct contact between the sinusoidal lumen and the space of Disse. Only larger particles, such as chylomicrons, and cells are excluded. Sinusoidal endothelial cells differ from normal vascular endothelium in several additional ways, including the absence of factor VIII–related antigen (except in inflammatory conditions) and high endocytic activity. Endocytosis of immune complexes and some proteoglycans are major functions. They also synthesize molecules that affect vascular tone such as nitric oxide, endothelins, and prostaglandins.

Kupffer cells *are specialized macrophages located in sinusoidal lumens,* mainly at branch points. Once thought to be "fixed," it is now known that they can migrate along the sinusoid and into areas of tissue injury (Fig. 2-3). Kupffer cells may have a dual origin as they are derived, at least in part, from blood-borne monocytes, but they are also capable of local proliferation, particularly in inflammation. They are not efficient antigen presenters, but they are proficient phagocytes of apoptotic and necrotic cells, particulates, and microorganisms; consequently, the liver is a major "filtering organ" for the body. There are species differences in the efficiency of this process. Clearance of particulates, and endotoxin in particular, is accomplished more effectively by Kupffer cells in dogs, humans, and laboratory rodents than in ruminants, horse, pig, cats, and whales, species that have a significant population of intravascular macrophages in the pulmonary vasculature. Kupffer cells can phagocytose a variety of gut-derived materials; bacteria, various biologically active bacterial components, including lipopolysaccharides, lipoteichoic acids, and peptidoglycans, without stimulating inflammation. Activated Kupffer cells can secrete tumor necrosis factor-α and other cytokines, and nitric oxide; these contribute to peripheral vasodilation and hypotension in systemic inflammatory response syndromes initiated by bacterial components. Other secreted cytokines, such as interleukin-1 (IL-1) and IL-6, mediate the acute-phase response and some aspects of the immune and liver regenerative responses. However, there can be a balance in proinflammatory and anti-inflammatory signaling as there are distinct differences in the signaling repertoire of different Kupffer cells. Some Kupffer cells are more likely to secrete IL-10, which can suppress macrophage activation and cytokine secretion. Cytokine responses of Kupffer cells are believed to be important in regulating the extent of adaptive immune response or tolerance to potentially antigenic macromolecules that can reach the liver through the portal blood.

The liver contains large numbers of **lymphocytes,** comprising ~5% of the entire cell population of the liver, with an organ-specific lymphocyte distribution characterized by the enrichment of elements of the innate immune system, including natural killer T lymphocytes (NKT cells), natural killer (NK cells), and innate lymphocytes, in addition to the Kupffer cells previously mentioned. Elements of the acquired immune system, CD8+ T cells, are also increased when compared with peripheral blood. The majority of intrahepatic lymphocytes are involved in innate immune responses rather than acquired immunity. Hepatic NK cells constitute ~40% of hepatic lymphocytes and are distinct phenotypically and functionally from blood NK cells. Hepatic NKT cells reside in the space of Disse, are considered large granular lymphocytes, and were previously referred to as pit cells. Intrahepatic NK cells have important functions in defense against foreign antigens released from the gut, viral infections, metastatic tumors, hepatocellular carcinoma, and modulation of hepatic fibrosis. The liver also contains the largest population of γδ T cells in the body. Although the precise function of these diverse lymphocyte types is not currently understood, their large number alone suggests that they must be involved in immunologic homeostasis and respond to immunologic challenges, indicating that the liver can be considered a lymphoid organ.

Hepatic dendritic cells play an important role in the induction and regulation of immune responses. These antigen-presenting cells have only recently been studied in the liver. There are several other antigen-presenting cells in the liver, including the sinusoidal endothelial cells and Kupffer cells. Unlike cells that reside within the sinusoid, hepatic dendritic cells are found within the portal tract. Hepatic dendritic cells are considered to be functionally immature compared to the dendritic cells of the spleen and bone marrow, and they may be involved in immune tolerance in the liver.

Hepatic stellate cells (HSC), originally described by Boll and von Kupffer in the 1870s, were neglected until the 1950s, when they were described in detail by Ito. They have also been known as *lipocytes, Ito cells, or fat-storing cells.* HSC reside in the space of Disse, but there are other populations of similar cells with the ability to produce ECM and to transform into a myofibroblast phenotype within the connective tissue of the portal tract and centrilobular veins. There are 4 key functions of HSC: (1) storage and homeostasis of retinoids, including vitamin A; (2) maintenance and remodeling of the sinusoidal ECM in health and disease; (3) production of growth factors, such as hepatocyte growth factor and various cytokines; and (4) regulation of sinusoidal diameter by contraction of cellular processes. This may be in response to adrenergic stimulation, as all HSC are in contact with autonomic nerve fibers. HSC can become greatly distended with lipid in carnivores on some diets.

Activation of HSC has been extensively studied because of their importance in hepatic fibrosis. In the transition from quiescence to activation, HSC lose their characteristic lipid droplets, possibly catabolizing the lipid to support their

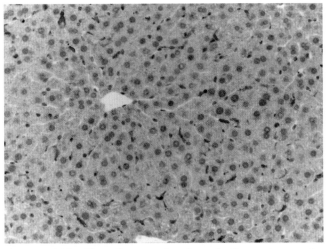

Figure 2-3 Kupffer cells, stained with antibodies against myeloperoxidase, line the sinusoids at regular intervals.

activation. They then develop a myofibroblast phenotype characterized by the expression α–smooth muscle actin. Pro-inflammatory cytokines released primarily by Kupffer cells, such as transforming growth factor-β released in response to tissue injury, stimulate HSC to increase the deposition of ECM, including collagen type I, III, and IV, and laminin. This new ECM transforms the sinusoid to a less permeable capillary, lined by a basement membrane–like layer and without fenestrations in the sinusoidal endothelium, reducing transfer of macromolecules between hepatocytes and the blood. The acquired contractility of the HSC during fibrogenesis is increased because of an increase in the contractile stimulus of endothelin-1 and a reduction in vasodilation driven by diminished nitric oxide generation. In severe chronic injury leading to cirrhosis, the increased expression of contractile proteins within activated stellate cells can further restrict sinusoidal blood flow as a primary effect, rather than a consequence of nodule formation and fibrosis. Peribiliary fibrosis arises from activation of the circumferential fibroblasts of the bile ducts that undergo a phenotypic transformation similar to that of the HSC along the sinusoids. Fibrosis of the portal tracts and the central vein connective tissue develops from activation of myofibroblasts resident in these areas as well. It is also possible that epithelial-mesenchymal transition of hepatocytes, biliary epithelial cells, or HSC can contribute to hepatic fibrosis during chronic injury.

Mast cells are abundant in the liver, particularly in dogs. They typically occupy a perivenous location, where they may influence vascular tone and respond to various potentially injurious substances or organisms. Degranulation of mast cells in the liver leads to contraction of the spiral smooth muscle, restricting blood outflow from the canine liver. This is a feature of shock in dogs.

Hematopoiesis in the fetal life of mammals occurs mainly in the perisinusoidal compartment of the liver sinusoids. Post-natally, hepatic hematopoiesis declines but can return as *extramedullary hematopoiesis* in conditions of increased demand (Fig. 2-4). Because the liver is an early site of hematopoiesis, the environmental conditions and cells, including resident populations of appropriate stromal cells and, possibly hematopoietic stem cells, remain supportive for the initiation or reactivation of a stem cell niche. The degree of hepatic extramedullary hematopoiesis in larger species can have diagnostic significance, but in laboratory rodents and other small animals, it can be an incidental observation.

Further reading

Crawford JM, Burt AD. Anatomy, pathophysiology and basic mechanisms of disease. In: Burt AD, et al., editors. Macsween's Pathology of the Liver. 6th ed. New York: Churchill Livingstone; 2012. p. 2-77.
Malarkey DE, et al. New insights into functional aspects of liver morphology. Toxicol Pathol 2005;33:27-34.

DEVELOPMENTAL DISORDERS
Hepatic cysts

Serous cysts are occasionally found attached to the capsule on the diaphragmatic surface in calves, lambs, and foals (Fig. 2-5). These cysts are usually small and multiple, but some are isolated and very large. Cyst walls are composed of connective tissue lined by flattened or cuboidal epithelium. The content is clear and serous. Their origin is not known, but it is variously postulated that they are serosal inclusion cysts, part of congenital polycystic biliary anomalies, or of endodermal origin. They do not contain bile. The declining incidence of these anomalies with age suggests that a large proportion of them involute in the early postnatal period.

Solitary biliary cysts—single round cysts lined by a flattened single layer of biliary epithelium—are uncommon and may be congenital or acquired. **Multiple hepatic peribiliary cysts** putatively arising from peribiliary glands have been reported in a 6-month-old pig.

Hamartomas

Von Meyenburg complexes (biliary microhamartomas) are developmental malformations arising from persistent embryonic ductal plate remnants. These are discrete, usually subcapsular, fibrotic areas containing small, irregularly shaped, often dilated, U-shaped or branching, bile duct–like structures lined by low cuboidal epithelium (Fig. 2-6).

Mesenchymal or **mixed liver hamartomas,** rare benign tumor-like lesions characterized by disorganized hepatocellular and/or biliary structures embedded in a mucinous primitive mesenchyme have been reported in 2 equine fetuses.

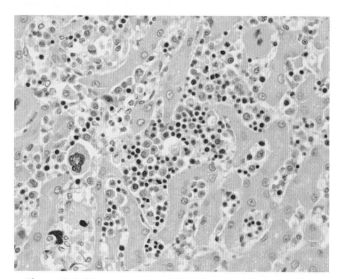

Figure 2-4 Hepatic **extramedullary hematopoiesis** in a dog.

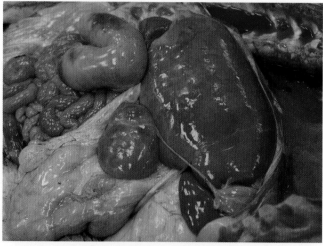

Figure 2-5 Serous cyst attached by a stalk to the hepatic capsule in a 3-day-old Holstein calf. (Courtesy J.L. Caswell.)

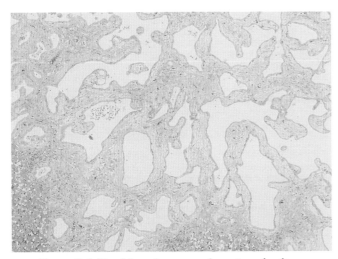

Figure 2-6 Von Meyenburg complexes in a dog liver.

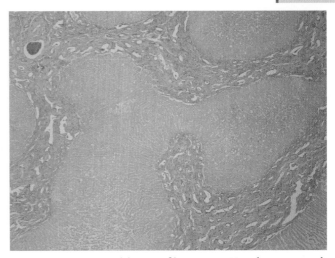

Figure 2-7 Congenital hepatic fibrosis in a Himalayan cat with polycystic kidney disease.

Ductal plate malformations

Persistence and/or aberrant remodeling of the embryonic ductal plate can give rise to a spectrum of cystic biliary diseases. **Congenital hepatic fibrocystic diseases,** part of the group of hepatorenal fibrocystic disease that includes the polycystic kidney diseases, *are a product of ductal plate malformations occurring at different levels of the biliary tree.* Analysis of the underlying genetic basis of the human hepatorenal fibrocystic diseases has identified defective protein components in primary cilia and associated basal bodies. These mechanotransducer organelles are involved in environmental monitoring, signal transduction, and cell proliferation, and are important in the normal development of the biliary system in the liver, as well as renal tubules. As such, many of these diseases are now considered "ciliopathies."

In human hepatopathology, the hepatorenal fibrocystic diseases can be grouped into 3 descriptive categories: (1) **polycystic liver disease** (often seen in association with autosomal dominant polycystic kidney disease of adults), characterized by isolated microscopic to macroscopic unilocular or multilocular cysts in a fibrous stroma, with no continuity with the intrahepatic biliary tree, thought to originate from von Meyenburg complexes in the most peripheral branches of the biliary tree; (2) **congenital hepatic fibrosis** (often seen in association with autosomal recessive polycystic kidney disease of childhood), characterized by defective remodeling of the ductal plate at the level of interlobular ducts, with excess abnormally shaped embryonic bile ducts retained in the primitive ductal plate configuration, abnormal portal veins, and progressive fibrosis of the portal tracts; and (3) **Caroli disease,** characterized by non-obstructive saccular or fusiform dilation of medium- and large-sized intrahepatic bile ducts, with maintenance of continuity with the biliary system. Caroli syndrome refers to Caroli disease co-occurring with congenital hepatic fibrosis. In veterinary medicine, a similar classification of the liver lesions has been proposed: **adult polycystic disease** (including von Meyenburg complexes), **juvenile polycystic disease/congenital hepatic fibrosis,** and **congenital dilation of the large and segmental bile ducts** (resembling Caroli disease).

Congenital cystic lesions involving the hepatic biliary system and kidneys have been reported in juvenile dogs, cats, pigs, goats, and foals, and have been compared to congenital hepatorenal fibrocystic disorders of humans. Cysts may also be found in the pancreas or other organs. Animals may die from progressive renal insufficiency, and/or from hepatic dysfunction and portal hypertension associated with hepatic fibrosis. Hepatic fibrosis and cysts are present in a significant proportion of cats with *polycystic kidney disease,* inherited in Persian cats, exotic shorthaired, and other related breeds as an autosomal dominant C→A transversion mutation in exon 29 of the feline *PKD1* gene, resembling the adult form of polycystic kidney disease in humans. The liver lesions have been more difficult to classify, and may appear as multiple large cysts resembling adult-type polycystic disease, as congenital hepatic fibrosis characterized by portoportal bridging fibrosis with excess abnormally formed bile ductules (Fig. 2-7), or as combinations of both lesions. Polycystic kidney and liver disease reported in West Highland White and Cairn Terrier litters resembles the autosomal recessive polycystic kidney disease of children. *Congenital hepatic fibrosis* has been described in dogs. Affected animals are presented at or before a year of age with clinical signs of liver disease, including ascites, microhepatica, and *extrahepatic portosystemic shunts.* Histologically, these dogs had livers with extensive bands of portal bridging fibrosis containing numerous small irregular, tortuous bile ducts, often accompanied by absent or hypoplastic portal veins and compensatory arteriolar proliferation, and with no evidence of nodular regeneration and minimal inflammation, allowing differentiation of this congenital condition from acquired chronic liver disease. Congenital hepatic fibrosis has also been reported in aborted and neonatal calves, in the latter case accompanied by cyst formation in the kidney and lung. Congenital hepatic fibrosis with cystic bile ducts has been described in Swiss Freiberger foals (Fig. 2-8) and is seen occasionally in other breeds, with generalized portal bridging fibrosis containing many small, irregularly formed and occasionally cystic bile ducts. Macroscopic congenital dilation of the large and segmental bile ducts and diffuse cystic kidney disease, resembling *Caroli disease,* has been reported in dogs.

Extrahepatic biliary anomalies

Cats occasionally have divided or bipartite gallbladders. Reduplication of the gallbladder has also been reported in swine. Other anomalies of the extrahepatic biliary system include *agenesis of the gallbladder* reported in dogs, and *absence or*

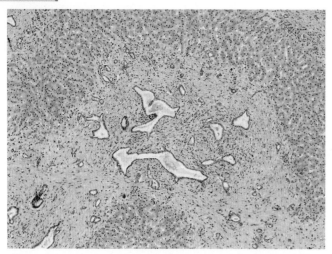

Figure 2-8 Congenital hepatic fibrosis in a Swiss Freiberger foal.

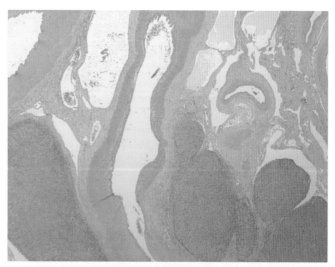

Figure 2-10 Congenital intrahepatic arterioportal fistulae with thick-walled anastomosing vessels and atrophy of adjacent parenchyma in a dog.

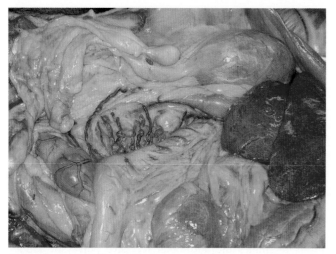

Figure 2-9 Multiple **acquired portosystemic vascular shunts** in a dog with chronic liver disease.

atresia of one or more ducts, reported in lambs, calves (eFig. 2-1), foals, a cat, a dog, and a pig. In carnivores, bile duct atresia may lead not only to jaundice, but also to vitamin D–deficiency rickets, because of their inability to absorb fat-soluble vitamins. Congenital atresia may be associated with defects in the developmental morphogenesis of bile ducts, or in utero vascular, inflammatory, or toxic insults to the biliary tree that culminate in the obliteration of the lumen.

Choledochal cysts arising from the cystic or common bile duct have been described in cats.

Congenital vascular anomalies

These include congenital portal vein aneurysms, hepatic arteriovenous malformations, congenital portosystemic shunts between the portal vein and other systemic veins, and primary hypoplasia of the portal vein. *Extrahepatic* **congenital** *portosystemic shunts are readily distinguished from shunts that are* **acquired** *during portal hypertension, as acquired shunts are typically multiple, thin-walled, tortuous collateral venous connections between the portal vein or its tributaries and caudal vena cava, renal vein, or azygos vein* (Fig. 2-9). Although multiple acquired shunts do not develop in the presence of congenital PSS, they

can arise with other congenital abnormalities, such as arteriovenous malformations or hypoplasia or dysplasia of portal veins, as a consequence of portal hypertension. Acquired shunts resulting from portal hypertension secondary to liver injury and repair are discussed later in the section Vascular factors in hepatic injury and circulatory disorders.

Portal vein aneurysms, both congenital and acquired as a consequence of concurrent liver disease, have been described in dogs. Extrahepatic aneurysms were always located at the level of the gastroduodenal vein insertion. All were asymptomatic, although predisposed to portal vein thrombosis.

Hepatic arteriovenous malformations have been reported in dogs and cats. These are congenital or, in some instances, acquired communications between branches of the hepatic artery, and more rarely, the gastroduodenal artery and left gastric artery and portal vein. Mixing of higher-pressure arterial blood with venous blood results in retrograde flow into the portal vein, arterialization of the portal circulation, and development of portal hypertension, with the opening of vestigial, low-resistance, collateral, extrahepatic portosystemic communications (acquired extrahepatic shunts). The fistulae may be macroscopic or microscopic, are typically multiple, and may involve one or more lobes of the liver. The hepatic parenchyma of affected lobes may be atrophied, with dilated, tortuous, pulsatile vessels visible on the capsular surface. Histopathologic findings include hyperplasia and anastomoses of arterioles and venules (Fig. 2-10). Affected vessels have irregularly thickened walls with intimal hyperplasia consisting of smooth muscle proliferation and deposition of elastin fibers, focal subintimal fibromuscular proliferation, and smooth muscle hyperplasia of the tunica media. Degenerative changes characterized by deposition of mucinous material and mineral in the intima and media of arterioles, as well as thrombosis and recanalization of portal veins, are also observed. Adjacent hepatic parenchyma may be atrophic, with periportal fibrosis, and bile duct hyperplasia, arteriolar proliferation, and relative collapse of portal vein branches within portal tracts. Arteriovenous fistulae may also be acquired, developing subsequent to abdominal trauma, rupture of hepatic artery aneurysms, and secondary to hepatic vein obstruction or cirrhosis with extreme portal hypertension.

Congenital portosystemic vascular anomalies *are typically single anomalous vessels that directly connect the portal venous system with the systemic venous circulation, bypassing the hepatic sinusoids and hepatic parenchyma.* They occur in dogs and cats, and, rarely, in pigs, foals, goats and calves. These portosystemic shunts (PSS) may be either intrahepatic or extrahepatic in location. The most common **intrahepatic shunt,** located in the left hepatic division, is a *persistent patent ductus venosus* (Fig. 2-11). Central and right divisional intrahepatic shunts have also been described in dogs and cats. The major types of **extrahepatic shunts** include direct shunting from the portal vein or major tributary (typically left gastric or splenic veins, less commonly the gastroduodenal or mesenteric veins) to the caudal vena cava (portocaval shunt) (Fig. 2-12, eFig. 2-2) or to the azygos vein *(portoazygos shunt),* or connection of the portal vein to the caudal vena cava, which itself shunts to the azygos vein. Extrahepatic portosystemic shunts may also have hypoplasia of the portal vein distal to the origin of the shunt. Large-breed dogs typically have intrahepatic shunts, usually a patent ductus venosus, but sometimes other large intrahepatic communications. Small-breed dogs and cats usually have single large extrahepatic shunts between the portal vein and vena cava or azygos vein. An inherited basis is suspected for several breeds, including Irish Wolfhounds, Maltese, Yorkshire Terriers, and Australian cattle dogs.

Affected dogs are usually presented in adolescence with failure to thrive or with the neurobehavioral manifestations of hepatic encephalopathy. Often, there is a clinical history of depression, convulsions, and other nervous signs that are exacerbated by a high-protein diet, and may be alleviated by dietary control. *Because there is no cause of portal hypertension, these dogs do not develop ascites.*

The liver that has been bypassed by a congenital shunt is hypoplastic, largely because of diversion of hepatotrophic factors, including insulin, glucagon, and epidermal growth factor that originate in the intestine and pancreas. Affected livers may be smooth surfaced with normal color and texture. Histologically, hepatocytes and hepatic lobules are small with close and irregular spacing of portal triads. Larger portal veins may be inapparent or appear collapsed and empty of circulating blood elements; portal veins in smaller triads may be small, collapsed, absent, or indistinguishable. Hepatic arterioles are often more prominent, and may be multiple and tortuous (Fig. 2-13), related to increased compensatory arterial perfusion. Numbers of arteriolar structures within triads may also appear increased, as small caliber and usually inapparent arterioles become evident histologically after compensatory hypertrophy. A proliferation of small caliber bile ducts (ductular reaction) has been confirmed in some cases by cytokeratin 19 immunohistochemistry. Dilated vascular structures devoid of blood, presumably small- and large-caliber lymphatics, are often prominent in the periphery of some portal triads. Dilated lymphatics may also be present in the connective tissue surrounding hepatic veins. In dogs, the spiral smooth muscle in the wall of the hepatic vein may be more prominent in dogs with shunts than normal dogs. There may be increased deposition of fibrous connective tissue surrounding portal triads and hepatic veins. Hepatocytes may contain cytoplasmic lipid droplets, and multiple small lipogranulomatous foci with hemosiderin and ceroid in Kupffer cells, and macrophages are typically present throughout the liver, especially in animals >1 year of age.

Primary portal vein hypoplasia (PVH) has been reported in dogs, particularly Cairn and Yorkshire Terriers, and

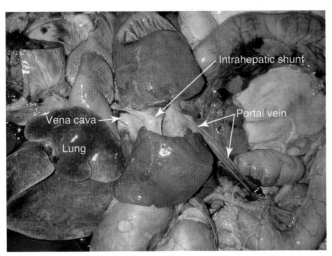

Figure 2-11 Congenital intrahepatic shunt, **persistent patent ductus venosus** in a dog. (Courtesy J.L. Caswell.)

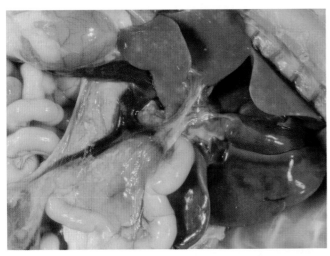

Figure 2-12 Congenital extrahepatic **portocaval shunt** in a cat.

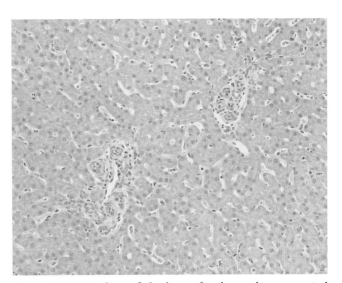

Figure 2-13 Histology of the liver of a dog with a **congenital portocaval shunt.** Closely spaced portal triads contain multiple sections of hepatic arterioles and lack discernable portal veins.

occasionally in cats, affecting either the extrahepatic or intra-hepatic portal vein, or both. Intrahepatic portal vein hypoplasia is considered to be the underlying lesion in conditions previously described as *microvascular dysplasia, hepatoportal fibrosis,* and *idiopathic noncirrhotic portal hypertension* in some young dogs. Depending on the level of the abnormality and extent of involvement of the lobes of liver, *PVH may be accompanied by portal hypertension, ascites and the development of multiple collateral portosystemic shunts.* Histologically, there is hypoplasia or absence of portal vein radicles, secondary arteriolar proliferation, and atrophy of hepatocytes. Moderate to marked portal fibrosis may also be present, with biliary hyperplasia. These changes represent stereotypic sequelae to under-perfusion and thus can be indistinguishable histologically from congenital portosystemic shunts; however, development of portal hypertension is a distinguishing feature of PVH.

Macroscopic PSS and microscopic portosystemic vascular anomalies may co-occur in dogs, as evidenced by a lack of resolution of clinical signs, and persistence of histologic changes in additional liver biopsies subsequent to macroscopic shunt ligation. Decreased tolerance of complete surgical shunt attenuation has been associated with lack of identifiable portal veins and the presence of a ductular reaction in biopsies taken during the initial surgical shunt attenuation procedure, although an earlier study showed no association of severity of several histologic findings, such as arteriolar proliferation, biliary hyperplasia, and fibrosis, with survival time after shunt attenuation.

Further reading

Berent AC, Tobias KM. Portosystemic vascular anomalies. Vet Clin North Am Small Anim Pract 2009;39:513-541.

Brown DL, et al. Congenital hepatic fibrosis in 5 dogs. Vet Pathol 2010;47:102-107.

Cullen JM, et al. Morphological classification of circulatory disorders of the canine and feline liver. In: Rothuizen J, et al., editors. WSAVA Standards for Clinical and Histological Diagnosis of Canine and Feline Liver Diseases. Philadelphia: Saunders Elsevier; 2006. p. 41-59.

Lee KCL, et al. Association between hepatic histopathologic lesions and clinical findings in dogs undergoing surgical attenuation of a congenital portosystemic shunt: 38 cases (2000-2004). J Am Vet Med Assoc 2011;239:638-645.

van den Ingh TSGA, et al. Morphological classification of biliary disorders of the canine and feline liver. In: Rothuizen J, et al., editors. WSAVA Standards for Clinical and Histological Diagnosis of Canine and Feline Liver Diseases. Philadelphia: Saunders Elsevier; 2006. p. 61-76.

DISPLACEMENT, TORSION, AND RUPTURE

The position of the liver should be observed as soon as the abdomen is opened at postmortem examination. Caudal displacements resulting in extension of the margins of the liver beyond the costal arch may be the result of hepatic enlargement or of displacement of the diaphragm secondary to pleural effusion or other space-occupying lesions in the thorax. Congenital or acquired displacements associated with ventral and diaphragmatic hernias are common. Individual lobes or the entire organ may be displaced into the subcutis, pleural cavity, or pericardial sac, often along with other viscera; lobar

blood supply may not always be compromised; however, individual displaced lobes may be severely congested and may rupture, or, given time, become indurated.

Partial or complete **liver lobe torsions** have been reported in pigs, dogs, cats, and horses. The left lateral lobe may be predisposed because of its mobility, large size, and relative separation from other lobes; however, torsions of other lobes, in particular the left medial lobe, as well as double-lobe torsions have been reported in dogs and horses. Other predisposing causes include absence of or damage to the ligamentous attachments that provide spatial support for the liver, trauma, or the presence of a mass lesion in the affected lobe. Torsed lobes undergo various degrees of ischemia, culminating in infarction caused by venous occlusion or venous and/or arterial thrombosis, and affected animals may die because of shock, hemorrhage, or development of septic peritonitis. Ischemia may favor overgrowth of *Clostridium* spp. with development of necrosis and emphysema. Subacute cases may develop hepatic abscessation, and if the animal survives, fibrosis and chronic inflammation.

Rupture *of the liver occurs commonly as the result of trauma because the organ is fragile relative to its mass.* Fatal liver rupture may be produced by the sudden accelerations and pressures of vehicle collisions without much evidence of trauma to other parts of the body. Large tears may be obvious in the liver capsule and hepatic parenchyma after trauma; however, anastomosing linear patterns of fine shallow capsular fissures may be concealed in part by clotted blood. Liver rupture is often clinically occult, because quite large ruptures may not disturb liver function unless severe enough to cause rapid exsanguination, or unless the biliary tract is involved. Intrahepatic bile duct rupture results in bile extravasation into the hepatic parenchyma or beneath the hepatic capsule, forming bile lakes or bile infarcts, areas of hepatocyte degeneration, and necrosis surrounded by reactive macrophages; larger accumulations of bile may be walled off by a pseudocapsule, forming biliary pseudocysts. Rupture of major bile ducts or the gallbladder results in yellow-stained *bile peritonitis,* which may remain sterile and become chronic, or may be fatal, particularly if infected by enterohepatic circulation of bacteria such as clostridia.

The liver is more likely to rupture after trauma in young animals. Fatal ruptures occur in foals during parturition, sometimes concurrently with costal fractures, and in the smaller species subject to energetic emergency resuscitation. Diffuse hepatic conditions with enlarged friable parenchyma (e.g., acute hepatitis, amyloidosis, severe congestion, severe lipidosis, and infiltrating neoplasms) are more likely to rupture, sometimes spontaneously, and the clinical consequences are related to the extent of hemorrhage. Parasites that penetrate the capsule cause numerous small ruptures but seldom lead to significant hemorrhage.

Further reading

Banz AC, Gottfried SD. Peritoneopericardial diaphragmatic hernia: a retrospective study of 31 cats and eight dogs. J Am Anim Hosp Assoc 2010;46:398-404.

Hinkle SG, et al. Liver lobe torsion in dogs: 13 cases (1995-2004). J Am Vet Med Assoc 2006;228:242-247.

Tennent-Brown BS, et al. Liver lobe torsion in six horses. J Am Vet Med Assoc 2012;241:615-620.

HEPATOCELLULAR ADAPTATIONS AND INTRACELLULAR ACCUMULATION

The liver must be highly adaptable to balance function with changing demand. Increases in the size of hepatocytes *(hypertrophy)* and their numbers *(hyperplasia)* collectively bring a larger mass of hepatocytes into service. Such adaptations in hepatic volume and function result from alterations in the expression of many genes. These responses are more evident in smaller species, notably in laboratory rodents that have a very pronounced liver growth response after exposure to various xenobiotics. The liver can also adapt to reduced demand or oxygen supply by a combination of *cellular atrophy* and *apoptosis*. Hepatocytes can be lost by apoptosis in substantial numbers, with minimal elevation in serum enzymes of hepatic origin such as alanine aminotransferase.

Hepatocellular atrophy

Hepatic mass readily adapts to metabolic demands, and *the liver can undergo marked atrophy during illness and/or starvation without much evidence of impaired hepatic function.* During prolonged starvation, some hepatocytes are removed by apoptosis without replacement, but most of the atrophy is explained by loss of cytoplasmic mass. Atrophic livers, as seen, for example, in old grazing herbivores with poor teeth, are dark and small, and the capsule may appear too large for the organ, showing fine wrinkles on handling. These livers may even appear to be firmer than normal because of condensation of normal stroma. Histologically, portal triads and hepatic venules are closer together, and lobules contain increased numbers of smaller hepatocytes with scanty cytoplasm (Fig. 2-14). *Hepatocellular mass can be rapidly lost by autophagy and apoptosis* (see later section on Types and patterns of cell death in the liver).

Hepatic atrophy, rather than hepatocellular atrophy, can also result from impaired replication of hepatocytes. Most adult hepatocytes are replicatively competent, although mitotic figures are infrequent because healthy hepatocytes have a relatively long life-span of several months. Diminished portal blood flow not only limits oxygen, but also trophic factors that act to regulate replication and mass of the liver. These trophic factors include several polypeptide growth factors, including hepato-cyte growth factor and insulin-like growth factors, and many hormones, including insulin, glucagon, and catecholamines.

Atrophy of only a part of the liver may be a response to pressure or to impairment of blood or bile flow. The histologic features of this atrophy are similar to those of starvation atrophy. However, the functional consequences of focal hepatic atrophy are minor because the remaining liver can compensate and adapt by a process that involves replication and enlargement of hepatocytes. Local pressure atrophy occurs adjacent to space-occupying lesions in the liver, or as a result of chronic pressures from neighboring organs, such as distended rumen in the ox. It has been suggested that *right hepatic lobe atrophy*, reported in horses, results from long-term compression from abnormal distension of the right dorsal colon and base of the cecum (eFig. 2-3). Chronic diffuse diseases of the biliary tract, such as sporidesmin poisoning and fascioliasis, are likely to cause atrophy of the left lobe in ruminants, possibly as a result of the greater difficulty in maintaining adequate biliary drainage from this lobe, whose bile ducts are longer than those of the right in these species. The atrophy of biliary obstruction is complicated by some degree of superimposed inflammation and fibrosis.

Hepatocellular hypertrophy

Hypertrophy is the term used for the increase in liver size caused by an increase in hepatocyte volume that may result from expansion of one or more organellar components of the hepatocytes. *Exposure to various xenobiotics can induce the expression of many genes, leading to expansion of the smooth endoplasmic reticulum (SER), resulting in hepatocyte hypertrophy.* Agents that elicit this response act via nuclear receptors, such as the arylhydrocarbon-activated receptor, the constitutive androstane receptor, or the pregnane X receptor. Phenobarbital, for example, is a potent inducer of the various enzyme systems of the SER, including several cytochromes P450 (CYPs). Hypertrophy may occur in defined lobular regions, typically the centrilobular region or may affect the entire lobule in more advanced cases, depending upon the activity and dose level of the xenobiotic (Fig. 2-15). Even when it is restricted to the centrilobular region, hypertrophy usually enlarges the entire liver. Although hepatocellular hypertrophy is most often associated with preferential increase in SER,

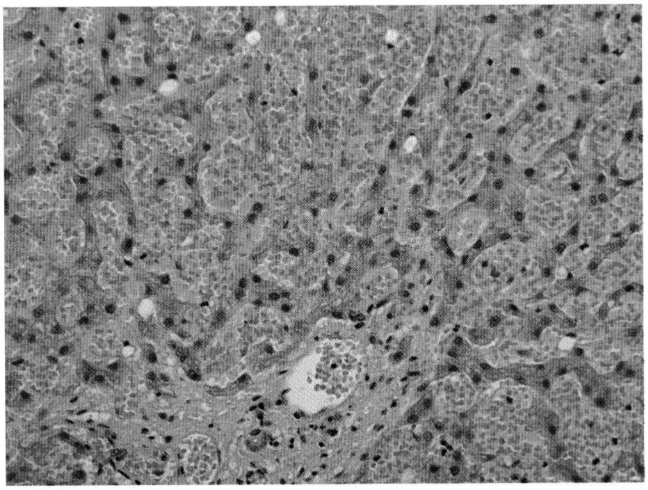

Figure 2-14 Hepatocellular atrophy in a dog with chronic right-sided heart failure.

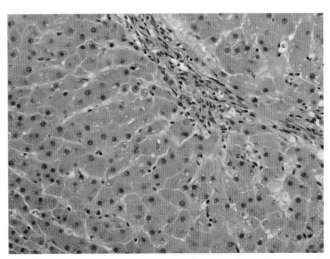

Figure 2-15 Increased cytoplasmic volume resulting from **smooth endoplasmic reticulum induction** in a dog treated chronically with phenobarbital.

proliferation of peroxisomes, or mitochondria can also cause hepatocellular hypertrophy. The light microscopic appearance of hypertrophy upon routine hematoxylin and eosin (H&E) staining will sometimes suggest the selective involvement of one organelle. If total SER volume is increased, the cytoplasm will typically have an eosinophilic ground-glass appearance upon light microscopy. If total peroxisomal volume is increased, the cytoplasm is often noted to have an eosinophilic granular appearance. The response can be seen within a few days after exposure to various drugs and other xenobiotic compounds. Accordingly, the liver becomes grossly enlarged. This induction of SER or peroxisomes is reversible, and after discontinuation of exposure to the inducing agent, the expanded SER or excess peroxisomes are removed by autophagy, and many hepatocytes undergo apoptosis. Although these changes are considered physiologic adaptations, there are potential adverse sequelae; accordingly, this response has toxicologic significance, and will be dealt with later in the section on Toxic hepatic disease.

Polyploidy and multinucleation

Most mature mammalian hepatocytes are tetraploid or octaploid, whereas many immature and replicating hepatocytes are diploid. The relative proportion of polyploid hepatocytes varies among species, and polyploidy increases with age. Polyploidy is more common in rodents and is believed to result from asynchrony of cell division in which binucleated diploid cells undergo a second round of DNA replication, giving rise to 2 tetraploid daughter cells. Impaired replication can also increase the number of polyploid cells. The term **megalocytosis** was first used to describe the changes of liver cell cytoplasm and nucleus that occur in pyrrolizidine alkaloid poisoning. This form of megalocytosis has some specific features and is described in the later section on Chronic hepatotoxicity. Impaired regeneration, atrophy and >4N polyploidy can also be produced by other DNA-damaging agents such as aflatoxins. A feature of these patterns of atrophy with polyploidy is the persistence of larger replicatively impaired polyploid hepatocytes amid regenerating smaller diploid hepatocytes, hepatocellular nodules, and hyperplastic bile ductules.

Most hepatocytes are mononuclear, but a variable proportion is binucleated, especially in young or regenerating livers of small animals. Multinucleation by more than 2 nuclei of non-neoplastic hepatocytes is a rare phenomenon in domestic mammals, and its diagnostic or pathogenetic significance is usually unclear. Multinucleation can result from incomplete cell division or cell fusion, but this distinction is difficult to determine. Hepatocytes can fuse during severe steatosis, but the degree of multinucleation in fatty livers is hard to discern because the plasma membrane perimeters of fatty hepatocytes are ill defined. Syncytial multinucleation of hepatocytes has been observed in various degenerative and regenerative conditions. In protoporphyria of Limousin cattle, small clusters of hepatocytes contain 4-10 or more closely packed nuclei, but it is not clear whether this represents fusion or multiple nuclear divisions. Syncytial hepatocytes are a characteristic of postinfantile giant cell hepatitis of children, and similar hepatocyte multinucleation can be observed in association with some forms of hepatitis in newborn cats, foals, and piglets (see Inflammatory diseases of the liver and biliary tract). Multinucleated hepatocytes have been described in young cats with thymic lymphomas, and in cats with experimental dioxin poisoning.

Intranuclear inclusions

In addition to the various nuclear inclusions associated with some viral infections, *3 types of inclusions may be found in hepatocyte nuclei.*

1. Spherical, apparently hollow globules within the body of the nucleus are *membrane-bound entrapped nuclear membrane invaginations* that ultrastructurally contain cytoplasmic components such as glycogen and mitochondria. These inclusions are infrequent in otherwise normal livers but are more often seen in chronically injured livers, especially in chronic pyrrolizidine alkaloid poisoning, in which polyploid nuclei are more likely to indent and invaginate.
2. Eosinophilic block-like intranuclear inclusions with a regular crystal lattice (*"brick inclusions"*) are common in hepatocytes and renal proximal tubular epithelium. They are more numerous in old animals, particularly dogs. Their composition and pathogenesis are still unknown, but they evidently have little effect on the health of the cells in which they occur, even when they are large enough to distort the nucleus. They do not contain heavy metals and can be distinguished from the acid-fast, noncrystalline intranuclear inclusions observed in renal epithelial cells and occasionally in hepatocytes in lead poisoning.
3. *Lead inclusions* consist of a lead-protein complex and have a characteristic furry electron-dense ultrastructure.

Pigmentation

Congenital melanosis occurs in calves and occasionally in lambs and swine. The melanin deposits may be numerous, and vary in size from flecks, to irregular, blue-black areas 2 cm or more in diameter. The melanin is confined to the capsule and the stroma. These deposits are sharply defined in young animals, but become more diffuse and fade with age (eFig. 2-4).

A condition known as **acquired melanosis** is the massive accumulation of black pigment (not melanin) in hepatocytes and Kupffer cells of mature sheep and, less frequently cattle, after prolonged grazing on extensive unimproved pastures in inland eastern Australia, the Falkland Islands, and Scandinavia. The condition in Norway has also been described as *hepatic lipofuscinosis.* The color of the affected livers ranges from a dull gray to uniform black, and there is usually a prominent acinar pattern. In severe cases, there is also pigmentation of the hepatic lymph nodes, lungs, and renal cortex. Histologically, the pigment is present as granules in lysosomes in periportal and midzonal hepatocytes and macrophages of the liver, the proximal tubular epithelium of the kidneys, and in alveolar and interstitial macrophages in the lung. There is no evidence of liver dysfunction, even in the blackest livers. The source of this pigment is not known, but the epidemiologic features of its occurrence indicate that it is derived from a component of the diet that is sequestered within lysosomes.

Bile pigmentation may impart an olive-green color to the liver in diffuse or segmental obstructive biliary disease or intrahepatic cholestasis. Histologically, conjugated bile pigments may distend bile canaliculi, visible microscopically as golden-brown linear streaks arrayed in a chicken wire-like pattern between the hepatocytes (Fig. 2-16). In this case, the identity of the pigment is obvious, but when it is present in granular form in Kupffer cell cytoplasm, it may easily be confused with hemosiderin and hematin. Bile pigment is encountered infrequently in hepatocyte cytoplasm, almost never in

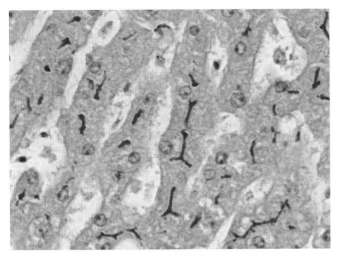

Figure 2-16 Bile plugs distend bile canaliculi in a horse with intravascular hemolysis following ingestion of red maple leaves.

dogs, except in rare cases with dramatic cholestasis. Death of individual hepatocytes releases the canalicular plugs into the space of Disse and the sinusoids, where they may be phagocytosed by Kupffer cells.

Lipofuscin *is the term given to small, golden, granular cytoplasmic deposits derived from the lipid component of membranous organelles,* more obvious in hepatocytes near the centrilobular areas. Lipofuscin accumulates in hepatocellular lysosomes and indicates senility, atrophy, or increased turnover of membrane lipids. The pigment is particularly common in the centrilobular regions of the liver of cats after they reach maturity. **Ceroid** is a yellow pigment similar to lipofuscin and is associated with *peroxidation of fat deposits.*

Black pigment also accumulates in hepatocellular lysosomes of mutant Corriedale sheep with hyperbilirubinemia. These sheep have a condition resembling the human Dubin-Johnson syndrome, in which there is mutation in the canalicular transporter in the organic anion-transporting polypeptide family. This suggests that retention of the pigment might be a sequel to a hepatic excretory defect.

In **congenital erythrocytic protoporphyria** (ferrochelatase deficiency) of Limousin and Blonde d'Aquitaine cattle, a dark golden-brown lipofuscin-like lysosomal material is present in portal areas, Kupffer cells, and sinusoidal endothelial cells, and is heavily concentrated in the cytoplasm of hepatocytes.

Acquired protoporphyria (Fig. 2-17A, B) with liver injury has been described in German Shepherd dogs as an idiopathic syndrome and in a group of Beagle dogs treated with an experimental drug. Grossly, affected German Shepherd dogs had dark livers that contained multiple regenerative nodules. Histologically, there was abundant bridging portal fibrosis and typical orange birefringent protoporphyrin crystals in hepatocytes. Photosensitization was not evident. Hepatic vacuolation and nodule formation has also been described in a cat with porphyria.

Hemosiderin deposits are seldom sufficient to give gross discoloration, but when this occurs, the color is dark brown. The pigment is detected microscopically as yellow or brown crystals chiefly in the Kupffer cells, although small amounts may be found in hepatic cells. The ferric iron component of this pigment can be demonstrated by *staining with Prussian blue;* otherwise, it can easily be confused with lipofuscin. *Most hemosiderin deposits are punctate Prussian blue staining*

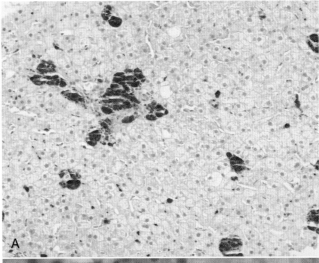

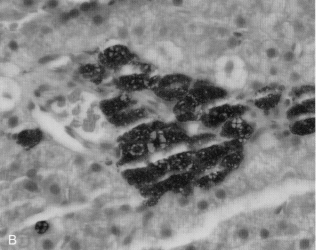

Figure 2-17 A. Dark golden-brown **protoporphyrin crystals** in the liver of a dog. **B.** Protoporphyrin crystals with bright red **Maltese cross** birefringence when viewed under polarized light.

aggregates in Kupffer cells but can also be seen as finer particles in hepatocytes. Diffuse hemosiderin deposits in Kupffer cells occur quite commonly in all species, and its presence is usually *suggestive of excess hemolytic activity* relative to the rate of reutilization of iron. Thus it is seen in hemolytic anemia, anemia of copper deficiency, in cachexia, and after blood transfusions or iron injections. It may be seen in Kupffer cells of the centrilobular zones in severe chronic passive congestion of the liver. Localized hemosiderin deposition occurs in areas of hemorrhage. Hemosiderin is normally present in the liver in the early neonatal period, when fetal hemoglobin is being replaced by mature hemoglobin.

Hemosiderin should be distinguished from **hematin,** which is produced by the action of formic acid on hemoglobin following a prolonged postmortem interval, and is usually regarded as a *histologic artifact.* Hematin is also an iron-containing pigment, but the iron is in the reduced ferrous state and does not stain with ferricyanide. It takes the form of crystalline brown deposits that are birefringent under polarized light, mainly within hemoglobin-rich areas such as blood vessels. Hematin is darker than hemosiderin and occurs in irregular clumps, often extracellularly. Hematin may, however, be found in Kupffer cells and macrophages in small amounts.

Hepatic iron overload has previously been divided into **hemosiderosis** when there is only an excess accumulation of hepatocellular iron and **hemochromatosis** when the excess iron storage has produced fibrosis and inflammation and hepatic injury, although this terminology is not used consistently. Hemochromatosis, as an inherited disorder is relatively common in humans with specific mutations. Iron overload is common in some birds, such as mynahs, and in lemurs, but rare in domestic mammals. A form resembling heritable hemochromatosis has been reported in Salers or Salers-cross cattle. Affected animals develop a wasting disease at ~1-2 years of age, have a 30-100 fold increase in liver iron content, with dark-brown discolored, firm livers, hemosiderin accumulation in hepatocytes, and periportal and perivenular bridging fibrosis with nodular regeneration. Hemosiderin also accumulates in Kupffer cells, lymph nodes, kidney, pancreas, spleen, and other organs.

Iron overload from dietary excess has been observed in sheep and cattle exposed to *high levels of iron in pasture and water.* The liver is enlarged and brown with diffuse fine nodularity, and the hepatic and adjacent lymph nodes are also darkened. Large amounts of iron are present in the hepatic parenchyma, the biliary epithelium, and the cortex of lymph nodes, and lesser amounts are present in the broad fibrous septa. The iron is stored predominantly in lysosomes. Brown discoloration of bone marrow resembles the osseous pigmentation of porphyria. The pathogenesis of nutritional iron overload is unknown. Iron overload has also been described in horses, with animals displaying signs of liver failure and neurologic impairment. The microscopic lesions in the livers of these animals are similar to those for other species.

Brown crystalline deposits of **2,8-dihydroxyadenine (2,8-DHA)** have been described in hepatocytes and in other tissues in slaughtered cattle with no evidence of other disease. These accumulations are strongly birefringent under polarized light, and are seen in the cytoplasm of hepatocytes and macrophages of hepatic lymph nodes and as extracellular deposits in portal stroma and renal tubular lumens. Grossly, the portal stroma stands out as a green network, and affected lymph nodes were enlarged, and the medullary sinusoids were distended with green pasty material. The crystals were identified as 2,8-DHA by a panel of crystallographic methods and mass spectrometry. The pathogenesis is unknown.

Pigments of parasitic origin are particularly associated with flukes. Heavy deposits of *black iron-porphyrin compound* are formed around the cysts and migratory pathways of *Fascioloides magna.* Lesser amounts of similar pigment are deposited in bile ducts infested by *Fasciola hepatica* (see later section on Helminthic infections). The presence of this pigment in the hilar nodes should suggest otherwise inapparent infestations by flukes. In schistosomiasis, the liver may be gray because of the accumulation of black pigment in Kupffer cells.

Vacuolation

The term "**vacuolar hepatopathy**" *has been used to denote multifocal or diffuse zonal hepatocellular cytoplasmic vacuolation* before a more specific term can be applied, for example, before contents of vacuoles are identified. Specific forms of hepatocyte vacuolar change include hydropic swelling, glycogenosis, and steatosis (lipidosis). **Hydropic degeneration** can only be appreciated in carefully controlled experimental circumstances and is an early cytoplasmic ballooning seen after various toxic and metabolic insults, hypoxia, and cholestasis. Water and sodium ion influx expands membranous

compartments of mitochondria, lysosomes, and endoplasmic reticulum (ER). The term **feathery degeneration** is applied to the type of hydropic change that occurs in hepatocytes in which there has been prolonged cholestasis. The cells are swollen and vacuolated and crisscrossed by a fine protoplasmic network that is brown with bile pigments (Fig. 2-18). This change is uncommon in cats and dogs.

Hepatic glycogenosis or **glucocorticoid hepatopathy**, often referred to as **steroid-induced hepatopathy,** is probably the most severe example of hepatocellular vacuolar change in dogs. *It involves glycogen accumulation induced by hyperadrenocorticism, because of either functional adrenocortical or pituitary tumors, or to treatment with glucocorticoids.* The liver is enlarged and pale tan. Hepatocytes are swollen, and the cytoplasm appears as fine, diaphanous strands that enclose multiple spaces with poorly demarcated edges. Vacuolar change may range from mild to severe, with swelling of hepatocytes from 2-10 times normal size and displacement of the nucleus and organelles to the cellular periphery (Fig. 2-19). The zonal distribution may be very variable and may become diffuse in long-standing cases or with higher doses. Single-cell drop-out, multifocal small aggregates of neutrophils along sinusoids, and

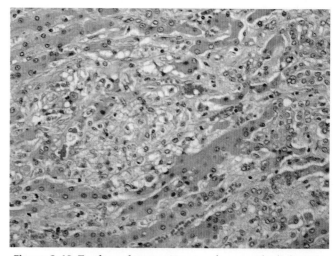

Figure 2-18 **Feathery degeneration** in a horse with cholestasis.

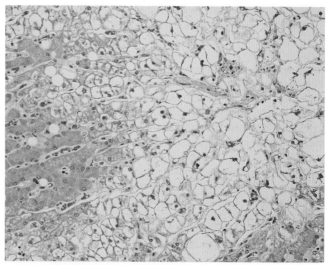

Figure 2-19 **Prominent vacuolation of hepatocytes** following **glucocorticoid administration** in a dog.

scattered small foci of extracellular hematopoiesis are also commonly observed. The ill-defined vacuolar boundaries in steroid hepatopathy are readily distinguishable from spherical lipid vacuoles in hepatic steatosis. *The pathogenesis of this condition is uncertain,* because glycogen storage alone does not fully explain the influx of fluid, and possible perturbations in hepatocellular ion channels or aquaporins have not been assessed. The amount of glycogen remaining in affected cells is widely variable, a function of the original glycogen concentration, recent catabolism, and postmortem dissolution. Glycogen content can best be demonstrated in frozen section, followed by staining with periodic acid–Schiff, and can be confirmed as glycogen by its sensitivity to digestion with diastase. Livers affected by glucocorticoid hepatopathy maintain normal hepatocyte functions, but the condition can be confirmed by the induction and *serum increase of glucocorticoid-inducible alkaline phosphatase,* with minor or negligible increases in alanine aminotransferase. Similar vacuoles may be created by other adrenocortical steroids, possibly progestins, as occasionally seen in older, female dogs that appear to have overproduction of adrenal cortical hormones other than cortisol and alkaline phosphatase elevation, although the specific pathogenesis is unknown. Some drugs, such as the chelator D-penicillamine, can produce similar vacuolation.

Loss-of-function mutations in hepatic and renal glucose-6-phosphatase resulting in increased hepatic glycogen storage have been reported in Maltese puppies or related crossbred dogs, and these dogs serve as an animal model of **glycogen storage disease (glycogenosis) type Ia.** These dogs have severely debilitating problems in maintaining their blood glucose because dephosphorylation of glucose-6-phosphate is a key step in both glycogenolysis and gluconeogenesis. The condition is typified by severe hepatocellular glycogenosis. Livers are markedly enlarged, pale, and have diffuse vacuolation of hepatocytes with large amounts of glycogen and small amounts of lipid. Hepatic fibrosis and nodular regeneration can develop with time. Renal tubular epithelium is also vacuolated. Glycogen storage disease **type III,** with hepatic glycogen storage, has been reported in dogs, predominantly German Shepherd dogs. **Type IV** glycogenosis has been reported in Norwegian Forest cats, although this disorder causes pale blue granules in hepatocellular cytoplasm rather than clear vacuoles.

Characteristic hepatocellular vacuolation is also described in dogs with end-stage nodular livers presented clinically with *hepatocutaneous syndrome.*

Hepatocellular steatosis (lipidosis)

Hepatocellular steatosis *is the term used to describe fatty livers of animals. However, the terms steatosis, lipidosis, and fatty change tend to also be used interchangeably.* All of these terms refer to the *visible accumulation of triglycerides (triacylglycerols) as round globules in the cytoplasm of hepatocytes.* The threshold for application of these terms is vague because triglyceride storage and transport are normal hepatic functions, but they are appropriate when the amounts are greater than would normally be seen. Hepatocellular steatosis can be physiologic or pathologic. Any circumstance in which hepatic uptake of lipids exceeds oxidation or secretion can lead to hepatocellular steatosis. Increased mobilization of triglycerides during *late pregnancy or heavy lactation in ruminants* is associated with hepatocellular steatosis. The lipid represents increased transit of triglycerides in an otherwise healthy liver, so there is little diagnostic significance in mild degrees of hepatocellular

steatosis in lactating cows. In some of these animals, severe energy deficiency can also lead to clinical ketosis with metabolic acidosis. In addition, severe steatosis occurs in high-producing dairy cows fed diets in which either the mix of available fatty acids is incorrect or lipids are oxidized and rancid.

Hepatocellular steatosis is common in injured hepatocytes because the normal high throughput of fatty acids and triglycerides can be readily impeded at various points in the complex pathway of hepatic lipid metabolism and secretion of very-low-density lipoproteins (VLDLs). Hepatocytes obtain some fatty acids from albumin and other carrier proteins in the portal blood, but most is hydrolyzed by sinusoidal endothelial hepatic lipase from triglyceride in chylomicrons or VLDL in plasma. Very-long-chain fatty acids are initially oxidized by acyl–coenzyme A oxidase in peroxisomes to shorter acyl–coenzyme A that can be transported via a carnitine-dependent process into mitochondria for further oxidation. Although some fatty acid is used for energy in hepatic mitochondria, most from dietary or adipose sources is converted to triglycerides that are further processed into lipoproteins in the hepatocyte ER and actively secreted into the plasma as VLDL. Endothelial lipoprotein lipase in muscle and adipose tissue hydrolyzes triglycerides in the VLDL, and the fatty acids released are used locally by β-oxidation in mitochondria of muscle or re-esterified into triglyceride in adipocytes. The depleted VLDLs are returned by receptor-mediated endocytosis to hepatocytes, where their constituents are catabolized and recycled.

The synthesis and export of VLDL in hepatocytes are energy- and resource-dependent, so any disturbance of the supply of apoproteins (apoprotein B primarily), phospholipids, cholesterol, or ATP, or physical disruption of the organelles involved in synthesis, assembly, and secretion, has the potential to inhibit lipoprotein synthesis or secretion. Fatty acids can continue to enter hepatocytes, allowing triglyceride globules to accumulate in the hepatocyte cytoplasm. In some species, damage to peroxisomes reduces the initial peroxisomal oxidation step for catabolism of long-chain fatty acids and also upregulates various genes regulated by peroxisome proliferator–activated receptor-α. Lipoproteins in the ER, Golgi, and membrane-bound secretory vesicles can also accumulate if there is selective damage to the distal secretory apparatus. Damage by various toxic and hypoxic insults will not lead to triglyceride accumulation in hepatocytes if supplies of mobile triglycerides from adipose tissue or the diet are low.

The microscopic appearance of triglyceride globules in hepatocytes ranges from small discrete microvesicles to large coalescing macrovesicles. Microvesicular lipid vacuoles are smaller than the nucleus and tend not to displace the nucleus (Fig. 2-20). **Microvesicular steatosis** can be a hallmark of more severe hepatic dysfunction than macrovesicular steatosis. This pattern can occur in several toxic hepatopathies causing mitochondrial injury, including some drug toxicities, such as antiviral nucleosides, aspirin in Reye's syndrome, and excessive tetracycline administration, all of which can be fatal. These toxicities tend to target: mitochondria, disrupting energy production; the normal electron transfer chain, causing oxidative injury; and interfere with β-oxidation of lipids. Partially oxidized lipids typically have a lower surface tension than triglycerides and therefore form smaller vesicles in the aqueous medium of the cytoplasm. Uncontrolled diabetes mellitus and feline fatty liver syndrome can produce microvesicular hepatic

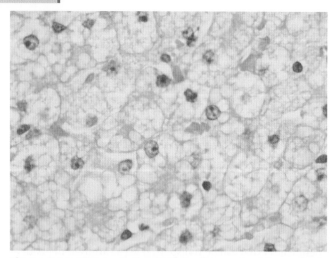

Figure 2-20 Microvesicular lipid is characterized by multiple round, clear vacuoles that are smaller than the nucleus and do not displace the nucleus.

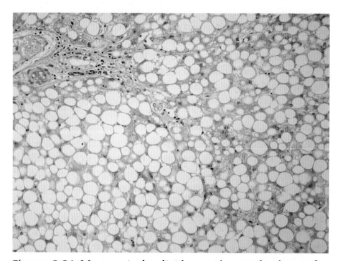

Figure 2-21 Macrovesicular lipid vacuoles in the liver of a donkey. Vacuoles are larger than the nucleus and tend to displace it to the periphery of the cell.

steatosis or a mixture of microvesicular and macrovesicular steatosis. Acute steatosis with predominantly microvesicular accumulation tends to result in a modestly enlarged pale liver without much change in texture, whereas macrovesicular hepatic steatosis more often produces an enlarged liver.

In some more protracted toxic injuries, smaller lipid globules can coalesce into large central **macrovesicles** *that displace the nucleus.* The pathogenesis of the larger globules is not well understood, but it involves some alteration of the globule-cytoplasm interface that normally prevents coalescence of the small micellar globules, possibly the greater hydrophobicity of the triglycerides. These fatty livers tend to be more yellow and enlarged, and the texture is more friable than livers with microvesicular steatosis. Each hepatocyte usually contains one large globule (macrovesicle) that alters the contour of the cell and displaces the nucleus (Fig. 2-21). The sinusoids are compressed and appear under-perfused, and the tissue at low magnification resembles adipose tissue. In severe degeneration, the liver is moderately or greatly enlarged, with a uniform light yellow color. The edges are rounded, and the surface is

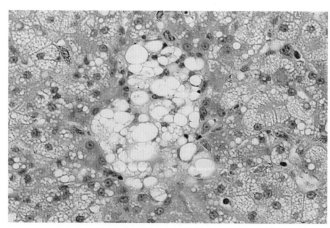

Figure 2-22 Fatty cyst in the liver of a dog.

smooth (eFig. 2-5). The cut surface has a diffuse greasy appearance or a red and yellow lobular pattern if there is also hepatic congestion or zonal necrosis. *In severe diffuse hepatic steatosis, the parenchyma is less dense, and portions will float in water or fixative.*

Assessment of the functional significance of steatosis depends on the differentiation of physiologic steatosis caused by increased mobilization by otherwise normal hepatocytes from pathologic changes that represent some degenerative change in hepatocytes. However, *fat accumulation is a sensitive response to hepatocellular injury and can occur in the absence of other obvious alterations in hepatic structure or function.* The triglyceride globules themselves are not harmful to hepatocytes, so the amount of fat present is more an indicator of the duration of insult and triglyceride supply than of the severity of hepatic injury. Steatosis is usually reversible, although a liver that has been fatty for some time is more likely to have concurrent damage, including fibrosis, pigment accumulation, and nodular hyperplasia, mostly attributable to ongoing peroxidative damage, cell turnover, and activation of stellate cells.

Hepatocellular steatosis is now recognized as a more significant indicator of potential, more severe liver injury than previously appreciated. In ruminants, the association between hepatic steatosis, ketosis, and displaced abomasum are well recognized. Infectious diseases, such as metritis and mastitis, may be more likely or prolonged. Neutrophil function is suppressed, as is interferon production by lymphocytes, and endotoxin clearance is also reduced. Hepatocytes become more sensitive to injury following exposure to cytokines such as tumor necrosis factor-α or endotoxin as well. Consequently, *fatty livers are more vulnerable to a wide range of toxic and nutritional insults,* so other necrogenic insults and responses can be concurrent. Increased levels of fatty acids in the liver increase the oxidative stress and contribute to membrane lipid peroxidation, reduced hepatocyte life-span, and some local repair responses.

When lipid accumulates in large amounts, there is a tendency for *groups of the fat-laden cells to rupture or fuse and eventually form a multinucleated rim about a foamy mass of lipid.* This epithelial structure is known as a **fatty cyst** (Fig. 2-22). The next stage, which occurs when released lipid is picked up by macrophages that form foamy aggregations in sinusoids, in the stroma of portal tracts, and hepatic venules is termed a **lipogranuloma**. Subsequent peroxidation of the less saturated fatty acids and covalent modification and

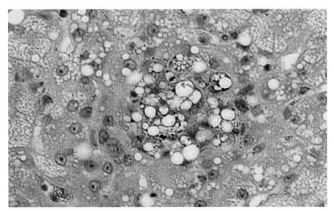

Figure 2-23 Pigment granuloma (lipogranuloma) in the liver of a dog.

polymerization of oxidized lipids form a complex of lysosomal residues known collectively as **ceroid**. This material is only slightly soluble in lipid solvents and is periodic acid–Schiff positive, diastase resistant, variably acid fast, and autofluorescent. In histologic sections, ceroid pigment appears as colorless or yellow irregular fragments associated with the lipid globules in macrophages and, to a lesser extent, hepatocytes. Affected portal lymph nodes become slightly enlarged, yellow-green, and rather oily on section. If iron accumulates along with the ceroid, the lesion is more correctly termed a **pigment granuloma** (Fig. 2-23). These are discrete perisinusoidal clusters of macrophages, containing cytoplasmic lipid vacuoles, lipofuscin, and hemosiderin, and often contain lymphocytes or plasma cells. They accumulate and congregate with age and hepatocellular turnover, but have no known clinical significance.

Some chronic changes commonly seen in the *livers of old dogs* can be associated with fatty liver; these include lipogranulomas, fatty cysts, and ceroid accumulation. Occasionally, there can be found sharply defined, fibrous, stony, hard masses, usually close to the surface, sometimes as much as 3-4 cm in diameter. These masses are usually sufficiently mineralized to show up distinctly on clinical radiographs. The mineral appears to be deposited on a matrix of degenerate collagen, laid down about perivascular foci of foamy macrophages and accumulations of cholesterol. The fibrous tissue may be laid down in response to the continued presence of fat, ceroid, or cholesterol, but no reason is apparent for the strictly localized distribution of the reaction. There are no recognizable hepatocytes in these lesions.

Physiologic steatosis (fatty liver) *occurs in late pregnancy and heavy lactation, particularly in ruminants and llamas.* In this circumstance, the lipid is typically macrovesicular, with large, round, clear vacuoles that tend to displace the nucleus. Obvious steatosis is also seen in neonates, especially in those species whose milk is relatively rich in fat. These livers are fatty enough to be pale to the naked eye. The high rate of mobilization of triglycerides from body fat stores is mainly responsible for fatty liver in lactating ruminants. However, fatty liver is a concern because lipid mobilization also increases when the dietary energy intake is insufficient relative to the production demands that are greatest in early lactation of high-producing cows. Insufficient dietary intake by an animal with adequate fat reserves depletes hepatocellular glycogen and initiates a heavy demand for triglycerides from adipose tissue. When hepatic triglyceride concentrations exceed 10%

on a wet weight basis, severe or clinical fatty liver ensues. At this time, urinary ketones are elevated, and body weight loss and appetite depression can occur. In severe cases, cattle can suffer from hepatoencephalopathy. It is estimated that in the first month after parturition 5-10% of dairy cattle severe fatty liver, and 30-40% have moderate fatty liver (5-10% liver triglyceride by wet weight basis). The liver depends primarily on fatty acid oxidation for its own considerable energy needs. It must also synthesize a large amount of protein and phospholipids for lipoprotein export to other tissues, and this can be rate limiting, resulting in accumulation of triglyceride in the cytoplasm. In starvation, the reduced availability of protein and lipotrope cofactors, such as choline, can exacerbate the bottleneck. The liver is the main supplier of glucose for the brain and milk saccharides, and it adapts by converting fatty acid metabolites to glucose (gluconeogenesis) and ketones.

Acute **ketosis** of lactating dairy cows with intake insufficiency or secondary to abomasal displacement is usually associated with fatty liver with a predominantly diffuse microvesicular pattern. *Cows are more tolerant of ketosis associated with lactation than are pregnant ewes that can die from starvation-induced* **pregnancy toxemia** *and ketoacidosis.* In cows, hepatic steatosis is predominantly centrilobular, whereas it is most severe in the periportal zone in pregnancy toxemia of sheep. The hepatic changes reflect increased mobilization of triglycerides from adipose tissue rather than hepatic disease per se. In cows and ewes with increased mobilization of triglycerides, there may be indistinct foci of white discoloration of abdominal fat that tend to be obscured when adipose tissue solidifies postmortem.

Fatty liver of **diabetes** *occurs when insulin is deficient or inactive* because of *lack of functioning receptors.* Reduced insulin-dependent glucose uptake by cells leads to accelerated lipolysis from adipose tissue in much the same way as when energy intake is limiting. The liver is thus presented with a large load of fatty acids, and the rate by which this moves through the liver can be impeded in various ways. Insulin deficiency alone will produce fatty liver. Some cases in carnivores are also complicated by concurrent exocrine pancreatic insufficiency, so protein malabsorption can be a contributing influence on diabetic hepatic steatosis. The centrilobular hepatocytes usually show the greatest degree of steatosis, but in advanced long-standing diabetes, the change is often diffuse and marked.

Lipoprotein synthesis and transport are dependent on oxidative metabolism, so **hypoxia** of hepatocytes leads to triglyceride accumulation. The 2 most common causes of hepatocellular hypoxia are *anemia* and reduced sinusoidal perfusion in *passive venous congestion.* In these situations, hepatic steatosis is most severe in the centrilobular zone, provided that the adipose and dietary supply of triglyceride is sufficient. Hepatic steatosis can be grossly visible as a yellow zonal pattern in chronic passive congestion of the bovine liver, but is less obvious in carnivores with passive hepatic congestion.

Local hypoxia is probably the basis for another example of fatty liver. Small, sharply demarcated patches of intense fatty infiltration are often seen in bovine livers at or adjacent to sites of capsular fibrous adhesions—so-called **"tension lipidosis."** These patches are neither swollen nor shrunken, usually extend <1 cm into the parenchyma, and are of the same consistency as normal liver (Fig. 2-24). The acinar structure of these lesions is undisturbed, but the hepatocytes therein show

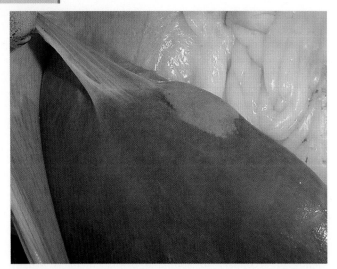

Figure 2-24 Subcapsular focal fatty change ("tension lipidosis") associated with capsular ligamentous attachment in an ox. (Courtesy A.P. Loretti.)

pronounced steatosis, presumably related to interference with local perfusion caused by tensions transmitted to the parenchyma by the adhesion.

Hepatic steatosis caused by **intoxication** is common. There are several stages of the cycle of hepatic lipid metabolism that can be affected selectively by various toxins to produce fatty liver. For example, it is possible experimentally to cause triglyceride accumulation by interfering with mitochondrial fatty acid oxidation with sublethal doses of cyanide, or by inhibiting apolipoprotein synthesis by administration of orotic acid. Most toxins that cause fatty liver in naturally occurring situations, however, also produce a greater or lesser degree of hepatocellular necrosis. Fatty liver occurring as a manifestation of toxic hepatic disease will be further discussed in the later section on Toxic hepatic disease, but the generalization may be made here that most important veterinary hepatic intoxications cause widespread membrane damage and/or disturbance of protein synthesis. These cause lipid accumulation in the hepatocyte by interfering with lipoprotein synthesis and export, as well as with fatty acid oxidation. *Steatosis requires time and a negative energy balance to develop, so it is more likely to occur in toxicoses with a longer clinical course.* However, if adipose reserves are depleted, there is less lipid available to accumulate in the liver.

Although fatty liver in domestic animals is more frequently associated with generalized interferences with energy metabolism, there are some specific **nutritional deficiencies** that will produce fatty liver. These have usually been defined under experimental conditions. *Choline deficiency*, in conjunction with deficiency of other lipotropic factors, such as *L-methionine* and *vitamin B$_{12}$*, rapidly produces fatty liver, largely as a result of reduced synthesis of phosphatidylcholine, a component of secreted lipoproteins. Fatty liver in experimental choline deficiency involves lipid peroxidation and increased hepatocellular turnover, leading to cirrhosis and neoplasia. It is unlikely that primary choline deficiency occurs in domestic animals, but other lipotrope deficiencies have been reported.

Ovine white-liver disease, first described in lambs in New Zealand, also occurs in southern Australia, the United Kingdom, and continental Europe. Goats are also susceptible. Ovine white-liver disease is characterized by a syndrome of ill-thrift to emaciation, anorexia, and mild normocytic normochromic anemia, occasionally with photosensitization and icterus. The condition is associated with low liver cobalt levels and low plasma concentrations of vitamin B$_{12}$, and the disease has been shown to be *cobalt and vitamin B$_{12}$ responsive.* Lambs up to 1 year of age are more commonly affected than ewes, and pastures are likely to be adequate at the times of peak incidence in late spring and early summer.

In the early stages, the liver changes consist of vacuolar accumulation of triglyceride in hepatocytes, usually most severe in the centrilobular zones. In addition, ceroid pigment is present in all cases, early in hepatocytes and later also in sinusoidal cells and macrophages. The fatty change may be very severe in the early stage, the liver being grossly swollen. A moderate degree of bile ductular proliferation is also a consistent feature, and the epithelium of the smaller ductules in the triads is dysplastic. Spongy degeneration of cerebral white matter, typical of the hyperammonemia of hepatic failure, is present in some cases.

Experimental feeding of a diet low in cobalt to sheep resulted in reduced growth rate, anorexia, lacrimation, alopecia, emaciation, and marked reduction in plasma and liver vitamin B$_{12}$ concentrations. At autopsy, livers were pale, swollen, and fatty. Histologically, livers with severe fatty degeneration were characterized by widespread hepatocyte disassociation, accumulation of lipid droplets, eosinophilic inclusions and lipofuscin in hepatocyte and Kupffer cell cytoplasm, nuclear lipid inclusions, ductular proliferation, and hepatocyte apoptosis. These lesions are characteristic of spontaneous cases of ovine white-liver disease. Ultrastructurally, degeneration of mitochondria and proliferation of the smooth endoplasmic reticulum are evident. The disease can be produced in cobalt-deficient sheep fed diets high in propionate precursors, which may help explain the explosive nature of outbreaks on lush pasture.

Hepatic lesions similar to lipotrope-deficient forms of experimental nutritional cirrhosis have been reported in sheep, goats, cattle, deer, and pronghorn antelope from Texas, New Mexico, and northeastern Mexico. *Hard yellow-liver disease, or* **hepatic fatty cirrhosis,** *is a progressive, chronic disease characterized by weight loss and hepatic encephalopathy* (eFig. 2-6). The disease typically appears in years following above-average winter rains, followed by drought conditions in the summer months. Grossly visible liver lesions in sheep begin in the subcapsular hepatic parenchyma along the porta hepatis as pale yellow, firm areas, spreading peripherally to involve ~80% of the liver in the final stages of the disease. Microscopic changes include accumulation of fine cytoplasmic lipid droplets in centrilobular hepatocytes, later involving the entire lobule, with rupture and formation of fatty cysts. Centrilobular fibrosis accompanies the ruptured fatty cysts, progressing to widespread bridging centrilobular fibrosis, with islands of regenerating hepatocytes. Kupffer cells and macrophages in regional lymph nodes, spleen, and lung contain abundant ceroid. The etiology of this condition is unknown, although unidentified hepatotoxins, possibly altering lipoprotein synthesis and secretion, combined with nutritional stress, have been postulated.

Equine hyperlipemia *is almost exclusively a disease of donkeys, miniature horses, and ponies,* and among these, the Shetland breed predominates. The syndrome is characterized by marked elevation of serum triglyceride concentration, predominantly very-low-density lipoprotein (VLDL), but other lipid fractions are also elevated, with visible prominent lipemia and hepatic steatosis. The condition is usually fatal after about a week. A negative energy balance is a key feature. Pregnant or lactating mares are most likely to develop the disease, particularly if they are older, excessively fat, and have recently suffered reduced feed intake because of onset of parturition, conditions such as laminitis or parasitism, or other causes of stress. The clinical course is marked by somnolence, complete anorexia, and colic, progressing to mania in some cases, although most simply become progressively more depressed. Some ponies develop ventral subcutaneous edema and most develop moderate diarrhea. Metabolic acidosis is a consistent feature in animals that die.

The liver at autopsy is severely fatty and may have ruptured; the steatosis also extends to heart and skeletal muscle, kidney, and adrenal cortex. *The hepatic steatosis is remarkable only by its severity;* there may be some focal hepatocellular necrosis, and there is consistent prolongation of bromosulfophthalein retention times and elevation of serum alkaline phosphatase levels. Evidence of disseminated intravascular coagulation is seen as serosal hemorrhages and microscopic thrombi in various organs, and even gross infarction of myocardium and kidney. *Small lipid emboli* may be detected in frozen sections of lung, myocardium, and brain in these animals; their relationship to the microthrombosis is uncertain.

The pathogenesis of this disease is obscure. Because the excess lipid in liver and blood is in the form of triglyceride, the implication is that the liver is capable of esterifying fatty acid mobilized from depot fat. The triglyceride thus formed is presumably then exported to the plasma as VLDL. It is believed that the primary cause of hyperlipemia is increased production via an increased rate of adipocyte lipolysis, leading to fatty acids and glycerol being released into the bloodstream and the increased hepatic synthesis of triglyceride as VLDL, rather than reduced clearance of VLDL from the serum. Another possibility is that there is an inability on the part of all tissues other than the liver to use fatty acids from VLDL at the normal rate, whereas triglyceride synthesis from fatty acids continues in the liver. In any event, at this stage lipids begin to accumulate in hepatocytes.

It has been proposed that an underlying cause of pony hyperlipemia is a *comparative resistance to insulin* in susceptible animals, and that this is compounded in stressful episodes by *increased levels of circulating cortisol.* Various steroid hormones, including glucocorticoids, have been shown to interfere with insulin action, and hyperlipemic ponies often have elevated plasma insulin levels, which suggests reduced function of insulin receptors. However, plasma ketones are much less consistently elevated, which appears to be characteristic of equids; this suggests that the increased ketogenesis that one might expect in insulin resistance is not a typical feature in horses.

Hepatic steatosis is common in *companion animals.* Following periods of stress or fasting, toy-breed dogs can develop profound hypoglycemia and a striking microvesicular hepatic steatosis. This may be the result of poor homeostasis of blood glucose levels. Most often, affected pups die from cerebral complications of hypoglycemia, but significant liver dysfunction also occurs. Dogs eating diets deficient in vitamin E may develop severe hepatic steatosis, but there are many circumstances in companion animals where the exact cause for individual cases of steatosis cannot be determined.

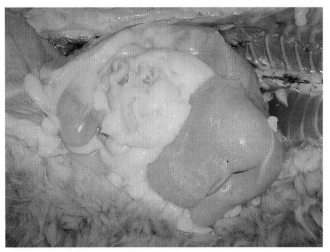

Figure 2-25 Hepatomegaly resulting from **hepatic steatosis** in a cat (Courtesy A.P. Loretti.)

The syndrome of feline hepatic steatosis *most commonly occurs in obese, nutritionally stressed female cats, which display vomiting, anorexia, weakness and weight loss, jaundice, and hepatomegaly* (Fig. 2-25). Neurobehavioral signs indicative of hepatic encephalopathy, other than drooling and depression, are rarely reported. Affected cats generally have hyperbilirubinemia, and a significant increase in serum alkaline phosphatase activity, in the face of normal or modest increases in γ-glutamyltranspeptidase activity, a key diagnostic feature of this syndrome. Untreated, the mortality rate is high. The liver has diffuse, macrovesicular or microvesicular steatosis, by definition affecting >50% of hepatocytes. Focal or zonal lipid accumulation in <50% of the parenchyma is considered more likely to be physiologic, or associated with other systemic abnormalities, rather than idiopathic feline hepatic steatosis. Bile pigment accumulates in canaliculi or Kupffer cells and can be confused with lipofuscin and ceroid.

The pathogenesis of hepatocellular triglyceride accumulation in this disease is obscure, and likely multifactorial, involving increased mobilization and uptake of nonesterified fatty acids by the liver, alterations in formation and release of VLDL, and impaired oxidation of fatty acids within hepatocytes. Ultrastructural studies have demonstrated decreased numbers and abnormal morphology of hepatic peroxisomes as well as mitochondria, both of which are important in the oxidization of fatty acids, but whether these changes are significant or simply adaptive responses is unknown. Starvation may reduce the availability of proteins, choline, and other precursors necessary for lipoprotein synthesis.

Severe hepatic steatosis can also develop in cats, *concurrent with or secondary to other major medical problems* such as diabetes mellitus, which alter metabolism of fat. Acute pancreatitis appears to be an important predisposing disease to secondary hepatic steatosis in cats—an association with clinical significance as it has a poorer prognosis than uncomplicated idiopathic hepatic steatosis. Secondary hepatic steatosis has also been reported with concurrent inflammatory liver disease, such as cholangitis, renal disease, small intestinal disease, neoplasia, and hyperthyroidism.

Familial hyperlipoproteinemia has been described in cats, associated with *congenital lipoprotein lipase deficiency.* The condition is characterized by lipid vacuoles and ceroid accumulation in liver, spleen, lymph nodes, kidney and adrenal glands, multifocal xanthomas, and focal arterial degenerative changes. An autosomal recessive mode of inheritance is suspected. **Primary idiopathic hyperlipidemia** has also been reported in Miniature Schnauzer dogs and Beagles, although the metabolic defect has not been identified. Affected dogs have fasting lipemia, elevated plasma VLDL, and may have hyperchylomicronemia. Affected animals may develop severe vacuolar hepatopathy associated with both glycogen and triglyceride accumulation, with eventual stromal collapse and regenerative nodule formation. There is also an association between hyperlipidemia and gallbladder mucocele.

An incompletely characterized condition known as **hepatic lipodystrophy** has been recognized in pedigree Galloway calves since 1965. Calves initially appear normal but develop lethargy, tremors, and opisthotonos, and die by 5 months of age. On postmortem examination, affected calves have an enlarged, pale, mottled liver. Histologically, there is marked hepatic steatosis with portal fibrosis and ductular reaction (Fig. 2-26). Vacuolar changes in the white matter of the brain are consistent with hepatic encephalopathy. A metabolic defect has been proposed.

Lysosomal storage diseases

In common with other tissues in animals with a heritable deficiency of specific lysosomal enzymes, liver cells may accumulate substrates normally catabolized by the missing enzyme. These lysosomal stores can be less obvious in the liver than in other tissues such as the central nervous system, and although they are unlikely to affect hepatic function, they can sometimes be recognized in liver biopsies (eFig. 2-7). However, *hydropic and fatty changes in hepatocytes can obscure or lead to misidentification of lysosomal storage vacuoles.* Kupffer cells and bile duct epithelium may be more severely affected than hepatocytes, which have additional catabolic and excretory pathways, including the ability for lysosomal exocytosis into the bile canaliculi. In animals with ceroid lipofuscinosis, lysosomal storage is minimal in hepatocytes compared to that in the brain. Examples of storage disorders associated with hepatomegaly and abnormal hepatic or Kupffer cell lysosomal inclusions include *GM$_1$ gangliosidosis* (β-1-galactosidase deficiency) in cats, *mucopolysaccharidosis type I* (α-L-iduronidase

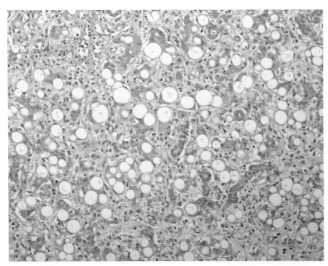

Figure 2-26 Hepatic steatosis, portal fibrosis, and bile duct hyperplasia resulting from **hepatic lipodystrophy** in a Galloway calf. (Courtesy M.J. Hazlett.)

deficiency) in dogs, and *α-mannosidosis* in cats. These and others are discussed in more detail in Vol. 1, Nervous system.

Hepatic **phospholipidosis** is an excessive accumulation of phospholipids within the cytoplasm of hepatocytes. This condition is an acquired storage disorder caused by some therapeutic drugs and chemicals, including amiodarone and chlorphentermine. Despite the diversity of agents capable of causing phospholipidosis, most of these are cationic amphipathic molecules. Mechanistically, phospholipidosis is caused by cationic amphipathic molecules binding to cellular phospholipids and inhibiting complete digestion by lysosomal phospholipase A1, A2, or C within lysosomes; although less often, direct inhibition of phospholipase can occur, as in the case of gentamicin. This leads to an accumulation of lysosomal phospholipids that can develop acutely or only following long-term drug administration. The histologic appearance of phospholipidosis can be quite variable, but typically, hepatocellular and Kupffer cell cytoplasm contains numerous round clear vacuoles that are smaller than the diameter of the nucleus or larger, imparting a foamy appearance to the cytoplasm. Fine vacuoles are most often apparent adjacent to canaliculi. Zonal distribution can vary depending on the type of drug or chemical. Biliary epithelium can also be affected, with or without hepatocellular involvement. The clear vacuoles can be confused with microvesicular steatosis, and in most cases, ultrastructural examination is needed to identify phospholipidosis with certainty. At the ultrastructural level, there is a characteristic multilaminated whorl of material with a "fingerprint" pattern, termed *myeloid bodies*, within affected lysosomes.

Amyloidosis

In most species, *hepatic amyloidosis is usually part of generalized amyloidosis.* **Systemic amyloidosis** of domestic animals is typically associated with overproduction of amyloid A (AA), an amino-terminal fragment of serum amyloid A, a highly inducible acute-phase protein in most species. In humans, AA amyloidosis occurs either as a familial trait (familial Mediterranean fever), or secondary to a sustained acute-phase reaction in chronic inflammatory or neoplastic diseases. Amyloid infiltration of the liver occurs sporadically in cattle, horses, dogs, and cats as a secondary response to chronic disease or tissue-destructive process. In horses, hepatic amyloidosis occurs chiefly as a result of chronic inflammation and has been well recognized in horses used for the production of hyperimmune serum. Horses may develop icterus and other signs of hepatic failure, but cattle die first of the primary disease or from uremia resulting from concurrent renal amyloidosis. Dogs and cats typically develop signs of renal dysfunction, although cats may be presented with spontaneous hepatic rupture. **Familial AA amyloidosis** is recognized in Chinese Shar-Pei dogs. The condition resembles familial Mediterranean fever in humans, and is characterized by febrile episodes, swollen hock syndrome, and the development of renal and sometimes hepatic amyloidosis. Familial AA amyloidosis is also recognized in Abyssinian cats and suspected in Siamese and Oriental cats.

Affected livers in horses are pale, enlarged with rounded edges, friable, and prone to fracture; in cattle, affected livers may be firm. Affected livers in all species are predisposed to rupture and bleeding (eFig. 2-8). Amyloid is deposited first in the parenchyma about the portal tracts and appears gray and waxy. Amyloid is deposited in the perisinusoidal space between the sinusoidal lining and hepatocytes and is sometimes found in the walls of the afferent vessels. The surrounded

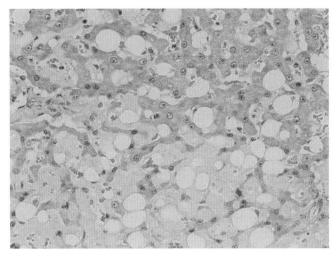

Figure 2-27 **Amyloid** in spaces of Disse compressing hepatocytes in a cat.

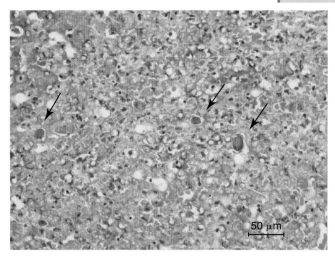

Figure 2-28 Three **apoptotic hepatocyte**s (arrows) in a region of injury in the liver of a dog.

hepatocellular cords atrophy. On H&E staining, amyloid appears as *homogeneous eosinophilic amorphous extracellular material* (Fig. 2-27). Staining with Congo red results in apple-green birefringence when viewed with polarized light. Thioflavine T stain produces yellow-green fluorescent staining of amyloid when viewed under ultraviolet light.

Further reading

Armstrong PJ, Blanchard G. Hepatic lipidosis in cats. Vet Clin North Am Small Anim Pract 2009;39:599-616.

Bobe G, et al. Invited review: pathology, etiology, prevention, and treatment of fatty liver in dairy cows. J Dairy Sci 2004;87:3105-3124.

Macleod NS, Allison CJ. Hepatic lipodystrophy of pedigree Galloway calves. Vet Rec 1999;144:143-145.

Mogg TD, Palmer JE. Hyperlipidemia, hyperlipemia, and hepatic lipidosis in American miniature horses: 23 cases (1990-1994). J Am Vet Med Assoc 1995;207:604-607.

O'Toole D, et al. Hepatic failure and hemochromatosis of Salers and Salers-cross cattle. Vet Pathol 2001;38:372-389.

Xenoulis PG, Steiner JM. Lipid metabolism and hyperlipidemia in dogs. Vet J 2010;183:12-21.

TYPES AND PATTERNS OF CELL DEATH IN THE LIVER

Irreversible damage leads to cell death that is evident histologically as long as the affected animal survives for a sufficient period of time, usually hours. Although all cells in the liver are susceptible, most interest and evaluation has been directed toward hepatocytes, biliary epithelium, and sinusoidal endothelium. The 2 predominant types of cell death are **necrosis,** also termed **oncotic necrosis,** and **apoptosis,** although there are other less common forms of cell death. These types of cell death can be separated mechanistically and histologically to a certain extent.

Types of cell death

In routine diagnostic settings, the terms apoptosis and necrosis can be based on descriptive criteria recognized in routine H&E-stained sections of liver. There have been attempts to refine the terminology and criteria for cell death in the liver, but this is still hindered by our incomplete understanding of different cell death pathways and cellular responses in various diseases.

Apoptosis

Apoptosis *is a form of programmed cell death that permits removal of cell debris without much leakage of cell contents or inflammation. Key features of apoptosis include retention of plasma membrane integrity until the later stages of the process; proteolysis of intracellular cytoskeletal proteins by aspartate-specific proteases, leading to collapse of subcellular components; chromatin condensation and marginalization; nuclear fragmentation; plasma membrane bleb formation; and eventual cell fragmentation into smaller apoptotic bodies bound by intact plasma membrane* (Fig. 2-28). *These bodies are rapidly phagocytosed and degraded by neighboring hepatocytes or Kupffer cells.* The rapid disappearance of these fragments means that very few apoptotic bodies in a section can indicate a rapid rate of hepatocellular death and turnover. Biochemically, apoptotic cells are characterized by phosphatidylserine on the outer surface of the cell membrane, increased mitochondrial permeability with release of internal proteins and activation of caspases.

Apoptosis is the main means of physiologic removal of damaged and aged cells and for remodeling of tissue. Liver mass is maintained by a balance of mitosis and apoptosis. Experimental support for the importance of this balance comes from studies of mutant mice deficient in the principal mediator of apoptosis, the receptor Fas (Fas/CD95), which develop prominent hepatocellular hyperplasia over time.

Apoptosis can be initiated by extrinsic or intrinsic events involving the death receptors or mitochondria, respectively. *Extrinsic mechanisms* can be activated via cell surface receptors termed death receptors when they bind their cognate ligands. Death receptors include Fas, tumor necrosis factor-α (TNF-α) receptor and death receptor 4 (DR4) and 5 (DR5). The main signaling molecules in the liver are the Fas ligand (FasL), TNF-related apoptosis-inducing ligand (TRAIL), and TNF-α. When the membrane-bound death receptors bind their ligand, they trigger formation of a multiprotein complex, the death-inducing signaling complex (DISC). Conformational changes in this complex trigger the activation of caspase 8, the key mediator of apoptosis and subsequent activation of the effector caspases: caspases 3, 6, and 7. More details on hepatocellular apoptosis are available in recent reviews.

Intrinsic mechanisms involve mitochondrial injury with release of proapoptotic factors. Activators of the latter pathway include oxidative stress, DNA damage, toxins, endoplasmic reticulum (ER) stress, including the unfolded protein response, lipid peroxidation, ultraviolet and γ-irradiation, and deprivation of growth factors. All of the pathways initiated by these agents converge on the mitochondria, leading to mitochondrial outer membrane permeabilization (MOMP). Mitochondrial membrane permeability is effected either through direct membrane damage, or more commonly by opening of regulated transmembrane pores by *bax* and other proapoptotic members of the *Bcl-2 family*. Cytochrome C and other intermembrane mitochondrial factors released from the mitochondrion form an apoptosomal complex in the cytoplasm that activates the distal caspase pathways, including caspase 9, that execute many of the cell fragmentation events. Alternatively, MOMP can be triggered by another mechanism involving multiprotein channels within the mitochondria, leading to swelling and release of proapoptotic molecules.

Functional classification of cell death has been developed on the basis of chemical rather than the histologic-morphologic criteria because different pathways can lead to similar morphologies. For example, intrinsic pathways can be divided into caspase-dependent and caspase-independent pathways.

Injury to the ER via oxidative stress, hypoxia, calcium depletion, inflammation, and altered glycosylation, among other mechanisms, leads to the *"unfolded protein response (UPR)"* that can also activate the distal caspase pathway by a separate mechanism. Hepatocytes are also susceptible to an intrinsic mechanism of apoptosis that is active after removal of hepatotrophic influences, including those that function via the constitutive androstane receptor, and other nuclear receptors. In addition, lysosomes can undergo selective membrane permeabilization, leading to a partial release of their contents in response to death signaling mediated by oxidative stress, some lipid mediators, and by Bcl-2 family members. Release of lysosomal proteases can cooperate with the caspase cascade or act in a caspase-independent fashion.

Both extrinsic and intrinsic pathways lead, in turn, to disruption of the cytoskeleton and nucleus primarily through the activation and direct action of caspases 3, 6, and 7. *An important feature of apoptosis is the requirement for adenosine triphosphate (ATP) to initiate the execution phase.* If the degree of mitochondrial damage is sufficient to exhaust ATP stores, membrane ion homeostasis deteriorates and leads to a mechanism of cell death more consistent with necrosis. For example, although mild to moderate oxidative stress may initiate intrinsic pathways of apoptotic cell death, processes leading to marked oxidative stress typically cause cell death by necrosis, not only resulting from the severity of mitochondrial damage, but also by direct inhibition of the proapoptotic caspase cascade.

Loss of cell anchorage to the extracellular matrix can activate a form of programmed cell death related to apoptosis that is termed **anoikis**. Detached cells can die intact, as in exfoliation, or undergo typical fragmentation into apoptotic bodies. Hepatocyte survival in vitro depends on their integrins that adhere to the extracellular matrix, but it is still unknown how loss of these contributes to cell death of hepatocytes in the intact liver.

Phagocytosis of apoptotic fragments follows flipping of phosphatidylserine from the inner leaflet of the plasma membrane to the outer leaf, where it can then be recognized by the phosphatidylserine scavenger receptor. Various assays can be used to detect portions of these pathways in hepatocytes; caspase-cleaved cytokeratin 18 can be recognized by antibodies to an internal domain, whereas chromatin fragmented by a calcium-activated endonuclease generates double-strand breaks that can be tagged by the terminal deoxynucleotide transferase-mediated dUTP nick-end labeling (TUNEL) technique. However, there are still few diagnostic situations in which these indicators have been shown to be useful. Increased numbers of apoptotic hepatocytes can be more readily assessed with a suitable cytologic marker. *In routine sections, a previous increase in apoptosis can be suggested by increased amounts of lysosomal debris and pigment in Kupffer cells, but this is not specific for apoptosis.*

Rapid phagocytic removal of apoptotic hepatocyte fragments can minimize secondary inflammation in cases of minor injury. However, phagocytosis of apoptotic bodies by Kupffer cells and hepatic stellate cells is not innocuous and can engender inflammation and fibrosis. Kupffer cells and resident macrophages express several ligands (TNF-α, TRAIL, and Fas ligand) that lead to increased hepatocyte apoptosis. Similarly, hepatic stellate cells are stimulated to release profibrotic cytokines and type 1 collagen following phagocytosis of apoptotic bodies. In addition, apoptotic cells release nucleotides ATP and uridine triphosphate (UTP), which can bind to purinergic receptors on macrophages and hepatic stellate cells and which may provide additional stimulus for fibrosis and inflammation. Excessive apoptosis is currently viewed as a driver of hepatic inflammation and fibrosis.

Necrosis

Necrosis *is morphologically recognizable by initial cell swelling and subsequent loss of plasma membrane integrity, leading to large organelle-free blebs and cell lysis.* Some authors prefer the term **"oncosis"** to emphasize the cell swelling response in necrosis to contrast with cell shrinkage in apoptosis (Fig. 2-29). Necrosis occurs when cells are depleted of ATP and

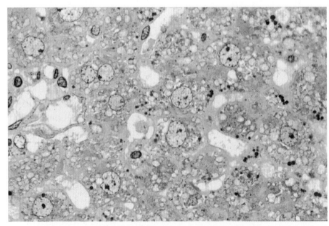

Figure 2-29 Necrosis of hepatocytes is initiated by cell swelling evident in this toluidine blue–stained section of liver. (Courtesy V. Meador)

lack sufficient energy to maintain membrane associated ionic pumps, leading to swelling and gross calcium influxes that result in disruption of the mitochondrial and plasma membranes, including release of lysosomal enzymes. Oncosis *is generally regarded as a severe injury to cell membrane integrity or other vital functions*, leading to enzyme leakage, inflammation, and tissue repair. *Release of cellular contents typically elicits a secondary inflammatory response and provides the serum enzymes that are useful clinically to detect liver necrosis.* However, these sequelae can also occur after hepatocyte apoptosis, either because the capacity for phagocytic removal of dead cells is exceeded, or because the insult worsens such that necrosis may supervene.

Necrosis is often a consequence of profound loss of mitochondrial function involving the opening of the membrane permeability transition (MPT) pore, a megachannel composed of inner- and outer-membrane proteins. This results in mitochondrial depolarization and ATP depletion because of inhibited oxidative phosphorylation. Poly-ADP-ribose polymerase (PARP) is a DNA repair enzyme that can deplete injured cells of available ATP when it is activated to repair the multitude of DNA strand breaks induced by cell damage. Conversely, PARP is swiftly cleaved in apoptosis to maintain ATP levels. Much of the ATP in hepatocytes is used for membrane homeostasis of Na^+, K^+, and Ca^{2+} ions. ATP depletion or physical damage to membranes of the cell surface, mitochondria, and ER leads to loss of ion homeostasis, altered cellular volume regulation, and increased intracellular calcium ion concentrations. Activation of calcium-dependent endonucleases, proteases (e.g., calpains), and phospholipases is responsible for the terminal events in necrosis. The source of calcium may influence the type of cell death, as calcium influx from the plasma membrane is associated with necrosis, but calcium released from the ER is more likely to trigger apoptosis. Newer evidence suggests that necrosis is not entirely a passive process. For example, necrosis can be initiated via cell surface receptor–driven processes when TNF is present in high concentrations.

The term **coagulative necrosis** *may be applied to groups or zones of intact, but dead hepatocytes that have shrunken slightly, stain intensely with eosin, and may have visible but distorted nuclei* (Fig. 2-30). These cells may also be dehydrated but,

unlike apoptosis, the removal of water is not an active process, and the affected cells do not undergo spontaneous fragmentation. It seems that coagulative necrosis, which is often seen in acute hepatotoxicity, is the *result of sudden and catastrophic denaturation of cytosolic protein*, which imparts a rather dense, rigid texture to the dead cells, somewhat preserving their shape. *The term* **lytic necrosis** *has been used for areas of necrosis in which the hepatocytes are disintegrating, usually in the presence of infiltrating phagocytes, especially neutrophils.* This is consistent with the later stages of postnecrotic inflammation that follow necrosis rather than apoptosis.

One might expect that the different types of cell death might be informative in relation to causes and pathogenesis. However, apoptosis, necrosis, and mixed responses are common in liver injury in vivo. Many insults can initiate either necrosis or apoptosis of hepatocytes; these include hypoxia, reactive oxygen metabolites, hepatotoxic chemicals, viral infections, bacterial toxins, and inflammation. Some of the molecular events are common to both. Mitochondrial damage and several other activation responses are common to apoptosis and necrosis, and programmed cell death responses can be activated before they are overwhelmed by more intense injury responsible for necrosis. Susceptibility therefore depends on many factors, including the level and duration of insults, replication status, and integrity of the various homeostatic and cytoprotective functions. Indeed, review of caspase-cleaved substrates reveals that different toxic drugs do not cause a uniform pattern of caspase activation and that it is likely that there are distinct pathophysiologic pathways of apoptosis. Clearly, apoptosis is not a consistent and stereotypic response.

There are important misconceptions regarding differences between apoptosis and necrosis and their effects on the liver. It is often assumed that apoptosis, unlike necrosis, leads to a "clean" death that does not provoke inflammation or elevation of transaminases and other markers of inflammation. However, there is evidence that phagocytosis of apoptotic bodies, termed *efferocytosis*, particularly by Kupffer cells can, in fact, activate the Kupffer cells and stimulate additional cell death. Various inflammatory markers are elevated in both acute and chronic apoptosis. The view that apoptosis, because it involves release of intact membrane bodies, does not lead to transaminase elevation has been shown to be incorrect in several studies. Injection of Fas ligands has been shown to produce significant increases in serum transaminases within hours and that this response is blocked in Bcl-2 transgenic mice. In addition, deletion of anti-apoptotic proteins results in elevated transaminase levels.

Other forms of cell death

There are a number of other forms of cell death. These include autophagy, pyroptosis, necroptosis, entosis, netosis, and parthanatos, which can be identified by biochemical means and specific forms of inhibition. A complete description is beyond the scope of this text.

Tissue patterns of cell death
Focal necrosis

Focal necrosis is very common in autopsy material. The lesions are microscopic or barely visible to the naked eye and are usually numerous. Their designation as focal depends on their size and on a random distribution relative to the lobules. There

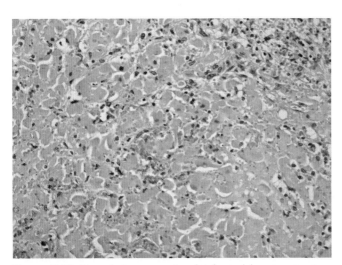

Figure 2-30 Coagulative necrosis of infarcted hepatocytes in a cat resulting from compression by an adjacent mass.

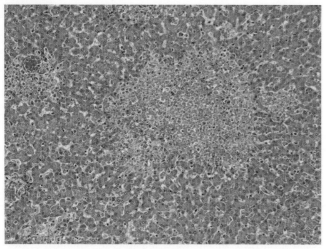

Figure 2-31 Focal necrosis caused by canid herpesvirus 1 in a dog.

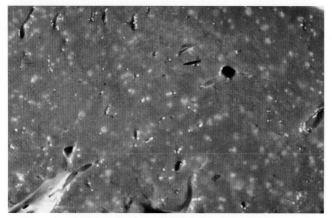

Figure 2-32 Focal hepatitis—the so-called **"sawdust liver"** of cattle.

may be a tendency for focal necrosis to occur nearer to the portal vessels than to the periphery of the circulatory fields, and to be concentrated in some lobular agglomerates rather than others.

Focal necrosis occurs in many infections, parasitic migrations, and instances of biliary obstruction, and in these, the designation **focal hepatitis** will often be more appropriate, because most are attended by some degree of focal inflammation. The infectious causes may be viral (Fig. 2-31) or bacterial. Many septicemic bacterial infections consistently produce focal hepatic lesions; examples are salmonellosis, tularemia, pseudotuberculosis, listeriosis in the fetus and newborn, and *Mannheimia haemolytica* septicemia in lambs. The focal necrosis may be the outcome of a Kupffer cell reaction, as in salmonellosis, or of bacterial embolism. The cause can usually be determined by histologic examination.

In cattle, focal necrosis in a few or many visible foci is common at autopsy and is common enough to be important at slaughter; it is responsible for the descriptive appellation *"sawdust liver"* (Fig. 2-32). The pathogenesis is not known and probably varies, but it may be caused by organisms from the gut that reach the liver in the portal blood. *The lesion is not specific and consists of focal parenchymal necrosis with disruption of reticulin fibers and infiltration of neutrophils and lymphocytes;*

frank suppuration does not occur. This lesion is said to be more frequent in livers from feedlot-fattened cattle.

Focal necrosis in biliary obstruction follows rupture of distended canaliculi or smaller cholangioles, with the formation of small bile lakes. Necrosis of larger bile ducts caused by neutrophilic cholangitis or destructive cholangitis can also release bile. The yellow pigment is readily visible microscopically and provokes small granulomas with giant cells.

Focal necrosis is of very little functional significance for the liver, even when numerous. The lesions heal with some scarring, but this too probably disappears in time. They are of diagnostic importance in some diseases such as salmonellosis, and as indicators of possible bacteremia for meat inspectors.

Lobular necrosis

Although various terms are used, the simplest way to visualize these patterns of necrosis is by using the hepatic lobule concept.

The time-honored designation "centrilobular necrosis" is a common lesion in response to intoxication or hypoxia. **Centrilobular (zone 3) necrosis** *is the most common form of zonal necrosis in domestic animals.* The hepatocytes in the centrilobular zone are particularly vulnerable to necrosis, in part because they are farthest from incoming arterial and portal venous blood bearing oxygen and essential nutrients. They also contain the greatest concentration of cytochromes P450 that activate various exogenous compounds into reactive metabolites capable of injuring or killing hepatocytes (see later section on Toxic hepatic disease).

Severe viral infections, such as canine adenovirus 1 and Rift Valley fever virus, can produce centrilobular necrosis, and the reasons for the increased susceptibility of the hepatocytes of this zone in these diseases are not established. Plausible explanations include zonal expression of entry receptors used by viruses to infect hepatocytes or ischemia-related hepatocellular swelling and sinusoidal damage because of virus-induced endothelial injury that reduce effective perfusion of the centrilobular hepatocytes.

Centrilobular degeneration and necrosis are seen commonly in animals that have died rather slowly. It is assumed that, in the agonal period, the hepatocytes in this zone are disproportionately affected by tissue hypoxia as a result of the failing circulation. This necrosis is more extensive if the animal is anemic. Centrilobular necrosis is also seen in passive venous congestion of the liver, most often in cases of acute and dramatic decompensation of cardiac function, as atrophy of hepatocytes is a more common outcome.

In the liver with centrilobular necrosis, there is usually a prominent zonal pattern, which takes the form of a fine, regular, pallid network of surviving, often fatty, hepatocytes in the periportal zone, which stands up above the red, collapsed areas adjacent to the hepatic venules (Fig. 2-33). The zonal necrotic insult frequently affects the sinusoidal endothelium, allowing erythrocytes to enter the perisinusoidal space and contribute to the redness of the necrotic zones. Histologically, necrosis is confined to the centrilobular region (Fig. 2-34), although bridging can occur in more severe cases (Fig. 2-35). Necrotic cells that are removed can be replaced by stagnant blood, at least in the acute phase. However, this red-on-yellow zonal pattern is difficult to interpret grossly because hepatic steatosis may also have a zonal distribution without having significant necrosis.

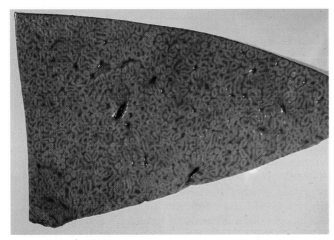

Figure 2-33 **Enhanced zonal pattern** of hepatocellular necrosis in a horse. (Courtesy R. Panciera.)

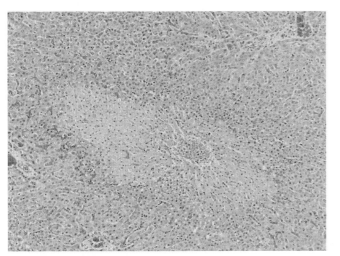

Figure 2-34 **Acute centrilobular necrosis** in an ox.

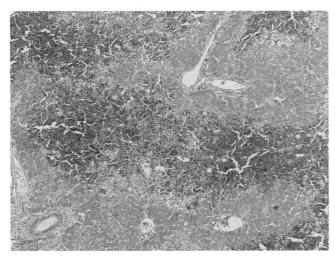

Figure 2-35 Bridging centrilobular **hemorrhagic necrosis** caused by *Xamia* sp. poisoning in a sheep.

However, vascular influences on the susceptibility to necrosis mean that segments of the lobule can be differentially affected. Frequently, the areas of necrosis are joined to one another, thus cutting the conventional lobules into segments, and at the same time, outlining the periphery of the

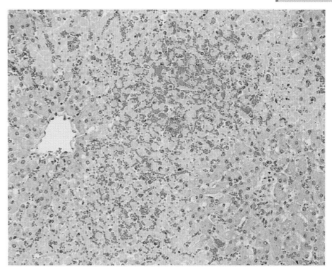

Figure 2-36 Acute **midzonal necrosis** in a foal.

circulatory fields of the hepatic lobules. Some of these areas of necrosis extend up to larger portal triads, because the periphery of some lobules may lie against the larger portal tracts. Often, the hepatocytes between the necrotic and more normal zones show hydropic degeneration or fatty change.

If the insult is of short duration, quite extensive centrilobular necrosis may be followed by phagocytic infiltration and hepatocellular proliferation and complete restoration of normal structure and function within a few days. Severe centrilobular necrosis may be followed shortly by proliferation of bipotential progenitor cells found near cholangioles, termed the ductular reaction, and mature bile duct epithelia that also respond to the regenerative stimulus. With restitution of the normal complement of hepatocytes, the proliferative response in the progenitor cells and biliary tract subsides unless the original insult is continuous or repeated.

Some intoxications can produce selective **midzonal (zone 2) necrosis,** affecting only a narrow, sharply defined band of hepatocytes (Fig. 2-36). It may be more diffuse within the lobule, so that periportal or centrilobular degeneration may be superimposed on the more severe midzonal lesion.

Periportal (zone 1) necrosis *is also an uncommon lesion,* perhaps more often seen than midzonal necrosis, and can be caused by direct-acting hepatotoxins that do not require metabolism by the cytochromes P450 to produce toxic moieties. More than one pattern of zonal necrosis can be found in the same liver. The various forms of zonal necrosis cannot reliably be distinguished from one another grossly, but one may expect to see in periportal necrosis a reversal of the pattern seen in centrilobular necrosis; that is, in periportal necrosis, the surviving hepatocytes about the hepatic venules may appear as pale, raised islands within a regular network of red, collapsed periportal tissue. Careful scrutiny may reveal the smallest hepatic venules at the center of the pale islands.

Paracentral necrosis, *a form of coagulative necrosis, occurs when an isolated portion of the centrilobular region of the lobule (or complete hepatic acinus of Rappaport—perhaps visualized more easily as an entire acinus) dies and is viewed in transverse section* (Fig. 2-37). It is possibly an ischemic lesion or infarct produced by an occlusion of a terminal portal venule, such as may occur in disseminated intravascular coagulation. Its appearance in certain of the acute hepatotoxicities probably

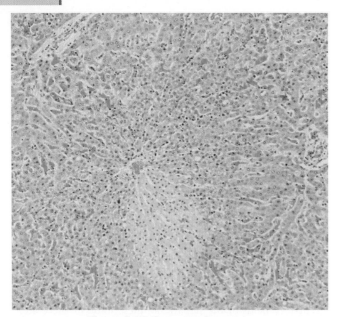

Figure 2-37 Paracentral necrosis.

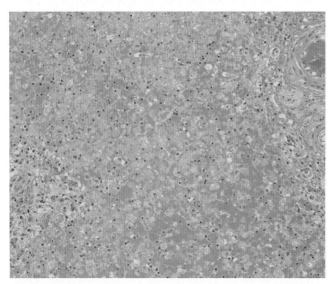

Figure 2-38 Massive necrosis with destruction of the periportal limiting plate and ductular reaction caused by *Amanita* poisoning in a cat.

represents the death of a single complete acinus as a result of local vascular insufficiency, although, theoretically, high local microsomal enzyme activity or local deficiency of hepatocellular protective factors may play a part. Occlusion and rupture of a bile ductule or cholangiole are other potential causes of paracentral necrosis.

Massive necrosis

Massive necrosis refers to necrosis of an entire hepatic lobule, not necessarily necrosis of the liver as a whole. By accepted definition, *every cell in the affected lobule is dead, including the hepatocytes of the limiting plate* (Fig. 2-38). Without surviving parenchyma to support regeneration, affected lobules collapse, so that portal areas and hepatic venules are approximated and the intervening stroma is condensed. Such a liver must regenerate from surviving hepatocytes in other, less severely affected lobules or by proliferation of progenitor cells that mature into hepatocytes. The distribution of massive hepatic necrosis

often relates to the distribution of larger vessels. Collapse, condensation, and subsequent scarring are characteristic, the end result being known as **postnecrotic scarring.** The liver is not uniformly involved typically. Large areas of parenchyma remain intact, and these enlarge amid scarring areas during compensatory regeneration.

A liver that is the seat of massive necrosis may be of normal size or smaller. Fine red threads of fibrin may be present on the surface, especially in the grooves between the lobes. There is a surface mosaic appearance of red, gray, or yellow areas intermingled with areas of dark red. The gray or yellow areas of parenchyma, representing surviving tissue, form irregular, coalescing patches that may be <1.0 cm in diameter. *The intermingled red areas represent areas of necrosis, hemorrhage, and collapse, and these are depressed a few millimeters below the surface.* In the healing stage, the depressed areas of hemorrhage and necrosis are condensed, shrunken, and scarified so that the surface of the liver is traversed by fine or heavy scars that separate large nodules of regenerative hyperplasia. Further acute episodes may be superimposed so that the presented lesion may be a mixture of acute massive necrosis and postnecrotic scarring.

Hepatosis dietetica *of swine is a now uncommon syndrome of massive hepatic necrosis in association with its immediate or late effects, namely "yellow-fat disease," degeneration of skeletal and cardiac muscle, serous effusions, ulceration of the squamous mucosa of the stomach, and fibrinoid necrosis of arterioles.* These lesions may occur alone or in any combination, although all seldom occur in one animal. They are known to be of nutritional origin, and the fact that the various lesions can occur separately indicates the complexity of the pathogenesis. Experimental observations have revealed the *need for concurrent deficiencies of sulfur-containing amino acids, tocopherols, and trace amounts of selenium if hepatic necrosis is to develop.* Selenium protects efficiently against the hepatic necrosis and massive effusions, and tocopherols are probably protective against other lesions that occur as part of the syndrome. The pathogenesis is incompletely understood, but is in part related to the generation of free radicals, exacerbated by deficiency of free-radical scavengers such as vitamin E, and selenium, protective against reactive oxygen radicals through its role in glutathione peroxidase and some other selenoproteins. Hepatosis dietetica occurs in rapidly growing pigs fed diets largely of grain and containing protein supplements lacking in either quality or quantity. There is some evidence that in pigs that are nutritionally predisposed, a cold and damp environment or some other stress may precipitate the disease. Death usually occurs without signs of illness or after a short period of dullness. Melena, dyspnea, weakness, and trembling may be observed in some cases. Jaundice is indicative of a relapsing course.

Affected pigs are usually in good condition. The carcass may be anemic if ulceration of the gastric mucosa has occurred, and, in these cases, free and digested blood may be found in the stomach and intestine. Jaundice is not common, but *yellow staining of adipose tissues (yellow-fat disease)* is. In relapsing cases, hemorrhagic diathesis may occur, manifested mainly by hemorrhage into and about joints. Protein-rich fluid collects in the serous cavities in small volume. Fine strands of fibrin are present in the peritoneal cavity.

Pulmonary edema accompanies myocardial lesions that consist of intramural and subendocardial hemorrhages with focal areas of hyaline degeneration. The changes in the liver dominate the autopsy findings. The massive hepatic necrosis

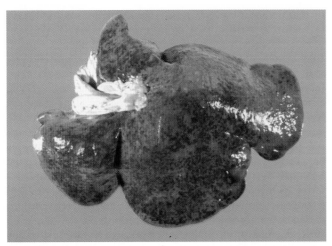

Figure 2-39 Hepatosis dietetica in a pig. (Courtesy University of Guelph.)

is of the typical appearance described earlier, and in a number of cases, both acute and chronic lesions are found (Fig. 2-39). The sites of severest injury are the dorsal parts on the diaphragmatic surface. The right lobe may escape and later undergo marked hypertrophy. The gallbladder is often edematous.

The histologic changes that occur in this syndrome are described elsewhere with the particular organs involved. Briefly, centrilobular necrosis of the liver is typical (eFig. 2-9). Additionally, fibrinoid degeneration of small arteries occurs in some cases. The arterial degeneration may occur in any organ or in most organs but is relatively common in only the small vessels of the mesentery, gut, and heart (see Mulberry heart disease, in Vol. 3, Cardiovascular system).

Piecemeal necrosis

Models of *immune-mediated hepatocyte necrosis* have emerged from studies of human viral hepatitis and some forms of drug-induced chronic hepatitis. *This pattern of necrosis amid sites of more active inflammation at the limiting plate of hepatocytes immediately adjacent to the edge of the portal tract is referred to as piecemeal necrosis.* The mechanisms may involve either direct damage to hepatocytes by the uptake of antigen-antibody complexes, or cooperation between macrophages and T lymphocytes. These may cause cell-mediated destruction of hepatocytes that have taken up these complexes or, perhaps, native antigen or virus. Whatever the agency, the mode of cell removal in this sort of injury often takes the form of *single-cell necrosis or apoptosis*, which may be directly triggered by immunologically competent cells. This type of liver injury, in which *inflammation characteristically disrupts the limiting plate*, giving an irregular appearance to the periportal zone, is discussed further in the section on Chronic hepatitis.

Necrosis of sinusoidal lining cells

Injury to the endothelium of hepatic sinusoids can develop in a variety of forms. The sinusoidal endothelial cells may lose their typical fenestrae or pores, limiting contact between plasma and hepatocellular microvilli, and if there is an increased deposition of extracellular matrix (ECM) beneath the altered endothelium, the alteration is termed "capillarization of sinusoids," leading to reduced hepatic function. Sinusoidal endothelial cells may relax their connections to the fine

meshwork of the hepatic "reticulin" or detach completely forming microemboli in the sinusoid downstream. In addition, the residual, exposed space of Disse has an increased risk of sinusoidal thrombosis. Acute endothelial injury can occur as a result of ischemia-reperfusion injury, acetaminophen or pyrrolizidine toxicity, and effects of endotoxin, all of which can lead to localized ischemia and necrosis. Other endothelial toxins include ngaione poisoning and microcystin-LR, a highly toxic cyclic heptapeptide produced by *Microcystis aeruginosa*, an aquatic cyanobacterium (blue-green alga). Microcystin-LR is selectively injurious to hepatic sinusoidal endothelial cells by inhibiting protein phosphatases. When the cytoskeleton becomes hyperphosphorylated, endothelial cells undergo apoptosis, leading to hemorrhagic necrosis.

Some forms of peliosis hepatis may develop following endothelial necrosis. More chronic injury can produce fibrosis, leading to diminished or disrupted sinusoidal blood flow. Alteration of the sinusoidal blood flow can be a primary event leading to hepatocyte hypoxia with liver dysfunction and disruption of the portal circulation. Secondary endothelial cell injury can result when hepatocytes are being destroyed by the elaboration of toxic molecules within their cytoplasm, it is to be expected that the *sinusoidal lining cells may also suffer should the products of these biotransformations spill into the space of Disse.* Erythrocytes increase in the perisinusoidal space and, when endothelial damage is severe, the regions of necrosis are hemorrhagic. Necrosis of sinusoidal endothelial cells is seen very early in the course of many hepatotoxicities.

Sinusoidal phagocytes are sometimes vulnerable to necrosis by virtue of their role in clearing the portal blood of particulate or colloidal material; should these particles be toxic or infectious, Kupffer cell necrosis may occur alone, but more usually, there is damage to surrounding hepatocytes as well.

Necrosis of bile duct epithelium

It is unusual for the bile duct epithelium to be singled out by specific lethal insults, but this is seen in intoxication by *sporidesmin* (see section on Toxic hepatic disease). Usually, there is accompanying portal inflammation. Some experimental toxicants, such as α-naphthylisothiocyanate, are lethal to bile duct epithelia and elicit a local inflammatory cholangitis. Idiosyncratic drug-induced destructive cholangitis can lead to acute cholangiolar injury as well as chronic cholestasis with damage and loss of bile ducts (*destructive cholangitis*). Treatment with sulfonamides, other drugs, and viral infection have been linked to this response (Fig. 2-40).

Further reading

Guicciardi ME, et al. Apoptosis and necrosis in the liver. Compr Physiol 2013;3:977-1010.

Luedde T, et al. Cell death and cell death responses in liver disease: mechanisms and clinical relevance. Gastroenterol 2014;147:765-783.

RESPONSES OF THE LIVER TO INJURY

The liver is a remarkably versatile organ. Given its central position in the body, supplied by blood draining the gastrointestinal tract, and the fact that it is the key organ involved in detoxification of exogenous (xenobiotics) and endogenous compounds (endobiotics), the liver must respond to injury, including metabolic, infectious, and hemodynamic insults.

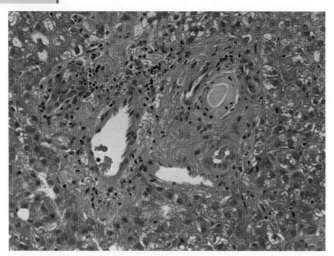

Figure 2-40 Acute necrosis of biliary epithelium in a dog following exposure to trimethoprim-sulfa.

This section describes the 3 main categories of liver response to injury: regeneration, fibrosis, and ductular reaction (biliary hyperplasia).

Hepatic regeneration

Mild injury involving the hepatocytes, biliary epithelium, endothelial cells, and mesenchymal elements typically is completely resolved quickly through regeneration. This is particularly true in younger animals, as the vigor of regeneration diminishes with age. Even in cases of massive hepatocellular necrosis, complete recovery is possible if the reticulin framework of the liver persists and surviving hepatocytes have sufficient time to regenerate and replace the lost hepatic mass.

In adulthood, the liver is a stable organ with limited replication of mature hepatocytes, biliary epithelium, and other cells in the liver. However, loss of hepatic mass through injury, such as infections, toxic insult, or surgical removal, will transform the mature hepatocytes, biliary epithelium, and/or bipotential progenitor cells, as well as hepatic stellate cells and endothelial cells, into actively proliferating cells until normal functional mass has been replaced. *As much as 70% of the normal liver can be removed surgically without clinical insufficiency, and in the course of a few weeks, it is back to its normal mass.* Depending on the nature of the injury, regeneration occurs via one of 2 pathways. In cases of moderate injury, cell loss is replaced by proliferation of mature hepatocytes or biliary epithelium, providing swift replacement of parenchymal loss. In cases of more severe injury, or conditions that inhibit replication of mature cells, there is proliferation of bipotential progenitor cells, called a ductular reaction. These cells reside in the periportal region of the lobule at the level of the canals of Hering, the site where bile canaliculi and biliary epithelial cells first join and form the beginning of the epithelium-lined biliary tree. They are recognized histologically as small, basophilic cells that form single-cell arrays or ductules with narrow lumens. Depending on the differentiation pathway that is followed, they can mature into hepatocytes or bile duct epithelium.

Regeneration of mature hepatocytes following surgical removal is well known. An example from Greek mythology is Prometheus, punished for giving fire to the mortals, daily had his liver partially eaten by an eagle (a symbol of Zeus), only to regrow and be eaten again. Although the mythical *daily* regrowth of hepatic mass is more prodigious than the real-world response, hepatic regeneration is nonetheless remarkable. In rodents, partial hepatectomies can be repeated more than 10 times, followed by restoration of normal hepatic mass. Individual hepatocytes are able to replicate up to 70 times. Simple replacement of missing hepatocytes alone does not truly constitute regeneration because normal liver microscopic architecture is essential to maintain normal hepatic function. Although new lobes are not regenerated following hepatectomy, the remaining lobes enlarge, and the proliferated hepatocytes and other cellular elements progress through a series of steps that involve interaction of hepatocytes and angiogenic processes to restore the normal relationships between the hepatocytes and the sinusoids.

Regeneration of mature hepatocytes is stimulated by several factors. These include polypeptide growth factors, such as hepatocyte growth factor, epidermal growth factor, transforming growth factor-α (TGF-α), and insulin-like growth factors. Hepatocyte growth factor is the most potent mitogen and is released by hepatic stellate cells to stimulate hepatocytes in a paracrine fashion. This growth factor can also be embedded in the ECM to be released by proteases. Hepatic regeneration is also enhanced by nutrition, with fasting slowing and dietary protein promoting regeneration. In addition, catecholamines and a broad variety of hormones support regeneration, with insulin, glucagon being the most significant. Cytokines, such as IL-6, produced by TNF-α–stimulated Kupffer cells, are other important effectors. When IL-6 binds its receptor, it stimulates mitogenic intracellular signaling and potentiates signaling by other growth factors. These effectors are examples of the important role of the innate immune system in hepatic regeneration. The autonomic nervous system also plays a role in hepatic regeneration, as denervation of the liver can significantly limit hepatic regeneration.

Following hepatocyte proliferation, normal liver architecture must be preserved to maintain hepatic function. Several cell types are involved in this process. Following partial hepatectomy, the initial proliferation creates aggregates of hepatocytes 10-14 cells thick. These aggregates are penetrated by endothelial buds that eventually establish sinusoidal channels. Ingrowth of the endothelial cells is driven by regulators of angiogenesis, such as vascular endothelial growth factor (VEGF) and platelet-derived growth factor (PDGF). Hepatic stellate cells replicate and synthesize ECM within ~4 days of partial hepatectomy and help establish normal hepatocyte-matrix interactions.

Once the needed hepatic mass has been replaced, the regenerative process must be regulated to terminate cell proliferation. TGF-β and related family members, including *activin*, are the best known mediators responsible for curtailing hepatocyte proliferation. These mediators are produced primarily by the hepatic stellate cells. They can increase ECM production as well as suppress hepatocellular replication, are downregulated during proliferation, and increase once appropriate hepatic mass has been achieved.

In severe, often toxic, liver injury, mature hepatocytes cannot replace damaged hepatic mass, and *bipotential progenitor cells* are engaged to restore the hepatic mass. At the interface of the portal tract connective tissue and the hepatic parenchyma, and in the vicinity of the canals of Hering, there is a compartment that serves as the site of quiescent progenitor cells. Proliferation of these cells gives rise to the "ductular

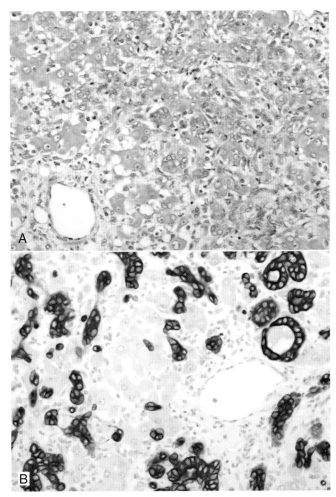

Figure 2-41 A. Ductular reaction in an injured liver. **B.** Cytokeratin 7 stain.

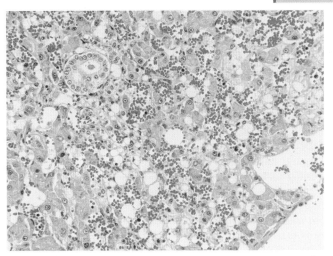

Figure 2-42 Ductule formation in the centrilobular region of a dog with chronic right-sided heart failure.

reaction," characterized by ductular structures lined by cuboidal, basophilic cells (Fig. 2-41A). The relationship between the "oval cells" described in rodents and the ductular reaction still requires some clarification, but it is likely that the same cell type is involved. In addition, there may be progenitor cells among the mature biliary epithelial cells, and others may be marrow derived and blood-borne to the liver. Immunohistochemical staining of these cells in humans and rodents reveals that they contain cytokeratin markers of biliary epithelium and, simultaneously, hepatocyte markers such as albumin (Fig. 2-41B). Similar cells are present in animals as well. There are several circumstances that can trigger the ductular reaction other than massive necrosis, although this is the best recognized form. Both cholestasis and hypoxia can drive the ductular reaction causing proliferation in the periportal region for the former, and in the centrilobular region in the latter instance. The ability of these cells in the ductular reaction to differentiate into mature biliary or hepatocellular phenotypes is well established. It should be appreciated that in most clinical circumstances, hepatic regeneration is a less orderly process than that which occurs in healthy experimental animals. *Regeneration requires normal arterial and venous inflow as well as venous and biliary drainage.* Without a supportive environment, hepatic regeneration of hepatocytes, biliary epithelium, and nonparenchymal cells may be quite variable within different regions of the liver. Following massive necrosis, all

remaining hepatocytes are likely to initiate a replicative response, whereas random focal necrosis will engender a local proliferation of hepatocytes. Scattered individual cell necrosis is repaired almost imperceptibly. In the more common pattern of centrilobular necrosis, seen in many toxic insults, complete repair is usually evident with a 24-48 hour period. Chronic or repetitive injury often results in nodule formation as discussed in the section on Fibrosis.

Ductular reaction (bile duct hyperplasia)

Ductular reaction (biliary hyperplasia) is a characteristic reaction of the liver to various types of insult involving proliferation of bile duct epithelium, hepatic progenitor cells, and possibly metaplasia of mature hepatocytes. The histologic hallmark of the ductular reaction is the formation of new, irregular, and tortuous ductules or chains of cells formed from flattened or cuboidal basophilic epithelium.

There are 3 main types of ductular reactions. (1) A common association with acute *bile duct obstruction* is proliferation of preformed bile duct epithelium, creating a rapid increase in bile duct surface area. This can protect hepatocytes from bile acid buildup through a recirculation process termed *cholehepatic recirculation.* (2) In cases of serious injury to hepatocytes, particularly when mature hepatocytes are not able to replicate, there is a prominent ductular reaction originating from *hepatic bipotential progenitor cells (or oval cells).* The bipotential nature of these cells is supported by the detection of biliary epithelial cytokeratins 7 and 19 in cells with an otherwise hepatocellular phenotype. A dramatic presentation of ductular proliferation is often evident in animals that succumb several days after a fatal hepatic intoxication or in horses with Theiler's disease. (3) Ductular reaction may also result from metaplasia of mature hepatocytes in regions of hypoxia.

Ductular reaction may also develop secondary to *local portal inflammation and fibrosis.* Ductular formation can also occur in areas of hypoxia. Such ducts formed by metaplasia of mature hepatocytes can be found in centrilobular areas in animals with chronic heart failure and passive congestion, for example (Fig. 2-42).

However, reabsorption of bile constituents by biliary epithelium leads to a neutrophilic inflammatory reaction and local edema formation, which can be confused with a bacterial infection. With persistence, the ductular reaction can contribute to portal and periportal fibrosis as the ductular cells secrete profibrogenic growth factors, cytokines, and chemokines.

Illustrative examples from natural disease are provided by the toxicoses of phomopsin, pyrrolizidine alkaloids, and aflatoxin, and by equine serum hepatitis and ovine white-liver disease.

Fibrosis

Hepatic fibrosis is a potentially reversible form of wound healing in which there is an accumulation of various ECM components. *In cases of acute or self-limited injury, fibrosis may resolve completely and normal liver architecture can be restored, but when damage is too extensive to be repaired, a scar may be permanent, and if the injury is persistent, there is progressive deposition of ECM, leading to the "final common pathway" and ending in fibrosis and cirrhosis.* In normal liver, the ECM exists in a state of dynamic balance, with synthesis and degradation occurring in balance to maintain normal levels of all constituents. It is found in the portal tracts, along the sinusoids in the space of Disse, around the central vein and in Glisson's capsule. Normally, the hepatic ECM constitutes only 3% of the relative areas on a tissue section and only 0.5% of the total liver wet weight. The main constituents of the hepatic ECM are collagen, proteoglycans, laminin, fibronectin, and matricellular proteins. In the space of Disse, the matrix is composed primarily of collagens IV and VI. Following injury, however, fibrillar collagens I and III as well as fibronectin are deposited. These deposits disrupt the normal structure and function of the sinusoids, leading to *capillarization of sinusoids,* discussed later. The ECM is not merely scaffolding for the liver. It also functions as a repository for various growth factors and metalloproteinases in latent form, and it can bind a variety of survival factors, such as hepatocyte growth factor and TNF-α, that may protect the growth factors and inhibit hepatocyte apoptosis. In addition, interactions between cells and the ECM can affect the phenotype of the hepatocytes and stellate cells and the composition of the ECM. Thus the process of hepatic fibrosis is distinct from the condensation of the hepatic reticular framework that can be seen following hepatocyte loss.

The process of ECM production in the injured liver is initiated by a process that *activates hepatic mesenchymal cells into myofibroblasts.* These mesenchymal cells constitute a prototypical mesenchymal cell type that mediates injury and repair in a number of tissues, including the kidney, skin, lung, and bone marrow. All of these cell types have the ability to produce ECM, and have contractile ability. The best recognized group in this family is the *hepatic stellate cells,* but there are other important groups in this family, including portal fibroblasts, bone marrow–derived cells, and, via epithelial-mesenchymal transition, hepatocytes that can acquire a mesenchymal phenotype. *Portal fibroblasts,* particularly those surrounding the bile ducts, are an important source of ECM formation in the portal tracts. This is particularly evident in cases of biliary tree injury. Portal fibroblasts/myofibroblasts are distinct from stellate cells based on distinct protein markers.

Hepatic stellate cells are found in the space of Disse, often between hepatocytes. In normal circumstances, these cells store lipid, primarily vitamin A (retinyl esters), in characteristic large round vacuoles. In injured liver, hepatic stellate cells become activated. A principal morphologic change involves the loss of the lipid vacuole and transformation into a spindle-shaped myofibroblast. In some species, stellate cells contain immunohistochemically detectable α–smooth muscle actin before activation, and in other species, activation is required for expression of this protein. When activated, they replicate robustly at sites of injury and are the main source of collagen and other ECM components, such as proteoglycans, fibronectin, and hyaluronan, lining the space of Disse. Activated stellate cells also release proinflammatory, profibrogenic, and promitotic cytokines. Other features of stellate cells include the ability to present antigen and their consistent contact with individual fibers of autonomic nerve endings.

Hepatic blood flow can be significantly modified by activated stellate cells. Blood flow through sinusoids can be restricted by the contraction of the stellate cells that extend processes around the sinusoidal endothelial cells. In health, there is a balance between the nitric oxide–stimulated vasodilation and endothelin-1–driven vasoconstriction. During active fibrosis and cirrhosis, there is an increase of endothelin-1, produced by sinusoidal endothelial cells causing contraction of the stellate cell–derived myofibroblasts.

Fibrosis can form within portal tracts expanding their area, or as septa extending into the parenchyma and eventually bridging between portal tracts or central veins. Fibrosis in the portal tracts is primarily generated by the activity of portal fibroblasts, rather than hepatic stellate cells. Biliary injury leads to a rapid proliferation of periductular myofibroblasts derived from portal fibroblasts and ECM production. The volume of the portal tracts is increased by the generation of the ECM, ductular proliferation, myofibroblast proliferation, and edema.

Fibrosis can be less florid and more insidious when it lines the space of Disse, disrupting the normal exchange between the plasma and hepatocyte microvilli. The essential microvascular unit of the liver is the sinusoid, lined by fenestrated endothelial cells, and separated from the hepatocytes by the space of Disse. A porous basal membrane–like matrix in the space of Disse helps to maintain the differentiated states of the hepatocytes and hepatic stellate cells that inhabit the space of Disse. When there is excess ECM lining the space of Disse, the adjacent sinusoidal endothelial cells lose their characteristic fenestrations, and *the sinusoids are transformed functionally into capillaries.* This process is known as **capillarization** and leads to significantly impaired exchange between the hepatocytes and the plasma. This causes diminished hepatic function when the lesion is extensive. The cells responsible for the ECM deposition are primarily in the myofibroblast family, including hepatic stellate cells.

Because collagen has a finite half-life, and as hepatic fibrosis exists in a balance of synthesis and removal, it is potentially reversible. Elimination of the source of injury or successful therapy can lead to stellate cell apoptosis and a reduction in the synthesis of inhibitors of the enzymes responsible for the degradation of the collagen and other ECM elements, primarily matrix metalloproteinases. This has been demonstrated in rodent models of hepatic fibrosis produced by bile duct ligation, and models using carbon tetrachloride. However, over time, collagen can mature and fibrils can cross-link and become resistant to enzymatic degradation, leading to permanent fibrosis. Long-term or permanent fibrotic changes can also be caused by severe acute injury that leads to an initial focus of fibrosis and is so severe that it affects local vascular supply.

The *distribution of fibrosis* in the liver can reflect the pathogenesis of the injury responsible.

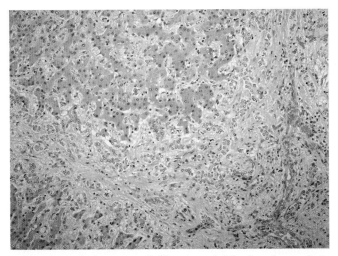

Figure 2-43 Bridging portal fibrosis and bile duct hyperplasia secondary to bile duct obstruction in a horse.

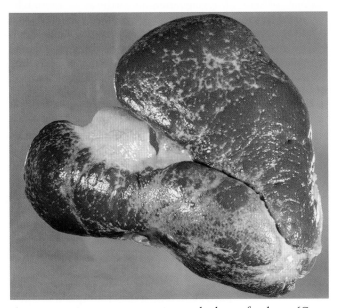

Figure 2-44 Postnecrotic scarring in the liver of a sheep. (Courtesy P. Stromberg)

- Inflammatory disorders that produce piecemeal necrosis of hepatocytes, typically viral hepatitis in humans and often an idiopathic disorder in veterinary species, can evolve to form portal-to-portal, or portal-to-central, fibrous septa.
- In the event of *inflammation or obstruction involving the bile ducts*, proliferation of periductular myofibroblasts and prominent ductular reaction can lead to **biliary fibrosis** or a pattern of portal-to-portal bridging termed **biliary cirrhosis** when accompanied by nodular regenerative proliferation of hepatocytes (Fig. 2-43).
- **Postnecrotic scarring** *occurs after massive necrosis*, where large areas of parenchyma are destroyed. The reticulin network collapses and condenses and portal areas converge, resulting in broad, irregular bands of scar tissue with variable irregular areas of parenchymal regeneration interspersed (Fig. 2-44).
- **Diffuse hepatic fibrosis** is the outcome of *chronic parenchymal injury*, such as prolonged inflammation or multiple episodes of zonal necrosis. The fibrosis throughout the

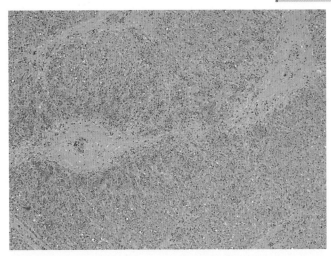

Figure 2-45 Centrilobular fibrosis (cardiac fibrosis), most severe at the center of the lobe in chronic passive congestion in a dog.

lobules bridges connective-tissue tracts in portal areas and hepatic venules to produce *pseudolobulation*, in which small areas of parenchyma are separated by a pattern of fibrosis on the scale of true lobules. This pattern of fibrosis can lead to capillarization of sinusoids, or intrahepatic bypass of portal and arterial blood, both of which can reduce the influences of growth factors and nutrients on liver regeneration. The accompanying hypoxia is important in the genesis of the hepatocellular atrophy that is almost always concomitant with diffuse hepatic fibrosis.

- **Centrilobular (periacinar) fibrosis** is the most common pattern *following zonal necrosis in hypoxic and toxic injury*. Good examples are seen in animals with prolonged passive venous congestion of the liver, especially when this is caused by extracardiac sources of increased venous pressure, rather than to congestive heart failure (Fig. 2-45). Otherwise, this pattern of fibrosis is a response to toxic injury; poisoning by pyrrolizidine alkaloids may cause it in ruminants, and extraordinary development of periacinar fibrosis may follow accidental exposure to nitrosamines in several species.

Cirrhosis

Cirrhosis has several definitions, and consensus regarding the essential features is difficult to obtain. In general, it is agreed that cirrhosis is not merely an end stage of ECM accumulation in the liver, but, in fact, is a multifaceted distortion of hepatic parenchymal architecture and hepatic vascular anatomy. By one definition, cirrhosis is "a diffuse process characterized by fibrosis and the conversion of normal liver architecture into structurally abnormal nodules." The key features are the formation of regenerative nodules of hepatocytes surrounded by fibrous septa and vascular disorders that often integrate both central veins and portal tracts. Other than dogs, most veterinary species develop diffuse hepatic fibrosis following chronic injury, but do not develop regenerative nodules. *Chronically injured canine livers often have a robust formation of regenerative nodules separated by fibrous septa typical of cirrhosis* (Fig. 2-46A-C). Portosystemic shunts and venous occlusion may result, interfering with hepatic function and driving portal hypertension. *Note that not all nodular livers are cirrhotic.* Clinically, *cirrhosis results in hepatic insufficiency*, mainly in the form of ascites and hypoproteinemia rather than excretory

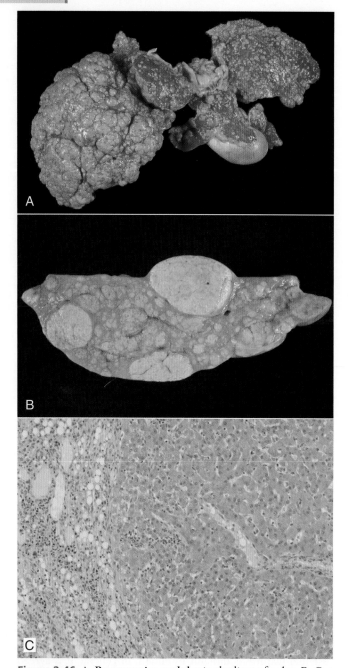

Figure 2-46 **A. Regenerative nodules** in the liver of a dog. **B.** Cut surface of the liver. **C.** Microscopic appearance of the regenerative nodule and adjacent septum.

dysfunction and icterus, although, in advanced cases, all manifestations of fatal liver failure can occur. The *hallmarks of cirrhosis* are:

1. *Bridging fibrous septa*, ranging from delicate bands to broad scars that replace multiple adjacent lobules. These fibrous septa contain vascular channels, originating from sinusoids in collapsed parenchyma or angiogenesis that allow a considerable portion of blood to bypass hepatocytes. These microvascular channels in fibrous septa resist flow more than normal sinusoids. This factor, as well as the relative increase in flow in these vessels shunting around the nodules, contributes to portal hypertension.
2. *Impaired exchange* between hepatocytes and sinusoidal blood, because of the increase in perisinusoidal ECM.

3. *Parenchymal nodules*, created by the regenerative attempts of entrapped hepatocytes, and varying in size from <3 mm in diameter (micronodular) to several centimeters in diameter (macronodular). These nodules are composed of trabeculae that are typically 2 or more cells thick, with relative reduction of sinusoidal space. Some expanding nodules may compress the vessels within fibrous septa, contributing to portal hypertension. Nodule formation is prominent in dogs, but significantly less so in most other domestic species.
4. *Ongoing damage and reorganization* of the hepatic connective tissue, sometimes with areas of portal and arterial thrombosis and segmental ischemia is typical, but not always present.

   Cirrhosis is usually the end result of several pathogenic processes, namely, cell death (necrosis or apoptosis) and active inflammation with chronic fibrosis. Cirrhosis is not a synonym for chronic hepatic fibrosis, although some insults that cause chronic diffuse fibrosis in the liver can lead to cirrhosis. The nodular pattern of regeneration in cirrhosis is caused by expanding islands of surviving parenchyma entrapped between bands of scar tissue. At the point of liver failure, these regenerative attempts are insufficient to restore function. Despite the increased hepatocellular mass, the inability to restore normal function is attributed to altered circulation through the bridging scar tissue, portal hypertension and shunting, deposition of ECM in the perisinusoidal space, reduced supply of portal growth factors, inhibition of proliferation of ECM, and toxic inhibition of hepatocellular proliferation. The characteristic fibrovascular septa that bridge portal and central vascular tracts are readily observed in liver sections, but the portal-hepatic shunting therein can be difficult to identify. Clinical evidence for portosystemic shunting, such as impaired ammonia or bile acid clearance, can reflect acquired portocaval shunts that often develop as a result of portal hypertension from chronic hepatic fibrosis.

Acquired portosystemic shunting

Any chronic liver disease that causes sufficient fibrosis or atrophy to restrict portal blood flow significantly and produce portal hypertension has the potential to cause the development of collateral portosystemic shunts. These are described later in the section on Vascular factors in hepatic injury and circulatory disorders.

Further reading

Desmet VJ. Ductal plates in hepatic ductular reactions. Hypothesis and implications. III. Implications for liver pathology. Virchows Arch 2011;458:271-279.

Hernandez-Gea V, Friedman SL. Pathogenesis of liver fibrosis. Annu Rev Pathol 2011;6:425-456.

Michalopoulos GK, DeFrances MC. Liver regeneration. Science 1997;276:60-66.

HEPATIC DYSFUNCTION

Hepatic failure is a syndrome that results from inadequate hepatic function. The liver provides numerous essential processes, and liver failure can affect metabolic, synthetic, catabolic (detoxification), and immune functions. There is no specific point at which diminished function can clearly be defined as "failure," given the various functions of the liver, but it is best understood as the point at which liver function is not capable of sustaining life. The liver is an organ with very large functional capacity and regenerative potential. Signs of insufficiency do not develop until the reserves in production, supply, and recovery are exhausted. *The central role of the liver in many systemic functions means that liver disease can be manifested as lesions or dysfunctions elsewhere, for example, in the brain, skin, blood, and gut.* Failure may develop suddenly, frequently following exposure to toxic compounds, or failure may develop in a slow inexorable fashion as a chronic disease processes. Hepatic failure, particularly chronic liver failure, may not affect all processes equally, and one or more features of liver failure may predominate in individual cases.

Acute liver failure is uncommon, and is clinically evidenced as a severe and rapid liver injury. There are a number of causes. The consequences are also multiple and varied, including abrupt loss of normal metabolic and immunologic functions, as well as hepatic encephalopathy, coagulopathy, jaundice, photosensitization (in herbivores), and possibly dysfunction of other organs. In humans, there are recognized viral infections that can cause acute liver failure, but there are currently no known animal viruses capable of causing this syndrome, although recent studies suggest that equine serum hepatitis (Theiler's disease) may be caused by an equine pegivirus. Toxin-induced acute liver failure is likely the most common form in veterinary medicine. The toxic injury may come from natural sources, such as those found in plants and fungi, or from overdose of or idiosyncratic reactions to therapeutic drugs. Hyperthermia from environmental heating or prolonged seizure activity can also cause acute hepatic failure. Acute ischemic injury from profound hypotension secondary to sepsis or cardiac failure may also occur.

Chronic liver failure results from progressive destructive processes, such as fibrosis or inflammation, or a combination of the two. The hallmarks of chronic liver failure in dogs are fibrosis and nodular regeneration, but other species are more prone to a fibrotic response alone. The progressive loss of critical functional hepatic mass caused by ongoing hepatocyte injury, shunting of portal blood within fibrous septa bypassing hepatocytes, and abnormal bile drainage, lead to a terminal stage of hepatic insufficiency.

Chronic liver failure can be subdivided into 2 forms: end-stage liver, the typical fibrotic liver with progressive loss of functional hepatic mass, and "acute on chronic failure," a circumstance in which a patient with compensated chronic liver disease acutely develops failure. The causes for the acute transition to failure are not certain, but the buildup of various toxins, such as aromatic amino acids, benzodiazepines, and ammonia, among others, may be involved. Other theories include increased bacterial or fungal translocation from the gut, leading to hepatic infection and sepsis.

Liver failure, whether acute or chronic, affects a number of critical processes. These disturbances include hepatic encephalopathy, cholestasis and jaundice, hepatogenous photosensitization, hemorrhagic diathesis, hepatorenal syndrome, ascites, and hepatocutaneous syndrome.

Hepatic encephalopathy (HE)

The neurologic manifestations of hepatic failure are variable and nonspecific; they range from dullness, through complete unawareness and compulsive aimless movement, to mania and generalized convulsions. There is considerable variation in the clinical signs of hepatic encephalopathy between different species. Sheep rarely show more than dullness and central blindness, with perhaps some compulsive chewing movements and tremor. The picture in cattle is similar, but mania and aggression may also be seen, whereas frenzy is more often recorded in horses. The closer clinical observation of cats and dogs may reveal more subtle behavioral changes, and inappetence and vomiting are commonly reported in carnivores with portosystemic shunts. Ptyalism is common in cats with HE.

The clinical context in which HE occurs can be important. *In animals with acute hepatic disease, HE is a serious sign, usually indicating imminent death.* However, in animals with more chronic conditions, such as portosystemic shunting or deficiency of a urea cycle enzyme, neurologic signs can be intermittent for many months, and may disappear after appropriate dietary modification. The pathogenesis of HE involves more than just neurons, as astrocyte and glial cell responses are now evident. Older literature, particularly in vitro studies, which did not take all of these features into account, will likely need reinterpretation.

Ammonia toxicity is regarded as the major part of the clinical signs and the brain lesions; however, there are a number of other factors that may play a role. Blood ammonia is largely of dietary origin, derived from protein and urea by microflora in the large bowel. Ammonia is also derived from hepatic deamination of amino acids and from metabolism of glutamine in peripheral tissues. Ammonia is normally removed in the first pass of portal blood through the liver, wherein it is incorporated with carbon dioxide into carbamoyl phosphate that enters the urea cycle. In shunting or hepatic failure, ammonia that bypasses hepatic clearance accumulates in the circulation. Ammonia is able to cross the blood-brain barrier, and initially, this influx leads to astrocyte injury. Astrocytes are the site of ammonia detoxification in the brain, and they eliminate ammonia by the synthesis of glutamine through amidation of glutamate by the enzyme glutamine synthetase. Elevated blood ammonia increases the accumulation of glutamine in astrocytes, resulting in osmotic stress and astrocyte swelling caused by cytotoxic edema. Affected astrocytes that are adjacent to endothelium cannot maintain the blood-brain barrier, and this permits increased ammonia entry into the brain. Direct ammonia-induced effects on brain endothelial cells are also possible. Briefly, the consequences of increased ammonia in the brain include a net decrease in energy metabolism within the brain, increased edema formation because of astrocyte dysfunction, and injury to neurons, leading to an imbalance in neurotransmitters that emphasizes neural inhibition.

The pathogenesis of HE may vary depending on the type of liver failure—acute or chronic—that produces the cerebral injury. Also, not all parts of the brain are affected in a similar fashion. In acute hepatic failure, cerebral edema may be the leading cause of death because of increased intracerebral pressure with possible herniation. The increase in intracranial pressure is, however, linked to brain ammonia levels. Currently, it is thought that swollen astrocytes release vasogenic factors, such as nitric oxide, causing intracerebral hyperemia, and that this leads to edema formation. Systemic inflammatory responses can enhance the severity of HE. Neuroinflammation, mediated by microglia, is evident in acute liver failure and tends to increase with increasing duration of HE. Synergetic interactions between increased ammonia and systemic or neuroinflammation can increase the severity of HE.

However, the specific mechanisms by which systemic inflammation triggers neuroinflammation are not currently known.

In chronic hepatic failure, ammonia and neuroinflammation are likely to contribute synergistically to HE. Ammonia plays a role as a directly neurotoxic agent, altering neurotransmission, and potentially contributing to cerebral energy failure through inhibition of α-ketoglutarate dehydrogenase, a rate-limiting enzyme in the tricarboxylic acid cycle. Chronic increase in brain ammonia is associated with disrupted neural transmission involving all of the different neurotransmitter systems of the brain. The main neurotransmitter systems affected involve neuropeptides, with an evolution toward an increase in the inhibitory γ-aminobutyric acid (GABA)ergic system, and downregulation of the excitatory glutaminergic system. Increased intracerebral ammonia leads to an increase in extracellular glutamate, which will initially drive upregulation of N-methyl-D-aspartate (NMDA) receptors, causing neuronal damage, but eventually, there is a reduction in NMDA receptors and glutaminergic signaling, leading to neuroinhibition. In addition, increased ammonia alone has been linked to neuroinflammation, possibly through direct activation of microglia, which also interferes with normal neural transmission.

Newer studies in animal models have demonstrated that agents acting on specific targets in the brain, including phosphodiesterase 5, type A GABA receptors, and mitogen-activated kinase (p38), can improve cognitive function in mild forms of experimental hepatic encephalopathy. Survival can be increased by treatment with NMDA receptor agonists. Studies have also implicated alterations in inhibitory and excitatory neurotransmitters, including endogenous benzodiazepines, and serotonin, as well as their receptors. Although infusion of ammonia or hyperammonemia caused by deficiency of urea cycle enzymes reproduces similar neurologic signs and vacuolar lesions, other noxious substances in the alimentary tract are also believed to contribute to hepatic encephalopathy resulting from liver failure. These include *variably toxic amines, captans, thiols, and short-chain fatty acids,* which are normally removed from the portal blood in one passage through the liver after production in the large bowel. Thus there are many factors to consider in the pathogenesis of HE.

The microscopic lesions of HE are subtle and variable, likely because postmortem examinations of the brain are performed at various time points of chronicity and clinical severity. There are also significant differences in the microscopic lesions between species. In humans, *the hallmark of HE is Alzheimer type II astrocytosis, in which astrocytes are enlarged with swollen nuclei, margination of chromatin, and prominent nucleoli.* These can be found in large animals, particularly horses. In dogs, Alzheimer type II changes are rare if they occur at all, but vacuoles in gray matter, particularly in brain stem nuclei, predominate. Lesions in cats have features of both the dog and the horse (see Vol. 1, Nervous system). These changes can be observed best in animals with chronic liver disease and portosystemic shunts; the brain lesions can be minimal in animals with acute liver failure.

Cholestasis and jaundice

Cholestasis is the term for impaired bile secretion and flow as well as a failure to secrete organic and inorganic components of bile, with accumulation of these elements in blood. Normal bile formation and flow is dependent on the activity of a series of membrane transporters found in enterocytes,

hepatocytes, and biliary epithelium. In rare cases, hereditary mutations can lead to cholestasis, but more often, cholestasis is caused by exposure to injurious drugs, hormones, proinflammatory cytokines, or obstruction. Clinically, cholestasis leads to increased levels of bilirubin and bile acids in the blood because of retention. Injury to the biliary tree leads to increases in serum alkaline phosphatase. Disturbance of bile flow can originate from altered function of hepatocytes, termed hepatocellular cholestasis, or because of obstruction of the biliary tree, termed obstructive cholestasis. *Hepatocellular cholestasis* can be attributed to impaired uptake, metabolism, secretion, or transport of bile constituents. *Obstructive cholestasis* is related to obstruction of bile flow at the level of the major bile ducts or gallbladder.

Jaundice (icterus) occurs when the tissues, particularly the sclerae, are pigmented yellow because of an excess of bile pigments, primarily bilirubin, in the plasma. Jaundice can arise from hepatocellular cholestasis or obstructive cholestasis and, in addition, from prehepatic causes, such as an overproduction of bilirubin from heme catabolism in hemolytic diseases (Fig. 2-47). The associated hypoxia caused by anemia may facilitate cholestasis in hemolytic diseases.

Histologically, both forms of cholestasis share common features, but there are additional lesions associated with duct obstruction in the portal tracts and bile ducts. The main histologic manifestation of cholestasis is accumulation of homogeneous waxy brown bile pigment in bile canaliculi. Bile regurgitated from hepatocytes can also be found in Kupffer cells following phagocytosis. Bilirubin can be found in the hepatocellular cytoplasm in most species, especially if frozen sections are examined, but it is quite rare for bile to be evident in canine hepatocytes. Bile accumulation is more severe in the centrilobular regions of the lobules, but can extend to the periportal regions in severe cases. With time, canalicular plugs are cleared, and they may not be evident in more chronic cases of cholestasis. Hepatocyte rosettes, collections of 2 or more hepatocytes surrounding a dilated canaliculus are common. Hepatocellular degeneration may also be evident, sometimes with bile staining of the cytoplasm of injured hepatocytes. Scattered apoptotic cells may be present, although significant

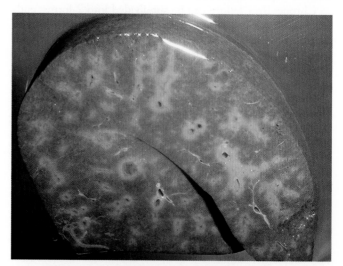

Figure 2-47 Deeply bile-stained liver from a jaundiced dog with immune hemolytic anemia and cholecystitis. (Courtesy A.P. Loretti.)

necrosis is not usually a feature of cholestasis. In more severe cases of obstructive cholestasis, confluent areas of bile-stained hepatocellular necrosis, termed **bile infarcts,** can develop. Bile infarcts are rare in dogs and cats, but can be found in other species. *Cholate stasis* refers to hepatocellular degeneration in the periportal region, often accompanied by a proliferation of small-caliber bile ducts (ductular reaction). Affected hepatocytes have swollen pale cytoplasm, and they may contain copper granules. This lesion is most common in horses with obstruction and rare in dogs. In hepatocellular cholestasis, there are no distinctive lesions in the portal tracts. However, in obstructive cholestasis, there are a number of distinctive changes. Initially, there is edema in the portal tract and an inflammatory infiltrate that is most often predominantly neutrophilic. There is an accompanying proliferation of small-caliber bile ducts arranged in an apparently haphazard fashion (ductular reaction). There may be degeneration or proliferative changes in pre-existing interlobular bile ducts, often associated with inflammation, depending on the cause of the obstruction. Ductal ectasia may also be present. With time, there is an increase of fibrosis that expands the portal tract outline and can bridge between portal tracts in cases of severe obstruction. In addition, there is concentric fibrosis surrounding the bile ducts. Proliferation of bile ducts, termed ductular reaction, is a constant feature. Mixed inflammatory cells, usually with fewer neutrophils than that seen in acute cholestasis, as well as macrophages containing pigment found in the portal tract.

Hepatocellular cholestasis arises when there is a disturbance in 1 or more of the 3 main steps involved in bile excretion. They include failure (1) to take up bilirubin, bile acids, or other bile constituents; (2) to conjugate bilirubin, bile acids, or other constituents; and (3) to transport and excrete conjugated bilirubin, bile acids, or other bile constituents into canaliculi. Most of these bile metabolism issues are mediated by a series of hepatobiliary transporters, molecular pumps involved in the transport of bilirubin, bile acids, and other organic ions in hepatocytes, canaliculi, and biliary epithelium, although some pumps serve to export substances as well. Hepatocellular uptake of unconjugated and conjugated bilirubin, like other organic ions, is mediated by members of the organic anion-transporting polypeptide (OATP) family found on the basolateral aspects of hepatocytes. Bilirubin is conjugated by uridine diphosphate–glucuronyl transferase in the endoplasmic reticulum of hepatocytes. From there it is transported into the bile. Bile acids are imported from the plasma by the Na$^+$-taurocholate cotransporting polypeptide (NTCP). Transport of bile acids, the main osmotic driving force for bile formation (bile acid–dependent flow), into the canaliculus is performed by the bile salt export pump (BSEP). Aquaporin channels facilitate the movement of water into the canaliculus in response to the osmotic forces produced by the bile acids. Movement of bilirubin into the canaliculus for excretion is accomplished by the multidrug-resistance–associated protein-2 (MRP-2). Reduced glutathione is also a substrate for MRP-2, and it is reduced glutathione and bicarbonate that are the main elements of the bile acid–independent portion of bile flow, the second most significant force in bile flow. Bile is continually modified by transporter-driven processes of secretion and absorption during its transit to the duodenum.

In hepatocellular cholestasis, drugs or endotoxin-induced proinflammatory cytokines interfere with the activities of molecular pumps or inhibit their synthesis. Endotoxin exposure both reduces activity of OATP and NCTP, but also interferes with the activity of BSEP and MRP-2.

Hepatocellular cholestasis can also occur through disruption of the structural integrity of the canaliculi, as discussed later for *Lantana camara* toxicity. Poisons such as phalloidin and cytochalasin, which disrupt the polymerization cycle of pericanalicular actin microfilaments, are cholestatic because these contractile filaments are required for propelling bile along the canaliculi. In horses, fasting can cause plasma bilirubin increases and jaundice. The mechanism may be the impaired uptake of bilirubin from the plasma or possibly impaired conjugation of bilirubin when energy supplies are low. Rarely, cholestasis and its indicators can occur in the absence of significant hepatocellular damage and other signs of liver failure. This can occur in toxicity by *L. camara* in ruminants and as an idiosyncratic reaction to some drugs.

In **obstructive cholestasis,** the activities of NTCP and OATP transporters are both reduced, causing bile acids and bilirubin to accumulate in the blood. Transport of bile acids out of the hepatocyte and into the canaliculus is maintained by BSEP. The regulation of transcription of the various transporters in hepatocellular or obstructive cholestasis is controlled by the interaction of bilirubin or bile acids with several nuclear receptors, primarily PXR (pregnane X receptor) and, to a lesser extent, others, such as CAR (constitutive androstane receptor) and FXR (farnesoid X receptor). During cholestasis, nuclear receptors orchestrate protection of hepatocytes from injury by reducing the expression of basolateral uptake transporters and increasing the expression of basolateral export pumps, as well as reducing new bile acid synthesis and increasing the rate of intrahepatic metabolism of bile acids. However, these adaptive responses are not always sufficient to prevent cholate-induced hepatotoxicity.

Severe diffuse liver necrosis obviously impairs bile excretion at various levels, but *the severity of cholestasis or of jaundice depends on the amount of liver affected, the chronicity, the supply of heme for catabolism, and nonhepatic routes of bilirubin excretion.* Focal liver injury can have substantial local cholestasis, but clinically detectable cholestasis does not occur because bilirubin can be cleared by unaffected parts of the liver. Similarly, segmental duct obstructions that spare some parts of the liver can lead to cholestasis but not jaundice. This can occur in anorexic or dehydrated cats, in which bile may become dehydrated and viscous, causing ductal obstruction.

Some of the various transporters and conjugating enzymes involved in bilirubin excretion can be genetically defective. *Congenital hyperbilirubinemia in mutant Southdown sheep* is the result of impaired hepatic uptake of unconjugated bilirubin. These animals have few liver lesions, but eventually develop chronic renal disease, the reason for which is not clear. Unconjugated bilirubin levels in the plasma are consistently elevated, but sufficient excretion takes place to prevent them from becoming icteric. They become photosensitized, indicating that excretion of phylloerythrin (phytoporphyrin) is less efficient than that of bilirubin.

Hyperbilirubinemia in mutant Corriedale sheep is a defect in excretion of conjugated bilirubin similar to Dubin-Johnson syndrome in humans and mutant rat strains. In humans and rats, there is a mutation in Mrp-2 causing hypofunction and a similar mutation is likely in affected sheep. Affected sheep have an elevation of plasma bilirubin (just over half of which is conjugated), but there is no obvious jaundice. Nevertheless, phylloerythrin (phytoporphyrin) excretion in these

Corriedale sheep is also sufficiently impaired to produce photosensitization. There is impaired excretion of other conjugated metabolites, and there is dark pigmentation of the liver by polymerized residues of retained catecholamine metabolites. This pigment, resembling lipofuscin, accumulates in lysosomes in the pericanalicular cytoplasm.

The recognition of jaundice at postmortem sometimes involves differentiation of bile staining of tissues from the yellow staining caused by accumulation of carotenoid pigments. These latter are limited to fat depots and are to be expected in certain species such as horses; sometimes there are breed influences, as seen in the yellow fat of Channel Island breeds of dairy cattle. The yellow discoloration of fat depots of older cats is less well understood. In animals fed ox liver, carotenoids may again be responsible, and in others, there may be some contribution by ceroid-type pigments. Distinction of the fatty pigments from bile depends on the absence of the former from pale, nonfatty tissues, such as periosteum and dermal collagen.

Photosensitization

Photosensitization is the term applied to inflammation of skin (usually unpigmented) because of the action of ultraviolet light of wavelengths 290-400 nm on photodynamic compounds that have become bound to dermal cells. In **primary photosensitization,** these compounds may have been deposited unchanged in the skin after ingestion, before the normal liver is capable of excreting the native compound. This is seen, for example, after ingestion of hypericin in St. John's wort *(Hypericum perforatum).* Photodynamic agents may also be produced by aberrant endogenous metabolism. This can occur, for example, in congenital erythropoietic protoporphyria caused by ferrochelatase deficiency in Limousin and Blonde d'Aquitaine calves.

Hepatogenous photosensitization almost always accompanies cholestasis of more than a few days' duration in herbivores that are kept in sunlight and that have been eating green feed. *Phytoporphyrins* (formerly termed phylloerythrins) are green photoactive catabolites of plant porphyrins (mainly chlorophyll) that are generated by the alimentary microflora of herbivores. Some phytoporphyrin is absorbed and normally excreted in the bile by the transporters that eliminate bilirubin. Cholestasis in herbivores can increase retention of phytoporphyrin in the blood, and it can result in photosensitive dermatitis of unpigmented areas of skin exposed to sunlight for several days (Fig. 2-48). It is possible, however, for mild photosensitization to appear in the absence of gross or microscopic evidence of cholestasis in animals grazing alfalfa, *Paspalum,* pangola, or *Panicum* grasses; however, it is unclear if these are related to phytoporphyrin or other photoactive products of these forages. Absence of serum biochemical evidence for cholestasis or liver damage is used to differentiate primary from secondary photosensitization in these circumstances.

If no hepatic changes can be discerned in photosensitized animals, the possibility of primary photosensitization must be considered, but hepatogenous photosensitization cannot be excluded unless adequate liver function tests are performed.

Hemorrhage and liver failure

Hemorrhagic diathesis characterized by widespread ecchymoses and petechiae can occur when the liver is injured and becomes the site of significant clotting factor consumption. However, recent investigations suggest that clinically

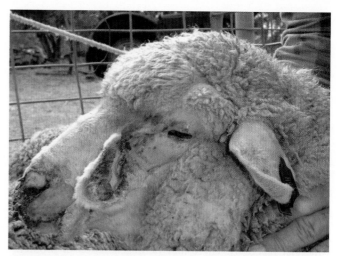

Figure 2-48 Hepatogenous photosensitization caused by *Panicum miliaceum* (French millet) in a sheep. (Courtesy P. Hoskin.)

significant hemorrhage is not common in acute liver failure. The liver is the source of plasma proteins involved in the clotting cascade, but these are normally supplied in substantial excess, and can be induced as part of the acute-phase response to inflammation. Thus *coagulopathy with hemorrhage is most likely to occur when there is acute liver necrosis,* for example, in acute canine infectious hepatitis or xylitol toxicity. Under these conditions, there is significant intrahepatic consumption of clotting factors at sites of endothelial necrosis in the damaged liver. Although the damaged liver also fails to resupply the clotting factors, consumption is probably a minor contributing influence. In more chronic liver diseases with hypoproteinemia, coagulation tests may be prolonged, but hemorrhagic diathesis is unlikely, unless there is an additional demand for hemostasis, for example, during the trauma of surgery. Although production of clotting factors is often reduced in liver failure, there is a commensurate reduction in anticoagulant synthesis as well. Portal hypertension and endothelial cell dysfunction may also be a contributing cause for bleeding in chronic liver disease. Overall, the pathogenesis of hemorrhagic tendencies in chronic liver disease is complex, multifactorial, and incompletely understood. Consumption of clotting factors can also occur in septic diseases that affect the liver and other tissues.

Nephropathy

Acute liver failure may be accompanied by oliguria and biochemical indications of renal failure. **Hepatorenal syndrome** is a complication of advanced cirrhosis in humans, characterized by renal failure in which there are no intrinsic renal morphologic or functional causes. The pathogenesis of hepatorenal syndrome is related to *deterioration in effective arterial blood volume because of splanchnic arterial vasodilation and reduced venous return and cardiac output.* Intense compensatory vasoconstriction of the renal circulation results in decreased glomerular filtration and resultant renal failure. In addition, some hepatic toxins such as acetaminophen may produce injury in the nephrons as well.

Edema and ascites

Ascites (retention of excess low-protein peritoneal fluid) is a feature of chronic liver failure, but is more frequently associated with systemic venous congestion (e.g., right-sided heart failure) or hypoproteinemia secondary to protein-losing renal or alimentary tract conditions. *It is likely that ascites in advanced liver disease is influenced by both mechanical and dynamic influences on blood flow through a damaged liver.* Reduced synthesis of albumin and globulins by the failing liver can reduce vascular oncotic pressure, but edema resulting from this mechanism is generalized. Experimentally, restriction of blood flow from the liver leads to a swift increase in sinusoidal plasma within the space of Disse, leading to increased lymph flow into the thoracic duct and through the hepatic capsule. This explains rapid ascites formation in cases of hepatic outflow obstruction or veno-occlusive diseases.

There are several theories that explain the complicated process of ascites formation in chronic liver disease. The theory that best encompasses the known circulatory changes is known as the *peripheral arteriolar vasodilation hypothesis.* In end-stage livers, there is progressive sinusoidal and portal vein hypertension with collateral vein formation and acquisition of shunting vessels to the systemic vasculature. Sinusoidal hypertension appears to be an important feature as ascites rarely develops with prehepatic portal hypertension. *The main factor leading to ascites formation is splanchnic vasodilation.* In chronic liver failure, there is increasing portal vein hypertension and a local release of vasodilators, such as nitric oxide, leading to splanchnic arterial dilation. With progression, the extent of the arterial vasodilation increases to the point that effective arterial volume and pressure drops, leading to activation of vasoconstrictor and antinatriuretic factors, including activation of the renin-angiotensin-aldosterone system and the sympathetic nervous system, promoting retention of sodium and fluid. Intestinal capillary pressure and permeability are increased as a result of the increased portal vein hypertension, promoting excess fluid transit to the abdominal cavity. Over time, sodium retention by the kidneys is insufficient to compensate for the progressive arteriolar vasodilation as well as the movement of sodium and fluid to the extracellular space of the abdomen. This movement is enhanced by hypoproteinemia caused by reduced synthesis by the liver and dilution secondary to fluid retention. Consequently, there is persistent activation of antinatriuretic systems, and fluid continues to accumulate. There is evidence that increased venous return caused by reduced peripheral arterial vasodilation stimulates endogenous natriuretic substances, but this response is insufficient to counteract the more significant release of antinatriuretic signals.

Retention of peritoneal fluid can also sometimes result from mechanical obstructions to mesenteric and peritoneal lymphatics by inflammatory or neoplastic lesions. Peritoneal fluids with a higher protein and cell content that accumulate in various abdominal inflammatory conditions are considered exudates (see section on Peritonitis in Vol. 2, Alimentary system and peritoneum).

Hepatocutaneous syndrome

An *idiopathic vacuolar hepatopathy with parenchymal collapse and nodular regeneration* has been reported in dogs and cats that have been presented clinically with hepatocutaneous syndrome *(necrolytic migratory erythema, superficial necrolytic dermatitis).* The skin disease resembles necrolytic migratory erythema in humans, a well-defined paraneoplastic syndrome typically associated with hyperglucagonemia secondary to glucagon-secreting pancreatic neoplasia, but also reported in individuals with hepatitis, cirrhosis, celiac disease, chronic malabsorption, and inflammatory bowel disease. *In dogs, hepatocutaneous syndrome is most commonly associated with liver disease,* including severe vacuolar hepatopathy, idiopathic hepatocellular collapse, and hepatopathy secondary to anticonvulsant drug administration, and more rarely with glucagonoma and gastric carcinoma.

Clinical presentation is typically because of the dermatitis; skin lesions include erythema, crusting, exudation, ulceration, and alopecia, affecting footpads, periocular, perioral, anogenital regions, and pressure points. The dermatologic lesions are described more fully in Vol. 1, Integumentary system. Affected dogs have depressed plasma amino acid concentrations, inconsistent elevations of plasma glucagon levels, and may also become diabetic. The liver of affected dogs is usually grossly nodular, resembling cirrhosis (eFig. 2-10A); however, histologically, there is typically moderate to severe vacuolation of hepatocytes, with parenchymal collapse accompanied by nodular regeneration (eFig. 2-10B). Inflammation, necrosis, and fibrosis are not usually prominent. Although some studies report fibrosis typical of cirrhosis, more characteristically, there is a network of reticulin and fine collagen fibers representing the remnants of collapsed hepatic lobules, with proliferation of bile ductules. The vacuolated hepatocytes stain with oil red O for lipids. *The hepatic lesions have been suggested to support an underlying metabolic, hormonal, or toxic etiology.* In humans, persistent hyperglucagonemia stimulates prolonged gluconeogenesis, resulting in secondary hypoaminoacidemia. Although hepatic insufficiency can increase glucagon levels in animal models, in dogs, the link between liver disease and hypoaminoacidemia remains unclear. A hypermetabolic state with exaggerated amino acid catabolism has, however, been suggested. Other biologically active molecules that are normally cleared by the normal liver or generated by a damaged liver should also be considered.

Further reading

Bernal W, et al. Acute liver failure. Lancet 2010;376:190-201.

Mullen KD, Prakash RK. Hepatic Encephalopathy. New York: Humana Press; 2012.

Quinn JC, et al. Secondary plant products causing photosensitization in grazing herbivores: their structure, activity and regulation. Int J Mol Sci 2014;15:1441-1465.

Tripodi A, Mannucci PM. The coagulopathy of chronic liver disease. N Engl J Med 2011;365:147-156.

POSTMORTEM AND AGONAL CHANGES IN LIVER

The liver, rich in nutrients for bacteria and freely exposed to agonal invaders from the intestine, *undergoes postmortem decomposition very rapidly.* Gas bubbles generated by anaerobic saprophytes form first in the hepatic blood vessels, but soon suffuse large portions of the organ. The vessels and adjacent parenchyma are stained by hemoglobin. The substance of the organ becomes soft and clay-like, and the formation of putrefactive gases may make it foamy. On the capsular surface, irregular, pale foci are visible; they superficially may resemble infarcts or fatty areas but can be observed to increase in size during the postmortem interval, and microscopically are without cellular reaction. Bacilli are present in large numbers in such foci. Green-black pigmentation of the capsule and superficial parenchyma occurs where the liver is in contact with gut, and the lobes surrounding the gallbladder become stained by bile.

Microscopic structural changes occur in the liver, approaching and immediately following death. Shrinkage of liver cells, possibly because of a period of anaerobic catabolism of glycogen, and widening of centrilobular (periacinar) sinusoids because of hepatic congestion, are seen after death. *Dissociation of liver cells* may be complete, with every cell in every cord separated and free from adjacent cells, so architectural patterns are lost. The early expression of this change affects centrilobular cells, which become detached, rounded in contour, condensed, and hyperchromatic. The dissociation is particularly evident in feline panleukopenia and leptospirosis, related in part to antemortem changes.

VASCULAR FACTORS IN HEPATIC INJURY AND CIRCULATORY DISORDERS

Hepatic artery

The hepatic artery delivers approximately ⅓ of the afferent hepatic blood supply, but ~40-50% of the oxygen. Hepatic artery flow responds to alterations in portal vein flow to sustain overall perfusion of the liver at a nearly consistent level via what is termed the *hepatic arterial buffer response*. Hepatic arterial flow is believed to be regulated via adenosine levels in the space of Mall. Adenosine is produced at a constant level, but with decreased portal flow less adenosine is washed out, raising local concentrations and causing the hepatic artery to dilate and increase arterial flow. Other mediators of arterial flow are recognized, and they include hydrogen sulfide, nitric oxide, and the autonomic nervous system.

Complete loss of arterial flow can be, after a brief period of injury, compensated for via the portal flow because the liver normally only extracts ~40% of the oxygen supplied by the portal vein. Within the liver, branches of the hepatic artery form several patterns, including (1) a peribiliary plexus, (2) a vasa vasorum for the portal vein, or (3) an array of terminal hepatic arterioles that drain directly into the sinusoids. In addition, the hepatic artery provides branches to supply the liver capsule. The peribiliary plexus surrounds intrahepatic bile ducts and likely plays a role in an exchange of bile constituents and vasoactive factors. Hepatic arterial occlusions occur rather commonly in animals but usually involve small intrahepatic branches and are of little consequence. Large segments of the liver may be necrotic in cats as a result of thrombosis of the aorta and hepatic artery. Verminous arteritis may occlude the hepatic artery in horses. The extent of necrosis depends on how completely the obstruction excludes collateral circulation and also on the oxygen tension of the portal blood. Ischemic areas of liver can be sequestered, but in some instances, bacteria such as clostridia and other anaerobes can flourish and release potent toxins with systemic effects.

Portal vein

The portal vein drains the large and small intestine, stomach, pancreas, gallbladder, and spleen and normally contributes ⅔ of hepatic blood flow. Because the portal vein collects blood from the abdominal viscera, the rate of flow is variable, depending on physiologic factors such as eating, which increases, or stress, which decreases, portal flow. Portal venous blood has considerably more oxygen than most systemic venous blood and contributes ~60% of the liver's oxygen needs. The portal vein branches successively until the finest branches, the terminal portal venules, drain into the sinusoids via side branches, the inlet venules. Entry of blood into the sinusoids is regulated via sphincters in the terminal inlet venules. Portal blood flow is likely streamlined, rather than turbulent, but there is little agreement regarding existence of specific patterns of flow. Streamlining may account for the different regional distributions sometimes observed with metastatic tumors and infections. The umbilical vein usually drains to the left lobe, so hematogenous umbilical infections tend to localize in the left lobe.

The liver cannot regulate portal venous flow, so hepatic blood flow is largely balanced by arterial supply that varies with the portal venous supply to maintain a relatively consistent hepatic perfusion. Hepatic microcirculation is well regulated at the level of inflow by sphincters in the finest branches of the portal venules, the inlet venules, as well as the terminal branches of the hepatic arterioles and at the level of outflow by sphincters that regulate passage of blood from the sinusoids to the terminal hepatic venules. In dogs, the spiral smooth muscle that invests the wall of sublobular hepatic veins can contract and alter hepatic venous outflow in various conditions, particularly in shock, where contraction leads to acute congestion and pooling of blood in the liver and the organs that drain into the portal vein. Hepatic blood thus flows evenly through the sinusoids under a very-low-pressure gradient. The liver receives ~25% of the cardiac output, even though it represents only ~2.5% of body mass. Approximately 25% of the weight of the liver in situ is blood.

Obstruction of the portal vein, if sudden and complete, can produce a condition akin to strangulation of the gut, and death occurs quickly without significant hepatic change; however, surgical diversion of the portal vein into the vena cava produces only transient injury to the liver. Obstruction of a large branch of the portal vein in cattle, sheep, and cats leads to acute ischemia of a wedge of tissue in which necrosis may be zonal or massive. Obstruction of many small portal radicles is common, with necrosis of many lobules. It is evident that if a collateral supply develops and oxygenation remains adequate, obstruction of portal radicles will have no immediate effect on the hepatic parenchyma, save perhaps to make it more sensitive to toxic injury. The parenchyma in the affected lobe, deprived of hepatotrophic factors, loses much of its regenerative power and atrophies fairly rapidly, allowing condensation and scarification of the stromal tissues. Loss of portal venous inflow and obstruction of hepatic venous outflow, a double-hit insult, can lead to complete infarction of the liver as seen in hepatic lobe torsion. Arterial supply can be obstructed as well in this situation.

Acute increase in pressure in the portal vein may occur in any severe episode of widespread acute hepatic necrosis; the cause appears to be simple obstruction of the sinusoidal flow by thrombosis and actual sinusoidal disruption. In such animals, there is severe acute congestion of the liver, slight ascites, free fibrin accumulations in the abdomen (not the firm capsular adhesions seen in passive congestion), and distended portal lymphatics.

Obstruction of the extrahepatic portal vein is quite uncommon. External compression may occur because of adjacent abscesses or neoplasms. **Portal vein thrombosis** may be caused by damage to the portal vein by local inflammatory processes

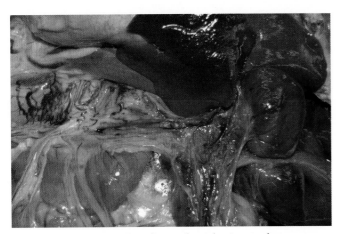

Figure 2-49 Portal vein thrombosis in a dog.

or be associated with states of hypercoagulability or retrograde intravascular growth of hepatic neoplasms. In dogs, thrombosis of the portal vein has been associated with distant neoplasia, immune-mediated hemolytic anemia, protein-losing nephropathy and enteropathy, pancreatitis, peritonitis, and corticosteroid administration (Fig. 2-49). Portal vein obstructions of slow development are expected to lead to portal hypertension and its consequences. Atresia or hypoplasia of the extrahepatic portal vein can be demonstrated in some cases of primary portal vein hypoplasia and is discussed previously in the section on Developmental disorders.

Obstruction of intrahepatic portal vessels is a consequence of progressive fibrosing lesions of primary hepatic disease centered on the portal triads. The small portal vessels may be obliterated in the proliferative portal lesions, and new connections may be established, including small functional arteriovenous communications. Regenerative hepatic nodules and neoplasms may deform and compress portal vessels in some locations.

Portal hypertension is defined as increased blood pressure within the portal vein caused by resistance to normal flow rates. Portal hypertension can arise from disturbances of venous blood flow in any of the following 3 sites: *prehepatic, intrahepatic, and posthepatic.*

Prehepatic portal hypertension is relatively uncommon and occurs when blood flow through the portal vein is impaired before it enters the liver. The most common cause is portal vein thrombosis. Intrahepatic portal hypertension arises from increased resistance to blood flow at the level of the hepatic parenchyma. Intrahepatic portal hypertension can be subdivided into 3 forms: *presinusoidal* (including intrahepatic portal vein hypoplasia, intrahepatic arterioportal fistulae, periportal neoplastic or inflammatory infiltrates, and periportal fibrosis), *sinusoidal* (cirrhosis or long-term inflammatory disease with fibrosis and capillarization of sinusoids, amyloidosis, neoplastic infiltrations), and *postsinusoidal* (perivenular fibrosis, veno-occlusive disease).

Posthepatic causes of portal hypertension are uncommon, but can result from increased resistance to blood flow in the major hepatic veins, caudal vena cava, or right heart. Causes include partial or complete thrombosis of the hepatic veins, which is very rare; obstruction of the hepatic veins by neoplastic occlusion (e.g., pheochromocytoma); and kinking of the caudal vena cava, associated with abdominal trauma. Congestive heart failure can also lead to portal hypertension.

Regardless of cause, *persistent portal hypertension can lead to acquired portosystemic shunts* (discussed later), with the exception of passive congestion, which rarely, if ever, results in the development of shunt vessels. These shunts are usually numerous and composed of distended thin-walled veins, which may connect the mesenteric veins and the caudal vena cava. Ascites is common in conditions that develop acquired shunts because of the associated portal hypertension.

Efferent hepatic vessels

Efferent flow begins in the sinusoids and passes through terminal hepatic venules and larger hepatic veins to the vena cava. In the sinusoidal network, flow is interconnected in many directions. However, in normal conditions, lobule outflow is closely matched to inflow. In dogs, hepatic veins have substantial spiral smooth-muscle sphincters that regulate outflow, but these are not evident in other domestic species. Splanchnic engorgement during anesthesia and anaphylaxis is an indication that these smooth muscles control canine hepatic outflow in a dynamic manner. Obstruction at the level of the large hepatic veins can occasionally occur because of suppurative phlebitis, hepatic abscesses, neoplasms, or other physical obstacles that impinge on the hepatic veins. Similar space-occupying lesions in or around the vena cava in the diaphragm or mediastinum can also affect hepatic outflow, along with systemic venous return.

The amount and arrangement of conventional connective tissue around the terminal hepatic veins and larger hepatic veins influence the patterns of fibrosis observed in various patterns of centrilobular injury. Hypoxia from anemia, heart failure, or shock can cause centrilobular necrosis, as can many toxic agents that are preferentially injurious to zone 3 hepatocytes. Necrosis at this level elicits a tissue repair response involving the fibrous connective tissue along the terminal hepatic venules. Tissue fibrosis can increase the resistance of the hepatic parenchyma and slow local outflow. This can redirect sinusoidal blood to alternative less-affected venules, unless the necrosis is extensive. **Hepatic veno-occlusive disease** *is the obliteration of small intrahepatic veins that may begin with damage to the sinusoidal endothelium, accumulation of red cells and fibrin in the subintimal space, and subsequent subendothelial fibrosis.* This pattern of postnecrotic fibrosis can contribute to the development of portal hypertension. Veno-occlusive disease is a feature of pyrrolizidine toxicosis in humans ingesting these alkaloids in so-called bush tea. In domestic animals, occlusive changes in terminal venules are notable in poisoning by ragwort (*Senecio jacobea*) in cattle and also in dogs treated experimentally with the pyrrolizidine alkaloid monocrotaline. Veno-occlusive disease has also been reported as a consequence of prolonged chemotherapy, radiotherapy, and bone marrow transplantation in humans, and similarly in dogs treated with irradiation or busulfan. Idiopathic veno-occlusive disease with perivenular fibrosis around central and sublobular veins, causing Budd-Chiari–like syndrome (see later), has also been reported as a rare occurrence in the dog and cat. Total or subtotal obliteration of central hepatic or sublobular veins by subintimal accumulation of collagen and fibrous tissue has also been reported in captive snow leopards and cheetahs.

Passive congestion of the liver develops when the blood pressure in the hepatic veins increases relative to that of the hepatic portal veins and can occur in any species. *It is almost always the consequence of cardiac dysfunction,* including acute and chronic heart failure, pericardial disease, and processes

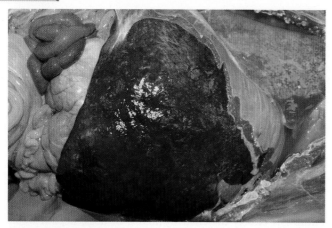

Figure 2-50 **Acute passive congestion** of the liver in a cria with a congenital heart defect.

that obstruct the flow of blood into or out of the heart, such as abscesses, heartworm disease, and local neoplasia. Right-sided heart failure, in particular, produces elevated pressure within the caudal vena cava that later involves the hepatic vein and its tributaries.

Acute passive congestion of the liver occurs when there is sudden cardiac decompensation, particularly on the right side of the heart, or shock. Grossly, there is slight enlargement of the liver, which is typically dark red, and blood flows freely from any cut surface (Fig. 2-50). The intrinsic lobular pattern of the liver may be slightly more pronounced, particularly on the cut surface, because centrilobular areas are congested (dark red) in contrast to the more normal color of the remainder of the lobule. The microscopic picture in acute passive congestion is initially characterized by distention of central veins and adjacent sinusoids, with accompanying distention of lymphatics in the stroma of hepatic veins, portal triads, and the capsule. The appearance of the liver differs with the duration and severity of the congestion. Fatty change, trabecular atrophy, and necrosis of centrilobular hepatocytes with retention of the perisinusoidal reticulum framework develop quickly. Erythrocytes tend to move into the perisinusoidal spaces left by the lost hepatocytes, and may be seen trapped there when blood drains from sinusoids and veins in freshly fixed sections. The intrahepatic network of lymphatics at this stage becomes very distended and may form extensive cavernous channels about hepatic veins and venules, in portal triads, and just beneath the capsule. With increased venous pressure, transudation of red blood cells and high-protein-content edema can develop, leading to polymerization of released fibrinogen on the capsular surface that yields a fibrin coating of the capsule and blood-tinged abdominal fluid. Distension of the space of Disse may be seen, but rarely, if ever, in tissue well fixed soon after death, and is best regarded as a postmortem artifact. By comparison, perisinusoidal edema is more obvious in hepatic congestion associated with shock or inflammatory conditions.

In **chronic passive congestion,** the amounts of fibrous connective tissue in the liver increase in various patterns that differ among species. The capsular surface becomes thicker and more opaque, and can develop a finely nodular texture with the formation of capsular plaques (eFig. 2-11A). In dogs and cats, the edges of the central lobes become rounded, whereas the margins of lateral and caudate lobes are sharpened by peripheral atrophy and fibrosis. If the cause of the

congestion is still present, there is usually copious ascites at this stage. In species in which fibrosis is more pronounced, a chronically congested liver has a distinct reticulated acinar pattern, often more obvious beneath the capsule than in deeper parenchyma. This pattern is known as **"nutmeg liver"** and is *the result of the contrast of red centrilobular zones of congestion with loss of hepatocytes, among pale swollen periportal parenchyma composed of viable hepatocytes that are fatty* (eFig. 2-11B). This classic pattern of chronic passive congestion is most obvious in ruminants and horses. The "nutmeg" pattern can be mimicked by some forms of toxic periacinar necrosis or fatty change but should always be distinguishable from them by the presence of fibrous plaques in Glisson's capsule in the passively congested liver. The pale lobular pattern is less obvious in carnivores and should not be expected in animals that have insufficient adipose reserves for mobilization. Over longer periods, *centrilobular fibrosis links terminal hepatic venules with one another and with the larger portal triads in a pattern known as* **cardiac fibrosis.**

Inflammatory changes in the outflow veins are sometimes observed. Acute inflammation and thrombosis of sublobular veins are typical of acute salmonellosis in many species, but these changes are terminal and not associated with hepatic dysfunction. Inflammatory cell infiltrates are occasionally observed in the larger hepatic veins, and have been described in dogs with parvoviral myocarditis. Muscular hypertrophy of walls of hepatic veins has been described in dogs with arteriovenous fistulae. Fibrous remodeling of these veins has been associated with nitrosamine intoxication in domestic animals.

The term **Budd-Chiari syndrome** is used to describe the clinical features associated with hepatic venous outflow obstruction caused by thrombosis of the main hepatic veins in humans. **Hepatic vein thrombosis** is a rare occurrence in dogs and cats. In veterinary medicine, it is more appropriate to use specific morphologic diagnostic terms to describe pathologic changes that develop in response to various mechanical causes of postsinusoidal obstruction of hepatic venous flow, resulting in development of *hepatomegaly, postsinusoidal portal hypertension, high-protein ascites, and acquired portosystemic collateral shunting.* Causes include obstruction of flow caused by tumors (e.g., intraluminal leiomyosarcoma or other sarcoma, adrenal pheochromocytoma with extensive invasion into the caudal vena cava in the dog) or abscesses in the liver or caudal vena cava, hepatic venous or vena caval thrombosis, congenital malformation (fibrous web), kink or acquired stricture occluding the lumen of the vena cava or hepatic veins (intrahepatic postsinusoidal venous obstruction), or cardiac abnormalities impairing right atrial function (cor triatrium dexter, neoplasia). Histologic changes include distension of the hepatic veins and perivenous sinusoidal congestion, which, with chronicity, leads to perivenous fibrosis typical of chronic passive congestion.

Thrombosis of the caudal vena cava has been described in detail in cattle, where rupture of a hepatic abscess into the caudal vena cava is the most common etiology (Fig. 2-51). Sequelae include pulmonary emboli, endoarteritis, multifocal pulmonary abscessation, and chronic suppurative bronchopneumonia.

Acquired portosystemic shunts

Congenital shunts have been described previously in the section on Developmental disorders. *Acquired portosystemic shunts within and external to the liver can develop in association*

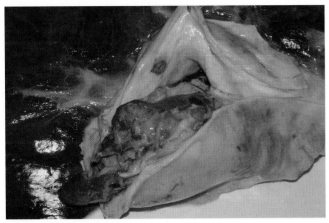

Figure 2-51 Thromboembolism of the caudal vena cava in an ox. (Courtesy K.G. Thompson.)

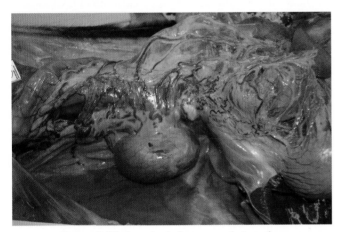

Figure 2-52 Acquired shunt vessels in a dog.

with various chronic liver diseases that lead to portal hypertension. These shunts tend to be multiple, small, and tortuous (Fig. 2-52). They may be difficult to identify postmortem when they are collapsed. They are easily destroyed by routine dissection, so they must be noted before removal of the abdominal viscera. Acquired shunts can be associated with evidence of portal hypertension, such as distension of the portal veins and ascites, but when shunts are multiple and well established, portal hypertension is somewhat relieved. *It is important to distinguish these varicose dilations that develop in response to portal hypertension from true congenital portosystemic shunts.* Acquired shunts arise in vestigial nonfunctional portosystemic communications that dilate and become functional in response to portal hypertension. They tend to develop between mesenteric veins and the caudal vena cava, right renal vein, or gonadal veins, and are multiple, taking the form of a plexus of tortuous, thin-walled vessels. Esophageal shunts and varicosities are common in humans with cirrhosis, but are much less important in domestic animals. This may be related to postural differences such that shunts are more likely to enter the vena cava, where central venous pressure is least. In dogs, acquired shunts are most numerous along the caudal mesentery.

Peliosis hepatis/telangiectasis

Peliosis hepatis is a term used to designate a hepatic vascular disorder characterized by cystic, blood-filled spaces in the liver. The distinction between telangiectasis and peliosis hepatis is subtle at best, and both conditions can be considered together.

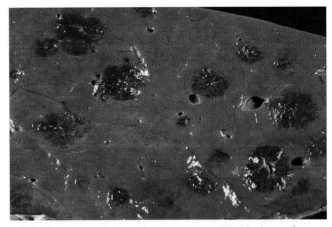

Figure 2-53 Peliosis hepatis (telangiectasis) in the liver of an ox. (Courtesy K.G. Thompson.)

There are 2 forms of peliosis hepatis, although both can appear in the same animal. Intrinsic weakness of the local reticulin framework leading to sinusoidal dilation is the hallmark of the *phlebectatic form of peliosis hepatis*, and the other form is characterized by death of hepatocytes and sinusoidal distention *(parenchymal type)*. Peliosis hepatis lesions occur throughout the liver as dark red areas, irregular in shape but well circumscribed, and ranging from pinpoints to many centimeters in size (Fig. 2-53, eFig 2-12). Sectioned or capsular surfaces are depressed after death, and on cutting, they appear as cavities from which the blood drains to reveal a delicate network of residual stroma. The histologic lesion is characterized by multiple, dilated, blood-filled spaces sometimes surrounded by fibromyxoid stroma. The blood-filled cystic spaces may be lined by endothelium. In humans, these lesions have an idiosyncratic association with administration of various drugs, including anabolic and contraceptive steroids. Infectious peliosis hepatis caused by *Bartonella henselae* or *B. quintana* infection has also been described in immunosuppressed human patients.

Peliosis hepatis has been reported in cattle, dogs, and cats, but the pathogenesis is unknown. B. henselae DNA has been identified by PCR from the liver of a single canine case, but does not seem to be involved in the feline disorder. Bovine hepatic peliosis hepatis (telangiectasis) and human peliosis hepatis have been suggested to share a similar pathogenesis. Primary alteration of the sinusoidal barrier, with rupture of the reticulin fibers and increased deposition of basement membrane components in the perisinusoidal region and fibrosis, may alter oxygen and substrate exchange between hepatocytes and the blood, leading to hemodynamic imbalance, hepatocyte atrophy, and eventually to sinusoidal disruption. Peliosis hepatis in livers is quite common in older cats and cattle (Fig. 2-54). There is no evidence clinically of related liver dysfunction. In cats, the cavities are rather more frequent in the subcapsular zone and rarely exceed 2-3 mm in size. There are often other senile changes in these livers, such as chronic fatty change, nodular hyperplasia, and chronic hepatitis.

A specific condition termed *"peliosis"* develops in cattle poisoned by plants of *Pimelea* spp. This form *begins as diffuse periportal sinusoidal dilation.* Because these changes are also found in these animals in the spleen and in other organs with sinusoidal microcirculation, it seems that the lesions may be adaptive to progressive and dramatic increases in total blood volume. In the late stages of the intoxication by *Pimelea,* the

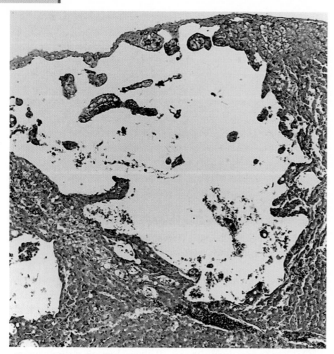

Figure 2-54 Histologic appearance of **peliosis hepatis** in a dog.

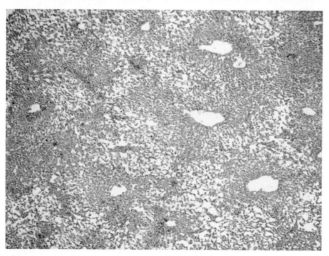

Figure 2-55 **Periportal sinusoidal dilation** resulting from chronic *Pimelea* poisoning in an ox. (Courtesy R. Kelly.)

liver may resemble a huge, blood-filled sponge (Fig. 2-55). The animals eventually die of a combination of hemodilutional anemia and circulatory failure.

Further reading

Crawford JM, Burt AD. Anatomy, pathophysiology and basic mechanisms of disease. In: Burt AD, et al., editors. Macsween's Pathology of the Liver. 6th ed. New York: Churchill Livingstone; 2012. p. 2-77.

Eipel C, et al. Regulation of hepatic blood flow: the hepatic arterial buffer response revisited. World J Gastroenterol 2010;16: 6046-6057.

INFLAMMATORY DISEASES OF THE LIVER AND BILIARY TRACT

The inflammatory response in the liver is unusual for 3 main reasons. First, *hepatic microvasculature is structurally and functionally different from tissues with capillary vasculature.*

Microvascular permeability to plasma proteins, a hallmark of acute inflammation in most tissues, is a normal property of the fenestrated sinusoidal endothelium of the liver. Thus sinusoidal edema is not a prominent feature of acute parenchymal inflammation, although edema can be observed in the capsule, portal tracts, connective tissue of the terminal and sublobular hepatic veins (particularly in dogs), and in the wall of the gallbladder. Microvascular blood flow in hepatic sinusoids is also less responsive to the actions of various vasoactive mediators that alter blood flow in most other acutely inflamed tissues. Second, resident *Kupffer cells play an important and complex role in liver inflammation, injury, and repair.* Kupffer cells function in the innate immune response, acting as the final component of the gut barrier by phagocytosing pathogens, immunoreactive material, and endotoxin entering the liver via the portal circulation. However, Kupffer cells also exhibit a range of different activated phenotypes, depending on the local metabolic and immune environment. Classically activated macrophages secrete proinflammatory cytokines, including tumor necrosis factor-α, interleukin-1 (IL-1), IL-6, IL-12, and inducible nitric oxide synthase (iNOS), influencing cell populations in the liver and elsewhere, whereas alternatively, activated macrophages express anti-inflammatory mediators, including IL-10 and contribute to resolution of inflammation and promote repair. Dysregulation of the complex control of inflammatory responses in Kupffer cells can contribute to chronic inflammation in the liver. Third, *the liver has central regulatory influences on many proinflammatory insults and inflammatory mediators.* As the major source of acute-phase proteins, including secreted pathogen recognition receptors (PRRs), short pentraxins, components of the complement system, and regulators of iron metabolism, hepatocytes are essential constituents of innate immunity and largely contribute to the control of a systemic inflammatory response. The liver is also the site of degradation of most soluble plasma proteins, and Kupffer cells are the main site of clearance of immune complexes from the circulation, playing an important role in the development of immunotolerance to potential antigenic substances absorbed from the intestine. A full discussion of immune surveillance, and the complex innate and adaptive immune responses involved in initiation and regulation of liver inflammation, is beyond the scope of this chapter, and readers are directed to current review articles on the subject.

These unusual aspects of the inflammatory response in the liver can make it more difficult to differentiate certain degenerative and inflammatory conditions in this organ. Ongoing cell death and repair can appear inflammatory, and acute leukocyte responses can cause necrosis and apoptosis in the liver. *The term* "**necroinflammatory**" *is convenient when the underlying pathogenetic mechanisms of necrosis and inflammation are unknown.*

Increased numbers of leukocytes (**sinusoidal leukocytosis**) are observed in hepatic sinusoids in many acute or subacute bacteremias, as well as in conditions of steroid excess in dogs. This change can be diagnostically useful but does not constitute evidence of hepatitis unless there is obvious infiltration of granulocytes, monocytes, or lymphocytes into the perisinusoidal space. **Extramedullary hematopoiesis** can also appear as focal aggregates of myeloid cells in the perisinusoidal compartment. This change can be distinguished from inflammatory infiltrates by the presence of immature myeloid cells. Occasionally, hematopoietic cells from the splenic red pulp can be artifactually extruded into the portal vasculature and appear in the liver, usually as nucleated cell aggregates in the larger portal veins.

Infectious agents capable of causing hepatitis include viruses, bacteria, fungi, protozoa, and helminths. Autoimmune and idiosyncratic drug responses also occur, but often the etiology of acute or chronic hepatitis cannot be determined.

Hepatic inflammation

The liver is subject to infectious and degenerative insults that elicit inflammatory responses in various patterns, for which the general term *hepatitis* is appropriate. The term **hepatitis** *is used for focal or diffuse hepatic conditions that are either caused by infectious agents or characterized by a leukocytic infiltrative inflammatory response, irrespective of the cause.* This definition allows inclusion of viral infections that are hepatotropic, even though the lesions are mainly characterized by hepatocellular necrosis or apoptosis rather than by the inflammatory response to the agent. The term hepatitis is also used for responses to some hepatic toxicants, metals, or drug metabolic idiosyncrasies in which there is a prominent leukocytic response to damaged cells. However, in responses in which single necrotic hepatocytes elicit a mild neutrophilic or histiocytic response, the term hepatitis is less appropriate because the pattern of injury is primarily degenerative. **Cholangitis** *refers to inflammation of the biliary tree.* More specifically, **choledochitis** refers to inflammation of the bile ducts, and **cholecystitis** refers to inflammation of the gallbladder. **Cholangiohepatitis** *applies to hepatic inflammation centered on the biliary tract and extending into adjacent hepatic parenchyma.*

Patterns and character of inflammation in hepatitis vary according to causative agent, severity and stage of disease, the route of entry into the liver, and pathogenesis of liver injury. Some viral pathogens, such as canine adenovirus 1, can cause acute and diffuse hepatitis, with centrilobular to widespread hepatocellular necrosis, mixed leukocyte infiltrates, sinusoidal congestion, and edema. By comparison, most infectious causes of hepatitis, for example, toxoplasmosis, various herpesviruses, and various bacteria, produce a more patchy pattern of inflammation with focally intense leukocyte and Kupffer cell responses in the vicinity of areas of necrosis. The distribution, character, and chronicity of these focal lesions are important diagnostically, but they typically do not damage enough functional hepatic parenchyma, ducts, or vasculature to produce systemic signs of liver failure. Foci of hepatitis with necrosis are common incidental findings, and these are assumed to reflect localized responses to bacteria that arrive via the portal system. Occasionally, such focal necroinflammatory lesions are large and numerous, for example, in cattle with rumenitis.

Acute hepatitis

Hallmarks of acute hepatitis typically include a combination of inflammation, typically a granulocytic inflammatory cell infiltrate, foci of hepatocellular apoptosis and necrosis, and in some instances, evidence of regeneration. Leukocyte infiltrates in acute diffuse hepatitis tend to accumulate mainly in the vicinity of the portal tracts, around major bile ducts, or sometimes in the capsule and around the central veins. Small but important numbers of neutrophils and mononuclear cells, including lymphocytes, are usually seen in the perisinusoidal space and among hepatocytes, and are often focally concentrated in sites of necrosis, or adjacent to infectious organisms. Edema is an unusual feature of acute hepatitis, but is seen in severe injury, for example, in infectious canine hepatitis. Grossly, hepatic edema is most obvious in the gallbladder,

large extrahepatic bile ducts, hepatic lymph nodes, and sometimes in the capsule. Microscopically, edema is also evident in the portal triads, in the connective tissue of the terminal and sublobular veins, and sometimes by an increase in the perisinusoidal space.

Kupffer cells are key participants in the acute inflammatory responses in the liver. They can enlarge and accumulate vacuoles and lysosomal debris during regular phagocytic removal of microorganisms, cell debris, and extravascular erythrocytes. They can also be activated to secretory histiocytes that release various cytokines and other mediators that induce hypertrophic or proliferative responses of hepatocytes, stellate cells, and endothelium. Activated Kupffer cells are larger and more prominent or numerous in sections, their nuclei are larger and vesicular, and their cytoplasm is basophilic and may contain vacuoles or ingested particulate matter. In overwhelming infections, many of the Kupffer cells and adjacent sinusoidal endothelial cells and hepatocytes undergo necrosis.

Chronic hepatitis

Chronic liver disease in domestic animals has historically been classified into several different entities based on morphologic criteria, but fibrosis is a consistent feature. In human medicine, classification of chronic hepatitis has been simplified, and morphologic divisions such as chronic active hepatitis and chronic persistent hepatitis, originally defined in specific clinical contexts, have been abandoned because of problems of evolving definitions and application, and lack of correspondence with prognosis. The single designation "**chronic hepatitis**" is now used for *chronic necroinflammatory disease lasting more than 6 months,* further modified by specifying the etiology, type and severity of inflammation, and degree and distribution of apoptosis and/or necrosis (**disease activity or grade**), and the degree of fibrosis (**disease chronicity or stage**). Numerous systems for *grading and staging chronic hepatitis* have been developed. In human medicine, chronic hepatitis is usually the result of chronic infection with hepatotropic viruses, and, less commonly, autoimmune, drug-induced, or associated with inherited metabolic diseases, such as Wilson disease. In veterinary medicine, chronic liver disease may develop following chronic bile duct obstruction, infection with hepatotropic infectious agents, familial or hereditary metabolic diseases, or may be toxic, drug-induced, or possibly autoimmune in origin. However, *the majority of chronic liver disease is idiopathic,* reflecting deficiencies in our current level of understanding of the etiologic, pathophysiologic, and clinical implications of the patterns of inflammation and necrosis seen in domestic animals.

Regardless of the etiology, *initial acute liver damage will not progress to fibrosis or cirrhosis unless the inflammation and damage are protracted,* for example, by ongoing hepatocellular injury mediated by immunologic mechanisms, including antibody- and lymphocyte-mediated cytotoxicity, or ongoing oxidative damage. Clinical signs are nonspecific in the early stages, but as the disease progresses to involve more of the liver and impair regeneration, icterus, ascites, and hepatic encephalopathy may develop as typical correlates with hepatic insufficiency.

Chronic hepatitis of humans has several characteristic lesions. These are also evident in animals, although not always to the same degree or frequency as described in the various forms of viral, immune-mediated, and idiosyncratic hepatitis in humans. The first is **periportal interface hepatitis,** sometimes referred to as *"piecemeal necrosis"* (Fig. 2-56). *This*

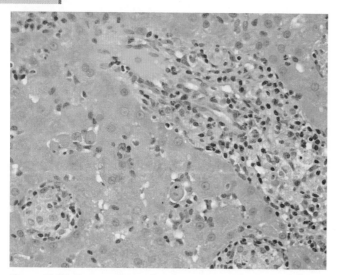

Figure 2-56 **Periportal interface hepatitis** in chronic hepatitis in a dog.

necroinflammatory change initially destroys the limiting plate of periportal hepatocytes, and may continue to erode into the hepatic parenchyma, expanding the portal areas. Portal inflammation is variable in intensity, and includes infiltration by lymphocytes and plasma cells. Bridging necrosis, with tracts of necrosis dissecting across the hepatic lobule between portal triads or between portal areas and central veins, may also develop. Degenerative changes affecting hepatocytes in areas of interface hepatitis include cell swelling and apoptosis. Bile duct degeneration, multifocal necrosis, and hepatocellular regeneration, in the form of 2-cell–thick hepatic plates and mitotic figures, may also be seen. Deposition of collagen and basement membrane material in the space of Disse leads to capillarization of hepatic sinusoids. Single or small groups of hepatocytes may be isolated and entrapped in expanded portal areas. Fibrosis may progress to bridge portal tracts and central veins, disrupting hepatic lobular architecture and culminating in the development of cirrhosis.

Further reading

Beighs V, Trautwein C. The innate immune response during liver inflammation and metabolic disease. Trends Immunol 2013;34:446-452.

Bode JG, et al. Hepatic acute phase proteins—regulation by IL-6 and IL-1 cytokines involving STAT3 and its crosstalk with NF-kB-dependent signaling. Eur J Cell Biol 2012;91:496-505.

Dixon LJ, et al. Kupffer cells in the liver. Compr Physiol 2013;3: 785-797.

Goodman ZG. Grading and staging systems for inflammation and fibrosis in chronic liver diseases. J Hepatol 2007;47:598-607.

Knolle PC, Thimme R. Hepatic immune regulation and its involvement in viral hepatitis infection. Gastroenterol 2014;146:1193-1207.

Szabo G, Csak T. Inflammasomes in liver diseases. J Hepatol 2012; 57:642-654.

Chronic hepatitis in dogs

Chronic hepatitis is a relatively common diagnosis in dogs, characterized by hepatocellular apoptosis or necrosis, a variable mononuclear or mixed inflammatory cell infiltrate, evidence of regenerative attempts, and fibrosis of variable extent and pattern. Although various infectious etiologies and drug- and toxin-induced chronic hepatic disease have been described, *the majority remains idiopathic, although excess hepatic copper accumulation is the best characterized cause of chronic hepatitis in the dog.* Breeds of dogs reported to be at increased risk for chronic hepatitis include the Bedlington Terrier, Doberman Pinscher, West Highland White Terrier, Labrador Retriever, American and English Cocker Spaniel, Skye Terrier, Standard Poodle, Dalmatian, and English Springer Spaniel. Hepatic copper accumulation in association with chronic hepatitis has been documented in most of these breeds, but apart from the recognized genetic mutation in the *COMMD1* gene in Bedlington Terriers, leading to a primary copper storage disease with impaired copper excretion, the pathogenesis of the breed-related copper accumulation remains unclear.

In the dog, disease grade is correlated with increasing hepatocellular apoptosis, proliferation, expression of nitric oxide synthase isoforms, and total hepatic iron, whereas disease stage is correlated with increasing α-smooth muscle actin–labeled periductular myofibroblasts and perisinusoidal stellate cells, CK7-positive ductular cells, the extracellular matrix protein tenascin-C, and expression of genes important in the production and regulation of hepatic fibrosis, including platelet-derived growth factors PDGFB and PDGFD, thrombospondin 1, transforming growth factors β1 and β2 (TGFB1 and TGFB2), matrix metalloproteinase 2 and tissue inhibitor of matrix metalloproteinase 1, and the collagen genes *COL1A1* and *COL3A1.*

Given the importance of autoimmune hepatitis in human medicine, several studies have evaluated the possible contributions of immune mechanisms in dogs. Upregulation of major histocompatibility complex class II antigen expression in hepatocytes has been demonstrated in Doberman hepatitis in association with lymphocyte infiltration, and it has been proposed that hepatocytes presenting a putative major histocompatibility complex class II molecule–associated autoantigen could be targets for T-cell–mediated immune attack. An association with specific major histocompatibility complex DLA class II haplotypes has been described in Doberman Pinschers and English Springer Spaniels with subclinical or clinical hepatitis, and it has been suggested that the highly polymorphic DLA genes may be involved in altered susceptibility to chronic hepatitis. However, a primary autoimmune pathogenesis has yet to be demonstrated.

The presence, mechanism, and role of **hepatic copper** accumulation in dogs continues to generate ongoing interest. Although copper is an essential metal cofactor for cuproenzymes, free copper ions can catalyze the formation of reactive hydroxyl radicals capable of causing oxidative injury (see the Copper section later in Toxic hepatic disease). The liver is central to copper homeostasis, and biliary excretion is the major route for regulating levels of copper in the body. Hepatic copper accumulation can arise (1) as the result of a primary metabolic defect in hepatic copper metabolism, (2) secondary to abnormal hepatic function with cholestasis and altered biliary copper excretion, or (3) as a consequence of excess dietary copper intake. Secondary copper accumulation occurs in the majority of human patients with primary biliary cirrhosis, prolonged extrahepatic bile duct obstruction, or chronic liver disease; however, dogs appear to be relatively resistant to hepatocellular copper accumulation as a result of cholestasis, at least in experimental studies following ligation of the common bile duct.

In the dog, the reference range for hepatic copper is generally considered to be ≤400 µg/g dry weight (DW);.concentrations >1,800-2,000 µg/g DW are considered pathogenic. *In primary genetic copper storage disorders and excess copper intake, copper accumulation appears at least initially to be primarily centrilobular, extending throughout the lobule as the condition progresses*, with hepatic copper concentrations usually >2,000 µg/g DW. *In copper storage secondary to abnormal hepatic function, copper usually accumulates in smaller amounts in the periportal parenchyma or without a consistent pattern*, in concentrations typically <2,000 µg/g DW.

When the hepatic concentration of copper surpasses 400 µg/g DW, the excess begins to accumulate within lysosomes. These copper-laden lysosomes become consistently demonstrable by the histochemical stains rubeanic acid and rhodanine, at copper concentrations exceeding 400 µg/g DW (Fig. 2-57), although some studies note visible copper granules at hepatic copper concentrations as low as 200 µg/g DW. A reasonable estimate of copper burden can be made from stained sections; however, biochemical determination of copper is more reliable and can be useful to follow the effectiveness of copper chelation therapy. Care should be taken when collecting liver for copper levels, as once the normal lobular architecture is lost because of injury and regenerative nodule formation, copper distribution within the liver becomes heterogeneous. Hepatocytes in regenerative nodules often have relatively low levels of copper, possibly as an adaptation that facilitates their ability to proliferate and form nodules, or as a function of inadequate time for significant copper accumulation in the hepatocytes forming nodules. The intervening areas of parenchymal collapse may contain an abundance of copper. Because of this regional variation, small samples, such as those taken from needle biopsies, are often inaccurate, and larger samples are required.

Regardless of the reasons for copper accumulation, lysosomal copper can exceed a threshold or be released when hepatocytes die, and thereby contribute to the development of hepatitis. *Hepatic pathology does not typically occur at concentrations <2,000 µg/g DW*, although higher values can still be found in some dogs with normal liver histology, and other factors, such as antioxidant levels and other oxidative stress from drugs or other factors, may influence the relationship between copper concentration and injury.

A hereditary, autosomal recessive copper-associated hepatopathy associated with impaired biliary copper excretion and progressive accumulation of copper within hepatocytes has been well documented in **Bedlington Terriers.** The majority of affected Bedlington Terriers have been found deficient in a protein, COMMD1 (copper metabolism MURR1 domain protein 1), caused by deletion of exon 2 in the *COMMD1* gene, although there are other less common mutations that can also occur. Although its function is not fully understood, the COMMD1 protein has been shown to interact with the copper transporter ATP7B, important in Wilson disease, a copper storage disorder in humans, and its absence in affected dogs may impair ATP7B-mediated copper export from hepatocytes into the canaliculus. Homozygous affected dogs have the highest copper levels. *Bedlington Terriers are the only breed to date shown to accumulate copper continuously throughout life*, and hepatic copper concentrations in these animals may be very high; as much as 12,000 µg/g DW has been recorded, and levels >5,000 µg/g are common. Affected dogs are usually presented with signs of progressive liver failure, including ill-thrift, wasting, ascites, and signs of encephalopathy. An acute form may occur in some dogs, with acute hepatic necrosis and release of copper into the systemic circulation, where it provokes a hemolytic crisis and rapidly developing anemia and icterus (eFig. 2-13). The initial histologic lesion is multifocal centrilobular hepatitis, with foci of macrophages, lymphocytes, plasma cells, and neutrophils among the copper-laden hepatocytes in zone 3. Apoptotic hepatocytes, some containing copper granules, appear at the periphery of some foci. Copper levels >3,000 µg/g DW result in widespread massive necrosis in some dogs. Survivors may progress to develop postnecrotic cirrhosis. Grossly, the livers in later stages are fibrotic, pale, and finely nodular.

Chronic hepatitis is well documented in **Doberman Pinschers.** The disease is more common in middle-aged female dogs. Histologic changes in the livers of dogs exhibiting clinical signs of advanced hepatic disease include piecemeal necrosis of periportal zone 1 hepatocytes, with a mixed inflammatory cell infiltrate, as well as necrosis of zone 3 hepatocytes with bridging necrosis crossing the lobule (Fig. 2-58). Copper accumulation is evident in centrilobular hepatocytes, with various degrees of portal fibrosis, bile duct proliferation, bridging fibrosis, and development of cirrhosis in the most severely affected dogs. Intrahepatocyte bile pigment accumulation and intracanalicular bile stasis are present in periportal zones, along with iron accumulation in Kupffer cells and macrophages.

Elevated concentrations of hepatic copper have been reported in many, but not all, Doberman Pinschers with chronic hepatitis, and *the significance of increased hepatic copper concentration in this breed remains controversial*. A recent investigation into the possibility of impaired copper excretion in affected Doberman Pinschers reported that 5 dogs with elevated liver copper and persistent subclinical hepatitis but without demonstrable cholestasis had comparable rates of plasma copper clearance to control dogs, but reduced rates of biliary excretion of ^{64}Cu, suggesting that impaired copper excretion may play a role in disease in this breed. Significantly reduced levels of mRNA of various proteins involved in copper binding, transport, and excretion, including ATP7A, ATP7B, ceruloplasmin, and metallothionein, have been documented in Dobermans with clinical hepatitis with high hepatic

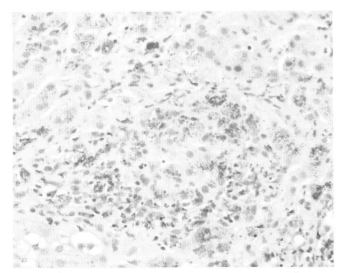

Figure 2-57 Copper staining (rhodanine) in the liver of a West Highland White Terrier.

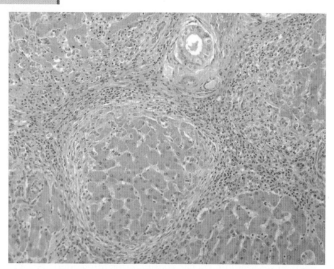

Figure 2-58 Periportal interface hepatitis with mixed inflammatory infiltrates and bridging portal fibrosis in a Doberman Pinscher dog.

copper concentrations, along with a reduction in gene expression of components of the antioxidant defense system, including SOD1, catalase, as well as reduced levels of glutathione, so continued investigations are needed to further clarify the pathogenesis of chronic hepatitis in Dobermans.

West Highland White Terriers are at increased risk of developing chronic hepatitis and cirrhosis. There is evidence to support *familial* hepatic copper accumulation in some West Highland White Terriers, although the mode of inheritance is not completely understood. Hepatic copper accumulates in zone 3 hepatocytes, up to ~8 months of age, with concentrations rarely >2,000 μg/g DW. Clinical illness directly attributable to copper hepatotoxicity (concentrations >2,000 μg/g DW) in West Highland White Terriers is, however, apparently uncommon. *Idiopathic chronic hepatitis progressing to cirrhosis does also occur in this breed,* and may be distinguished on the basis of a different zonal location and morphology of the inflammatory lesions. In the idiopathic disease, inflammatory foci are smaller, composed of a single apoptotic hepatocyte or fragments of cells accompanied by a few lymphocytes and plasma cells, and are commonly localized to zone 1, or may be random in distribution. In dogs with copper toxicosis, foci of inflammation and necrosis were larger, always found around the central vein among copper-laden hepatocytes, and were composed of debris-filled macrophages, lymphocytes, plasma cells, and scattered neutrophils, with occasional apoptotic hepatocytes around the periphery. *Distinguishing between copper toxicosis and idiopathic chronic hepatic disease may be difficult in cirrhotic livers,* which, irrespective of the underlying cause, may have reduced copper burdens because of connective-tissue displacement of hepatic parenchyma, and typically lower concentrations of copper in regenerative nodules.

Chronic hepatitis been reported in genetically related Skye Terriers, accompanied by modest and somewhat inconsistent hepatic copper accumulation. Lesions ranged from hepatocellular degeneration and necrosis with mild inflammation in zone 3, to chronic hepatitis and cirrhosis with marked intracanalicular cholestasis. Hepatic copper concentrations ranged from 800-2,200 μg/g DW, and copper-containing hepatocytes were found predominantly in zone 3.

Copper-associated chronic hepatitis has been described in **Labrador Retrievers,** characterized by centrilobular infiltrates of macrophages containing intracytoplasmic copper and hemosiderin, fewer neutrophils, mononuclear inflammatory cells, as well as scattered foci of hepatocellular necrosis, lobular collapse, periacinar to bridging fibrosis, nodular regeneration, and in some cases cirrhosis. Hepatic copper concentrations in one study were typically >2,000 μg/g, whereas mean hepatic copper concentrations in a separate study were also found to be significantly higher in affected dogs (614 μg/g, range 104-4,234 μg/g) compared to age- and sex-matched control dogs (299 μg/g, 93-3,810 μg/g). A concurrent general increase in hepatic copper concentrations in a study population of Labrador Retrievers spanning 30 years was postulated to be associated with increased dietary copper availability, the result of a change in the form and bioavailability of supplemental copper added to commercially produced dog foods. A positive association between dietary copper levels and hepatic copper concentrations has been demonstrated, and high dietary copper has been suggested as a risk factor for development of copper-associated hepatitis in susceptible animals within the breed. Concurrent renal proximal tubular dysfunction with glucosuria, and increased renal copper has been described in some Labrador Retrievers with copper-associated hepatitis, and sporadically in other breeds.

Chronic liver disease associated with elevated hepatic copper concentrations has also been reported in **Dalmatians.** A range of necroinflammatory changes has been reported, including multifocal, piecemeal, centrilobular to massive hepatic necrosis, and cirrhosis, although, in one study of 10 dogs, various degrees of piecemeal necrosis and bridging fibrosis were the most common histologic change, with either primarily lymphocytic or neutrophilic inflammatory infiltrates. Morphologic or biochemical evidence of cholestatic liver disease was not prominent. Hepatic copper concentrations ranged from 745-8,390 μg/g DW (mean 3,197 μg/g) in one report of 10 dogs, aged 2-10 years, with a variable zonal distribution. Three previous cases in young Dalmatians reported hepatic copper concentrations of 7,940 μg/g DW, 1,916 μg/g wet weight, and 2,356 μg/g wet weight, and 2 of these reports describe diffuse positive staining for copper in all hepatocytes, with the strongest staining observed in centrilobular hepatocytes.

Chronic hepatitis has been reported in **American and English Cocker Spaniels** *and* **English Springer Spaniels,** characterized clinically in the later stages by ascites, weight loss, and icterus. Affected dogs develop chronic hepatitis and cirrhosis, and, at postmortem, livers are typically small and firm, with multiple small regenerative nodules (Fig. 2-59). Histologically, there is moderate to severe portal hepatitis, with inflammatory infiltrates of predominantly lymphocytes, plasma cells, and fewer neutrophils, and variable degrees of portal fibrosis and bridging fibrosis. One study of American Cocker Spaniels reported diffuse fibrosis typical of lobular dissecting hepatitis in 7 of 13 affected dogs, in addition to patterns of fibrosis more typical of cirrhosis. Piecemeal necrosis and limiting plate destruction have been reported in Cocker Spaniels, whereas in English Springer Spaniels, hepatocyte necrosis and apoptosis in areas of inflammatory infiltrates in both portal areas and scattered throughout the hepatic parenchyma was more typical. Biliary hyperplasia or marked ductular reaction was noted in affected Cocker Spaniels. Hepatic copper staining is variable, and hepatic copper accumulation is not a consistent feature.

α1-Antitrypsin (α1-AT) deficiency *has been suggested to play a role in chronic hepatitis in some dog breeds, including English Cocker Spaniels,* although whether this is an

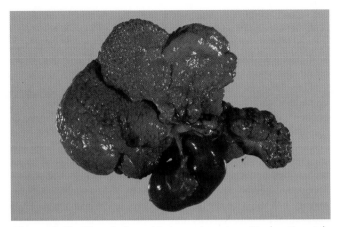

Figure 2-59 **Chronic hepatitis** in an American Cocker Spaniel.

epiphenomenon or cause of chronic liver disease has not yet been proven. α1-AT, a plasma glycoprotein synthesized mainly by hepatocytes, is a member of the serine proteinase inhibitor (serpin) superfamily, and is a potent inhibitor of neutrophil elastase. Hereditary α1-AT deficiency in humans is associated with mutations that perturb the protein's tertiary structure and promote polymerization. These misfolded forms of α1-AT accumulate within the rough endoplasmic reticulum of hepatocytes, forming PAS-positive globules. α1-AT deficiency has been associated in humans with neonatal hepatitis, juvenile cirrhosis, and adult hepatocellular carcinoma.

Lobular dissecting hepatitis, associated with predominantly sinusoidal inflammation and fibrosis, has been described in young dogs with ascites and acquired portosystemic shunts. The liver is usually small, pale with a predominantly smooth surface, and occasional hyperplastic nodules (eFig. 2-14). The histologic lesion is characterized by dissection of lobular parenchyma by reticulin and fine collagen fibers into individual and small groups of hepatocytes, accompanied by a variable, mixed inflammatory infiltrate of lymphocytes, plasma cells, and lesser numbers of neutrophils and macrophages (Fig. 2-60A, B). Activated fibroblastic cells, likely hepatic stellate cells, may also be prominent along sinusoids. Hepatocytes form rosettes or pseudoductular structures, and regenerative nodules may be present. Portal inflammation and periportal fibrosis are not conspicuous features of this disease. The etiology of this disorder remains unknown.

Chronic hepatitis in other species

Copper-associated liver disease has also been described in domestic cats. A hepatopathy with excess hepatic copper (4,074 μg/g DW) was first reported in a Siamese cat, characterized by enlarged, finely vacuolated, and individual necrotic hepatocytes with centrilobular and midzonal copper accumulation. Chronic hepatitis and cirrhosis, with marked accumulation of stainable copper in macrophages in fibrous septa and with sparser staining in regenerative nodules, was reported in a European Shorthair cat with similarly elevated liver copper concentrations (4,170 μg/g DW; the upper reference range limit for hepatic copper concentration is cats is <180 μg/g DW). A recent retrospective study described an additional 11 cats with presumed primary copper-associated hepatopathy, characterized by elevated hepatic copper concentrations (>700 μg/g DW), diffuse or centrilobular and intermediate zone copper staining, without any other co-occurring cholestatic disorders. Affected cats had hepatocyte vacuolation

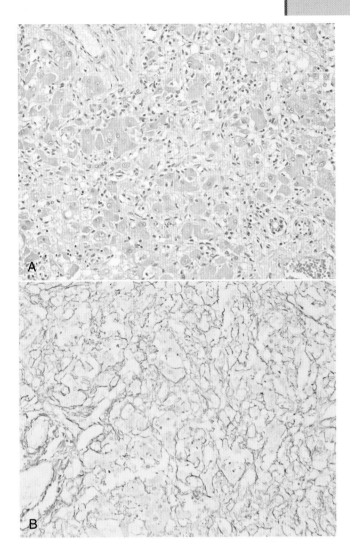

Figure 2-60 **A. Lobular dissecting hepatitis** with diffuse fine interstitial fibrosis isolating hepatocytes in a juvenile Golden Retriever dog. **B.** Reticulin stain demonstrating pattern of lobular dissection.

consistent with glycogen accumulation, fibrillar collagen in the perivenular region, and variable mild parenchymal collapse, with bridging fibrosis in one cat. Cats also accumulate copper in the liver secondary to other cholestatic hepatobiliary disorders, such as chronic cholangitis/cholangiohepatitis, or extrahepatic bile duct obstruction, although copper staining in these cases is principally in hepatocytes in portal and intermediate zones.

Chronic hepatitis seen as end-stage livers occurs in horses (eFig. 2-15) and ruminants, particularly cattle, and is often assumed to be associated with ingestion of hepatotoxins, such as pyrrolizidine alkaloids in forage, or a consequence of prolonged administration of hepatotoxic therapeutics, although in the absence of specific histologic lesions and/or a corroborative clinical history, the underlying causes are rarely discovered.

Further reading

Bexfield NH, et al. Chronic hepatitis in the English springer spaniel: clinical presentation, histological description and outcome. Vet Rec 2011;169:415-419.

Favier RP, et al. Copper-induced hepatitis: the COMMD1deficient dog as a translation animal model for human chronic hepatitis. Vet Q 2011;31:49-60.

Fieten H, et al. Canine models of copper toxicosis for understanding mammalian copper metabolism. Mamm Genome 2012;23:62-75.

Hoffman G. Copper-associated liver diseases. Vet Clin Small Anim 2009;39:489-511.

Hurwitz BM, et al. Presumed primary and secondary hepatic copper accumulation in cats. J Am Vet Med Assoc 2014;244:68-77.

Johnston AN, et al. Hepatic copper concentrations in Labrador Retrievers with and without chronic hepatitis: 72 cases (1980-2010). J Am Vet Med Assoc 2013;242:372-380.

van den Ingh TSGAM, et al. Morphological classification of parenchymal disorders of the canine and feline liver. In: Rothuizen J, et al., editors. WSAVA Standards for Clinical and Histological Diagnosis of Canine and Feline Liver Diseases. Chapt. 7. Philadelphia: Saunders Elsevier; 2006. p. 85-101.

Miscellaneous inflammatory liver disease

Nonspecific reactive hepatitis refers to hepatic inflammation characterized by light inflammatory infiltrates, primarily in the portal tracts, without any evidence of hepatocellular necrosis. It is often observed during inflammation of the splanchnic organs and is a reactive response, rather than primary inflammation of the liver.

Giant cell hepatitis *is an uncommon lesion in animals, but is recorded in cats, calves, and foals* (Fig. 2-61). There is evidence for maternal leptospirosis in some cases reported in foals. Two cases are reported in young cats with concurrent thymic lymphomas. The liver is deeply bile stained. Histologically, the acinar structure is effaced, and the blood vessels engorged. Hepatocytes are large and syncytial and may contain 10 or more nuclei. The pale or ballooned cytoplasm contains bile pigments, and cytoplasmic invaginations into hepatocyte nuclei are common. Inflammatory cells are not conspicuous. Liver parenchymal giant cell transformation occurs in humans in a wide variety of congenital and neonatal liver disorders, including bile duct obstruction associated with biliary atresia, viral and bacterial infections, some metabolic disorders such as galactosemia, some cases of Down syndrome and other genetic disorders, as well as in idiopathic neonatal hepatitis, a cholestatic condition of undetermined cause. Although giant

cells were originally suggested to be a marker of infantile obstructive cholangiopathy in humans, their association with a wide range of disorders supports an *alternative conclusion that giant cell formation represents a nonspecific reaction of the infant's hepatocytes to various types of injury.*

Hypertrophic hepatic cirrhosis in calves is described from Germany and occasionally observed elsewhere. Death may occur in liver failure within a few days to weeks of birth, or the disease may be discovered at slaughter for veal. The liver is moderately enlarged with rounded borders, very firm but smooth on the surface, and gray. Histologically, there is some biliary hyperplasia, but the lesion is dominated by diffuse fibrosis infiltrated in the early stages by mononuclear inflammatory cells. No cause has been identified. Similar lesions of **congenital hepatic fibrosis** may be found in unborn or aborted calves.

Systemic granulomatous disease has been reported in cattle grazing *hairy vetch (Vicia villosa)*. The disease is characterized clinically by dermatitis, pruritus, diarrhea, wasting, and high mortality. Histologic lesions include infiltration of skin and internal organs, including portal areas of the liver, by monocytes, lymphocytes, plasma cells, eosinophils, and multinucleated giant cells. The pathogenesis is unknown, although the inflammatory reaction has characteristics of a type IV hypersensitivity reaction. Alternatively, vetch lectin may act to activate T lymphocytes directly to initiate the cellular response.

Further reading

Suzuki K, et al. Giant cell hepatitis in two cats. J Vet Med Sci 2001;63:199-201.

Inflammatory diseases of the biliary tract

Inflammation of the gallbladder is termed **cholecystitis**. *Inflammation of the large bile ducts is* **cholangitis**, *whereas inflammation of the smallest intrahepatic bile ductules is termed* **cholangiolitis**. Cholangiolitis is uncommon in animals, and occurs mainly in conjunction with inflammation of larger ducts. Destructive cholangiolitis has been observed in dogs, and is associated with adverse drug reactions in humans.

Cholecystitis

Cholecystitis is uncommon and is often associated with concurrent cholelithiasis, although acalculous cholecystitis has been reported in the dog, with a single case report in a pig. *Cholecystitis is thought to be caused by reflux of intestinal bacteria into the gallbladder via the bile ducts, or to hematogenous entry of bacteria from the adjacent hepatic circulation.* Aerobic gram-negative bacteria are the most frequent isolates from canine cases, although occasionally anaerobic bacteria such as clostridia have been cultured. *Campylobacter jejuni* has been isolated from 2 dogs with bacteremia and cholecystitis. Occasionally, parasites, such as flukes that colonize the bile ducts, can enter the gallbladder and cause cholecystitis. Canine cholecystitis has been associated with various systemic disorders, including diabetes mellitus, severe enteritis, biliary stasis, septicemia, as well as with the use of immunosuppressive drugs, each of which may promote bacterial colonization of the gallbladder. In the acute lesion, histologic changes include neutrophilic inflammatory infiltrates in the wall and lumen of the gallbladder, with focal erosion or ulceration, and edema.

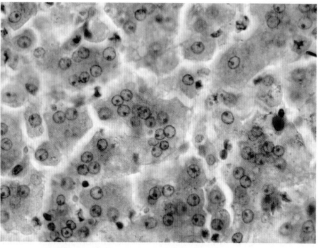

Figure 2-61 Giant cell hepatitis in a cat.

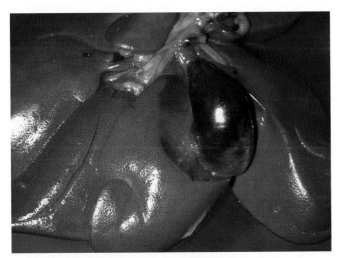

Figure 2-62 Infarcted gallbladder in a dog.

More chronic stages develop typical mixed inflammatory infiltrates, with fibrosis. Occasionally, the infiltrate may be predominantly lymphoplasmacytic, with formation of lymphoid follicles within the mucosa.

Gallbladder infarction characterized by transmural coagulative necrosis of the gallbladder wall with intravascular fibrin thrombi has been reported in dogs (Fig. 2-62). The arterial blood supply to the gallbladder is the cystic artery, a branch of the hepatic artery, and occlusion may cause partial or complete infarction. Predisposing factors have not been identified; however, the lack of significant concurrent inflammatory response suggests that this is not simply a sequela to underlying cholecystitis.

Gallbladder mucocele is discussed further under Ectopic, hyperplastic, and metaplastic lesions.

Cholangitis/cholangiohepatitis

Although pure cholangitis does occur, extension of inflammation from the ducts into the adjacent hepatic parenchyma can occur, and such lesions can quite accurately be regarded as cholangiohepatitis.

Bile contains various antimicrobial factors, including β-defensins and bile acids that are inhospitable to most bacteria, except for some species with particular capsule adaptations. Bacterial cholangiohepatitis is usually caused by common opportunists of enteric origin, such as coliforms and streptococci. Some bacteremic organisms, including some *Salmonella*, can be cultured from the bile, but the mechanism by which they get there is unknown. Salmonellosis is a distinctive cause of fibrinous cholecystitis in cattle, especially calves.

The *pathogenesis of bacterial cholangitis/cholangiohepatitis* depends on various predisposing conditions, similar to those involved in the pathogenesis of pyelonephritis. These include infection by bacteria that reach the ducts hematogenously, facilitated by localization in the peribiliary plexus or by extension from sinusoidal Kupffer cells or foci of necrosis. Descending cholangitis is occasionally observed in cattle with suppurative hepatitis with extension from abscesses directly into the ducts or via the portal lymphatics. Cholangiohepatitis of this origin may be restricted in its distribution to biliary fields, but in some cases, it does become quite diffuse in the biliary system. Alternatively, bacteria can ascend the ducts from the intestine, facilitated by bile stasis caused by

mechanical or functional obstructions. The inflammatory and proliferative responses in cholangitis further interfere with bile flow and exacerbate the ductular spread of bacterial infections once they are established. Again, these lesions can be quite regionally variable, and may be missed on hepatic biopsy if only small areas are sampled.

The course and pathologic changes in cholangiohepatitis vary greatly, from fulminating suppurative infection to persistent mild inflammation that, over a period of months or years, leads to hepatic fibrosis of biliary distribution. *Severe suppurative cholangiohepatitis* may follow a short course to death, the effects being those of the infection itself, which may become septicemic, rather than of hepatic injury. At autopsy, the liver is swollen, soft, and pale, and its architecture is blurred. Few or many suppurative foci may be visible beneath the capsule and on the cut surface (eFig. 2-16). They are small, sometimes miliary in distribution, and not encapsulated. Lesions in other organs may be those of septicemia and jaundice. Microscopically, the larger ducts contain purulent exudate, and the smaller ones are disintegrated. Dense masses of neutrophils, liquefied or not, are present in the portal triads and infiltrate the degenerate parenchyma.

In *subacute and chronic cholangiohepatitis*, the inflammation is more proliferative than exudative. The liver is enlarged and may be of normal shape, or distorted because of irregular areas of atrophy and regenerative hyperplasia. Its surface may be smooth or finely granular; the capsule is thickened and may bear fibrous tags or be adherent to adjacent viscera. Within areas of duct obstruction, retention of bile pigments can be found in the regions served by the occluded ducts, but systemic icterus (or photosensitization in herbivores) is unlikely unless a large portion of liver is affected. On cut surface, the enlarged portal tracts are easily visible and accentuate the architecture of the organ. Eventually, the new fibrous tissue replaces the parenchyma, and in chronic diffuse cases in which the original infection persists, continuous fibroplasia may produce hepatic enlargement, the organ becoming huge, gray, and gristly. This spectrum of liver changes is typical of alsike clover poisoning ("big-liver disease") in horses (discussed in the later section on Toxic hepatic disease). Alternatively, the chronic fibrosis may occur in wedge-shaped areas oriented to a small bile duct. The enlarged interlobular ducts may be readily visible and frequently contain plugs of inspissated secretion and debris.

Microscopically, the reaction remains centered on portal tracts. These are expanded in subacute cases by infiltration of leukocytes and macrophages and the proliferation of small ducts and, in chronic cases, chiefly by organizing fibrous tissue and proliferating bile ducts. Encroachment on the parenchyma is minimal but inevitable. Continued degeneration of the periportal parenchyma is probably an additional stimulus to local fibroplasia, which, as well as thickening the smallest portal triads, extends along their length and links up with neighboring triads, thus subdividing the acini into segments. The hepatic venules and sublobular veins are involved. Regenerative nodules are not a prominent feature of cholangiohepatitis unless large areas of parenchyma have been destroyed, in which case the least damaged lobes are expanded by coarse nodules.

Neutrophilic cholangitis (suppurative or exudative cholangitis/cholangiohepatitis) *is a relatively common disorder of cats and, much less commonly, dogs.* This condition has been suggested to be the result of acute inflammation in the biliary

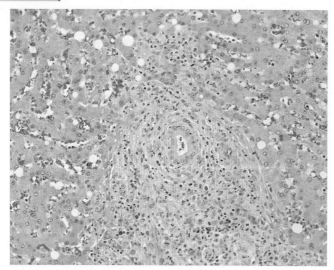

Figure 2-63 Neutrophilic bile duct inflammation with portal edema, early fibrosis, and a mixed infiltrate of neutrophils, lymphocytes and plasma cells extending across the limiting plate in a case of **subacute cholangiohepatitis** in a dog.

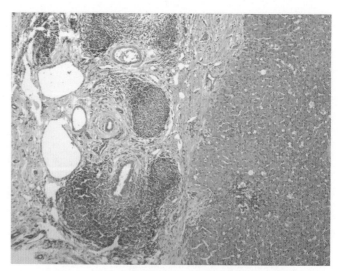

Figure 2-64 Lymphocytic cholangitis in a cat.

tree associated with ascending bacterial infection, and in cats, the condition often occurs in conjunction with other disorders, including *acute extrahepatic bile duct obstruction, pancreatitis, or inflammatory bowel disease.* In the cat, the biliary and pancreatic ducts share a common entry to the duodenum, and simultaneous infectious inflammation of these systems is common. *Escherichia coli* is the most frequent bacterial isolate; however, *Bacteroides, Klebsiella,* hemolytic *Streptococcus,* and clostridia have also been reported. The acute stage is characterized by edema and neutrophilic portal infiltrates, inflammation and degeneration of bile ducts with neutrophils in ductular lumens and emigrating through the ductular epithelium. Some cases may progress to cholangiohepatitis, with infiltration of inflammatory cells into hepatic lobules and periportal hepatocellular necrosis. Areas of suppuration and hepatic abscessation may occur. Mixed cholangiohepatitis, with neutrophils, lymphocytes, and plasma cells infiltrating portal areas accompanied by bile duct proliferation, biliary epithelial degeneration, and various degrees of periportal to bridging fibrosis, may represent the subacute stage (Fig. 2-63), whereas concentric periportal fibrosis and pseudolobule formation may represent the most chronic stage of the disease.

An apparently distinct condition of cats, **lymphocytic cholangitis** (lymphocytic portal hepatitis, nonsuppurative cholangitis/cholangiohepatitis) *is a slowly progressive disease characterized by lymphocytic infiltrates within the portal area, with variable degrees of bile duct or oval cell proliferation and peribiliary, portal-to-bridging fibrosis* (Fig. 2-64). An immune-mediated pathogenesis has been proposed, and in one study, most cats with lymphocytic cholangitis had T-cell–predominant portal infiltrates, often with accompanying portal B-cell aggregates. The presence of various degrees of lymphocytic targeting and infiltration of bile ductules with concurrent degenerative changes in ductular epithelium, destructive cholangitis leading to ductopenia, and portal lipogranulomas may be useful in distinguishing this condition from hepatic lymphoma in the cat, along with T-cell receptor clonality assays.

Destructive cholangitis has also been described in dogs, and is characterized by destruction and loss of bile ducts in the smaller portal tracts, with subsequent inflammation composed of pigment-laden macrophages, neutrophils, and/or eosinophils, and in some instances, fibrosis. The extent of injury may be sufficient to cause marked icterus and acholic feces because of marked intrahepatic cholestasis. The pathogenesis of this lesion is unclear; however, toxic injury, idiosyncratic drug reactions (see Fig. 2-40) and infection by canine distemper virus have been implicated in some cases.

Biliary tract obstruction

Cholelithiasis *(gallstone formation) is seldom observed in animals.* The choleliths usually form in the gallbladder and are composed of a *mixture of cholesterols, bile pigments, salts of bile acids, calcium salts, and a proteinaceous matrix.* Choleliths of mixed composition are yellow-black or green-black and are friable. *Pigment stones,* composed of calcium bilirubinate, and *cholesterol stones* have also been reported in dogs. There may be hundreds of small stones or a few large ones. The large stones are usually faceted. The origin of these mixed gallstones is uncertain, but their development is probably secondary to chronic mild cholecystitis and related to disturbances of the resorptive activities of the gallbladder, whereby the bile salts are removed faster than the stone-forming compounds. Gallstones are usually asymptomatic. Occasionally, they lodge in and obstruct bile ducts and cause jaundice. The larger stones may cause pressure necrosis and ulceration of the mucosa, local dilations of the bile ducts, and saccular diverticula of the gallbladder. Calculi seldom form in the ducts, although calcareous deposits often do so in fascioliasis of cattle. Calcium bilirubinate calculi have been reported in the bile ducts of horses (Fig. 2-65), associated with intermittent jaundice.

Occasionally, particles of solid ingesta may find their way into the gallbladder; sand has been seen in sheep, and seeds in pigs.

Biliary obstruction is rarely caused by impacted gallstones. Usually, it is *the result of cholangitis or cholecystitis,* the obstruction being produced by masses of detritus and biliary constituents, parasites, or cicatricial stenosis of the ducts. Adult ascarids may cause mechanical obstruction. Inspissated bile-stained friable plugs are occasionally responsible for obstructions in segments of the liver in horses. Tumors of the pancreas and duodenum, and tumors and abscesses of the hilus of the liver and portal nodes, may cause compression stenosis of the ducts. Edematous swelling of the papilla in enteritis may also be of

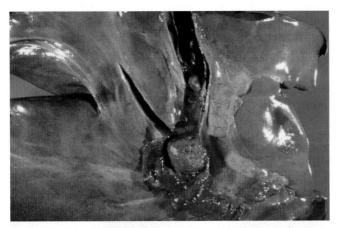

Figure 2-65 **Cholelith** obstructing the bile duct in a horse.

significance. Biliary obstruction by abnormal intraluminal mucoid secretion *(gallbladder mucocele)* has been reported in dogs (see later section on Ectopic, metaplastic, and hyperplastic lesions).

The consequences of biliary obstruction depend on the site and duration of the obstruction. When the main duct is involved, there is jaundice. When one of the hepatic ducts is involved, there is no jaundice, and depending on the efficiency of biliary collaterals, there may be no pigmentation of the obstructed segments of liver. Increases in serum γ-glutamyltranspeptidase and alkaline phosphatase usually occur when a sufficiently large amount of the duct system is affected. The ducts undergo progressive cylindrical dilation, which may be extreme. The smallest interlobular ducts and the cholangioles proliferate. There is inflammation in the walls of the ducts and the portal triads, and this is probably due in part to chemical irritation by bile acids but is largely caused by secondary bacterial infections. These infections may be acute and purulent, or low grade; in these cases, bacteria may not be easily cultured. The cholangiohepatitis that almost inevitably follows has been described previously.

Rupture of the biliary tract or the gallbladder causes steady leakage of bile into the peritoneal cavity, the omentum being unable to seal even small defects. The bile salts are very irritating and may cause *acute chemical peritonitis.* The peritoneal effusion that follows may remain sterile; more often it is infected by enteric bacteria, and severe diffuse peritonitis ensues. This may be rapidly fatal, particularly if clostridia are involved. Many perforations of the biliary tract are traumatic in origin; however, in dogs, cholecystitis, gallbladder necrosis/infarction, and gallbladder mucocele have all been associated with gallbladder rupture.

Further reading

Callahan Clark JE, et al. Feline cholangitis: a necropsy study of 44 cats (1986-2008). J Feline Med Surg 2011;13:570-576.

Center SA. Diseases of the gallbladder and biliary tree. Vet Clin North Am Small Anim Pract 2009;39:543-598.

Holt DE, et al. Canine gallbladder infarction: 12 cases (1993-2003). Vet Pathol 2004;41:416-418.

van den Ingh TSGAM, et al. Morphological classification of biliary disorders of the canine and feline liver. In: Rothuizen J, et al., editors. WSAVA Standards for Clinical and Histological Diagnosis of Canine and Feline Liver Diseases. Philadelphia: Saunders Elsevier; 2006. p. 61-76.

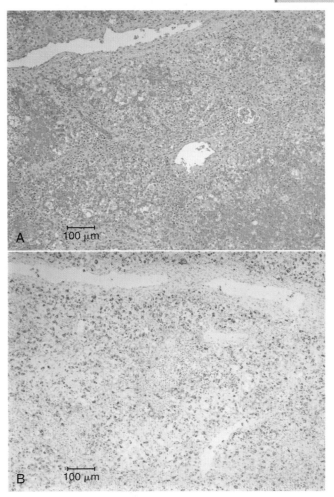

Figure 2-66 **A.** Hepatitis caused by **porcine circovirus 2 (PCV-2)** infection in a pig. **B.** Immunohistochemical stain for PCV-2 antigen. (Courtesy J. DeLay.)

Warren A, et al. Histopathologic features, immunophenotyping, clonality and eubacterial fluorescence in situ hybridization in cats with lymphocytic cholangitis/cholangiohepatitis. Vet Pathol 2011;48: 627-641.

INFECTIOUS DISEASES OF THE LIVER
Viral infections

Various systemic viral diseases may affect the liver. Adenoviral infections of lambs, calves, and goat kids can cause multifocal hepatic necrosis and cholangitis, in addition to pneumonia. Lymphohistiocytic hepatitis, with jaundice and various degrees of apoptosis of hepatocytes, disorganization of hepatic plates, and perilobular stromal condensation, is seen in some cases of porcine circovirus 2–associated disease (Fig. 2-66A, B). Canid herpesvirus 1 infection in puppies and, more rarely, in adult dogs causes disseminated focal necrosis and hemorrhages in parenchymal organs, including the liver, with formation of amphophilic intranuclear inclusion bodies in epithelial cells of kidney, lung, and liver. Similar microfoci of hepatic necrosis sometimes occur in aborted or newborn foals with congenital equid herpesvirus 1 infections (Fig. 2-67), in neonatal calves infected with bovine herpesvirus 1, in piglets with suid herpesvirus 1 infections, and in feline fetuses following

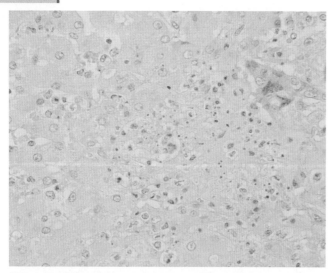

Figure 2-67 Focal hepatic necrosis with intranuclear inclusion bodies and syncytial cells in **congenital equid herpesvirus 1 infection** in a foal.

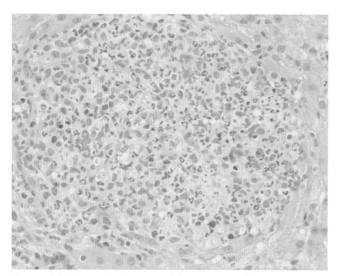

Figure 2-68 Pyogranulomatous hepatitis caused by **feline infectious peritonitis virus** infection.

intravenous feline herpesvirus 1 inoculation of the pregnant queen. Feline coronavirus infection can cause granulomatous hepatitis in some infected cats, as part of feline infectious peritonitis (Fig. 2-68). Multifocal hepatic necrosis has been described in large felids and domestic cats infected with highly pathogenic influenza A virus H5N1. Hepatocellular and Kupffer cell necrosis with mild mononuclear portal inflammation was reported in outbreaks caused by virulent systemic strains of feline calicivirus in cats in the United States and United Kingdom. Systemic cowpox virus infection with foci of hepatic necrosis containing immunoreactive cowpox viral antigen has been reported in a cat.

The viral diseases discussed in more detail later are those in which the liver is the major target organ, causing substantial hepatic injury that sometimes culminates in hepatic failure. Unlike humans, in which several pathogenic hepatitis viruses from various families are well described, few viruses that specifically target the liver have been identified in the major domestic mammals. Hepadnaviruses have been found in members of the squirrel family, including woodchucks and various species of ground squirrels and arctic ground squirrels,

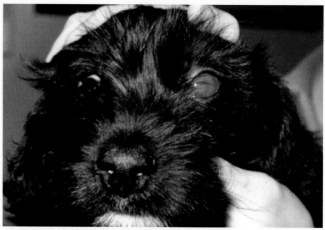

Figure 2-69 **Infectious canine hepatitis.** Corneal edema or "blue-eye." (Courtesy North Carolina State University CVM.)

as well as in birds, including some species of ducks, geese, and herons. Infection with hepatitis E virus (HEV) genotypes 3 and 4 is common in domestic and wild pigs, and although clinical disease is not apparent in infected swine, they may serve as reservoirs for this potentially zoonotic pathogen. Lesions of mild multifocal lymphoplasmacytic hepatitis with focal hepatocellular necrosis have been reported in pigs experimentally inoculated with HEV, but lesions in natural infections are not recognized. Flaviviruses, including a nonprimate hepacivirus and a GB-virus–like virus (pegivirus) have recently been described in horses, although their potential clinical significance is unknown. A second novel pegivirus species of horses, Theiler's disease–associated virus, is described in more detail later.

Infectious canine hepatitis

Canine adenovirus 1 (CAdV-1) infection is the cause of infectious canine hepatitis, a severe liver disease in dogs; other canids, including coyotes, foxes, wolves; and in bears. Vaccination has made the disease rare in many countries in which it was endemic. Deaths from infectious canine hepatitis are usually sporadic, although small outbreaks can occur among young dogs in kennels. Fatalities seldom occur among dogs >2 years of age. In areas where the disease is not controlled by vaccination, it is probable that most dogs in the general population contact CAdV-1 in the first 2 years of life and suffer either inapparent infection or mild febrile illness with pharyngitis and tonsillitis.

In more severe cases, there is vomiting, melena, high fever, and abdominal pain. There may be petechiae on the gums; the mucous membranes are pale and occasionally slightly jaundiced. Nonspecific nervous signs occur in a few cases. There is also a peracute form of the disease in which the animal is found dead without signs of illness, or after an illness of only a few hours. In convalescence, there may be a unilateral or bilateral opacity of the cornea caused by corneal edema (so-called blue eye, a type III hypersensitivity reaction with immune-complex–mediated corneal injury) (Fig. 2-69), which disappears spontaneously.

CAdV-1 has special tropism for endothelium, mesothelium, and hepatic parenchyma, and it is injury to these that is responsible for the pathologic features of edema, serosal hemorrhage, and hepatic necrosis. The histologic specificity of the lesions depends on the demonstration of large, solid intranuclear inclusion bodies in endothelium or hepatic parenchyma

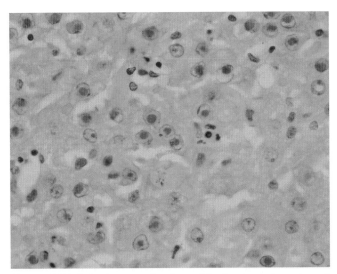

Figure 2-70 Infectious canine hepatitis (canine adenovirus 1 infection). Intranuclear inclusion bodies in numerous hepatocytes. (Courtesy University of Guelph.)

(Fig. 2-70). Inclusions are occasionally observed in other differentiated cells but always have the same morphologic and tinctorial features, being deeply acidophilic with a blue tint.

The morbid picture of spontaneously fatal cases is usually distinct enough to allow a diagnosis to be made at gross postmortem. Superficial lymph nodes are edematous, slightly congested, and often hemorrhagic. Blotchy or paintbrush hemorrhages may be present on intestinal and gastric serosae, and there is usually a small quantity of clear or blood-stained fluid in the abdomen. Jaundice, if present, is slight. The liver is slightly enlarged, with sharp edges, and is turgid and friable, sometimes congested, with a fine, uniform, yellow mottling (eFig. 2-17A). Red strands of fibrin can be found on its capsule, especially between the lobes. In the majority of cases, the wall of the gallbladder is edematous (eFig. 2-17B), and may have intramural hemorrhages; when edema is mild, it may be detected only in the attachments of the gallbladder.

Gross lesions in other organs are inconstant. Small hemorrhagic infarcts may be found in the renal cortices of young puppies. Hemorrhages may occur in the lungs, and occasionally, there are irregular areas of hemorrhagic consolidation in the caudal lobes. Hemorrhages in the brain occur in a small percentage of cases, typically only grossly visible in the midbrain and brainstem. Hemorrhagic necrosis of medullary and endosteal elements occurs in the metaphyses of long bones in young dogs, and the hemorrhages are readily visible through the thin cortex of the distal ends of the ribs.

At low magnification, the histologic changes in the liver are of centrilobular (periacinar) zonal necrosis, resembling the zonal pattern of some acute hepatotoxicities. *The susceptibility of centrilobular parenchyma to necrosis in this disease is as yet unexplained.* Close to the portal triads, the hepatocytes may be nearly normal in appearance, except for loss of basophilia and the presence of a scattering of inclusion bodies. In spontaneously fatal cases, most of the parenchyma of the peripheral and central portions of the lobules (acini) is dead, the hepatocytes having undergone coagulative necrosis, and in some of these, ghosts of inclusion bodies may be detectable. The margin between necrotic parenchyma and viable tissue is usually quite sharp, although in the viable tissue, there are many individual hepatocytes undergoing apoptosis, most of them without inclusion bodies. Fatty change is common. The

dead cells do not remain long, so the sinusoids become dilated and filled with blood. The reticulin framework remains intact, an observation in keeping with the fact that, *in recovered cases, restitution of the liver is complete.* Massive necrosis with collapse does not occur. As is typical of severe centrilobular necrosis, the necrotic zones, initially eccentric areas about hepatic venules, extend and link up to isolate portal units. Intranuclear inclusions can be found in Kupffer cells in variable numbers. Many of the Kupffer cells are dead, others are proliferating, and others are actively phagocytic in the removal of debris. Leukocytic reactions in the liver are mild and are directed against the necrotic tissue; mononuclear cells are present, but neutrophils, many degenerating, predominate. There is some collection of bile pigment, but it is moderate, in keeping with the short course of the disease.

Microscopic lesions in other organs are largely the result of injury to endothelium. Inclusion bodies in endothelial cells can be difficult to find and are looked for, with most profit in renal glomeruli, where endothelium is concentrated. Occasionally, they are found in the epithelium of collecting tubules. When areas of hemorrhagic consolidation of the lungs are present, there is hemorrhage, edema, and fibrin formation in the alveoli, and in these consolidated areas, inclusions are often common in alveolar capillaries and even in dying cells of the bronchial epithelium. Changes in the brain are secondary to vascular injury. Hemorrhages, if present, are from capillaries and small venules, and inclusions in endothelial nuclei can usually be found in vessels that have bled. Other endothelial and adventitial cells are hyperplastic and mixed with a few lymphocytes. Small foci of softening or demyelination may be present in relation to the hemorrhages. Lymphoreticular tissues are congested, and inclusions may be found in reticulum cells of follicles, in the red pulp of the spleen, and in macrophages anywhere.

Following natural oronasal exposure, viral multiplication occurs in the tonsils and leads to tonsillitis, which may be quite severe with extensive edema of the throat and larynx. Fever accompanies the tonsillitis and precedes the viremic phase, which lasts 4-8 days, accompanied by leukopenia. Hepatic necrosis develops at about day 7 of experimental infection; however, an immune response with adequate neutralizing antibodies may clear the virus from the blood and limit the extent of hepatic damage. *In surviving animals, hepatic regeneration occurs rapidly, and there do not appear to be any significant residual lesions.* Small foci of hepatocellular necrosis may still be present at 2 weeks, and foci of proliferated Kupffer cells may be detectable for another week or 2. Progressive hepatic injury does not seem to follow the acute phase of the natural disease, although chronic hepatitis has been experimentally reproduced in partially immunized dogs challenged with the virus. Adenoviral antigen has been detected immunohistochemically in occasional Kupffer cells in 5 dogs with a range of chronic hepatic inflammatory lesions and in one dog with a patent ductus venosus; however, a retrospective study of formalin-fixed paraffin-embedded liver from 45 dogs with chronic hepatitis or cirrhosis failed to reveal CAdV-1 by either PCR or immunohistochemistry, although the possibility that the virus initiates hepatic damage by provoking self-perpetuating hepatitis could not be excluded. Focal interstitial nephritis occurs commonly, and the cellular infiltrates are persistent but not functionally significant. They consist of interstitial lymphocytic accumulations, especially about the corticomedullary junction and in the stroma of the pelvis.

Corneal edema is a late development, corresponding temporally to increasing neutralizing antibody titer. It may occur as early as day 7 of infection, but is usually delayed to between 14 and 21 days. Viral antigen can be detected in these eyes by fluorescent techniques, but not in the corneal structures. Inflammatory edema is present in the iris, ciliary apparatus, and corneal propria, and inflammatory cells are abundant in the filtration angle and iris. The infiltrates are principally plasma cells, and there is evidence that the ocular lesion is a hypersensitivity reaction to circulating immune complex deposition, with complement fixation, inflammatory cell chemotaxis, and corneal endothelial damage resulting in an anterior uveitis with corneal stromal edema.

Originally, it was assumed that the widespread tendency to hemorrhage in this disease was because of leakage from damaged vascular endothelium, coupled with an inability on the part of the damaged liver to replace clotting factors. Although these effects play a role, it is now known that *the exhaustion of clotting factors is in large part the result of their accelerated consumption, as the widespread endothelial damage is a potent initiator of the clotting cascade.*

Wesselsbron disease

This disease is caused by **Wesselsbron virus**, an arthropod-borne flavivirus that, according to serologic surveys, is widespread in Africa in various species of animals and birds. Various *Aedes* mosquitoes are the vectors. Humans are also susceptible to clinical and inapparent infection. *The virus produces outbreaks of abortion and perinatal death in sheep.* Susceptible adults rarely show clinical signs but may have a biphasic febrile response to infection; other clinical signs, when present, are of hepatitis and jaundice.

The lesions in lambs dying within 12 hours of birth consist mainly of widespread petechiae and gastrointestinal hemorrhage; longer survival allows jaundice to develop, and the liver becomes orange-yellow, enlarged, friable, and patchily congested. The bile in the gallbladder becomes thick and dark in some cases, but this may be due more to hemorrhage into the gallbladder than to hemolysis. Lymph nodes are rather constantly enlarged, congested, and edematous.

The most characteristic histologic changes are seen in the liver. There are randomly scattered foci of necrosis, with apoptosis and proliferation of sinusoidal lining cells (Fig. 2-71). Mononuclear cells and pigment-filled macrophages accumulate in the portal stroma as well as in the sinusoids. In a variable proportion of cases, *hepatocyte nuclei may contain eosinophilic, irregular inclusions.* These are not accompanied by as much margination of nuclear chromatin as that associated with conventional viral inclusions, and their significance is obscure. Wesselsbron viral antigen can be demonstrated in necrotic acidophilic and degenerating hepatocytes and rarely in the inclusions. In jaundiced animals, there may be considerable canalicular cholestasis; whether or not this is the result of hemolysis does not appear to have been determined. Hepatocellular proliferation is apparent in the less acute cases. Lymphoid follicles in lymph nodes and spleen show pronounced lymphocyte necrosis and stimulation of lymphoblasts.

Rift Valley fever

This is an *arthropod-borne viral infection of ruminants and humans,* in many respects similar to Wesselsbron disease. **Rift Valley fever virus** (RVFV) is, however, responsible for greater

losses. Morbidity and mortality may occur in adult sheep; death sometimes occurs in adult cattle, but it is chiefly a disease of the young, causing *heavy mortality among lambs, kids, and calves, and abortion in ewes, does, and cows.* The infection in enzootic form is widespread in eastern and southern Africa, but it has, in plague-like proportions, extended to West Africa, Egypt, and the Arabian Peninsula. RVFV is a member of the *Phlebovirus* genus, 1 of the 5 genera in the family *Bunyaviridae.* It is transmitted by many species of mosquito of the genera *Culex* and *Aedes,* in which transovarial passage can occur. Mosquitoes, once infected, remain so, and in them, the virus is not pathogenic. High levels of viremia occur in sheep and cattle and are maintained for up to 5 days. During epizootics, the virus may be spread by fomites, aerosols, and mechanically by other biting insects.

In endemic situations, the disease in adults is usually mild, but in epidemics in sheep and goats, severe illness occurs with fever, mucopurulent nasal discharge, and dysentery. The mortality rate is then very high, reaching 90-100% in lambs and 10-30% in adults. The disease in cattle is less severe, but pregnant animals abort, and the mortality rate in adult animals is 5-10%, whereas in calves it may reach 70%.

As in Wesselsbron disease, *the gross postmortem picture is dominated by widespread hemorrhage, ranging from serosal petechiae to severe gastrointestinal bleeding.* The liver in the acute cases in neonatal lambs is similar to that in cases of Wesselsbron disease, being yellow, swollen, soft, and patchily congested or hemorrhagic. In older animals and in less acute cases, however, the liver tends to be darker and shows scattered pale foci of necrosis 1-2 mm in diameter. There may be fibrinous perihepatitis, edema of the gallbladder wall, and moderate, blood-tinged ascites. Experimental infection of calves produced encephalomyelitis in an animal that survived the initial viremic stage.

Within 12 hours of experimental infection of lambs, there are *randomly distributed foci of hepatocellular necrosis in the liver.* These foci include aggregates of inflammatory cells and prominent apoptotic bodies and initially involve about a half dozen hepatocytes (eFig. 2-18). Within a few hours, however, these primary foci enlarge and may become almost confluent. In the meantime, the remaining parenchyma may rapidly undergo necrosis that spares only a small rim of periportal hepatocytes. In naturally infected calves, the primary foci of necrosis undergo lysis more rapidly than the surrounding parenchyma; these foci thus have a striking "washed-out" appearance. Where the expanding foci of necrosis include portal triads, there may follow fibrinous vasculitis and thrombosis. Fibrin deposition in sinusoids is common, and so is mineralization of necrotic hepatocytes. Cholestasis is apparent in sections but is not a prominent feature.

Eosinophilic intranuclear inclusion bodies, often elongated, are sometimes seen in degenerate hepatocytes; there is associated nuclear vesiculation and chromatin margination. There is necrosis in germinal centers of lymphoid follicles in lymph nodes and spleen similar to that seen in Wesselsbron disease. Renal glomerular hypercellularity and necrosis have been described in the experimental disease. By immunohistochemistry, RVFV antigen can be detected in focal areas in cytoplasm of degenerating and necrotic hepatocytes but not in nonparenchymal cells.

Ultrastructural studies have shown condensation of degenerate hepatocytes, abundant apoptosis, and the presence of membrane-bound fragments of hepatocellular cytoplasm, but

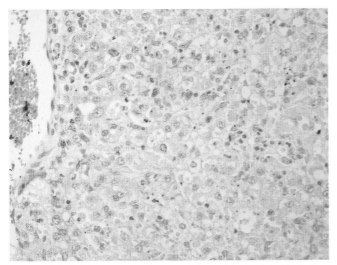

Figure 2-71 Focal necrosis and apoptosis in Wesselsbron disease in a lamb. (Courtesy S. Youssef.)

sinusoidal lining cells are not notably damaged; the Kupffer cells instead participate in the uptake of the necrotic and apoptotic hepatocytes. There is abundant fibrin in sinusoids in the vicinity of the primary foci of necrosis. *The intranuclear inclusions are composed not of recognizable viral particles but of filaments.* Virus is occasionally discernible in the cytoplasm, associated with tubular membranes.

It seems that the primary infection of the liver produces the primary necrotic foci, from which more virus spreads to damage neighboring parenchyma; the virus clearly has a marked preference for hepatocytes. The hemorrhagic component of the syndrome is probably related to consumption of clotting factors; there is no direct evidence for the endothelial damage seen in infectious canine hepatitis.

In summary, Rift Valley fever is characterized by obvious focal hepatic necrosis, on which is superimposed an extensive centrilobular and midzonal necrosis; cholestasis is not as prominent as it is in Wesselsbron disease. The liver lesions in the latter disease consist of smaller, randomly distributed foci of hepatocellular necrosis, more active reaction by the sinusoidal lining cells, and more obvious cholestasis.

Equine serum hepatitis (Theiler's disease)

Equine serum hepatitis is a common cause of acute hepatic failure in horses. The disease was originally described in 1919 by Arnold Theiler, in horses passively immunized with equine serum against African horse sickness, and was later recognized in horses passively immunized against anthrax, tetanus, and equine encephalomyelitis. Various injectable biologics of equine origin have been associated with the disease, including *Clostridium perfringens* toxoids, tetanus antitoxin, and equine herpesviral vaccines prepared from equine fetal tissue and pregnant mare serum. However, although such an association holds for the majority of cases, there are many, usually sporadic, cases in horses that have not received any injections. It is unknown how many exposed horses get subclinical disease, because the condition is seldom diagnosed before the onset of hepatic failure. However, some horses do recover after transient illness with jaundice, and some can survive with residual neurologic problems.

Recent metatranscriptomic analysis of serum from 2 index clinical cases in an outbreak of serum hepatitis in horses passively immunized against botulism, as well as from the equine hyperimmune plasma product administered before the outbreak, identified a previously unknown and highly divergent member of the *Flaviviridae* family, designated "*Theiler's disease–associated virus*" (TDAV). In this outbreak, 8 of 22 horses developed serum biochemical evidence of liver injury, although only the 2 index cases developed clinical signs of acute hepatic insufficiency. A qRT-PCR–based assay found evidence of TDAV in serum from 15 of 17 horses treated with the botulinum antitoxin, as well as in 1 of the 3 donor horses used to produce the antitoxin, whereas 20 in-contact untreated horses and 20 additional horses from a separate premises were assay negative. Viral load did not, however, appear to be predictive of biochemical or clinical extent of hepatic injury. One of 4 horses experimentally inoculated with the virus developed elevated serum liver enzymes. Four of the original 17 horses continued to be asymptomatically positive for TDAV 1 year later, demonstrating chronic infection, whereas horses that tested negative initially continued to test negative at 1 year, suggesting that horizontal transmission is inefficient. Although Koch's postulates remain to be fulfilled, *TDAV appears to be a plausible candidate viral cause of this disease.* Further research is necessary to establish the precise role of this virus in the disease.

The incubation period of disease is typically 42-60 days, sometimes up to 90 days. Onset of the typical clinical syndrome is sudden, with death occurring in 6-24 hours. Clinically, there is lethargy; jaundice; photosensitivity; hyperexcitability, often with mania; continuous walking and pushing; apparent blindness; and ataxia. Death occurs suddenly without a period of prostration.

At autopsy, icterus is present, with moderate ascites; the spleen is normal or congested, and there may be petechial hemorrhages on serous membranes and renal cortices, and some congestion of the intestine with hemorrhage into its lumen. Grossly, the liver usually appears atrophic, small, and flabby because of the acute loss of many hepatocytes (Fig. 2-72A). The liver may be stained by bile pigments, and its surface mottled with a few strands of fresh fibrin. The mottling is more evident on the cut surface, which may be severely congested with an apparent zonal pattern, and sometimes fatty (Fig. 2-72B).

Microscopically, the hepatic lesion is considerably older than the clinical course would suggest. *There may be a few surviving swollen and vacuolated periportal hepatocytes or sometimes complete depletion of parenchymal cells in the section.* In less-affected regions in animals with adequate dietary or adipose reserves to mobilize, there is severe macrovesicular fatty change in most remaining hepatocytes. Acute necrosis is typically not seen, and there is no significant hemorrhage. Variable numbers of apoptotic hepatocytes are expected. In the periphery of the acini, severely ballooned cells undergo dissolution to leave scattered fatty cysts, but most of them disappear to leave either sinusoids that are dilated and filled with blood or a condensed and distorted reticulin framework. Extensive deposits of bile pigments are present in Kupffer cells and hepatocytes. Leukocytes, including lymphocytes, plasma cells, histiocytes, and a few neutrophils, may infiltrate diffusely, but not in large numbers. There is diffuse but very slight fibroplasia, especially in the portal units. In some livers, there is a ductular reaction, with small irregular clusters of proliferating ductular cells evident in the portal areas.

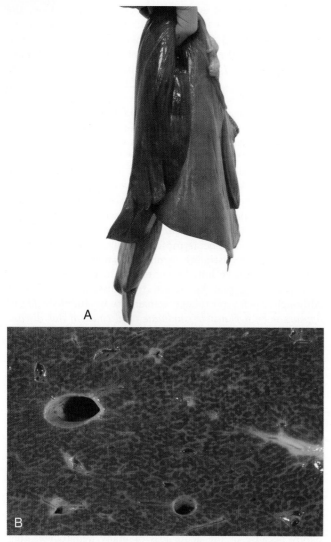

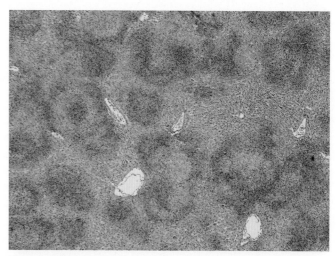

Figure 2-73 Multifocal hepatitis caused by *Listeria monocytogenes* infection in a calf. (Courtesy J.L. Caswell.)

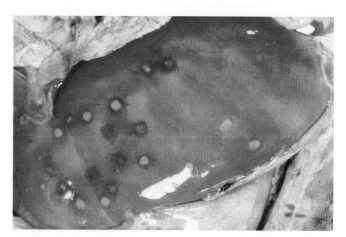

Figure 2-74 *Campylobacter fetus* infection in an ovine fetus. (Courtesy P. Stromberg.)

Figure 2-72 **Equine serum hepatitis (Theiler's disease). A.** Small, limp and flaccid "dishrag" liver. **B.** The reticular pattern in this slice of liver suggests zonal necrosis.

Bacterial infections

Bacterial hepatitis is common, but, with a few important exceptions, is usually focally distributed and of little clinical significance. Bacteria may gain entrance to the liver in various ways: by direct implantation, for example, by foreign-body penetration from the reticulum; by invasion of the capsule from an adjacent focus of suppurative peritonitis; hematogenously via the hepatic artery or portal and umbilical veins; or via the bile ducts.

Excepting peracute septicemias, *there are few specific bacterial infections that have a sustained or repeated bacteremic phase without producing hepatic lesions.* There are, in addition, many cases of nonspecific bacteremia, especially those originating in the drainage field of the portal vein, in which focal hepatitis occurs. Because their differential diagnosis is of some importance, it is probably useful to list here those specific bacterial diseases in which focal hepatitis is expected or characteristic, but not constant. The specific infections may occur as fetal or perinatal infections. The list includes *Listeria monocytogenes* in fetal and neonatal lambs, calves, foals, and piglets (Fig. 2-73); *Campylobacter fetus* in fetal and neonatal lambs (Fig. 2-74); *Actinobacillus equuli* in foals; *A. suis* in pigs; *Yersinia pseudotuberculosis* in lambs and occasionally in dogs and cats;

Further reading

Chandriani S, et al. Identification of a previously undescribed divergent virus from the *Flaviviridae* family in an outbreak of equine serum hepatitis. Proc Natl Acad Sci U S A 2013;110:E1407-E1415.

Ikegami T, Makino S. The pathogenesis of Rift Valley fever. Viruses 2011;3:493-519.

Marschall J, Hartmann K. Avian influenza A H5N1 infections in cats. J Fel Med Surg 2008;10:359-365.

Moeller RB, et al. Systemic *Bovine herpesvirus 1* infections in neonatal dairy calves. J Vet Diagn Invest 2013;25:136-141.

Odendaal L, et al. Sensitivity and specificity of real-time reverse transcription polymerase chain reaction, histopathology, and immunohistochemical labeling for the detection of Rift Valley fever virus in naturally infected cattle and sheep. J Vet Diagn Invest 2014;26: 49-60.

Resendes AR, et al. Apoptosis in postweaning multisystemic wasting syndrome (PMWS) hepatitis in pigs naturally infected with porcine circovirus type 2 (PCV2). Vet J 2011;189:72-76.

Francisella (Yersinia) tularensis in lambs and cats; *Mannheimia haemolytica* and *Histophilus somni (Haemophilus agni)* in lambs; *Salmonella* spp. in all hosts; *Clostridium piliforme* (Tyzzer's disease) in foals and dogs; *Nocardia asteroides* in dogs; and the mycobacteria in all hosts (Figs. 2-75, 2-76A, B).

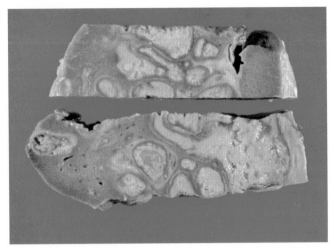

Figure 2-75 Tuberculosis in a bovine liver. (Courtesy University of Guelph.)

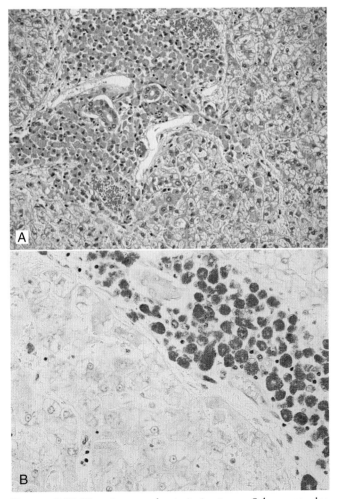

Figure 2-76 Hepatic mycobacteriosis in a Schnauzer dog **A.** H&E. **B.** Acid-fast stain. (Courtesy J.L. Caswell.)

Hepatic abscess

Hepatic abscesses, quite apart from the lesions of the specific infections just given, *are common*, especially in cattle. They may arise by direct implantation of a foreign body from the reticulum or by direct invasion of the capsule from a suppurative lesion of traumatic reticulitis and may be single or multiple, but in either case, they are often preferentially distributed to the left lobe. They may be hematogenous from portal vein emboli, or by direct extension of omphalophlebitis. Arteriogenic abscesses via the hepatic artery may occur in pyemias but are quite uncommon.

Omphalogenic abscesses are more common in calves than in other species but occur in all. The bacterial flora is frequently mixed, but *Arcanobacterium pyogenes, Fusobacterium necrophorum*, streptococci, and staphylococci usually predominate. Hepatic abscesses are not inevitable sequelae to omphalitis or even to omphalophlebitis, but they do not develop from navel infections in the absence of omphalophlebitis. As there is no flow of blood in these vessels after birth, involvement of the liver is by direct growth along the physiologic thrombus. Omphalophlebitis can be quite severe without extension to the liver. Hepatic abscesses of omphalogenic origin are often restricted to the left lobe (Fig. 2-77), but they may be restricted to the right or be generalized in their distribution.

Hepatic abscesses are also common and of economic importance in feedlot cattle. They are usually found at slaughter but, when numerous, may be fatal after a few days of vague digestive illness. Their pathogenesis and character are discussed with rumenitis, to which they are a sequel (see Vol. 2, Alimentary system and peritoneum). Liver abscesses in feedlot sheep likely have a similar pathogenesis, with *F. necrophorum* as the primary isolate. A second category includes parasitic granulomas populated by various opportunistic bacteria.

Hepatic abscesses of biliary origin occur in all animals. They occur in pigs in which ascarids have migrated into the bile ducts. Cholangitic abscesses in horses, dogs, and cats are usually caused by enterobacteria as part of a fulminating ascending cholangiohepatitis that is fatal after a short course.

The *sequelae* of hepatic abscessation are variable. Usually, they are insignificant and asymptomatic. Sterilization of the focus with either resorption and complete healing or encapsulation is common. Those near the surface of the liver regularly produce fibrinous and then fibrous inflammation of the capsule and adhesion to adjacent viscera. They seldom

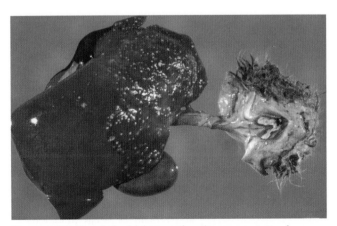

Figure 2-77 Omphalophlebitis with **miliary metastatic abscesses** in the left lobe of the liver in a calf.

perforate the capsule but do commonly break into hepatic veins to produce any one or a combination of thrombophlebitis of the vena cava, endocarditis, or pulmonary abscesses or embolism. Acute extension of a hepatic abscess into the major hepatic vein can lead to pulmonary embolism that can be acutely fatal. In adults, death may occur if the hepatic abscesses are multiple and fresh, and especially if they are necrobacillary in origin; death is probably the result of toxemia.

Hepatic necrobacillosis

Occasionally, *F. necrophorum* infection of the liver is observed following *omphalophlebitis in lambs and calves*, or as a complication of *rumenitis in adult cattle*. In feedlot cattle, both *F. necrophorum* subsp. *necrophorum* (biotype A) and subsp. *funduliforme* (biotype B) have been isolated. The hepatic lesions are multiple slightly elevated, rounded, dry areas of coagulative necrosis, sometimes a few centimeters in diameter (eFig. 2-19) and surrounded by a zone of intense hyperemia. Affected neonates seldom live long enough for the necrotic foci to liquefy and assume the appearance of ordinary abscesses, but this may be seen in adult cattle. *The histologic appearance of the foci in the stage of coagulative necrosis is quite characteristic.* The necrotic amorphous central area is bordered by a zone of wholesale destruction of leukocytes, whose nuclear chromatin is dissipated in a finely divided form, and among which the filamentous fusobacteria are mostly concentrated. Outside this zone, there is severe hyperemia and hemorrhage, and thrombosis of local vessels is common. The lesion in neonatal lambs is to be distinguished from that caused by *Campylobacter fetus*.

The pathogenic mechanisms of *F. necrophorum* involve various toxins, in particular, a high-molecular-weight leukotoxin specifically toxic to ruminant neutrophils. This unique toxin activates neutrophils and induces their apoptosis, consistent with the remarkable abscess-inducing propensity of *F. necrophorum* in ruminants. However, other toxins, endotoxic lipopolysaccharide (LPS), and hemagglutinins are also implicated as virulence factors. Mixed infections are frequent, and synergism between *F. necrophorum* and other pathogens, such as *Arcanobacterium pyogenes*, may also play a role in the pathogenesis of liver necrosis and abscessation.

Necrotic hepatitis (black disease)

Organisms of the genus *Clostridium* are notably circuitous in their means of producing disease. This is true of **C. *novyi*;** *type B strains, which produce potent exotoxins and are the cause of black disease (infectious necrotic hepatitis).* The alpha toxin of *C. novyi* is related to the large clostridial cytotoxins produced by *C. difficile* and *C. sordelli*. These toxins enter cells by receptor-mediated endocytosis and inhibit ras and rho guanosine triphosphatases by glycosylation. The beta toxin is a necrotizing and hemolytic phospholipase C (lecithinase). Black disease occurs in nonimmune animals when these exotoxins are released by *C. novyi* within an anaerobic focus in the liver. These anaerobic sites, which provide a suitable environment for germination of *C. novyi* spores, are most commonly a result of migrating liver flukes.

C. novyi is widely distributed in soil, and the spores are continually ingested by grazing animals in areas where black disease occurs. Some spores cross the mucous membranes, probably in phagocytes, and remain as latent infections in macrophages, mainly in the liver, spleen, and bone marrow. The duration of latency in tissue is not known, but it can be

many months. In endemic areas, many healthy sheep, cattle, and dogs harbor latent infections in their livers. *Black disease is principally an acutely fatal disease of sheep in regions where the inciting helminths are endemic.* The disease is most commonly initiated by migrating larvae of the common liver fluke *Fasciola hepatica*. In Bessarabia and France, it is endemically related to the distribution of *Dicrocoelium dendriticum*, the lancet liver fluke. Sporadic cases may be related to *Cysticercus tenuicollis* infection or may be idiopathic.

Deaths in sheep from black disease occur rapidly and usually without warning signs. Illness, if observed, is brief and characterized by reluctance to move, drowsiness, rapid respiration, and quiet subsidence. Affected animals are usually in good nutritional condition. Postmortem decomposition occurs rapidly. *The name of the disease is derived from the appearance of flayed skins, the dark coloration being caused by an unusual degree of subcutaneous venous congestion.* Frequently, there is edema of the sternal subcutis, and airways contain stable foam. Serous cavities contain an abundance of fluid that clots on exposure to air. The fluid is usually straw colored, but that in the abdomen may be tinged with blood. The volume of fluid in the abdomen and thorax may vary from about 50 mL to 1.5 L. The pericardial sac is distended with similar fluid in amounts up to ~300 mL. Subendocardial hemorrhages in the left ventricle are almost constant. Patchy areas of congestion and hemorrhage may be present in the pyloric part of the abomasum and in the small intestine.

The typical and diagnostic lesions occur in the liver and are always present. They are usually clearly evident on the capsular surface, the diaphragmatic surface especially, but the organ may have to be sliced carefully to find them. The liver will be the seat of either the acute traumatic hemorrhagic lesions of acute fascioliasis, the cholangiohepatitis of the chronic disease, or both. *The lesion of black disease, and occasionally there are several, is a yellow-white area of necrosis 2-3 cm in diameter, surrounded by a broad zone of intense hyperemia, roughly circular in outline, and extending hemispherically into the substance of the organ.* There may be a coagulum of fibrin on the capsular surface overlying the necrotic area. Occasionally, the essential lesions are rectilinear in shape or very irregular. The lesions appear homogeneous on the cut surface, but some contain poorly defined centers of soft or caseous material.

The histologic evolution of the hepatic lesions begins with the necrotic and hemorrhagic tracts caused by wandering immature flukes. These are sinuous tunnels ~0.5 cm in diameter that contain blood, necrotic hepatic cells, and the leukocytes, chiefly eosinophils, attracted by the flukes. About the tunnels is a narrow zone of coagulative necrosis, also produced by the flukes. As usual, the necrotic tissue is demarcated by a thin zone of scavenger cells, chiefly neutrophils. If latent spores are present in the necrotic areas, they quickly vegetate and are visible in sections as large, gram-positive bacilli. In nonimmune animals, the vegetative organisms elaborate exotoxins that cause necrosis of the surrounding tissue, including the eosinophils of the fluke tunnel. As the area of necrosis expands, the bacterial proliferation keeps pace so that bacilli can be found in all parts of the necrotic focus but not in the surrounding viable tissue. *Usually, bacteria are concentrated at the advancing margin of the lesion*, just inside a zone of infiltrated neutrophils. At about the time of death and immediately afterward, the bacilli scatter in the liver and to other organs.

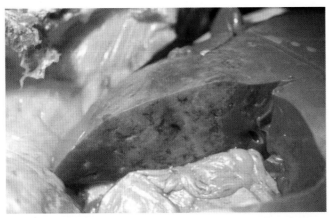

Figure 2-78 Large focus of hepatic necrosis in an ox with **bacillary hemoglobinuria.** (Courtesy University of Guelph.)

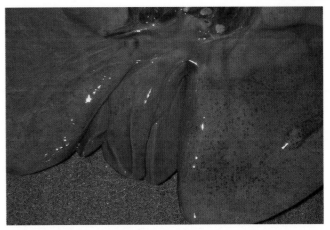

Figure 2-79 Foal liver with multifocal hepatitis in *Clostridium piliforme* infection **(Tyzzer's disease).**

Bacillary hemoglobinuria

Bacillary hemoglobinuria is a counterpart of black disease. The cause is **Clostridium haemolyticum,** which is closely related to *C. novyi.* Both species produce the *beta toxin,* a necrotizing and hemolytic lecithinase (phospholipase C). The pathogenesis of the 2 diseases is comparable, as both depend on a focus of hepatic injury within which latent spores can germinate. *Bacillary hemoglobinuria as an endemic disease exists only in areas where* Fasciola hepatica *abounds, and it is probable that flukes are the primary cause of the initiating lesion.* The disease does occur sporadically where there are no flukes and may be prompted by other parasites or other diverse focal lesions, which are smudged out in the expanding areas of necrosis. There is scant information on the ecology of the organism, but it is clear that it has its own environmental requirements, and the disease will not persist in areas where these requirements are not met. The spores will remain in the livers of cattle for several months after removal from pastures where the disease is endemic. Spores may persist in the bones of cadavers for 2 years. Spores of this and other sporulating anaerobes can frequently be demonstrated in the liver, where they are probably retained in Kupffer cells.

Bacillary hemoglobinuria occurs in *cattle and sheep.* It is characterized clinically by *intravascular hemolysis with anemia and hemoglobinuria,* but, perhaps reflecting variety in exotoxins between strains of the organism, hemolysis may not be a feature. The essential lesion is hepatic and similar to that of black disease but is much larger and usually single (Fig. 2-78). It has been described as an infarct secondary to portal thrombosis, and although this may occur in isolated cases, it is scarcely a creditable pathogenesis for a disease of endemic occurrence. Thrombosis does occur in the affected areas but can be a result, rather than a cause, of the initial lesion and is found more frequently in the hepatic venules than in branches of the portal vein. There is severe anemia, the kidneys are speckled red or brown by hemoglobin, and the urine is of port-wine color. Peritoneal vessels are injected, and in some cases, there is severe, dry, fibrinohemorrhagic peritonitis.

Clostridium piliforme *infection*

Clostridium piliforme (formerly *Bacillus piliformis*) infection has long been known as **Tyzzer's disease,** a cause of severe losses in laboratory rodents; however, it has also been reported in *foals, calves, dogs, and cats.* Although the disease is probably initiated by an intestinal infection, lesions in the gut are less specific and constant than those in the liver, which consist of *focal hepatitis and necrosis.*

Affected foals usually die between the ages of 1-4 weeks; often they are found dead after a short illness. The liver shows pale foci up to a few millimeters across (Fig. 2-79); these are represented microscopically by randomly distributed foci of coagulative necrosis with moderate neutrophilic infiltrate (Fig. 2-80A). This lesion is not diagnostic in itself; its specificity depends on the presence of the causal organism in hepatocytes in the periphery of the necrotic zones. At present, *C. piliforme* can only be isolated with difficulty on artificial media, so diagnosis is usually based on demonstration of the large, long bacilli in the cytoplasm of degenerate and also otherwise apparently normal hepatocytes at the periphery of the necrotic zones. The organisms are gram negative and are best delineated with silver impregnation techniques, such as that of Warthin-Starry, but they may be seen with routine stains, such as Giemsa, particularly when the material is fresh. Differentiation from other organisms, including postmortem saprophytes, can be achieved by immunohistochemistry or immunofluorescence. *The bacilli tend to lie in sheaves or bundles* (Fig. 2-80B). There may also be colitis sufficiently severe to cause diarrhea, but not as severe as that seen in rabbits with this disease.

Fewer cases of Tyzzer's disease have been reported in dogs and cats. The liver lesions are essentially the same as those in foals and rodents, and there is also enteritis or enterocolitis. Immunodeficiency predisposes to the disease because it occurs sporadically in dogs that have undergone immunosuppressive or anticancer therapy. Such cases may be complicated by concurrent viral, mycotic, or protozoal infections.

Leptospirosis

Leptospirosis is a systemic disease characterized by acute jaundice, cholestatic liver injury, and renal failure in dogs, and is discussed in more detail in Vol. 2, Urinary system. The hepatic lesions described following acute experimental infection of dogs with *Leptospira kirschneri* serovar *grippotyphosa* include mixed perivascular periportal infiltrates of neutrophils, lymphocytes, and plasma cells, with mild hepatic lipidosis, dissociation of hepatocytes, and intracanalicular bile plugs evident by day 12 postinfection, along with increased hepatocellular mitotic activity. *Clinical icterus has been attributed to cholestasis caused by dissociation of hepatocytes* (eFig. 2-20). Dogs experimentally infected with *Leptospira interrogans* serovar *pomona*

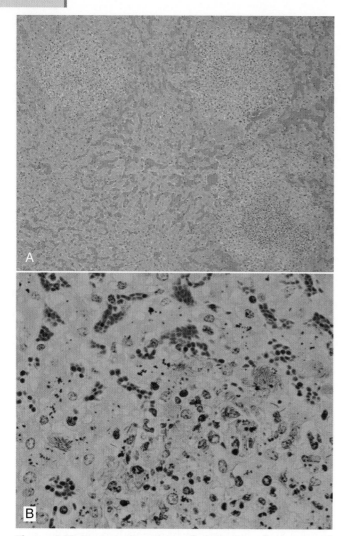

Figure 2-80 **Tyzzer's disease** in a foal. **A.** Foci of necrosis and suppurative inflammation. **B.** *Clostridium piliforme* bacilli in bundles in hepatocytes at margin of lesion. Warthin-Starry silver stain.

developed pulmonary and renal petechial hemorrhages, and friable livers with multifocal 1-2 mm raised white foci corresponding to periportal inflammatory infiltrates of lymphocytes, plasma cells, neutrophils, and macrophages; small foci of hepatic necrosis; and bile plugs in canaliculi, in addition to renal, pulmonary, and cardiac lesions. Organisms were identified by immunohistochemistry at the brush borders of renal proximal convoluted tubules as well as at the luminal surface of bile duct epithelium. In a retrospective study of dogs with supportive clinical signs and microscopic agglutination test titers of ≥320 for one or more serovars tested, including *autumnalis, bratislava, canicola, grippotyphosa, icterohaemorrhagiae,* and *pomona,* histologic lesions in the liver were subtle, with sinusoidal neutrophil margination, Kupffer cell hypertrophy, and low levels of hepatocellular single-cell necrosis and mitoses. Some livers had diffuse interstitial lymphocytic hepatitis, with mitotic figures, anisokaryosis, binucleation, and some degree of lobular collapse. Chronic hepatitis has also been experimentally produced by leptospiral infection in dogs; however, clinical cases are rarely documented.

Other bacteria

A single case of clinical disease associated with **Helicobacter canis** has been reported in a 2-month-old puppy with peracute disease causing weakness and vomiting before death. Multiple coalescing yellow foci in the liver up to 1.5 cm in diameter consisted of hepatocellular coagulative necrosis with infiltrating mononuclear cells and neutrophils. Spiral bacteria were visualized by Warthin-Starry silver stains in area of necrosis, within bile canaliculi, and occasionally in bile duct lumens. This organism has previously been identified in the blood of diarrheic children, and in the feces of 4% of dogs in an epidemiologic study examining the incidence of *Campylobacter-like* organisms in 1,000 dogs.

Bartonella spp. infection has been associated with a wide variety of granulomatous syndromes and peliosis hepatis in humans, often in association with immunosuppression. *Bartonella henselae* and *B. clarridgeae* are associated with self-limiting illness and persistent intravascular infection in cats; mild lymphocytic cholangitis/pericholangitis and lymphocytic hepatitis have been reported with experimental infection of cats with *B. henselae. B. henselae* has been identified in liver tissue by PCR from a single case of peliosis hepatis in a Golden Retriever and granulomatous hepatitis in a Basset Hound, whereas *B. clarridgeae* DNA was identified in liver tissue from a Doberman Pinscher with histologic lesions of Doberman hepatitis, however, the extent to which infection induces disease in dogs is currently unknown.

Further reading

O'Toole D, et al. Tularemia in range sheep: an overlooked syndrome? J Vet Diagn Invest 2008;20:508-513.

Rissi DR, Brown CA. Diagnostic features in 10 naturally occurring cases of acute fatal canine leptospirosis. J Vet Diagn Invest 2014;26: 799-804.

Tadepalli S, et al. *Fusobacterium necrophorum*: a ruminal bacterium that invades liver to cause abscesses in cattle. Anaerobe 2009;15: 36-43.

Helminthic infections

Various helminths, including cestodes, nematodes, and trematodes, as well as the larval pentastome *Linguatula serrata,* can produce inflammation of liver and bile ducts. Those parasites that have the biliary system as their final habitat will be discussed in detail later. The others produce hepatic lesions in the course of their natural or accidental migrations, and are discussed under the organ (for most of them, the gut) that is their final habitat. It is useful, however, to describe briefly here the lesions produced by larvae in transit.

The initial lesion produced by wandering larvae is traumatic. Sinuous tunnels permeate the parenchyma and often breach the capsule. In the tunnels, there are free red cells, degenerating hepatocytes, and leukocytes, chiefly eosinophils, which react to the parasites. Bordering the tunnel is a narrow zone of coagulative necrosis of parenchyma with neutrophils at its margin. Eosinophils also infiltrate the portal triads. The necrotic parasitic tracts heal by scarification, and the fibroblastic tissue, infiltrated with eosinophils, is eventually incorporated into the portal units. Most larvae escape from the liver, but some eventually become encapsulated in the liver in abscesses containing numerous eosinophils. The abscesses may caseate and come to resemble tubercles, and eventually many are heavily mineralized to form permanent pearly nodules. In sheep, the most common cause of this type of hepatitis (aside from liver fluke) is **Cysticercus tenuicollis** in its wandering phase. Lambs may die of severe hemorrhagic hepatitis (Fig.

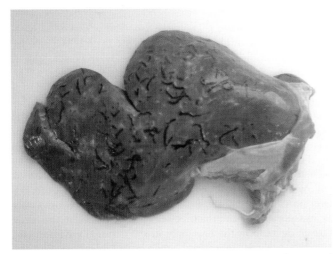

Figure 2-81 **Hemorrhagic subcapsular migration tracks** caused by *Cysticercus tenuicollis* in a lamb. (Courtesy A. Rehmtulla.)

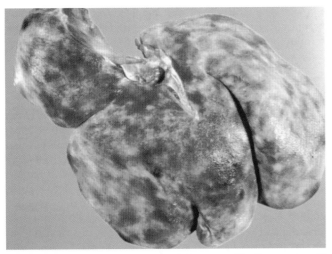

Figure 2-82 **Multifocal interstitial hepatitis** ("milk-spot liver") caused by *Ascaris suum* migration in a pig.

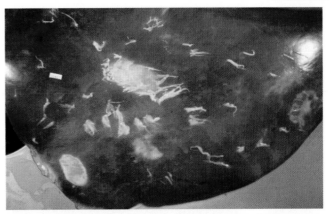

Figure 2-83 **Fibrous tags** on the diaphragmatic surface of an equine liver. (Courtesy University of Guelph.)

2-81) caused by very heavy infections of this parasite, and in pigs, an aberrant host, *C. tenuicollis* can produce a very intense inflammatory reaction.

In pigs, larvae of ***Ascaris suum*** and ***Stephanurus dentatus*** produce similar but distinct patterns of focal interstitial hepatitis. The ascarids produce their distinctive accentuation of the stroma *("milk spots")* (Fig. 2-82) when quite small larvae are immobilized by the host's inflammatory reaction; thus the foci are relatively small. The fibrotic lesion produced by *S. dentatus* larvae, on the other hand, is less focal and more in the nature of a track, and there are usually small, inflamed, capsular craters where the larvae have emerged from the liver to migrate to their preferred perirenal site. There will be obvious portal phlebitis at the hepatic hilus when infection by *S. dentatus* has been by the oral route, and in these livers, the parenchymal lesion is more severe in this vicinity.

Migration tracks left by **larval strongyles** can be found under the liver capsule in young horses, and historically, these have been thought to relate to the dense, discrete, capsular fibrous tags and plaques that are almost universally found on the diaphragmatic surface of the liver of mature horses. However, these hepatic fibrotic lesions remain common in horses even after the widespread use of effective anthelmintics, and their precise etiology remains unknown (Fig. 2-83).

Parasites can produce hepatic lesions by other means. The hydatid intermediate stages of *Echinococcus* encyst in the liver and may destroy much of it; the larvae of *Ascaris suum* in cattle add to the usual insult by causing portal phlebitis and small areas of infarction; the adults of *Ascaris* in all species, but especially in pigs, may migrate into the bile ducts; and the eggs of schistosomes enter in the portal blood to lodge in the intrahepatic portal vessels and provoke granulomatous inflammation.

Cestodes

Stilesia hepatica and ***Thysanosoma actinioides,*** the "fringed tapeworm," are the only cestodes that inhabit the bile ducts. They are parasites of ruminants, *Stilesia* occurring in Africa, *Thysanosoma* in North and South America. The life cycles of the parasites are not completely known but may involve oribatid mites as intermediate hosts. *T. actinioides* may also be found in the pancreatic ducts and small intestine. Usually, the infestations are light but, even when heavy, are not of much significance (eFig. 2-21). Very heavy infestations by *S. hepatica* occur without signs of illness, although the bile ducts may be nearly occluded, slightly thickened, and dilated. Saccular dilations of the ducts may occur and be filled with worms. The fringed tapeworm is perhaps more pathogenic, and unthriftiness may accompany heavy infestations.

Echinococcus granulosus hydatid cysts occur most commonly in the liver of ruminants in endemic areas (Fig. 2-84) but have been reported as incidental postmortem findings in the liver of pigs and horses. The cysticerci and hydatids, which in the intermediate stages invade the liver, are discussed further in Vol. 2, Alimentary system and peritoneum.

Echinococcus multilocularis is found in Europe, parts of northern Asia, and North America, where it has a sylvatic life cycle. Red and arctic foxes are the most important definitive hosts, although coyotes, raccoon-dogs, and wolves can also be infected. In North America, there are few documented cases of intestinal infection by *E. multilocularis* tapeworms in domestic dogs and even fewer in cats. The adult tapeworm is small, 5 mm, and infective eggs are shed in the feces to be ingested by the intermediate host, which in temperate areas are typically various species of rodents, including voles, lemmings, and deer mice. The hexacanth embryo is released from the egg, travels through the intestinal wall, and migrates to the liver via the hepatic portal circulation. The metacestode

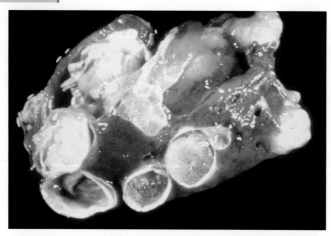

Figure 2-84 **Hydatid liver disease** (*Echinococcus granulosus* infestation) in a sheep. (Courtesy University of Guelph.)

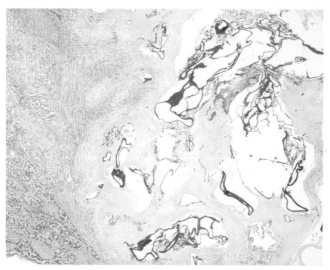

Figure 2-85 *Echinococcus multilocularis* **cysts with acellular laminated membranes** in the liver of a dog. PAS stain. (Courtesy A. Brooks.)

stage is an *alveolar hydatid cyst*, composed of numerous small vesicles lined by a PAS-positive acellular laminated membrane or cuticle layer and a layer of germinal epithelium from which protoscolices develop. Some infections in dogs do not progress to form protoscolices, and instead form irregular large cysts with a PAS-positive laminated membrane (Fig. 2-85). Additional exogenous budding results in spread of the metacestodes to other internal locations. The life cycle is completed when the infected intermediate host is consumed by a definitive host, where the protoscolices attach to the intestinal wall and mature. Other species can occasionally act as aberrant intermediate hosts, including pigs, horses, and humans; *human alveolar echinococcosis is a serious zoonosis*. Dogs can simultaneously act as definitive and intermediate hosts for this parasite. Cases of hepatic alveolar hydatid cysts have been reported in dogs from highly endemic areas in Belgium, Germany, Switzerland, and most recently in Canada (British Columbia, Ontario). Affected dogs display progressive abdominal enlargement, intermittent inappetance, and vomiting, and the cysts may be found in the liver, omentum, abdominal cavity, or lungs.

Nematodes

Calodium hepaticum (*Capillaria hepatica*) is the one nematode that in the adult phase inhabits the liver. It is a slender worm, morphologically resembling the whipworms, and it lives in the parenchyma rather than in the bile ducts. The usual hosts of the adult stage are rodents, but sporadic infestations are observed in dogs. These worms are *not highly pathogenic*. The adults provoke some traumatic hepatitis, and the eggs, which are deposited in clusters, provoke the development of localized granulomas. The eggs are readily recognized by their ovoid shape and polar caps. The granulomas can be seen through the capsule or in the substance of the liver as yellow streaks or patches. The eggs cannot escape from the liver unless a predator eats them. Predators, however, act only as transport hosts, and the ingested eggs are passed in the feces. Larvae develop in the eggs only in the external environment, and the cycle is completed when a suitable host eats the mature larvae in the eggs.

Trematodes

Various trematodes (flukes) are parasitic in the livers of animals. They belong to the families *Fasciolidae (Fasciola hepatica, F. gigantica, Fascioloides magna)*, *Dicrocoeliidae (Dicrocoelium dendriticum, D. hospes, Platynosomum concinnum)*, *Schistosomatidae (Heterobilharzia americana)*, and *Opisthorchiidae* (including *Metorchis* spp., *Opisthorchis felineus, Clonorchis sinensis, Pseudamphistomum truncatum*). The diseases produced are known collectively as **distomiasis.**

Fasciola hepatica, the common liver fluke of sheep and cattle, is the most widespread and important of the group. Patent infestations can develop in other wild and domestic animals and in humans. These flukes are leaf shaped and ~2.5 cm long in sheep and slightly larger in cattle. *They are found in the bile ducts.* Being hermaphroditic, only one fluke is necessary to establish a patent infestation, and each adult may produce 20,000 eggs per day. The longevity of the adult flukes is amazing and is potentially as great as or greater than that of the host; they have been known to survive for 11 years, and it seems that they can produce eggs all this time. The eggs are eliminated in bile, and on pasture, in conditions of suitable warmth and moisture, hatch a larva (miracidium) in ~9 days. If the environmental temperature is low, the incubation period may be delayed for some months. The miracidium can survive only in moisture. It is actively motile and penetrates the tissues of the intermediate host, which is an aquatic snail. Different snails serve this purpose in different countries, but all of them belong to the genus *Lymnaea*.

Each *miracidium*, on penetrating a snail, develops into a mother *sporocyst* that reproduces, probably parthenogenetically, giving rise to a small number of the second generation, the *redia*. Each redia produces either redia or *cercariae*, or to the 2 successively. Cercariae, the larval stage of the third (sexual) generation, first appear 1-2 months after the miracidium penetrates. Cercariae continue to escape daily for the life of the snail, but even so, total cercarial production is only 500-1,000. They actively escape from the snail and are attracted to green plants, where they encyst and become infective metacercariae in 1 day. These can remain infective for 1 month in summer and up to 3 months in winter. The developmental events from egg to this stage take 1-2 months under favorable conditions.

Infestation occurs by ingestion. Excystment occurs in the duodenum. The young flukes penetrate the intestinal wall and cross the peritoneal cavity, attaching here and there to suck blood and penetrate the liver through its capsule; a few no doubt pass in the portal vessels or migrate up the bile duct. They wander in the liver for a month or more before settling down in the bile ducts to mature, which they do in 2-3 months. Some may, by accident, enter the hepatic veins and systemic circulation to lodge in unusual sites; intrauterine infestations are on record. *Lesions caused by aberrant flukes are quite common in bovine lung.* They consist of resilient nodules just under the pleura of the peripheral parts of the lung. They range in diameter from ~1 to many centimeters and consist of thinly encapsulated abscesses situated at the ends of bronchi. The content is slightly mucoid, unevenly coagulated brown fluid; in some lesions, the reaction is predominantly caseous. The location of the lesion suggests that it begins as a peripheral bronchiectasis that later becomes sealed off. The fluke persists in the debris, but is small and hard to find.

The essential *lesions* produced by *F. hepatica* occur in the liver and may be described, first, as those produced by the migratory larvae, and second, as those produced by the mature flukes in the bile ducts; the two often intermingle (eFig. 2-22). There is the further incidence of peritonitis, which is produced by the young flukes on their way to the liver and, perhaps also, by some that break out through the capsule.

Usually, there is no obvious reaction to the passage of young flukes through the intestinal wall and across the peritoneal cavity, except for small hemorrhagic foci on the peritoneum, where the flukes have been temporarily attached. Few or many parasites may be found in any ascitic fluid and attached to the peritoneum of the diaphragm and the mesenteries. When the infestations are heavy and repeated, such as may be observed in sheep, cattle, and swine, *peritonitis* occurs. The young flukes at this stage are <1.0 mm long. The peritonitis may be acute and exudative or chronic and proliferative. It is usually concentrated on the hepatic capsule, especially its visceral surface, but may be restricted to the parietal peritoneum or to the visceral peritoneum, including the mesenteries of the gut. In acute cases, there are fibrinohemorrhagic deposits on the serous surfaces, and in chronic cases, there may be fibrous tags, with adhesions or a more or less diffuse thickening by connective tissue. Many young flukes can be found microscopically in the fibrinous deposits, and in the diffuse peritoneal thickenings, there are tortuous migration tunnels containing blood, debris, and the young parasites. In cases with involvement of the visceral peritoneum, young flukes can be found in enlarged mesenteric lymph nodes.

The acute lesions in the liver caused by the wandering flukes are basically traumatic, but there is an element of coagulative necrosis, which is possibly related to toxic excretions of the flukes. The migratory pathways are tortuous tunnels that appear on cross-section as hemorrhagic foci 2-3 mm in diameter. If a tunnel is followed, a young fluke <1.0 mm long can be found at the end. When the infestation is heavy, the liver may appear to be permeated by dark hemorrhagic streaks and foci. Older tunnels from which the debris has been cleared may appear as light yellow streaks because of infiltration of eosinophils. Microscopically, fresh tunnels are filled with blood and degenerate hepatocytes and are soon infiltrated by eosinophils. Later, macrophages and giant cells arrange themselves about the debris and remove it, and healing occurs by granulation tissue, which is rich in lymphocytes and eosinophils. In light infestations, the scars may disappear, but in heavy infestations, they may fuse with each other and with portal areas to produce

moderate irregular fibrosis. There may, as yet, be no change in the bile ducts. Probably, *most of the young flukes reach the bile ducts, but some do not and become encysted in the parenchyma.* One or more flukes may be present in each cyst, which consists of a connective-tissue capsule and a dirty brown content of blood, detritus, and excrement from flukes. The cysts ultimately caseate and may mineralize or are obliterated by fibrous tissue. These cysts are most frequent on the visceral surface, where they cause bulging of the capsule.

Heavy infestations by immature flukes may cause death at the stage of acute hepatitis. Such an outcome is not common, but occurs in sheep. It is estimated that 10,000 metacercariae ingested over a short period are necessary to produce acute death in sheep. Death may occur suddenly or after a few days of fever, lassitude, inappetance, and abdominal tenderness. This is also the stage of the parasitism in which *black disease* occurs.

Mature flukes are present in the larger bile ducts and cause cholangitis. The relative importance of different factors in their pathogenicity is not known, but they cause mechanical irritation by the action of their suckers and scales, cause obstruction of the ducts with some degree of biliary retention, predispose to bacterial infections, suck blood, and probably produce toxic and irritative metabolic excretions.

The *biliary changes* occur in all lobes but are usually most severe in the left, and the right may be moderately hypertrophied. From the hilus, *the bile ducts on the visceral surface stand out as white, firm, branching cords* that in extreme instances may be 2 cm in diameter and allow detectable fluctuation over extended segments or in localized areas of ectasia. This dilation of the ducts in sheep, swine, and horses is largely mechanical and is caused by *distension by masses of flukes and bile.* It is permitted by the relative paucity of new connective-tissue formation in the walls of the ducts in these species; this in turn is probably related to the rather mild catarrhal type of inflammation in the lumina of the ducts. In *cattle,* desquamative and ulcerative lesions in the large bile ducts are more severe than in other species, and there is a correspondingly greater proliferation of granulation tissue in and about the walls of the ducts (Fig. 2-86). The walls of the ducts in cattle are, in consequence, much thickened, and the lumen is irregularly stenotic and dilated and lined largely by granulation tissue. This contributes the typical *"pipe stem"* appearance to the ducts in cattle; the connective tissue may be, in addition,

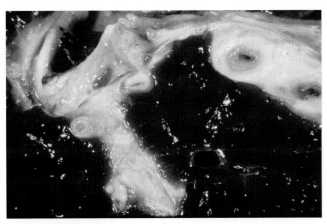

Figure 2-86 Thickened, dilated bile ducts, caused by ***Fasciola hepatica*** infection in an ox. (Courtesy J.L. Caswell.)

mineralized, sometimes so heavily that it cannot be cut with a knife. The bile ducts contain dirty dark brown fluid of a mucinous or tough consistency, formed from degenerate floccular bile, pus, desquamated cells and detritus, clumps of flukes, and small masses of eggs in dark brown granular aggregates (eFig. 2-23).

Although the lesions are most obvious in ducts large enough to contain the flukes, there is, with time and severe or repeated infestations, *progressive inflammation in the smaller portal units* because of direct irritation by the flukes, superimposed infections, and biliary stasis. The course of events is as described earlier for subacute and chronic cholangitis. The proliferating connective tissue and bile ductules in individual portal areas extend to join each other and the scars left over from the migratory phase, so that inflammatory fibrosis may obliterate parenchyma in many foci. In such livers, the left lobe, which is the one most severely affected, may be atrophied, indurated, and irregular.

The development of cholangitis of the degree described depends on long-standing or heavy infestations. Lesions of lesser severity, or those less fully developed, are associated with light infestations of short duration. They may then be recognized only by local dilations of the ducts, or even these may not be readily apparent. In such mild infestations, the fact of past or present parasitism may only be suggested by the detection of characteristic black iron-porphyrin pigments, grossly visible in the hilar nodes. It also contributes to the character of the biliary contents.

Chronic debility with vague digestive disturbances is common in chronic fascioliasis, and deaths are common among sheep. Clinically and at postmortem, there are, in addition to the essential lesions, more or less severe anemia, moderate anasarca, and cachexia. Jaundice is seldom seen.

Fasciola gigantica displaces *F. hepatica* as the common liver fluke in many parts of Africa and in nearby countries, southeast Asia, and the Hawaiian Islands. It is 2 or 3 times as large as *F. hepatica*, but its life cycle and pathogenicity are comparable.

Fascioloides magna is the large liver fluke of North America; cervids are the definitive hosts. It is a parasite of *ruminants* and lives in the hepatic parenchyma, not in the bile ducts, although in tolerant hosts (cervids) the cysts in which it localizes communicate with the bile ducts to provide an exit for ova and excrement. The life cycle of this parasite generally parallels that of *Fasciola hepatica*. The young flukes are very destructive as they wander in the liver. In cattle, they wander briefly, producing large necrotic tunnels before becoming encysted. The cysts, enclosed by connective tissue, do not communicate with bile ducts but form permanent enclosures for the flukes, their excreta, and ova. *The cysts, which may be 2-5 cm in diameter, are remarkable for the large deposits of jet black, sooty iron-porphyrin pigment they contain* (eFig. 2-24), and except for the flukes and soft contents, they superficially resemble heavily pigmented melanotic tumors. Commonly, these flukes pass from the liver to the lungs of cattle, to produce lesions of similar character. In sheep, this parasite wanders continuously in the liver, producing black, tortuous tracts, which may be 2 cm in diameter, and extensive parenchymal destruction. Even a few flukes may kill a sheep. There is a single case report of natural infection in a horse.

The **dicrocoelid flukes** inhabit both biliary and pancreatic ducts. *Eurytrema pancreaticum* prefers the pancreas (and is described with that organ) but in heavy infestations can be found in the bile ducts. *Dicrocoelium* and *Platynosomum* prefer the bile ducts. These are small, narrow flukes, 0.5-1.0 cm long, and may easily be mistaken for small masses of inspissated bile pigment. They are not highly pathogenic, and even in heavy infestations, there may be no signs of the toxemia observed in infestations by *F. hepatica*. These flukes may occur as mixed infestations.

Platynosomum fastosum is a small fluke inhabiting the biliary ducts and gallbladder of *cats* from southern North America, Central and South America, Malaysia, and the Pacific Islands. The life cycle includes *Sublima octona* snails as the first intermediate host, and *Anolis* spp. lizards, marine toads *(Bufo marinis)*, geckos, and various arthropods as second intermediate or paratenic hosts. Cats become infected after ingestion of the second intermediate or paratenic hosts, the cercariae are released into the upper digestive tract, enter the biliary tree, and complete their life cycle. Mature flukes are found in the gallbladder and bile ducts, and after 8-13 weeks, eggs are shed into the feces (Fig. 2-87). Although the majority of infections are subclinical, heavy infestations may cause anorexia, vomiting, lethargy, jaundice, and death. Severely affected livers are enlarged, friable, and may be bile stained, with thickened, distended gallbladders, dilated and/or thickened common bile ducts and cystic ducts, and dilated intrahepatic ducts. Histologically, there are various degrees of chronic cholangitis, fibrosing cholangiohepatitis, and cholecystitis, with dilated and hyperplastic ducts surrounded by lymphocytes, plasma cells, and eosinophils, and in some cases neutrophils, with fluke eggs within or adjacent to ducts. Eggs and adults may be difficult to find. Infection has been reported to co-occur with cholangiocarcinoma in some cats.

Dicrocoelium hospes is found in *cattle* in countries south of the Sahara. Little is known of it, but it is presumed to be comparable in all respects to the better-known *D. dendriticum*, which is common in Europe and Asia and sparsely distributed in the Americas and North Africa. *Dicrocoelium* spp. are found in dry lowland or mountain pastures, whereas *Fasciola* spp. occur in wetter habitats, so the prevalence of *Dicrocoelium* is increasing with desertification. This fluke is no more fastidious in its choice of final hosts than many other species of fluke, and, depending on opportunity, it can infest all domestic species, with the possible exception of cats. It is, however, of most importance as a parasite of sheep and cattle, in which it

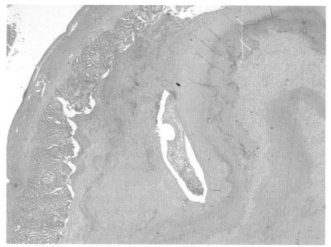

Figure 2-87 Dicrocoelid fluke in the gallbladder of a cat. (Courtesy Purdue University CVM.)

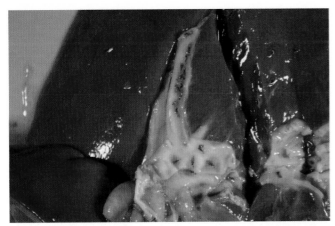

Figure 2-88 *Dicrocoelium dendriticum,* the lancet fluke, in the bile ducts of a sheep.

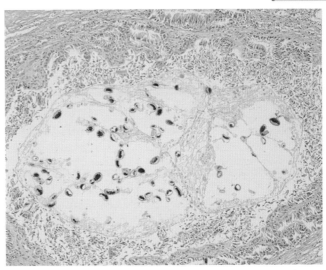

Figure 2-89 *Dicrocoelium dendriticum* with embryonated eggs in the bile duct of a sheep.

inhabits the bile ducts. Other domestic species and rodents are important as reservoirs.

The life cycle of **Dicrocoelium dendriticum,** the lancet fluke or small liver fluke, differs in some details from that of *F. hepatica*. The eggs are embryonated when laid and do not hatch until swallowed by one of the many genera of land snails that are the first intermediate hosts. In the snails, the mother sporocyst produces a second generation of daughter sporocysts, which in turn produce cercariae. The cercariae leave the snail in damp weather and are expelled from the snail's lung, clumped together in slime balls. The slime balls are not infective until the cercariae are swallowed by, and encyst in, the ant *Formica fusca*; other ants may be involved in different countries. The cycle is completed when the definitive hosts swallow the ants. The route of migration of the larvae from the gut to the liver is probably via the bile ducts from the duodenum.

The pathologic changes in the liver produced by *D. dendriticum* are those of cholangiohepatitis that is less severe than that produced by *Fasciola hepatica* (Fig. 2-88, eFig. 2-25). The severity and diffuseness of the hepatic lesion are determined by the number of lancet flukes present, and they may be in the thousands. The flukes and their eggs darken the dilated ducts. Even in early infestations, there may be some scarring of the organ at its periphery. In heavy infestations of long standing, there is extensive biliary fibrosis, producing an organ that is indurated, scarred, and lumpy and that at the margins may bear areas that are shrunken and completely sclerotic. The histologic changes are the same as those in fascioliasis, with perhaps more remarkable hyperplasia of the mucous glands of the large ducts (Fig. 2-89).

Heterobilharzia americana, a trematode in the family *Schistosomatidae*, is the causative agent of *canine schistosomiasis* in North America, primarily reported from the south Atlantic and Gulf Coast states. Raccoons are the most common definitive hosts, although in addition to dogs, several other diverse mammalian species may become naturally infected, including domestic horses. Eggs shed in feces hatch in water and release motile miracidia, which penetrate the tissues of the intermediate host, lymnaeid freshwater snails. Larval stages multiply in the snail, and free-swimming cercariae are released into freshwater. These penetrate the intact epidermis of the definitive host, migrate to the lung, and finally the liver, where they mature, move to the mesenteric and intrahepatic

portal veins to mate, and release eggs that migrate through mesenteric venules, crossing into the bowel lumen by means of proteolytic enzymes. Aberrant migration of eggs results in multifocal eosinophilic and granulomatous inflammation in intestines, pancreas, and liver. Adult trematodes may occasionally be found in hepatic vessels. Clinical signs in affected dogs include diarrhea, vomiting, weight loss, and lethargy, and ~50% of cases in dogs are associated with hypercalcemia, thought to be the result of unregulated calcitriol synthesis by macrophages in the granulomatous lesions. In horses, multiple small fibrosing granulomas scattered throughout the liver, with rare intact or fragmented eggs, are typical and are usually clinically inapparent.

The **opisthorchid flukes** are parasites in the bile ducts of *carnivores*. They may also occur in swine and humans, and one species, *Clonorchis sinensis (Opisthorchis sinensis)*, is an important human parasite. The life cycles, where known, include mollusks as the first intermediate hosts and freshwater fish as the second.

Metorchis conjunctus *is the common liver fluke of cats and dogs in North America and is important as a parasite of sled dogs in the Canadian Northwest Territories.* The first intermediate host is the snail *Amnicola limosa porosa*, and the second is the common sucker-fish *Catostomus commersonii*. The cercariae actively burrow into the musculature of the fish to encyst and become infective. The immature flukes crawl into the bile ducts from the duodenum and mature in ~28 days. Infestations may persist for more than 5 years. *Metorchis albidis* has been described in a dog from Alaska, *Parametorchis complexus* in cats in the United States, and *Amphimerus pseudofelineus* in cats and coyotes in the United States and Panama; the life cycles are not known but are presumed to include fish. *Metorchis bilis* has been reported in red foxes and occasionally in cats from Germany.

Opisthorchis felineus *(O. tenuicollis) is the lanceolate fluke of the bile ducts of cats, dogs, and foxes in Europe and Russia.* It is particularly common in eastern Europe and Siberia and is more sparse in other areas. **Clonorchis sinensis,** the Oriental or Chinese liver fluke is an important human pathogen endemic in Japan, Korea, southern China, and southeast Asia; dogs, cats and swine can act as reservoir hosts. There are additional, less well-known, species of *Opisthorchis* in humans and

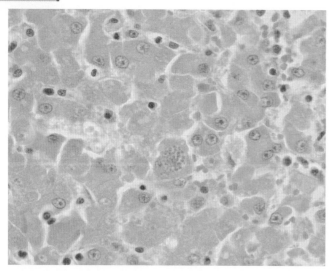

Figure 2-90 *Toxoplasma gondii* cyst in the liver of a cat.

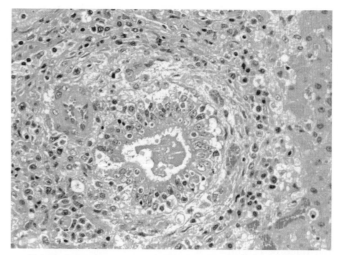

Figure 2-91 Hepatic coccidiosis in the bile duct of a pig.

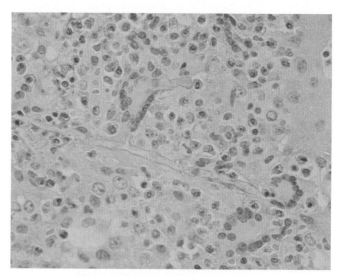

Figure 2-92 Fungal hepatitis in a pig.

animals. The first intermediate hosts for the miracidia of O. *felineus* and *C. sinensis* are snails of the genus *Bithynia*, and several genera of cyprinid fishes can act as second intermediate hosts.

Pseudamphistomum truncatum occurs in carnivores and humans sporadically in Europe and Asia. Its life cycle is as for *Opisthorchis*.

The opisthorchid flukes, so far as known, resemble *Dicrocoelium* in migrating up the bile ducts to their habitat. This may be the reason that they are more numerous in the left than in the right lobes of the liver. They can probably live in the liver for as long as the host lives. The pathologic effects are comparable to those of *D. dendriticum*. Light infestations may be asymptomatic, and heavy infestations may cause jaundice, chronic cholangiohepatitis, and severe biliary fibrosis. Both in humans and animals, adenomatous and carcinomatous changes of the biliary glands have occurred in association with these parasites; the association is probably more than coincidental.

Protozoal infections

Protozoal hepatitis is due mainly to infection with *Toxoplasma* (Fig. 2-90), *Neospora*, and *Leishmania*. Granulomatous hepatitis has been described in dogs associated with systemic infections by *Hepatozoon canis*. Vascular occlusion by enlarged monocytes bearing *Cytauxzoon felis* merozoites can be found in the liver of infected cats. *Sarcocystis neurona* schizonts were reported in the liver of a dog with systemic, multi-organ infection, and schizonts from an unspeciated *Sarcocystis* were observed in hepatocytes in a horse with suppurative and necrotizing hepatitis.

Hepatic coccidiosis causing acute cholangiohepatitis similar to that in mink and rabbits has been observed in isolated cases in the goat, calf, and dog (Fig. 2-91). These infections are usually considered aberrant, and often coincide with intestinal coccidiosis. Coccidial meronts and, in some cases, gamonts are present within the cytoplasm of biliary epithelium. The organisms are presently unclassified.

Fungal infections

Fungal infections of the forestomachs with hematogenous dissemination to the liver occur occasionally in cattle and sheep, usually as a complication of rumenitis. Lesions in the liver are typically hemorrhagic infarcts initially or granulomatous with chronicity, and are associated with infection by *Aspergillus fumigatus* and various members of the class Zygomycetes (Fig. 2-92).

Granulomatous hepatitis associated with disseminated fungal or algal infections has also been reported in dogs and cats. The species involved include *Histoplasma capsulatum* (eFig. 2-26), *Cryptococcus* spp., *Coccidioides immitis*, *Sporothrix schenckii*, *Aspergillus* spp., and *Prototheca* spp.

Further reading

Andrade RLFS, et al. *Platynosomum fastosum*-induced cholangiocarcinomas in cats. Vet Parasitol 2012;190:277-280.

Corapi WV, et al. Multi-organ involvement of *Heterobilharzia americana* infection in a dog presented for systemic mineralization. J Vet Diagn Invest 2011;23:826-831.

Corapi WV, et al. Natural *Heterobilharzia americana* infection in horses in Texas. Vet Pathol 2012;49:552-556.

Dubey JP, et al. *Sarcocystis neurona* schizonts-associated encephalitis, chorioretinitis, and myositis in a two-month-old dog simulating toxoplasmosis, and presence of mature sarcocysts in muscles. Vet Parasitol 2014;202:194-200.

Hoon-Hanks LL, et al. Hepatic neosporosis in a dog treated for pemphigus folicaceus. J Vet Diagn Invest 2013;25:807-810.

Peregrine AS, et al. Alveolar hydatid disease *(Echinococcus multilocularis)* in the liver of a Canadian dog in British Columbia, a newly endemic region. Can Vet J 2012;53:870-874.

TOXIC HEPATIC DISEASE

Hepatic susceptibility

The liver is particularly vulnerable to toxic injury because it is exposed to virtually everything that is absorbed. The portal vein that drains the stomach and intestines flows directly to the liver. This facilitates high hepatic concentrations of ingested foreign chemicals or drugs termed **xenobiotics,** as well as many naturally occurring substances with toxic potential. Most xenobiotics are unable to directly enter the hepatocyte and require specific transporters to pass through the lipid bilayer of the hepatocyte membrane. The uptake of exogenous and endogenous compounds from the sinusoidal blood is facilitated by a number of basolaterally located transporters. These transporters are members of a large group of sodium-independent solute transporters known as *organic anion transporting polypeptides* (OATP). Xenobiotics may be concentrated in hepatocytes to various degrees by mechanisms that remain obscure, but which are associated with special binding proteins of hepatocytes, attachment to enzymatic sites where metabolic conversions occur, and inhibition of export into the bile. The liver is exposed to high concentrations of toxic metabolites because of its role as the primary site of biotransformation for many therapeutic agents and endogenous substances. Some metabolites may produce hepatocellular injury, and others may cause biliary injury once they are transported into the canaliculi. Certain drug metabolites may be reabsorbed in the enterohepatic circulation in a fashion similar to bile acids, facilitating repeated exposure to the drug in question. In addition, many drug administration regimens may achieve relatively high millimolar concentrations, resulting in depletion of conjugating cofactors such as glutathione, which can reach the lower limits required for other cytoprotective roles.

Role of hepatic biotransformation in hepatotoxicity

An understanding of hepatic biotransformation is essential for an appreciation of the hepatotoxic potential of foreign compounds. *Hepatocytes are the major site of metabolism of endogenous substances and xenobiotics, including plant- or fungal-derived secondary metabolites consumed in food, environmental chemicals and drugs.* Given the numerous enzymes and the magnitude of their expression, the liver easily exceeds the metabolic capacity of all other organs. A major metabolic function of the liver is to transform lipophilic substances, including endogenous steroid hormones and most xenobiotics, into more water-soluble polar molecules to be excreted in bile or urine. Relevant hepatic enzymes involved in biotransformation and their associated activities can be grouped into 3 *major categories.*

- Phase 1 reactions promote oxidation, reduction, hydrolysis, cyclization, and decyclization of the parent compounds. This is typically accomplished through addition of oxygen or removal of hydrogen, carried out by mixed-function oxidases that are usually CYP enzymes (also known as cytochrome P450 monooxygenases), using NADPH and O_2. Most of these phase 1 enzymes are found in the *smooth endoplasmic reticulum* of the hepatocyte.

- Phase 2 reactions are typically *conjugation reactions* in which a polar molecule, such as glucuronic acid, sulfate, or glutathione, is added to carboxyl, hydroxyl, amino, or sulfhydryl groups on phase 1 metabolites, making them typically less toxic and more water soluble. Most of these enzymes are found in the *cytosol.*

- In phase 3 reactions, conjugated molecules are transported by various *transporter molecules* across the modified hepatocyte membrane that lines the canaliculus.

Phase 1 reactions may either increase (bioactivate) or eliminate the biological activity of the xenobiotic substrate. However, bioactivation of molecules poses a potential risk. Although this step is necessary to prepare the substrate to form a covalent bond with polar compound in phase 2, it creates, if only transiently, reactive intermediates, such as free radicals and epoxides. These reactive intermediates can bind to cellular macromolecules, such as the CYP enzymes, that produced them, other cellular enzymes or structural proteins, or RNA and DNA, leading to hepatocyte injury, death, or neoplastic transformation. The CYPs can be found in all parts of the hepatic lobule, but the hepatocytes of centrilobular region have a higher content than those of the periportal region, which apparently accounts for the *centrilobular predominance of injury produced by compounds metabolized by this system,* including carbon tetrachloride and acetaminophen. In contrast, *hepatocytes in the periportal zone are more susceptible to direct-acting toxicants, such as metal salts,* because of their proximity to incoming portal and arterial vascular flow.

So-called "drug-drug" interactions can arise when 2 drugs are metabolized by the same CYP, so that metabolism of one or both of the compounds is altered by competition or interference with the relevant CYP enzyme function.

Phase 2 reactions inactivate the phase 1 metabolite through conjugation with a polar molecule and facilitate its export by transforming the lipophilic molecule into a water-soluble molecule that can be transported out of the hepatocyte and into the bile or the circulation for removal via the kidney. Reduced glutathione is a major substrate for phase 2 reactions mediated by glutathione S-transferases. Active metabolites of many compounds, including acetaminophen are detoxified by conjugation with glutathione. Depletion of glutathione can greatly enhance the toxicity of many compounds. Hepatic glutathione is also important in the removal of various free radicals and reactive oxygen species generated by normal metabolic processes as well as detoxification pathways through the action of glutathione peroxidase. Different species and different breeds of animals possess a divergent array of phase 1 and phase 2 types with differing levels of activity and target substrates that contribute to the differences in metabolism and toxicity of xenobiotics observed in different species. Acetaminophen toxicity in the cat is a relevant example. Felids have limited phase 2 metabolism caused, in part, from diminished activity of uridine diphosphate (UDP)-glucuronosyl transferase, an enzyme involved in glucuronidation of bioactivated molecules. Limited glucuronidation of acetaminophen metabolites leads to saturation of other detoxification pathways and depletion of glutathione. The lack of glutathione then enables a highly toxic metabolite of acetaminophen, N-acetyl-para-benzoquinoneimine (NAPQI) to bind to cellular proteins and membranes, causing cell injury and death. NAPQI is also responsible for the prominent methemoglobinemia seen in intoxicated cats. *Toxic hepatic injury depends on the balance between the production of reactive metabolites and their detoxification by conjugation and other protective mechanisms.*

The enzyme complex involved in bioactivation is not limited to metabolism of foreign substances, but is also involved in the metabolism or synthesis of a number of lipophilic endogenous substances. The principal endogenous substrates include arachidonic acid, eicosanoids, cholesterol, bile acids, steroids, and vitamin D.

Phase 3 reactions involve movement of conjugated substrates across the membrane of the canaliculus. As with the processes involved in uptake of substances from the plasma, several transporters embedded in the canalicular membrane are responsible for the movement of the water-soluble conjugated substrates from the cytoplasm into the lumen of the canaliculus. These transporters have a range of occasionally overlapping substrates, including bile acids and conjugates of glutathione, glucuronate, and sulfonate. These water-soluble metabolites are excreted in the bile via members of the ATP-binding cassette (ABC) superfamily of transport proteins located on the apical canalicular membrane. These include the most significant transporter in humans, the multidrug-resistance protein-1 (MDR1). Multidrug-resistance–associated protein-2 (MRP2) is responsible for export of glutathione conjugates, such as bilirubin conjugates, and shows a striking species difference in expression, with very low expression in the dog and very high expression in the rat. This influences biliary excretion of drug conjugates from the liver and may influence toxicity in the liver or elsewhere.

The mechanism by which xenobiotics and some endogenous substances can cause CYP enzyme induction in the liver, as well as induction of phase 2 reactions, and hepatocellular hypertrophy is mediated by the activation of nuclear receptors that function as transcription factors. These transcription factors include aryl hydrocarbon hydroxylase receptor (AHR), constitutive androstane receptor (CAR), pregnane X receptor (PXR), and peroxisome proliferator–activated receptor-α (PPAR-α). These nuclear receptors are also important mediators of hepatocellular metabolism, including hepatic lipid metabolism, bile acid homeostasis, as well as liver regeneration, inflammation, fibrosis, cell differentiation, and tumor formation. Each of these receptors may be directly activated by the binding of the xenobiotic (or its metabolite) to the receptor, although some activators of CAR do not bind to the receptor but rather phosphorylate the receptor, which results in nuclear translocation. The nuclear receptor genes vary among species, and there are many species differences and gene polymorphisms that affect the receptors or the genes that they stimulate.

In summary, a broad variety of factors can influence the mechanisms and extent of **drug-induced liver injury** (DILI), the term for hepatic injury from xenobiotics. There is a variety of alternative pathways for metabolism, supported by a variety of isoforms of different gene families, particularly the CYP enzymes and the many genetic polymorphisms within individual alleles that code for the different isoforms. Other factors such as age, nutritional status, sex, diet, prior or concurrent exposure to environmental compounds, or intercurrent disease all influence the response to toxic injury. Some of these variables contribute to the variations seen in responses among species and individuals to liver injury.

Role of inflammation in hepatotoxicity

The extent of liver injury following exposure to xenobiotics is not, however, determined by the chemistry of drug metabolism alone. Following exposure to injurious compounds, the inflammatory response, particularly the innate immune response, can significantly influence the extent of hepatocellular injury. Studies using acetaminophen have provided most relevant information on this issue; however, the effects of inflammation are complex, and not all studies are in agreement. There are conflicting studies demonstrating either pro-inflammatory or anti-inflammatory effects of Kupffer cells following drug-induced injury. Some clarification of this controversy has been facilitated by the identification of subsets of intrahepatic macrophages following injury. In addition to the resident Kupffer cells, a population of infiltrating macrophages can be detected quite soon (within 12 hours) after acetaminophen intoxication. There are 2 major phenotypes of intrahepatic macrophages. **M1 macrophages** are proinflammatory, a source for tumor necrosis factor-α, interleukin-1β (IL-1β) and nitric oxide, which stimulates hepatocellular injury, and these macrophages constitute the majority of the Kupffer cell population. **M2 macrophages** are anti-inflammatory, secreting IL-10-, IL-6- and IL-18–binding proteins, which modulate inflammation, and comprise the majority of the infiltrating macrophages. Stimulation of other members of the innate immune system, such as natural killer and natural killer T cells can accentuate acetaminophen toxicity. Neutrophils recruited to the liver by the release of damage-associated molecular pattern (DAMP) molecules from necrotic hepatocytes also augment tissue injury. Thus it is clear that *altered inflammation can influence drug-induced hepatic injury*, but the subtleties remain to be unraveled.

Mechanisms of injury

There are many mechanisms underlying hepatotoxicity. These include (1) covalent binding of cellular proteins by bioactivated metabolites, which leads to intracellular dysfunction manifested by loss of normal intracellular ionic gradients altering intracellular calcium homeostasis, by actin filament disruption, and by cell membrane damage, such as cell blebbing or swelling and total disruption. A consequence of actin filament disruption can be cholestasis because of the loss of pulsatile contractions that drive canalicular bile flow; (2) drug-induced disruption of canalicular transport pump function, leading to cholestasis and jaundice; (3) inhibition of cellular enzyme pathways of drug metabolism because of covalent binding of CYPs by bioactivated metabolites; (4) covalent binding of the drug to cell proteins, which creates new adducts that serve as immune targets for cytotoxic T-cell attack or antibody formation when transported to the cell surface in vesicles, inciting an immunologic reaction; (5) programmed cell death (apoptosis), occurring through tumor necrosis factor and Fas pathways; and (6) inhibition of mitochondrial function, limiting β-oxidation of fat and ATP generation, leading to accumulation of reactive oxygen species and lipid peroxidation, microvesicular fat accumulation, lactic acidosis, and inability to generate ATP. These are discussed in detail in other texts. The liver is composed of several cell types, not only hepatocytes, and similar types of injury can also affect the biliary epithelium and sinusoidal endothelium, and to a lesser extent, hepatic stellate cells, Kupffer cells, and other immune cells.

Classification of hepatotoxins

Hepatotoxins can be classified as intrinsic or idiosyncratic, and these categories apply as well to the types of drug-induced hepatotoxicity that are observed in humans and animals. The effects of **intrinsic hepatotoxins** *are considered to be dose related, predictable, and reproducible in experimental animals, and the underlying mechanisms are typically at least partially understood.* Intrinsic hepatotoxins can cause liver injury in overdose situations in most normal recipients but are also capable of inducing similar liver damage at lower doses in individuals with genetic or acquired abnormalities in drug metabolism. The majority of intrinsic hepatotoxicants are converted to *reactive metabolites,* including lipoperoxidative free radicals.

The analgesic **acetaminophen** represents a well-characterized example of an intrinsic hepatotoxin, with species differences in metabolism and associated susceptibility to oxidative and hepatic injury. Dogs and cats can tolerate doses within therapeutic levels; however, higher doses may saturate the glucuronidation and sulfation detoxification pathways, resulting in increased formation of the reactive benzoquinone-imine metabolite NAPQI via a third cytochrome P450–mediated pathway. These can be scavenged by glutathione conjugation; however, massive doses can cause lethal acute hepatic failure, associated with overproduction of reactive metabolites, and depletion of hepatic and erythrocyte glutathione. As discussed previously, clinical toxicity occurs at lower doses and is more severe in cats because they express fewer hepatic isoforms of glucuronyltransferase as part of phase 2 hepatic metabolism and are unable to accelerate excretion of excess metabolites through glucuronide conjugation. This is compounded by a propensity for hemoglobin oxidation, resulting in methemoglobinemia. Toxicity results when reduced glutathione levels drop below a threshold level, resulting in marked oxidative stress, and allowing reactive metabolites to bind covalently to cellular macromolecules.

By comparison, **idiosyncratic hepatotoxins** *are typically less dose related (although there is likely a minimum threshold), more unpredictable, and importantly, occur in only a very small proportion of exposed individuals (i.e., <1 in 10,000-100,000).* The mechanisms of idiosyncratic hepatotoxicity are generally not known, but reflect an unusual susceptibility of individual recipients to effects that are unrelated to the drug's therapeutic action or overdose toxicity. Idiosyncratic hepatotoxicity is more likely a series of rare drug-related toxicities with different forms of pathogenesis than a single entity. There are 2 main categories of idiosyncratic hepatotoxicity recognized in humans: *hypersensitivity-related drug-induced liver injury (drug allergy) and toxic metabolite-dependent drug-induced liver injury.*

Hypersensitivity-related idiosyncrasies are characterized by a latency period before toxicity is evident and reoccur promptly upon re-exposure. Typically, they involve immune-mediated hypersensitivity responses to the drug metabolites that covalently bind to liver proteins, forming neoantigens that may be recognized as foreign by the immune system, with further liver injury resulting from the ensuing specific immune response or upregulation of components of the innate immune system. In humans, a genetic component to hypersensitivity-related idiosyncratic hepatic toxicity is strongly suspected. Single nucleotide polymorphisms in the human leukocyte antigen (HLA) region or particular HLA haplotypes have been associated with idiosyncratic drug toxicity in humans for several drugs, reflecting the development of pharmacogenomics.

Toxic metabolite-dependent idiosyncrasies involve excessive generation of a regular toxic metabolite, or altered metabolism to unusual hepatotoxic metabolites. There is accumulating evidence of considerable genetic diversity (polymorphisms) in hepatic drug metabolism among individual humans and domestic animals, and these may explain many unusual responses to drugs. This variation could be qualitative, with the production of a toxic metabolite not normally produced, or quantitative, with overproduction of a normally minor hepatotoxic metabolite.

Morphology of toxic injury to the liver

The morphologic forms of hepatic injury produced by hepatotoxins are varied. *Acute toxic injury to the liver can be cytotoxic (hepatocellular), cholestatic, or mixed.* **Cytotoxic hepatocellular injury** results in hepatic degeneration, zonal necrosis, focal and nonzonal necrosis (apoptosis), or lipidosis, accompanied by the clinicopathologic features of acute hepatic injury. In general, necrosis produced by intrinsic hepatotoxins is zonal. *Acute cytotoxic injury is often manifested as steatosis (lipidosis),* a result of impairment of movement of triglycerides through the liver, interference with very-low-density lipoprotein synthesis or transport, or impaired hepatic consumption of fatty acids by mitochondrial oxidation. **Cholestatic injury** is a reflection of failure of bile excretion associated with biliary epithelial or canalicular injury or other alteration of bile secretion, and displays the features of obstructive jaundice. The typical histologic manifestation consists of bile casts in canalicular spaces, with variable parenchymal injury. An exception to this pattern can be seen in some plant intoxications, such as those produced by steroidal sapogenins and *Lantana* spp., which can cause cholestasis with minimal evidence of canalicular plugging. **Mixed toxic insults** display the morphologic and clinical features of both hepatocellular and obstructive injury. Chronic toxic injury to the liver may be manifested as chronic hepatitis, with fibrosis progressing to cirrhosis; vascular injury, such as veno-occlusive disease; and neoplasia.

The histologic changes in **acute toxic hepatic injury** are rather stereotyped. They range from apoptosis, through confluent coagulative and zonal necrosis, to massive hemorrhagic destruction that includes sinusoidal lining cells (Fig. 2-93). The histology of these acute intoxications is often characterized by *centrilobular necrosis,* usually coagulative (Fig. 2-94). Rarely, the pattern of necrosis may be periportal or midzonal. Depending on the nutritional status of the animal, there may be variably severe fatty or hydropic change in hepatocytes adjacent to the necrotic zones. The necrotic cells may accumulate calcium. Variations on the general process of hepatocellular necrosis have little diagnostic or pathogenetic specificity. In sublethally injured cells, there may be prominent but nonspecific clumping of smooth endoplasmic reticulum, particularly in the centrilobular zones.

The *clinical and gross characteristics of fatal acute intoxications* that destroy liver parenchyma are rather consistent, regardless of the origin of the toxin. The animal dies after a brief period of dullness, anorexia, colic, and various neurologic disturbances, including convulsions; these are attributed to hepatic encephalopathy. Postmortem examination reveals a slight excess of clear, yellow abdominal fluid, which contains

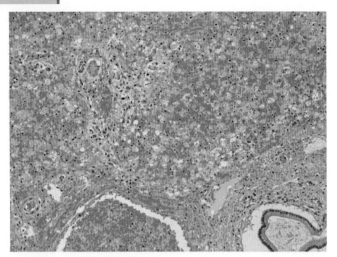

Figure 2-93 Massive necrosis following ingestion of *Amanita phalloides* by a cat.

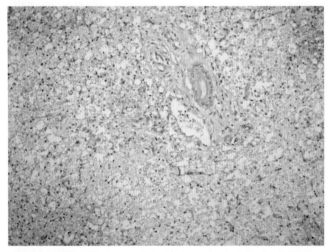

Figure 2-94 Acute centrilobular hepatic necrosis following ingestion of *Cycad* sp. in a dog. (Courtesy J. Cooley.)

sufficient fibrinogen to form a loose, nonadherent clot. The appearance of the liver depends on the severity and stage of the injury. Severe acute toxicity that destroys endothelium typically results in a hemorrhagic zonal pattern, in which case the liver may be deep red-purple and obviously swollen and turgid. In less severe injury without hemorrhage, the liver tends to be lighter brown because of a combination of edema (exclusion of sinusoidal blood), destruction of cytochrome pigments, and accumulation of bile pigments and/or fat. If the animal survives for several days, the liver develops a typical zonal yellow fatty change as triglyceride accumulates in sublethally injured hepatocytes.

In acute fatal hepatotoxicities, there may be widespread hemorrhage resulting from lack of coagulation factors. Petechiae and ecchymoses are seen most consistently on serous membranes, especially on the epicardium and endocardium and abdominal viscera. Diffuse hemorrhage into the gut, particularly the duodenum in ruminants, is also common, as are hemorrhages into the wall of the gallbladder. Hemorrhages are largely the result of excessive consumption of clotting factors and platelets within the areas of necrosis in the liver, although the concurrent failure of the damaged liver to replace those coagulation

factors undoubtedly becomes important when these factors are consumed. Gross lesions, such as icterus, and photosensitization, which reflect failure of biotransformation or excretion of endogenous materials, develop too slowly to be a feature of acutely fatal hepatotoxicities. However, the rate of accumulation of bilirubin increases when hemorrhage occurs in the necrotic liver or as a consequence of coagulopathy.

Chronic hepatotoxic injury *may manifest in many patterns,* as previously described. These include areas of necrosis with primarily mononuclear inflammatory infiltrates, steatosis, cirrhosis, atrophy with nodules, hepatic vein thrombosis, venoocclusive disease, peliosis hepatis, cholangitis, ductular reaction (biliary hyperplasia), and carcinogenesis. In contrast to the acute intoxications, chronic hepatotoxicities are more likely to display a mix of these responses, and this can provide more diagnostic specificity. For example, agents that impair hepatocellular regeneration might not be potent necrogens but tend to produce hepatic apoptosis and atrophy, fibrosis of various patterns, compensatory bile duct hyperplasia, nodular regeneration, some degree of cholestasis, and frequently megalocytosis (polyploidy). Such hepatotoxins are potential carcinogens because they favor the selective growth of hepatocellular nodules that are resistant to mitoinhibitory effects.

Clinical signs of chronic hepatotoxicity are usually problems resulting from inadequate detoxification and excretion; these include jaundice, photosensitization, and hepatic encephalopathy. Most of the toxins responsible for chronic hepatotoxicity may produce acute nonspecific zonal or massive necrosis if experimentally administered at dose rates higher than those to which animals are likely to be exposed in the field, although such acute toxicity is only occasionally observed in field cases of the diseases.

Toxic agents

The range of substances that can cause hepatotoxicity is so broad that it encompasses virtually all categories of natural and synthetic chemicals. These include metals (iron, copper), drugs (e.g., acetaminophen), plant components (phytotoxins), fungal metabolites (mycotoxins), bacterial products (e.g., cyanobacterial microcystin-LR), and various industrial products (especially aromatic solvents). Many drugs are also hepatotoxic. Differences in individual susceptibility to hepatotoxic responses likely occur for all classes of chemicals that are metabolized in the liver.

In the following sections, toxic hepatic disease will be separated into drug- or pharmaceutical-induced hepatotoxicity (so-called adverse drug reactions), and hepatotoxicity associated with exposure to plant or environmental toxins, including metals. The latter have been somewhat arbitrarily divided into acute and chronic, and although it is recognized that the difference between acute and chronic hepatotoxicity is often simply a matter of dose rate, it is convenient to categorize the sources according to the syndrome of liver damage that they most commonly produce. Various plants and moldy feeds are hepatotoxic, and some phytotoxins (e.g., pyrrolizidine alkaloids) and mycotoxins (e.g., aflatoxins) are notorious hepatotoxins and hepatocarcinogens. Many phytotoxins and mycotoxins target other organ systems or have physiologic rather than pathologic effects. Some of those that cause diagnostic lesions are discussed under the respective target tissues elsewhere. Generally, these areas of toxicology are better accessed in comprehensive references on phytotoxins or mycotoxins.

Adverse drug reactions: drug-induced liver injury (DILI)

The definition of an adverse drug reaction is any injurious or unintended response to a drug that occurs at a normal dose for normal use. DILI is the most common form of adverse drug reaction in humans, and although hepatotoxic drug reactions are recognized in dogs and cats, the true prevalence of DILI in domestic animals is unknown. DILI should not be considered as a single disease, given the diverse array of drugs that can trigger injury.

Acute hepatic disease has been attributed to adverse reactions to a wide variety of therapeutic drugs, particularly in companion animals. Submassive to massive hepatic necrosis and cholestatic hepatitis have been reported in dogs as an idiosyncratic reaction to **trimethoprim-sulfonamide** combination therapy and the related sulfonamide-based anticonvulsant drug **zonisamide**, although zonisamide is in a different chemical category, is less likely to form toxic adducts, and is not likely to share a similar pathogenesis of liver injury. Severe lobular to massive hepatic necrosis may occur in cats associated with repeated oral administration of **diazepam** at recommended doses. Severe centrilobular hepatic necrosis has been associated with use of the anthelmintic **mebendazole** in dogs. Hepatotoxicity has been reported in 4 dogs treated with **amiodarone**, a class III antiarrhythmic agent. This is one of the more commonly reported adverse effects of amiodarone in humans and is related to the drug's effect on lipid metabolism. Administration of the anabolic steroid **stanozolol** has also been associated with elevated alanine aminotransferase, coagulopathy, and development of hepatic lipidosis with cholestasis in cats. Adult beef cattle testing positive for stanozolol in urine also had hepatic changes, including cholestasis, periportal fibrosis and inflammation, and focal necrosis, although the changes could not conclusively be attributed to anabolic steroid administration. Other pharmacologic agents associated with acute hepatic injury include **thiacetarsemide, methoxyflurane, halothane, oil of pennyroyal,** intravenous injection of **manganese chloride** and inadvertent subcutaneous injection of intranasal *Bordetella bronchiseptica*/canine parainfluenza vaccine in dogs, **methimazole, glipizide,** and the photodynamic therapy agent **aluminum phthalocyanine tetrasulfonate** in cats.

Xylitol is an artificial sweetener used commonly in baked goods or chewing gum intended for use by diabetics or dieters. Although high doses can be tolerated by most species, there is a particular sensitivity in dogs. Dogs that ingest >0.5 g/kg can be at risk to develop acute severe hepatic necrosis. Dogs exposed to fatal doses have centrilobular to massive lytic necrosis of hepatocytes and widespread hemorrhage. Affected dogs also develop hypoglycemia and hyperinsulinemia. There may be an element of idiosyncratic toxicity involved as dogs have tolerated higher doses in experimental settings, so there may be breed-related or other factors influencing acute toxicity. The mechanism of toxicity is not currently known, but intracellular ATP depletion and generation of reactive oxygen species have been suggested as possible mechanisms for hepatocyte injury.

Carprofen is a nonsteroidal anti-inflammatory drug used in the treatment of degenerative joint disease and management of acute pain in dogs primarily. Diffuse and massive hepatocellular injury, characterized by hepatocellular vacuolar change, lytic necrosis, apoptosis, and bridging necrosis, with mild secondary inflammation and cholestasis, has been reported in dogs administered therapeutic dosages of carprofen. The injurious response is likely to be idiosyncratic as a chronic experimental study did not produce injury. A related nonsteroidal anti-inflammatory drug, diclofenac, causes idiosyncratic liver injury in humans.

The anticonvulsant drugs **primidone, phenytoin,** and **phenobarbital** have been associated with the development of *chronic hepatic disease and cirrhosis in dogs*. These drugs, used either alone or in combination, can cause biochemical and clinical signs of hepatic dysfunction in up to 14% of dogs treated for >6 months, but only a small percentage of cases progress to cirrhosis and hepatic failure. Currently, monitoring blood levels and adjusting dosages of these drugs to a nontoxic level has significantly reduced the incidence of liver injury. The most consistent histologic finding in the majority of dogs treated with phenobarbital is *proliferation of the hepatocellular smooth endoplasmic reticulum resulting from induction of microsomal enzymes*, including various subfamilies of cytochrome P450. This results in hepatocellular swelling with fine diffuse granularity, a so-called "ground-glass" appearance to hepatocyte cytoplasm. This histologic change is an adaptive response, reflected clinically by increases in serum concentrations of alkaline phosphatase, alanine aminotransferase, and γ-glutamyl transpeptidase, but is not indicative of hepatocellular injury. Actual hepatotoxicity may represent an idiosyncratic reaction in a small percentage of treated dogs, although the possibility of dose-dependent intrinsic hepatotoxicity with long-term treatment has not been ruled out. It is also possible that the enzyme induction associated with anticonvulsant therapy may alter the ability of the liver to detoxify other nonspecified compounds that could be the effectors of liver damage. Certainly, enzyme induction may alter the pharmacokinetics of other co-administered drugs. *Chronic hepatitis associated with anticonvulsant therapy is characterized by bridging portal fibrosis, biliary hyperplasia, nodular regeneration, and mild inflammatory cell infiltrates*. A separate syndrome of *cholestatic hepatotoxic injury with jaundice* has also been described in dogs receiving high doses of phenytoin in combination with primidone or phenobarbital. This is characterized by intrahepatic cholestasis, with hepatocellular swelling, vacuolation, and small multifocal areas of hepatocellular necrosis, and has been suggested to represent a metabolic disturbance rather than direct cytotoxic hepatocellular injury. **Hepatocutaneous syndrome** (*superficial necrolytic dermatitis*) associated with typical hepatic pathology of parenchymal collapse, vacuolation, and nodular regeneration has also been reported as a separate syndrome in dogs with a history of chronic phenobarbital therapy.

Acute and chronic hepatic disease, characterized by periportal hepatitis, periportal fibrosis, and biliary hyperplasia, have been reported in dogs treated with **oxibendazole-diethylcarbamazine** combination therapy for prevention of hookworm and heartworm. Chronic hepatic disease has also been reported following administration of **mibolerone, methotrexate** and **CCNU** (1-(2-chloroethyl)-3-cyclohexyl-1-nitrosourea) in dogs, **ketoconazole** in dogs and cats, and **megestrol acetate** and **griseofulvin** in cats.

Hepatotoxic plants

Hepatotoxic plants occur in botanical families as diverse as the relatively primitive *Cycadaceae* through the *Compositae* and *Solanaceae*. The evolutionary relationships between herbivores and toxic plants are complex; in some situations, consumption of plants by herbivores has competitive or neutral advantage for the plant, especially those that are lush and prolific, so toxicity is counterproductive or unnecessary. However, in arid or semiarid habitats, plants must put up more resistance to herbivores that could obliterate them. Indigenous herbivores are typically reluctant to do this, and are either resistant or reluctant to graze some plants. Plants sometimes protect critical parts at particular stages of growth. For example, *Xanthium pungens* (Noogoora burr) concentrates its toxin in the cotyledons. The seeds are rarely eaten, even by cattle, but intoxications can occur when this plant is eaten shortly after germination. Phytotoxic liver disease is therefore more frequently encountered in animals grazing pastures at particular times of the year, with limited choice or supply, or when hungry animals are introduced to plants for which their natural or induced resistance is low. The patterns of liver disease resulting from consumption of toxic plants are for the most part quite consistent in comparison with what is seen with exposure to other classes of hepatotoxins. An exhaustive review of the toxicity of all such plants would be repetitive. However, some plants that do produce more distinctive patterns of liver lesions will be discussed in more detail.

Further reading

Adams DH, et al. Mechanisms of immune-mediated liver injury. Toxicol Sci 2010;115:307-321.

Dunayer EK, Gwaltney-Brant SM. Acute hepatic failure and coagulopathy associated with xylitol ingestion in eight dogs. J Am Vet Med Assoc 2006;229:1113-1117.

Holt MP, et al. Identification and characterization of infiltrating macrophages in acetaminophen-induced liver injury. J Leukoc Biol 2008;84:1410-1421.

Kaplowitz N, DeLeve LD. Drug-Induced Liver Disease. 3rd ed. New York: Academic Press; 2013.

Kumar V. NKT-cell subsets: Promoters and protectors in inflammatory liver disease. J Hepatol 2013;59:618-620.

Miller ML, et al. Apparent acute idiosyncratic hepatic necrosis associated with zonisamide administration in a dog. J Vet Intern Med 2011;25:1156-1160.

Raekallio MR, et al. Evaluation of adverse effects of long-term orally administered carprofen in dogs. J Am Vet Med Assoc 2006;228:876-880.

Acute hepatotoxicity: plant-derived and environmental toxins

Cyanobacteria (blue-green algae)

These primitive highly toxic microorganisms can flourish as a seasonal bloom on lakes and ponds that have accumulated phosphates and nitrates as runoff from fertilized soils. Outbreaks of poisoning are not common, but they occur in many countries and may be responsible for heavy mortality among mammals or birds that drink from affected bodies of water. Most well-documented cases have involved *Microcystis aeruginosa,* which may poison stock after the bloom has been piled by wind against the shores of expanses of water. Other toxic species are included in the genera *Anabaena* and *Aphanizomenon.* Some deaths are too sudden to be caused by liver damage and are probably the result of the *"fast-death factor"* that has been found in some blooms. The syndrome is one of collapse and prostration, with hyperesthesia that may be

manifested as convulsions and death within a few minutes; there are no specific lesions in this form of the toxicosis.

The most well-understood cyanobacterial hepatotoxin is *microcystin-LR, a highly potent cyclic heptapeptide protein phosphatase inhibitor.* Other species of cyanobacteria, such as *Nodularia spumigenia* found in New Zealand and the Baltic region, contain different, but still potent toxins such as *nodularin.* Ruminants are most commonly poisoned, but poisoning has been reported in horses, sheep, dogs, and domestic poultry. The cyanobacterial toxin is released when the microorganisms disintegrate, which may occur spontaneously in bodies of water or after the application of copper sulfate for algae control, or in the rumen or stomach after ingestion. Microcystin-LR is very stable and persists in water at typical ambient conditions, with a 10-week half-life. It is stable following boiling as well. The toxin is taken into hepatocytes by organic anion-transporting polypeptide (OATP) membrane transporters and causes cell damage by inhibiting cytoplasmic protein phosphatase 1 and 2A. This leads to disorganization of hepatocyte and endothelial cytoskeletal actin filaments, and disruption of their shape and integrity, leading to necrosis, apoptosis, and perisinusoidal hemorrhage. The distribution of the necrosis is usually centrilobular to massive. The pattern may vary within the individual liver and from case to case. In subacute intoxications, the liver is severely fatty, and necrosis is limited to individual hepatocytes or small groups, rather than being zonal. Phagolysosomes and bile pigments accumulate in the cytoplasm, and there is slight biliary proliferation and fibrosis. Necrosis of the renal tubules can also occur. Diagnosis can be made by detection of microcystin in vomitus or liver.

Toxic fungi

Amanitins are potent hepatotoxins found in several mushroom genera, including *Amanita, Galerina,* and *Lepiota.* The genus **Amanita** contains several species, including *A. phalloides, A. verna, A. virosa,* and *A. ocreata,* which are considered extremely toxic. These mushrooms are mycorrhizal with various species of deciduous and coniferous trees, and may be found in urban, suburban, and rural areas. The amanitins are *bicyclic octapeptides,* ingestion of which is responsible for gastroenteritis, hypoglycemia, and fulminant liver failure in humans, dogs, cats, cattle, and other animals. They are stable compounds and persist in the acid environment of the stomach and following cooking. Amanitin is transported from the systemic circulation to hepatocytes by a specific OATP transporter on the hepatocyte surface. Toxicity is accentuated by enterohepatic circulation of the toxin, causing repeated hepatic exposure. Amanitin inhibits nuclear RNA polymerase II, thus interfering with transcription and inhibiting protein synthesis, resulting in cell death. Dogs or cats dying after ingestion of *Amanita* spp. have massive hepatocellular necrosis with focal areas of hemorrhage (see Fig. 2-93). Surviving periportal hepatocytes have vesicular nuclei with loss or fragmentation of nucleoli, consistent with ultrastructural reports of chromatin condensation, dissolution of the nucleolus, and decline in nucleolar RNA content. Necrosis of the proximal convoluted tubules often accompanies the hepatic injury and can aid in the index of suspicion for amanitin intoxication. Because the histologic lesions are nonspecific, and previously, it was difficult to obtain a definitive diagnosis of amanitin intoxication, under-diagnosis was likely. Confirmatory testing is available, and the liver, bile, and kidney are the preferred organs for testing.

Cycadales

Members of this order have been responsible for chronic hepatotoxicity and neurotoxicity in cattle. Acute hepatotoxicity has been reported in cattle and sheep that have eaten the seeds or young leaves of species of *Cycas* or *Zamiaceae*. Dogs are intoxicated by eating the seeds of *Cycas* spp. usually raised as ornamental plants in warmer climates. The toxin responsible is *methylazoxymethanol, which is the aglycone of various nontoxic glycosides, including cycasin and macrozamin,* in these plants. The toxin is split from the glycoside by bacterial metabolism in the gut, and its hepatotoxicity is the result of further metabolism by hepatic CYPs; the pattern of necrosis is thus centrilobular (see Fig. 2-94). The metabolites of the aglycone are apparently *potent alkylating agents,* and the chronic liver lesions reflect this; there is megalocytosis (which is not as persistent as that of pyrrolizidine alkaloid poisoning), nuclear hyperchromasia, cholestasis, fatty change, and various degrees of diffuse fibrosis. There is fairly consistent acute renal tubular injury. Chronic exposure leads to cancer development in the liver, kidney, and intestinal tract of laboratory rodents.

Cycads also produce a *neurotoxic amino acid, β-N-methylamino-L-alanine* (BMAA). BMAA is excitotoxic, activating neurotransmission mediated by glutamate receptors, which in excess can lead to cytotoxic influx of calcium ions. Chronic cycad poisoning of cattle causes a chronic nervous disorder characterized by a progressive proprioceptive deficit. This is the result of axonopathy in upper spinocerebellar and lower corticospinal tracts. The axonopathy, morphologically subtle at first, may eventually progress to frank Wallerian degeneration.

Solanaceae

Toxic species of the genus **Cestrum** (jessamine) include *Cestrum diurnum,* a cause of enzootic calcinosis in cattle attributed to active vitamin D analogs; the other known toxic species all produce similar hepatic disease. Speciation within the genus is uncertain, partly because of hybridization; however, the species named as hepatotoxic are *C. parqui, C. laevigatum,* and *C. aurantiacum.*

Cestrum spp. cause acute hepatotoxicity in the field in South America, southern and central Africa, and Australia. Cattle are more frequently poisoned than other species, but sheep and goats are susceptible, and fowl may be if they eat the fruit. The young leaves and unripened berries are the most toxic parts of the plant. In acute hepatotoxicity, there is marked centrilobular and midzonal coagulative necrosis and hemorrhage. There are no records of chronic liver disease caused by this plant, and photosensitization is rarely seen. The toxin is water soluble and has been identified as an *atractyloside.*

Compositae/Asteraceae

Xanthium pungens (Noogoora burr) in Australia and *Xanthium strumarium* (rough cocklebur) in the United States, as well as *X. cavanillesii,* (the cocklebur) in Brazil and South Africa, have been reported to be hepatotoxic while in the seedling stage because the toxins are concentrated in the cotyledons. The burrs are also toxic, and although usually too coarse to be grazed, they can be consumed if ground into feeds. Cattle, swine, and sheep are susceptible, and toxicosis typically occurs following a period of feed scarcity, after flooding or rain has allowed germination. The clinical signs and lesions are not specific, being those described for acute hepatotoxins in general. The toxic principle is a *diterpenoid glycoside, carboxyatractyloside,* although there may be other closely related toxic glycosides in some plants. **Wedelia glauca** also contains atractyloside and causes acute hepatotoxicity in cattle and sheep in Uruguay and Argentina. The condition has been reproduced experimentally in sheep and cattle and rats.

Atractyloside toxins inhibit exchange of ATP from the mitochondria with adenosine diphosphate (ADP) in the cytosol, a process essential for oxidative phosphorylation. Atractylosides inhibit the ADP/ATP carriers (AACs), including the form expressed in the liver. Carboxyatractyloside blocks exchange by binding to a cationic functional domain of bovine AAC1. Lack of ATP and mitochondrial pore leakage lead to apoptosis and necrosis, with ion pump failure, lipid peroxidation, and glutathione depletion. The extent of necrosis depends on dosage. In lethal poisoning with hepatic failure, there is typically midzonal vacuolation and centrilobular necrosis, but it can be panlobular.

Other plants produce similar lesions, but the toxins have not been identified. *Helichrysum blandowskianum* is hepatotoxic to cattle and sheep in southern Australia and has caused sudden deaths with centrilobular necrosis. The condition has been reproduced experimentally. High mortality with acute centrilobular liver necrosis has been reported in cattle grazing sprouting plants of *Vernonia rubricaulis* in Brazil. Similar lesions were reproduced with 3 g/kg of sprouting plants. Various species of *Asteraceae* in South Africa, including *Asaemia axillaris, Athanasia trifurcata, Lasiospermum bipinnatum, Hertia pallens,* and *Pteronia pallens,* have been associated with field outbreaks of acute hepatotoxicity in grazing sheep or cattle. Similar liver lesions have been reproduced experimentally. Experimental intoxications by all of these species have, in some animals, produced centrilobular as well as midzonal necrosis. *Asaemia axillaris, Athanasia trifurcata,* and *Lasiospermum bipinnatum* are also associated with more chronic liver toxicity with photosensitivity.

Ulmaceae

Trema tomentosa (T. aspera), the poison peach, has caused severe losses of cattle in Australia. Similar disease has been reported in goats and horses ingesting *Trema micrantha* in Brazil, and hepatotoxicity has been reproduced in rabbits. The syndrome is acute, there is no photosensitization, and mildly intoxicated animals may recover completely. The toxic principle is a glycoside, designated *trematoxin.* The pattern of necrosis is consistently centrilobular and is identical in appearance to that of *Cestrum* and *Xanthium* poisoning.

The gross and microscopic pathology of experimental poisoning by *Trema, Xanthium pungens,* and *Cestrum parqui* has been shown to be identical in all morphologic respects in the same group of sheep.

Myoporaceae

Hepatotoxic species of *Myoporaceae* so far incriminated are **Myoporum deserti,** *M. acuminatum, M. insulare,* and *M. tetrandum* of Australia, and *M. laetum* in New Zealand, southern Brazil, and Uruguay. The toxic oils are contained in the leaves and branchlets, but within the species, there is variation in the chemical characters and toxicity of the oils; not all strains of toxic species are toxic. There is some delay between ingestion and absorption of the *furanosesquiterpenoid oils,* the best

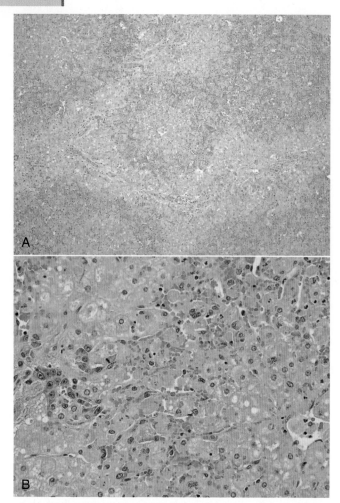

Figure 2-95 Midzonal necrosis caused by ingestion of *Myoporum* sp. in a donkey. **A.** Low-power view. **B.** Higher magnification. (Courtesy R. Kelly.)

known of which is *ngaione*, which are responsible for intoxication. Twenty-four to 48 hours may elapse before signs of toxicity appear. Gross lesions include widespread hemorrhage and a pale yellow liver. Histologically, the pattern is unusual, as the injury to the hepatocytes occurs in periportal or midzonal regions accompanied by biliary hyperplasia (Fig. 2-95A, B). Some animals live long enough to become photosensitized; others may die much more rapidly, with pulmonary edema. The edema appears to be a direct effect of the toxin after its metabolism by the club cells (formerly Clara cells) of the airway.

Livers from intoxicated sheep may show a striking, broad pattern of variable congestion and even infarction, which is superimposed on the more regular lobular pattern of periportal necrosis. Sections of these livers reveal acute fibrinoid necrosis of portal vessels, which suggests that the coarser lesions may have a vascular basis.

Sawfly larvae

Sawfly larval poisoning is an acute hepatotoxicosis documented in cattle and to a lesser extent sheep and goats in various locations, including Australia, Denmark, and South America. Ingestion of the larval stage of the "sawfly," 1 of 3 insect species that are members of the order Hymenoptera and the suborder Symphyta, produce hepatic injury. In Aus-

tralia, the insect species is *Lophyrotoma interrupta (Pergidae)* or *L. zonalis (Pergidae)*; in Denmark the insect is *Arge pullata (Argidae)*, and in South America a third species, *Perreyia flavipes (Pergidae)*, is incriminated. In parts of northeastern Australia, the larvae are parasitic on the leaves of the tree *Eucalyptus melanophloia*, and heavy infestations may occur. *L. zonalis* has been introduced to Florida to control the spread of *Melaleuca quinquenervi*. In Denmark, sawfly larvae feed on birch trees. There is a short clinical course following ingestion, and often, affected cattle are found dead. Animals that survive typically develop icterus and secondary photosensitization. At postmortem examination, ascites, petechiae, and ecchymoses are evident. The liver is enlarged with an accentuated lobular pattern. Mural edema of the gallbladder may be apparent. Sawfly larvae can be found in the rumen and, on occasion, through to the abomasum. Histologically, there is centrilobular to massive acute hepatic necrosis. Outbreaks tend to be seasonal, related to the life cycle of the insects. The toxic principle is believed to be D-amino acid–containing peptides. The major toxin is an octapeptide, *lophyrotomin*, present in the in the larvae of Australian and Danish sawflies. There is a different toxin in the South American sawflies, identified as the heptadecapeptide *pergidin*.

Halogenated hydrocarbons

Various halogenated hydrocarbons, such as *carbon tetrachloride* (used historically as a fasciolicide), *bromobenzene, hexachloroethane, tetrachloroethylene*, and *chloroform*, are activated by cytochromes P450 to hepatotoxic or nephrotoxic metabolites. They have similar hepatotoxic properties, but these agents are little used now, so few animals encounter them in toxic doses. However, some of these chemicals have been used experimentally to investigate the mechanisms of hepatotoxicity, so they warrant brief consideration here. Carbon tetrachloride is metabolized to trihalomethane, a necrogenic free-radical metabolite, and reactive oxygen radicals are concurrently generated. Centrilobular hepatic necrosis with midzonal hydropic change caused by membrane peroxidation occurs within 30 hours of experimental exposures, but lethal toxicity occurs later, when steatosis and the early stages of tissue repair responses are manifest.

Phosphorus

White phosphorus has historically been used for vermin control, and has been implicated in the accidental exposure and deaths of wild waterfowl. It may be present in some incendiary devices such as fireworks. As a rodenticide, it is mixed with fat to promote absorption, and much of the dose is transported to the liver shortly after ingestion. A small amount may be lost by vomition, as elemental phosphorus is directly irritating to the gastrointestinal tract. The mechanism of phosphorus hepatotoxicity is uncertain. It is apparent that metabolism to a toxic intermediate is not necessary, but there is some dispute on the involvement of lipoperoxidation in the hepatocellular injury. There is evidence that protein synthesis is impaired early and that this is responsible for the lipid accumulation that is a prominent feature. A few hours after ingestion of phosphorus, there is severe colic and vomition. If the animal survives this acute phase, there may be apparent recovery for a few days, followed by jaundice and other signs of liver failure, and death by about the fifth day. At postmortem, there is severe icterus and fatty liver, the latter sometimes being predominantly periportal in distribution. Hepatocellular necrosis is not often a prominent feature histologically, notwithstanding the evidence of liver failure. Fatty change is also seen in the myocardium and distal nephrons.

Iron

Iron-dextran complexes have been widely used in the prevention and treatment of anemia in suckling swine. Very occasionally, *severe losses may occur in animals with marginal vitamin E–selenium deficiency;* in these cases, there is, apparently, iron-catalyzed lipoperoxidation in hepatocytes and muscle. The result is sudden massive hepatic necrosis similar in many respects to that of hepatosis dietetica. Large amounts of potassium escape into the circulation from the liver and muscle, and sudden death may result from the cardiotoxicity of this ion. At postmortem, there is staining of subcutaneous tissues and lymph nodes near the site of injection, and there are lesions in the liver or skeletal muscles. The liver is of normal size and of normal color or pale, depending on whether or not the animal is anemic. The presence of underlying necrosis may be indicated only by the numerous small or large hemorrhages present on the capsular and cut surface. Insoluble iron compounds with the staining reactions of hemosiderin are found in mesenchymal cells in many tissues, the largest amounts being in macrophages of the local lymph nodes and in Kupffer cells. Death in piglets from hepatic necrosis occurs ~10 hours after administration. Saccharated iron may produce acute widespread muscle necrosis at ~24 hours, rather than hepatic necrosis in piglets with marginal vitamin E–selenium status. The myocardium is not affected.

Acute hepatotoxicity was reported in young *foals* because of administration of a proprietary paste of iron and yeast products, given as a dietary supplement within a few hours of birth. Not all foals so treated became sick, but those that did developed severe acute centrilobular hepatocellular necrosis, resembling the disease in piglets, and dramatic ductular reaction (biliary hyperplasia).

Acute iron intoxication has also been reported in young *cattle* administered injectable hematinics containing elemental iron, and rarely in adult *horses* administered oral vitamin supplements containing ferrous fumarate or ferrous sulfate. Oversupplementation, low vitamin E or selenium concentrations, or concurrent disease may have contributed to these cases. Consumption of *elemental iron* produces a periportal or panlobular pattern of necrosis.

Chronic hepatotoxicity: plant-derived and environmental toxins

Aflatoxin

The **aflatoxins** are a group of *bisfuranocoumarin compounds* produced as metabolites mainly by *Aspergillus flavus, A. parasiticus,* and *Penicillium puberulum.* The metabolites are designated by the blue or green color they fluoresce when viewed under ultraviolet light and migration patterns during chromatography, and the major ones are B_1, B_2, G_1, and G_2. A less toxic metabolite, M_1 is found in milk and other dairy products from cattle that ingest B_1. Many others may be produced in minor amounts in fungal colonies or as metabolic products of the major toxins in animals. *The most significant and best studied of the aflatoxins is B_1* because of its relative abundance and its potency as a hepatotoxin.

Strains of ***Aspergillus*** differ in the varieties and amounts of individual toxins produced, indicating that the biosynthesis of the toxins is genetically determined. The production of toxins also varies under different conditions of fungal growth, which is influenced by the quality of the substrate, temperature, relative humidity, moisture content of the substrate, and microbial competition. Thus the toxicity of moldy feedstuffs is impossible to assess without measurement of toxin production. Aflatoxins can be produced on growing crops in the field, but much greater levels are likely to accumulate in *stored or unharvested mature grains,* particularly if they are damaged by moisture. Various feeds other than grains, ranging from legume stubbles to bread, may be the substrate in outbreaks of aflatoxicosis. Contaminated grain has been incorporated into commercial dog food, leading to outbreaks of acute toxicity.

Aflatoxins are metabolized by the hepatic mixed-function oxidase system to various toxic and nontoxic metabolites, the proportions of which vary with the species and age of the animal involved. The most potent of these is the 8,9-epoxide metabolite of aflatoxin B_1; this binds to a variety of cellular proteins causing acute toxicity, and its carcinogenic activity derives primarily from adduct formation with guanine in nucleic acids in sensitive species that lack adequate glutathione S–transferase–mediated resistance. The mutational consequence is a G to T transversion. Acute toxicity is most evident in dogs, rats, ducks, guinea pigs, and calves, and each species may be fatally intoxicated by a dose rate of <1.0 mg/kg body weight. Although cats are also sensitive, they rarely ingest contaminated food. Acute, fulminating liver necrosis is sometimes seen in dogs that eat contaminated bread, dog food, or garbage, which may contain very high concentrations of the toxin. Younger animals of all species are much more susceptible and may die within a few hours. The gross postmortem picture is dominated by widespread hemorrhage and massive hepatic necrosis, changes also seen at the microscopic level (eFig. 2-27). Large animal species rarely are exposed at sufficient doses by normal dietary intake to develop acute toxicity. Sheep and adult cattle are quite resistant to the toxin.

Prolonged exposure to low concentrations of the toxin is a more common problem than acute toxicity in large animal species, and may merely produce reduced growth rates and moderate enlargement of the liver without any significant hepatic signs. The enlargement may be partly the result of hypertrophy of hepatocellular smooth endoplasmic reticulum and some degree of fatty change. As the level of aflatoxin in the ration increases (in young pigs, e.g., to 1.0 mg/kg ration), the liver may show all or none of the following changes: pallor, enlargement, bile staining, increased firmness because of fibrogenesis, and fine nodular regenerative hyperplasia. There may also be edema of the gallbladder and bile-tinged ascites in more severe cases. Even under experimental conditions, some individuals may show minimal liver lesions, whereas others, under the same levels of exposure, die of liver failure. Histologically, affected livers show obvious increase in size of some hepatocytes and their nuclei (megalocytosis) with focal necrosis or apoptosis. Bile ductules proliferate early, and reticulin and collagen deposition occurs throughout the acinus according to no distinct pattern (Fig. 2-96). Fatty change in affected livers is variable in extent and occurrence, and bile pigments accumulate in canaliculi and hepatocytes in more severely affected livers. Minor degrees of megalocytosis may be seen in proximal tubular epithelium in the kidney. *The changes produced resemble those of pyrrolizidine alkaloid toxicosis.* This can be attributed to the fact that aflatoxin and pyrrolizidine alkaloids *inhibit hepatocellular regeneration* such that nodules

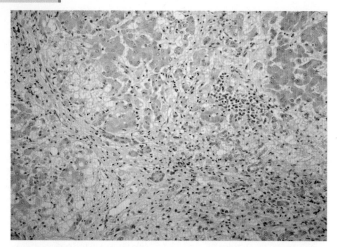

Figure 2-96 Hepatocellular steatosis and ductular proliferation in canine **chronic aflatoxicosis.**

and ductules regenerate as the liver becomes atrophic. These are also *genotoxic* and *carcinogenic*, so they might be involved in the occurrence of liver cancers in animals, as they are in humans.

At higher dose rates of aflatoxin, most centrilobular hepatocytes disappear and are replaced by a mixture of inflammatory cells, fibroblasts, and primitive vascular channels. The liver may be much smaller than normal, particularly in young animals, presumably because of mitotic inhibition, and focal hepatocellular necrosis is more obvious or may be supplanted by zonal (centrilobular) necrosis. Fatty change in these livers may be severe and uniformly distributed.

Fumonisin

Fumonisin B_1, a mycotoxin elaborated by certain strains of **Fusarium verticillioides** (previously *moniliforme*) and ***F. proliferatum*** in infected corn, induces a pulmonary edema syndrome in pigs, hepatocellular carcinomas in laboratory rats, and leukoencephalomalacia. Hepatotoxicity occurs in horses and swine. Hepatic toxicity has also been reported in sheep and baboons. In horses, hepatoxicity occurs less often than leukoencephalomalacia. The clinical course is relatively short, with death likely within 5-10 days of the onset of clinical signs, such as anorexia, depression, icterus, and edema of the head. Bilirubin and liver enzymes are typically elevated. At postmortem, the liver is typically firm, yellow, and small, with an accentuated lobular pattern. Histologic lesions include abundant apoptosis that may progress to centrilobular necrosis and variable amounts of fibrosis in the portal tracts. Cardiotoxicity is also evident in swine and horses.

Fumonisin B_1 is also a *primary hepatotoxin in pigs*. Experimental feeding trials with pigs have shown dose-related differences in pathology. Pigs intubated with a minimum of 16 mg fumonisin B_1/kg body weight per day developed interlobular edema, variable hydrothorax, and pulmonary edema, whereas pigs intubated with 8 mg/kg per day for 7-8 days, or fed diets containing 200 mg fumonisin B_1/kg of feed for 21 days, developed marked icterus. Histologic changes included hepatocellular necrosis without a zonal distribution, depletion of centrilobular hepatocytes, lobular disarray, and megalocytosis characterized by large numbers of swollen hepatocytes with abundant granular eosinophilic cytoplasm and occasional large nuclei, randomly interspersed with small angular hepatocytes and scattered necrotic cells. These pigs showed no

evidence of pathologic changes in the lungs, whereas pigs given higher doses showed *hepatic necrosis in addition to pulmonary edema*. The liver changes appear to be reversible upon cessation of exposure. Gilts fed low levels of fumonisin B_1 for 90 days developed hepatic nodular hyperplasia, along with hyperkeratosis and parakeratosis and hyperplasia of the distal esophageal mucosa. Fumonisins are inhibitors of sphingosine and ceramide synthetase, leading to inhibition of sphingolipid biosynthesis. As a consequence, there is an accumulation of bioactive intermediates of sphingolipid metabolism (sphinganine and other sphingoid bases and derivatives), as well as the depletion of complex sphingolipids, which interfere with the function of some membrane proteins and may be involved in the toxic hepatic effects.

Phomopsin

There are 2 distinct manifestations of toxicity associated with *Lupinus* spp.; discussed here is the condition formerly known as *"lupinosis," which is a true mycotoxic liver disease.* The teratogenic and neurotoxic effects of some of the isoquinoline alkaloids from the plants themselves are discussed in Vol. 1, Bones and joints and Vol. 1, Nervous system.

The fungus **Diaporthe toxica** *(formerly Phomopsis leptostromiformis)* is parasitic on green *Lupinus* plants, but it becomes saprophytic after the host plant dies. Phomopsins (A or B) are produced if the lupin stubble is moistened, and such stubbles may remain toxic for months. Additional toxins are suspected. Severe acute liver damage has been described in sheep on very toxic stubbles in Western Australia, but in many of these cases, it has been difficult to separate the toxicity of the lupins from that of copper, which in this area is often concentrated in ovine livers (see later section on Copper).

The usual syndrome of phomopsin poisoning is subacute to chronic. Inappetence occurs soon after experimental administration of the toxin is begun; liver damage is clinically inapparent for several days. The gross pathologic abnormalities of acutely intoxicated sheep include icterus and modest ascites. The main abnormalities are evident in the liver, which varies from a yellow discoloration because of lipidosis in more acute cases, to a variable ochre to orange discoloration with a firm texture with increasing chronicity (Fig. 2-97A). Histologically, there is early hepatocyte swelling and accelerated cell death among hepatocytes. Increased mitotic activity is soon apparent, although by this time, the liver has become smaller. The mitotic activity is in fact largely ineffectual, as close examination reveals that many mitotic figures are abnormal. There is either clumping or dispersal of chromatin, and *there appears to be mitotic arrest at late metaphase* (Fig. 2-97B-D). Remaining hepatocytes swell, their cytoplasm becomes granular, and their nuclei vesicular and may contain vesicular intranuclear pseudoinclusions. There is variably severe fatty change, dependent to a large degree on the fat reserves of the animal. There is also accumulation of complex pigment in macrophages in portal stroma and about hepatic venules; this granular material contains lipofuscin, ferric iron, and copper at least. Bile duct proliferation is also a prominent feature of the chronic disease. With progression, hepatic fibrosis occurs, predominantly diffuse in distribution, and by this stage, there is usually clinical icterus and anorexia.

The liver continues to shrink, presumably as a result of continued mitotic inhibition and progressive fibrosis. The organ is small, tough, and has a finely granular surface and texture. It is pale gray-orange but usually retains its shape. Fibrosis is

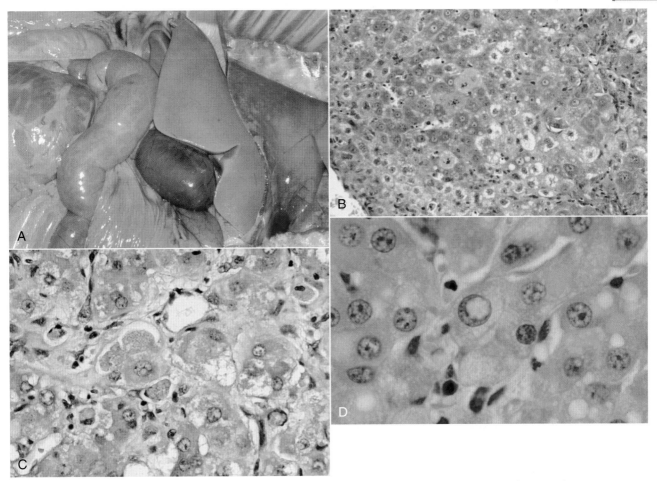

Figure 2-97 Phomopsin poisoning (lupinosis) in sheep. **A.** Affected sheep have pale livers with prominent icterus. **B.** Numerous, and **abnormal, mitotic figures** in subacute phomopsin poisoning. **C. Brown pigment** within Kupffer cells. **D.** Clear **intranuclear pseudoinclusions** can be found in affected hepatocytes. (Courtesy J.G. Allen.)

initially portal to periportal, but central areas can also become fibrotic. Bridging fibrosis between portal areas and portal to central regions can develop. In naturally occurring cases, however, discontinuous intake of the toxin may produce a liver grossly distorted by asymmetrical nodular regeneration and fibrosis. The atrophic changes are most severe in the left lobe.

Photosensitization occurs in phomopsin-poisoned sheep; it may be severe if the animals have access to green feed while under the influence of the toxin. Lupinosis in sheep has also been experimentally observed to induce mild skeletal myopathy, resembling nutritional myopathy.

Phomopsin poisoning in cattle causes most losses when the animals are lactating or heavily pregnant; in these animals, the syndrome is essentially one of ketosis, to which such cows would be predisposed by the anorexia that is an obvious clinical feature of this intoxication. Pregnant sheep are less likely to have access to toxic lupin roughage during late gestation; otherwise, ketosis triggered by phomopsin would be expected just as often as in cattle.

Chronic hepatic fibrosis with fine, nodular regeneration may occur infrequently in cattle as the result of chronic phomopsin poisoning. Similar liver changes may also be seen in horses, in which there may also be hemolytic anemia of unknown pathogenesis.

Sporidesmin

The mycotoxin *sporidesmin* is produced by the fungus **Pithomyces chartarum** and concentrated in the conidia (spores); the most important substrate is dead ryegrass *(Lolium perenne)* that has been moistened in warm weather. Intoxication causes *chronic liver damage and severe hepatogenous photosensitivity ("facial eczema")* and is a serious cause of loss of sheep and, to a lesser extent, cattle, goats, and farmed deer on the North Island of New Zealand. Sporadic and subclinical intoxication occurs irregularly on the South Island, in southern Australia, and South Africa. Although the fungus is found throughout the world, toxigenic strains appear to be limited to New Zealand. Sporidesmin intake in conjunction with ingestion of *Tribulus terrestris* causes another hepatogenous photosensitivity *(geeldikkop)*; this is similar to but distinct from facial eczema, and is described later.

Sporidesmin is concentrated in the fungal spores, and the toxigenicity of pasture is related to the density of the spores in it. Sporidesmin is not specifically hepatotoxic. Administration of the toxin does produce rapid disorganization of hepatic cell organelles and triglyceride accumulation, but these are mild and nonspecific changes. If administered in suitable dosage, the toxin causes permeability alterations in many tissues and will, for example, produce corneal edema on local application. *The hepatobiliary lesions are caused by the excretion of unconjugated sporidesmin in bile, where its concentration may initiate oxidative injury,* likely mediated by the production of a hydroxyl radical. Sporidesmin is also excreted in urine, and if the dose is high enough, edema and mucosal hemorrhage occur in the bladder. The hepatic lesion is the result of irritation of mesenchymal tissues in the portal triads and surrounding the bile ducts. A high concentration of sporidesmin can injure biliary epithelium, allowing diffusion of the bile duct contents. Release of toxin, possibly accentuated by the release of bile acids as well, produces irritative lesions and necrosis in the adjacent blood vessels.

The liver in acute forms of the disease is enlarged, with rounded edges, and is finely mottled and discolored yellow-green by retained bile pigments, although the discoloration may be blotchy. There is mild edema and congestion of the wall of the gallbladder, which may be distended with bile of normal quality or with mucin (white bile). The extrahepatic ducts are thickened and prominent, and there is edema of the adventitia. The ductal changes may extend to the papilla of Vater and can be traced by the naked eye deeply into the parenchyma. In more chronic cases, alterations of size and pigmentation of the liver are variable. Pale areas of capsular thickening, which may be elevated or depressed, are visible. On cut surfaces, they extend deeply as wedge-shaped areas in which biliary fibrosis has produced an exaggerated acinar pattern, and the parenchyma is pale and atrophic; these areas are related to occluded bile ducts.

The liver is firm and cuts with increased resistance. The medium and large caliber intrahepatic ducts are conspicuous. There is irregular stenosis of their lumens, some are occluded by cellular debris and inspissated bile or mucin, and in some, cicatrization of the new fibrous tissue causes complete atresia. Occlusion of the ducts causes the parenchyma served by them to undergo atrophy, necrosis, and fibrosis (Fig. 2-98). The livers of animals that have survived an attack of cholangitis of this genesis are distorted in shape and size by large nodules of regeneration and persistent areas of atrophy and fibrosis. The atrophy and fibrosis may affect either lobe, but usually, the left is most severely affected.

Histologically, the changes are those of *acute cholangitis or cholangiohepatitis* to which there is minimal leukocytic reaction. There is extensive necrosis of the lining of the larger intrahepatic ducts and the extrahepatic ducts, the epithelium being cast off as debris mixed with a few leukocytes. There is

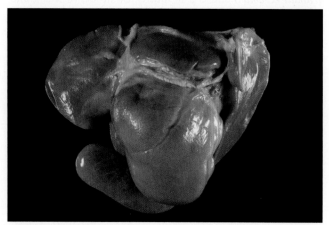

Figure 2-98 Chronic sporidesmin intoxication ("facial eczema") in sheep. Liver lobe atrophy and fibrosis. (Courtesy K.G. Thompson.)

edema of the adventitia of the ducts, with active fibroplasia and scarring. Inflammatory cells are present, but not in large numbers, and they are chiefly lymphocytes and histiocytes. Injury to the smaller radicles of the bile ducts is less severe, but fibrosis is active. The portal tracts are enlarged by fibrous tissue and by the active generation of new bile ducts that follows and which is more prominent in chronic intoxication (eFig. 2-28). Affected camelids appear to be susceptible to florid hyperplasia of the bile ducts.

In more severe intoxications, there may be *coagulative necrosis of blood vessel walls in the portal triads;* when this is incomplete, the most damaged segment of the vessel tends to be that adjacent to the nearest injured bile duct. Both arteries and veins may be affected, and it is possible that necrosis is related to vascular insufficiency as well as to impaired bile drainage. Changes in the hepatic parenchyma are minimal and secondary to those in the portal triads. In acute cases, there may be extensive pigmentation of hepatocytes and Kupffer cells by bile pigments, but this is irregular in distribution in the liver. Inspissated bile can be found in the bile ducts and canaliculi. There is some necrosis of hepatocytes adjacent to inflamed portal areas, and other areas of necrosis, focal in type and distribution and probably the result of biliary obstruction, may be numerous.

Other morbid alterations include great enlargement of the adrenals produced by cortical hypertrophy; sclerotic intimal plaques in the arteries, veins, and lymphatics in the hilus of the liver; and a tendency for the newly formed bile ductules to recanalize occluded ducts.

Pyrrolizidine alkaloids

Pyrrolizidine alkaloids have been identified in nearly 3% of all plant species, from >6,000 species of 3 families: the *Asteraceae (Compositae), Leguminosae (Fabaceae),* and *Boraginaceae.* The main genera responsible for plant toxicoses in domestic mammals are **Senecio, Crotalaria, Heliotropium, Cynoglossum, Amsinckia, Echium,** and **Trichodesma,** and are widely distributed around the world. Intoxication is relatively infrequent because most plants containing pyrrolizidines are unpalatable. Contamination of baled or cubed forage with toxic plants is a common route of exposure. The seeds are also toxic, and the small seeds of *Amsinckia* and *Crotalaria* may, depending on harvesting technique, heavily contaminate other harvested grains used in prepared pig and poultry feeds. More than 350 pyrrolizidine alkaloids have been identified chemically, and most of the toxic plant species contain more than one of the alkaloids. So far, only a small proportion of the known alkaloids have well-characterized toxicity; these are all esters of 1 of 3 amino alcohol bases (necines) or acids (necic acids). The *retronecine group* includes *monocrotaline, retrorsine, retronecine, ridelliine, senecionine, and jacobine,* and the *heliotridine group* includes *lasiocarpine and heliotrine.* These toxins must be metabolized to more reactive forms for toxicity. Cytochromes P450 mediate the N-oxidation of the necine bases. They can also mediate the 2-step hydroxylation of the necine bases at the C3 and C8 positions; this is followed by spontaneous dehydration to the *highly reactive dehydropyrrolizidine (DHP) alkaloids.* The toxic DHP alkaloids are electrophilic and can bind covalently to amino acids, proteins, and nucleic acids at guanine and adenine residues. Acute toxicity derives from damage to cellular proteins. Antimitotic effects can be exerted via damage to microtubules. The DNA-binding activity is responsible for genotoxicity; the DHP-derived

DNA adducts are a common pathway for carcinogenic activity of pyrrolizidine alkaloids. The DHP metabolites can be detoxified by glutathione conjugation by glutathione S–transferases. Ester linkages at the C7 and C9 positions can be hydrolyzed by carboxylesterases to generate the necine or acid moieties; this is generally considered to be a detoxification pathway.

The toxicity of a pyrrolizidine alkaloid-containing plant depends on many factors. The content of toxin varies by species of plant; the stage of growth, as new growth tends to have more toxin in general; and the time of year and environmental factors such as rainfall. For an individual pyrrolizidine alkaloid, toxicity depends on the amount of alkaloid that can be converted to reactive metabolites, the rate of cytochrome P450–mediated generation of the DHP, and the efficiency of detoxification by glutathione conjugation. Toxicity also depends on the species exposed, age and sex of the animal intoxicated, and the metabolic activity and the mitotic stage of its target cells. Young animals are generally much more susceptible than adults. Grazing animals are more likely to consume plants that contain pyrrolizidine alkaloids, but because the toxins are produced by the plants to deter herbivores, it is unusual for an animal to consume large amounts. Ruminants, especially sheep and goats, are much less susceptible than pigs, in part because the toxins can be degraded in the rumen. However, sheep can graze out stands of *Senecio* that would be lethal to cattle. Horses and cattle have similar, intermediate susceptibilities. *Most pyrrolizidine alkaloids are hepatotoxic because they are metabolically activated to DHPs in the liver.* There are 3 common morphologic expressions of pyrrolizidine poisoning. First, *acute centrilobular to massive necrosis* occurs in animals ingesting large amounts of these alkaloids. Because the plants responsible are unpalatable, naturally occurring outbreaks of acute poisoning are generally restricted to circumstances where animals face starvation, such as grazing pastures affected by prolonged drought. Ingested dosages in grazing circumstances are usually too low for acute effects; however, acute hemorrhagic centrilobular necrosis has been described after experimental exposures to high doses of pyrrolizidine alkaloids. The centrilobular pattern of necrosis produced is similar to that caused by many other hepatotoxins that are bioactivated by hepatic cytochromes P450. Second, phasic (usually seasonal) repetitive exposure to these alkaloids leads to *hepatic atrophy with formation of regenerative nodules. This is the most common expression of field exposure to pyrrolizidine alkaloids, and affected livers show a characteristic pattern of hepatocellular polyploidy known as* **megalocytosis** (Fig. 2-99). Third, prolonged exposure exclusively to *Heliotropium* induces *firm, fibrotic atrophic livers without nodular regeneration.* If seasonal exposure to these toxic alkaloids declines, then a remarkable degree of recovery is possible.

Pyrrolizidine alkaloids inhibit DNA synthesis and mitosis in hepatocytes, but some are able to replicate their DNA without undergoing mitosis, resulting in greatly enlarged hepatocytes with large convoluted polyploid nuclei. Some enlarged nuclei have cytoplasmic invaginations that can become entrapped as intranuclear inclusions. However, many hepatocytes in an affected liver do not become megalocytic. Those that are completely inhibited do not replicate DNA at all, whereas those that are more resistant can replicate more normally and give rise to nodular populations of smaller, more normal hepatocytes. Inhibited hepatocytes and megalocytes are long lived but eventually many undergo apoptosis.

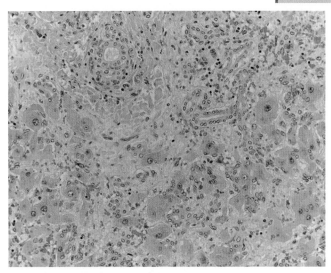

Figure 2-99 **Megalocytosis** in *Senecio* ragwort poisoning in an ox.

In *chronic pyrrolizidine alkaloid poisoning,* the liver can become atrophic as hepatocytes are lost faster than they can be replaced. The atrophy can be compensated to various degrees by megalocytosis and regeneration of small, less inhibited hepatocytes that proliferate in a nodular pattern. Concurrently, there is *usually proliferation of bile duct epithelial cells (termed ductular reaction) in the portal triads.* This is largely explained by the propensity of hepatic progenitor cells to proliferate forming ductules when adult hepatocytes cannot respond to the regenerative stimuli that prevail when liver mass is inadequate. *There may also be some periportal fibroplasia that varies with species and exposure; typically, it is minimal in sheep, moderate in horses, and may be marked in cattle* (eFig. 2-29). In **cattle,** the fibrous tissue can infiltrate along the sinusoids to dissect lobules, separate individual cells, and link up with the walls of efferent veins. In acute poisoning, in which there is centrilobular necrosis, fibrosis can also develop in a "veno-occlusive" pattern around and sometimes obliterating the hepatic venules. There is evidence that pyrrolizidine metabolite injury is not restricted to hepatocytes and that endothelial cells are also involved, leading to additional vascular insult and fibrosis in the liver. Direct endothelial injury from pyrrolizidines may occur, but an alternative explanation proposes a form of "bystander" injury, where toxic metabolites are formed in hepatocytes but are able to damage adjacent endothelial cells. This pattern of fibrosis may occur in some field cases in cattle, but is more commonly observed in humans exposed to pyrrolizidine alkaloids in herbal preparations or "bush teas," and it can be produced experimentally after sublethal acute experimental hepatotoxicity. In fatal cases in cattle, the livers are very tough and nodular, and the nodules have variably efficient biliary drainage and cytochrome expression, so there may be a very striking color pattern, ranging from fatty yellow through green and brown. Hepatic fibrosis can result in portal hypertension with ascites, severe mesenteric edema, and diarrhea. Excretory insufficiency with moderate jaundice and photosensitization can also occur.

The disease in **sheep** is always protracted as a consequence of the relative resistance of this species; indeed, clinical signs may not be seen until after a second season of exposure. The plants most often implicated are *Heliotropium europaeum* and *Echium plantagineum.* The shape of these failed livers is normal, but they are small, gray-yellow, fairly smooth, and toughened by condensation of normal stroma rather than by fibroplasia. If the liver copper content was high before intoxication, toxicity can culminate in copper release and an episode of intravascular hemolysis. In this case, the carcass will be intensely jaundiced, and the kidneys are stained with methemoglobin and bilirubin. The relationship of chronic copper poisoning to pyrrolizidine alkaloid poisoning is discussed later.

Horses are susceptible to both acute and chronic toxicosis, and liver failure produced in horses by these alkaloids is similar to that seen in cattle. Horses are more likely to manifest signs of hepatic encephalopathy with head-pressing and compulsive walking; in some places, these nervous signs give rise to colloquial names such as "walkabout" and "walking disease." Administration of a high dose of *Cynoglossum officinale* resulted in severe liver disease within 7 days after dosing, with elevated serum enzymes, altered bile acid metabolism, and extensive hepatocellular necrosis with minimal periportal fibrosis and biliary hyperplasia, and little or no megalocytosis. Edema and infarction of the cecum and colon were also present at postmortem. Administration of a low dose to horses for 14 days resulted in transient clinical depression and weight loss, transient elevations of serum enzymes and bile acids, and minimal periportal hepatocellular necrosis with fibrosis, developing extensive megalocytosis by week 14. The megalocytosis became the most prominent change 6 months after exposure.

Metabolites of pyrrolizidine alkaloids are formed by any cells with adequate cytochrome P450 activity. Although the liver is the main site of bioactivation, other cells such as proximal convoluted renal tubules and club cells (formerly termed Clara cells) in the lung can generate metabolites that cause local injury. Death in some instances may be the result of renal damage and in others the result of pulmonary vascular and interstitial lesions. Variation in the source of the toxin and in the species-based metabolic differences in the affected animals account for the differences in susceptibility of the different tissues. Alkaloids from *Crotalaria* affect the widest range of tissues in most animals; most notably, monocrotaline causes diffuse lung injury, leading to pulmonary edema progressing to fibrosis. Respiratory difficulty has been described in horses eating *C. dura,* and *C. crispata* produces similar lesions. Sheep develop pulmonary signs after eating *C. globifera* and *C. dura,* and pigs after eating *Senecio jacobaea.* The experimental feeding of *C. spectabilis* to rats or the injection of monocrotaline, extracted from the plant, produces progressive pulmonary disease, pulmonary hypertension, and cor pulmonale, with necrotizing vasculitis of the pulmonary arterioles. Emphysema occurs in pigs and is an outstanding feature of the pulmonary disease of horses. The essential reactive lesion is diffuse fibrosis of alveolar and interlobular septa, with patchy epithelialization occurring more slowly.

Lantana camara

Lantana camara is an attractive ornamental shrub native to the Americas and Africa that grows readily in tropical and subtropical habitats. It contains various *toxic pentacyclic triterpenes,* the most abundant of which are lantadene A, lantadene C, and icterogenin, although metabolites may also be toxic. Lantadene A appears to be the most toxic; at high doses experimentally, it causes severe acute centrilobular necrosis of the liver. The mechanism of toxicity is not known, but may be related to the effects of lantadene A on mitochondrial energetics.

However, *L. camara* poisoning in grazing animals is manifested as *subacute or chronic cholestasis, characterized by severe icterus and photosensitization,* most commonly seen in cattle, but rarely in sheep, goats, and horses. Goats are quite susceptible to the toxin, but are less likely to eat the plant. Neonatal ruminants appear resistant suggesting the rumen may retain the plants and provide longer exposure to the toxins.

Photosensitization is usually severe after 2 days, but jaundice is more severe in chronic cases. Heavily intoxicated cattle can die within 2 days, but most fatal cases run a course of ~2 weeks. Ruminal stasis and anorexia appear early, and the large bowel contains dark, dry feces. The rumen is a reservoir of toxin that remains active and can perpetuate the intoxication after access to the plant is curtailed. The liver is enlarged, pale, and stained yellow, orange, or green-gray by bile pigment. The gallbladder is greatly distended with pale, sometimes slightly mucoid, bile.

The severity of the liver changes may be much less than expected from the intensity of the icterus and photosensitization. The most consistent histologic finding in the liver is hepatocellular enlargement and fine cytoplasmic vacuolation, together with some degree of bile accumulation in canaliculi, hepatocyte cytoplasm, and Kupffer cells. The canalicular cholestasis is usually more severe in the centrilobular zones, whereas the cytoplasmic vacuolation is often more pronounced in the periportal hepatocytes. There is usually some bile duct proliferation, and in some cases, there will be a high incidence of periportal apoptosis, focal coagulative necrosis, or hepatocellular dissociation.

Electron microscopy reveals an apparent increase in volume of smooth endoplasmic reticulum and a quite characteristic form of collapse of many bile canaliculi. Other canaliculi are distended and have damaged microvilli. Because much of the bilirubin that accumulates in the plasma of such animals is conjugated, it seems that the cholestasis is due in large measure to direct interference with canalicular transport of bile. The mechanisms of cholestasis have not been determined, but damage to the contractile pericanalicular cytoskeleton or its associated cell adhesion molecules required for canalicular integrity are plausible targets (see previous section on Cholestasis and jaundice).

Animals are usually polyuric because of acute tubular injury, resulting in severe dehydration, in part related to a disinclination to drink. The kidneys are slightly enlarged and wet on section, and, especially in the more chronic cases, the cortex is pale and the medulla hyperemic. The renal lesion is nonspecific acute tubular injury, ranging in severity from mild vacuolar change to patchy tubular necrosis and extensive tubular cast formation. The role of the hyperbilirubinemia in the production of the renal damage has not been assessed. Severe myocardial necrosis can be produced in sheep by *Lantana* poisoning, and may be responsible for the early deaths in cattle.

Intoxication by steroidal sapogenins: tribulosis and related toxicoses

Consumption of **Tribulus terrestris,** particularly by the grazing of young wilted plants or sometimes hay, causes cholangitis and photosensitization in sheep. This plant has caused enormous loss of sheep in South Africa, where the toxicosis is known as **geeldikkop** ("yellow bighead," because of icterus and marked edema of ears and face). The disease has been reproduced by oral administration of crude extracts of *steroidal* *sapogenins or their glycosides, saponins, of T. terrestris,* but which of the various saponins in the plant are responsible for the disease is unknown. The disease has also been reproduced experimentally by co-administration of sporidesmin and *T. terrestris,* but the liver lesions are histologically distinct from those produced by sporidesmin alone (facial eczema).

In geeldikkop, the most characteristic gross finding is the presence of a white, semifluid accumulation of fine, crystalline material that can be expressed from the cystic duct and larger intrahepatic ducts. The gallbladder mucosa is also partly covered with a fine, crystalline deposit. The gross lesions of geeldikkop are similar to those of facial eczema in that there is generalized icterus, and the liver is discolored by bile pigment and either slightly swollen or distorted, according to the duration of the disease.

In poisoning by sporidesmin alone, however, there is more obvious edema and fibrosis of bile ducts, and bile infarcts in the parenchyma are more common. The acute lesion consists of swelling and feathery vacuolation of hepatocytes, and marked hyperplasia of Kupffer cells that may show similar cytoplasmic changes. In these acute cases, the presence of acicular crystals may be very difficult to detect (Fig. 2-100A, B). *With more chronic intoxication, the most consistent histologic abnormality is the presence in bile ducts of various amounts of crystalline material* (Fig. 2-100C). The crystals are fine, flat, and are deposited in affected ducts, and, less commonly, in hepatocytes themselves and in renal tubules. There may be associated bile ductular proliferation in severe cases, but often the degree of histologic hepatocellular damage is mild compared to the severity of the photosensitization. The cholestasis is not solely the result of mechanical obstruction by the crystals, because photosensitization can occur in such outbreaks in animals whose livers show very little cholangitis and contain very few crystals. The severity of peribiliary fibrosis is more variable and probably depends on the relative contribution of sporidesmin to the intoxication. There is some hepatocellular degeneration and apoptosis, and there is fairly uniform swelling of cytoplasm. Bile pigment accumulates in Kupffer cells and hepatocyte cytoplasm, but not to any marked extent in canaliculi. Focal necrosis of the gallbladder mucosa is often present. The severity of the hepatic lesion increases with the duration of exposure.

The biliary crystals from sheep with geeldikkop have been determined to be composed principally of *calcium salts of steroidal sapogenins* present in *T. terrestris.* Plant saponins are metabolized in the rumen and liver to episapogenin glucuronides, which in the presence of calcium may precipitate, forming the characteristic biliary crystals. Cholestasis is likely related to reduced bile acid secretion into the lumen of the canaliculi, rather than biliary occlusion by these plant sapogenins. This explains the evidence of cholestasis before crystals can be seen histologically. Other unidentified plant components may also play a role in hepatocellular and biliary injury. It has also been suggested that the toxins responsible may act primarily on the membranes of the bile canaliculi, in a manner similar to that of *Lantana* poisoning. *Hepatocellular damage likely also plays a role in phytoporphyrin (phylloerythrin) retention.*

Switchgrass (*Panicum virgatum*), Kleingrass (*P. coloratum*), and other **Panicum** species are associated with hepatogenous photosensitization in grazing animals, including sheep, goats, and horses in the United States, Australia, and other areas of the world. The toxic agent(s) are steroidal sapogenins, and

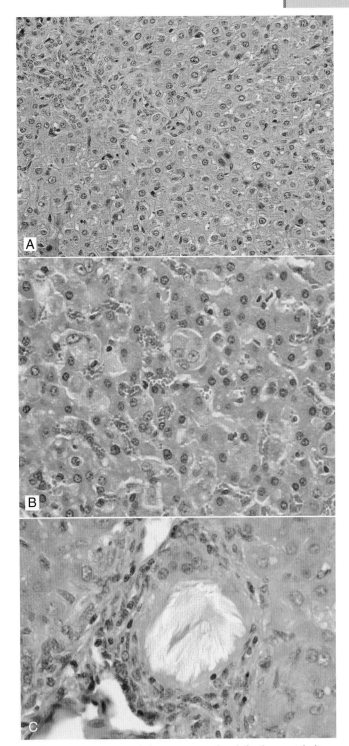

Figure 2-100 A. Crystal deposition within bile duct epithelium in a goat grazing **Panicum** sp. B. **Foamy material within macrophages** in an ox ingesting **Brachiaria** sp. (Courtesy R. Kelly.) C. Fine crystalline material in **expanded Kupffer cells** in a goat grazing **Panicum** sp.

their type and concentration vary with the part of the plant (highest concentrations being in the young growing leaf) and with the environmental conditions. Hot and dry conditions, have been associated with outbreaks. Younger animals appear to be more susceptible. Crystals may be produced in the biliary tree, hepatocytes, sinusoids, or Kupffer cells.

Crystal-associated cholangiohepatopathy is not specific for *Tribulus* or *Panicum* spp. intoxication. Similar changes occur in the hepatogenous photosensitivity disease, **alveld,** in sheep grazing pastures in Norway, the British Isles, and in the Faeroe Islands containing *Narthecium ossifragum*. Similar disease has been reported in ruminants intoxicated by *Agave lecheguilla*, *Nolena texana*, and the pasture species *Brachiaria decumbens* (signal grass) in Brazil. In New Zealand, crystal deposition in the biliary tree of cattle has been reported following ingestion of *Phytolacca octandra* (inkweed). In those cases studied *(T. terrestris, P. dichotomiflorum, P. schinzii, Narthecium ossifragum)*, the characteristic crystalloid material deposited in the bile is principally composed of calcium salts of steroidal sapogenins. In some cases, crystal formation may not be apparent in bile ducts, and affected Kupffer cells and macrophages are more evident. There may be differences in the histologic responses of cattle and sheep grazing various sapinogenin-containing plants. Foamy Kupffer cells and hepatocytes along with foamy macrophages in mesenteric and hepatic lymph nodes may be a more common response in cattle versus crystal formation within bile ducts in sheep (Fig. 2-101). To complicate diagnostic efforts, foamy macrophages in the mesenteric and hepatic lymph nodes are also found in healthy cattle and sheep grazing *B. decumbens* in Brazil. With the exception of *Nolena texana*, steroidal sapogenins have been demonstrated in all of these plants. As with *T. terrestris*, extracts of *B. decumbens* containing steroidal saponins produced typical lesions of cholangitis with crystal deposition when orally administered to lambs, with *Pithomyces chartarum* spore counts below detectable levels. Similarly, analysis of samples of *B. decumbens* and *P. dichotomiflorum* on which cattle and goats had recently been photosensitized showed only low levels of *P. chartarum* spores, and all isolates obtained failed to produce sporidesmin. Despite this, it is also apparent that neither *Tribulus* nor *Panicum* stands are at all times dangerous. Levels of saponins have been shown to vary greatly within a species from site to site, and with the age of the plant. Additionally, the role of sporadic environmental conditions, such as wilting, which might concentrate the saponins or other unidentified toxins, or the synergistic involvement of endophytic fungi, remains to be determined.

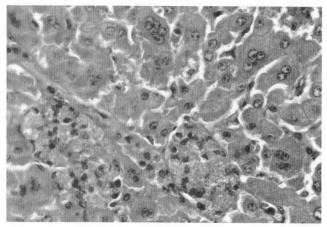

Figure 2-101 Chronic cholangitis and plugging of bile duct by lipophilic **crystalloid material,** in photosensitivity disease of sheep grazing **pangola grass.** Similar to reaction seen in geeldikkop. (Courtesy J.G. Allen.)

Other plants reported occasionally to produce unexpected photosensitivity include *Digitaria* spp., *Cooperia pedunculata*, *Nidorella foetida*, and *Chloris* spp., and such valuable pasture genera as *Medicago*, *Trifolium*, *Avena*, and *Biserrula pelecinus*, although the latter species may cause primary photosensitization.

Nitrosamines

Epizootics of poisoning by **dimethylnitrosamine** occurred in Norwegian cattle, sheep, and fur-bearing animals, from 1957-1962. The toxin was present in herring meal and was thought to be a *reaction product of trimethylamine and other lower amines with sodium nitrite,* added as a preservative, the reacting amines being products of decomposition. Animals consumed several pounds of the toxic meal each day before becoming ill. *This intoxication has little importance in livestock now that it is easily prevented.*

At postmortem, there was moderate anasarca and signs of hemorrhagic diathesis. Livers affected acutely were enlarged and firm, with mottled discoloration and sometimes a nutmeg appearance. In chronic intoxication, the liver was small, granular, and very firm. A number of cases recovered after prolonged convalescence, and in these, there was atrophy and fibrosis of the left and caudate lobes, and the right lobe was hyperplastic and hemispheric. Histologically, in acute cases, there was widespread hemorrhagic centrilobular necrosis and an unusual degree of intimal and subendothelial reaction in sublobular and hepatic veins. The chronic lesion was dominated by extensive centrilobular fibrosis, with obliterative changes in many central and sublobular veins. Sporadic cases of portal hypertension in Greyhound dogs have been recognized where hepatic veno-occlusive disease is the predominant lesion. In these cases, a history of feeding meat treated with large amounts of nitrites or sulfites in an attempt to preserve the color of fresh meat is common, but a causal relationship has not been established.

The *hepatocellular changes are not specific* for dimethylnitrosamine or other hepatotoxic nitrosamines. Nitrosamines are metabolized in the liver and other tissues to reactive alkyl groups that bind covalently to various macromolecules, especially guanine in nucleic acids. Hepatotoxicity develops more slowly than in response to toxicants that induce membrane peroxidation, as many hepatocytes with DNA damage undergo apoptosis when stimulated to replicate. There is some megalocytosis, nuclear vesiculation and nucleolar prominence, cytoplasmic intranuclear inclusions, and variable fatty change and cytoplasmic bile accumulation. The typical effects of chronic experimental nitrosamine hepatotoxicity, such as hepatocellular fibrosis, nodules, and neoplasms, have not been evident in the accidental poisonings. Dimethylnitrosamine-induced hepatotoxicosis in dogs has been proposed as a model of toxin-induced progressive hepatic disease in this species.

Indospicine

Legumes of the genus **Indigofera** have long been known to contain the toxic amino acid indospicine (6-amidino-2-hexanoic acid), which is a structural analogue of arginine, and which was shown in early experimental work to be hepatotoxic for rats and other species. The dose rates necessary to cause chronic liver injury in these species were, however, quite high, and field cases of intoxications were only seen in cattle grazing *I. spicata*, which has the highest naturally occurring concentrations of indospicine. In Australia, a serious outbreak of fatal liver disease occurred in dogs that had been fed meat from horses that had been grazing *I. linnaei*, a plant native to the arid zones of Australia that has been known to produce, in horses, a chronic neurologic disorder known as "Birdsville horse disease." The disease in horses is not associated with liver damage, although these animals do accumulate indospicine in most tissues, including muscle.

Dogs fed indospicine-contaminated meat for several weeks may develop *progressive liver damage.* Affected livers may be small, firm, and pale, or they may be nodular because of hypertrophy of surviving hepatocytes (eFig. 2-30A). Histologically, lesions begin as vacuolation of a narrow band of centrilobular hepatocytes, followed shortly by accumulation of mononuclear inflammatory cells in this zone and in the stoma of the hepatic venules (eFig. 2-30B). Progression of the lesion is marked by scattered necrosis of a widening zone of centrilobular hepatocytes, disorganization, vacuolation because of fatty change, and accumulation of ceroid pigment in macrophages. Moderate centrilobular fibrosis is seen in later stages, as well as pronounced canalicular cholestasis. By this stage, affected animals begin to show icterus, inappetance, and depression. Bile ductular proliferation is not a marked feature. Death is attended by the usual signs of hepatoencephalopathy and tendency to bleed spontaneously. There is no evidence of direct neurologic damage as is seen in horses. More recently, dogs ingesting canned commercial camel meat developed serious and sometimes fatal liver disease. This may be a concern for dogs with food allergies that are fed nonstandard protein sources in special diets.

This intoxication is remarkable by virtue of its unpredictability. Experimental intoxication by pure indospicine has validly been shown to reproduce the naturally occurring intoxication caused by horsemeat feeding; however, liver failure can be produced by either means in only a small proportion of dogs so exposed. On the other hand, milder degrees of liver damage are reliably produced by both methods. Thus it seems an idiosyncratic response is superimposed upon a more consistent effect of the toxin; the nature of the accompanying inflammatory response suggests that the former may be immunologically mediated. This has yet to be established, as has the proposal that the mechanism of the intoxication is the result of competitive inhibition of arginine.

Senna (Cassia) occidentalis

Ingestion of large amounts of seeds from *Senna occidentalis* in the family *Leguminosae* can produce acute hepatic necrosis in cattle, pigs, goats, and horses. Hepatic injury is characterized by lesions ranging from vacuolation, to scattered apoptosis and centrilobular necrosis. In all species, except for horses, there is significant cardiac and skeletal muscle injury and myoglobinuria that are the predominant lesions, rather than hepatic injury. The toxic agent is not known currently.

Trifolium hybridum (alsike clover)

Alsike clover is a legume that grows well on wet clay soils in North America, where it is sometimes responsible for outbreaks or single cases of *cholangitis in horses* that consume it as pasture or hay. *The toxic principle has not been isolated,* but it likely is in highest concentrations in the flowering stage used for hay. However, there are evidently contributing factors because, although alsike clover is widespread in cultivation, *toxicity is rare.* Toxicity usually occurs when alsike clover is a

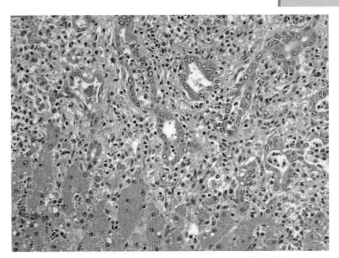

Figure 2-102 Chronic cholangiohepatitis caused by **alsike clover poisoning** in a horse.

major component of pastures or hay, but some horses are believed to graze it selectively in a mixed pasture.

Clinical signs of poisoning initially include mild colic, ill-thrift, and anorexia, with increasing occurrence of signs of hepatotoxicity with cholestasis. In some there can be icterus and photodynamic dermatitis. Exposure to the plant can occur for a year or more before signs of hepatic insufficiency develop, but cholestatic liver disease can be detected biochemically before horses become ill. More severely affected horses display neurologic disturbances, either excitement or mania in irregular episodes, or long periods of extreme dullness, anorexia, apparent blindness, forced wandering, head pushing, and yawning. Clinical problems related to hypoproteinemia, such as coagulopathy or ascites, are not a feature of this disease, probably because most of the hepatocytes are not directly affected.

The lesions of alsike clover poisoning are those of *diffuse subacute to chronic biliary hyperplasia (ductular reaction) and fibrosis,* with the major lesions within and adjacent to all intrahepatic biliary tracts (Fig. 2-102). The liver may be enlarged, sometimes greatly so, or shrunken, pale, and tough or rubbery in consistency. The surface is smooth, but its appearance is mottled. The mottling is clear on the cut surface and is caused by bands of gray fibrous tissue, distinctly visible to the naked eye, surrounding and compressing each lobule. Near the margins of the liver and in some other areas, scar tissue may completely replace the parenchyma. Areas of parenchymal atrophy may occur upstream of some occluded ducts. Microscopically, there is pronounced proliferation of fibrous tissue in and around the portal tracts associated with hyperplasia of well-formed bile ducts (ductular reaction). Some areas have prominent neutrophil infiltration into ducts, but in many areas this does not occur. In the early stages, the proliferation of bile ducts is often greater than the proliferation of the fibrous tissue, but later the proportions are reversed. The proliferating tissue extends slowly to connect adjacent portal triads, circumscribing areas that correspond to conventional lobules. The fibrous tissue does not permeate along the sinusoids, and there is gradual and uniform constriction of the parenchyma.

The distribution of liver lesions suggests that the harmful factor in alsike clover is excreted into the bile in a form that damages the ducts. However, the biliary proliferation and fibrosis is similar to that observed in areas of the liver that are drained by chronically obstructed bile ducts, so it seems likely some of the later changes are secondary to cholestasis. Agents that interfere with bile excretion have the potential to interfere with elimination of various potentially injurious substances. Thus it is possible that alsike clover ingestion might increase toxicity of other factors in the forage.

Tephrosia cinerea

Tephrosia cinerea is a member of the *Leguminosae* family and is found in Brazil. Prolonged ingestion causes chronic liver disease characterized clinically by wasting, and dramatic ascites in affected sheep. Hydrothorax and hydropericardium can also be present. Livers are pale with multiple small, ~1-mm diameter nodules. The livers are firm, and there is gallbladder edema. Histologically, there is portal fibrosis and biliary hyperplasia that is typically more severe in the subcapsular region. Most hepatocytes are enlarged because of vacuolation. Scattered individual necrotic cells are present, and focally, there is evidence of bile stasis. Inflammation is modest.

Brassica rapa

Turnip *(Brassica rapa)* or other *Brassica* family forage ingestion by cattle on the North Island of New Zealand is incriminated as a cause of hepatogenous photosensitization and biliary injury. The injury can mimic sporidesmin toxicity clinically with elevated γ-glutamyl transferase (GGT) and phytoporphyrin plasma levels. Histologically, bile ducts of smaller caliber than those injured by sporidesmin may be affected following turnip forage ingestion.

Copper

The heavy-metal copper is an essential trace element that plays an important role in numerous essential biological processes, including mitochondrial respiration (cytochrome C oxidase), connective-tissue maturation cross-linking (lysyl oxidase), antioxidant defense (superoxide dismutase), melanin synthesis (tyrosinase), iron metabolism (ceruloplasmin), and neurotransmitter biosynthesis (dopamine β hydroxylase). However, *copper is toxic at excess concentrations because of its 2 redox states that can mediate free-radical production, resulting in direct oxidation of cellular components.* The liver is the major organ involved in the regulation of copper levels, and homeostasis is maintained by the balance of dietary intake and copper excretion via the bile. Dietary copper is taken up by the enterocytes of the small intestine by dedicated transporters, divalent metal transporter (DMT1) and copper transporter 1 (Ctr1), and conveyed in the portal blood bound to carrier proteins ceruloplasmin and transcuprein, or in a non-specific fashion to albumin, to the liver for uptake. In the hepatocyte, copper is sequestered in metallothionein or glutathione. Excretion into the bile or blood is regulated by a series of specific chaperone proteins, such as the copper-transporting ATPase ATP7A. Excess copper is stored in lysosomes. Copper-induced injury is produced by oxidative processes that initially reduce available glutathione and eventually damages lipids, proteins, and nucleic acids. Cellular metabolism, structural integrity, and energy generation are affected. *Hepatic copper toxicosis can result from a primary metabolic defect in hepatic copper metabolism, altered hepatic biliary excretion of copper, or from excess dietary intake of the element.*

There is significant variation in species susceptibility to copper toxicosis. Sheep as a species are most prone to copper poisoning, because of reduced biliary excretion of copper. Some sheep breeds are more susceptible than others, reflecting differences in the efficiency of intestinal absorption of copper, rather than differences in efficiency of biliary excretion. Altered biliary excretion of copper in sheep does not appear to be associated with alteration in the structure or expression of the gene for ATP7B, the copper transporting P-type ATPase that is defective in Wilson disease, the human autosomal recessive disorder of hepatic copper metabolism.

Excessive hepatic copper accumulation is important in chronic hepatitis in dogs, and is discussed in further detail in the section Chronic hepatitis in dogs.

In cases of chronic hepatitis caused by copper accumulation, the liver is usually small, often with an accentuated lobular pattern; severely affected livers are characterized by architectural distortion, which ranges from a coarsely nodular texture to an end-stage liver. Chronic hepatitis, depending on the duration of inflammation and injury, is characterized by portal and periportal mononuclear cell inflammation and fibrosis of portal areas that may extend into adjacent periportal areas of the lobule, leading to the prominent lobular pattern. Small aggregates of pigmented macrophages, containing copper and lipofuscin, surrounded by mononuclear inflammatory cells are a reliable feature of copper excess. With progression, hyperplastic nodules and bridging fibrosis develop.

In dogs and sheep, toxic amounts of copper can accumulate in the liver, although dietary copper levels are not excessive by standards for other species. Copper poisoning does occur in cattle and pigs, but in these species, it is because of abnormally high intake of the element. Acute copper poisoning can occur following either the ingestion or injection of excess copper, and *animals deficient in vitamin E or molybdenum appear especially susceptible to acute copper poisoning.*

Chronic copper toxicosis in sheep occurs as a result of the presence of 3 environmental factors acting alone or in concert. First, *excessive copper intake* may occur as a result of contamination of water (naturally occurring or through the use of copper piping or fixtures), pasture or prepared feed; the latter is difficult to avoid when feed mills are preparing rations for different species and is probably partly responsible for the observation that housed sheep are more prone to copper poisoning than animals at pasture. Second, increased copper accumulation occurs as a result of increased availability of dietary copper; this happens when *dietary levels of molybdenum are unusually low.* Molybdenum, in the presence of sufficient sulfate, forms insoluble complexes with copper in the gut and liver, making the copper biologically inert. Subterranean clover growing on calcareous soils in southern Australia may be relatively deficient in molybdenum, and in these areas, British breeds of sheep are known to be more susceptible than Merinos to chronic copper poisoning. *Other hepatotoxins* constitute the third environmental factor that predisposes sheep to outbreaks of chronic copper poisoning. The most important of these are pyrrolizidine alkaloids (from *Heliotropium* or *Echium*) in eastern Australia, and phomopsin from lupins in western Australia and, possibly, South Africa.

The basis for chronic copper poisoning in sheep is the peculiar avidity of the liver for copper, coupled with the very limited rate at which this species can excrete the element in the bile. After intraportal injection of a copper isotope, practically all the radioactivity is removed during the first passage through the liver. Most of the copper is sequestered in hepatocellular lysosomes, where it does little damage at concentrations of up to 200-300 µg/g dry weight. As the concentration rises, there is presumably more interaction between other cell components and the copper. There is some evidence that lysosomal membranes lose integrity and allow copper and lysosomal hydrolases to damage the rest of the cytoplasm. By the time the liver copper concentration has reached 300 µg/g or more, there is a histologically apparent increase in hepatocellular turnover, with single hepatocytes undergoing apoptosis within a dense knot of neutrophils. At still higher copper levels, the apoptotic rate increases, while all cells become swollen and their nuclei vesicular. The mitotic rate increases, presumably to keep pace with the accelerated loss of hepatocytes, and large macrophages appear in the sinusoids and stromal spaces about the vessels. These cells contain eosinophilic or somewhat brown, granular debris, which consists of copper-containing lipofuscins.

Sheep with liver copper concentrations >1,000 µg/g may be clinically and hematologically normal, so long as the increasing mitotic rate produces enough new hepatocytes to take up the copper released by dying cells. At this stage, however, there will be elevated levels of liver-specific enzymes in the plasma. If the rate of hepatocellular loss exceeds the capacity of the liver to phagocytose and sequester cell debris quickly, the plasma copper levels can rise to levels that are high enough to damage circulating erythrocytes, and intravascular hemolysis ensues. *The effect of the hemolysis and anemia on the liver is to accelerate the rate of hepatocellular necrosis; thus copper enters the circulation at an increasing rate and acute copper toxic crisis is manifest.* The lethal clinical syndrome is then one of *paroxysmal intravascular hemolysis and liver failure,* in which a sheep may pass from apparent good health to death within ~6 hours. Stresses, such as brief starvation, may also precipitate the crisis in susceptible sheep, but the mechanisms involved are unknown. During the hemolytic crisis, some of the copper is lost from the disintegrating liver; some passes into the urine, and kidney copper concentration rises to 1,000 µg/g or more. *Blood or kidney copper levels* therefore give a truer indication of a prior hemolytic crisis caused by chronic copper poisoning than does elevation of liver copper alone.

The *gross lesions* of fatal chronic copper poisoning are those of acute copper toxicity. The carcass is discolored by marked icterus, superimposed on which is the red color imparted by free hemoglobin. Often, there is a brown hue as well, because a proportion of the hemoglobin is oxidized to methemoglobin. The spleen is engorged, dark, and soft. The kidneys are deep red-brown to black and the urine deep red, as a result of hemoglobinuria with oxidation to methemoglobin, and concurrent icterus. The liver is often slightly soft and swollen, and deep orange, but if the condition arises after long-term liver injury, atrophy and fibrosis may be evident. The spectrum of liver lesions can be complicated by other causes of liver necrosis, including hypoxia caused by anemia, heart failure, and shock.

A breed of sheep from the Hebridean island of North Ronaldsay has apparently adapted to a seaweed diet low in both copper and molybdenum but rich in zinc. *Zinc is also capable of interfering with copper uptake,* and these sheep, although avoiding copper deficiency, are exquisitely susceptible to chronic copper poisoning when transferred to normal pasture. Hepatic disease associated with copper toxicity in this breed appears to differ morphologically from other domesticated sheep breeds. Copper accumulation begins in periportal hepatocytes, accompanied by a mixed inflammatory infiltrate and cholangiolar proliferation. Characteristic pericellular fibrosis, initially confined to the portal tracts and periportal zones, later extends to diffuse fibrosis and cirrhosis, associated ultrastructurally with numerous hepatic stellate cells. North Ronaldsay sheep have been proposed as a possible animal model for human non-Wilsonian hepatic copper toxicosis and cirrhosis of infancy, and for investigation of copper-associated hepatic fibrogenesis.

The events described in sheep also occur in **chronic copper poisoning in pigs and cattle,** and acute intravascular hemolysis may be seen, especially in calves. Usually, however, there is less of the acute terminal chain reaction in these species, and there is more evidence of chronic liver damage with extensive portal fibrosis and biliary hyperplasia within the triads.

Acute copper poisoning *is most often seen in ruminants after accidental administration of single large doses of copper,* by either the oral or parenteral routes. Iatrogenic copper toxicosis has been induced by administering copper oxide boluses to neonatal calves, and by injection with copper disodium edetate in weanling calves. Doses of 20-100 mg/kg can produce acute poisoning in sheep. Copper toxicosis has also been reported in veal calves fed milk replacer supplemented with various copper-containing hematinics. Affected animals develop severe gastroenteritis, abdominal pain, diarrhea, and dehydration. The liver lesion varies with chronicity of exposure, from nonspecific acute centrilobular necrosis, to cholangiohepatitis with periportal fibrosis. Intravascular hemolysis may occur if plasma copper levels are sufficiently elevated.

Acute bovine liver disease

Acute bovine liver disease is a poorly understood entity that occurs in southern Australia. Outbreaks occur primarily in the spring and the autumn, and all ages of cattle can be affected. Sudden death or photosensitization may occur. There is an association with ingestion of *Cynosurus echinatus* (rough dog's tail). The characteristic histologic lesion involves a periportal hepatocellular necrosis with bile duct proliferation (eFig. 2-31). The presence of mycotoxin(s) produced by the fungus *Dreschlera biseptata* growing in some plants has been suggested to be the principal toxicant or cofactor in the syndrome.

Further reading

Aslani MR, et al. In vitro detection of hepatocytotoxic metabolites from *Drechslera biseptata*: a contributing factor to acute bovine liver disease? Aust J Exper Agric 2006;46:599-604.

Bandarra PM, et al. *Trema micrantha* toxicity in horses in Brazil. Equine Vet J 2010;42:456-459.

Brum KB, et al. Intoxication by *Vernonia rubricaulis* in cattle in Mato Grosso do Sul. Pesq Vet Bras 2002;22:119-128.

Cerqueira VD, et al. Colic caused by *Panicum maximum* toxicosis in *Equidae* in northern Brazil. J Vet Diagn Invest 2009;21:882-888.

Cesar ASJ, et al. Toxic hepatopathy in sheep associated with the ingestion of the legume *Tephrosia cinerea*. J Vet Diagn Invest 2007;19:690-694.

Collett MG. Bile duct lesions associated with turnip (*Brassica rapa*) photosensitization compared with those due to sporidesmin toxicosis in dairy cows. Vet Pathol 2014;51:986-991.

Collett MG, et al. Photosensitisation, crystal-associated cholangiohep-atopathy, and acute renal tubular necrosis in calves following inges-tion of *Phytolacca octandra* (inkweed). N Z Vet J 2011;59:147-152.

Cruz C, et al. Experimentally induced cholangiohepatopathy by dosing sheep with fractionated extracts from *Brachiaria decumbens*. J Vet Diagn Invest 2001;13:170-172.

Ferguson D, et al. Survival and prognostic indicators for cycad intoxica-tion in dogs. J Vet Intern Med 2011;25:831-837.

Fu PP, et al. Pyrrolizidine alkaloids—genotoxicity, metabolism enzymes, metabolic activation, and mechanisms. Drug Metab Rev 2004;36:1-55.

Garcia AF, et al. Comparative effects of lantadene A and its reduced metabolite on mitochondrial bioenergetics. Toxicon 2010;55:1331-1337.

Haywood S, et al. The greater susceptibility of North Ronaldsay sheep compared with Cambridge sheep to copper-induced oxidative stress, mitochondrial damage and hepatic stellate cell activation. J Comp Pathol 2005;133:114-127.

Lockhart PJ, et al. Cloning, mapping and expression analysis of the sheep Wilson disease gene homologue. Biochim Biophys Acta 2000;1491:229-239.

Oelrichs PB, et al. Isolation and identification of the toxic peptides from *Lophyrotoma zonalis* (Pergidae) sawfly larvae. Toxicon 2001;39:1933-1936.

Oliveira-Filho JP, et al. Hepatoencephalopathy syndrome due to *Cassia occidentalis (Leguminosae, Caesalpinioideae)* seed ingestion in horses. Equine Vet J 2013;45:240-244.

Quinn JC, et al. Secondary plant products causing photosensitization in grazing herbivores: Their structure, activity and regulation. Int J Mol Sci 2014;15:1441-1465.

Simola O, et al. Pathologic findings and toxin identification in cyano-bacterial *(Nodularia spumigena)* intoxication in a dog. Vet Pathol 2012;49:755-759.

Stegelmeier BL. Pyrrolizidine alkaloid–containing toxic plants (*Senecio, Crotalaria, Cynoglossum, Amsinckia, Heliotropium,* and *Echium* spp.). Vet Clin North Am Food Anim Pract 2011;27:419-428.

Tan ET, et al. Determination of hepatotoxic indospicine in Australian camel meat by ultra-performance liquid chromatography-tandem mass spectrometry. J Agric Food Chem 2014;62:1974-1979.

Thiel C, et al. The enterohepatic circulation of amanitin: kinetics and therapeutic implications. Toxicol Lett 2011;203:142-146.

Tokarz D, et al. Amanitin toxicosis in two cats with acute hepatic and renal failure. Vet Pathol 2012;49:1032-1035.

Voss KA, Riley RT. Fumonisin toxicity and mechanism of action: over-view and current perspectives. Food Safety 2013;1:2013006-2013006.

Wisløff H, et al. Accumulation of sapogenin conjugates and histologi-cal changes in the liver and kidneys of lambs suffering from alveld, a hepatogenous photosensitization disease of sheep grazing *Narthecium ossifragum*. Vet Res Commun 2002;26:381-396.

HYPERPLASTIC AND NEOPLASTIC LESIONS OF THE LIVER AND BILE DUCTS

Remarkably, *the occurrence of fatal liver malignancies is rather uncommon in aged dogs and cats;* this suggests that they are either less exposed, or they are more resistant to the etiologic agents responsible for liver neoplasms in humans. Domestic species are not subject to significant chronic oncogenic viral infections, such as the hepatitis B and hepatitis C viruses that account for the majority of human hepatocellular carcinoma.

Ectopic, metaplastic, and hyperplastic lesions

Ectopic and metaplastic lesions in the gallbladder have been reported. Ectopic tissue includes hepatocyte nodules attached to or within the wall, and pancreatic islands, which may include islets of Langerhans. Gastric ectopia, readily distin-guishable by the presence of chief and parietal cells, may form plaques or large polyps. Ectopia of cardiac or pyloric mucosa is mimicked by metaplastic changes.

Nodular hyperplasia of hepatocytes is common in old dogs, but rare in other species. The lesions in dogs do not have a breed or sex predisposition, but their incidence increases sharply with age. Hyperplastic nodules typically develop in livers of normal mass, whereas **regenerative nodules** arise as a result of compensatory hyperplasia of surviving hepatocytes in a background of hepatic injury, atrophy, and fibrosis (see Responses of the liver to injury).

Nodular hyperplasia often occurs as multiple randomly distributed masses throughout the lobes. The grossly visible nodules are spherical, well circumscribed, varying in size from 2 mm to 3 cm or more, and may bulge from the capsular surface or be entirely hidden within the parenchyma (Fig. 2-103). They may be sharply distinct from the surrounding parenchyma because of color differences, either lighter than the surrounding liver because of increased lipid or glycogen content within hepatocytes comprising the nodule, or darker because the sinusoidal vessels are distended with blood. Some nodules are the same color as the surrounding tissue and can only be identified by examination of a washed or blotted slice under a strong light.

The larger hyperplastic nodules grow expansively; they do not induce a fibrous capsule, but they can compress the sur-rounding parenchyma. The hepatocytes comprising nodular hyperplasia are often phenotypically different from those in adjacent parenchyma (Fig. 2-104). Old canine livers often have microscopic focal hyperplasia of similarly altered hepa-tocytes that can be distinguished from the surrounding paren-chyma, but they evidently grow more slowly and do not compress their boundaries. These can be regarded as examples of the numerous atypical focal hyperplasias that arise as altered foci, nodules, plaques, or polyps in various tissues of old dogs. In more prominent paler nodules, hepatocytes can be enlarged and vacuolated with lipid or glycogen accumula-tion. Mitotic figures are uncommon. The sinusoids of the

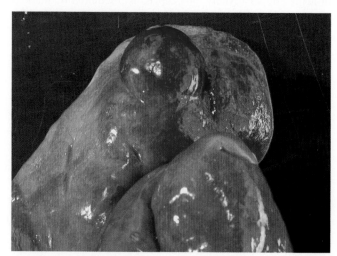

Figure 2-103 Nodular hyperplasia in the liver of a dog.

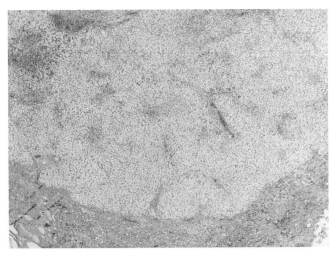

Figure 2-104 Nodular hyperplasia in the liver of a dog. These nodules have a discrete border with adjacent parenchyma and often are vacuolated.

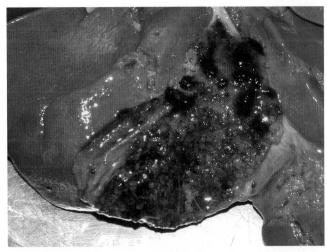

Figure 2-105 Cystic mucinous hyperplasia of the mucosa of the gallbladder in a dog.

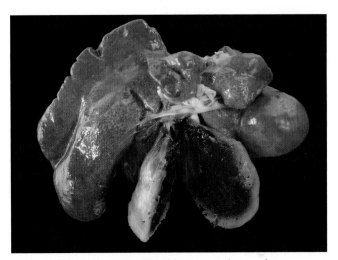

Figure 2-106 Gallbladder mucocele in a dog.

nodules are often dilated, and foci of hematopoiesis are occasionally observed. Necrosis and hemorrhage in hyperplastic nodules are rare.

The significance of hyperplastic nodules in old dogs is usually negligible. After acute liver necrosis, these atypical hepatocytes within pre-existing hyperplastic foci and nodules may have phenotypic alterations that confer a survival advantage, and can survive and flourish as larger nodules amid regions of necrosis, so in these instances, they can be beneficial. Although hyperplastic nodules rarely progress to lesions with detrimental impact, they are often found during liver imaging, laparotomy, or biopsy and need to be differentiated from other focal lesions of more significance. Because they are atypically differentiated, they are the potential source of secreted products of clinical or diagnostic significance, but their potential in this regard is unexplored. *The hallmark of nodular hyperplasia, in contrast to the hepatic adenoma and hepatocellular carcinoma, is that it largely retains normal liver architecture, including a modified lobular structure with recognizable central veins and portal triads.* However, this feature may be difficult to appreciate in small biopsies. The biological distinction between atypical hyperplasia and neoplasia is sometimes equivocal; in the latter, continued growth that is independent of promoting influences is responsible for enlargement, and the designation of adenoma should apply to lesions that are enlarging.

Cystic mucinous hyperplasia *of the mucus-producing glands in the mucosa of the gallbladder* has been reported as an incidental lesion in dogs and sheep. These cystic hyperplastic nodules are often numerous, may be sessile or polypoid, and contain mucin (Fig. 2-105).

Dilation of the gallbladder with accumulated mucoid secretion **(gallbladder mucocele)** has been reported in dogs and infrequently in cats. Histologically, affected gallbladders display proliferated mucosa with characteristic projecting fronds of epithelium that extend into the lumen of the gallbladder, as well as formation of mucus-filled cysts. Severely affected gallbladders are distended with abnormal semisolid accumulations of mucus or other secretions, and the wall may undergo ischemic necrosis and rupture (Fig. 2-106). Bile-laden mucus may also extend into the cystic, hepatic, and common bile ducts, resulting in variable degrees of extrahepatic biliary obstruction. The etiology of this condition is unknown, and

may be related to decreased gallbladder motility, bile stasis, and altered bile composition and viscosity.

Mucosal hyperplasia in the large bile ducts is frequently observed in the long-standing mild cholangiohepatitis of fluke infestation. The hyperplasia is of microscopic dimensions, but in some instances, it appears histologically to be atypical. Localized, polypoid foci of cystic hyperplasia are specific changes in cattle poisoned by highly chlorinated naphthalene.

Hepatocellular tumors

Primary epithelial neoplasms of the liver include tumors of either hepatocellular or cholangiocellular origin, and they are uncommon in most species, representing <1% of all neoplasms in cats and dogs. Pot-bellied pigs are a possible exception. *Proportionately, hepatocellular neoplasms are more common in dogs, whereas cholangiocellular tumors predominate in cats.* Unlike the situation in humans, there are no clear associations in domestic animals between hepatocellular tumors and viruses, chemical carcinogens, mycotoxins, or drugs, such as synthetic steroids. With the exception of the occasional association of liver tumors with certain flukes or tapeworm larvae, and the rare adenoma seen in the bovine liver with chronic pyrrolizidine poisoning, *hepatobiliary tumors in domestic*

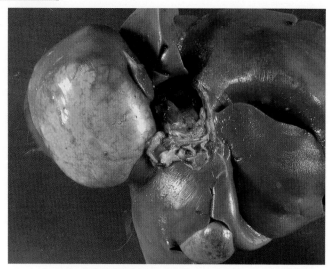

Figure 2-107 Hepatocellular adenoma in a dog.

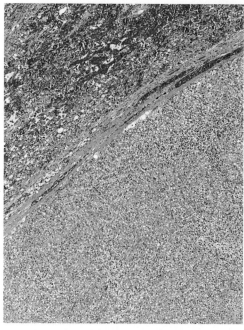

Figure 2-108 Histologic appearance of a canine **hepatocellular adenoma.** Compression of the adjacent parenchyma is apparent, and a capsule is evident at this site.

animals are not obvious successors to recognized antecedent liver diseases.

Hepatocellular adenomas are benign neoplasms of hepatocytes. Hepatocellular adenomas are reported in dogs, cats, cattle, sheep, and pigs, but likely occur in all species. They are rarely of any clinical significance. Hepatocellular adenomas are typically solitary, but they can be multiple. They range from 2-12 cm in diameter and are roughly spherical masses. Typically, they are well demarcated from the adjacent parenchyma because of the compression caused by their expanding growth, but not encapsulated. Hepatocellular adenomas often bulge from the capsular surface, or they can be pedunculated, and in some instances, they may be found entirely within the hepatic parenchyma. The color of hepatocellular adenomas varies from yellow-brown to dark mahogany red. Paler adenomas contain lipid or glycogen, and these lesions often have a soft and friable consistency compared to normal liver (Fig. 2-107).

Histologically, the hepatocytes in hepatic adenomas do not differ markedly from normal hepatocytes or those in hyperplastic nodules, and often contain lipid, glycogen, or occasionally protein secretory vacuoles. Minimal anisocytosis and increased basophilia of the cytoplasm and prominence of nucleoli can be seen, but mitotic figures are uncommon. *Cells are arranged in cords or trabeculae that may be several cells thick, but the width tends to be consistent. There is a discrete well-defined border with adjacent parenchyma* (Fig. 2-108). *Adenomas lack normal lobular architecture.* Essentially all of the blood supplying adenomas comes from the hepatic artery. As a consequence, rather than portal tracts, isolated arteries, bile ducts, and hepatic veins can be found coursing through the mass. *Usually, no more than a single portal tract may be present, likely entrapped by the expanding hepatocyte population.* Extramedullary hematopoietic foci may sometimes be found in the adenomas, as well as ectatic vascular spaces. Focal necrosis may occur.

Hepatocellular carcinomas are uncommon, but occur in all veterinary species; they may be single and massive, nodular or diffuse. Several features suggest malignancy, including the absence of pedunculation or clear demarcation from the adjacent parenchyma and the presence of varied coloration of the cut surface produced by hemorrhage and necrosis (eFig. 2-32). *Venous invasion is typical of the hepatocellular tumors,* and

intravascular spread may extend to the large hepatic veins and vena cava. Carcinomas occasionally penetrate the capsule to implant on the peritoneum. Metastasis is uncommon in all domestic species but, when present, may be evident in the hepatic lymph node most often. Hematogenous metastases occur first in the lungs. Spontaneous rupture is common and may cause fatal blood loss. This consequence is a much more frequent cause of morbidity and mortality than metastatic disease. Some hepatocellular carcinomas in cattle are scirrhous, hard, and white. Paraneoplastic hypoglycemia may occur in animals with hepatocellular carcinoma.

Hepatocellular carcinomas may be quite variable in histologic appearance, and multiple patterns may occur within a single neoplasm. *Trabecular carcinomas are the most common histologic pattern* (Fig. 2-109). Neoplastic cells resemble normal liver, and grow in irregularly thick plates or trabeculae that vary from few to many cells thick. Necrosis may be present, and sinusoids may be dilated, and there may be large ectatic blood-filled spaces. Other patterns include *pseudoglandular (adenoid) carcinomas,* characterized by lobular arrangement of neoplastic hepatocytes within scant connective-tissue stroma, and *solid carcinomas,* characterized by solid sheets of poorly differentiated, often pleomorphic cells that do not form sinusoids (Fig. 2-110A, B). A scirrhous variant has been described in dogs, characterized by multiple foci of cytokeratin 19-positive ductular structures embedded in abundant fibrous stroma (Fig. 2-111A, B). A feature of some hepatocellular tumors is the presence of giant cells, quite conspicuous by virtue of a large nucleus, multilobed nuclei, or multiple nuclei. Mitotic figures are more frequent in carcinomas than adenomas, but may not be a prominent feature of well-differentiated carcinomas. Immunohistochemical staining using antibodies that bind a hepatocyte specific antigen, HepPar1, identifies a large proportion of canine and feline hepatocellular carcinomas. However, more aggressive forms of canine hepatocellular carcinoma may not stain with HepPar1, but instead >5% of

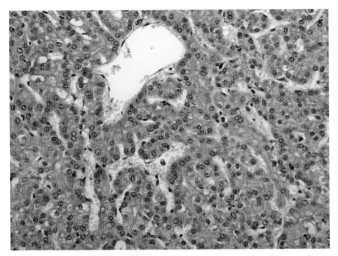

Figure 2-109 **Trabecular hepatocellular carcinoma** from a dog.

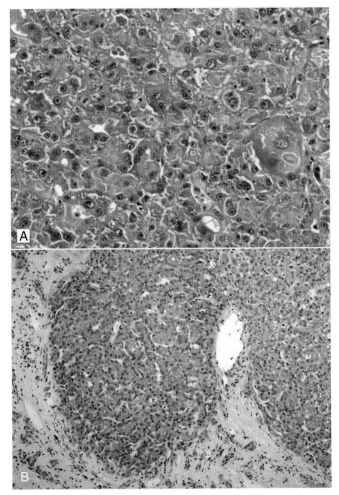

Figure 2-110 **A.** A **solid pattern** in a poorly differentiated **hepatocellular carcinoma** from a dog. **B.** Invasion at the margin of a hepatocellular carcinoma in the liver of a dog.

the cells can be stained with antibodies that recognize cytokeratin 19, a marker of hepatic progenitor cells, immature hepatocytes, and biliary epithelial cells. These canine hepatocellular carcinomas have an aggressive growth pattern, including a markedly increased incidence of intrahepatic and extrahepatic metastasis.

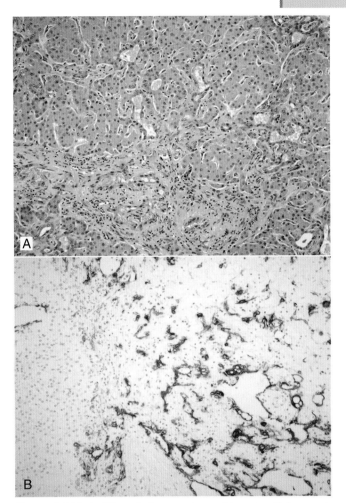

Figure 2-111 **A.** The **scirrhous variant of hepatocellular carcinoma** has areas of ductular proliferation and abundant connective tissue within areas of neoplastic hepatocytes. **B.** Ductular structures staining with cytokeratin 19.

Hepatoblastomas, rare benign tumors putatively originating from primitive hepatic precursor cells, have been reported most often in horses, but also in sheep, dogs, cats, and a llama. Hepatoblastomas in humans are neoplasms of infancy and childhood. Cases in domestic species have been reported in both young and adult animals, but are most frequently reported in foals. Hepatoblastomas are typically single, firm, lobulated masses with areas of necrosis and hemorrhage. Compression of adjacent parenchyma is evident and, on occasion, invasion can be seen. The histologic patterns of hepatoblastomas can be epithelial, either fetal or embryonal, or mixed epithelial and mesenchymal. *Fetal hepatoblastomas* are composed of large, polygonal cells, approximately the size of adult hepatocytes, with round to oval nuclei and granular to vacuolated, eosinophilic to amphophilic cytoplasm (Fig. 2-112A). *Embryonal hepatoblastomas* form ribbons or rosettes of smaller basophilic cells with scant cytoplasm (Fig. 2-112B). *Mixed epithelial-mesenchymal hepatoblastomas* contain variable amounts of fibrous connective tissue or other mesenchymal tissues, including cartilage or bone, in addition to epithelial cells. Combinations of these patterns are common. Portal tracts are absent. Immunohistochemical staining for α-fetoprotein is typically positive, and HepPar-1 staining is

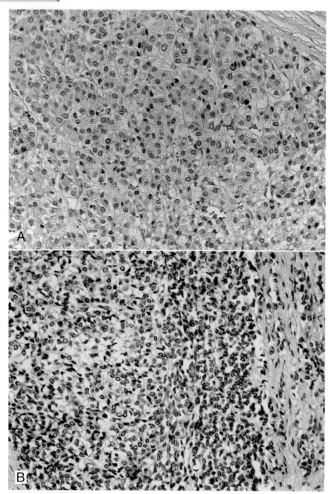

Figure 2-112 A. Hepatoblastoma with a **fetal pattern** from a foal. **B.** Hepatoblastoma with an **embryonal pattern** from a foal.

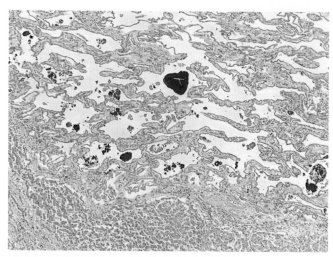

Figure 2-113 Biliary adenomas are composed of uniform arrays of well-differentiated biliary epithelium forming uniform small tubules.

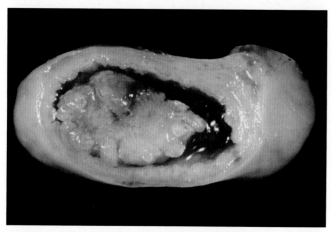

Figure 2-114 Gallbladder adenoma in a dog. (Courtesy J. Tobias.)

usually absent, supporting the view that they arise from precursor cells.

Cholangiocellular tumors

Cholangiocellular adenomas are uncommon benign neoplasms of biliary epithelium. Cholangiocellular adenomas are usually solitary, pale gray to white, and well-circumscribed roughly spherical masses that tend to grow by expansion. They may distend the normal outline of the liver, although they can occur as intrahepatic masses. Cholangiocellular adenomas are composed of tubules lined with a single layer of well-differentiated biliary epithelium and a moderate amount of intervening stroma. The tubules may have narrow lumens, and there can be variable amounts of stroma within the mass (Fig. 2-113). Adjacent hepatocytes are usually compressed at the margins, but are not found between tubules. The tubules contain a clear watery to viscous fluid. Cuboidal or flattened neoplastic biliary epithelial cells have a moderate amount of pale eosinophilic cytoplasm. Nuclei are round to oval, vesicular, and oriented centrally. Nucleoli are small or inapparent. There are typically no mitotic figures.

Extrahepatic cholangiocellular adenomas are rare, with the exception of gallbladder adenomas reported in abattoir surveys of cattle and rarely in domestic carnivores (Fig. 2-114). The smaller specimens may be solid on cut surface and white, but the large specimens, and many of the small ones, are cystic.

Lesions formerly termed *biliary cystadenomas,* a subtype commonly seen in cats and occasionally in dogs, are most likely developmental anomalies of the embryonal biliary tree, termed **ductal plate anomalies,** which is more clearly appreciated when biliary cysts are coincident with cystic renal developmental lesions, although either lesion may occur independently. The ductal plate anomalies can be multilocular and lined by bile duct epithelia that may be flattened by pressure, or in some areas papillary. The septal stroma is collagenous. Their development later in life may be the result of progressive secretion by the lining epithelial cells, creating cysts only when sufficient fluid has been produced. Entrapped hepatocytes are often present.

Cholangiocarcinomas (cholangiocellular carcinomas) are reported in dogs, cats, sheep, cattle, horses, and goats. Affected livers are usually otherwise normal, with no suggestion as to an underlying cause, although there are associations with chronic fluke infestations in humans and rarely in carnivores.

Cholangiocellular tumors can usually be distinguished from the hepatocellular variety by their multiplicity, firmness, pale beige color produced by more or less abundant stroma, and the typical umbilicate appearance of those that involve the capsule (Fig. 2-115). The central depressed area can be the result of necrosis or cavitation-associated collapse of tumor vessels in the

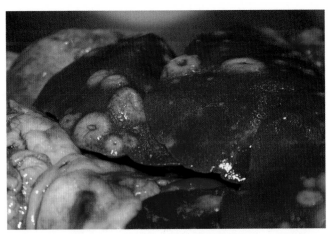

Figure 2-115 A cholangiocarcinoma in the liver of a dog. **Umbilication** is prominent. (Courtesy J.L. Caswell.)

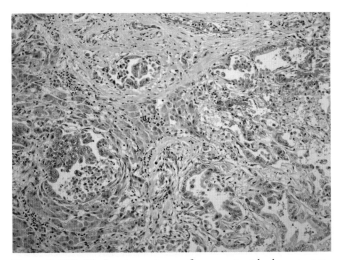

Figure 2-116 **Cholangiocarcinoma** from a cat with characteristic crude acini and tubules separated by abundant connective tissue.

central parts of the tumor nodules. Even multiple nodules may not cause much enlargement of the liver. In dogs and cats, the tumors are almost always multiple or diffuse. The multiple nodules of tumor might represent intrahepatic lymphogenous metastases, but the possibility of multicentric origin must be entertained. Hematogenous metastases are unusual, but metastases to the regional nodes are common. In cats especially, there is a tendency to invade Glisson's capsule and implant on the peritoneum; the diffuse variety may cause great enlargement, although with retention of shape.

Microscopically, cholangiocellular carcinomas form ductules and acini, and sometimes papillary formations within the lumen of the neoplastic ducts (Fig. 2-116). The cells are cuboidal or columnar, with a small amount of clear or slightly granular cytoplasm. The nuclei are small and fairly uniform, and nucleoli are not prominent. Mitotic figures are often abundant. The tubules do not contain bile, but in well-differentiated specimens may contain mucins. The epithelial components are separated by fibrous connective-tissue stroma, which may have pronounced collagen deposition, the so-called *scirrhous response* that gives the tumor a firm texture. In poorly differentiated cholangiocarcinomas, pleomorphic to anaplastic cells can be observed. It is not uncommon to encounter areas

of poorly differentiated cells within a mass that is predominantly well differentiated. *Cholangiocellular carcinomas have a highly invasive growth pattern*, and frequently metastasize to hepatic lymph nodes, lungs, and the peritoneal cavity.

Primary intrahepatic cholangiocellular carcinoma can be difficult, and often impossible, to distinguish from metastatic adenocarcinomas, especially those of pancreatic or mammary epithelial origin. Mucus secretion and intrasinusoidal permeation are more typical of biliary origin. Distinction from hepatocellular carcinoma of adenoid pattern may be assisted by demonstration of mucin, abundant mitotic figures, and presence of a prominent connective-tissue stroma.

Extrahepatic cholangiocellular carcinoma (or biliary cholangiocarcinoma) of the gallbladder or extrahepatic bile ducts is much less frequent than the intrahepatic form, but has been reported in dogs, cats, cattle, and swine.

Mixed hepatocellular and cholangiocellular carcinomas

Rare hepatic carcinomas have the histologic and cytologic characteristics of both hepatocellular carcinoma and cholangiocellular carcinoma. These tumors likely arise from bipotential hepatic progenitor cells. The hepatocytic nature of some tumor cells can be confirmed with the monoclonal antibody HepPar-1, and cells of biliary phenotype can be stained by immunohistochemistry using antibodies that bind to cytokeratin 7, a typical intermediate filament of biliary epithelium (Fig. 2-117A-C).

Hepatic carcinoids

Hepatic carcinoids, presumably arising from the diffuse neuroendocrine cell population found among the biliary epithelium and possibly within the hepatic parenchyma, have been reported in dogs, cats, and cattle. They may arise within the liver, in the extrahepatic bile ducts or within the gallbladder. The gross pathologic appearance of carcinoids is typically that of disseminated pale gray to tan small masses within the liver, but on some occasions, only a single mass is formed (eFig. 2-33). Like other neuroendocrine tumors, *hepatic carcinoids typically form nests of cells separated by a fine fibrovascular stroma*. The cells are oval to spindle shaped, and may form a rosette or pseudolobular pattern (Fig. 2-118). Mitotic figures are usually frequent. Argyrophilic cytoplasmic granules may be detected by silver impregnation stains; more precise identification of carcinoids may require immunohistochemical stains for neurosecretory products, such as neuron-specific enolase or serotonin. These are aggressive neoplasms, with frequent intrahepatic spread, and metastasis to local lymph nodes, peritoneum, and lung.

Mesodermal tumors

Primary mesenchymal tumors of the liver are quite uncommon. Of the mesenchymal tumors, primary **hemangiosarcomas** are likely the most frequent. Primary hepatic hemangiosarcomas occur in dogs, cats, cattle, and sheep. Hemangiosarcoma of the liver should always be considered metastatic until proven otherwise by diligent search. Some of these tumors are solitary, large, and gray-white, with scattered hemorrhagic areas, and others are ill defined and cavernous (Fig. 2-119). The latter may rupture into the peritoneal cavity to produce severe hemorrhage. Microscopically, hepatic hemangiosarcomas resemble those found in other sites; however, it may be impossible to find malignant cells in or lining cavernous areas. At

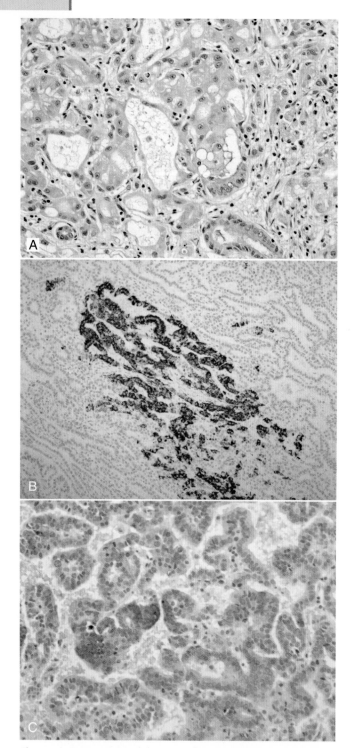

Figure 2-117 A. Mixed hepatocellular and biliary carcinomas contain neoplastic cell populations with both biliary and hepatocellular phenotypes. H&E. **B.** HepPar1-stained cells. **C.** Cytokeratin 7–stained cells.

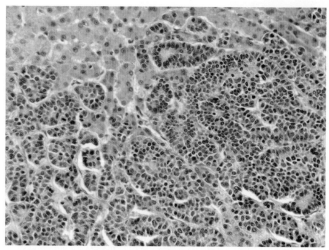

Figure 2-118 Hepatic carcinoid from a cat with characteristic islands and rosettes separated by fine fibrovascular stroma and characteristic invasive behavior.

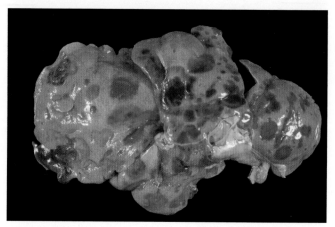

Figure 2-119 Hepatic **hemangiosarcoma** in the liver of a dog. Careful examination is required to distinguish primary from metastatic disease.

the margins of the tumor, there is a distinctive pattern or growth in which small, solid nodules of malignant cells may be found, or these cells can be found forming capillary structures or invading along pre-existing sinusoids. The latter phenomenon is particularly characteristic. As the cells invade along the sinusoids, perhaps in single file, they initially produce little distortion of the hepatic cords. Behind them, the sinusoids are spread widely apart, and individual hepatocytes or portions of cords are isolated and appear to be floating freely, surrounded by a thin layer of connective tissue and neoplastic cells. Differential diagnoses other than metastatic lesions include the syndrome of telangiectasia in Pembroke Welsh Corgi dogs, telangiectatic lesions in older animals, and vascular hamartomas in cattle. Hepatic **hemangiomas** have been reported in dogs and a pig.

Leiomyomas are occasionally observed in the gallbladder of dogs and cattle. **Leiomyosarcomas** and **fibrosarcomas** have been reported in the liver of cats and dogs, hemangiopericytoma and fibrosarcoma in cattle, and a single case of botryoid-type embryonal rhabdomyosarcoma in a cat. Other rare mesenchymal tumors reported in either dogs or cats include lymphangioma, plasmacytoma, osteosarcoma, nerve sheath tumor, liposarcoma, and chondrosarcoma.

The **myelolipoma** is an unusual tumor that develops in the livers of domestic cats and wild felids. The tumor develops as multiple growths, 0.5-5 cm diameter, in one or more lobes; if they project above the surface of the liver, they are irregularly nodular. Myelolipomas are friable, and yellow to orange because of their high fat content. The neoplasm is composed

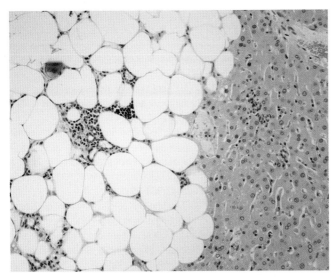

Figure 2-120 **Myelolipoma** of the liver of a dog.

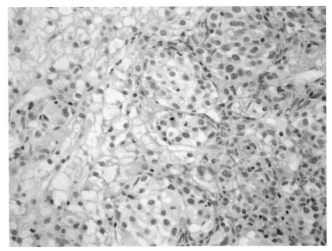

Figure 2-121 **Histiocytic sarcoma** in the liver of a dog.

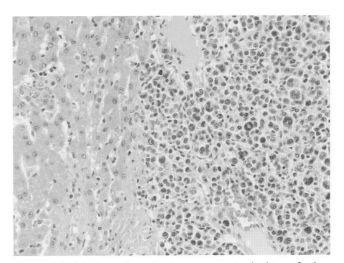

Figure 2-122 **Primary hepatic plasmacytoma** in the liver of a dog.

of normal-appearing, mature adipocytes with a variable admixture of myeloid cells, including both mature and immature cells of the granulocytic, erythrocytic, and megakaryocytic series (Fig. 2-120). In captive wild cats, similar lesions have been seen in the spleen. These were judged to be separate developments of the same process. Metastasis to other organs has not been reported.

Metastatic neoplasms

The liver is particularly "fertile soil," as metastatic lesions markedly outnumber primary hepatic neoplasms. Metastatic solid neoplasms may be multiple, but are usually not numerous and usually do not elicit clinical or biochemical evidence of hepatic injury or dysfunction. Malignancies arriving via the portal vein, such as pancreatic or gastric carcinoma or hemangiosarcomas, may practically replace the liver before producing clinical signs, one of which may be icterus caused either by extrahepatic bile duct obstruction, or by intrahepatic cholestasis, or both. In dogs, the most common metastatic hematopoietic, mesenchymal, and epithelial neoplasms are lymphoma, hemangiosarcoma, and pancreatic carcinoma, respectively. Some of the carcinomas (e.g., thyroid, mammary), melanoma, and sarcomas from more remote sites also metastasize to the liver via the lungs and hepatic artery, and some (e.g., ovarian carcinoma, mesothelioma) implant on the capsular surface from within the peritoneal cavity.

The hepatic perisinusoidal and periportal compartments are hospitable to various hematopoietic neoplastic cell types. Accordingly, malignant histiocytosis, myeloid and erythroid leukemias, and mast cell tumors often localize in the liver along hepatic sinusoids. Some lymphomas, histiocytic sarcomas (Fig. 2-121), plasmacytomas (Fig. 2-122), and mast cell tumors also produce solid sarcoma masses in the liver as primary or metastatic lesions. *Lymphoma in the liver is common*, especially when the spleen is involved, and occasionally, the liver appears to be the major or primary site affected. Typically, lymphoma is most apparent in the portal tracts, and the connective tissue surrounding the central veins can also be infiltrated, but late in the course of disease, the sinusoids are affected (eFig. 2-34). There are occasional exceptions to this pattern. Hepatosplenic γδ T-cell lymphomas (also CD3+ and CD11d+) in dogs demonstrate preferential involvement of the liver and spleen, and neoplastic lymphocytes are most common within the sinusoids. Hepatocytotrophic lymphoma is a T-cell lymphoma variant (CD3+, CD11d−) that invades hepatocytes. Diffuse infiltration of the liver in myeloproliferative disorders and mast cell leukemia may also cause extreme enlargement of the organ; the infiltrates localize preferentially in and around the sinusoids (Fig. 2-123). Hepatic infiltration may be in discrete nodules 2 cm or more in size, particularly lymphoma in horses, but it is usually diffuse in the connective tissues of the portal triads.

Melanomas and hemangiosarcomas have characteristic gross features in the liver, but most metastatic tumors cannot be distinguished by their gross appearance. Sarcomas do tend to form a few large, smooth-surfaced nodules, and carcinomas do tend to form more nodules and to be umbilicate when in contact with Glisson's capsule. Hemangiosarcomas come from the spleen, usually, and may virtually replace the liver with small, blood-filled caverns. Their microscopic appearance is the same as that of the primary tumors.

A non-neoplastic condition, *hepatic splenosis*, a rare condition in which normal splenic tissue becomes implanted into the liver, can be confused with metastatic disease. Normal

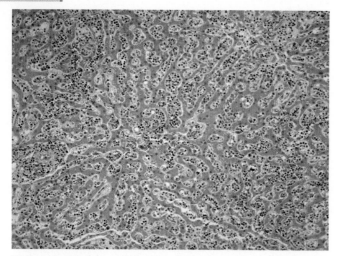

Figure 2-123 Monomyelocytic leukemia cells typically array along the hepatic sinusoids as seen in this dog.

spleen enters the liver, often via the portal vein after surgery or trauma to the spleen and multiple soft red masses up to ~4 cm in diameter can develop. Histologically, the masses resemble splenic tissue.

Further reading

Beeler-Marfisi J, et al. Equine primary liver tumors: a case series and review of the literature. J Vet Diagn Invest 2010;22:174-183.

Charles JA, et al. Morphological classification of neoplastic disorders of the canine and feline liver. In: Rothuizen J, et al., editors. WSAVA Standards for Clinical and Histological Diagnosis of Canine and Feline Liver Diseases. Philadelphia: Saunders Elsevier; 2006. p. 117-124.

Gamlem H, et al. Canine vascular neoplasia—a population-based clinicopathologic study of 439 tumours and tumour-like lesions in 420 dogs. APMIS Suppl 2008;125:41-54.

Knostman KA, et al. Intrahepatic splenosis in a dog. Vet Pathol 2003;40:708-710.

Patnaik AK, et al. Hepatobiliary neuroendocrine carcinoma in cats: a clinicopathologic, immunohistochemical, and ultrastructural study of 17 cases. Vet Pathol 2005;42:331-337.

van den Ingh TSGAM, et al. Morphological classification of biliary disorders of the canine and feline liver. In: Rothuizen J, et al., editors. WSAVA Standards for Clinical and Histological Diagnosis of Canine and Feline Liver Diseases. Philadelphia: Saunders Elsevier; 2006. p. 61-76.

van Sprundel RG, et al. Classification of primary hepatic tumours in the dog. Vet J 2013;197:596-606.

(i) *For more information, please visit the companion site: PathologyofDomesticAnimals.com.*

CHAPTER 3

Pancreas

Kenneth V.F. Jubb • Andrew W. Stent

■ ACKNOWLEDGMENTS

This update of the Pancreas chapter is based on previous editions by Drs. Ken Jubb, Peter Kennedy, Nigel Palmer, and Jennifer Charles, and we gratefully acknowledge their contributions.

GENERAL CONSIDERATIONS

The pancreas is seldom carefully scrutinized at routine autopsy or subject to microscopic examination. Biopsy examinations are largely restricted to dogs and carry significant risk of provoking acute inflammation. However, the pancreas is subject to intense research activity, reflecting the importance of the endocrine pancreas and particularly diabetes mellitus in human public health. Moreover, investigation of the development of the exocrine tissue is providing valuable insight into the effects of nutrition on fetal and postnatal development, as well as uncovering important influences on the pathogenesis of pancreatic carcinoma. It is important to note that the current understanding of pancreatic ontogeny and physiology is based upon in vivo and ex vivo investigations with a limited range of species, predominantly rodents and chick embryos. These studies often fail to acknowledge the immense interspecies variability in prenatal and postnatal development and maturation of the pancreas, and the relevance of published data to domestic animals may be questionable, particularly as findings are often inconsistent among species and even individuals.

Functional and structural changes in the normal pancreas are not self-initiated, but rather occur in response to systemic metabolic activity, although in practice the relationship between cause and effect is often obscure. Pancreatic function is largely controlled by entero-endocrine hormones derived from the gastrointestinal mucosa, but also influenced by stimuli from the endocrine component of the pancreas. The endocrine tissue constitutes ~1-2% of the pancreatic mass and is uniquely arranged in islets distributed throughout the exocrine lobules, although extra-islet endocrine cells are sometimes located individually or in small clusters, particularly in cats, dogs, and horses. *There is an important interdependence between the endocrine and exocrine elements* of the organ, and the hormones produced by islets are important for the regulation of exocrine tissue. The complex structural and functional interrelationship between the endocrine and exocrine pancreas is mediated most importantly by insulin and somatostatin. *Both insulin and pancreatic polypeptide are trophic for acinar tissue; somatostatin and glucagon are inhibitory.* The paracrine effects of these molecules are facilitated by an insulo-acinar portal circulatory system, wherein afferent vessels predominantly flow through the islets before supplying the exocrine tissue, although this varies with species and even within individual pancreatic lobules. Notwithstanding the intimacy of relationships between endocrine and exocrine systems of the pancreas, pragmatism allows the systems to be described separately while noting that the combination of endocrine and exocrine secretory functions in one organ is specific to vertebrates.

Further reading

Barreto SG, et al. The islet-acinar axis of the pancreas: more than just insulin. Am J Physiol Gastrointest Liver Physiol 2010;299: G10-G22.

Bockman DE. Toward understanding pancreatic disease: from architecture to cell signaling. Pancreas 1995;11:324-329.

EXOCRINE PANCREAS

Early **organogenesis** is best described in the mouse and not in domestic species, but it is a reasonable assumption that, except for timing of events, there will be similarities with other mammals. Initially, the endoderm of the gut tube is organized regionally into distinct organ fields by a series of incompletely understood cranial-to-caudal and dorsal-to-ventral patterning events. The incipient pancreas first emerges as a bud from the dorsal gut endoderm, shortly followed by ventral buds that form both pancreatic and bile ducts. Coiling of the gut tube brings the buds into proximity. As progenitor ducts project into the mesenchyme under the influence of epidermal growth factor, remodeling distinguishes future duct and acinar regions (Fig. 3-1A). Proliferation of the buds and formation of ducts

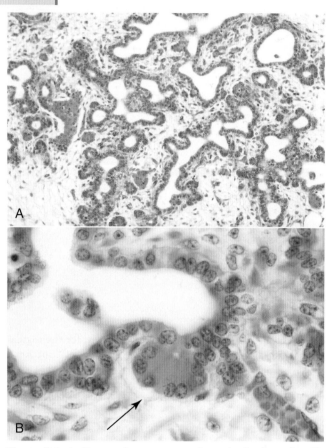

Figure 3-1 A. Pancreatic organogenesis in the lamb at day 48. Ductal epithelium invades through the mesenchyme, with scattered colonies of islet-like tissue distributed throughout. **B.** Detail of (A). **Incipient acinar tissue** budding from embryonic ductular epithelium (arrow).

may, in part, result from progressive branching, but the remarkable ability of the pancreas to regenerate from loss of substance suggests that the ductular architecture may be more interlinked than this model implies. Collateral connections have been demonstrated in the dog and several other species, in which the ductal architecture is described as a continuous branching system, circuitous and anastomotic. Acinar cells arise from the tips of the proliferating epithelium and rapid growth is achieved by splitting and duplication of acinar tips (Fig. 3-1B). In species suitably examined, the ductal systems of the 2 pancreatic anlagen form a fused network, with the proliferating dorsal bud giving rise to the left lobe and the accessory pancreatic duct, whereas the ventral bud produces the pancreatic duct and the right lobe.

There are **differences within and between species** as to which of the embryonic ducts serves as the main conduit in the developed pancreas. The accessory pancreatic duct, derived from the ventral anlage and entering the duodenum at the minor duodenal papilla, does not persist in small ruminants and the majority of cats; it is the major duct in the dog, the lesser duct in the horse, and the only duct in the pig and ox. The pancreatic duct develops from the dorsal anlage and is the only duct in small ruminants as well as the majority of cats and is the main duct in horses; in dogs, it is the lesser duct and is occasionally absent. It opens into the duodenum at the major papilla, with or immediately adjacent to the bile duct.

Innervation of the pancreas is important for regulating exocrine secretion. Parasympathetic autonomic stimulation derived from the vagus nerve promotes secretion of pancreatic juice, mediated by ganglion cells within the interstitial tissue. The ganglion cells are also innervated by the enteric nervous system acting independently of central systems to coordinate secretory control by gastrointestinal hormones. *Pacinian corpuscles* are normally prominent in the interlobular connective tissues of the pancreas of the cat, and may be grossly visible as discrete nodules 1-3 mm in diameter.

By weight and volume the pancreas is predominantly composed of acinar tissue. The organ lacks a conventional capsule but is organized into lobules interspersed by septa derived from a thin condensation of surrounding connective tissue that also invests the ductal system. The lobules are composed of glandular acini that are distributed along the smaller ducts. Each acinus forms about an evagination of the ductal system that is called the *intercalated duct*. The intercalated duct is lined by cuboidal centroacinar cells, distinguishable in histologic sections by clear unstained cytoplasm. Ductular epithelium progressively becomes more columnar along intralobular and interlobular ducts, and there is a corresponding alteration in epithelial secretory profile, with decreased bicarbonate secretion and increased production of mucins. Both enteric and pancreatic endocrine cell populations are also present within the ductular epithelium, although their importance remains unclear.

*The major **function of the exocrine pancreas** is the synthesis and secretion of digestive enzymes.* Acinar cells secrete trypsin, chymotrypsin, collagenase, phospholipase, elastases, and carboxypeptidases as inactive proenzymes, whereas amylase and lipase are secreted in their active forms. The proenzymes and enzymes are packaged within acinar cells into membrane-bound zymogen granules. Entry of gastric acid and fatty acids into the duodenum causes local release of secretin, which in turn stimulates secretion of water and bicarbonate by pancreatic ductal epithelium, particularly by the centroacinar cells. The bicarbonate contributes to neutralization of gastric acid in the duodenum. However, this is not essential for maintaining a neutral pH, suitable for optimal activity of the digestive enzymes, as the duodenal mucosa itself has an enormous capacity to secrete bicarbonate and absorb hydrogen ions. The presence of undigested lipid and amino acid peptides in the duodenal lumen promotes release of cholecystokinin by mucosal endocrine cells; this secretagogue promotes rapid discharge of digestive enzymes from zymogen granules into the ducts and also has a direct, rapid, and substantial trophic effect on acinar cells.

Within the duodenum, exocrine secretions also inhibit bacterial proliferation, exert a trophic effect on the mucosa, and contribute to the normal degradation of exposed mucosal brush-border enzymes. The exocrine pancreas also produces *intrinsic factor*, which is essential for the absorption of cobalamin (vitamin B_{12}) in the ileum. In addition, the organ plays an important role in zinc homeostasis, accumulating zinc absorbed from the intestines and secreting excess into pancreatic juice. This function is partly mediated by the zinc-binding protein, metallothionein, which is present in acinar cells and exocrine secretions.

The exocrine pancreas is a labile organ. It synthesizes much more protein on a weight-for-weight basis than does any other tissue and consumes a correspondingly large amount of precursor substrate, but the mechanisms responsible for homeostatic regulation of pancreatic tissue remain poorly understood. A degree of zonal variability and peri-islet hypertrophy is often observed in acinar tissue, reflecting exposure to trophic hormones secreted into the islet-acinar portal system.

The response of the exocrine pancreas to changes in nutrient intake is rapid, and adaptation to new diets can produce dramatic alterations in the composition of pancreatic juice. Secretion of proteases is a reflection, in part, of dietary protein levels; amylase secretion is influenced by the level of dietary carbohydrate and by plasma levels of cortisol and insulin. The dietary influence on lipase secretion is less clear but secretion is to some extent dependent on dietary protein levels. Acinar cell hypertrophy and hyperplasia leading to organ enlargement occurs in response to diets rich in protein and energy. When these substrates are withdrawn, the organ reverts to normal mass via autophagy and apoptosis. If dietary protein and energy become suboptimal, acinar cells and the exocrine organ atrophy.

Maternal malnutrition during gestation and lactation may retard maturation of the exocrine pancreas of the offspring. Paradoxically, the enzyme content of the pancreas may increase in the offspring; whether this increase enhances the ability of the offspring to resist malnutrition remains unclear. The exocrine pancreas is normally functionally immature at birth, and synthesis of some digestive enzymes may not commence postnatally for several weeks. Enzymatic activity of milk and proximal intestinal secretions compensate for this insufficiency in suckling animals. The weight of the pancreas increases rapidly during the immediate postnatal period, chiefly because of an increase in the number rather than size of acinar cells. Colostrum, which contains growth-promoting factors such as epidermal growth factor and insulin-like growth factors, plays a role in this early organ growth. Release of endogenous gut hormones such as gastrin that have trophic effects on the pancreas may contribute to this early development, and glucocorticoids also promote maturation of the acinar cells. At weaning, dietary and hormonal changes combine to cause abrupt increases in pancreatic enzyme synthesis and secretion. In animals weaned early, the surge in circulating glucocorticoids is considered to be more important than the dietary changes in triggering the alterations to enzyme output.

Acinar, ductal, and islet cells are all capable of **regeneration**, and restoration of the exocrine parenchyma typically proceeds rapidly following acinar destruction. Regeneration of exocrine components proceeds via the facultative progenitor potential of ductular epithelium, as well as proliferation of mature acinar cells through the formation of metaplastic ductular intermediates. The progenitor capabilities of the ductular epithelium are broad, and hepatocellular differentiation occasionally may be observed in regenerating pancreas. β-cell regeneration appears to occur largely via mitotic division of the mature β-cell population, together with expansion of redifferentiated ductular tissue. Adult stem cells are not currently thought to play a major role in the regenerative process, although this remains an area of active debate.

The regenerative capacity of the exocrine tissue is exemplified in cerulein toxicosis. Cerulein, an analogue of cholecystokinin, causes dose-dependent dissolution of the acinar cells in rodents that, even if total, can be fully repaired in a week or so. Slower regeneration of both exocrine and endocrine elements follows partial surgical ablation. Complete restitution of exocrine parenchyma by mitotic division and hypertrophy

of viable acinar cells may follow minor cell loss. Extensive or persistent parenchymal injury may provoke proliferation of ductular epithelium and connective tissues.

Stellate cells akin to those of the liver have been identified in the normal pancreas in a periacinar location and appear to be the major mediators of pancreatic fibrogenesis. In the quiescent state, pancreatic stellate cells express desmin but not α-smooth-muscle actin. Following activation by injury, these cells acquire a myofibroblastic phenotype and synthesize fibrillar collagens, including collagen type I.

Further reading

Egerbacher M, Bock P. Morphology of the pancreatic duct system in mammals. Microsc Res Tech 1997;37:407-417.

El-Gohary Y, et al. Three-dimensional analysis of the islet vasculature. Anat Rec (Hoboken) 2012;295:1473-1481.

Gallo LA, et al. Maternal adaptations and inheritance in the transgenerational programming of adult disease. Cell Tissue Res 2012;349:863-880.

Gittes GK. Developmental biology of the pancreas: a comprehensive review. Dev Biol 2009;326:4-35.

Mossner J. New advances in cell physiology and pathophysiology of the exocrine pancreas. Dig Dis 2010;28:722-728.

Pan FC, Wright C. Pancreas organogenesis: from bud to plexus to gland. Dev Dyn 2011;240:530-565.

Developmental anomalies of the exocrine pancreas

Complex movements amongst embryonic tissues provide abundant opportunities for pancreatic abnormalities including systemic developmental errors.

Agenesis or **aplasia** (complete absence) of the pancreas may be associated with more generalized and severe malformations incompatible with survival.

Pancreatic hypoplasia occurs sporadically in calves. The defect is in the exocrine tissue; the islets are normal in number and morphology. The hypoplastic organ is small, pale, and loosely textured. Its margins are poorly defined, but the parenchyma is centered on a normal duct system. Microscopically, acinar tissue is present as small scattered clusters of cells in glandular array. Some of the cells may appear well differentiated and contain zymogen granules, but most are small, basophilic, and of indifferent type.

Variations in the disposition of the ducts are common in dogs. Most dogs have 2 separate ducts opening into the duodenum, with interductal anastomoses within the pancreas, and with the accessory pancreatic duct the major conduit. A small percentage of dogs may have only an accessory duct entering the duodenum, and some may have 3 functional openings into the intestine.

An **annular pancreas**, characterized by a thin flat ring of normal pancreatic tissue completely encircling the duodenum, has been observed in dogs and piglets; the annulus may cause duodenal stenosis. This anomaly probably reflects failure of normal embryonic rotation of the duodenal anlagen.

Congenital stenosis or **cystic dilation of a pancreatic duct** is occasionally reported in domestic animals, and congenital intrapancreatic cysts lined by squamous or low cuboidal epithelium are occasionally seen in lambs. Cystic dilation of intralobular and interlobular pancreatic ducts accompanied by polycystic kidneys and cystic intrahepatic bile ducts is reported in cats, piglets, and goat kids. Saccular ductal distension to form a structure resembling a gallbladder and termed a **pancreatic bladder** has been described in cats and may be congenital or acquired. Such structures are usually asymptomatic, but large cysts may compress the bile duct to cause jaundice. True congenital **duplication of the gallbladder** with the accessory organ arising from the ventral pancreatic bud has also been observed in cats.

Ectopic or **accessory pancreatic tissue** forming small pancreatic nodules may be found in the submucosa, muscularis or serosa of the stomach or intestine (especially in the duodenum), the mesentery, gallbladder, spleen, lymph node, or liver. The ectopic rests are of normal morphology, although islets are not always present. Ectopia may result from dislocation of portions of the duodenal buds during development, from persistence of an anlage that would normally regress, or from activation of pancreatic transcription factors within pluripotential endodermal epithelium.

Splenic organogenesis occurs in close proximity to the developing pancreas within the dorsal splanchnic mesenchyme, and the organs continue to be connected in some reptiles and fish. In domestic species they may be linked by a mesenteric band or, occasionally in dogs and cats, ectopic acinar tissue or islets may be found in the substance of the spleen.

Intrapancreatic hepatocytes are occasionally observed as an incidental finding, especially in neonates. Hepatocytes may also appear in the adult pancreas during attempted regeneration after massive lobular injury, reflecting pluripotency of regenerating ductular epithelium.

Further reading

Cano DA, et al. Pancreatic development and disease. Gastroenterol 2007;132:745-762.

Shen CN, et al. Molecular basis of transdifferentiation of pancreas to liver. Nat Cell Biol 2000;2:879-887.

Regressive changes of the exocrine pancreas

Nonspecific degenerative changes are frequently observed within the exocrine tissue and should not be confused with **autolysis**, which occurs rapidly within the pancreas because of postmortem release and activation of digestive enzymes. Autolyzed pancreata are often discolored dark red to brown, and hemorrhage within the pancreatic interstitium and peripancreatic tissue may occur after death, particularly in dogs and horses. Histologically, the distribution is often patchy. The cells separate, acinar tissue may appear smudged, and affected areas are poorly staining and display slate gray coloration with hematoxylin and eosin.

Insult to either the acinar or ductular epithelium frequently manifests in vacuolar hydropic change, reflecting dysregulation of cellular volume resulting from mitochondrial fluid accumulation. Microvesicular steatosis occasionally is observed in the cytoplasm of acinar epithelium as an early nonspecific pathologic degeneration. Substrate accumulation occurs in lysosomal storage disorders such as α- and β-mannosidosis and galactosialidosis. Vacuolation of ductal epithelium because of glycogen accumulation is a feature of diabetes mellitus. **Pancreatic lipofuscinosis** is occasionally seen in dogs deficient in vitamin E. Accumulation of lipofuscin causes khaki to brown discoloration of the pancreas and of intestinal smooth muscle

grossly; the urinary bladder and mesenteric lymph nodes may also be affected. The golden-brown pigment granules in the basal cytoplasm of pancreatic acinar cells and intestinal myocytes are periodic acid-Schiff–positive, sudanophilic, and weakly acid-fast. Microscopic pigment accumulation may occur in other tissues, including the pigmented epithelium of the retina.

Lipomatosis of the pancreas occurs occasionally in cats, pigs, and cattle, usually as part of generalized obesity but sometimes restricted to the pancreas. Adipose tissue accumulates in the interstitium and disperses the parenchyma to create a false microscopic impression of diminished exocrine mass with fatty replacement. Although there may be some pressure atrophy of the parenchyma, *lipomatosis is not functionally significant.*

Exocrine degeneration and necrosis

Necrosis of individual acinar cells or local groups occurs in various local and systemic disorders, including febrile states, viral infections (most commonly those displaying epitheliotropism, including canine distemper, foot-and-mouth disease, and a number of adenoviruses), intoxications, and in hypovolemic or septic shock. Associated inflammation is often minimal. In most cases the lesions are incidental to the course of the systemic disease.

Multifocal degeneration and necrosis also may be seen in many **intoxications**, including trichothecene mycotoxicosis of pigs resulting from consumption of T-2 toxin, deoxynivalenol (vomitoxin), or diacetoxyscirpenol (anguidine) produced by *Fusarium* species. These mycotoxins may also cause pancreatic interstitial edema, hyperplasia of ductular epithelium, and necrosis of islet cells. Selenium excess may cause degenerative change in the exocrine pancreas, with experimental toxicosis in pigs producing acute pancreatic edema, hemorrhage, and acinar necrosis. Ingestion of *Cassia occidentalis* also has been reported to cause pancreatic necrosis in pigs.

Acute intoxication by **anticholinesterases** is also recognized to cause exocrine degeneration in both humans and domestic species, manifesting as ballooning necrosis of acinar cells, together with interstitial edema and vasculitis. These lesions are theorized to reflect inhibition of pancreatic pseudocholinesterase, resulting in excessive secretory stimulation of exocrine tissue as well as increased intraductal pressures. Cats appear relatively resistant to this form of toxicity because of deficiency of pseudocholinesterase. Although reports of pancreatic damage following anticholinesterase intoxication are rare in the literature, extensive use of these chemicals as pesticides within the veterinary field suggests that this phenomenon may be under-recognized.

Zinc toxicity causes striking pancreatic lesions in several species, including domestic animals and humans. There are numerous opportunities for exposure to zinc, and narrow margins between safe and unsafe levels of exposure. Metallic zinc is available in alloys and galvanized products, zinc compounds are widely available in pesticides and herbicides, and zinc salts are occasionally used in the treatment of dermatologic conditions in cattle and sheep.

Zinc is an essential element for a multitude of biochemical processes in plants and animals, but the biologic and physiologic roles and homeostatic mechanisms are not well understood. It follows that the hierarchy of functions affected by deficiency or excess may be subject to modulating factors that influence the expression of zinc toxicity in individuals

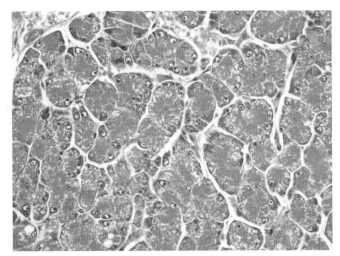

Figure 3-2 Zinc toxicity in a dog. In the acute phase, there is basilar vacuolar degeneration within the acinar cells.

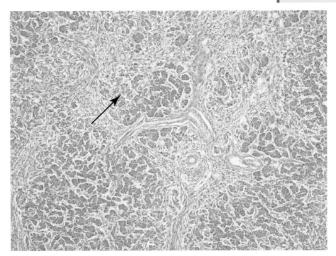

Figure 3-3 Zinc toxicity in a dog. With chronicity the pancreas becomes markedly fibrotic with minimal associated inflammation and sparing of islets (arrow).

and the organs principally affected. The most consistent expressions of zinc toxicity in animals are in pancreas, liver, kidney, and blood, the latter expressed as Heinz body hemolytic anemia. The pancreas is the major route of zinc excretion, and this may explain the comparatively high vulnerability of the pancreas to toxicity. Susceptibility of the pancreatic structures to zinc toxicity varies among domestic species, with the ductular elements affected first in sheep and other ruminants, whereas acinar tissue is most vulnerable in pigs. The pathogenesis of the pancreatic response is unclear, in part because of the variable response to excess zinc among domestic animal species, and also because of the rapidity of the regenerative response producing a mix of degenerative and regenerative features. Generally, *microvesicular degeneration and necrosis of acinar elements dominate early and are followed by acinar atrophy and fibrosis.* The islets are usually unaffected. There are associated changes in tissue concentrations of copper, iron, and manganese that raise the possibility that the hemolytic anemia and the hepatic necrosis, which is sometimes massive, may be caused by impaired capture of free radicals by various dismutases, rather than by the direct effects of zinc itself.

In acute zinc intoxication, the pancreas is enlarged and pale with prominent lobulation. The interlobular connective tissues are widened by slightly viscous edema fluid that may be stained by free hemoglobin. The liver may be reduced in size with a surface mosaic of prominent fatty degeneration and dark sunken areas of necrosis and collapse. Renal lesions such as tubular dilation and necrosis may not be present in acute intoxications. Histologically, the acinar cells are enlarged with vacuolated cytoplasm, and zymogen granulation may be prominent as an early change (Fig. 3-2). There is no or minimal inflammatory cell presence.

Progression of the pancreatic toxicity is marked by shrinkage and nodularity of the organ, some lobules being normal and others shrunken. The interstitial edema is replaced by prominent fibrosis (Fig. 3-3). Histologically, damaged lobules are uniformly affected. Acinar cells may be necrotic and exfoliated, the acinar lumen enlarged, and the lining cells flat and atrophic producing a pseudoacinar or tubular arrangement. Late in the disease progression, the liver may show postnecrotic scarring and there may be renal tubular degeneration

affecting especially the straight ascending and descending limbs of the loops of Henle.

Although toxins may directly exert deleterious effects on exocrine tissue, recent observations suggest that *many chemicals, including ethanol, act via production of free radicals or other redox reactive molecules.* The exocrine pancreas already generates a large free radical load during normal metabolic processes, and an additional burden produced by exogenous sources may overwhelm regulatory antioxidant pathways. Moreover, the exocrine acinar cells possess latent cytochrome P450 activity, and the oxidative damage of some pancreatic toxins may be amplified following biotransformation within the exocrine tissue. Agents that induce the cytochrome P450 pathway, including corticosteroids and even feeds rich in C18:2 fatty acids, such as corn oil, may potentiate pancreatic toxicity. Cytochrome P450 is also induced by chronic pancreatitis, thereby increasing the susceptibility of an already-damaged organ to toxic insult.

Further reading

Foster JR. Toxicology of the exocrine pancreas. In: Ballantyne B, Marrs TC, et al., editors. General and Applied Toxicology, vol. 3. 3rd ed. John Wiley and Sons, Ltd.; 2009.

Graham TW, et al. A pathologic and toxicologic evaluation of veal calves fed large amounts of zinc. Vet Pathol 1988;25:484-491.

Mikszewski JS, et al. Zinc-associated acute pancreatitis in a dog. J Small Anim Pract 2003;44:177-180.

Pang VF, et al. Myocardial and pancreatic lesions induced by T-2 toxin, a trichothecene mycotoxin, in swine. Vet Pathol 1986;23:310-319.

Acute pancreatic necrosis. *Acute pancreatic necrosis is the more common of the pancreatic diseases in dogs and also occasionally occurs in cats.* It may manifest as an acute and potentially life-threatening syndrome or as a chronic intermittent or relapsing syndrome, often subclinical, that may culminate in exocrine pancreatic insufficiency and diabetes mellitus caused by progressive destruction of functional tissue. *Clinicians tend to use the term pancreatitis with reference both to this condition and to diseases that are primarily inflammatory* and centered on the ducts and interstitial tissues, often qualifying only on the basis of whether clinical disease is acute or chronic. Even in the scientific literature, the terms are often used interchangeably. This is understandable because clinical expressions of these disorders overlap substantially and distinction is often impossible without inspection of the organ. However, these disorders have different causes, pathogenesis, and histologic characteristics.

Early descriptions of pancreatic necrosis were derived from dogs fed a diet high in fats (lard) and low in protein for unrelated experimental purposes. Pancreatic lesions similar to those in spontaneous cases regularly developed after some weeks of exposure to the diet and were described as dissimilar to the lesions seen in human pancreatitis. *The earliest lesions in acute pancreatic necrosis occur in the adipose tissue of the peripancreatic mesentery* and are visible grossly as yellowish flecks or small plaques of necrosis and saponification of adipocytes. This is followed by necrosis of the marginal acinar cells (those lying at the surface of the lobule), and is identifiable by smudging of cytoplasmic detail that strongly suggests autodigestion of pancreatic tissue by activated enzymes. Disease progresses with necrosis and reactive inflammation concentrated at the periphery of affected lobules together with more or less extensive involvement of adjacent adipose and other connective tissues. The duct system and centrilobular parenchyma are unaffected in the early stages of the disease.

In many cases, the **inciting cause** of the pancreatic necrosis is obscure. Because the periphery of the pancreatic lobule is also the periphery of the circulatory field, *hypoperfusion and possibly reperfusion may be important in the pathogenesis of necrosis* and could account for its occasional onset after prolonged hypotension, following abdominal surgery, or in conjunction with gastric dilation-volvulus. Abdominal trauma may be the trigger in some animals, and the condition also has been associated with the use of such drugs as azathioprine. Nutritional factors, especially the quantity and quality (in terms of fatty acid composition) of lipids and degraded protein appear, circumstantially, to be important, suggesting that lipid peroxidation damage may be a precipitating insult. Alternatively, high-fat diets may promote excessive release of cholecystokinin and hyperstimulation of the exocrine pancreas. Pancreatic parenchyma also exhibits drug-metabolizing activity and a capacity to produce toxic free radicals, which may subsequently trigger damaging lipid peroxidation cascades.

Diffusion of enzymes from the exocrine tissue is thought to be responsible for the early fat necrosis. Lipase and amylase are secreted in an active form, and there is some evidence that amylase may be largely responsible for initial injury to adipocyte cell membranes. Premature intracellular activation of zymogen-bound proenzymes also occurs in exocrine cells early in the disease process, and is strongly associated with a persistent increase in intracellular calcium. Normal enzyme secretion is stimulated by rapid spiking of cytoplasmic calcium concentrations, but when the calcium increase is sustained—as occurs with hypoxia, hypercalcemia, hyperlipidemia, and other cellular insults—ATP production is blunted and the energy-intensive process of zymogen secretion is suppressed. Calcium then stimulates the fusion of lysosomes with zymogen granules within the Golgi apparatus, resulting in intracellular activation of trypsinogen, which in turn activates other proenzymes such as proelastase and prophospholipase. Activated elastase and phospholipase A appear to be particularly important in expanding the area of pancreatic necrosis. Trypsin, phospholipase A, elastase, lipase, and colipase damage the

walls of local blood vessels, inducing vasoactive amine release, increased vascular permeability, edema, hemorrhage, and thrombosis; enzymatic tissue necrosis may therefore be compounded by *superimposed ischemic necrosis*. There is local activation of the complement cascade and release of cytokines such as tumor necrosis factor-α (TNF-α), interleukin-1 (IL-1), IL-6, IL-8, and platelet-activating factor (PAF). Some of these molecules promote chemotaxis of leukocytes into the area. The leukocytes amplify the pancreatic damage via the generation of oxygen-derived free radicals and additional cytokines.

Under normal circumstances, the exocrine pancreas possesses robust **defenses against autodigestion**. Intracellular hydrolases are capable of degrading retained zymogen granules, and protease inhibitors such as pancreatic secretory trypsin inhibitor and α_1-antitrypsin are co-secreted with digestive enzymes to prevent premature activation. In acute pancreatic necrosis, these defense mechanisms appear to be overwhelmed, and experimental supplementation of these enzymes has been shown to ameliorate disease progression.

*Middle-aged to older **dogs** that are overweight or obese are at increased risk of acute pancreatic necrosis.* Miniature Schnauzers, Yorkshire and Silky Terriers, nonsporting and nonworking breeds, and perhaps Miniature Poodles are predisposed, and female dogs are more likely to be affected than males. These observations and the predisposition of Miniature Schnauzers with idiopathic hyperlipidemia to the disease may be a consequence of the elevating effect of hypertriglyceridemia on cytosolic ionized calcium levels in acinar cells. Dogs with hyperadrenocorticism, hypothyroidism, hypercalcemia, or uremia also may be at increased risk of acute pancreatic necrosis.

The intensity of inflammation associated with acute pancreatic necrosis may produce devastating **systemic consequences**. Recruitment of large numbers of leukocytes results in systemic release of proinflammatory mediators such as TNF-α, IL-1, and chemokines such as IL-8, and this cytokine storm induces the systemic inflammatory response syndrome and multiple organ dysfunction. Animals with acute pancreatic necrosis are highly susceptible to disseminated intravascular coagulation because of activation of clotting factors combined with widespread endothelial damage. Mortality rates of 27-42% are reported in dogs with acute pancreatic necrosis, although most dogs with mild disease clinically recover within a few days. Although the extent of necrosis may well influence the outcome in dogs, secondary infection of the organ occurs rarely in this species. Other factors that have been associated with mortality in affected dogs have included obesity, concurrent diabetes mellitus, hyperadrenocorticism, hypothyroidism, epilepsy, and prior gastrointestinal disease.

Although most dogs survive an episode of acute pancreatic necrosis, *it is doubtful whether complete resolution of the pathologic process ever occurs.* Rather, the necrotizing process typically smolders continuously and often asymptomatically until there is almost complete destruction of the pancreas. There is seldom any difficulty in finding microscopic areas of acute necrosis in chronically affected organs. Whether the apparently relentless course is due to persistence of the primary pathogenetic mechanism or a self-perpetuating property of the lesion is not known. The initial lesion is often localized to one portion of the organ, whereas the smoldering foci are often multiple, of random distribution, affect the periphery of

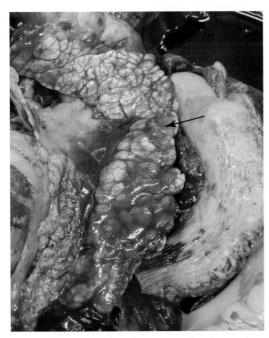

Figure 3-4 **Acute pancreatic necrosis** in the dog with peripancreatic hemorrhage, edema, and a focus of fat necrosis (arrow).

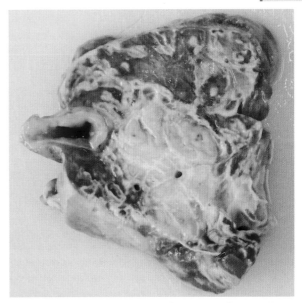

Figure 3-5 **Cross-sectional view of pancreas from a dog with recurrent pancreatic necrosis.** Note the variegated appearance of the pancreas caused by hemorrhage, necrosis, dystrophic mineralization, and fibrosis. Duodenum is at left of tissue.

the organ remnants, and tend to avoid any surviving parenchyma in the original focus, the latter being identifiable by fibrosis and atrophy. Clinical signs of exocrine and endocrine insufficiency may develop as a consequence of continued destruction of the organ, and pancreatic necrosis is a common cause of diabetes mellitus in dogs.

Grossly, in fatal cases of acute pancreatic necrosis, a small volume of turbid serous fluid containing free lipid droplets is usually present in the peritoneal cavity. Petechial and ecchymotic hemorrhages may be present in the pancreas and adjacent omentum and mesenteries, but extensive hemorrhage is not usually a feature. Numerous small white chalky areas of fat necrosis, each with an intensely hyperemic border, are present adjacent to the pancreas and in the mesentery. In some cases foci of necrotic fat are widely distributed throughout the peritoneal cavity and may be detectable as far away as the ventral mediastinum, to which digestive enzymes have been conveyed by lymphatics. The entire pancreas may be edematous, swollen, and soft (Fig. 3-4) or edema may be confined to localized areas. The necrotizing process may be confined to the central pancreas or one wing. Fibrin strands pass from the affected surface of the pancreas to the omentum, mesenteries, and the visceral surface of the liver. The cut surface of the pancreas has a variegated appearance caused by merging of white areas of fat necrosis and gray-yellow areas of parenchymal necrosis; one or other appearance may predominate (Fig. 3-5). The texture is unusually greasy. Areas of parenchymal necrosis are soft and may liquefy.

Histologically, there is necrosis of peripancreatic adipose tissue and pancreatic parenchyma, edematous separation of the interstitium, mural necrosis, and thrombosis of blood vessels and reactive inflammation (Fig. 3-6). Infiltrating leukocytes, chiefly neutrophils and macrophages, congregate at the boundary of necrotic and viable tissue. The necrotic fat saponifies and may undergo mild dystrophic mineralization. The initial parenchymal lesions at the periphery of the lobules

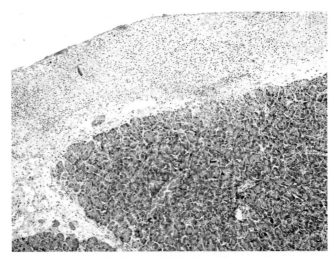

Figure 3-6 Early stages of **acute pancreatic necrosis** in a dog, displaying perilobular hemorrhage, edema, and leukocyte infiltration, with sparing of pancreatic parenchyma.

are composed of small foci of coagulative necrosis in which the acinar cells become shrunken and acidophilic. These foci rapidly expand and liquefaction of the necrotic tissue leaves large lakes of debris. The collagenous stroma resists digestion for some time. Much fibrin may be precipitated in the edematous interstitium, and capillaries at the margins of necrotic areas may be occluded by fibrin thrombi. Phlebothrombosis, which may be associated with phlebitis or mural necrosis, may be apparent both adjacent to and distant from the parenchymal lesions; similar changes may occur in the small arteries, but these vessels are less susceptible to injury. With development of DIC, microvascular thrombosis may be apparent in multiple organs.

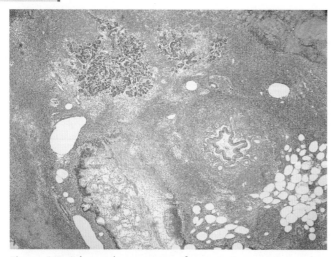

Figure 3-7 Advanced progression of **pancreatic necrosis** in a dog, resulting in destruction and condensation of acinar tissue, extensive fat necrosis, and interstitial fibrosis.

Infrequently, inflammatory masses such as abscesses, pseudocysts, or phlegmon may develop in the pancreas in the aftermath of acute necrosis. These lesions are discussed later, in the section on Pancreatitis.

The *duration of the disease influences the gross appearance of the pancreas*. With chronicity, the organ may be irregular in conformation and knobby or reduced to a few distorted lobules adjacent to where the ducts enter the duodenum. In some cases the remnants of the organ are too small to be visibly appreciated but they may still be palpable in areas indicated by a slight puckering of the mesentery. Scar tissue is usually not extensive and adhesions are absent or minor. Microscopically, a few small rounded lobules remain and these are compressed and atrophic (Fig. 3-7). Interstitial tissue is increased but this is probably as much the result of condensation of stroma as by fibrosis. Blood vessels and nerves are also condensed into the small area of the pancreatic remnant. Islets often cannot be identified. Lesions of diabetes mellitus or intestinal abnormalities typical of exocrine pancreatic insufficiency also may be present in advanced cases.

A minority of dogs with pancreatic necrosis may develop **multifocal necrotizing panniculitis**, and comparable subcutaneous lesions have been experimentally induced in cats by ligation of the pancreatic ducts. Release of activated enzymes, particularly phospholipase A, lipase, amylase, and trypsin, into the systemic circulation has been incriminated in the pathogenesis. In humans, the tendency to develop panniculitis in association with pancreatic necrosis is associated with a decrease in the serum concentration of α_1-proteinase inhibitor or α_2-macroglobulin. A similar association has yet to be demonstrated in small animals.

Acute pancreatic necrosis in **cats** is not readily distinguished clinically from chronic interstitial pancreatitis; the distinction is morphologic, with the necrotizing lesion being similar to that in dogs. Older domestic shorthaired cats are most commonly affected and there is no sex predisposition. The condition has been reported after abdominal trauma (including that associated with falling from a great height) and in cats with lipodystrophy, acute hypercalcemia, ductal reflux of duodenal contents, and organophosphate poisoning. Serious complications of acute pancreatic necrosis in cats are as described in dogs, but hepatic lipidosis, often severe, also may develop in affected cats.

Pancreatitis

Multifocal necrosis of the exocrine pancreas with minimal response from inflammatory cells is common in systemic infections with epitheliotropic viruses but is incidental to the course of the systemic disease. Bacterial embolism to the pancreas is not uncommon in cats and dogs with septic peritonitis.

Acute pancreatitis, in which the process is initially of centrilobular and periductal distribution, is occasionally observed in cats, horses, and dogs. In cats, the lesion is often associated with systemic toxoplasmosis; causative associations in dogs are only sporadically identified and predisposing factors are uncertain. It is likely that in affected dogs the initiating event is reflux of infection or activated digestive enzymes and bile salts from the duodenum into the main pancreatic duct to cause ductal necrosis. Reflux may be encouraged by increased luminal pressures during severe vomiting. The initial periductal parenchymal lesions rapidly enlarge and may become confluent to involve most of the pancreas. The organ is initially edematous and hyperemic, and the parenchyma becomes friable and hemorrhagic. The extensive hemorrhage may obscure the parenchyma and necrotic foci in adjacent adipose tissue. Apart from the intensity of accompanying hemorrhage, this stage may show some histologic overlap with the more common pattern of acute pancreatic necrosis that commences at the periphery of the organ.

Aside from the dog, **chronic interstitial pancreatitis** is the pattern of inflammation that is usually seen in domestic animals. The lesion is frequently identified at autopsy of mature cats, is occasionally observed in horses, and is rare in other species. *Chronic interstitial pancreatitis usually arises by extension of an inflammatory process that commences in the ducts.* The cause is usually an ascending infection involving intestinal bacterial flora or migration of flukes.

In chronic interstitial pancreatitis, the organ may be enlarged or reduced in size. In horses, the tendency is for enlargement and the parenchyma may be replaced by a tough mass of scar tissue with adhesions to adjacent structures. Flattened remnants of pancreatic tissue may be visible near the surface of the mass. Incision reveals tortuous and eccentrically dilated ducts that may contain purulent exudate or a large volume of slightly viscid mucus.

In **horses**, chronic interstitial pancreatitis may be provoked by the larvae of *Strongylus equinus* or, less commonly, *S. edentatus* that pass part of their developmental cycle in and about the pancreas. More typically, the disease in horses is associated with acute bacterial duodenitis and extension to the pancreatic ducts. Cholangitis also may develop in affected horses.

Initial reports of chronic interstitial pancreatitis in **cats** suggested the Siamese may be predisposed, but subsequent case studies have not supported this. The common biliary and pancreatic drainage in cats means that the pancreas is susceptible to extension of cholangitis. Agents such as *Toxoplasma gondii* and *Eurytrema procyonis* flukes have been sporadically implicated in feline pancreatitis, as has feline infectious peritonitis virus. There is also an association between feline pancreatitis and inflammatory bowel disease.

In **cats,** the pancreas is usually reduced in size and is firm, gray, and multinodular (Fig. 3-8). Clear retention cysts are often visible through the capsule and particularly on the cut

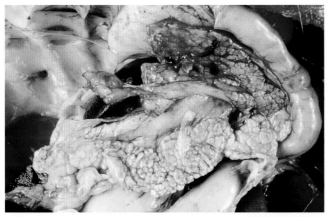

Figure 3-8 Chronic interstitial pancreatitis in a cat. The pancreas is pale with prominent nodularity.

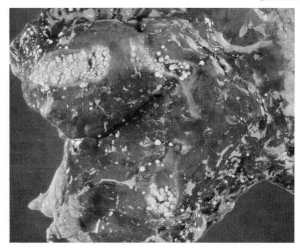

Figure 3-10 Ductal pancreatolithiasis in a cow.

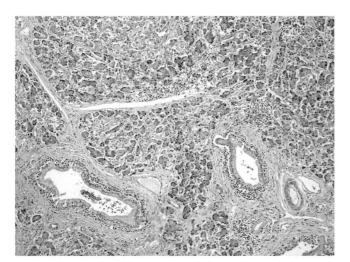

Figure 3-9 Histologic appearance of **chronic interstitial pancreatitis** in a cat. There is extensive interstitial and periductal fibrosis, and aggregates of lymphocytes that infiltrate through the acinar tissue.

surface. Fibrosis may not be recognizable on gross inspection but is typically extensive throughout the interlobular and intralobular septa. In exceptional cases, the whole organ may be converted into a shrunken, distorted, fibrous remnant. Histologically, the ducts may contain catarrhal exudate and are often enveloped by dense fibrous tissue (Fig. 3-9). Localized ductal stenoses and cystic dilations may occur. The epithelium of the ducts is hyperplastic and there may be squamous metaplasia. Fibrous tissue extends from around the ducts to the interlobular stroma and subdivides many of the lobules. The interstitial tissues are permeated by leukocytes, chiefly lymphocytes and plasma cells. Acinar parenchyma atrophies as a consequence of fibrosis and ductal obstruction, but the islets are usually well preserved.

Inflammatory masses involving the pancreas and peripancreatic tissues are potential sequelae of chronic pancreatitis. A **pancreatic phlegmon** is a solid mass of indurated pancreas and adjacent tissues that results from inflammation, edema, and necrosis. A phlegmon may develop within a few days of onset of necrosis and typically resolves spontaneously within 2-3 weeks, after the necrotizing process subsides. Necrosis may cause some cavitation of a phlegmon.

Pseudocysts are intrapancreatic or peripancreatic, fluctuant pockets of pancreatic enzyme secretions, necrotic debris, inflammatory exudates, and blood. They are more common than abscesses as sequelae of acute or chronic pancreatic necrosis. Pseudocysts may develop within days to weeks of onset of pancreatic necrosis. Disruption of pancreatic ducts by inflammation (or necrosis) and duct occlusion contribute to their development. Pseudocysts are usually solitary and unilocular and may reach 10 cm in diameter, the wall formed by granulation tissue that matures to fibrous scar tissue. Unlike true cysts, there is no epithelial lining.

Pancreatic abscesses are pockets of purulent exudate and necrotic debris within the pancreas or adjacent tissues. Sterile abscesses may form within areas of intense liquefactive necrosis of parenchyma. Larvae of *Stephanurus dentatus*, migrating from the liver across the peritoneum to the perirenal area in pigs, may encyst in the pancreas and provoke abscessation. Septic abscesses may result from secondary infection of necrotic parenchyma or, less often, a pseudocyst. They can also arise by direct extension from a neighboring focus of infection, as they occasionally do from septic peritonitis and from perforated esophagogastric ulcers in pigs. Some may contain chyle as a result of lymphatic leakage, and gas bubbles occasionally may be present in abscesses.

Systemic **granulomatous infections** may involve the pancreas, but lesions are usually microscopic and less important than those in other viscera. Chronic sclerosing and granulomatous pancreatitis owing to zygomycotic fungi has been reported in dogs, and pyogranulomatous pancreatitis occurs in feline infectious peritonitis. Disseminated cryptococcosis may occasionally involve the pancreas of cats, but is usually only associated with mild pyogranulomatous inflammation. Destructive granulomatous and eosinophilic pancreatitis can be a feature of multisystemic eosinophilic epitheliotropic syndrome of horses; a proportion of these cases are examples of enteropathy-associated lymphoma.

In **pancreatolithiasis**, concretions form within the pancreatic duct system. The calculi are occasionally detected in cattle at slaughter, being slightly more common in cattle >4 years of age, but are rare in other species. The calculi are usually hard, white, numerous, and small, often resembling sand grains, and are chiefly composed of carbonates and phosphates of calcium and magnesium (Fig. 3-10). The calculi are associated with and may be a consequence of ductal inflammation, including that provoked by flukes, but are typically incidental findings, and rarely cause complete duct obstruction.

Further reading

Bostrom BM, et al. Chronic pancreatitis in dogs: A retrospective study of clinical, clinicopathological, and histopathological findings in 61 cases. Vet J 2012;195:73-79.

De Cock HEV, et al. Prevalence and histopathologic characteristics of pancreatitis in cats. Vet Pathol 2007;44:39-49.

Frick TW. The role of calcium in acute pancreatitis. Surgery 2012; 152:S157-S163.

Johnson PJ, et al. Conditions of the equine pancreas. Equine Veterinary Education 2009;21:26-29.

Mansfield C. Acute pancreatitis in dogs: advances in understanding, diagnostics, and treatment. Top Companion Anim Med 2012;27: 123-132.

Mansfield C. Pathophysiology of acute pancreatitis: potential application from experimental models and human medicine to dogs. J Vet Intern Med 2012;26:875-887.

Mansfield CS, Jones BR. Review of feline pancreatitis part one: the normal feline pancreas, the pathophysiology, classification, prevalence, and aetiologies of pancreatitis. J Feline Med Surg 2001;3: 117-124.

Mohr AJ, et al. Acute pancreatitis: a newly recognised potential complication of canine babesiosis. J South Afr Vet Assoc 2000; 71:232-239.

Exocrine atrophy

Although exocrine pancreatic atrophy may be secondary to other disorders of the pancreas or its ducts, primary pancreatic atrophy is also a common and significant consequence of nutrient deprivation, especially in those species genetically selected for rapid growth, and in populations subject to marasmic nutritional cycles. Acinar atrophy occurs in starvation, prolonged anorexia, cachexia, protein-caloric deficiency, and maldigestive and malabsorptive syndromes. In protracted anorexia or starvation, the pancreas may be reduced to <10% of normal mass; other tissues, particularly the liver, will also be reduced in mass in these conditions.

The susceptibility of the exocrine pancreas to anatomic and functional atrophy is dependent on 2 characteristics. First, the turnover of protein in the pancreas is of a high order, similar to that of intestine, skin, and liver, and together with other tissues of high turnover, is subject to catabolic loss of acinar cell proteins as required to compensate for nutritional shortfall. Second, the pancreas is a passive intermediary in gastrointestinal digestive processes and thereby subject to the influences of many peptides of neurogenic and endocrine origin in the gastrointestinal mucosa, and to the loss of such stimulation.

The protein deficient condition of **kwashiorkor** in childhood in equatorial countries, and protein-calorie malnutrition in adult humans, provide an elegant demonstration of the remarkable plasticity of the acinar pancreas. Under conditions of protein deficiency, but with adequate caloric intake, rapid and profound reduction of exocrine pancreatic tissue occurs. Synthesis of amylase, lipase and trypsin is depressed but returns promptly to normal if nutritional state is improved. The loss of enzymes in secretion is sequential. Lipase is reduced and disappears first, followed by trypsin; amylase is reduced but not lost entirely. Morphologic studies

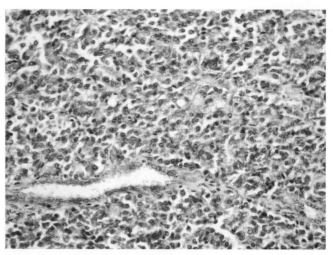

Figure 3-11 Exocrine pancreatic atrophy caused by starvation in a pig. Acinar cells are small and poorly granulated, and there is widespread dissociation of acinar architecture.

of the pancreas in human cases of kwashiorkor and protein-calorie malnutrition in domestic species are sparse, but changes equivalent to those in human malnutrition have been induced in rats and mice. Experimentally in mice, pancreatic mass has been shown to decrease by >75% in as little as 4 days, without corresponding reduction in DNA, indicating marked catabolism of nonessential cellular components without cell death. There is gradual disappearance of zymogen granules and reduced size of acinar cells, although early change may be subtle, with sparing of acini adjacent to islets. Virtually all cellular organelles are altered; endoplasmic reticulum is reduced, wide variation occurs in mitochondrial size and shape, and the number of lysosomes is increased. With progression, there is loss and disorganization of acinar architecture, and dissociation of acinar cells into loose arrangement (Fig. 3-11). At this stage, nutritional correction restores acinar function, but the manner in which cellular association and acinar architecture are rejuvenated is unclear. However, the regenerative process appears to be reliant on activation of the mammalian target of rapamycin (mTOR) signaling pathway. With chronicity, continuing autophagy ultimately results in acinar cell apoptosis and dissolution of the exocrine tissue with attendant fibrosis, indicating irreversible change.

Aside from generalized protein malnutrition, **selective nutritional deficiency** also may cause significant atrophy of the exocrine pancreas. Selenium deficiency with or without concurrent vitamin E deficiency causes atrophic pancreatic lesions in chicks and mice in as little as 2 weeks, presumably reflecting oxidative stress caused by depletion of glutathione peroxidase. Histologically, there is acinar cell shrinkage and luminal dilation, together with abundant interstitial and periductal fibrosis. Inadequate intake of zinc, copper, vitamin A, and essential amino acids also may cause various degrees of exocrine atrophy.

Rapid atrophy also results from **obstruction of ductal drainage**, whether resulting from compression by adjacent inflammation or neoplasia, or from luminal occlusion by parasites, inflammatory exudate, or pancreatoliths. Atrophy in these cases is typically coupled with retrograde ductal ectasia, as well as proliferation and hyperplasia of new ductules.

Further reading

Crozier SJ, et al. Molecular mechanisms of pancreatic dysfunction induced by protein malnutrition. Gastroenterol 2009;137:1093-1101.

Spoelstra MN, et al. Kwashiorkor and marasmus are both associated with impaired glucose clearance related to pancreatic β-cell dysfunction. Metabolism 2012;61:1224-1230.

Canine juvenile pancreatic atrophy. Pancreatic acinar atrophy of juvenile onset is a distinct subclass of exocrine insufficiency, which has in the past been designated erroneously as *pancreatic hypoplasia*. It was initially described in German Shepherd dogs and—based on limited genetic analysis—the pattern of inheritance was suggested to be autosomal recessive, but more recent testing suggests that it is a more complex genetic disorder. A familial predisposition has also been noted in Rough-Coated Collies, Chows, and English Setters. The condition is reported sporadically in other breeds, including Beagles and Greyhounds. Clinical onset varies among breeds, with English Setters presented within the neonatal period, and Beagles having more delayed onset with signs not present until animals are several months of age. The majority of cases do not display signs of exocrine pancreatic insufficiency until 6-12 months of age. This variability in the age of onset suggests that the genetic setting in different breeds may be diverse. In a significant proportion of dogs, the clinical onset is precipitated by intercurrent gastrointestinal illness or a change in the normal household environment or diet.

Atrophy of the exocrine parenchyma is attended by intense but patchy infiltration by T lymphocytes and the early stages of this process are sometimes referred to as *atrophic lymphocytic pancreatitis*. Cytotoxic CD8+ cells predominate over CD4+ cells in the pancreas as the disease progresses. The lymphocytes may be found both between and within acinar cells, and intraepithelial lymphocytes also may be observed within the ductal epithelium. Lymphoid follicles may form in the parenchyma, and plasma cells, macrophages, and eosinophils also may infiltrate. Plasma cells are more commonly observed in more advanced areas of parenchymal destruction. Reactive fibroplasia is not a significant feature of the process. *The nature of the lesion suggests that the condition may be an autoimmune cell-mediated process directed against acinar cells*, but there is currently no evidence to incriminate autoantibodies in the pathogenesis.

By the time clinical signs emerge, exocrine atrophy is advanced and there is usually little remaining evidence of the preceding degenerative and inflammatory events. At autopsy of clinically affected dogs, the intestines are distended by bulky ingesta. The peritoneal cavity is devoid of fat and transparency of the mesenteries allows the flimsy tissue of the atrophic pancreas to be recognized. The main ducts and their larger tributaries can be seen easily, and many of the smaller ducts are recognizable grossly with the aid of transillumination. The ducts are of normal size, length, and configuration. Surrounding them is a thin pink veil of residual acinar parenchyma (Fig. 3-12). Microscopically, any remnant pancreatic lobules are small and composed of small acinar cells that stain darkly and do not assume a glandular arrangement. Tubular complexes—ductule-like structures lined by agranular, atrophic acinar cells—may be identifiable within the residual lobules. Occasional isolated lobules of normal appearance may be present. There is increased prominence of the connective tissues, ducts, islets, blood vessels, and nerves of the pancreas

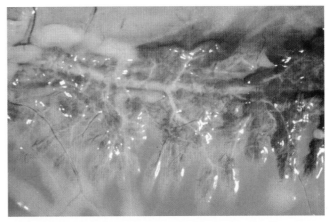

Figure 3-12 **Juvenile pancreatic atrophy** in a dog. Small remnants of parenchymal tissue surround prominent pancreatic ducts.

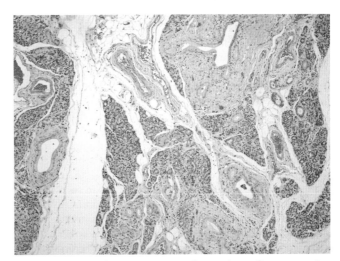

Figure 3-13 Histologic appearance of **juvenile pancreatic atrophy.** Pancreatic ducts are prominent among scant, atrophic exocrine tissue. Focal lymphocytic infiltrates are present within the interstitium.

owing to condensation (Fig. 3-13). Mild interstitial and periductal fibrosis may be present, but fatty replacement of the organ is more common.

The islets are usually histologically normal, but dual loss of both exocrine and endocrine components has been reported in Greyhounds, several of which exhibited insulin-dependent diabetes mellitus. Diabetes mellitus has also been reported in a German Shepherd with juvenile pancreatic atrophy. Haphazard distribution of various islet cell types, hyperplasia of pancreatic polypeptide and delta islet cells, and emergence of a profusion of nerve fibers immunoreactive for enkephalins and vasoactive intestinal peptide within islets have been noted in dogs with pancreatic acinar atrophy. The significance of these observations is uncertain.

Exocrine pancreatic insufficiency

Although the normal pancreas possesses substantial tissue reserve, significant impairment of exocrine function manifests in maldigestion and malabsorption of nutrients caused by reduced availability of pancreatic enzymes in the intestinal lumen. Exocrine insufficiency may occur as a consequence of congenital or acquired depletion of acinar tissue. The acquired form most commonly develops as a sequela to destruction of the exocrine pancreas, and may be induced by almost any pancreatic pathology of sufficient severity, including pancreatitis and pancreatic necrosis, toxic injury, localized and systemic infections, ductal disease (particularly in cases of obstruction), and neoplasia. Acquired exocrine insufficiency also may result from alterations in nutrient and neuroendocrine influences, reflecting the exocrine pancreas' heavy reliance on extrinsic signals for maintenance of functional mass. Physiologic activity of acinar tissue is dependent on a diverse range of stimuli—including vagal innervation, neuro-enteral signals from the gastrointestinal tract, and hormonal secretions from the pancreatic islets and the diffuse endocrine system of the gut—and withdrawal of these signals can leap to rapid decline in pancreatic function. Starvation or severe imbalances in protein, carbohydrate, and lipid intake may cause derangement of neuro-hormonal influences, as may structural or inflammatory disease of the gastrointestinal wall.

Progression to insufficiency may be slow or rapid, but clinical disease only manifests when ~90% of secretory power is lost. Developing deficiency may be compensated in part by salivary and other alimentary secretions and the clinical onset delayed.

Exocrine pancreatic insufficiency is observed commonly in dogs and is being recognized with increasing frequency in cats. Juvenile pancreatic atrophy is the most common form of exocrine insufficiency in dogs. Excluding this syndrome, reports of exocrine insufficiency in dogs generally involve older age ranges, and both females and household pets are overrepresented. These risk factors are likely to reflect the higher incidence of acute pancreatic necrosis in such animals. For cats although exocrine insufficiency is traditionally associated with chronic pancreatitis in older animals, recent reports suggest no breed or age predilection, with a number of cases detected at <6 months of age. Measurement of serum trypsin-like immunoreactivity is useful for clinical screening in dogs and cats; values <2.5 µg/L in dogs and <8 µg/L in cats are considered diagnostic, although there are occasional anomalous results. Isolated cases of exocrine insufficiency in horses are usually a result of chronic pancreatitis.

The most common clinical signs of exocrine insufficiency are loose feces and chronic weight loss despite a normal to voracious appetite. The hair coat may be of poor quality and marked muscle atrophy may be apparent in some animals. The feces are commonly pale, soft, voluminous, and malodorous but may occasionally be watery or even of normal appearance. Steatorrhea is not invariably present, but can lead to greasy soiling of hair of the tail and perineum, especially in cats. There may be a pot-bellied appearance caused by bulky intestinal contents, and affected dogs are at increased risk of intestinal accidents, especially mesenteric torsion. Hepatic steatosis also may develop in dogs and cats with exocrine pancreatic atrophy.

Malassimilation of nutrients is not simply caused by failure of intraluminal digestion by pancreatic enzymes. Pancreatic proteases normally cleave proenzyme forms of small intestinal microvillar membrane enzymes and also inactivate or degrade exposed brush border enzymes. In several species, exocrine pancreatic insufficiency is associated with increased activity of the jejunal brush border enzymes, sucrase and maltase, and an increase in high-molecular-weight microvillar membrane proteins, which are thought to be intestinal proenzymes. These alterations may impair the intestinal phase of digestion and

absorption. Concurrent intestinal syndromes causing mucosal villus atrophy may compound the malabsorptive effects, and this phenomenon is often observed in neonates because of immaturity of the exocrine tissue. Increased activity of enterocyte lysosomal degradative enzymes also occurs in exocrine pancreatic insufficiency, possibly to compensate for these changes. Protein synthesis by the jejunal mucosa is also reduced in affected dogs. The mechanism is unclear, but malnutrition and decreases in luminal trophic factors (e.g., pancreatic secretions and products of digestion) and humoral trophic factors (e.g., insulin, glucagon, and gastrin) may be implicated. Intestinal transport mechanisms for monosaccharides, disaccharides, fatty acids, and amino acids are also disturbed, contributing to malabsorption. These functional changes in the intestinal mucosa are not usually associated with histologic lesions. However, dietary sensitivity leading to inflammatory bowel disease is also a potential consequence of exocrine insufficiency as there is increased intestinal mucosal exposure to antigenic macromolecules because of the deficiency of pancreatic proteases.

Small intestinal bacterial overgrowth (SIBO) frequently occurs, reflecting both the increased volume of undigested nutrients within the alimentary tract, and also the loss of the antimicrobial influence of pancreatic juice. Changes in small intestinal flora are both quantitative and qualitative, and although poorly characterized in domestic animals, the major bacteria involved in the human form of the disease include *Escherichia coli*, *Streptococcus* spp., and anaerobes such as *Clostridium*, *Bacteroides*, and *Lactobacillus*. Diagnosis of SIBO is problematic, as there is considerable overlap between the flora in health and disease; fecal bacterial counts >10^5 are considered to suggest bacterial overgrowth. The osmotic effect of bacterial carbohydrate fermentation within the small intestine causes chronic or recurrent diarrhea, and this is often compounded by direct degradation of brush border enzymes such as lactase by bacterial proteases. Deconjugation of bile salts by aberrant intestinal flora impairs lipid processing, and the dysbiosis also may result in damage to the intestinal mucosa through induction of a mucosal immune response, as well as the direct effects of bacterial enzymes on enterocyte integrity. In humans, intestinal flora alterations are recognized to be an important factor in the development of inflammatory bowel disease, as well as having a wider influence on systemic immunity, and a similar relationship is likely in domestic animals.

Further reading

Brenner K, et al. Juvenile pancreatic atrophy in Greyhounds: 12 cases (1995-2000). J Vet Intern Med 2009;23:67-71.

Clark LA, Cox ML. Current status of genetic studies of exocrine pancreatic insufficiency in dogs. Top Companion Anim Med 2012;27: 109-112.

German AJ. Exocrine pancreatic insufficiency in the dog: Breed associations, nutritional considerations, and long-term outcome. Top Compan Anim Med 2012;27:104-108.

Sekirov I, et al. Gut microbiota in health and disease. Physiol Rev 2010;90:859-904.

Steiner JM. Exocrine pancreatic insufficiency in the cat. Top Companion Anim Med 2012;27:113-116.

Westermarck E, Wiberg M. Exocrine pancreatic insufficiency in the dog: historical background, diagnosis, and treatment. Top Companion Anim Med 2012;27:96-103.

Parasitic diseases of the pancreas

The pancreatic lesions of migratory larvae of *Strongylus equinus*, *S. edentatus*, and *Stephanurus dentatus* have been described in the preceding section.

Various **metazoan parasites** may be found within the pancreatic ducts of domestic animals. Their significance depends on the extent to which they occlude the ducts, either by direct physical obstruction or by provoking inflammation and periductal fibrosis. Ascarids may invade the ducts from the intestine in pigs, horses, and dogs. *Thysanosoma actinioides*, the fringed tapeworm, may spill from the bile ducts of ruminants into the pancreatic ducts and small intestine. In heavy infestations in herbivores and carnivores, trematodes such as *Dicrocoelium dendriticum*, *Opisthorchis tenuicollis*, *O. felineus*, *O. viverrini*, *Clonorchis sinensis*, *Platynosomum fastosum*, *Metorchis conjunctus*, and *Amphimerus pseudofelineus* may be found in both the pancreatic and bile ducts.

Dicrocoelid flukes of the genus **Eurytrema** may inhabit both the pancreatic and biliary ducts but prefer the former. *Eurytrema pancreaticum* is the most important species and is a common parasite of the pancreatic and bile ducts of ruminants and other herbivores throughout Asia and South America and is also reported in Madagascar and Russia. *E. coelomaticum* is common in Brazilian cattle, where nearly 50% of the population are infected, and is reported in ruminants in China. *E. tonkinese* is found in cattle in Vietnam. Snails act as the first and grasshoppers the second intermediate hosts. The flukes are presumed to gain access to the pancreatic ducts directly from the duodenum following ingestion of an intermediate host.

Other species of *Eurytrema* are found in carnivores, wild herbivores, and birds. Pigs may harbor *Eurytrema* flukes of either herbivore or carnivore origin. *E. procyonis* is a common parasite of the pancreatic ducts of raccoons in many parts of the United States, and has also been detected in red and gray foxes and domestic cats. In areas in which the fluke occurs, up to 14% of cats may be infected. The common garden snail, *Mesodon thyroidus*, and grasshoppers act as intermediate hosts. *E. procyonis* is infrequently reported in the bile ducts and gallbladder of cats.

Intraductal flukes may provoke only mild luminal and periductal inflammation, hyperplasia of the ductal epithelium, and periductal fibrosis. In some animals, however, there may be pronounced cording and dilation of the ducts and chronic interstitial pancreatitis, leading to near total loss of exocrine parenchyma and severe replacement fibrosis. Duct obstruction is thought largely to mediate the periductal fibrosis and the progressive atrophy of exocrine elements. Irritation of the ductal mucosa by the flukes and their ova and inflammation in response to dead flukes contribute to the progressive scarring.

E. pancreaticum preferentially targets the left pancreatic lobe in ruminants. Infestation of cattle with *E. pancreaticum* or *E. coelomaticum* may cause progressive wasting, and emaciation, recumbency, and death have been reported in sheep heavily infested with *E. pancreaticum*. Although islets are preserved in most cases, progressive destruction culminating in diabetes mellitus has been reported in sheep. Glucosuria has also been noted in raccoons harboring *E. procyonis*. In cats, *E. procyonis* is found in the small- and medium-sized ducts of both pancreatic lobes, but the tail of the pancreas is usually more severely affected than the head. Duct obstruction in cats is thought to be responsible for the significant reduction in the volume of pancreatic secretions and in the content of digestive enzymes and bicarbonate. With heavy infestations, the major pancreatic duct may be greatly dilated and much of the organ is shrunken, pale, and fibrotic. However, most cats are asymptomatic and diagnosis is by identification of typical dicrocoelid eggs with a single operculum in the feces.

Further reading

Bassani CA, et al. Epidemiology of eurytrematosis (*Eurytrema* spp. Trematoda: Dicrocoeliidae) in slaughtered beef cattle from the central-west region of the State of Paraná, Brazil. Vet Parasitol 2006;141:356-361.

Graydon RJ, et al. Mortalities and wasting in Indonesian sheep associated with the trematode *Eurytrema pancreaticum*. Vet Rec 1992;131:443.

Rachid MA, et al. Chronic interstitial pancreatitis and chronic wasting disease caused by *Eurytrema coelomaticum* in Nelore cow. Arq Bras Med Vet Zootec 2011;63:741-743.

Hyperplastic and neoplastic lesions of the exocrine pancreas

Unsurprisingly in an organ undergoing constant morphologic adaptation to nutritional influences, *hyperplasia is commonly encountered in the exocrine pancreas*, particularly in older dogs, cats, and cattle.

Exocrine hyperplasia typically occurs in multiple variably sized discrete nodules throughout the pancreatic parenchyma (Fig. 3-14). Their gray-white color and firm consistency contrasts grossly with the color and texture of normal pancreas. The lesions are incidental findings, and in most cases there is no evidence of a preceding pancreatic insult. *Histologically, the hyperplastic tissue is nonencapsulated and does not compress surrounding parenchyma, differentiating it from an adenoma.* There may be a mosaic of normal and hyperplastic tissue within affected lobules. There is considerable variability in the morphology of the hyperplastic cells, but they are typically uniform within a single nodule (Fig. 3-15). Cells may be large and stain more intensely acidophilic than their normal counterparts, or alternatively may be small and poorly staining. The cells are often vacuolated and there may be apparent loss of acinar architecture. Islet tissue is not affected, although exocrine hyperplasia may be particularly marked in areas adjacent to islets, indicating a role for trophic factors.

Hyperplasia of ductular epithelium is occasionally seen, often in an environment of chronic pancreatitis, exocrine parenchymal atrophy, and interstitial fibrosis, or within foci of nodular hyperplasia of the exocrine parenchyma. It is also reported as an aging phenomenon. The hyperplastic lining

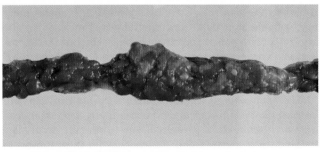

Figure 3-14 Nodular pancreatic hyperplasia in a cat.

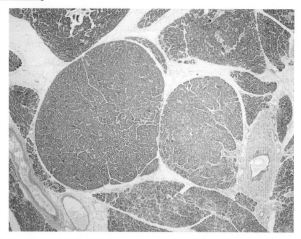

Figure 3-15 Nodular pancreatic hyperplasia in a cat. Acinar cells within the nodules are less intensely stained than the surrounding tissue, and are diffusely enlarged with increased zymogen granulation.

epithelium may protrude as papillae into the duct lumina, and the affected ducts may be dilated.

Exocrine pancreatic adenomas are rare, and some of those reported in older dogs, cats, and cattle may have been hyperplastic nodules. Adenomas are incidental findings at autopsy and their rarity suggests that they do not give rise to pancreatic adenocarcinoma. Adenomas may protrude from the surface of the pancreas, and grossly they more closely resemble normal parenchyma than do hyperplastic nodules. Expansive growth causes compression of adjacent parenchyma from which the tumor is usually separated by a thin fibrous capsule. The histologic pattern of an adenoma may be predominantly tubular or rarely acinar. In the tubular type (which is thought to be derived from ductal epithelium), small or large cystic spaces are lined by cuboidal or columnar epithelial cells and may contain mucin. Mitoses are rare. Multiple recurrent pancreatic cysts suggestive of cystadenomas have been associated with exocrine atrophy and eventual development of diabetes mellitus in a cat, presumably because of compression atrophy occurring in the adjacent parenchyma.

Exocrine pancreatic adenocarcinoma *is uncommon in all domestic animals,* but has predominantly been observed in dogs and cats. The malignancy is largely one of older age but some affected dogs have been only 3 years of age. Female dogs may be at slightly greater risk than males.

Several factors have been implicated in the pathogenesis of pancreatic adenocarcinoma, although there is little work specific for domestic animals. Nitrosamines are found in a variety of foodstuffs, particularly processed meat containing nitrite preservatives, and their carcinogenic potential with regard to the pancreas is well established in humans and a range of animal models. Concurrent disease processes are also associated with pancreatic carcinogenesis. There is a weak link between chronic pancreatitis and pancreatic malignancy, and an association with diabetes mellitus has been suggested in the literature, but is yet to be proved unequivocally.

The most common clinical signs in dogs and cats with this neoplasm are nonspecific: anorexia, weight loss, depression, lethargy, and vomiting. As a result, diagnosis typically occurs late in the disease course. There is a tendency for these tumors to arise centrally within the gland or in the duodenal wing; these

may provoke early clinical signs of biliary obstruction. Pancreatic panniculitis, a multifocal necrotizing steatitis presumed to reflect systemic release of lipase, has been observed in dogs with adenocarcinoma, although the syndrome may be seen with other pancreatic disease processes. Although the name suggests specificity for the subcutaneous adipose tissue, in reality lesions may be distributed throughout the body. A rare syndrome of paraneoplastic alopecia affecting the ventrum, legs, and usually the face also has been observed in cats with pancreatic adenocarcinoma. The stratum corneum of the affected skin is markedly atrophic and hypokeratotic, and there is attenuation of the follicular bulbs, resulting in a distinctive shiny appearance on gross examination. However, the lesion is not pathognomonic for pancreatic adenocarcinoma, as this condition may also develop with cholangiocellular carcinomas. Pseudohyperparathyroidism leading to hypercalcemia has been reported in a dog with pancreatic adenocarcinoma, and progressive destruction of normal pancreatic tissue may eventually result in the development of diabetes mellitus or exocrine pancreatic insufficiency.

Pancreatic adenocarcinoma may appear as a solitary, discrete, circumscribed mass or there may be multiple masses throughout the organ. The neoplasm is usually firmer than the adjacent pancreas. Some carcinomas are highly scirrhous and cannot be distinguished grossly from postinflammatory scarring. The cut surface of the neoplasm is typically heterogeneous and yellow to gray-white; areas of necrosis, hemorrhage, and mineralization may be obvious. Necrotic foci are often found in adipose tissue within and adjacent to primary and metastatic nodules and there may be adhesions of the pancreas to adjacent tissues. Some tumors may contain mucin-filled cysts.

Four main morphologic patterns of pancreatic adenocarcinoma are recognized histologically: **small tubular** (*the most common form*), **large tubular**, **acinar**, and **hyalinizing** (Fig. 3-16A-C). In the tubular forms, glandular structures resembling pancreatic ducts are formed by mucus-secreting cuboidal or columnar cells. Some tumors may contain localized ductular arrangements of well-differentiated cells that may be difficult to distinguish from the ductular response to incomplete obstruction. Well-differentiated acinar tumors are composed of small cells arranged into acini mimicking normal parenchyma. The hyalinizing form has been identified in the dog and is characterized histologically by the presence of large aggregates of PAS-negative hyaline material amidst variable tumor architecture.

The *histogenesis* of pancreatic adenocarcinoma has not been elucidated in domestic animals. Traditionally, the tubular forms have been considered to be derived from ductal epithelium whereas tumor cells containing brightly eosinophilic zymogen granules have been interpreted to be of acinar origin. This distinction is often arbitrary and the histologic pattern may vary considerably within a single tumor. Moreover, pluripotent ductular epithelium or endodermal stem cells could give rise to both tubular and acinar forms.

Undifferentiated carcinomas that do not form acinar or ductular structures are also seen. Some of these may be entirely composed of sheets of small anaplastic cells. Poorly differentiated tumors usually have a higher mitotic index and a more pronounced fibrous stroma.

The tendency of pancreatic adenocarcinomas to form tubules or acini usually permits their distinction from islet cell tumors, but a single case of mixed acinar-endocrine cell neoplasia has been described in a dog displaying intermittent

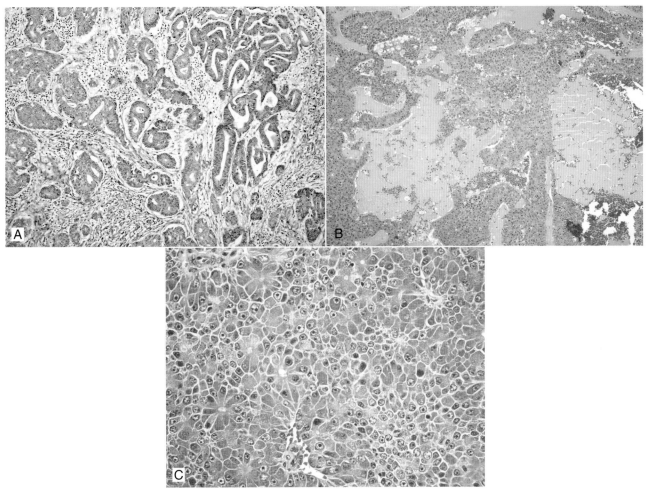

Figure 3-16 A. Small tubular form of exocrine pancreatic carcinoma with prominent scirrhous architecture. **B. Hyaline form** of exocrine pancreatic carcinoma displaying prominent interstitial aggregates of hyaline material. **C. Acinar form** of exocrine pancreatic carcinoma with formation of atypical acinar structures.

hypoglycemia. Detection of eosinophilic granules in tumor cells permits distinction of pancreatic adenocarcinoma from invasive or metastatic adenocarcinoma of gastrointestinal or biliary origin. Electron microscopy or immunohistochemical analysis for secretory products may be needed to clarify the origin of poorly differentiated tumors, with most exocrine neoplasms in dogs displaying reactivity for amylase and carboxypeptidase. Expression of the claudin-5 tight junctional protein by acinar cells is also lost in cases of canine exocrine adenocarcinoma, suggesting this may be a prerequisite of malignancy.

The prognosis with pancreatic adenocarcinoma is grave, as tumors metastasize widely and readily. Local invasion into the wall of the duodenum is common, and there may be obstruction of pancreatic or bile ducts. Neoplastic invasion of blood vessels and lymphatics may be obvious histologically in the pancreas, with tumor cells often tracking in the perineural lymphatics. The most common sites of metastasis are the liver, lungs, and regional lymph nodes, although dispersal to other organs, including the spleen, kidneys, heart, pleura, ovaries, and gastrointestinal tract has been reported. Peritoneal implantation is also common and there is also a propensity to extend along visceral nerves to the dorsal ganglia. Prediction of metastatic behavior from histological appearance is problematic, as

well-differentiated tumors can metastasize widely. A small subset of cats survived for an extended period (>1 year), but there was no correlation between survival and the histologic appearance of the tumor. The large tubular form is, however, reported to metastasize less readily than the other forms, and the hyalinizing form is also reported to be less aggressive.

Hepatopancreatic ampullary carcinoma has been reported in a single cat, as well as within multiple rhesus macaques from a single colony. Such tumors may cause obstruction of either or both ducts. In the cat, the tumor arose from the junction of the common bile duct and main pancreatic duct within the wall of the duodenum. The tumors affecting the macaques were typically aggressive, with duodenal invasion and metastasis to lungs, lymph node, liver, and colon.

Nonepithelial neoplasms rarely arise in the pancreas. Those reported include fibrosarcoma, hemangiosarcoma, liposarcoma, neurofibroma, and neurofibrosarcoma.

Metastasis to the pancreas from malignancies arising elsewhere appears to be rare but the paucity of reports may reflect lack of systematic examination and sampling of the organ at necropsy. The organ may become involved in hematopoietic malignancies and disseminated lymphoma. Neoplasms arising in the bile ducts, stomach, or duodenum, including intestinal lymphoma, may directly invade the pancreas.

Further reading

Belshaw Z, et al. Pancreatic mixed acinar-endocrine carcinoma in a dog. Vet Comp Oncol 2005;3:145-148.

Dennis MM, et al. Hyalinizing pancreatic adenocarcinoma in six dogs. Vet Pathol 2008;45:475-483.

Jakab C, et al. Expression of claudin-5 in canine pancreatic acinar cell carcinoma—an immunohistochemical study. Acta Vet Hungarica 2011;59:87-98.

Lindermann MJ, et al. Feline exocrine pancreatic carcinoma: A retrospective study of 34 cases. Vet Comp Oncol 2013;11:208-218.

ENDOCRINE PANCREAS

In pancreatic phylogeny, insulin-secreting β cells dominate the sequential evolutionary changes and the establishment of an endocrine pancreas precedes that of the exocrine pancreas. In insects, concentrations of trehalose (a glucose homolog) in hemolymph are regulated by insulin-like and glucagon-like reactivities located exclusively within the brain. In more evolutionarily complex organisms, such as the protochordate lancelets, the cells that produce insulin-like peptide depart from the brain for the embryonic gut, accompanied by dispersed populations of other hormone-producing cell types. In the most primitive vertebrates—exemplified by hagfish—β cells have migrated completely from the gut tube to form islet-like structures in the lateral plate mesoderm supporting the gut tube, leaving behind the distributed population of other endocrine cell types. These dispersed cells in the gastrointestinal epithelium form the diffuse neuroendocrine system and are of physiologic significance and occasional clinical significance in domestic animals when neoplastic. Of particular relevance to the pancreas are the glucagon-like peptides produced by enteroendocrine L cells within the intestinal mucosa. These peptides, in particular GLP-1, are released in response to nutrient passage, providing trophic stimulation for β cells and transiently stimulating the release of insulin to maintain euglycemia. It is likely that these effects are mediated by the enteric nervous system.

In higher vertebrates, the distribution of islet-like colonies within the embryonic mesentery coincides with the regions of the gut tube involved in the budding of the biliary and pancreatic anlagen. Residual small clusters of islet cells may be seen in the gut and bile ducts in some mature animals as a reflection of this embryogenesis.

There appears to be a general consensus that growth and maturation of the pancreas in higher vertebrates, including ductular, acinar, and endocrine tissues, results from the differentiation of a common PDX1-positive endodermal stem cell, refuting the evolutionary evidence of a neural crest origin for pancreatic endocrine cells. Involvement of neural crest tissue is thought to be confined to influencing the healthy differentiation of adjacent endoderm into insulin-secreting β cells. The basis of the current view comes from the failure of chick-quail chimeras to confirm neural crest lineage, together with a wide variety of ex vivo procedures that induce varieties of endocrine cell differentiation in pancreas, gut, and liver, but not the full array of major islet hormones.

As a broad definition for vertebrates, *an islet is a discrete glomerular organ perfused by capillary blood flow and sustaining a variety of immunophenotypically distinct cells that produce specific endocrine, paracrine, and intracrine hormones.* The distribution of islets in the pancreas is not uniform in relation to the lobes or lobules or interstitial tissue. In general, circulation within the pancreas initially flows through the islets in a portal system before supplying the adjacent acinar tissue. Exocrine parenchyma distant to this portal system or within lobules lacking islets is perfused directly from systemic circulation, as is the ductal system. The portal vascular arrangement facilitates perfusion of the local acinar tissue with trophic factors from the islet, and this is reflected histologically in the quality of acinar cells adjacent to islets. Insulin provides the predominant exocrine trophic stimulus, with pancreatic polypeptide providing lesser influence; glucagon and somatostatin are inhibitory. The distribution of islet cells around the vessels and the regulation of blood flow in the islet are unclear but may vary under different physiologic conditions. Islet capillaries are highly permeable, with 10 times more fenestrations than those in exocrine tissue, and blood flow is regulated at the precapillary level by gastrointestinal hormonal influences and physiologic states such as hyperglycemia. With the exception of amyloidosis, pathologic changes related to the intra-islet vessels are not routinely sought, but specific responses to disease have been observed in the islet vasculature, such as the upregulation of endothelial cell adhesion molecules during type 1 diabetes.

There are 5 main **cell types** in the pancreatic islets identified by the hormones they produce. The **β cells** that produce insulin and amylin (islet amyloid polypeptide) are the only ones present in all islets, and comprise 60-70% of the islet cell population. The other types include **α cells** that produce glucagon, **δ cells** that produce somatostatin, **PP cells** that produce pancreatic polypeptide and adrenomedullin, and **ε cells** that produce ghrelin. A range of other minor hormones, such as vasoactive intestinal peptide, are also variably produced in the islets of domestic species.

The effects and interactions of the pancreatic hormones are complex (Fig. 3-17). **Insulin** is the major regulator of serum glucose and is released in response to hyperglycemia. The hormone stimulates glucose uptake and glycogenesis by target cells, in particular hepatocytes, striated myocytes, fibroblasts, and adipocytes. Insulin has potent anabolic effects, promoting DNA, RNA, triglyceride and protein synthesis, as well as suppressing proteolysis. Insulin also promotes cellular growth and differentiation in common with the insulin-related growth factors.

The hypoglycemic effects of insulin are countered by **glucagon**, which promotes hepatocellular glycogenolysis and gluconeogenesis in response to low blood glucose, as well as stimulating lipolysis. Glucagon release is suppressed by **amylin**, which is co-secreted with insulin and also inhibits gastric secretory function and motility, as well as acting as a satiation signal. In contrast, **somatostatin** inhibits the release of glucagon, insulin, and pancreatic polypeptide, and is thought to play a role in regulating the magnitude of hormonal responses to neuronal and nutritional stimuli. **Ghrelin** is secreted by PD/1 cells in the gastric fundus as well as the islets, and although it is recognized as an important appetite stimulant, its primary role in the pancreas appears to be local suppression of insulin secretion. **Pancreatic polypeptide** antagonizes the effects of cholecystokinin by inhibiting exocrine pancreatic secretion and gallbladder contraction as well as delaying gastric emptying, whereas **vasoactive intestinal polypeptide** stimulates secretory activity within the exocrine pancreas, gallbladder, and intestine.

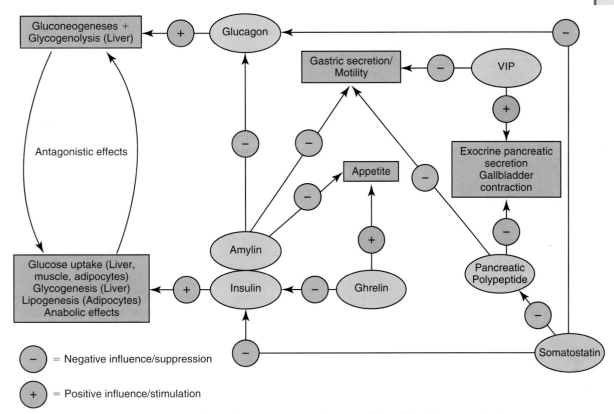

Figure 3-17 Diagram displaying the interactions and major effects of the dominant islet hormones. Hormones are denoted by blue ovals, physiological actions are indicated in purple boxes. See text for detailed descriptions. VIP, vasoactive intestinal peptide.

Synchronous islet response to secretory stimuli is largely achieved through a well-developed system of intercellular gap junctions that allows co-ordination of electrical signaling. This response is modified both qualitatively and quantitatively by a wide range of endocrine influences, including cholecystokinin, gastrin, and the gut-associated incretin, glucagon-like peptide 1. Vitamin D has been purported to promote insulin secretion, but the evidence remains inconclusive. Islet hormone secretion is also mediated by paracrine signals involving both the major islet hormones and other localized protein signals. Such intimate interaction is demonstrated by *parathyroid hormone related protein*, PTHrP, which all major endocrine cell types both bear receptors for and produce. Paracrine expression of PTHrP facilitates local calcium ingress, insulin secretion, and β-cell proliferation.

In addition to hormonal regulation of the endocrine pancreas, islet activity also may be modified by neuronal input. The islets are richly innervated by both adrenergic and cholinergic autonomic systems with the vagus nerve most prominent. Autonomic ganglia are distributed in the interstitial tissue and may contain islet tissue in a common capsule. The major neurotransmitters are acetylcholine and epinephrine with many peptides as co-transmitters. Insulin secretion is stimulated by the parasympathetic neurotransmitters and inhibited by sympathetic signals. In addition, the enteric nervous system, which is capable of independence from the central nervous system, may be important in enteropancreatic reflexes and exocrine secretion.

The arrangement of cells and their relative numbers are described for many vertebrate species, but there are inconsis-tencies in the descriptions between individuals and species that may reflect in part cellular plasticity, validity of immune reactants, or physiologic variability. Developmentally, islet cell distribution appears to reflect differential expression of cell adhesion molecules, in particular E-cadherin expression on β cells and neural cell adhesion molecule (N-CAM) expression on non–β cells. However, it is likely that a degree of architectural plasticity persists in adult life, and alterations in cellular composition may occur as adaptations to changing physiologic and pathologic demands. *Islet cells retain the ability to undergo mitotic division in adults*, although this function appears to be restricted to a small fraction of the islet population that progressively declines with age. New islet cells also may arise from ductular hyperplasia and transdifferentiation. Replication of β cells can be experimentally stimulated by exposure to glucose, D-mannose, essential amino acids, glucocorticoids, gastrin, CCK, GH, prolactin, IGF-1 and IGF-2, platelet-derived growth factor (PDGF), epidermal growth factor (EDF), and indeed by insulin itself via stimulation of the IGF-1 receptor.

The peculiarities of endocrine tissue distribution in different domestic species warrant discussion. In **dogs**, there are fewer islets in the left lobe and larger compact islets in the tail of the organ. Large islets of irregular size and shape are described in research colony Beagles as *nesidioblastosis*, although these animals are euglycemic with normal serum insulin concentrations. Most β cells are in islets, but ~25% are interstitial in acinar tissue, probably mixed with other unchar-acterized endocrine cells. The interstitial cells occur singly or in small clusters and may be sparse or abundant; their numbers

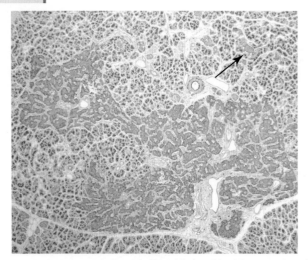

Figure 3-18 Large islet in a calf highlighted by blue-purple coloration. A small islet is present within the adjacent exocrine tissue (arrow). Aldehyde fuchsin stain.

and distribution may be correlated with systemic physiologic circumstances, but the distribution does not appear to be linked with abnormal insulin function.

In **cats**, the islets are large, of irregular shape and composed mainly of β cells. Encapsulated interlobular islets can be seen in connective tissues and in and adjacent to ganglia. Mixed cell types, solitary or in small clusters, may be seen in ductal lining epithelium, in ganglia and nerves, or abundantly in the interstitium of acinar tissue.

In **ruminants**, including cattle, sheep, goats, deer, and buffalo, there are 2 populations of islets, large and small, throughout fetal development and extending into mature life. The cellular composition of fetal islets has been reported for sheep and cattle, with features that suggest that islet ontogeny may differ among species. The large islets are of round or irregular shape, measuring between 200 and 1600 μm in fetal calves, and enmeshed in interlobular and periductal connective tissue without direct contact with acinar tissue (Fig. 3-18). They develop more or less concurrently with more regular small islets, but they do not appear to increase in size or number with natural postnatal growth. They are comprised almost entirely of β cells and are reminiscent of the initial β-cell organ of the embryonic gut tube in early vertebrates.

The small islets, which are usually <200 μm in size and are developmentally embedded in acinar tissue, contain β cells. They can be identified with granular cytoplasm at about the end of the first trimester in fetal lambs, but remarkably they degranulate in late gestation and remain so for 2-6 weeks thereafter when granulation is re-established. For several weeks postnatally, the small islets are difficult to distinguish from acinar tissue except by dense cellularity and indifferent cell character.

Many of the peculiarities of the ruminant endocrine pancreas are likely to reflect adaptation to different energy sources during fetal and postnatal life. Fructose is the most abundant hexose sugar in the fetal fluids of ungulate animals, including ruminants and pigs, but is negligible in humans and other species. Intravital exposure of the ovine fetus to either glucose or fructose in late gestation provokes minimal increase in plasma insulin, but postnatally, the fructogenic energy

substrate of the ovine fetus is quickly replaced by glucose resulting in altered activity of islet hormones, with an increase in insulin responsiveness to glucose and—at least initially—short chain fatty acids.

Like other endocrine glands, dysfunction of pancreatic hormones typically reflects excessive or insufficient secretion. In the case of the endocrine pancreas, excess typically occurs as a product of unregulated neoplastic disease, whereas insufficiency is applicable almost exclusively to insulin and the important syndrome of diabetes mellitus. It is now established that for some phenotypes of diabetes mellitus the thread of causation may stretch back to the pregnant uterus and that the intrauterine environment impacts the development of the endocrine pancreas and the β cells. Influences such as maternal obesity and increased glucocorticoid exposure have been shown to affect fetal islet development at different stages, with the common outcome of reduced islet size, reduced cell number, and altered responsiveness to higher glycemic levels at different gestational and postnatal ages. Furthermore, intrauterine growth retardation resulting from a number of causes has been linked to epigenetic alterations predisposing to both β-cell dysfunction and insulin resistance in peripheral tissues.

Further reading

Chen X, et al. Insulin-like growth factor and fibroblast growth factor expression profiles in growth-restricted fetal sheep pancreas. Exp Biol Med (Maywood) 2012;237:524-529.

Green AS, et al. Consequences of a compromised intrauterine environment on islet function. J Endocrinol 2010;205(3):211-224.

Heller RS. The comparative anatomy of islets. Adv Exp Med Biol 2010;654:21-37.

Ohira T, et al. A case of pancreatic nesidioblastosis with aberrant islet cell proliferation in a Beagle. J Toxicol Pathol 2004;17:55-68.

Rorsman P, Braum M. Regulation of insulin secretion in human pancreatic islets. Ann Rev Physiol 2013;75:155-179.

Son WC, et al. Spontaneously occurring extra-islet endocrine cell proliferation in the pancreas of young Beagle dogs. Toxicol Lett 2010;193:179-182.

Steiner DJ, et al. Pancreatic islet plasticity: interspecies comparison of islet architecture and composition. Islets 2010;2:135-145.

Diabetes mellitus

Diabetes mellitus is a metabolic syndrome characterized by sustained hyperglycemia, weight loss, polyphagia, and polyuria. Hyperglycemia may be the result of failure to synthesize or release adequate insulin if stimulated to do so by glucose, or reduced sensitivity of tissues to insulin, especially the liver, striated muscle (including cardiac myocytes) and adipose tissue. The failure of end organs to respond to insulin stimulation stems from inability to extract glucose from blood, reflecting a failure of target tissues to accept or respond to normal amounts of secreted insulin. In addition to impaired glucose entry into cells, hyperglycemia also reflects diminished glucose oxidation, increased glycogenolysis, and increased gluconeogenesis from amino acid sources. Diabetes mellitus is typically preceded by a period of impaired glucose tolerance, in which return to euglycemia after administration of glucose is slowed or incomplete. Early diagnosis and effective management of the prediabetic state is difficult to achieve in domestic animals, and unregulated chronic hyperglycemia is frequently associated with important degenerative changes in other organs.

The current classification of syndromes of diabetes mellitus places cases broadly into type 1, type 2, and other, defined as type S. These classifications acknowledge large levels of complexity in the pathogenesis of the diabetic syndromes in both humans and the non-obese mouse model, and the elasticity exercised in the interpretation of evidence. It should be kept in mind that human diabetes mellitus may represent a special case of the disease, and direct application of medical knowledge to veterinary cases may not be appropriate in all circumstances. Longitudinal studies investigating the clinically silent phase of the disease in domestic animals are lacking, and so causal factors and early pathogenesis in particular are poorly defined.

Type 1 diabetes mellitus is characterized by hyperglycemia and deficiency of insulin caused by primary immune-mediated or (rarely) idiopathic loss of β-cell mass; clinically, these cases are labeled as insulin-dependent diabetes mellitus (IDDM). In immune-mediated cases, β-cell destruction appears to be effected primarily by CD8+ T cells, through either the granzyme-perforin system or the Fas apoptotic pathway. There is strong circumstantial evidence that viral agents may trigger the initial immune response against β cells, although whether this is due to specific viral tropism for β cells or a form of molecular mimicry is uncertain. Genetic polymorphisms, particularly those involved in T-cell activation and antigen recognition, also appear to play an important role in the development of many cases of human, and presumably veterinary, type 1 disease.

Type 2 diabetes mellitus is a complex multifactorial disease, but is primarily characterized by a failure of appropriate glycemic control in the face of excess energy load. In humans, disease onset is strongly influenced by predisposing genetic and environmental factors, including obesity, inactivity, and micronutrient imbalances such as vitamin D deficiency. Many of these environmental impacts appear to be mediated through epigenetic effects, and this may provide an additional mechanism of heritability through intrauterine programming.

The pathophysiology of type 2 diabetes mellitus reflects both inadequate insulin secretion as well as increased resistance to insulinic effects in peripheral tissues; considerable controversy persists as to the relative importance and interdependence of these processes. Insulin resistance suppresses glucose uptake by tissues—in particular skeletal muscle—following eating, resulting in sustained hyperglycemia. The normal insulinic inhibition of gluconeogenesis within the liver is also impaired by insulin resistance, and continued production of glucose exacerbates the hyperglycemia. β cells attempt to compensate by boosting insulin secretion but eventually they become refractory to hyperglycemic stimuli, reflecting depletion of intracellular insulin reserves and release of incompletely processed proinsulin. Hyperglycemia also causes direct β-cell glucotoxicity by increasing oxidative stress, altering gene transcription and secretory signaling, and inducing inflammatory and apoptotic pathways. Increases in circulating fatty acids as a result of insulin insufficiency lead to aberrant lipid storage in nonadipose tissues, which if sufficiently severe this may result in lipotoxicity. This condition further suppresses insulin secretion by β cells and exacerbates insulin resistance in peripheral tissues, and may induce apoptosis through oxidative stress and generation of ceramides.

Type S includes those cases in which insulin action is antagonized by hormones and drugs, as well as instances of secondary β-cell destruction following extension of pancreatic inflammation, necrosis, or neoplasia.

Lesions associated with diabetes mellitus are widespread, reflecting the ubiquity of glucose dependence within the body. Muscle wastage occurs because of catabolism of proteins for glucogenic substrates, and insulin deficits also stimulate lipolysis and fatty acid mobilization from adipose tissue. Under normal circumstances these lipids are metabolized into lipoproteins within the liver, but in diabetic animals this energy-intensive process is impaired by the inability to use glucose effectively. Hepatic lipidosis and hypertriglyceridemia result, and steatosis also develops within the proximal renal tubular epithelium. Metabolic derangement also causes intracellular glycogen accumulation and vacuolation in many organs, particularly in rapidly progressing cases. Tissues affected include islet cells, renal tubules (especially the loops of Henle and distal convoluted tubules), and the pancreatic and biliary ductal epithelium (Figs. 3-19, 3-20). In the dog, hepatocytes may also display intranuclear glycogen vacuolation, and islets may become fibrotic. Cataracts develop rapidly in the dog and also sporadically in cats, reflecting osmotic stress within the lens caused by accumulation of the glucose metabolite

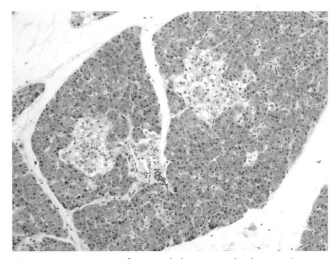

Figure 3-19 Pancreas from a diabetic cat displaying **glycogen vacuolation** within islets.

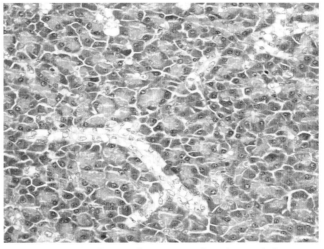

Figure 3-20 Vacuolation of pancreatic ductular epithelium in a dog with diabetes.

sorbitol. Osmotic diuresis and dehydration develop once the renal threshold for glucose resorption is exceeded, and loss of caloric stores through the urine contributes to the wasting effects of diabetes. Electrolyte disturbances, particularly hypokalemia, also may occur because of solute loss in the urine.

Chronic hyperglycemia induces a number of deleterious effects that may result in tissue damage. Hyperosmotic cytoplasmic swelling occurs because of intracellular accumulation of polyols such as sorbitol derived from excessive glucose metabolism. Hyperglycemia promotes glycation of tissue proteins, especially within myelin sheaths and blood vessels, resulting in demyelination and loss of vascular compliance. Advanced glycation end products also may induce expression of proinflammatory cytokines by endothelial cells and macrophages, promoting inflammation. Oxidative stress within tissues is increased with diabetes mellitus, and excess glucose also stimulates the proinflammatory protein kinase C signaling pathway. These effects of hyperglycemia appear to be particularly important in the pathogenesis of *diabetic neuropathy*. Up to 8% of diabetic cats display evidence of this disorder, typically manifesting as a symmetric plantigrade hindlimb stance that is reversible in mild cases, although if unchecked this may progress to permanent paraparesis, hyporeflexia, and proprioceptive deficits. *Diabetic nephropathy*, characterized by glomerulosclerosis, mesangial proliferation, and hyaline thickening of vascular basement membranes, also may develop as a response to hyperfiltration and derangement of local hemodynamic regulators such as nitric oxide and the renin-angiotensin-aldosterone pathway. *Diabetic retinopathy* is diagnosed infrequently in dogs and only manifests 5 years or more after onset of diabetes. The retinal vascular changes comprise venous dilation and tortuosity, saccular capillary microaneurysms, and focal hemorrhage, and are most severe at the posterior pole. These nonproliferative lesions in dogs resemble early stages of human diabetic retinopathy.

Significant morbidity and mortality attend the metabolic dysregulation of diabetes mellitus, and death may result from *ketoacidosis*, wherein ketones such as β-hydroxybutyric acid and acetone are generated by the liver as it attempts to provide an alternative lipid-derived energy source as a replacement for glucose. Insulin deficiency suppresses the use of ketones by peripheral tissues while also stimulating lipolysis and ketogenesis within the liver, resulting in the accumulation of ketones within circulation. This ketosis compounds the hyperosmolality and osmotic diuresis of diabetes, exacerbating dehydration, as well as causing marked acidosis and hypokalemia. If untreated, these physiologic derangements are frequently fatal, and disease progression is often exacerbated by renal failure, as well as thromboembolism caused by circulatory stasis and activation of clotting factors. In cases in which a low level of insulin efficacy persists, animals may become moribund in the absence of ketosis (nonketotic hyperosmolar diabetes), reflecting the hyperosmolar effects of marked hyperglycemia.

Diabetes mellitus in **cattle** has long been recognized in animals persistently infected by foot-and-mouth disease virus. Current reports also implicate bovine viral diarrhea virus in the pathogenesis of diabetes mellitus, and in view of the wide distribution of this infection and the high level of persistence, underreporting of diabetic sequelae seems likely. Regardless, these observations support a role for immunoparticipant factors in the pathogenesis of diabetes mellitus. Under the current classification system, the disease in cattle corresponds

to type 1 diabetes, with immunodestruction of β cells and retention of insulin responsiveness in tissues. Affected cattle are presented with progressive emaciation, polydipsia, polyuria, and persistent hyperglycemia, reduced glucose tolerance, and glucosuria. Histologically, the cellularity of islets is reduced, with hydropic change and decreased granularity particularly affecting the β cells. Lymphocytes infiltrate both small and large islets in all lobes in instances of early onset, along with a small population of macrophages and plasma cells. Mild interlobular and interacinar fibrosis accompanies atrophy of acinar cells and reduction of zymogen granulation. In more chronic cases, endocrine cells including β cells appear to be increased in periductal tissue, perhaps as a compensatory response.

Diabetes mellitus in the **horse** is rare and diagnosis is problematic because of marked variability in serum glucose and insulin concentrations in health. Insulin-dependent diabetes mellitus has been associated with a presumed autoimmune polyendocrine syndrome involving the pancreas, adrenal cortex, adrenal medulla, and thyroid gland. Chronic pancreatitis may reduce the islet-cell mass, resulting in insulin insufficiency and type S diabetes. Type S diabetes also has been described in association with granulosa-cell tumor of the ovary and pheochromocytoma. Diabetes mellitus is frequently associated with metabolic dysfunction in older horses arising from a functional adenoma within the anterior-intermediate lobe of the pituitary gland, but recent investigations of insulin sensitivity in these animals have been conflicting. Obese ponies and miniature horses are prone to develop hyperlipemia with associated insulin resistance.

Diabetes mellitus in the **cat** is relatively common. Most cases are type 2, and identified risk factors include Burmese breed genotype, obesity, male sex, drug treatments, and age, the majority of cases being >10 years of age. Other diseases may cause type S diabetes mellitus by decreasing β-cell numbers, especially pancreatitis and occasionally pancreatic neoplasia, or through marked insulin antagonism caused by excess of growth hormone in acromegaly or by hypersecretion of hormones from the adrenal cortex or thyroid.

In the cat, the gradual decline in function and number of β cells characteristic of the type 2 syndrome is potentially resolvable by dietary adjustment to high protein and low carbohydrate content. Synthetic and secretory exhaustion of β cells may not be a sufficient cause of the decline; glucotoxicity also may play a role, as exposure to excessive glucose promotes β-cell interleukin-1β secretion and apoptosis. *Amyloid in islets* (Fig. 3-21) is a useful marker of disturbed β-cell function in cats, and its detection in normoglycemic cats is indicative of a potential prediabetic state, but it is not obligatory as a cause of functional decline. Moreover, although a correlation exists between islet amyloidosis and feline diabetes, almost half of aged cats may display a degree of islet amyloidosis, and thus such changes should be interpreted with caution. The major constituent of the islet amyloid is *amylin*, produced by β cells and co-secreted with insulin. In a majority of diabetic cats, the deposition of amyloid within islets is associated with a decrease in β-cell numbers, suggesting that the substance may exert a toxic effect on β cells. A range of theories have been proposed to explain the toxic mechanism, including amyloid-induced alterations in cell membrane permeability, and induction of inflammatory mediators and β-cell apoptosis through intracellular accumulation of amylin oligomers.

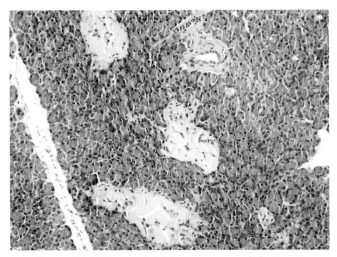

Figure 3-21 **Islet amyloid** deposition in a diabetic cat.

In **dogs**, early onset diabetes mellitus has been reported that is consistent with the type 1 classification. Onset at birth is described in the Keeshond as a probable recessive autosomal defect. Juvenile onset is also described in a family of Samoyeds and in a singlet Chow; these are classified as islet cell hypoplasia with diminished α and β cells. Diabetes mellitus with islet atrophy also occurs in some Greyhounds with juvenile pancreatic atrophy, discussed earlier. More typically insulin-dependent diabetes develops in older dogs, and a breed predisposition is present in Cairn and Tibetan terriers, Miniature Poodles, and Rottweilers, indicating that there is a genetic component to spontaneous cases. Specific allelic variants in major histocompatibility complex genes have been shown to increase susceptibility in affected breeds. There is evidence for immune-mediated destruction of β cells in these cases; ~50% of diabetic dogs with an undamaged exocrine pancreas have autoantibodies against β cells, but lymphocytic infiltrates are only occasionally observed within and surrounding the islets.

The most common cause of canine diabetes mellitus in the general population is loss of islets because of exocrine pancreatic disease, usually pancreatic necrosis or pancreatitis. Insulin resistance caused by antagonism by other metabolic regulators, such as glucocorticoids and progestagens derived from endogenous or exogenous sources is also well documented.

Diestrus- and gestation-associated diabetes occurs in the bitch in the latter half of pregnancy; it may be exacerbated if diets are high in fat content. Hormone profiles during diestrus, pseudopregnancy, and pregnancy are identical, but insulin insensitivity is more pronounced during pregnancy, suggesting that other factors are involved beyond pure hormonal antagonism. Nevertheless, progesterone from corpora lutea during pregnancy or pseudopregnancy indirectly alters insulin sensitivity through stimulation of pituitary growth hormone release and the development of mammary tissue.

Further reading

Ize-Ludlow D, Sperling MA. The classification of diabetes mellitus: a conceptual framework. Pediatr Clin North Am 2005;52: 1533-1552.

Koppieters KT, Von Herrath MG. Histopathology of type 1 diabetes: Old paradigms and new insights. Rev Diabet Stud 2009;6:85-96.

La Torre D, Lernmark A. Immunology of beta-cell destruction. Adv Exp Med Biol 2010;654:537-583.

Leahy JL. Pathogenesis of type 2 diabetes mellitus. Arch Med Res 2005;36:197-209.

Menzies-Gow N. Diabetes in the horse: a condition of increasing clinical awareness for differential diagnosis and interpretation of tests. Equine Vet J 2009;41:841-843.

Otzo M, et al. Diabetes from humans to cats. Gen Comp Endo 2013; 182:48-53.

Rand JS, et al. Canine and feline diabetes mellitus: nature or nurture? J Nutr 2004;134:2072S-2080S.

Rand JS. Pathogenesis of feline diabetes. Vet Clin Small Anim 2013;43:221-231.

Taniyama H, et al. Histopathological and immunohistochemical analysis of the endocrine and exocrine pancreas in twelve cattle with insulin-dependent diabetes mellitus (IDDM). J Vet Med Sci 1999;6: 803-810.

Hyperplastic and neoplastic diseases of the endocrine pancreas

Islet hyperplasia and nesidioblastosis

Islet hyperplasia in domestic animals is often subtle and difficult to distinguish from normal islet variability, but has been reported in humans and other primates, mice, rats, hamsters, and horses. Histologically, the islets are enlarged—in some cases comprising up to 40% of the pancreatic tissue—and may compress the surrounding exocrine parenchyma. The change is thought to represent a compensatory phenomenon, and in humans it may be observed in infants born of diabetic mothers, as well as those with hyperinsulinemic hypoglycemia, chronic pancreatitis, Zollinger-Ellison syndrome, and multiple endocrine neoplasia. In animals, the associations are less clear, although hyperplastic islets have been reported in pancreatic fibrosis. Hyperplasia is also documented in aged rats and horses, sedentary obese rats, and hamsters treated with corticosteroids.

Nesidioblastosis *is described as a non-neoplastic proliferation of islet and ductular tissue* and has been reported sporadically in domestic animals, particularly the dog. Newly formed islet cells appear to bud from proliferating epithelium of small intralobular ductules and thence migrate and organize into discrete islets. Occasionally the islet structures coalesce to form large aggregates, and these may appear identical to the large islets observed in ruminants. The majority of cells in the nesidioblastic foci are β cells, but the other major cell types also are represented to a variable degree. Although the pathogenetic pathway remains uncertain, the condition appears to be an aberrant regenerative response, and may be induced by a range of pancreatic insults, including partial pancreatectomy, ectopic autotransplantation of pancreatic tissue, and ductular occlusion. It may also be observed in animals without other apparent pancreatic disease. Experimental administration of *islet neogenesis-associated protein* (INGAP) induces similar changes in dogs and mice via activation of the RAS/MAPK signaling pathway. Unlike in humans, where hyperinsulinemic hypoglycemia is a common association, *nesidioblastosis in animals is typically an incidental finding.*

Pancreatic endocrine neoplasia

Pancreatic endocrine neoplasms are sporadically identified in domestic animals, particularly dogs, in which multiple tumors occasionally develop. They are also identified as part of the rare syndrome of **multiple endocrine neoplasia** in several species. Although many pancreatic endocrine neoplasms are functional and produce clinical signs of inappropriate hormone secretion, nonfunctional tumors also occur, typically presenting with an abdominal mass or metastatic disease. The true incidence of nonfunctional tumors remains unknown, however, as many remain clinically silent. Although insulinoma is the most commonly identified neoplasm in the endocrine pancreas, *functional pancreatic endocrine tumors often produce multiple hormones*, and fewer than 10% of tumors in dogs purely express a single hormone.

The tumors typically occur as small (<2 cm), solitary, well-circumscribed, homogeneous nodular masses with the pancreas, and may be missed on cursory examination. In accordance with the cooperative relationships between islets, many islets may be larger than the average in the organ and contain more nuclei, often clustered. Larger pancreatic endocrine neoplasms are unlikely to be functional. They are often lobular as a result of an expansive pattern of growth and may appear to be attached to adjacent structures. The main masses on cut surface are fibrotic or silky, firm, white, and may show yellow foci of necrosis. In cases of carcinoma, metastases may not be easily seen on inspection of the liver but, microscopically, they are expected to be widely distributed in the portal areas. Invasion of veins and lymphatics is best seen in marginal tissues. The tumors may spread from the local lymph node along perineural lymphatics to the sublumbar region.

The diagnosis of pancreatic endocrine neoplasm usually can be made on ordinary histologic examination, but identification of cellular phenotype requires additional histochemistry. Stains used to distinguish normal islet cell types such as Mallory-azan may be beneficial, but staining is inconsistent in neoplastic tissue. Immunohistochemistry may identify hormones normally produced within islets as well as others of ectopic origin. Additionally, more than one hormone is often identified in a tumor, but it is possible that not all hormones detected are expressed functionally. Most of the tumors in the canine pancreas are well differentiated, with sparse mitoses and relatively uniform nuclei containing a fine dusting of chromatin. Architecturally, there is a varied but characteristic organoid or pseudoalveolar pattern that, depending on orientation, may appear trabecular (Fig. 3-22A, B). Ductules may be present within the tumors, as well as aggregates of birefringent and congophilic islet amyloid polypeptide. Pancreatic endocrine tumors typically stain positively for chromogranin A and/or B, synaptophysin, and neuron-specific enolase. Distinguishing benign and malignant tumors may be difficult, and the classification is typically based on the presence of peripheral invasion and evidence of vascular or lymphatic metastasis. When present, large areas of necrosis, frequent mitoses, and marked cellular atypia are also useful indicators of malignancy. The following section describes the characteristics of pancreatic endocrine tumors with a singular hormonal phenotype, but it is important to note that the clinical presentation is determined by the specific balance of hormones produced.

Insulinomas are most prevalent in the dog, cat, and ferret. They also have been reported sporadically in horses and as incidental findings in cattle at postmortem (often in association with pheochromocytoma). Clinical disease largely reflects neuronal glucose deficiency (neuroglycopenia), with depression, weakness, seizures (typically brief, reflecting transitory hypoglycemia), and muscle fasciculation commonly reported. Polyphagia may occur as an adaptive response, and ptyalism

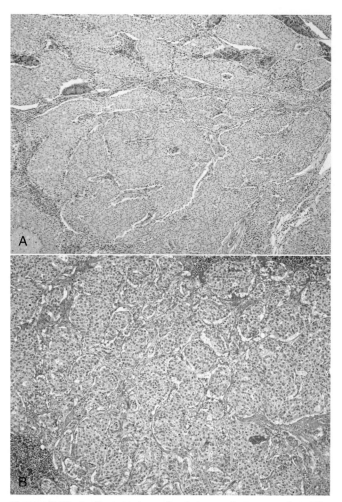

Figure 3-22 A. Pancreatic endocrine neoplasia in a dog. The tumor is composed of lobules of relatively uniform cells with pale acidophilic cytoplasm separated by fine fibrous septa. **B.** Higher magnification of (**A**).

is a frequent finding in ferrets. In dogs, weakness may be exacerbated by the development of paraneoplastic polyneuropathy, characterized by demyelination and axonal degeneration. Although the cause of the polyneuropathy is unidentified, an autoimmune pathogenesis has been proposed rather than metabolic deficiency resulting from hypoglycemia. Neuronal necrosis attributed to hypoglycemia has been observed in the superficial layers of the cerebral cortex of the dog.

Except for the ferret, in which the tumors are generally benign, insulinomas in domestic species are typically malignant and readily metastasize to regional lymph nodes or the liver. Prognosis largely depends on the clinical stage, with the overall mean survival time for dogs ranging between 12 and 18 months in different studies. Tumor characteristics associated with improved survival time include smaller tumor size, the presence of stromal fibrosis within the tumor, and low expression of Ki67 in tumor cells.

Functional **glucagonomas** may cause mild persistent hyperglycemia (type S diabetes mellitus) through stimulation of hepatic gluconeogenesis and glycogenolysis. The effects of glucagon on energy metabolism typically results in a variable degree of vacuolar hepatopathy, with severe cases displaying hepatocellular ballooning and widespread parenchymal extinction interspersed with nodular hyperplasia. In dogs, glucagonomas also are associated frequently with the development of *superficial necrolytic dermatitis*. Affected animals display erythema, hyperkeratosis, and superficial erosion affecting the foot pads, mucocutaneous junctions, and pressure points such as the elbow and hock. The pathogenesis of this disease is unclear, although it is likely to represent epidermal nutritional deficiency, with suggested causes ranging from zinc and fatty acid deficiencies to increased protein catabolism.

Gastrinomas are infrequently reported in the dog and cat, and although often located within the pancreas, the lineage of these tumors is controversial, as the pancreas is generally considered an ectopic location for gastrin production. However, the detection of progastrin within pancreatic tissue of multiple species (including cats and dogs) suggests that the gastrin gene is, in fact, expressed by low numbers of endocrine cells throughout the pancreas. Moreover, the immunophenotypic characteristics of pancreatic gastrinomas—in humans, at least—are distinct from those of enteral gastrinomas, with pancreatic tumors displaying positivity for pancreatic polypeptide, whereas those of duodenal origin express the sonic hedgehog marker. These observations suggest that the tumors are derived from intrinsic pancreatic endocrine tissue, rather than ectopic gastrointestinal G cells.

The primary presentation of gastrinoma is Zollinger-Ellison syndrome, wherein excess gastrin results in gastric acid hypersecretion, with attendant antral mucosal hypertrophy and gastroduodenal ulceration. Inactivation of pancreatic lipase and precipitation of bile salts at low pH in the duodenum may cause the development of steatorrhea. Gastrinomas typically metastasize early and, in contrast to other islet tumors, are often highly invasive histologically.

Pancreatic polypeptide-secreting islet neoplasia (PPoma) has been reported in a single dog with a presentation of chronic vomiting, inappetence, and upper gastrointestinal ulceration not unlike gastrinoma. Decreased bicarbonate production resulting from excess pancreatic polypeptide combined with mild acid hypersecretion is thought to result in gastrointestinal hyperacidity.

Somatostatinoma also has been reported rarely in dogs in association with multiple endocrine neoplasia, but the influence of several concurrent endocrine imbalances means the isolated clinical presentation is poorly characterized. However, development of these tumors has been associated with diabetes mellitus, cholelithiasis, weight loss, diarrhea, and anemia.

Further reading

Buishand FO, et al. Evaluation of clinico-pathological criteria and the Ki67 index as prognostic indicators in canine insulinoma. Vet J 2010;185:62-67.

Goutal CM, et al. Insulinoma in dogs: a review. J Am Anim Hosp Assoc 2012;48:151-163.

Hughes SM. Canine gastrinoma: Case study and review of the literature. New Zeal Vet J 2005;54:242-247.

Kiupel M, et al. World Health Organization Histological Classification of Tumors of The Endocrine System of Domestic Animals. 2nd Series. Washington, DC: Armed Forces Institute of Pathology.; 2008. p. 49-57.

O'Brien TD, et al. Islet amyloid polypeptide and calcitonin gene-related peptide immunoreactivity in amyloid and tumor cells of canine pancreatic endocrine tumors. Vet Pathol 1990;27:194-198.

Shaw DH. Gastrinoma (Zollinger-Ellison syndrome) in the dog and cat. Can Vet J 1988;29:448-452.

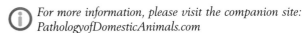 *For more information, please visit the companion site: PathologyofDomesticAnimals.com*

CHAPTER 4

Urinary System

Rachel E. Cianciolo • F. Charles Mohr

ACKNOWLEDGEMENTS

This update of the Urinary System chapter is based on previous editions by Drs. Ken Jubb, Peter Kennedy, Nigel Palmer, Grant Maxie, Shelley Newman, and John Prescott, and their contributions are gratefully acknowledged.

KIDNEY

GENERAL CONSIDERATIONS

The kidney is the central organ involved in the maintenance of a constant extracellular environment in the body. The vital homeostatic functions performed by the kidney include excretion of waste products, maintenance of normal concentrations of salt and water in the body, regulation of acid-base balance, production of a variety of hormones (erythropoietin, renin, prostaglandins), and metabolism of vitamin D to its active form, 1,25 dihydroxycholecalciferol ($1,25(OH)_2D_3$). *The essential requirements for normal renal function are adequate perfusion with blood (pressure >60 mm Hg), adequate functional renal tissue, and normal elimination of urine from the urinary tract.* Urinary tract disease is detected if any of these requirements are not met, and the outcome is always approximately the same: There is imbalance of salt and water, and of acids and bases, and there is retention of wastes. *The most commonly used index of failure is the amount of urea that is retained.* Urea itself is rather harmless, but if other urinary functions are sufficiently disturbed, a fairly consistent set of clinical signs emerges and the syndrome is called **uremia.**

Water and salt are the most important constituents of body fluids. The evolution of a terrestrial existence and homeothermy by mammals imposed a need to conserve water and salt and simultaneously excrete large quantities of metabolites. Nitrogenous wastes, and a multitude of other organic compounds and inorganic substances, impose a substantial load on the renal mechanism. Mammals excrete urea, which is highly soluble, diffusible, and osmotically active; excretion of wastes and conservation of water in mammals require concentrating mechanisms capable of raising the osmotic pressure of urine above that of blood. The extracellular fluid and plasma of the body are dialyzed through the kidney many times a day, producing copious amounts of filtrate, of which almost all is resorbed. Although this system effectively rids the body of wastes, it requires a large expenditure of energy and a dependable renal blood supply.

Renal blood flow is normally high, up to 25% of the cardiac output. Blood flow to the kidneys increases mildly after a high-protein meal and in certain systemic disease states, for example, fever. However, decreased blood flow causes injury more commonly. Whereas peripheral and splanchnic blood flow may be sacrificed in hypovolemia, renal blood flow is only diminished when it is necessary to preserve circulation to the heart and brain. Renal oxygen consumption equals about 10% of whole-body consumption. It is relatively small in relation to renal blood flow, but high compared to that of other tissues. Most of the oxygen consumed by the kidney is used in the resorption of essential solutes, which is predominantly a cortical function. Hence the consequences of reduced perfusion are largely borne by the cortex.

A unique feature of renal blood flow is that it varies little over a wide range of arterial pressures, thus ensuring a stable *glomerular filtration rate (GFR)*. The kidneys possess intrinsic mechanisms by which vascular resistance is varied to maintain constant glomerular filtration. Renal blood flow is normally directed predominantly toward the outer *cortical nephrons* rather than to the inner cortical, or *juxtamedullary nephrons*, but may be redistributed between the 2 areas. When reduction in renal perfusion occurs, it primarily affects the cortex. Depending on the severity and duration of the ischemic episode, it may lead to attenuation or atrophy of tubular epithelium, to necrosis of tubular epithelium, or to extensive necrosis of the renal cortex. Juxtamedullary nephrons are better at conserving water and concentrating urine. Therefore redirection of blood flow toward these nephrons helps maintain circulating blood volume and elimination of wastes during periods of poor perfusion.

The **glomerulus** produces ultrafiltrate as the net result of the difference between high capillary hydrostatic pressure and low hydrostatic pressure in Bowman's space. Additionally, the difference between osmotic pressures in these 2 compartments is also important in glomerular filtration. The glomerular basement membrane (GBM) is semipermeable, and dissolved substances and particles in suspension move across the glomerular capillary walls at rates determined by size, shape, and electrical charge. Malfunction of the glomerulus may result from inadequate glomerular blood flow and/or structural alterations that change its permeability.

After crossing the GBM, the ultrafiltrate enters the tubular lumens and is, in a strict sense, outside the body. Many of the filtered substances are retrieved by selective resorption, which requires special machinery and energy. If this function is defective, essential substances are lost in the urine. This occurs when enzymes are genetically deficient, tubular epithelial cells are injured, plasma levels of filterable substances are elevated, or the glomerulus has increased permeability. Myriad tubular functions are carried out sequentially, and the structure of the tubule varies along its length corresponding to the function to be performed.

The principal function of the kidney is the regulation of salt and water balance; this requires a system of monitors and feedbacks to achieve fine regulation. The hypothalamus and antidiuretic hormone (ADH, or vasopressin) control osmotic and volume regulation. The renin-angiotensin-aldosterone system (RAAS) is also involved in salt and water homeostasis and is described in more detail later.

Terrestrial mammals need to conserve water while eliminating high loads of waste and need to concentrate urine above the tonicity of plasma. This function is provided by the *loop of Henle;* juxtamedullary nephrons have long loops, extending into the deep medulla, whereas cortical nephrons have short loops. Some species have predominantly long loops and some predominantly short loops; species with a preponderance of long loops have greater concentrating ability. Although the deep or juxtamedullary nephrons are the first to develop and are active while development of the rest of the cortex is underway, neonatal nephrons have immature functional capacity and a relative inability to conserve sodium. Neonatal pigs, in particular, are thus very susceptible to dehydration. In contrast, renal functional capacity of calves approaches that of adult cattle within 2-3 days of birth.

According to the **"intact nephron"** hypothesis, nephron function is an all-or-none phenomenon. In progressive renal disease, the remaining nephrons respond by hypertrophy, because new nephrons cannot be formed in a mature kidney. Glomerular filtration and tubular function then increase concomitantly to maintain homeostasis. *All of the renal components are interdependent, and if one component is irreversibly damaged, function of the other components will be impaired.* Glomerular disease can cause decreased peritubular capillary perfusion and tubular atrophy, whereas tubulointerstitial disease can cause glomerular obsolescence. Interstitial inflammation and fibrosis may be primary events, but they also commonly accompany primary diseases of the glomeruli and tubules. *There is a tendency for chronic renal disease to affect multiple components of the kidney, resulting in chronic renal failure (CRF) and shrunken, scarred* **end-stage kidneys;** identification of the initiating cause may be impossible.

Anatomy

The *renal collecting system* is derived from the ureteral bud (metanephric duct), a diverticulum of the mesonephric (Wolffian) duct, and consists of *the ureter, pelvis, calyces, and collecting ducts.* Nephrons develop from the metanephric blastema and attach to the growing ends (ampullae) of the collecting system. The *uriniferous tubule* consists of the nephron and the collecting tubule. Renal calyces are the cup-shaped recesses of the pelvis that enclose conical masses of medullary pyramids. The apex of a pyramid is referred to as a *papilla*, and its tip is fenestrated by collecting ducts (area cribrosa). The fornix is the uppermost blind end of a calyx or pelvis.

Kidneys of domestic animals are classified as **unipyramidal** (unilobar) or **multipyramidal** (multilobar). *Cats, dogs, small ruminants, and horses have unipyramidal kidneys.* In cats, one lobe is present, and papillary ducts open into a calyx on a single renal papilla. In dogs, small ruminants, and horses, there is complete or partial fusion of several lobes and a single

crest-like papilla *(renal crest)*. *Pigs have multipyramidal kidneys* in which there are several distinct renal lobes, pyramids, and their respective papillae. Extensions of renal cortex between the pyramids are known as the *renal columns of Bertin*. Simple papillae occur in central pyramids, and compound papillae in pyramids at the renal poles; this is of pathogenetic significance because compound papillae are more susceptible to ascending infection. The *kidneys of cattle are also multipyramidal*, but have distinct external lobation, with each lobe having one pyramid. The renal calyces of cattle join directly to form the ureter without forming a pelvis. Note the difference between a renal lobe and a renal lobule. A *renal lobule* consists of a medullary ray and its associated nephrons. *Medullary rays* are seen histologically as lighter-staining linear areas in the cortex, and consist of collecting tubules, thick ascending limbs, and the terminal straight portions of the proximal tubules. Interlobular arteries course between lobules.

On sagittal section of a kidney, *subdivisions of cortex and medulla* may be distinguished, particularly in dogs and sheep. The *cortex* has a darker outer zone, and a paler inner zone, which in mature dogs often has prominent pale streaks because of the presence of fat in collecting ducts. Outer and inner zones may be seen in the *medulla* of canine kidneys, and the outer zone may be further subdivided into outer and inner bands (stripes), owing to the presence of the thick segments of the descending and ascending limbs of the loop of Henle in the outer zone and only the thick ascending limbs in the inner stripe, respectively. The inner zone of the medulla (papilla) contains the thin segments of the loop of Henle (Fig. 4-1). Mucous glands are large and prominent in the medulla of equine kidneys, and mucus and crystals are normally present in the equine renal pelvis.

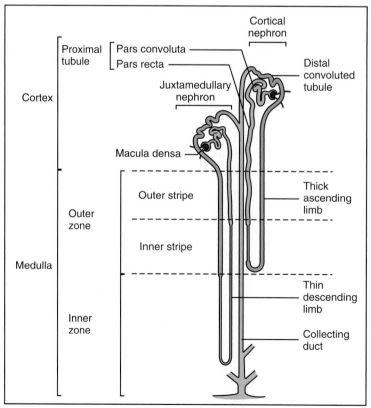

Figure 4-1 Diagram showing components of **cortical and juxtamedullary nephrons** and their location in zones of the kidney.

The functional unit of the kidney is the **nephron,** which consists of the *renal corpuscle, proximal tubule, loop of Henle, and distal tubule.* The glomerulus and Bowman's capsule comprise the renal corpuscle. The following approximate numbers of nephrons are present in each kidney—human, 200,000-1,800,000; cattle, 4,000,000; sheep, 650,000; pig, 1,250,000; dog, 400,000; cat, 200,000. The number of nephrons is fixed at birth in most mammals, although nephrogenesis may continue for several weeks after birth in animals with a short gestation period, such as dogs, cats, and pigs.

There are 4 main components of the kidney: blood vessels, glomeruli, tubules, and interstitium.

Vascular supply

Although the kidneys constitute only about 0.5% of body weight, *they receive 20-25% of cardiac output.* In multilobed kidneys, the *renal artery* divides in the pelvic region to form *interlobar arteries* that run in the renal columns between lobes up to the corticomedullary junction, where they branch to form *arcuate arteries.* These arteries run along the corticomedullary junction parallel to the capsule and terminate by becoming the radiating *interlobular arteries* in the cortex. Interlobular arteries give rise to prearterioles, which have a lumen diameter of <70 μm. The glomerular *afferent arterioles* (which are derived from the prearterioles) give rise to several glomerular capillary loops. The capillaries later rejoin to form the glomerular *efferent arteriole* and then divide again to form a peritubular capillary plexus. The efferent arterioles of the juxtamedullary nephrons branch to form *descending vasa recta* (straight vessels), which enter the medulla. The ascending vasa recta reform from the medullary capillary plexus and form a *countercurrent exchange system* with their closely associated descending vasa recta. The glomerular capillary tufts are perfused at a high pressure that favors filtration; the capillary bed rising from the efferent arterioles is low pressure, favoring resorption.

Because the renal artery and its branches are *end-arteries,* occlusion of any branch leads to infarction. Furthermore, interference with glomerular capillary flow markedly alters peritubular blood flow, especially in the medulla. The medulla is particularly sensitive to ischemia because of its relative avascularity and the low hematocrit in medullary capillaries.

Intrarenal blood flow and GFR are controlled by complex mechanisms, some of which are still being elucidated. The best understood regulatory mechanism is **tubuloglomerular feedback,** which is a negative feedback loop. It is mediated by the **juxtaglomerular apparatus (JGA),** which consists of the *macula densa* of the corresponding distal convoluted tubule, extraglomerular mesangial cells at the glomerular hilus between the arterioles, and the renin-containing juxtaglomerular cells in the wall of the afferent arteriole. The architecture of the JGA is important because it allows communication between cells of the distal tubule and the glomerular hilus. Briefly, low GFR results in decreased NaCl delivery to the distal tubule. This is detected by the macula densa cells (via a Na-K-2Cl cotransporter at their apical membrane), and the net result is contraction of the efferent arteriole with simultaneous dilation of the afferent arteriole. Increased GFR (or high NaCl) induces the opposite response. When macula densa cells detect low NaCl, they synthesize and secrete prostaglandin E_2 (PGE_2), which induces the release of renin from the afferent arteriolar juxtaglomerular cells. Renin acts on angiotensinogen (made by the liver) to generate angiotensin I in the kidney, which is then cleaved by angiotensin converting enzyme (ACE) into angiotensin II. This latter molecule is a potent vasoconstrictor, and has a greater effect on efferent than afferent arterioles. Angiotensin II also initiates adrenocortical synthesis of *aldosterone,* which, over the long term, increases resorption of sodium from the distal convoluted tubules and collecting ducts, resulting in water retention and expansion of the extracellular fluid volume. Angiotensin II also stimulates the secretion of ADH by the posterior pituitary, which helps raise the GFR by increasing water resorption through insertion of aquaporin-2 channels in the collecting duct. Other key mediators of tubuloglomerular balance include adenosine triphosphate (ATP), adenosine, nitric oxide (NO), myogenic control of afferent arteriolar tone, as well as other derivatives of angiotensin (angiotensin III, angiotensin IV, and angiotensin 1-7). Most of these additional mechanisms are involved in titrating the system so that GFR is kept within a narrow range. Interestingly, many angiotensin derivatives are vasodilatory, which underscores the complexity of this system. Detailed discussion of these mediators is beyond the scope of this chapter, and the reader is referred to relevant renal physiology texts.

The *renal venous system* begins with formation of venules from the peritubular vasa recta, and then closely parallels the arterial system. Veins in the outer cortex drain into stellate veins, which in cats are prominently visible on the capsular surface, and then into interlobular veins. Veins within the kidney have very thin walls and are susceptible to compression.

Lymphatics occur in the renal cortex and medulla. One set of lymphatics drains the cortical and medullary interstitium and follows the pattern of the vascular system; another set of lymphatics drains the capsular area. Lymphatic flow increases after urinary obstruction and in interstitial disease.

Glomerulus

The glomerulus is a vascular-epithelial structure designed for the ultrafiltration of plasma (Fig. 4-2). It develops embryologically by the invagination of a capillary-rich mesodermal mass into an epithelium-lined sac, which connects to the proximal tubule. The visceral epithelium (podocytes) covers the abluminal surface of glomerular capillaries, whereas the parietal epithelium lines the basement membrane of Bowman's capsule. This capsule encircles the urinary space that receives glomerular ultrafiltrate. The arterioles enter and leave the glomerulus at the *vascular pole,* and urine enters the proximal tubule at the *urinary pole* of the glomerulus. The *glomerular filtration membrane* (Fig. 4-3) consists of 3 layers: (1) capillary *endothelium* containing fenestrae of 50-100 nm diameter and coated by a thick glycocalyx on the luminal side; (2) *GBM,* which is 100-300 nm thick and consists of a central electron-dense lamina densa and peripheral electron-lucent layers, the lamina rara interna and externa; and (3) *podocytes.* The podocytes have complex interdigitating trabeculae whose *foot processes (pedicels)* are embedded in the lamina rara externa of the GBM. The pedicels are separated by 25-50 nm–wide *filtration slits,* which are bridged by thin *slit diaphragms* with pores of 6-9 nm in diameter. The GBM is produced continuously by the podocytes and endothelium, but does not completely encircle the glomerular capillaries. At the base of the capillary loop, the endothelial cells are in direct contact with mesangium. The GBM is a complex porous meshwork

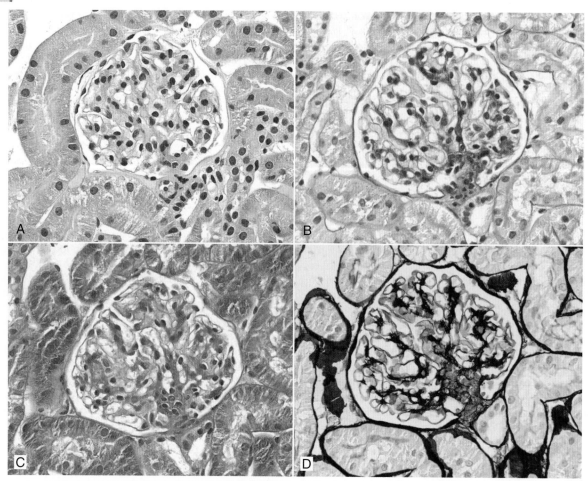

Figure 4-2 Normal canine glomerulus and macula densa, sectioned at 3-μm thickness. **A.** H&E stain. **B.** Podocytes can be clearly distinguished on the abluminal side of the delicate glomerular basement membrane, and mesangial zones contain <3 nuclei. Periodic acid–Schiff (PAS) stain. **C.** Mesangium at vascular pole may contain >3 nuclei. Masson trichrome stain. **D.** Note the smooth outer contour of the glomerular basement membrane. Jones' methenamine silver stain.

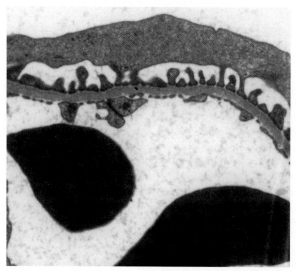

Figure 4-3 Transmission electron micrograph of a **normal canine glomerular filtration barrier,** consisting of the internal fenestrated endothelium, glomerular basement membrane (GBM), podocyte foot processes that are perpendicular to the GBM, and the podocyte cell body. Two erythrocytes are present in the glomerular capillary lumen.

composed of collagen (primarily type IV in mature glomeruli), laminin, polyanionic proteoglycans (mainly heparan sulfate), fibronectin, entactin, and other glycoproteins.

A large volume of glomerular ultrafiltrate is formed as a product of the high hydrostatic pressure of arteriolar blood, and the selective permeability of the filtration membrane. The entire plasma volume is filtered about 100 times per day. The GBM is a *size-dependent barrier* to filtration, prohibiting passage of particles with radius >3.5 nm. It is highly permeable to water and small solutes, but virtually excludes high-molecular-weight plasma proteins from the filtrate. The mechanism by which medium-to-large molecular weight proteins such as albumin cross the normal GBM is still under debate. The filtration barrier also excludes particles from filtration on the basis of *charge*. Thus anionic molecules are repelled by virtue of the presence of negatively charged sialoglycoproteins in the lamina rara interna and externa and the negatively charged glycocalyx of the endothelial cells. *Changes in porosity or charge of the filtration membrane alter glomerular permeability and can lead to proteinuria, a hallmark of glomerular damage.* The glomeruli of neonates are permeable to colostral protein for a few days.

The **mesangium** is the central region of the glomerulus that forms a supporting framework about which the glomerular capillaries ramify. *The mesangial matrix is basement-membrane–like periodic acid–Schiff (PAS)–positive glycoprotein, and the mesangial cells are phagocytic, contractile cells, which are derived from vascular smooth muscle cells.* These cells function in phagocytic removal of deposited macromolecules, removal of GBM, and may modulate intraglomerular blood flow; mesangial cells both respond to and produce a variety of cytokines. Mesangial cell hyperplasia and increased mesangial matrix are common changes in glomerular disease.

Tubules

The kidney functions by producing a large volume of glomerular filtrate from which the body resorbs the constituents it needs. Thus about 99% of the sodium chloride and water filtered are resorbed. This system effectively rids the body of wastes that are filtered by the glomeruli and not resorbed by the tubules. The *structure of a tubule segment is correlated with its function.* Thus cells of the proximal convoluted tubule have a well-developed brush border and numerous mitochondria. Energy for the sodium pump in this actively resorptive area is provided by mitochondrial oxidative phosphorylation; this area is especially vulnerable to hypoxia. Also, toxins are frequently resorbed by or secreted by the proximal tubule, causing chemical injury.

About 90% of the hydrogen ion excretion by the kidney occurs in the proximal tubule. The proximal tubule actively resorbs large quantities of sodium and chloride, and water passively follows, hence 60-80% of the glomerular ultrafiltrate that enters the proximal tubule is resorbed. *Tubules and peritubular capillaries are in close apposition to allow rapid removal of resorbed sodium chloride and water.* In addition to salt and water, proximal tubules resorb glucose, amino acids, calcium, phosphate, uric acid, proteins, and potassium. The movement of sodium ions down its concentration gradient into the proximal convoluted tubule provides energy to resorb glucose and amino acids via a cotransporter mechanism. The sodium concentration gradient is maintained by Na^+/K^+ ATPases located at the basal surface of these cells.

Many substances, such as glucose, amino acids, and water-soluble vitamins, are "threshold substances" that are almost completely resorbed until a certain concentration is reached in the glomerular filtrate. Above these threshold concentrations, the tubular transport maximum is exceeded, and the substance appears in the urine. For example, hyperglycemia of diabetes mellitus leads to glucosuria and **osmotic diuresis.** Proximal tubules are also involved in the trafficking of hydrogen ions, organic acids, p-aminohippurate, penicillin, and some iodinated radiopaque materials.

The long loops of Henle of the juxtamedullary nephrons penetrate deep into the medulla and assist in making the renal medullary tissue hypertonic. Urine concentrating ability is directly proportional to the length of the loop of Henle; desert-dwelling rodents have very long loops of Henle, whereas baby pigs have short loops and are thus very susceptible to dehydration. The loops of Henle serve as *countercurrent multipliers* and the capillaries as simple *countercurrent exchangers,* with the flow in each occurring in opposite directions. The countercurrent multiplier uses energy to produce a solute gradient that becomes greater toward the tip at the papilla and therefore is an active process. The gradient is passively preserved by vasa recta countercurrent exchange. Sodium chloride is actively pumped from the ascending limb of the loop of Henle into the interstitium, in turn drawing water

from the descending limb, and progressively increasing the solute concentration in the descending limb. The ascending limb is impermeable to water. Thus, as sodium chloride leaves and the fluid returns to the cortex, the degree of hypertonicity of luminal fluid lessens. More salt may be resorbed in the collecting ducts, further diluting the fluid.

Water diuresis occurs when a state of water excess exists or ADH is not released from the neurohypophysis. If water preservation is required, ADH is released and renders the epithelium of the collecting tubule highly permeable to water, producing concentrated urine, up to 3-4 times the blood osmolality (280 mosmol/L). The water resorbed in the medulla is passively transported into the ascending vasa recta to be delivered back to the systemic circulation. The solute concentration of the medulla consists of both sodium and urea. During antidiuresis, ADH renders the *cortical portions* of the collecting ducts permeable to water but not urea, thus increasing the urea concentration of the luminal fluid. ADH increases the permeability of the *medullary portions* of the collecting ducts to urea and water; urea then diffuses from collecting tubule to interstitium, and water follows. Tubules are not functionally mature in the kidneys of most neonates and cannot produce a medullary solute gradient to concentrate urine.

Either osmotic diuresis or water diuresis may result in **medullary solute washout** because of increased tubular flow rates and hence decreased efficiency of the countercurrent multiplier, the loop of Henle. The quantities of urea and sodium chloride resorbed are decreased as the result of increased tubular fluid transit time. Hence the medullary solute gradient decreases, as does urine concentrating ability. The same mechanism is operative in chronic renal disease in which there are high tubular flow rates in the small number of hypertrophic tubules present.

Although body buffers and pulmonary control of carbon dioxide excretion are the first lines of defense in protecting the pH of the extracellular fluids, *it is the action of the kidneys that ultimately corrects acid-base balance.* The kidneys excrete the excess alkali or acid responsible for the disturbance. Thus the kidneys can correct metabolic alkalosis by excreting alkaline urine containing the excess bicarbonate, and they can correct metabolic acidosis by increasing resorption of filtered bicarbonate, excreting titratable acids (secrete hydrogen ions), and by producing ammonia.

Interstitium

The interstitium normally contains peritubular capillaries, pericytes, and a few fibroblasts. Interstitial tissue is usually only obvious around interlobar, arcuate, and interlobular arteries. *Expansion of the cortical interstitium is abnormal* and may occur because of edema, cellular infiltration, or fibrosis. The glycosaminoglycan content of the medullary interstitium increases with age and ischemia. Specialized interstitial cells produce prostaglandins, particularly PGE_2 and $PGF_{2\alpha}$.

Examination of the kidney

Gross examination

The systematic gross inspection of a kidney entails observation of its *size, shape, color, and consistency.* The kidneys are usually equal in size and about 3 vertebrae long. Renal enlargement may occur because of addition of blood, edema, fat, urine in the pelvis or tubules, or swollen or hypertrophic nephrons.

Acute inflammation causes renal enlargement because of addition of fluid and cells, whereas chronic inflammation causes scarring and loss of parenchyma. The kidneys are usually bean- or horseshoe-shaped, although the bovine kidney is lobated externally. Focal lesions, such as those caused by infarction or pyelonephritis, may markedly distort the capsular surface, whereas more generalized diseases such as glomerulonephritis (GN) do not. The normal renal color is brown-red, except in mature cats, in which the cortices are yellow because of their high lipid content. The fat content in cats is apparently hormonally determined; pregnant females and sexually inactive old males have the most fat, pseudopregnant females and castrated males have somewhat less, estrous females and sexually active males have moderate amounts, and anestrous females have little or no renal fat. Kidneys autolyze fairly rapidly after death, particularly in fat animals in a warm environment. Pulpy kidneys, seen in clostridial enterotoxemia in sheep, may be difficult to distinguish from advanced autolysis.

The urinary system may be kept intact during examination, or the kidneys may be removed from the carcass. The kidney should not be severed from the ureter until the absence of hydronephrosis has been established. Each kidney is cut in the sagittal plane, and the cut surface is examined. The *normal cortex-to-medulla ratio* in this plane is about 1:2 or 1:3. *The cortex normally accounts for 80% of the renal mass*, a fact that is better appreciated in a coronal, than in a sagittal section. Diffuse diseases of the kidney usually respect the integrity of the medulla. Pyelonephritis involves the pelvis and papilla/medulla. Pallor of the cut surface suggests the deposition of fat or acute tubular necrosis (ATN); if the surface bulges

slightly when sectioned, diffuse tubular injury and interstitial edema are likely. Focal glomerular lesions do not cause glomerular prominence, but diffuse lesions, such as amyloidosis or diffuse GN, often do. *Removal of the renal capsule is essential for examination of the outer surface of the cortex.* The capsule should strip easily and leave a smooth surface underneath. Tearing of the cortex may indicate scarring, except in the horse, which normally has trabeculae attached to the capsule.

Histologic examination

The kidney must be trimmed so that a section from capsule to papilla is available. The section should first be examined subgrossly for evidence of localized lesions, for example, infarcts, abscesses, granulomas, pyelitis, mineralization, neoplasia, scars, medullary loss. The section is then scanned at low power. Glomeruli are normally distributed randomly throughout the cortex, with ~1-2 present per 40× field. Tubules should be tightly packed, with little intervening connective tissue (Fig. 4-4). In dogs, the diameter but not the number of glomeruli is significantly correlated to body surface area. This suggests that large-breed dogs have larger nephrons compared to small-breed dogs, as opposed to having more nephrons. Goat and sheep glomeruli are more cellular than those of most other species. Horses have the largest glomeruli of domestic animals (up to 200 μm diameter). Glomeruli in neonatal kidneys are small and hyperchromatic, particularly in the outer cortex (Fig. 4-5). Nephrons may be seen in the "S" stage of development in the outer cortex of fetuses and in neonates with ongoing renal development, such as dogs, cats, and pigs (eFig. 4-1).

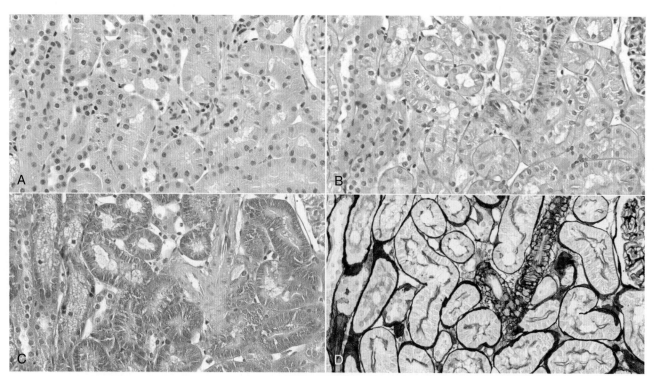

Figure 4-4 Normal canine tubulointerstitium, sectioned at 3-μm thickness. **A.** H&E stain. **B.** Apical brush border of proximal convoluted tubules is intact and stained pink, and peritubular capillaries are immediately adjacent to tubular basement membranes. PAS stain. **C.** Apical brush border of proximal convoluted tubules is blue, and interstitial fibrosis is not present. Masson trichrome stain. **D.** Jones' methenamine silver stain.

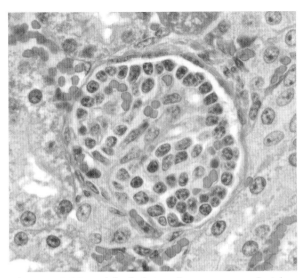

Figure 4-5 Normal fetal glomerulus in a neonatal piglet.

After scanning the section, the 4 basic elements of the kidney should be systematically examined, namely, glomeruli, tubules, interstitium, and blood vessels, to determine which structure is primarily injured.

Reactions of **glomeruli** to injury consist basically of combinations of cellular proliferation, mesangial expansion, leukocyte recruitment, remodeling of the GBM, and sclerosis. Epithelium of the proximal tubule may be present in the glomerular urinary space in acute tubular injury (ATI) or, more commonly, because of squeezing of the kidney during gross examination, especially if the kidney is autolytic; this change is termed *infraglomerular herniation or reflux*. Comparison of autolyzed feline kidneys to contralateral kidneys harvested immediately after euthanasia revealed that autolyzed kidneys weighed more and had increased glomerular diameters. However, the thickness of the GBM, the presence of intact foot processes, and the number of cells per glomerulus did not change after a 24-hour postmortem interval.

Tubules, especially proximal convoluted tubules, are the portions of the nephron that are most susceptible to ischemia and many toxins. Degenerative changes are nonspecific in character and usually not diagnostic of the causative condition. The proximal convoluted tubule is the longest cortical part of the nephron, and hence proximal tubules comprise the bulk of the cortex. Proximal tubules are more eosinophilic than the other tubules and have a brush border that may be seen in nonautolyzed specimens. The brush border can be easily seen as bright pink with the PAS stain (see Fig. 4-4B) and blue with Masson trichrome stain (see Fig. 4-4C). Delay in fixation leads to sloughing of apical cytoplasm into tubular lumina. Because cells of the distal tubule do not have a brush border and are flatter, the tubular lumina are larger. Interstitial fibrosis, particularly in areas of the interstitium lacking large blood vessels, is abnormal and indicates that tubular-capillary interactions are disrupted. Fibrosis may cause tubular obstruction and hence create retention cysts proximally.

Vascular changes may occur in various systemic states as in other organs, for example, arteriolosclerosis in hypertension and diabetes mellitus, arteritis in malignant catarrhal fever.

The **renal medulla** should be closely examined because this is the site of urine concentration and the accumulation of protein casts. Tubules and ducts in the medulla are normally separated by more connective tissue and ground substance than those in the cortex. Tubulointerstitial mineralization is common in renal disease and may be seen along with cortical mineralization in cases of hypercalcemic nephropathy. The papilla should be carefully examined for evidence of papillitis (an early lesion in pyelonephritis), for amyloid, and for papillary necrosis. Inclusion bodies can be prominent in pelvic urothelium of dogs; they may be nonspecific inclusions or could be canine distemper viral inclusions.

Renal biopsy

Renal biopsy is useful in evaluating renal disease in domestic animals, and *may be of particular use in cases of acute GN, nephrotic syndrome, asymptomatic proteinuria, and acute renal failure* (ARF). Biopsy techniques vary and include blind percutaneous, ultrasound-guided percutaneous, laparoscopic, surgical core, or surgical wedge procedures. In small animals, 16- or 18-gauge needles are appropriate, whereas use of 14 gauge has been reported to often include unwanted medullary tissue. Importantly, renal biopsy cores and wedges must be evaluated grossly to ensure that glomeruli are present in the sample. To do this, the tissue can be placed in a small Petri dish of physiologic saline and examined with a dissecting microscope or a magnifying glass. Small red dots are perfused glomeruli and should be easily visible in fresh biopsy tissue. Once an adequate sample has been obtained, a small piece (1-2 mm³) can be removed and placed in glutaraldehyde for possible ultrastructural evaluation. Alternatively, formalin-fixed tissue can be postfixed in glutaraldehyde and used for transmission electron microscopy (TEM). If immunofluorescence (IF) evaluation is desired, an unfixed core can either be immediately embedded in optimal cutting temperature compound (OCT) and quickly frozen, or a core can be placed in Michel's buffer for transfer to a service that specializes in nephropathology.

Although most renal biopsies are performed in small animals, recent studies have reported that the procedure has low morbidity in horses and can provide diagnostic tissue in >90% of cases. It is usually possible to obtain 10-20 glomeruli from an adult dog by using an automated spring-loaded biopsy instrument, such as the EZ core or Monopty biopsy needle. Of note, at least 20 glomeruli may be necessary to detect a focal glomerular disease process. The main hazard of the renal biopsy is arterial puncture and hemorrhage, which on rare occasions is fatal.

In addition to the usual hematoxylin and eosin (H&E) staining of paraffin sections of kidney, several other techniques are useful:

1. *Periodic acid–Schiff* (PAS) stain, which stains glomerular and tubular basement membranes, mesangial matrix, and Bowman's capsule basement membrane. Thin sections (3 μm) must be used. The PAS-methenamine silver technique is an improvement of this stain.
2. *Jones' methenamine silver* (JMS) stain, a methenamine silver-periodic acid stain, enables visualization of the GBM.
3. *Masson trichrome stain*, facilitates evaluation of interstitial scarring, and in some cases, immune complexes can be identified as red nodular material along the GBM.
4. *Other special stains for fibrin, amyloid, and lipids*. Microscopic resolution of glomerular lesions can be improved by the use of 1-μm thick methacrylate-embedded sections.

5. *Immunofluorescence* studies for localization of immuno-globulins, complement, fibrin-related compounds, and foreign antigens, especially in glomeruli.
6. *Immunoperoxidase* techniques, for localization of a wide variety of antigens.
7. *Transmission electron microscopy,* particularly for character-ization of immune deposits and abnormalities in podocytes, GBM, and mesangium.

Further reading

Burke M, et al. Molecular mechanisms of renal blood flow autoregula-tion. Curr Vasc Pharmacol 2014;12:845-858.

Cianciolo RE, et al. Pathologic evaluation of canine renal biopsies: methods for identifying features that differentiated immune complex mediated glomerulonephritides from other categories of glomerular diseases. J Vet Intern Med 2013;27:S10-S18.

Comper WD. Resolved. Normal glomeruli filter nephrotic levels of albumin. J Am Soc Nephrol 2008;19:427-432.

Jennette JC, et al. Heptinstall's Pathology of the Kidney. 6th ed. Phila-delphia: Lippincott-Raven; 2007.

Navar LG. Intrarenal renin-angiotensin system in regulation of glo-merular function. Curr Opin Nephrol Hypertens 2014;23: 38-45.

Peti-Peterdi J, Harris RC. Macula densa sensing and signaling mechanisms of renin release. J Am Soc Nephrol 2010;21:1093-1096.

Singh P, Thomson SC. Renal homeostasis and tubuloglomerular feed-back. Curr Opin Nephrol Hypertens 2010;19:59-64.

Vaden SL, et al. Renal biopsy: a retrospective study of methods and complications in 283 dogs and 65 cats. J Vet Intern Med 2005;19: 794-801.

Renal disease, renal failure, and uremia

Renal disease, which encompasses any deviation from normal renal structure or function, is usually subclinical. *Severe renal disease may lead to renal failure,* which is typically divided into acute and chronic forms. **Acute renal failure** (ARF) is charac-terized by rapid onset of oliguria or anuria and azotemia; it may result from acute glomerular or interstitial injury or from ATN, and is often reversible. **Chronic renal failure** (CRF) is the end result of many chronic renal diseases, is usually irre-versible, and is characterized by prolonged duration of signs of uremia. Importantly, the clinical syndrome of ARF can occur in the context of chronic renal disease, wherein subclini-cal injury progresses to a point that the patient displays clini-cal signs of renal disease with an abrupt onset.

Clarification of terminology is in order:

- **Uremia** literally means urine in the blood. It is a *clinical syndrome of renal failure,* caused by biochemical distur-bances, and is often accompanied by extrarenal lesions.
- **Azotemia** is a biochemical abnormality characterized by *elevation of blood urea and creatinine,* but without obliga-tory clinical manifestations of renal disease. Azotemia may be of renal or of extrarenal origin.
- **Prerenal azotemia** results from renal hypoperfusion, the result of conditions such as congestive heart failure, shock, or hemorrhage.
- **Postrenal azotemia** occurs because of urinary obstruction.

The evolution from normal renal function to uremia over the course of progressive renal disease occurs through *4 over-lapping stages:*

1. In the stage of **diminished renal reserve,** the GFR is about 50% of normal, and the animal is asymptomatic but has an increased susceptibility to additional renal insults.
2. At the stage of **renal insufficiency,** GFR is 25-50% of normal; the animal is azotemic.
3. In the stage of **renal failure,** GFR is only 20-25% of normal, the kidneys cannot maintain homeostasis, and uremia ensues, with its attendant gastrointestinal, cardiovascular, respiratory, and skeletal complications.
4. In **end-stage renal disease,** GFR is <5% of normal and the animal is in the terminal stages of uremia.

The biochemical disturbances of uremia reflect impair-ment in the kidney's regulation of fluid volume, regulation of electrolyte and acid-base balance, excretion of waste products, and metabolism of hormones. The clinical signs may be related to the renal disease itself, as with pyuria or renal pain; to the effects of reduced renal function, as with metabolic acidosis or dehydration; or to the compensatory responses to renal dysfunction, as with hyperparathyroidism.

Interference with **fluid volume regulation** may result in either dehydration or anasarca. *Dehydration* resulting from reduced renal concentrating ability may be related to lesions of the renal medulla and juxtamedullary nephrons. Vomition, and sometimes diarrhea, often exacerbates the dehydration. *Anasarca,* caused by reduction in the volume of glomerular filtrate in diffuse renal disease or by activation of the renin-angiotensin system, occurs infrequently. A more common cause of edema is hypoproteinemia resulting from loss of protein through injured glomeruli.

Disturbances in **electrolyte balance** include excesses and deficits of plasma sodium, potassium, and calcium. The han-dling of these substances by the kidney is complex, even in health; in disease it is often paradoxical and involves disor-dered tubular function, compensatory mechanisms, and endo-crine imbalances. Excesses of plasma sodium, potassium, and calcium contribute to anasarca, cardiotoxicity, and hypercal-cemic nephropathy, respectively, whereas deficits may cause dehydration, muscular weakness, tetany, and osteodystrophy.

Several aspects of the uremic syndrome contribute to **acid-base imbalance** and metabolic acidosis. Compensatory hyper-ventilation may occur. The main factors leading to acidosis in uremia are reduced capacity of distal and collecting tubules to produce ammonia, increased retention of hydrogen ions, and impaired resorption of bicarbonate ions at a time of increased utilization. The term **uremic acidosis** encompasses simultaneous azotemia, anion retention, and acidosis; **renal tubular acidosis** (discussed later in Specific tubular dysfunc-tions) describes acidosis without retention of urea or anions.

Failure to excrete metabolic wastes is the basis for tests of renal function; *elevated blood levels of urea and creatinine indi-cate reduced glomerular filtration.* However, azotemia occurs only after the loss of 75% or more of the GFR, and is thus an insensitive indicator of renal disease. Tests of concentrating ability, such as the water deprivation test, are also of limited usefulness because concentrating ability is not affected until at least two thirds of the renal mass has become nonfunctional.

Disturbances in endocrine function are important causes of signs and lesions in uremic animals. Retention of phosphate, resulting from reduced glomerular filtration, causes depression of ionized calcium, deficiency of $1,25(OH)_2D_3$, increased syn-thesis and secretion of parathyroid hormone (PTH), and development of secondary hyperparathyroidism (see section

Fibrous osteodystrophy; Vol. 1, Bones and joints). Reduced renal catabolism of PTH, and end-organ resistance to PTH, may contribute to hyperparathyroidism. Most uremic animals have hyperphosphatemia, and normocalcemia or hypercalcemia. Sometimes hypercalcemia and hypophosphatemia occur in uremic dogs, possibly because of lack of feedback inhibition of PTH release. Similar changes occur in some uremic horses and may be related to decreased renal excretion of calcium.

Nonregenerative **anemia** in uremic animals is of multifactorial pathogenesis and may result from a combination of factors, including decreased renal production of erythropoietin and possibly inhibitory effects of increased serum PTH concentrations (see Vol. 3, Hematopoietic system). Renal metabolism of vitamin D is sometimes impaired in animals with diffuse renal disease, and may add an element of osteomalacia to renal osteodystrophy. Abnormal glucose metabolism occasionally occurs in uremic dogs, and may be a result of peripheral resistance to insulin-mediated uptake of glucose or to reduced breakdown of insulin by diseased kidneys.

Uremic toxins can also impact protein catabolism and the various chemical and endocrine imbalances described previously. These toxins include low-, medium- and large-molecular-weight molecules. Low-molecular-weight molecules (<500 Da) include glomerulopressin, guanidines (e.g., creatine, creatinine), methylamines, myoinositol, oxalate, phenylacetylglutamine, phosphate, polyamines, pseudouridine, purines (e.g., uric acid), pyrimidines (e.g., thymine, uridine), trihalomethanes, and urea. "Middle molecules" range from 500-5,000 Da and include α- and β-chains of fibrinogen. Large molecules (>5,000 Da) include various peptides and cytokines, such as parathyroid hormone, β$_2$-microglobulin, granulocyte-inhibitory proteins, degranulation-inhibiting proteins, and chemotaxis-inhibiting protein. These various toxins are thought to be responsible for the profound malaise that characterizes the uremic syndrome. The *cause of death in uremia* varies from case to case. Metabolic acidosis, hyperkalemia, or hypocalcemia may be severe enough to be fatal.

Most forms of prerenal azotemia have a common basis of reduced renal blood flow and glomerular filtration. This occurs in a variety of circumstances, including severe dehydration, massive hemorrhage, especially into the upper intestinal tract, congestive heart failure, and shock of any cause. Reduced renal flow in these conditions is part of an adaptational mechanism that diverts blood to vital organs such as brain and heart. When the diversion is severe or prolonged, intrarenal mechanisms that divert blood flow away from cortical nephrons to juxtamedullary nephrons may produce patchy or diffuse cortical ischemia and necrosis (see Renal cortical necrosis and acute tubular necrosis). In such cases, prerenal azotemia may be followed by uremia of renal origin resulting from the cortical necrosis.

Postrenal azotemia is always the result of obstruction to the outflow of urine, and hence is oliguric or anuric. If obstruction is intermittent or incomplete, it may lead to hydronephrosis. If it is sudden and complete, it may lead to rupture or leakage of the lower urinary tract.

A form of extrarenal uremia, distinct from those mentioned, occurs in *newborn animals*, especially pigs, and is characterized by very high levels of blood urea. The kidneys of newborn pigs, dogs, and cats are functionally "immature" and incapable of producing hypertonic urine. Normally, this is of no consequence, because milk provides enough fluid to excrete, in hypotonic urine, the small amount of waste produced. However, when these newborn animals are anorectic, they lack both nutrients and fluid, and begin to catabolize tissue proteins and purines. Being unable to excrete the excess solute from protein and purine breakdown, their blood urea and uric acid reach very high levels. Because anorexia is usually associated with fever, vomition, or diarrhea, fluid loss is rapid. In pigs, the excess solute is deposited in the inner medulla as streaks of light-yellow urate precipitates (Fig. 4-6), which disappear during histologic processing. Pigs are apparently unique among mammals in that they do not resorb urates from glomerular filtrate; this accounts for their concentration in the medulla. It is not clear whether baby pigs also have an "immature" liver that fails to convert uric acid to allantoin.

The **nonrenal lesions of uremia** occur inconstantly and unpredictably, although they tend to be seen most often in dogs, especially those with chronic rather than ARF. Many animals dying with uremia are cachectic. This is probably caused by anorexia, vomition, and diarrhea as well as by body tissue catabolism to supply energy. Besides this general lack of condition, several distinctive lesions may develop in the gastrointestinal, cardiovascular, respiratory, and skeletal systems.

Ulcerative, necrotic stomatitis occurs in dogs and cats, and there is usually a foul-smelling brown film coating the tongue and buccal mucosa (Fig. 4-7). Like the gastrointestinal changes, oral lesions are more common in chronic than in acute uremia. The pathogenesis of the ulcers is not always clear, but some

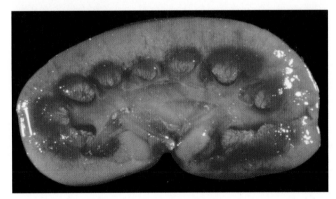

Figure 4-6 Urate calculi in renal medulla of a neonatal dehydrated piglet. (Courtesy K.G. Thompson.)

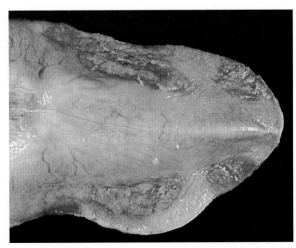

Figure 4-7 Ulcers on lateral margin and ventral surface of the tongue of a dog with **uremia.** (Courtesy M.K. Keating.)

are associated with fibrinoid necrosis of arterioles, and some are related to bacterial production of ammonia from urea in the saliva. Large areas of the *gastric mucosa* are often swollen, suffused with red-black blood, and may be mineralized and partly ulcerated (Fig. 4-8). This lesion, often called "gastritis," is initially noninflammatory, although opportunist bacteria may infect the ulcerated mucosa. Mucosal infarction occurs secondary to arteriolar necrosis. *Mineralization of the middle and deep zones of the gastric mucosa is common* (Fig. 4-9). Necrosis and mineralization of the muscular tunics are sometimes present. Intestinal lesions resemble those in the stomach, but they are less frequent, less severe, and without mineralization. Gastrointestinal lesions probably account for much of the vomition, diarrhea, and melena of uremic dogs. Intestinal intussusceptions sometimes develop in dogs with gastrointestinal lesions. Cats may have gastrointestinal lesions similar to dogs, but in uremic cattle, colitis is more common, and the stomach and proximal intestine are edematous. Hyperamylasemia and hyperlipasemia occur in some uremic dogs and may be the result of concurrent pancreatitis rather than the result of reduced renal clearance of the enzymes.

Systemic *arterial lesions* found in animals with acute renal insufficiency or with CRF are discussed elsewhere (see Vol. 3, Cardiovascular system). Lesions of various organs, such as uremic gastric infarction, may result from arterial injury and

thrombosis. Arteriolar lesions in the myocardium sometimes cause ischemia and necrosis. In chronic uremia, the left ventricle is often hypertrophied and dilated. *Hypertension* is common in canine kidney disease, and ventricular hypertrophy may be initiated or exaggerated by the hypertension. Lesions in the circulatory system are unusual, except in the dog, but arterial injury may occur in the intestines in cattle with acute tubular injury (ATI) and contribute to the colonic lesions of acute uremic syndromes in this species. In cattle with urethral calculi, pericardial effusion may be part of the anasarca. In dogs, hydropericardium with dull granulation of the pericardium may occur. Edematous distension of retroperitoneal tissue, expressed particularly as *perirenal edema*, occurs in pigs and cattle; the underlying renal lesion is usually ATN caused by ochratoxin or *Amaranthus retroflexus* in pigs, and oak poisoning in cattle (see Nephrotoxic tubular necrosis).

Most animals dying in uremia develop *terminal pulmonary edema*. The mechanism is unknown, and the edema is not always associated with significant pulmonary congestion; increased permeability of alveolar capillaries is the most likely pathogenesis. In a few animals, acute pneumonia develops terminally. It may be associated with aspiration of gastric content, and its fulminant nature is possibly related to the immunosuppression that develops in uremia. Pulmonary mineralization occurs in chronically uremic dogs. Mineral is deposited in the walls of the alveolar ducts and pulmonary arterioles. Dull granulations of the visceral pleura may be present over the cranial lobes. Occasionally in uremia, spectacular pulmonary lesions develop. They may be visible in radiographs as lines of increased density spreading out from the hilus, and these features are those of interstitial edema. At autopsy, the lung is edematous and resilient, and the alveolar spaces contain fibrin in the fluid. Leukocytes are present but may be a response to accidental superimposed infection. Mineralization is extensive, with deposition particularly on reticulin of alveolar walls that are widened (eFig. 4-2). The lesion is referred to as uremic lung or *uremic pneumonitis*; it is not common, and when it occurs, it may be patchy.

Perhaps the most constant lesion in the dog is *mineralization beneath the parietal pleura* in the intercostal spaces (Fig. 4-10). It is preceded by necrosis of the subpleural connective tissue with extension to intercostal muscle and overlying pleura. Once mineralization has occurred and the pleura repaired, the lesion appears as gray-yellow thickenings, horizontally wrinkled. The cranial intercostal spaces are involved first; when deposition is extensive, many more spaces may be affected.

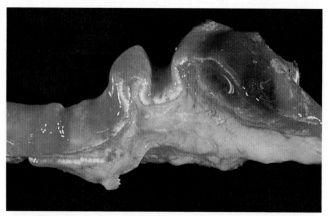

Figure 4-8 Uremic gastritis with hemorrhage and mineralization of the mucosa in a dog. (Courtesy M.K. Keating.)

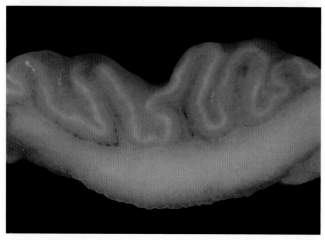

Figure 4-9 Marked **gastric mucosal mineralization** in a uremic dog. (Courtesy S. Jennings.)

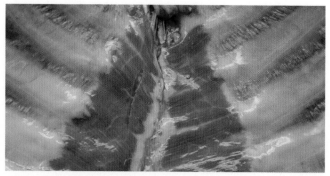

Figure 4-10 Necrosis and mineralization beneath the intercostal pleura between the ribs in a uremic dog.

The *pathogenesis* of diffuse tissue mineralization in uremia is not clear. There are at least 2 types of mineral deposit, and serum concentrations of calcium, magnesium, phosphate, and carbonate probably determine the type of calcium phosphate compound that is formed. When calcium is higher than magnesium, apatites are formed, whereas the opposite relationship favors deposition of amorphous calcium phosphate. The regularity with which certain tissues and organs are mineralized is no doubt related to local characteristics, such as tissue glycosaminoglycans, local pH, and cellular factors.

The effects of chronic uremia on the *skeleton* are discussed in Fibrous osteodystrophy, Vol. 1, Bones and joints. *Enlarged parathyroids* are common in dogs and cats with CRF; osseous lesions are less so.

Uremic encephalopathy is an uncommon complication of uremia in domestic animals. It has been reported in dogs, ruminants, and horses, and is expressed as white-matter spongiform degeneration that may be accompanied by reactive astrogliosis.

The **renal lesions of uremia** are varied, but if the syndrome is chronic, certain common changes tend to occur. *The end result is a fibrosed, mineralized kidney with globally sclerotic glomeruli, and a mixture of atrophic and hypertrophic tubules.* Often, this can only be diagnosed as **"end-stage kidney."** Severe mineralization occurs late in the course of renal failure and may diffusely involve glomerular and tubular basement membranes. According to the "precipitation-mineralization hypothesis," phosphorus absorbed from the intestines in excess of the excretory capacity of nephrons will induce precipitation of calcium phosphate microcrystals in tubular lumina, the interstitium, and renal capillaries. Dietary phosphate restriction may inhibit renal mineralization and its attendant inflammation, scarring, and loss of nephrons. Interstitial fibrosis and glomerulosclerosis are slowly progressive lesions that are common in the end stages of many renal diseases. *Progressive interstitial fibrosis is thought to be the final common pathway to CRF.* Hyperplasia and hypertrophy of tubules are inconstant compensatory changes that probably precede the onset of renal failure. Azotemia develops when glomerular filtration is reduced to 25% of normal. Until this time, adaptive changes in intact nephrons maintain renal function at an adequate level as other nephrons are lost. The glomerulus is probably the limiting factor in this compensatory mechanism, because it has a relatively limited ability to increase its function. It seems unlikely that uremia provides a suitable environment to permit or encourage compensatory hyperplasia, and it is likely that enlargement of nephrons is an early response to a reduction in renal mass rather than an adaptation to uremia.

Regardless of the initiating cause, **CRF tends to be progressive.** Progression occurs because of persistence of the primary disease problem and/or the addition of other renal insults or complications, such as urinary tract infection, systemic hypertension, and intrarenal deposition of mineral. As well, *endogenous factors* that often develop as compensatory mechanisms may contribute to perpetuation of renal failure. These factors include glomerular capillary hypertension and hyperfiltration, renal hypertrophy, increased renal oxygen consumption, and increased renal ammoniagenesis. Surviving nephrons may also be injured as a result of altered phosphate metabolism, altered lipid composition, and by increased activity of the coagulation system. High dietary protein intake may increase renal blood flow and GFR, possibly through the actions of mediators such as glucagon, growth hormone, prostaglandins, the renin-angiotensin system, and biogenic amines. Restricting protein intake may minimize renal hemodynamic changes and slow the progression of CRF. Glomerular hyperperfusion can lead to hypertrophy of the tuft and subsequent glomerulosclerosis with proteinuria.

Also to be considered when assessing renal disease in a mature or aged animal are **normal aging changes** that occur in the absence of any specific renal insult; these "background" changes may lead to decreased renal reserve, but usually not to renal failure. In aged dogs, for example, *renal weight is reduced* by 20-30% because of decreased size and number of nephrons. In humans, GFR decreases with age because the renal fraction of cardiac output decreases and because of intrarenal vascular changes, such as obsolescence of glomerular capillaries in juxtamedullary glomeruli and atrophy of arterioles of cortical glomeruli. Glomerular mesangial volume increases, proximal tubule volume and length decrease, and interstitial connective tissue increases. Changes in the ground substance of medullary connective tissue can reduce medullary hyperosmolality and hence renal concentrating ability. Aged animals with purely senescent renal changes have *decreased compensatory abilities*, such as hypertrophy, and are hence very susceptible to renal insults. Proteinuria may be taken as an indicator of increased glomerular permeability, but there is no sensitive and specific test for quantifying renal aging at present.

Renal transplantation is available in a number of centers as a therapeutic option for dogs and cats with end-stage renal disease. Various immunosuppressive protocols are used to prevent postoperative rejection of the transplanted kidney, particularly necessary when the donor is unrelated to the recipient. Surgical complications may be noted at autopsy, for example, avulsion of the renal vein, torsion of the vascular pedicle, retroperitoneal fibrosis. The various stages of rejection of renal allografts have been extensively categorized in human pathology (Banff criteria); however, small animals do not seem to fit into the same diagnostic categories. Histologic evaluation of >70 allograft feline kidneys revealed evidence of cyclosporine toxicity, necrotizing glomerulitis and vasculitis (suggestive of acute antibody-mediated rejection), and subcapsular and intralobular phlebitis. The latter feature is not described in the Banff scoring system, and its significance is unknown. Although a canine or feline renal transplant recipient may enjoy long-term (months to years) success, the pre-existing condition, for example, systemic hypertension, might persist and lead to failure of the transplanted kidney. *Complications* of immunosuppressive therapy in allograft recipients include a spectrum of infections, including a wide range of bacterial (*Mycobacterium, Actinobacillus*), yeast/fungal (*Candida, Penicillium, Encephalitozoon*), and protozoal (*Toxoplasma, Pneumocystis, Giardia*) diseases. In general, the uninephrectomized kidney donor survives well, and its remaining kidney hypertrophies to meet the body's needs.

Further reading

Bernsteen L, et al. Renal transplantation in cats. Clin Tech Small Anim Pract 2000;15:40-45.

Harison E, et al. Acute azotemia as a predictor of mortality in dogs and cats. J Vet Intern Med 2012;26:1093-1098.

Kaplan B, et al. Search for peptidic "middle molecules" in uremic sera: isolation and chemical identification of fibrinogen fragments.

J Chromatogr B Analyt Technol Biomed Life Sci 2003;796: 141-153.

Le Boedec K, et al. Pulmonary abnormalities in dogs with renal azotemia. J Vet Intern Med 2012;26:1099-1106.

McCarthy RA, et al. Effects of dietary protein on glomerular mesangial area and basement membrane thickness in aged uni-nephrectomized dogs. Can J Vet Res 2001;65:125-130.

Racusen LC, et al. The Banff 97 working classification of renal allograft pathology. Kidney Int 1999;55:713-723.

Vanholder RC, et al. Review on uremic toxins: classification, concentration, and interindividual variability. Kidney Int 2003;63: 1934-1943.

Juvenile, familial, and hereditary nephropathies

Although some consider **"juvenile nephropathy"** to be synonymous with **"renal dysplasia,"** the former is actually a broad all-encompassing term for noninflammatory, degenerative, or developmental, chronic renal disease of obscure pathogenesis in *young animals*, and is the preferred *clinical diagnosis* for renal insufficiency of undetermined etiology in these patients.

Familial nephropathy and **breed nephropathy** are more restrictive terms applied to renal disease observed in *families or breeds of animals*, particularly dogs. Of note, familial nephropathy can include genetic diseases as well as lesions observed in litters exposed to the same infectious agents or environmental stresses. **Hereditary nephropathy** *is the definitive term used once the inheritance of the nephropathy has been determined, through pedigree analysis, test matings, and eventually identification of underlying genetic abnormality.* A list of reported familial and breed nephropathies, many of which are suspected or proven to be hereditary, is provided in Table 4-1. This list will continue to change as inheritance of disease entities is defined; classifications will also be further refined as the

Table • 4-1

Suspected or proven familial and/or breed-related nephropathies in domestic species

Breed	Lesion	Gene/Inheritance
Abyssinian cat	Amyloidosis (medullary and glomerular)	Autosomal dominant with incomplete penetrance, suspected
Alaskan Malamute	Immature glomeruli and tubules; glomerular hypertrophy; glomerulocystic atrophy; glomerulosclerosis; adenomatoid tubular epithelia; mineralization of tubular basement membranes; severe interstitial inflammation in 2 of 3 dogs	Not identified
Basenji	Fanconi syndrome; histologic lesions are minimal and include tubular epithelial cell hypertrophy and karyomegaly	Not identified
Beagle	Glomerular and medullary AA amyloidosis affecting multiple dogs of a single litter	Not identified
	Primitive mesenchyme; persistence of metanephric ducts; asynchronous differentiation of nephrons and atypical tubular epithelium in related laboratory Beagles	Not identified
	Unilateral renal agenesis	Not identified
Bedlington Terrier	Increased interstitial connective tissue without inflammation; consolidated glomeruli and dilated, thickened Bowman's capsules; occasional cystic tubules	Not identified; only reported in 3 offspring of 2 litters from a single sire
Bernese Mountain dog	Immune-complex–mediated membranoproliferative glomerulonephritis with IgM and C3 deposition in glomeruli	Autosomal recessive, with an epigenetic influence by a sex-influenced genetic determinance
Boxer	Immature glomeruli and/or tubules; primitive mesenchyme	Not identified
	Small kidneys with cortical scars; nephron atrophy; paucity of glomeruli; glomerulocystic lesions; tortuous arteries with intimal thickening; immature glomeruli and/or metanephric tubules	Not identified
Brittany Spaniel	Membranoproliferative glomerulonephritis with IgG deposition, lacking C3, in glomeruli; part of hereditary canine C3 deficiency syndrome; dogs with recurrent systemic infections also have a predisposition to develop renal AA amyloidosis	Autosomal recessive caused by a deletion of a cytosine at position 2,136, resulting in a frame shift mutation that generates a premature stop codon
Bullmastiff	Uncharacterized glomerulonephropathy (segmental mesangial expansion and hypercellularity); small glomeruli, thickened Bowman's capsule, glomerulocystic atrophy; tubular atrophy: interstitial inflammation and fibrosis	Autosomal recessive (suspected)

Table • 4-1

Suspected or proven familial and/or breed-related nephropathies in domestic species—cont'd

Breed	Lesion	Gene/Inheritance
Bull Terrier	Polycystic kidney disease	Autosomal dominant caused by a missense mutation (G to A) in exon 29 of the *Pkd1* gene, which replaces glutamic acid with lysine in polycystin 1
	Basket weaving of the GBM, suggestive of Alport syndrome however, both α3(IV) and α5(IV) collagens are present; sometimes concurrent polycystic kidney disease	Autosomal dominant
Cairn Terrier	Polycystic kidney disease	Autosomal recessive (suspected)
Chow Chow	Immature glomeruli and glomerulocystic atrophy in radiating bands of interstitial fibrosis; compensatory glomerular hypertrophy in adjacent renal parenchyma	Not identified
Cocker Spaniel	Glomerulocystic atrophy; segmental accumulation of fibrocellular material in Bowman's space (suggestive of fibrous crescents); some Bowman's capsules contained an amorphous protein coagulum that variably stained positive for fibrinogen/fibrin in Bowman's space	Not identified; of note the lack of EM evaluation of the GBM precludes comparison of this familial nephropathy to that of English Cocker Spaniels
Dalmatian	Basket weaving of the GBM, suggestive of Alport syndrome; however, both α3(IV) and α5(IV) collagens are present	Autosomal dominant
	Urate calculi resulting from a transport defect in uric acid, which is generated during normal purine metabolism. This leads to hyperuricosuria and hyperuricemia	Autosomal recessive caused by a mutation in *SLC2A9*, a putative renal and hepatic urate transporter
Doberman Pinscher	Glomerulosclerosis; glomerulocystic atrophy; mesangial hypercellularity; EM of some dogs reveals lamination of the lamina densa rarely with intramembranous electron-dense material, whereas other dogs had material resembling fibrillar collagens within the GBM; IF studies revealed IgM staining in only 1 of 10 dogs	Not identified; affected females may have concomitant unilateral renal agenesis
Dutch Kooiker	Asynchronous differentiation of nephrons; persistent mesenchyme; persistent metanephric ducts; adenomatoid proliferation of the tubular epithelium	Not identified
English Cocker Spaniel	Proliferative and sclerosing glomerulopathy; basket weaving of the GBM	Single nucleotide substitution at 115 in *COL4A4*
Finnish Landrace sheep	Membranoproliferative glomerulonephritis with crescents; C3-dominant IF staining with variable IgM, IgA, and IgG IF staining	Autosomal recessive deficiency of complement factor C3
French Mastiff	Glomerulocystic atrophy; hypercellular glomeruli; thickened capillary walls without immune complexes	Possibly autosomal recessive
Gelbvieh cattle	Mesangial expansion and hypercellularity with glomerulosclerosis; affected calves also had a peripheral neuropathy	Unknown
German Shepherd dog	Renal cystadenocarcinomas; part of the renal cystadenocarcinoma/nodular dermatofibroma disease complex; bitches may also have uterine leiomyomas	Autosomal dominant
Golden Retriever	Radiating bands of interstitial fibrosis; glomerulocystic atrophy with or without primitive metanephric ducts and persistent mesenchyme	Not identified; not confirmed to be familial
Irish Terrier	Cystinuria and cystine calculi	X-linked
Japanese black (Wagyu) cattle	Chronic interstitial nephritis with zonal fibrosis; kidneys often have cystically dilated tubules and Bowman's capsules, resembling multicystic renal dysplasia	Autosomal recessive null mutation in *claudin-16*; 2 separate mutations have been identified
Keeshond	Cystic collecting ducts; glomerulocystic atrophy	Not identified

Continued

Table • 4-1

Suspected or proven familial and/or breed-related nephropathies in domestic species—cont'd

Breed	Lesion	Gene/Inheritance
Lhasa Apso	Radiating streaks containing immature and fetal glomeruli and tubules with paucity of collecting ducts and normal adjacent cortical parenchyma.	Not identified
Miniature Schnauzer	Radiating bands of immature glomeruli; sclerotic glomeruli; glomerulocystic atrophy; reduced number of glomeruli; mesangial cell hyperplasia; interstitial fibrosis and tubular atrophy	Not identified
Newfoundland	Glomerulosclerosis and glomerulofibrosis; EM revealed fibrillar collagen deposition in the mesangium and subendothelial space	Not identified
	Cystinuria and cystine calculi	Nonsense mutation in exon 2 of the *SLC3A1* gene
Norwegian Elkhound	Interstitial and periglomerular fibrosis; sacculations in distal tubules and collecting ducts	Likely autosomal dominant; mutations in *COL4A3* and *4A4* have been excluded as causes
Old English Sheepdog	Radiating bands of interstitial fibrosis; cystic tubules; glomerulocystic atrophy	Not identified; not confirmed to be familial
Pembroke Welsh Corgi	Telangiectasia	Not identified
	Glomerulosclerosis; glomerulocystic atrophy; interstitial fibrosis and tubular atrophy; interstitial inflammation; hyperplasia of collecting duct epithelium	Not identified
Persian cat	Polycystic kidney disease	Autosomal dominant inheritance; missense mutation (C to A) in exon 29 of *Pkd1* that results in a premature stop codon (at what would be position 3284 of the human polycystin 1 protein)
Rottweiler	Glomerulocystic atrophy; mesangial hypercellularity; glomerulosclerosis; lamination of the lamina densa	Not identified
Samoyed	Proliferative and sclerosing glomerulopathy; basket weaving of the GBM	X-linked; nonsense mutation in codon 127 of *COL4A5* that changes a glycine to a stop codon
Scottish Terrier	Cystine urolithiasis	Likely X-linked
Shar-Pei	Amyloidosis	Likely autosomal recessive inheritance; Gene not identified
Shih Tzu	Incomplete lobulation (gross); immature glomeruli and tubules; adenomatoid proliferation of tubular epithelium; metanephric tubules; cortical cysts; persistent mesenchyme and interstitial fibrosis	Likely autosomal recessive inheritance
Soft-coated Wheaten Terrier	Podocytopathy and segmental glomerulosclerosis	Podocytopathy is linked to mutations in *NPHS1* and *KIRREL2*
	Radiating bands of dense interstitial collagen; cystic tubules; sclerotic and immature glomeruli; affected dogs may also have podocytopathy with segmental sclerosis in bands of more normal parenchyma	Not identified
Standard Poodle	Immature glomeruli; glomerulocystic atrophy; interstitial fibrosis and tubular atrophy; interstitial inflammation	Not identified
West Highland White Terrier	Polycystic kidney disease; cysts also present in liver	Autosomal recessive

EM, electron microscopy; *GBM*, glomerular basement membrane; *IF*, immunofluorescence; *IgA, IgG,* and *IgM,* immunoglobulins A, G, and M, respectively.

pathogeneses of somewhat obscure familial and juvenile diseases are more fully characterized. Given greater knowledge of heritability, breed societies are able to undertake control programs.

Examples of specific familial and/or hereditary renal diseases abound, and will be discussed later under their respective sections of developmental defects, glomerular disease, tubular disease, and renal neoplasia. *In general, the canine familial renal diseases are characterized clinically by renal failure, in a group of related immature or young adult dogs.* For most breeds, only terminal clinical signs and end-stage lesions are described; inheritance, pathogenesis, and early morphologic changes are not reported. The age of onset of renal failure varies from a few weeks to several years but, in most cases, is 4-18 months. This wide age range and the lack of renal biopsies before end-stage disease hinder the diagnosis and investigation of pathogenesis. Therefore there is a danger that any case of ARF in a young dog of an appropriate breed will be misdiagnosed as being breed-related juvenile nephropathy. On the other hand, it is possible that some of the chronic interstitial nephritides formerly attributed to leptospirosis are familial renal diseases.

Many of the canine familial nephropathies have both glomerular and tubular lesions. There is also interstitial fibrosis, which may form radiating bands or generalized. Fibrotic regions often contain immature glomeruli. Importantly, glomeruli that appear to be immature must be evaluated cautiously, particularly when they are found in areas of scarring. Such "asynchronous differentiation" of nephrons may be the result of acquired scarring and mechanical inhibition of maturation. Furthermore, scattered rare immature glomeruli may be observed in kidneys that are otherwise normal in gross and microscopic appearance. Whether familial renal diseases are always expressions of dysplasia is a moot point. The sine qua non of dysplasia (primitive ducts, cartilage nodules [see Renal dysplasia]) is rarely met in affected kidneys; expanding the definition of dysplasia to include the presence of immature glomeruli greatly, and perhaps illegitimately, expands the number of affected cases of juvenile renal disease characterized as being "dysplastic." Until the etiopathogeneses of the lesions in young animals are clearly defined, they might better be termed "juvenile nephropathies."

Further reading

Bruder MC, et al. Renal dysplasia in beagle dogs: four cases. Tox Pathol 2010;38:1051-1057.

Casal ML, et al. Familial glomerulonephropathy in the bullmastiff. Vet Pathol 2004;41:319-325.

Chandler ML, et al. Juvenile nephropathy in 37 boxer dogs. J Small Anim Pract 2007;48:690-694.

Lavoué R, et al. Progressive juvenile glomerulonephropathy in 16 related French mastiff (Bordeaux) dogs. J Vet Intern Med 2010; 24:314-322.

McKay LW, et al. Juvenile nephropathy in two related Pembroke Welsh corgi puppies. J Small Anim Pract 2004;45:568-571.

O'Leary CA, et al. Renal pathology of polycystic kidney disease and concurrent hereditary nephritis in Bull Terriers. Aust Vet J 2002; 80:353-361.

Wakamatsu N, et al. Histologic and ultrastructural studies of juvenile onset renal disease in four Rottweiler dogs. Vet Pathol 2007;44: 96-100.

ANOMALIES OF DEVELOPMENT

The embryology of mammalian kidneys involves the sequential development of 3 successive but overlapping structures: the *pronephros, mesonephros,* and *metanephros.* The first 2 become vestigial, but act as inducers of the definitive kidney, the metanephros. Pronephric tubules, arising in the intermediate mesoderm of the cervical region, form the pronephric duct by fusion and extension of their caudal ends. This duct opens into the cloaca and, although the pronephric tubules are not functional in mammalian embryos, the use of their duct by the mesonephric tubules gives them potential significance in the genesis of renal anomalies. Mesonephric tubules develop from thoracic mesoderm caudad to the pronephros. The mesonephros is functional in mammalian embryos, but degenerates before birth. In males, some of the caudal tubules persist as efferent ducts of the epididymis, and the duct itself is used as the vas deferens. In females, cystic remnants of mesonephric tubules in the mesovarium may form the epoophoron and paroophoron, and remnants of the duct are known as Gartner's duct.

The formation of **the metanephros,** *the definitive kidney,* begins with the development of a *ureteral bud* from the mesonephric duct immediately cranial to its junction with the cloaca. The bud, accompanied by vessels and nerves, grows into a mass of mesenchymal cells, the *metanephric blastema.* Normal renal and ureteral development depends on the interaction of these 2 structures. As the bud grows into the blastema, it makes a specific number of successive, dichotomous divisions. The tubes formed by early divisions of the ureteral bud dilate and become the pelvis and calyces of the kidney. Tubes formed by later divisions develop into collecting ducts, and the last divisions give rise to collecting tubules. As the blind end of each collecting tubule, the ampulla, grows into the metanephric blastema, it induces compact masses of cells to form about it. These masses soon cavitate, become S shaped, and unite with the side of the ampulla, which continues to advance and divide.

The cavitated cell masses develop into *nephrons.* Connection of the lumens of the nephron and the collecting tubule occurs very soon after the cell mass cavitates. Glomerular development involves the formation of a lateral invagination in the S-shaped mass by mesenchymal cells that differentiate into endothelial and mesangial cells and become linked with the renal vasculature.

The complicated formation of the kidney provides for many patterns of malformation. The interaction of ureteral bud and metanephric blastema involves mutual inductions, and malformations of renal tissue are often accompanied by ureteral anomalies. Ectopic budding of the ureter from the mesonephric duct appears to be the primary event that precedes many congenital anomalies of the kidney and urinary tract. Ectopia results in hypoplastic kidney, ectopia of the ureterovesical orifice, urinary outflow obstruction, and/or reflux. The genes involved in navigating ureteric budding to the correct site often also regulate later developmental events of the kidney and urinary tract. Candidate genes have been proposed for a wide range of urinary developmental defects in humans and laboratory rodents.

The incidence of urinary tract anomalies is not known for most species. Survey results from large numbers of lambs suggest that anomalies occur more often than commonly believed.

Further reading

Greco DS. Congenital and inherited renal disease of small animals. Vet Clin North Am Small Anim Pract 2001;31:393-399.

Reidy KJ, Rosenblum ND. Cell and molecular biology of kidney development. Semin Nephrol 2009;29:321-337.

Stewart K, Bouchard M. Kidney and urinary tract development: an apoptotic balancing act. Pediatr Nephrol 2011;26:1419-1425.

Woolf AS, Davies JA. Cell biology of ureter development. J Am Soc Nephrol 2013;24:19-25.

Abnormalities in the amount of renal tissue

Lack of renal tissue may be complete *(agenesis)* or partial *(hypoplasia)*. Renal agenesis may be caused by developmental failure of the pronephros, mesonephros, or ureteral bud; by absence or complete unresponsiveness of the metanephric blastema; or by complete degeneration of the metanephric blastema. Partial degeneration, or partial responsiveness of the blastema to the inductive influences of the ureteral bud, probably produces renal dysplasia. The presence of even a fragment of recognizable metanephric tissue necessitates the diagnosis of dysplasia instead of agenesis.

Agenesis may be unilateral or bilateral. Bilateral agenesis is inconsistent with postnatal life. As is the case with all renal anomalies, agenesis may be associated with other urogenital deformities. Unilateral renal agenesis is compatible with normal life if the other kidney is normal; however, contralateral dysplasia, or even hypoplasia, may be present, in which case renal failure ultimately develops. The ureter may be absent or malformed with a blind end that terminates in connective tissue at the renal site. Renal agenesis occurs infrequently in all species, except when there is a *familial incidence*, as in some Beagles, Shetland Sheepdogs, and Doberman Pinschers, and in Large White pigs. Bilateral agenesis may account for some stillbirths, but this can only be assessed by careful examination of fetuses.

The small size of **hypoplastic kidneys** is the result of *a reduced number of histologically normal nephrons, lobules, and calyces*. Renal hypoplasia is a quantitative defect caused by reduced mass of metanephric blastema or by incomplete induction of nephron formation by the ureteral bud. When the amount of blastema is normal, but there is malfunction of the ureteral bud, renal dysplasia probably develops. Most of the small kidneys diagnosed as hypoplastic are actually probably dysplastic or scarred. The term "cortical hypoplasia" should be avoided because it is inconsistent with established concepts of renal embryology and anatomy. *Renal hypoplasia is rare.* It may be unilateral (Fig. 4-11) or bilateral. When unilateral, contralateral hypertrophy is expected.

Bilateral hypoplasia will likely lead to renal failure, and this often complicates or precludes the diagnosis because of the secondary changes that develop. Several forms of renal hypoplasia occur in humans but, because of the confusion of terminology, the variations and incidence of the condition in animals cannot be assessed. Kidneys suspected of being hypoplastic should be weighed along with their mate and examined for evidence of dysplasia and hypertrophy. In humans, in the absence of acquired disease, a decrease in size of one kidney by >50% or reduction of total renal mass by more than one-third is taken as evidence of hypoplasia.

Details regarding **excess renal tissue** are not well documented. *Duplication of ureters and kidneys occurs in cattle,*

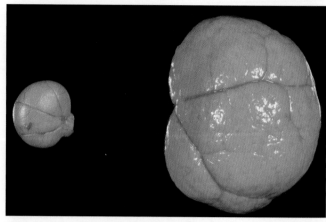

Figure 4-11 **Unilateral renal hypoplasia with contralateral compensatory renal hypertrophy** in a young cat. (Courtesy B. Harrington, C. Premanandan.)

pigs, and dogs, but it is not clear whether total renal mass is increased.

Further reading

McIntyre RL, et al. Developmental uterine anomalies in cats and dogs undergoing elective ovariohysterectomy. J Am Vet Med Assoc 2010;237:542-546.

Morita T, et al. Renal dysplasia with unilateral renal agenesis in a dog. J Comp Pathol 2005;133:64-67.

Taney KG, et al. Bilateral ectopic ureters in a male dog with unilateral renal agenesis. J Am Vet Med Assoc 2003;223:817-820.

Anomalies of renal position, form, and orientation

The kidneys develop in the pelvis and migrate to their sublumbar location, meanwhile rotating so that the ureter attains its normal orientation. During this movement, the blood supply shifts from the iliac arteries to the aorta. Various disruptions of this procedure may occur. Vitamin A deficiency in sows may cause anomalies such as those described later.

Malposition of the kidneys *(renal ectopia)* is observed more frequently in swine than in dogs or cats. Malpositioned kidneys are usually in the pelvic or inguinal location. One or both kidneys may be displaced. The kidneys may be normal or abnormally small. The renal arteries arise close to the bifurcation of the aorta or from the iliacs. The ureter is short, but may be kinked and thereby predisposed to hydronephrosis and pyelonephritis, or may empty into the genital tract, causing urinary incontinence. *Crossed renal ectopia* refers to malposition of a kidney that has crossed the midline; it may fuse with its contralateral partner.

Fusion of the kidneys may occur in utero. *Horseshoe kidney,* or *ren arcuatus,* seen in all species, results from fusion of the cranial or caudal poles of the kidneys (Fig. 4-12). The fusion may involve only a small portion of the capsule or parenchyma or be sufficient to produce a common pelvis. The ureters are not involved and their disposition depends on whether the cranial or caudal poles are fused. Such kidneys function normally.

Fetal lobulations, which are normal in embryos and cattle, may persist (eFig. 4-3) in other species if there is failure of

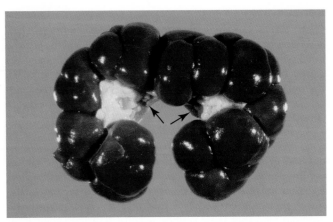

Figure 4-12 **Horseshoe kidney** in a calf. Ureters have been severed (arrows). (Courtesy University of Guelph.)

fusion of individual renal segments. They are not of pathologic significance.

Further reading

Jeong WI, et al. Renal and ureteral fusion in a calf with atresia ani. J Vet Med Sci 2003;65:413-414.

Shojaei B, et al. Morphological observation of a horseshoe (fused) kidney and its vascular pattern in a horse. Anat Histol Embryol 2012;41:388-391.

Renal dysplasia

Renal dysplasia is disorganized development of renal parenchyma because of anomalous differentiation. If normal development of the collecting duct system ("renal branching morphogenesis") is disrupted, then renal dysplasia can result. Transcription factors, growth factors, and cell surface signaling peptides are critical in regulation of renal branching morphogenesis. Renal lesions may be gross or microscopic. Renal dysplasia is *usually congenital.* But in cats, dogs, and pigs, which have an active subcapsular nephrogenic zone at birth, dysplasias may be caused by disease in the early neonatal period until differentiation of the nephrogenic tissue is completed. Dysplastic changes may be obscured by secondary compensatory, degenerative, and inflammatory changes.

The **causes** of renal dysplasia are ill-defined, but some may be *hereditary.* Cases of familial renal disease in several *dog* breeds often have dysplastic features (see Table 4-1). An autosomal dominant form of cystic renal dysplasia has been reported in *Suffolk sheep.* Many *human* cases of renal dysplasia are associated with intrauterine *ureteral obstruction,* and some animals probably have the same cause. Of note, rapid growth and the increased activity of the intrarenal renin-angiotensin system in the fetus may cause greater susceptibility to permanent renal injury if the fetus (or newborn, depending on the normal rate of maturation for that species) is exposed to a virus, toxin, or teratogen. Renal dysplasia in pigs has been attributed to *hypovitaminosis A;* formation of the trigonal wedge and proper insertion of the ureteral buds into the bladder, and hence proper renal development, are mediated by vitamin A and proto-oncogene Ret signaling pathways.

There is considerable variation in the appearance of those dysplastic kidneys that are grossly abnormal. Most of them are small, which accounts for their frequent misdiagnosis as hypoplastic. They are usually misshapen and fibrosed with thick-walled cysts and dilated tortuous ureters. One or both kidneys may be affected, and accessory vessels are occasionally identified (Fig. 4-13A). If the lesion is unilateral, the ipsilateral ureter should be examined for anomalous valves, diverticula, or atresia. If both kidneys are involved, scrutiny of the bladder and lower urinary tract is indicated. If the diagnosis rests on ultrasonographic and/or renal biopsy findings, then examination of the entire urinary tract via contrast imaging studies may help elucidate the pathogenesis and detect urinary reflux into the kidney. Some dysplastic kidneys may be only slightly irregular in contour or may appear normal, in which case microscopic examination is required for diagnosis. Considerable emphasis has been placed on the size of renal arteries in dysplasias, but changes should be interpreted with caution because degenerative lesions in the renal parenchyma may be accompanied by vascular remodeling. Extrarenal anomalies, such as imperforate anus and segmental ureteral agenesis, may occur in association with renal dysplasia.

The **microscopic criteria** of renal dysplasia are the presence of structures inappropriate to the stage of development of the animal or the development of structures that are clearly anomalous. Among the former are *areas of undifferentiated mesenchyme* in cortex or medulla, and *groups of immature glomeruli* (small glomeruli with peripheral nuclei and inapparent capillaries) in the cortex of adolescent or adult animals (Fig. 4-13B). Some lobules of the kidney may be devoid of glomeruli and/or tubules. Anomalous structures include *collecting tubules ending blindly* in cortical connective tissue, *atypical tubular epithelium,* and *primitive (metanephric) ducts* lined by cuboidal or columnar epithelium (Fig. 4-13C), sometimes surrounded by concentric layers of mesenchyme. *Dysontogenic (cartilaginous or osseous) metaplasia,* which occurs in some dysplastic human kidneys, is rarely present in dysplastic kidneys in domestic animals. There is some support for the opinion that only primitive ducts and cartilage nodules are prima facie evidence of dysplasia, on the grounds that all other lesions may be produced by acquired renal disease. Some of the more prominent gross lesions of dysplastic kidneys, such as cysts, dense medullary fibrosis, and fibrous wedges extending from pelvis to cortex, are probably regressive changes because of obstruction or infarction. Because *ureteral anomalies* are often concomitant, dysplastic kidneys are abnormally susceptible to pyelonephritis. Otherwise, there is little or no evidence of infection in the renal parenchyma.

Further reading

Bruder MC, et al. Renal dysplasia in Beagle dogs: four cases. Toxicol Pathol 2010;38:1051-1057.

Kolbjornsen O, et al. End-stage kidney disease probably due to reflux nephropathy with segmental hypoplasia (Ask-Upmark kidney) in young Boxer dogs in Norway. A retrospective study. Vet Pathol 2008;45:467-474.

Medina-Torres CE, et al. Bilateral diffuse cystic renal dysplasia in a 9-day-old Thoroughbred filly. Can Vet J 2014;55:141-146.

Philbey AW, et al. Renal dysplasia and nephrosclerosis in calves. Vet Rec 2009;165:626-630.

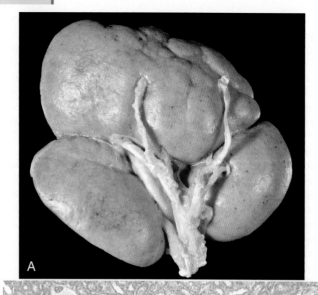

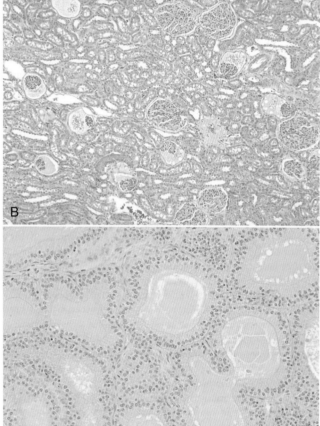

Figure 4-13 Renal dysplasia. A. Malformed kidney with **accessory vessels** in a young horse. (Courtesy E. Clark, P. Stromberg.) **B.** Numerous **fetal glomeruli with compensatory hypertrophy** of other glomeruli in a young dog with juvenile nephropathy. **C. Persistent medullary metanephric ducts** in a young dog.

Renal cysts

Cystic diseases of the kidney include various conditions characterized by one or more grossly visible cystic cavities in the renal parenchyma. No satisfactory classification of renal cysts exists, but location of cysts, mode of inheritance (or lack thereof), the presence of lesions in other organs, and the clinical course in affected animals are important aspects to consider.

Cysts can arise during organogenesis, and may be associated with histologic criteria of renal dysplasia. Cysts can also develop in nephrons and collecting tubules after the end of nephrogenesis. *Cysts can occur in any part of the nephron, including the glomerular space, or in the collecting system.* Analyses of their content indicate that *they are part of functional nephrons,* and that their activity is consistent with their location in the nephron.

Three **mechanisms,** which are not mutually exclusive, can lead to the formation of renal cysts:

1. Renal cysts may be caused by *obstructive lesions;* examples are the acquired retention cysts of chronic renal disease, some dysplastic cysts, and possibly those of glomerulocystic disease.
2. A fundamental change, of unknown origin, may occur in the *tubular basement membrane* and result in formation of saccular or fusiform dilations of the tubules. Some dilated segments may detach from the tubule and form spherical cystic structures. Likewise, detachment of the proximal tubule from the urinary pole will result in dilated Bowman's capsules and so-called "atubular glomeruli."
3. Disordered growth of tubular epithelial cells may lead to *focal hyperplastic lesions* and cyst formation.

Mutation of polycystic kidney disease (PKD) genes in humans may alter production of *polycystin* proteins, which are important in cell-cell and cell-matrix interactions; altered tubular epithelial growth and differentiation may lead to cyst formation. Renal cysts are seen in humans with primary aldosteronism or primary renal potassium wasting, perhaps as a consequence of chronic hypokalemia and tubular obstruction by proliferating tubular epithelial cells. Renal cysts are dynamic structures and their growth may be modified by pharmacologic means.

Many *chemicals,* such as long-acting corticosteroids, diphenylamine, polychlorinated biphenyls, 5,6,7,8-tetrahydrocarbazole-3-acetic acid, alloxan, diphenylthiazole, and nordihydroguaiaretic acid, cause renal cysts in experimental animals. Corticosteroids induce hypokalemia, and cyst formation can be prevented by injections of some potassium salts, but in general, the mechanisms of cyst development are not known. It seems possible that some of the therapeutic, prophylactic, and pollutant chemicals to which animals are exposed could be responsible for sporadic cases of renal cysts.

Renal cysts vary in size from the barely visible to structures that exceed that of the organ itself. Cysts are often more numerous in the cortex than medulla, this may simply reflect the relative volumes of the 2 regions. The cyst wall is clear or opaque, depending on the amount of surrounding connective tissue. The content is watery, and cysts are lined by flattened or cuboidal epithelium. A few cysts are more or less divided by thin trabeculae, but most are unilocular and roughly spherical, ovoid, or fusiform.

Simple renal cysts occur in all species but are most common in pigs and calves. There are different patterns of occurrence

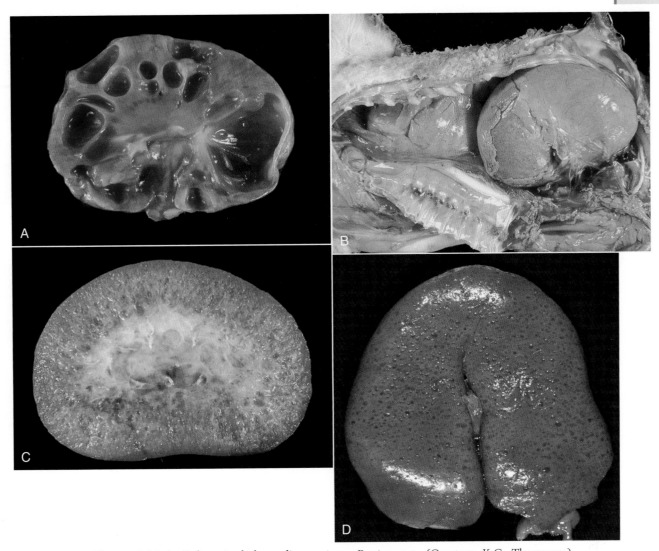

Figure 4-14 A. Polycystic kidney disease in a Persian cat. (Courtesy K.G. Thompson.) **B, C. Congenital polycystic disease** in a Perendale lamb. Kidneys are grossly enlarged by numerous parenchymal cysts. (Courtesy K.G. Thompson.) **D. Congenital polycystic kidney** in a 1-day-old foal. (Courtesy S.N. McGraw, B.G. Murphy.)

in pigs, but it is not clear whether similar patterns exist in other animals. The usual finding in pigs is one or a few unilocular cortical cysts, ~1-2 cm across, that bulge from the renal surface or are exposed when the kidney is sliced. They are usually bilateral and are incidental findings in young pigs. Affected kidneys are discarded in abattoirs. Although usually regarded as sporadic occurrences, these lesions may be examples of a cystic renal disease that is inherited as an autosomal dominant trait. Polygenic inheritance may determine the number of cysts in animals with the dominant gene. In this condition, few cysts are present at birth, but they gradually increase in number, and there may be 80-90 by 1 year of age. Signs of renal failure are not seen, but the condition has similarities to a human cystic disease in which renal failure develops in adults; a similar course in mature swine is conceivable.

Occasionally, areas containing many small cysts occur in one lobe of a bovine kidney or one pole of an equine kidney. They are not significant clinically.

Polycystic kidney disease (PKD) occurs in 2 major forms:
1. *Autosomal dominant* polycystic kidney disease (ADPKD), in Bull Terriers and Persian cats (Fig. 4-14), is similar to the *adult-onset* form of PKD in humans, which is linked to defects in genes *PKD1* and *PKD2*. Polycystin 1 and 2 are encoded by *PKD1* and 2, respectively, and localize to the primary cilia present on the apical surface of the tubular epithelial cells. There is one primary cilium per epithelial cell, and its purpose is to translate a physical event (fluid movement through the tubular lumen) into an intracellular calcium signal. The basal body of the primary cilium also plays a role in cell division, wherein the cilium is reabsorbed and serves as the centriole during mitosis, thereby linking the cilium to cell proliferation. Renal cysts develop bilaterally, are of proximal or distal tubular origin, grow progressively over time, and lead to chronic tubulointerstitial nephritis and renal failure in adult life. ADPKD in Persian cats (see Fig. 4-14), linked to a *PKD1* gene defect, is commonly accompanied by hepatic cysts and/or hepatic

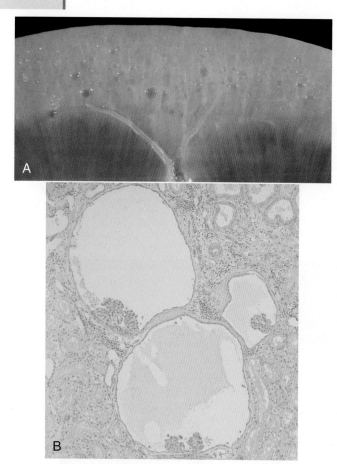

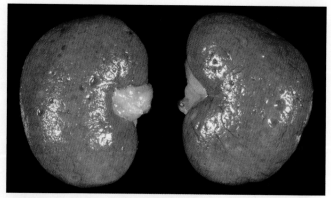

Figure 4-16 Multiple acquired cortical cysts in a dog. (Courtesy F. Aeffner, P. Stromberg.)

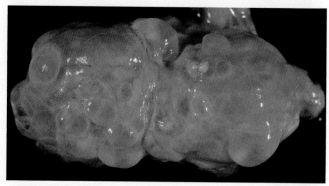

Figure 4-17 Capsular pseudocysts in a dog. (Courtesy S.N. McGraw, J.A. Luff.)

Figure 4-15 Glomerulocystic disease. A. Numerous cortical cysts in a goat, which were dilated Bowman's capsules. (Courtesy M. Buccellato, S. Weisbrode.) **B.** Multiple severely dilated Bowman's capsules in a dog. Glomerular tufts are compressed and atrophic.

fibrosis, and pancreatic cysts. Bull Terriers with ADPKD also have a mutation in *PKD1*, and some of the affected dogs may also have abnormal GBMs, as discussed later.

2. *Autosomal recessive* PKD (ARPKD), described in West Highland White and Cairn Terriers, and Perendale sheep, is similar to the *childhood* form of PKD in humans and may be accompanied by hepatic biliary cysts. In sheep, cysts are congenital and lambs die in utero or shortly after birth (see Fig. 4-14B, C). In humans, ARPKD has been linked to a mutation in *PKHD1* gene, which encodes another component of the primary cilia: fibrocystin. A genetic cause for the disease in domesticated species has not been identified.

Congenital PKD, of unknown inheritance, occurs in piglets, lambs, calves, goat kids, puppies, kittens, and foals. In humans, this variant is often diagnosed as *multicystic dysplasia*. There may be concurrent cystic bile ducts, bile duct proliferation, and sometimes pancreatic cysts. This form of PKD in domestic animals is manifested by stillbirths or death in renal failure during the first few weeks of life. Grossly, the kidneys are large and pale, and contain numerous 1-5 mm cysts that involve both cortex and medulla. Bile duct cysts range from barely visible up to 3 cm across, and the gallbladder and biliary system are often distended with bile that discolors the liver.

Glomerulocystic disease is the term used when cysts involve Bowman's capsules, and may be the result of

periglomerular fibrosis and hence stenosis of the glomerulo-tubular junction (Fig. 4-15). Although a few scattered dilated Bowman's capsules may not be clinically significant, renal insufficiency can be seen when many glomeruli are affected.

Acquired cysts of the kidney develop when tubules are obstructed by scar tissue. They are multiple and small, rarely exceeding 1.0 cm in diameter (Fig. 4-16). Most are located in convoluted tubules and Bowman's spaces. Hyperplastic collecting tubules are sometimes grossly visible as elongated cysts in the medulla of dogs with renal failure. These acquired cysts are distinguishable from primary cysts because they occur in kidneys with extensive scarring.

Perinephric pseudocysts occasionally develop unilaterally or bilaterally as a collection of fluid, which may be urine, blood, lymph, or transudate, in the space between the renal capsule and the renal reflection of the peritoneum (Fig. 4-17; eFig. 4-4A, B). It can be seen in any species but is most commonly observed in cats. *The space is not lined by epithelium* and is thus a pseudocyst. Potential causes include trauma, ureteral or lymphatic obstruction, venous congestion, and hypertension. Affected cats are usually old and have concomitant chronic renal disease.

Further reading

Bissler JJ, et al. Glomerulocystic kidney disease. Pediatr Nephrol 2010;25:2049-2056.

Gharahkhani P, et al. A non-synonymous mutation in the canine *Pkd1* gene is associated with autosomal dominant polycystic kidney disease in bull terriers. PLoS ONE 2011;6:e22455.

Johnstone AC, et al. Congenital polycystic kidney disease in lambs. Vet J 2005;53:307-314.

Lyons LA, et al. Feline polycystic kidney disease mutation identified in PKD1. J Am Soc Nephrol 2004;15:2548-2555.

Wilson PK. Polycystic kidney disease: new understanding in the pathogenesis. Int J Biochem Cell Biol 2004;36:1868-1873.

CIRCULATORY DISTURBANCES AND DISEASES OF THE BLOOD VESSELS

Renal hyperemia

Active hyperemia is seen in acute nephritis but especially in the acute septicemias and toxemias. Kidneys are swollen and uniformly dark, although in some cases, the hyperemia may be largely restricted to the medulla. Microscopically, all vessels, especially capillaries, are filled with blood. *Passive hyperemia (congestion)* follows the usual principles. Affected kidneys are enlarged and dark, and the capsular vessels are injected. On section, the corticomedullary junctional zone is dark and prominent, with engorgement of visible tributaries. Acute congestion with intertubular hemorrhages occurs in clostridial enterotoxemia of lambs and calves.

Renal hemorrhages

Hemorrhages are especially common in the renal cortex in a variety of bacteremias and viremias and sometimes in healthy slaughtered animals. Petechiae are very common in piglets dead of any cause. Many or few pinpoint hemorrhages occur beneath the capsule in classical swine fever (hog cholera), African swine fever, and porcine salmonellosis. In porcine erysipelas, the hemorrhages tend to be larger and more irregular in size and shape (Fig. 4-18). Severe hemorrhage in the wall of the renal pelvis and the medulla sometimes occurs in classical swine fever, in other acute infections of swine, and in the hemorrhagic diatheses; the hemorrhage occurs from rupture of the congested medullary vessels. Extensive subcapsular hemorrhage is not uncommon in clostridial enterotoxemia of calves; it produces a black cast molded to the shape of the cortex.

Renal infarction

Infarcts of the kidney are common lesions of localized coagulative necrosis produced by embolic or thrombotic occlusion of the renal artery or of one of its branches (Fig. 4-19). The sequelae depend on whether the obstructing material is septic or sterile and on the size and number of the vessels obstructed. Thrombi produce typical infarcts; septic thrombi produce abscesses that may heal, sequestrate, or discharge into the pelvis. Thrombosis of a trunk of a renal artery will produce total or subtotal necrosis of the kidney, the extent of the latter depending on the presence and efficiency of parahilar and capsular collaterals. If an arcuate artery is obstructed, then there is necrosis of

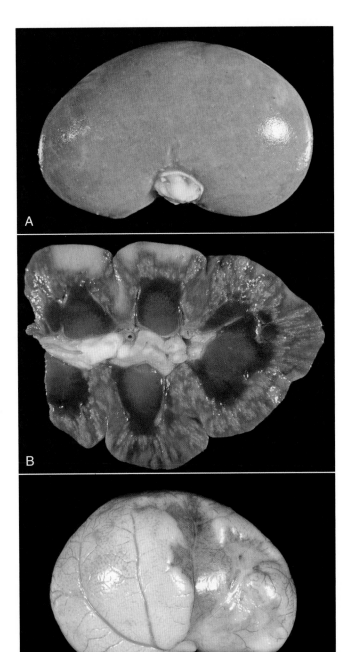

Figure 4-19 Renal infarction. A. Acute renal infarcts in a dog are raised and red as the result of hemorrhage and edema. (Courtesy B. Harrington, P. Stromberg). **B. Renal infarcts** in a cow associated with ascending pyelonephritis caused by nonhemolytic *E. coli* and *T. pyogenes.* (Courtesy M. Gramer, Univ of Minnesota.) **C. Chronic infarcts** and scarring in a cat. (Courtesy S. Chaney, P. Stromberg.)

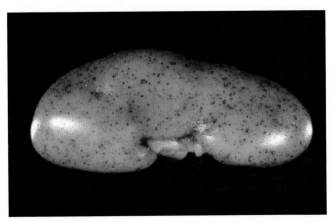

Figure 4-18 Renal cortical petechiae in a pig with erysipelas. (Courtesy P. Stromberg.)

a wedge of both cortex and medulla. If an interlobular vessel is involved, infarction is limited to the cortex. The ease and frequency with which the kidneys are infarcted result from their vascular architecture being of the "end-artery" type and the large volume of blood that continually traverses them. In cats, renal infarcts (see Fig. 4-19C) may serve as an indicator of underlying hypertrophic cardiomyopathy and distal aortic thromboembolism.

Soon after total obstruction of a vessel, the related wedge of tissue is swollen, intensely cyanotic, and congested by the blood that oozes into the vessels from collateral vessels. There is no sharp line between the infarcted zone and the adjacent normal tissue; instead there is a transition zone in which blood continues to ooze slowly toward the central region of the infarct. In the outer part of the marginal zone, the red cells survive and circulation may be re-established. This zone persists for the first 2-3 days; it has been referred to, erroneously, as the zone of reactive hyperemia (see Fig. 4-19). The extent of useful diffusion determines the actual limit of the infarct, and it is here that dehemoglobinization begins, neutrophils accumulate, and cells undergo necrosis. The dehemoglobinization begins at about 24 hours and may be complete by 2-3 days, when the infarcted area then becomes white. Before decoloration begins, the affected area is outlined by a thin but distinct white line of leukocytes.

The sequence of degenerative changes in the infarcted tissue reflects the specialization and sensitivity of the various structures. At the outer margins, only a few proximal tubules show epithelial necrosis. More centrally, every proximal tubule is dead and inside the zone of diffusion everything is dead. In the peripheral dead zone, there may be some revascularization within 1-2 weeks. The necrotic zone is progressively replaced by fibrous tissue, and healed infarcts persist as pale gray-white scars, wedge shaped, and depressed. The scars may be difficult or impossible to distinguish grossly from focal healed pyelonephritis.

Minute emboli that lodge in the glomerular or peritubular capillaries may produce small infarcts that are not detectable macroscopically. Because of the small size of such infarcts, there may be adequate diffusion across the infarcted zone so that leukocytes do not accumulate, epithelial necrosis is minimal and soon repaired, and circulation is re-established. Commonly, infarcts of various ages in a kidney indicate recurrent embolic episodes.

Primary vascular disease includes various processes, such as renal arteriosclerosis, arteriolosclerosis, arteriolar hyalinosis, and arteritis (eFig. 4-5), with "polyarteritis nodosa" and systemic diseases such as malignant catarrhal fever being examples of the latter category. A variety of degenerative proliferative arterial changes occur in chronic diffuse inflammatory diseases. Although they are probably secondary, they may be magnified by the *hypertension* that is expected to develop. Hypertension is common in canine and feline renal failure and can lead to further deterioration in renal function by causing additional glomerular and tubular damage. *Renal telangiectasia, aneurysms* or *pseudoaneurysms* are rarely reported to cause hematuria. Renal telangiectasia has been documented in related Pembroke Welsh Corgis.

Renal cortical necrosis and acute tubular necrosis

Acute tubular necrosis and renal cortical necrosis are grouped together here for purposes of discussion; acute tubular

necrosis (ATN) is also discussed in more detail later. These lesions occur infrequently in animals, but if severe may cause acute renal failure (ARF) and death. *Either variety of renal necrosis is usually a manifestation of hypoperfusion, or "shock,"* which may be classified as cardiogenic, hypovolemic, septic, or neurogenic. Outbreaks of renal cortical necrosis of unknown cause have occurred in kennels of dogs. Renal cortical necrosis and ATN occur in cattle in a variety of endotoxemic conditions, such as mastitis or metritis, and in gastrointestinal diseases, such as severe enteritis and grain overload. Bilateral cortical necrosis is a rare complication of esophagogastric ulceration in swine, and apparently results from hemorrhagic shock.

ATN, sometimes referred to as **acute tubular injury (ATI) or acute kidney injury (AKI),** is demonstrated by patchy necrosis of segments of both proximal and distal tubules; necrotic tubular epithelial cells become casts, which cause tubular blockage and oliguria. Other contributors to oliguria are tubular backleak through disrupted tubular basement membranes, compression of medullary tubules by edema and inflammation, reflex constriction of afferent arterioles, and decreased glomerular membrane permeability. In **renal cortical necrosis,** the whole or part of both cortices is involved, and there is destruction of both tubules and glomeruli. It appears probable that these lesions represent differences in degree and that they result from patchy or complete renal ischemia.

The usual balance between the renin-angiotensin and the eicosanoid systems that maintain fine regulation of intrarenal blood flow is disrupted during ischemia. During hypotension, perfusion of outer cortical nephrons is reduced, while perfusion of inner cortical nephrons is maintained; *intrarenal blood flow is redistributed toward the inner cortex and medulla.* This reaction occurs because the vasoconstrictive effects of angiotensin II and adrenergic stimulation are unopposed in the outer cortex, whereas in the inner cortex, prostaglandins modulate vasoconstriction; PGE_2 is produced in the medulla in response to ischemia, travels in tubular fluid to the area of the juxtaglomerular apparatus, and has a local vasodilatory effect on afferent arterioles of juxtamedullary nephrons.

The duration of ischemia is of obvious importance for the pathogenesis of necrosis. Complete ischemia of <2 hours duration can be expected to be followed by *good reflow* if cardiac output and blood pressure are restored to normal, whereas total ischemia of longer duration may be followed by patchy reflow or complete failure of reflow in the cortex, medulla, or both. Reflow is inhibited primarily because of vascular congestion by red cells swollen by plasma water uptake, and perhaps also by ischemia-induced swelling of endothelial cells of glomeruli, vasa recta, and peritubular capillaries. This *"no-reflow" phenomenon* may make an important contribution to renal ischemia and ARF. Severe ischemic injury can permanently alter peritubular capillary density, resulting in decreased urinary concentrating ability and predisposing to interstitial fibrosis. This progression might be mediated through local synthesis of *angiostatin*, a proteolytic cleavage product of plasminogen that inhibits angiogenesis, promotes endothelial cell apoptosis, and disrupts the integrity of capillaries.

Another mechanism by which renal cortical necrosis occurs is via the generalized Shwartzman reaction, an example of *disseminated intravascular coagulation*, which is often the result of gram-negative endotoxemia. Endothelial injury in glomerular and peritubular capillaries leads to microthrombosis and hemorrhagic renal cortical necrosis. This severe degree of renal damage is usually rapidly fatal, but milder lesions can be seen in a number of bacteremic diseases as petechiae or cortical hemorrhages.

The cellular destruction that occurs in ischemic renal injury begins with a decreased ability to produce ATP and hence an increase in membrane permeability that allows influx of calcium into the cell. Excess free cytosolic calcium activates phospholipases that further increase membrane permeability and lead to membrane disruption and generation of toxic lipid byproducts. Increased intracellular calcium also interferes with mitochondrial respiration and causes increased production of free radicals that further injure cell membranes and mitochondria. Unfortunately, reperfusion can be deleterious because reoxygenation increases the production of free radicals.

The **gross appearance** of the kidneys, other than those with hemorrhagic renal necrosis, varies considerably from case to case; it is determined by the severity, distribution, and duration of the ischemia and the quality of the reflow. In ATN, the cortices are finely mottled or flecked by small yellow foci of necrosis. In renal cortical necrosis, the cortices may be totally affected or the injury may be patchy; pigs tend to develop a "turkey egg" pattern marked by hemorrhagic glomeruli, but die before more extensive necrosis is evident (see Fig. 4-18), whereas cattle sometimes develop a distinctive patchy cortical necrosis (see Fig. 4-19B). The reaction is the same as for infarction given previously. A narrow subcapsular rim of viable tissue may remain. The affected areas of cortex are pale, almost white, slightly swollen, and stop sharply at the corticomedullary junction. The irregular areas of cortical infarction may be outlined by hemorrhage. The medulla may be normal, but in some cases, there is severe congestion of the inner stripe of the outer medulla or of the whole of the medulla so that it is swollen and resembles a blood clot.

The **histologic appearance** of a kidney with ATN includes irregular necrosis of the proximal tubules, with or without disruption of the tubular basement membranes. Hyaline and granular casts are present, particularly in distal tubules and collecting ducts. There can be interstitial edema as a result of tubular leakage. Preferential damage occurs to the pars recta and thick ascending limb because of their location in the poorly perfused outer medulla and because of their higher oxygen requirement. If the animal survives the ischemic episode, evidence of regeneration may be seen in ~1 week, namely, tubules lined by flattened epithelial cells with hyperchromatic nuclei and occasional mitoses. In cases of severe ischemia and renal cortical necrosis, various patterns of infarction may be seen, with glomeruli and vessels, as well as tubules, being necrotic. Microthrombi may be seen in capillaries, and hemorrhage may be present in glomeruli. The medulla is usually preserved.

Further reading

Basile DP, et al. Angiostatin and matrix metalloprotease expression following ischemic acute renal failure. Am J Physiol Renal Physiol 2004;286:F893-F902.

Bhargava R, et al. Acute lung injury and acute kidney injury are established by four hours in experimental sepsis and are improved with pre, but not post, sepsis administration of TNF-(antibodies. PLoS ONE 2013;8:e79037.

Hickey MC, et al. Concurrent diseases and conditions in cats with renal infarcts. J Vet Intern Med 2014;28:319-323.

Lien YH, et al. Pathogenesis of renal ischemia/reperfusion injury: lessons from knockout mice. Life Sci 2003;74:543-552.

Rosenberger C, et al. Renal parenchymal oxygenation and hypoxia adaptation in acute kidney injury. Clin Exp Pharmacol Physiol 2006;33:980-988.

Renal medullary necrosis

Under certain circumstances, medullary necrosis is the primary manifestation of renal injury. As noted previously, renal hypotension usually results in cortical necrosis because of redistribution of blood flow to juxtamedullary nephrons. However, medullary vessels are damaged when ischemia lasts longer than 2 hours. There might be failure of both medullary and cortical reflow after temporary ischemia, leading to both medullary and cortical necrosis. In the case of venous occlusion, the elevated intrarenal blood pressure maintains the patency of lower-resistance cortical vessels but not of higher-resistance medullary vessels, and hence medullary infarction predominates.

Toxic and hypoxic insults to the kidney are synergistic, and several protective mechanisms must be incapacitated to produce medullary injury. Prostaglandins are important autoregulators of renal perfusion. *Nonsteroidal anti-inflammatory drugs* (NSAIDs), such as aspirin, phenacetin, phenylbutazone, flunixin meglumine, ibuprofen, and meloxicam, inhibit cyclooxygenase, resulting in decreased production of PGE_2 and loss of its vasodilatory effect on arterioles of juxtamedullary nephrons. Additionally, NSAIDs may be directly toxic to renal medullary interstitial cells, and dehydration likely contributes to the pathogenesis. Papillary necrosis is characteristic of "**analgesic nephropathy**," such as renal crest necrosis in dehydrated horses treated with phenylbutazone (Fig. 4-20A, B; eFig. 4-6A, B).

Dehydration is involved in the pathogenesis of papillary necrosis in racing Greyhounds. Papillary necrosis occurs in lambs and calves that are dehydrated when treated with phenothiazine, and the necrosis is again apparently the result of *ischemia*. Accidental ingestion of a combination of monensin and roxarsone has caused renal medullary necrosis in normally hydrated dogs and pups.

Urinary obstruction, pyelonephritis, and amyloidosis can cause papillary necrosis in animals. Compression of thin-walled interstitial vessels is probably the mechanism by which all of these processes cause papillary necrosis. Specifically, outflow obstruction will cause collecting ducts to dilate, pyelonephritis will lead to significant interstitial inflammation and edema, and amyloid may be deposited directly in the medullary interstitium.

The *gross lesions* of medullary necrosis vary greatly in their extent and stage of development. Acute papillary infarction may be an incidental finding in an animal dead of other causes, such as dehydration and electrolyte imbalances in neonatal diarrhea. Massive medullary infarction would no doubt be part of ARF leading to death. In an animal that survives an episode of medullary necrosis, medullary scarring occurs, the papilla may slough, and secondary cortical scarring is seen. The sloughed papilla may remain in the pelvis and may become mineralized. *Microscopic lesions* cover the usual range of necrosis (see Fig. 4-20B) and scarring. *Sequelae* to medullary

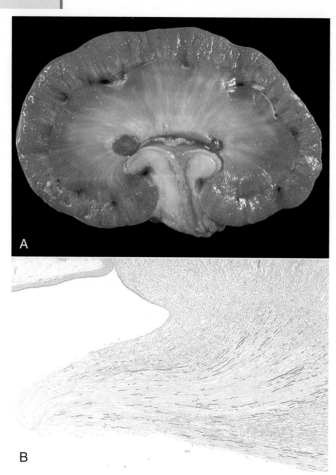

Figure 4-20 A. Renal crest necrosis in a dog caused by nonsteroidal anti-inflammatory drug (NSAID) toxicity. (Courtesy K.G. Thompson.) **B.** Histology reveals **coagulative necrosis with minimal inflammation** of the renal papilla of a cat with NSAID toxicity.

necrosis are based on the loss of the ability to concentrate urine, and include chronic renal failure and uremia.

Further reading

Brix AE. Renal papillary necrosis. Toxicol Pathol 2002;30:672-674.

Hao C, et al. Dehydration activates an NF(B-driven, COX2-dependent survival mechanism in renal medullary interstitial cells. J Clin Invest 2000;106:973-982.

MacAllister CG, et al. Comparison of adverse effects of phenylbutazone, flunixin meglumine, and ketoprofen in horses. J Am Vet Med Assoc 1993;202:71-77.

Rocha GM, et al. Direct toxicity of nonsteroidal antiinflammatory drugs for renal medullary cells. Proc Natl Acad Sci U S A 2001;98: 5317-5322.

Hydronephrosis

Hydronephrosis is dilation of the renal pelvis and calyces associated with progressive atrophy and cystic enlargement of the kidney (Fig. 4-21). The cause is some form of *urinary obstruction*, which may be complete or incomplete, existing at any level from the urethra to the renal pelvis. The obstruction may be caused by anomalous development of the lower urinary tract, or it may be acquired. *Acquired causes* include urinary

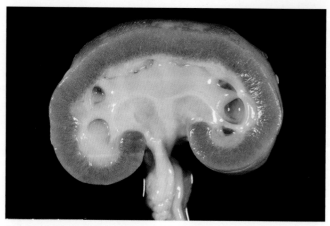

Figure 4-21 Hydronephrosis in a sheep. (Courtesy L. Himmel, C. Premanandan.)

calculi in any location; prostatic enlargement in the dog; cystitis, especially if it is hemorrhagic; compression of the ureters by surrounding inflammatory or neoplastic tissue; displacement of the bladder in perineal hernias; and acquired urethral strictures. Depending upon the site of obstruction, hydronephrosis may be unilateral or bilateral, and there may be some degree of hydroureter and dilation of the bladder.

The pathogenesis of hydronephrosis is based on the persistence of glomerular filtration in the presence of urinary obstruction, plus the development of ischemic lesions. Even with sudden complete obstruction, glomerular filtration continues because filtrate diffuses into the renal interstitium and perirenal spaces, where it is drained by lymphatics and veins. However, continued filtration creates increased pressure throughout the nephrons, collecting ducts, calyces, and pelvis. Pressure atrophy and apoptosis of tubular epithelium occur, diminishing tubular function and concentrating ability. Blood vessels are compressed, particularly hilar veins and inner medullary vessels, leading to *papillary ischemia and necrosis.* Interstitial inflammation is triggered by activated tubular epithelial cells and leukocytes releasing vasoactive factors, growth factors, and cytokines. Glomerular filtration eventually decreases because of intrarenal vasoconstriction. Nephrons atrophy and are replaced by progressive interstitial fibrosis.

The degree of development of hydronephrosis depends on whether or not it is bilateral, the completeness of the obstruction, and on other complications of obstruction. Bilateral obstruction, which includes obstruction localized to the bladder or urethra, results in early death from uremia. Unilateral obstruction produces the greatest degree of hydronephrosis, especially if the obstruction is incomplete or intermittent, because glomerular filtration can continue. If an obstruction is removed within about 1 week, renal function returns. After about 3 weeks of complete obstruction, or several months of incomplete obstruction, irreversible renal damage occurs. In unilateral hydronephrosis, the contralateral kidney can compensate if it is normal. Urinary stasis predisposes to infection; hence pyelonephritis might be superimposed on hydronephrosis.

Early *gross changes* consist of progressive dilation of the pelvis and calyces with blunting of the apices of the pyramids. Eventually, these may become excavated to form multilocular cysts communicating with the pelvis and separated by intricate ridges that represent original septa. In advanced cases, the kidney is transformed into a thin-walled sac with only a thin shell of atrophic cortical parenchyma.

Microscopically, there is dilation of the proximal convoluted tubules, followed shortly thereafter by dilation of distal and straight segments. The latter persists, with atrophy of the epithelium, but dilation of proximal tubules subsides. Instead, cortical tubules atrophy, and are separated or replaced by fibrosis. Much of the tubular atrophy may be through apoptosis. The glomeruli can persist for a long time. Various degrees of ischemia or infarction may develop in the cortex if the obstruction is sudden and complete; the infarcts are venous in origin. There is progressive destruction of the pyramids that spares the pelvic epithelium. Necrotic tissue is removed, and pyramids are gradually destroyed. Inflammatory response is often minimal to mild.

Further reading

Chandler KJ, et al. Hydronephrosis and renal failure in two Friesian cows. Vet Rec 2000;146:646-648.

Foster JD, Pinkerton ME. Bilateral ureteropelvic junction stenosis causing hydronephrosis and renal failure in an adult cat. J Feline Med Surg 2012;14:938-941.

Rousset N, et al. Unilateral hydronephrosis and hydroureter secondary to ureteric atresia, and uterus unicornis in a young terrier. J Small Anim Pract 2011;52:441-444.

GLOMERULAR DISEASE

Glomerular disease is important because interference with glomerular blood flow alters the formation of ultrafiltrate and impairs peritubular perfusion, which can lead to loss of the entire nephron.

- The term **glomerulonephritis** (GN) implies that secondary tubulointerstitial and vascular changes accompany the primary glomerular disease.
- The term **glomerulitis** is used when inflammation is restricted to glomeruli, as may occur in acute septicemias.
- **Glomerulopathy** refers to glomerular disease without inflammatory cells or with uncertain etiology or pathogenesis.
- Glomeruli may also be significantly affected in a variety of systemic diseases, such as **amyloidosis,** which is discussed later, bacterial endocarditis, and in various vasculitides.

Clinical presentations can be nonspecific and include hematuria, proteinuria, oliguria, hyposthenuria, and azotemia. Some dogs develop vascular thrombosis (i.e., pulmonary arteries or renal veins) because they are in a *hypercoagulable state* resulting from stimulation of production of acute-phase proteins, such as fibrinogen, while simultaneously losing low-molecular-weight anticoagulants, such as antithrombin III, into urine.

Proteinuria, occurring in the absence of urinary tract inflammation, is suggestive of glomerular damage, namely, as the result of increased glomerular permeability. Proteinuria is usually measured by calculating a ratio of the urine protein to the urine creatinine (UPC). This technique is preferable to only measuring urine protein at a single time point because it accounts for differences in urine concentration. A small amount of protein in a dilute urine sample is more clinically significant than the same amount of protein in a concentrated sample. Mild proteinuria (usually UPC 1-3) can be the result

of tubular injury. If the UPC is >3, then protein loss is likely glomerular in origin and might lead to development of the **nephrotic syndrome.** This syndrome is characterized by proteinuria, hypoalbuminemia, generalized edema, and hyperlipidemia, but edema is less common in dogs than in humans. In dogs, the nephrotic syndrome connotes a worse prognosis compared to patients with only proteinuria. Edema is the result of decreased plasma colloid osmotic pressure, stimulation of the renin-angiotensin-aldosterone system, and release of antidiuretic hormone (ADH) in response to hypovolemia. The hepatic response to hypoproteinemia is a generalized increase in production of proteins, including lipoproteins, leading to hyperlipoproteinemia and hypercholesterolemia.

Depending on the type or severity of the glomerular disease, there may be an increase in medium- and/or high-molecular-weight proteins in the urine. Additional biomarkers of glomerular disease include urinary albumin and urinary immunoglobulin G (IgG). Albumin is thought to indicate early kidney disease (and is sometimes referred to as microalbuminuria when it is mildly elevated), whereas the presence of large molecules, such as immunoglobulins, suggests a marked increase in glomerular permeability. Urinary protein electrophoresis can reveal "glomerular" or "tubular" patterns of injury, based on the size of the proteins in the urine. However, most dogs undergoing renal biopsy and serum protein electrophoresis fall into a "mixed glomerular and tubular" pattern because of the interaction of the 2 compartments.

The following terms are generally accepted for the description of glomerular disease:
- **Diffuse:** involves >50% of glomeruli
- **Focal:** involves <50% of glomeruli
- **Global:** involves the whole glomerular tuft
- **Segmental:** involves only part of the glomerulus
- **Mesangial:** affects primarily the mesangial area

Classification of GN in humans is relatively complex, based on extensive clinicopathologic correlations and responses to therapy. The following terms are currently used for the histologic description of GN in domestic animals:
- **Membranous:** GBM remodeling that is secondary to immune complex (IC) deposition on the abluminal surface of the GBM with normocellularity to mild hypercellularity (Fig. 4-22; eFig. 4-7)
- **Proliferative:** increased cellularity without significant alterations to the GBM; IC may or may not be identified (Fig. 4-23; eFig. 4-8)
- **Mesangioproliferative:** increased cellularity limited to the mesangium with evidence of IC deposition within the mesangium (Fig. 4-24; eFig. 4-9)
- **Membranoproliferative (mesangiocapillary) (MPGN):** proliferation (endocapillary and mesangial) with remodeling of the capillary loop resulting from IC deposition (usually between the endothelial cell and the GBM) (Fig. 4-25; eFig. 4-10)
- **Segmental glomerulosclerosis (GS):** segmental effacement of peripheral capillary loops by extracellular matrix; notably, GS can be superimposed on the above patterns or can occur as the sole pathologic process (Fig. 4-26; eFig. 4-11)
- **Global glomerulosclerosis (glomerular obsolescence):** tuft is shrunken, eosinophilic, and hypocellular (Fig. 4-27; eFig. 4-12)

There is an important distinction between the *patterns* of glomerular lesions and the *diagnostic terms*. For example, a

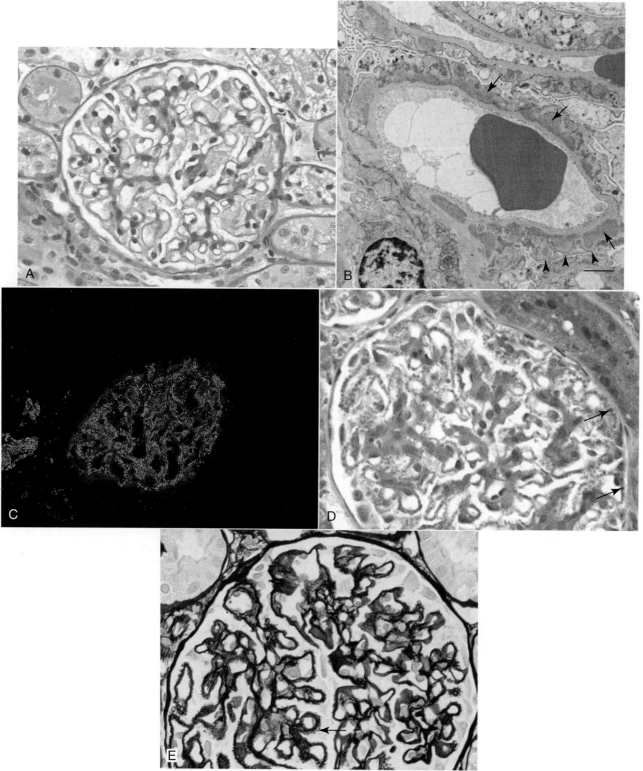

Figure 4-22 Membranous glomerulonephropathy (MGN) in a dog. GBM is thickened without associated hypercellularity. **A.** PAS stain. **B.** Transmission electron micrograph demonstrates regularly spaced electron-dense deposits (arrows) on the subepithelial surface. Some deposits are encircled by GBM (arrowheads). (Courtesy G. Lees, F. Clubb.) **C.** Immunofluorescence using an antibody against canine IgG reveals granular staining along capillary walls. (Courtesy G. Lees.) **D.** Masson trichrome stain from a different dog with MGN reveals numerous regularly spaced red nodules (arrows) on the abluminal (subepithelial) surface of the capillary loops. **E.** JMS stain reveals argyrophilic spikes (arrow) of GBM material between deposits and **holes** representing encircled deposits.

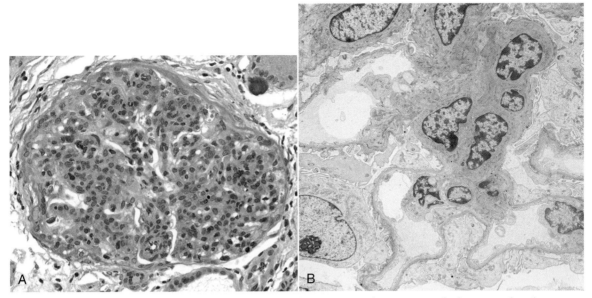

Figure 4-23 Proliferative glomerulonephropathy in a young dog. Note marked mesangial and endocapillary hypercellularity. **A.** PAS stain. **B.** TEM reveals mesangial hypercellularity. Note the absence of electron-dense deposits and the normal thickness of the capillary walls. (Courtesy G. Lees, F. Clubb.)

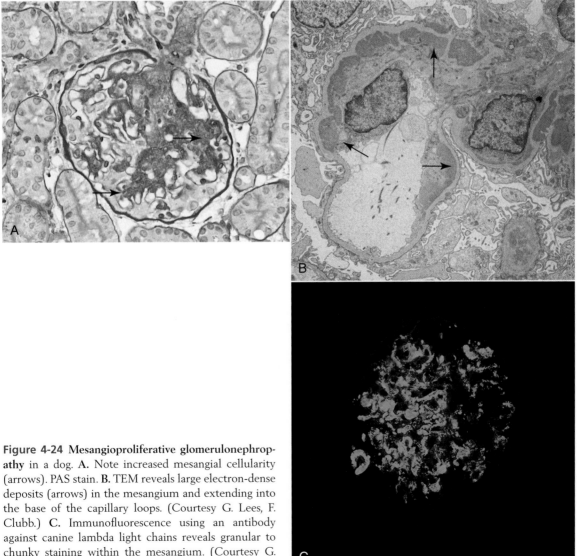

Figure 4-24 Mesangioproliferative glomerulonephropathy in a dog. **A.** Note increased mesangial cellularity (arrows). PAS stain. **B.** TEM reveals large electron-dense deposits (arrows) in the mesangium and extending into the base of the capillary loops. (Courtesy G. Lees, F. Clubb.) **C.** Immunofluorescence using an antibody against canine lambda light chains reveals granular to chunky staining within the mesangium. (Courtesy G. Lees.)

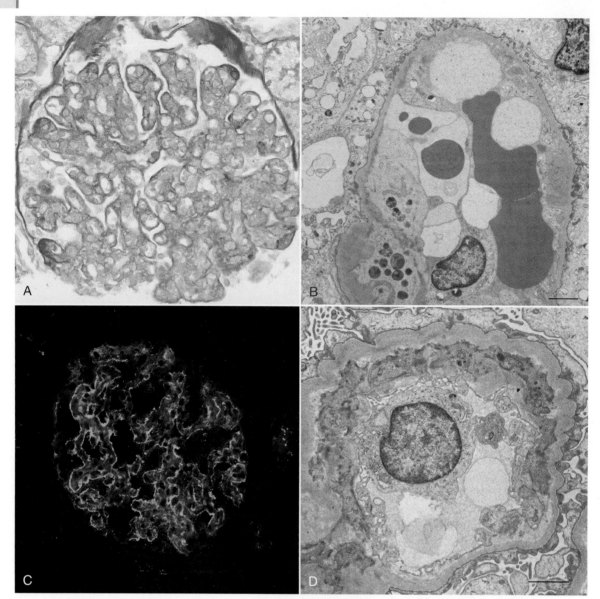

Figure 4-25 Membranoproliferative glomerulonephritis (MPGN) in a dog. A. PAS stain. (Courtesy G. Lees.) Note endocapillary endocapillary and mesangial hypercellularity. Double contours of the GBM are visible with PAS, Masson trichrome, and Jones' methenamine silver stains. **B.** TEM reveals small subendothelial electron-dense deposits, endothelial cell swelling and distortion of circulating red and white blood cells. (Courtesy G. Lees, F. Clubb.) **C.** Immunofluorescence using an antibody against lambda light chains reveals granular staining in the mesangium and along capillary walls. (Courtesy G. Lees.) **D.** TEM of a different dog with resolved MPGN, revealing circumferential mesangial cell interpositioning between the endothelial cell and the GBM within a capillary loop. (Courtesy G. Lees, F. Clubb.)

diagnosis of membranous glomerulonephropathy (MGN) in humans requires identification of IC on the abluminal surface of the GBM via IF, TEM, and/or special stains. In the early stages of the disease, the GBM may not be thickened at all, and deposits are only seen with TEM and IF. Furthermore, some diseases in humans (e.g., diabetes mellitus) result in severely thickened GBM that would never be diagnosed as MGN. This is because MGN does not simply refer to a histologic pattern of thickened capillary walls, but instead is a diagnosis of a specific type of **IC-mediated glomerulonephritis** (ICGN). Along the same lines, some glomerular diseases may have an "MPGN pattern" on histology because there is

hypercellularity and thickening of the GBM, but the lack of definitive immune complexes indicates that they are not true MPGN. Examples in dogs and humans include Alport syndrome and thrombotic microangiopathies, both of which are discussed in detail later.

A few veterinary nephropathology services offer routine TEM and IF evaluations, but it is still fairly limited to small animal renal biopsies. In autopsy specimens or cases with financial restrictions, one will almost always forego the advanced diagnostic modalities. In these situations, the pathologist can equivocate and merely provide a diagnosis of GBM thickening with or without hypercellularity. On the other

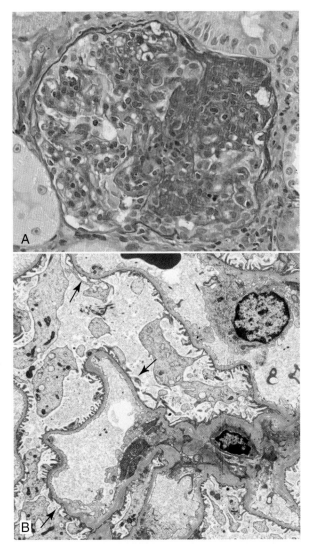

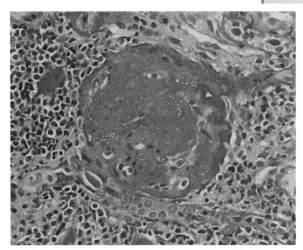

Figure 4-27 Global glomerulosclerosis (obsolescence) in a dog. PAS stain.

Figure 4-26 Focal segmental glomerulosclerosis (FSGS) in a dog; <50% of glomeruli in the biopsy were affected by this process. **A.** PAS stain. Note segmental effacement of the peripheral capillary lumens by extracellular matrix. This segment is adherent to Bowman's capsule (synechia). Although this glomerulus has mesangial hypercellularity, that feature is variable among cases of FSGS, with many sclerotic segments being hypocellular. **B.** TEM reveals segmental podocyte foot process effacement (arrows) and the absence of electron-dense deposits. (Courtesy G. Lees, C. Brown.)

hand, it is also useful to differentiate between ICGN and non-ICGN when advanced tests are performed on renal biopsy tissue. This helps the nephrologist make appropriate therapeutic decisions. Notably, epidemiologic studies based solely on histologic pattern without the use of advanced modalities to detect IC may skew impressions about common pathogeneses and prognoses of glomerular diseases.

Histologic changes in glomerulonephritis

Lesion development may be at different stages in glomeruli of the same kidney, and the type of glomerular reaction may not be uniform among glomeruli. Glomeruli commonly exhibit a spectrum of histologic changes. In view of the large renal reserve, it is important to correlate clinical and histologic findings to determine the clinical importance of glomerular changes. Glomeruli may be nonspecifically involved in renal diseases such as renal cortical necrosis, discussed previously, or they may be secondarily impacted by tubulointerstitial diseases such as pyelonephritis. Septic emboli frequently lodge in the glomerular and peritubular capillary beds, causing focal glomerulitis and focal interstitial nephritis in diseases such as porcine erysipelas and in actinobacillosis of foals. Diffuse glomerulitis, not necessarily associated with other renal changes, can be seen in acute septicemia and is characterized by increased endocapillary cellularity.

Cellularity of the glomerular tuft may be increased by proliferation of endothelial, epithelial, or mesangial cells. This assessment is usually subjective. Mesangial cells in glomeruli of dogs usually occur singly or in pairs, hence more than 3 mesangial cells must be in close proximity before the term *mesangial cell hyperplasia* is applied. Mesangial cell number in other species may vary. Proliferation of endothelial versus mesangial cells may be difficult to distinguish on standard hematoxylin and eosin (H&E) sections. Hypercellularity that is limited to the mesangium can often be easily distinguished using PAS or trichrome stains on thin (3 μm) sections. If there is still difficulty discerning the location of the increased cellularity, it is often assumed that at least some of the cells are inside capillary loops, distorting the architecture and effacing capillary lumens. In these scenarios, the term "endocapillary hypercellularity" can be used. Electron microscopy or 1-μm thick sections stained with toluidine blue can verify this assumption. Hypercellularity can be due to attraction of inflammatory cells or to hypertrophy or hyperplasia of native glomerular cells in situ (i.e., endothelial and mesangial cells). Additionally, mesangial cells may migrate out into the capillary loop (mesangial cell interpositioning), which will also contribute to the appearance of hypercellularity within a capillary loop. It is important to remember that mesangial hypercellularity and endocapillary hypercellularity can occur alone or together, and that the use of proper stains on appropriate sections can help the pathologist localize the source of the increased cellularity. If both are present, then both should be included in the histologic description. If, however, only mesangial cells are increased, then the correct morphologic diagnostic term is "mesangioproliferative."

Fibrin exudation into the urinary space (Fig. 4-28; eFig. 4-13), which occurs in severely damaged glomeruli with

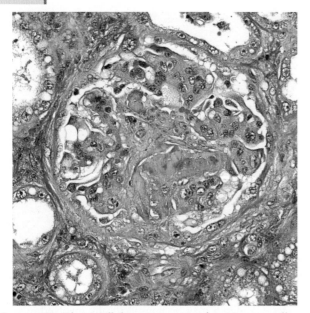

Figure 4-28 Fibrinocellular crescent in a dog. Masson trichrome (TRI). The material in Bowman's space stains lightly eosinophilic, pale pink on PAS, red to orange on TRI, and is nonstaining with the Jones' methenamine silver method. Crescents indicate rupture of a capillary wall. This dog had immune-complex–mediated glomerulonephritis, consistent with membranoproliferative glomerulonephritis.

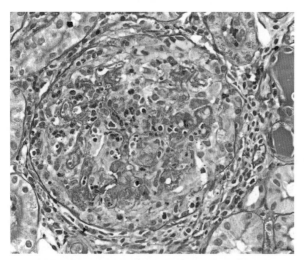

Figure 4-29 Glomerular cellular crescent in a dog. PAS stain. There are numerous inflammatory cells in Bowman's space. This dog had immune-complex–mediated glomerulonephritis, consistent with membranous glomerulonephropathy.

rupture of the GBM, leads to the proliferation of both visceral and parietal epithelial cells and often the infiltration of macrophages and neutrophils (Fig. 4-29; eFig. 4-14). These are the stages of a *glomerular crescent*. Some of the cells produce collagen, and fibroblasts from the interstitium can also invade Bowman's capsule. Experimental evidence implicates transforming growth factor-β as being integral in the transition from a "cellular" to a "fibrocellular" to a "fibrous" crescent. In humans, crescents are most commonly seen in cases of rapidly

progressive GN; however, they are only indicative of severe glomerular damage and not pathognomonic of any one disease. Crescents are fairly rare in cats and dogs, but may occur with some frequency in certain types of porcine GN.

The **swelling of foot processes** and their subsequent retraction is a reversible lesion in podocytes and is associated with protein leakage. Although it is often stated that podocytes do not replicate postnatally, multiple lines of evidence in humans and experimental glomerular diseases have questioned this concept. It is safe to say, at this juncture, that podocytes replicate slowly or infrequently. Severe injury can cause loss of podocytes and exposure of "bare" GBM, which can adhere to Bowman's capsule (synechiae) (see Fig. 4-26; eFig. 4-11). If the adhesion is extensive, the glomerular filtrate can diffuse into the interstitium surrounding the glomerulus.

Glomerular capillary walls may be thickened in H&E-stained sections because of endothelial or epithelial swelling and/or **thickening and/or remodeling of the GBM**. The GBM itself is not visible unless special techniques, such as PAS or JMS, are used on thin (1-3 μm) sections. Electron microscopy is required to characterize the morphology of the thickening GBM, which may be regular with a smooth outer contour or irregular because of deposition of electron-dense material in *subendothelial, intramembranous, or subepithelial* locations. *These electron-dense deposits are usually immune complexes.* Thickened peripheral capillary walls are particularly prominent in cases of MGN. Additionally, in MGN, subepithelial ICs are separated by projections *(spikes)* of basement membrane material, and eventually become encircled by and incorporated within the GBM, which can be visualized with PAS or JMS as *holes* in the GBM (see eFig. 4-7C). In MPGN, thickening of the GBM results from subendothelial IC deposition as well as mesangial cell interpositioning. This can be seen on the JMS as a characteristic *double-contoured GBM* or "tram-tracks" (see eFig. 4-10C).

As seen by light microscopy, **GS** is the accumulation of extracellular matrix that effaces the lumens of peripheral capillary loops and eventually results in consolidation of the tuft. **Hyalinosis** is often seen concurrently with GS and is defined as the presence of glassy PAS-positive material in the capillary wall (Fig. 4-30; eFig. 4-15). Hyalinosis indicates plasma insudation into the wall of the capillary loop. Both GS and hyalinosis are possible sequelae to IC-mediated GN. It is important to realize, however, that not all cases with GS have an underlying IC-mediated pathogenesis. Therefore TEM and IF are needed to correctly classify these cases. Primary GS is described in more detail later. Last, sclerosis limited to the mesangium is a frequent diagnosis in human glomeruli, most commonly seen in diabetic nodular GS. In these patients, the mesangial sclerosis has a very characteristic histologic appearance known as Kimmelstiel-Wilson nodules; this phenotype has only been demonstrated experimentally in diabetic rodents. Mesangial sclerosis without nodule formation was documented in uninephrectomized dogs that were made diabetic at 9 months of age. These dogs also had significant generalized thickening of the GBM compared to control dogs, which is another characteristic lesion of diabetic nephropathy in humans, noted on TEM. Glomerular lesions in spontaneously diabetic dogs are usually limited to mild mesangial expansion, occasionally associated with lipid in the mesangial matrix or cell cytoplasm.

Lesions in Bowman's capsule and Bowman's space may occur because of various combinations of hyperplasia of parietal epithelial cells in crescents, invasion by monocytes,

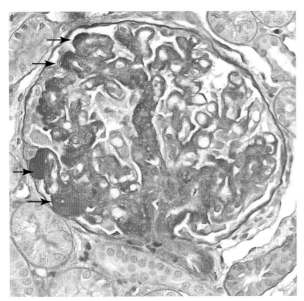

Figure 4-30 **Hyalinosis** of capillary walls in a dog. PAS stain. Most capillary walls are expanded by insudated plasma, which stains bright pink on PAS (arrows). Similar material is present in the wall of the afferent arteriole. This dog had immune-complex–mediated glomerulonephritis, consistent with membranoproliferative glomerulonephritis.

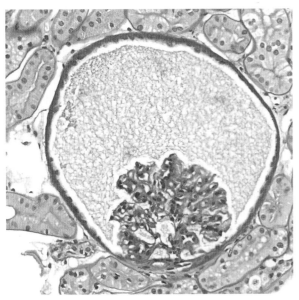

Figure 4-31 **Glomerulocystic atrophy** in a dog. PAS stain. Although this lesion can be a nonspecific finding in older dogs, these glomeruli are nonfunctional. Therefore, if they are common within a specimen, there may be renal insufficiency.

thickening of the basement membrane, and periglomerular fibrosis. Importantly, thickening and splitting of Bowman's capsule basement membranes can be a nonspecific lesion in older dogs (eFig. 4-16).

Glomerular cystic atrophy (Fig. 4-31; eFig. 4-17) may occur subsequent to tubulointerstitial scarring, which constricts tubules, inhibits or stops tubular fluid flow, and dilates Bowman's capsules. In humans and experimental animal models, this lesion is often referred to as "atubular glomeruli"; however, this latter term requires serial sections of entire

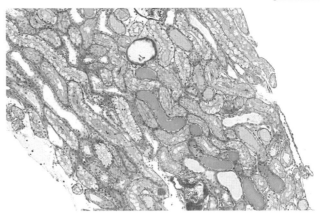

Figure 4-32 Tubulointerstitium from a proteinuric dog with focal segmental glomerulosclerosis. PAS stain. There are **bright pink intratubular casts of Tamm-Horsfall mucoprotein.** Additionally, there is vacuolar degeneration of tubular epithelial cells.

glomeruli to demonstrate the lack of a connection between Bowman's capsule and the proximal tubule. If glomerulocystic atrophy is diffuse and severe, small cysts can be seen grossly in the cortex and is called *glomerulocystic disease* (see Fig. 4-15).

Nonglomerular histologic changes in GN include *tubular protein casts* (Fig. 4-32). Proteinuria can damage and activate tubular epithelial cells, causing release of proinflammatory cytokines and growth factors that induce *interstitial fibrosis*. Indeed, the amount of tubulointerstitial fibrosis often correlates closely with the degree of chronic renal dysfunction in glomerulopathies. Histologic changes may also be of *ischemic origin* because of abnormal glomerular and peritubular blood flow—acute and chronic *inflammation and interstitial fibrosis*. Interestingly, in dogs and cats, there is often significant inflammation and ATI in acute MPGN. Advanced glomerular lesions are often concurrent with interstitial fibrosis and tubular atrophy, eventually producing the nonspecific histologic picture of *end-stage kidney*.

Pathogenesis of generalized glomerulonephritis

Glomerulonephritis may result from the deposition in glomeruli of circulating ICs, from formation in situ of antibodies against the GBM, or from activation of the alternative pathway of complement. Many types of GN are of unknown pathogenesis.

In **ICGN**, circulating antigen-antibody complexes of nonglomerular origin localize in glomeruli and are visible by IF or TEM within, or on either side of, the GBM. Causative antigens may be exogenous (e.g., bacterial or viral proteins) or endogenous (e.g., nucleic acid in systemic lupus erythematosus in humans). The classic experimental model of ICGN is intravenous injection of foreign protein resulting in IC deposition in glomeruli and a *characteristic granular pattern, as seen by IF.* With TEM, the complexes are seen as irregular electron-dense deposits in a subendothelial, subepithelial, or intramembranous location or within the mesangium. Immune complexes usually contain complement as well as antigen and antibody. In general, it is thought that IC deposition occurs during the period of equivalence of antigen and antibody concentrations or during slight antigen excess. An alternative view is that some antigens are capable of penetrating the GBM, where they bind antibody of low avidity. This antigen localization may be charge dependent. As well as forming traditional circulating IC, dirofilarial antigens may be deposited directly in basement membrane, inducing formation in situ of ICs and producing linear fluorescence. Candidates for "planted" antigens that may localize in glomeruli and result in the formation in situ of ICs include viral, bacterial, and parasitic products, drugs, and DNA. The relative importance of circulating soluble ICs versus in situ formation of complexes in causing ICGN is not resolved.

Chronic serum sickness is induced experimentally by giving repeated small doses of foreign protein to an animal, and circulating ICs are continually present. This condition models the continued antigenemia that occurs during various microbial and parasitic infections, such as feline leukemia virus infection and canine dirofilariasis, as well as during continued release of endogenous antigens, such as nucleoprotein in human systemic lupus erythematosus or tumor-associated antigens.

It is not completely straightforward to ascribe the cause of GN to ICs, as C3, C1q, and IgM are "sticky" molecules that may adhere to previously injured tissue. The significance of *circulating soluble ICs* is controversial, because they may be present without GN, and they may actually be markers for the disease rather than actual causative agents. Indeed, some investigators suggest that glomeruli damaged by other insults are susceptible to secondary IC deposition.

The reasons for *localization of immune complexes* in various glomerular sites, namely, subendothelial, intramembranous, subepithelial, or mesangial, are complex. Localization may be affected by the size, shape, charge, and chemical composition of the complexes. Penetration of the basement membrane by complexes may be aided by products of inflammation, such as IgE-mediated release of histamine and serotonin from platelets and basophils. The location of deposits may also change with time; subepithelial deposits separated by spikes of GBM may become surrounded by GBM and hence become intramembranous deposits.

Modification of glomerular IC occurs; they may be eliminated or they may enlarge. Complexes may be eliminated by solubilization, phagocytosis by neutrophils, macrophages, or mesangial cells, passage through the mesangium and egress at the vascular pole, degradation within the mesangial matrix, or by extracellular degradation by proteases. Thus, for example, removal of the source of persistent antigenemia in pyometra of dogs by ovariohysterectomy results in resolution of GN and cessation of proteinuria. Conversely, complexes may enlarge through combination with various blood-borne reactants, such as small amounts of antigen, free antibody, ICs of the same or different specificity, complement components, or antibodies against immunoglobulins or complement components (immunoconglutinin or C3 nephritic factor).

In **anti-GBM glomerulonephritis,** *antibodies are formed against intrinsic GBM antigens,* resulting in a *linear pattern of immunofluorescence* reflecting the uniform distribution of immunoglobulins and complement along the GBM. There is a notable lack of electron-dense deposits on TEM examination. In humans, this causes a severe crescentic GN without significant hypercellularity. Anti-GBM glomerulonephritis occurs as a component of Goodpasture syndrome in humans, which is the combination of anti-GBM antibodies together with antibodies against pulmonary capillaries, which can lead to acute pulmonary hemorrhage and death. Aside from humans, anti-GBM antibodies have only been documented in

a single horse. The lack of histologic lesions in that horse and the presence of linear IF staining in other horses without detectable anti-GBM antibodies suggest that spontaneous *anti-GBM disease* is limited to humans. It can be modeled in rats by injection of anti–rat kidney antibodies obtained from rabbits or ducks immunized with rat kidney tissue; this experimental model is also referred to as *nephrotoxic nephritis.* The animal model only acutely mimics the human form, because with time, the typical linear IF pattern is gradually converted to the granular pattern typical of ICGN. Ultrastructural evaluation reveals ICs in subepithelial and subendothelial locations.

Mechanisms of glomerular injury

Several mechanisms result in glomerular injury once ICs are formed in situ or deposited in glomeruli. The best-established mechanism is that of *complement fixation with resultant chemotaxis of neutrophils.* Complement components C3a, C5a, and C567 attract neutrophils, which, in the process of ingesting complexes, release lysosomal enzymes, arachidonic acid metabolites, and oxygen-derived free radicals, causing GBM damage. This is the *complement-leukocyte–dependent mechanism.* The terminal membrane attack complex of complement, C5b-9, can injure glomeruli by releasing oxidants, cytokines, and other mediators that damage podocytes, endothelial, and mesangial cells. Complement fragments cause release of histamine from mast cells, and hence cause increased capillary permeability, which may allow deposition of more ICs in the capillary wall.

Chemokines (chemotactic *cytokines*) produced by glomerular, mesangial, tubular, and interstitial cells activate circulating leukocytes bearing the respective surface receptors. Local attachment of leukocytes occurs through interaction of leukocyte integrins with adhesion molecules, such as intercellular adhesion molecule-1 and vascular cell adhesion molecule-1, on endothelial, mesangial, and interstitial cells. Activated leukocytes initiate their effector functions, such as respiratory burst, phagocytosis of IC, release of hydrolases and removal of matrix, cell debris, and apoptotic cells. Activated leukocytes also release additional mediators, chemokines, and cytokines in an amplification loop to recruit more leukocytes.

It is paradoxical that, although complement participates in glomerular injury, it also is capable of solubilizing ICs to facilitate their removal. Hence hereditary hypocomplementemia, as occurs in Finnish Landrace lambs, leads to persistence of ICs and glomerular injury. Interaction of complement fragments with platelets leads to coagulation, thrombosis, and fibrinolysis. Hageman factor links the complement, coagulation, and kinin-forming pathways. Fibrin and its degradation products are often present in inflamed glomeruli, and fibrinogen that leaks into the urinary space is a stimulus for monocyte infiltration, proliferation of parietal epithelial cells, and crescent formation. It is important to note that deposits composed solely of components from the complement system are not ICs. In humans, immune-mediated GN is subdivided into 2 main categories (*IC-mediated GN and C3 GN*). This division is important because it has etiologic, prognostic, and therapeutic implications. As discussed later, there is evidence to suggest a similar division of GN may be useful in veterinary species. Specifically, there are examples of breed-related/familial abnormalities in the complement system that can result in GN. However, in many veterinary cases, this type of classification system is purely academic.

Monocytes play a role in glomerular damage also, especially through their interaction with mesangial cells. Monocytes may be beneficial in removing ICs, but they also can cause enzymatic damage, as do neutrophils. There is evidence that they transform to cells of fibroblastic type in glomerular crescents.

The role of *mesangial cells* in the development of glomerular injury is increasingly recognized. Mesangial cells may initiate inflammation in the absence of leukocytes because they themselves can produce inflammatory mediators, including oxygen free radicals, interleukin-1 (IL-1), arachidonic acid metabolites, and a variety of growth factors. Likewise, mesangial cells can be stimulated to proliferate when macrophages and other immune cells release IL-1, β-endorphin, tumor necrosis factor, and platelet-derived growth factor (PDGF). In these scenarios, there is also an increase in mesangial matrix. Proliferating mesangial cells release autacoids, such as IL-1 and PDGF, producing an amplifying loop of inflammation. Transforming growth factor-β induces synthesis of mesangial matrix, and this can be countered by bone morphogenetic protein-7. Immunomodulatory peptides released by proliferating mesangial cells stimulate replication and activation of macrophages, which both amplify the inflammatory lesion and ameliorate it by the phagocytosis of ICs.

In addition to the immunologic causes of GN discussed previously, there are a number of *nonimmunologic causes of glomerular injury*. These include increased glomerular capillary pressure, coagulation in response to endothelial injury, serum lipid abnormalities, and glomerular hypertrophy, and they are discussed later.

Morphology of glomerulonephritis

Acute glomerulonephritis may not significantly alter the gross appearance of the kidney, which may be slightly or markedly enlarged, pale, soft, and edematous. Petechiae may be visible if bleeding has occurred from the inflamed glomeruli. In **subacute glomerulonephritis,** the kidney is often enlarged and pale tan with a smooth surface and nonadherent capsule. The capsule is tense, and the cut surface bulges. The pale tan cortex is well demarcated from a normal-colored medulla. This subacute phase is anatomically and developmentally arbitrary and progresses to the **chronic** phase, in which the kidney is shrunken and contracted with generalized fine granularity of the capsular surface (Fig. 4-33). When contraction is severe, it is grossly indistinguishable from diffuse chronic interstitial nephritis. The capsule may be adherent. On cut surface, the cortex is often uniformly narrowed, and the corticomedullary markings are obscured. Small cysts, which are obstructed tubules, are often present.

Histology reveals strikingly different lesions depending on the location of the ICs. In the **acute phase of proliferative GN or MPGN**, there is hypercellularity, usually because of influx of inflammatory cells. Neutrophils and/or monocytes marginate in the capillaries and, together with the swollen proliferating endothelial and mesangial cells, give a distinct impression of hypercellularity (see Fig. 4-25; eFig. 4-10). Occasionally, fibrin thrombi form in the capillaries, or there is fibrinoid necrosis of the tuft. This form of GN with the formation of fibrin thrombi is the usual picture seen in swine with petechiae. In **acute MGN,** glomeruli appear completely normal, in which case TEM and IF are needed to identify ICs. The tubulointerstitial compartment can be normal (most commonly in MGN) or characterized by edema, inflam-

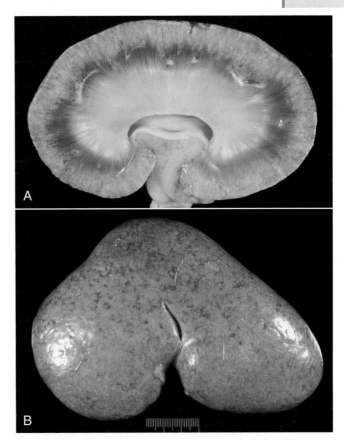

Figure 4-33 Chronic glomerulonephritis. A. In a dog. (Courtesy D. Russell, P. Stromberg.) **B.** In a horse. The cortical surface is pale tan and slightly irregular. (Courtesy L. Himmel, P. Stromberg.)

mation, or tubular epithelial injury (usually in acute proliferative or MPGN).

Although clinical signs can vary greatly, some can be anticipated. The swelling of the kidney can result in oliguria. If the concentrating capacity of the tubules is maintained, the urine is of high specific gravity. There is proteinuria, and there may be hyaline, granular, and/or red blood cell casts. In fact, RBC casts in urine are highly specific for active GN in humans. Although hematuria can be observed in many types of renal and lower urinary tract disease, the cast shape indicates an intrarenal source of the RBCs. RBC casts are occasionally seen in dogs and cats with severe acute glomerulonephritis (eFig. 4-18).

In the **subacute** phase, there is often mesangial hypercellularity and/or remodeling of the GBM. Subendothelial deposits will result in double contours of the GBM, whereas subepithelial deposits will induce spike formation between deposits. Repeat biopsies of the same patient might even reveal a change in the distribution of the deposits over time. Segmental GS and synechiae may be present. There is often increased tubulointerstitial scarring.

In the **chronic** phase, scarring of glomeruli occurs. There may be a reduction in the apparent number of glomeruli as obsolescent glomeruli blend with surrounding scar tissue. Although all glomeruli are usually involved, the degree varies somewhat so that many retain some function. The interstitial reaction initiated during the acute phase progresses with fibrosis and lymphocytic infiltration. Large numbers of tubules undergo atrophy and are replaced by scar tissue. The fibrosis becomes slowly self-perpetuating. Tubules that remain connected to functioning glomeruli may become dilated and develop epithelial hypertrophy and hyperplasia; these are responsible for the fine granularity of the surface and streakiness of the cut surface.

Renal failure can occur, with an increased volume of urine of low specific gravity. Albuminuria can vary and casts may be absent. The frequency with which GN leads to renal failure is not known. Therefore prospective studies in many species would help pathologists draw conclusions regarding prognosis. Furthermore, the anecdotal evidence about the success of immunosuppressive therapy in small animals with IC-mediated GN has led to the development of guidelines for immunosuppression in these patients.

Once the GFR has decreased to 30-50% of normal, progression to end-stage renal failure tends to be unavoidable. This occurs partly because of continuation of the primary glomerular disease, partly because of the addition of complicating factors such as hypertension, and partly because of adaptive changes in glomeruli in a failing kidney. These adaptive changes include hypertrophy and increased workload of the remaining nephrons, with resulting epithelial and endothelial injury and proteinuria. Mesangial cells respond by proliferating with production of extracellular matrix and eventual glomerulosclerosis. In any case, these further reductions of renal mass contribute to a vicious cycle of continuing GS.

Prevalence of glomerulonephritis

The frequency of diagnosis of GN in domestic animals has increased dramatically, mostly because of increased awareness and understanding of GN by clinicians and pathologists. Immune complexes commonly circulate throughout life, but few individuals develop significant lesions, so various factors such as genetic susceptibility or defective immune or other mechanisms may be operative in affected animals. Many associations of infectious and other diseases with GN have been identified. In essence, *any infection of low pathogenicity that is able to produce persistent antigenemia has the potential to cause IC disease.* The morphology of the glomerular lesion is of little assistance in identifying its cause, because many agents can cause the same type of lesion, and conversely, one agent can produce a spectrum of glomerular changes. Diseases known or suspected to induce immune-complex–mediated glomerulonephritis are listed in Box 4-1. Most cases in animals are *idiopathic*; those occurring in association with other diseases or in which glomerular lesions contain known antigens are referred to as *secondary*.

Dogs

Recent data suggest that almost half (48%) of the North American dogs that underwent biopsy for the clinical indication of proteinuria had ICGN, with GS and amyloidosis also being common glomerular diseases. In canine *pyometra*, ICGN may be less significant than tubulointerstitial lesions, the latter of which may be an age-related change, as opposed to being secondary to the pyometra. **Canine adenovirus 1** (CAV-1), *Dirofilaria immitis*, *Borrelia burgdorferi*, and *Leishmania infantum* (either singly or as coinfections) have all been associated with the development of ICGN. Experimental infections with CAV-1 have shown that the virus is present in glomerular endothelial cells within 4 days (as demonstrated by IF for anti-CAV antigen and viral inclusions on TEM). Histologically, endothelial cells are swollen and vacuolated. Within 7 days,

---

BOX • 4-1

Causes of immune-mediated glomerulonephritis in domestic animals

Viral
African swine fever virus
Aleutian mink disease virus
Bovine viral diarrhea virus
Canine adenovirus 1 (infectious canine hepatitis)
Classical swine fever virus
Equine infectious anemia virus
Feline leukemia virus

Bacterial/fungal
Borrelia burgdorferi
Canine pyometra
Campylobacter fetus
Encephalitozoon cuniculi
Septic valvular endocarditis

Protozoal
African trypanosomiasis
Babesia gibsoni
Leishmania infantum
Coccidiosis

Helminths
Dirofilaria immitis

Neoplasms
Various

Autoimmune
Multiple autoimmune diseases suspected

Hereditary
Abnormal complement system of Bernese Mountain dogs
Dense deposit disease of pigs
Hypocomplementemia of Brittany Spaniels
Hypocomplementemia in Finnish Landrace lambs

---

viral antigen, IgG, C3 staining, and electron-dense deposits can be detected in the mesangium but not at the periphery of capillary loops. At this stage, there are increased numbers of mesangial cells and infiltration of the tufts by neutrophils. Some glomeruli contain thrombi, and there may be segmental necrosis of the tuft.

Experimental chronic **dirofilariasis** was reported to cause either a strong immune response and clearance of microfilariae or a weaker response that cannot clear the microfilariae. In the strong response scenario, there was a strong granular pattern of IgG deposition in the mesangium, mesangial electron-dense deposits, and various degrees of mesangial hypercellularity. In the weaker response scenario, there were small electron-dense particles (<25 nm) distributed continuously along the GBM and in the mesangium. This correlated to a linear or pseudolinear staining pattern of IgG along capillary walls, whereas C3 had a granular pattern. Hypercellularity was mild and limited to the mesangium. Taken together, the

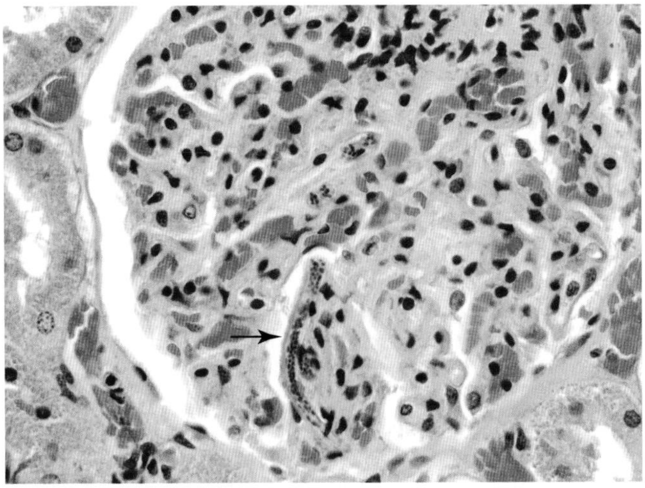

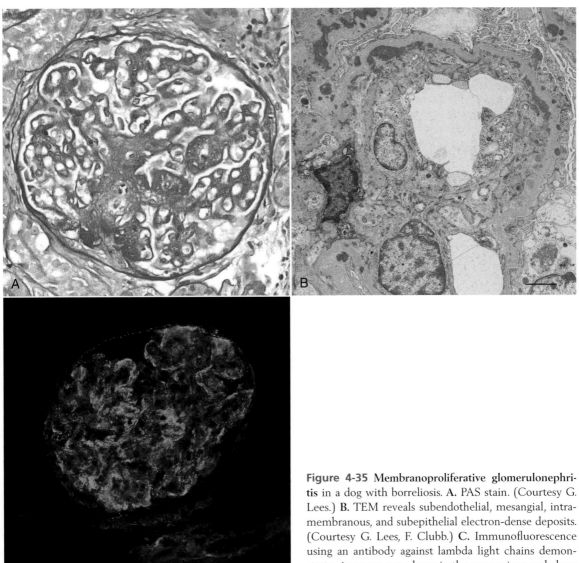

Figure 4-34 *Dirofilaria immitis* microfilaria (arrow) in a glomerular capillary of a dog.

authors suggested that uniform localization of filarial antigens along the GBM elicited an antibody response resulting in a linear (or "pseudolinear") appearance of the IgG. In addition to these phenotypes, MGN with subepithelial IC, mesangioproliferative GN with scattered mesangial and subendothelial IC, and focal segmental glomerulosclerosis without IC have all been reported in chronic experimental or spontaneous infections. Microfilariae may be observed in glomerular or peritubular capillaries (Fig. 4-34). More recent research suggests that dirofilariasis can modify the distribution and number of negatively charged macromolecules of the GBM, many of which are assumed to be proteoglycans, specifically heparan sulfate. This process might lead to proteinuria via a pathway that is not IC mediated. Importantly, spontaneous infections might not result in histologic glomerular lesions or only equivocal evidence of ICs.

A unique form of rapidly progressive MPGN (Fig. 4-35; eFig. 4-19) is putatively associated with infection by ***Borrelia***

Figure 4-35 **Membranoproliferative glomerulonephritis** in a dog with borreliosis. **A.** PAS stain. (Courtesy G. Lees.) **B.** TEM reveals subendothelial, mesangial, intramembranous, and subepithelial electron-dense deposits. (Courtesy G. Lees, F. Clubb.) **C.** Immunofluorescence using an antibody against lambda light chains demonstrates immune complexes in the mesangium and along capillary walls. (Courtesy G. Lees.)

burgdorferi, a spirochete transmitted by *Ixodes* ticks. Golden Retrievers and Labradors are predisposed, but it has been seen in many other breeds. Serologic tests for antibodies against the bacterial outer surface proteins (Osp) C and F or the recombinant protein C6 (which mimics the bacterial protein called variable major protein–like sequence, expressed) are often used as evidence of infection. Lyme nephritis has been reported to occur in <2% of serologically positive dogs, and <30% of the nephritic patients had concurrent or prior lameness. Definitive diagnosis of Lyme nephritis is difficult because *B. burgdorferi* organisms are not frequently found in the kidney, and disease is thought to be driven by IC containing a variety of antigens, including OspA, OspB, and/or flagellin. A validated consistent immunohistochemical test for these bacterial antigens is not commercially available, and elution of ICs from kidney tissue is not feasible as a routine diagnostic test. It has been reported that dogs with signs of Lyme disease have significantly more *B. burgdorferi*–specific IC in circulation compared to asymptomatic Lyme-positive dogs; however, there are nonclinical dogs that also have very high levels of circulating IC.

Renal biopsies of proteinuric dogs naturally infected with **Leishmania** spp. have demonstrated mesangioproliferative GN (with IC limited to the mesangium), MPGN (with subendothelial and mesangial IC), and GS without definitive IC deposition. Notably, biopsies 60 days after the initial biopsy rarely demonstrated a change in the severity of the glomerular lesion, suggesting that both progression and resolution are slow processes.

Deposition of **IgA** was reported 47 of 100 autopsied dogs in Japan with or without clinical renal disease, and IF labeling was considered moderate to marked in 22 dogs. The most common histologic lesion was mesangial expansion and hypercellularity with segmental sclerosis. Immunogold TEM demonstrated IgA deposits in mesangial locations. Although these lesions are strikingly similar to IgA nephropathy in humans, there are likely some differences in lesion pathogenesis. IgA in humans is the result of aberrant glycosylation patterns of the IgA1 isoform. Only primates are known to synthesize IgA1, whereas other species make the IgA2 isoform.

Proteinuria and azotemia together with MPGN (diagnosed via renal biopsy) were observed in a dog infected with **Babesia gibsoni.** Resolution of infection and restoration of renal function followed appropriate antibiotic therapy and a short course of immunosuppressive therapy. A 7-month-old dog that had been vaccinated once per month for 7 months with the distemper- hepatitis-leptospirosis-parainfluenza-parvovirus (DHLPPC) vaccine (without veterinary supervision) developed MPGN, and antigen from the vaccine was also detected in the glomeruli.

Canine familial glomerulonephritides. Familial glomerulonephritides associated with IC deposition have been rarely reported in dogs. In *Bernese Mountain dogs,* this condition is *autosomal recessive* and causes proteinuria and renal insufficiency in young adults. It is characterized as MPGN with concomitant tubulointerstitial nephritis. GBMs are duplicated, and there is mesangial interpositioning in GBMs and subendothelial deposits of IgM and C3.

Inherited deficiency of the third component of complement in *Brittany Spaniel dogs* leads to the development of MPGN. Affected dogs also have an increased susceptibility to infections. Interestingly, treatment of dogs with exogenous C3

resulted in increased proteinuria and more severe glomerular lesions.

Cats

Although most cat glomerulonephritides have been diagnosed as MGN, many have not been verified with TEM and/or IF. It is easy to mistake primary segmental GS for MGN with secondary sclerosis via light microscopy. Therefore caution should be used when interpreting the histologic lesion without TEM or IF. Even so, TEM- and IF-proven MGN and MPGN do occur in cats. Feline leukemia virus, together with hematopoietic tumors, has been associated with proliferative GN, with both subepithelial and subendothelial IC deposition.

Horses

Glomerulonephritis is observed in horses, but renal failure is rare. MPGN often occurs in horses with equine infectious anemia, and the renal lesions may be important. *Streptococcus equi* and herpesviral infections are suggested as causes of GN in horses. Transmission electron microscopy in horses with proliferative glomerulonephritis may reveal atypical ICs, which can vary from fibrillar to crystalline and rhomboid. In one horse, the ICs had a distinct fibrillar substructure. The outer diameters of the fibrils were 35-40 nm, and they contained a central pore. This appearance is similar to that of humans with immunotactoid glomerulonephritis and may imply a specific etiopathogenesis.

Swine

Acute fatal GN occurs sporadically in swine, but is of little economic importance. Deposition of ICs containing IgG and C3 is common in the mesangium of normal slaughter swine, but the mesangioproliferative GN is not of clinical significance. The *porcine dermatitis and nephropathy syndrome* (PDNS) in feeder pigs is associated with porcine circovirus 2 (PCV-2) infection and/or the antibody response to PCV-2 (Fig. 4-36). The systemic necrotizing vasculitis in PDNS appears to be immune mediated, and it results in proliferative GN, fibrin exudation in the tuft, cellular crescent formation, and interstitial nephritis. An autosomal recessive *hereditary*

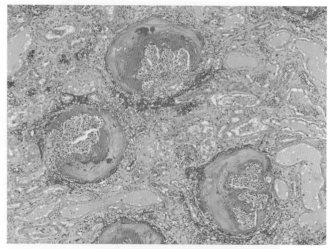

Figure 4-36 Crescentic proliferative glomerulonephritis in a pig with porcine dermatitis and nephropathy syndrome from porcine circovirus 2 infection. (Courtesy T. Clark.)

deficiency of factor H, a complement inhibitory protein, caused lethal dense deposit disease (also called MPGN type II) in Norwegian Yorkshire pigs; factor H deficiency led to massive glomerular deposition of complement, large sausage-shaped intramembranous dense deposits, and mesangial hypercellularity. Experimental infections with classical swine fever virus (hog cholera) led to proliferative ICGN with mesangial IgG deposits and intraglomerular viral antigen. Mesangial IC deposits, with fewer subendothelial and subepithelial deposits, were verified ultrastructurally. Glomerulonephritis of unknown pathogenesis was reported in 4 laboratory Göttingen minipigs. Because TEM and IF were not performed, the role of IC deposition is not known. Two pigs had protein in Bowman's space, resembling the early crescent formation that occurs in other swine breeds.

Ruminants

Immunologic evidence of GN is common in ruminants, but clinical disease is not. Glomeruli of sheep and goats are often hypercellular and have thick GBM, but the changes appear to have little clinical significance. An interesting exception is the *MPGN of* **Finnish Landrace sheep,** which is present at birth and is characterized by recessive inheritance of a deficiency of the complement component C3; in affected lambs, blood levels of C3 are about 5% of normal. This congenital deficiency contributes to the development of MPGN, probably because of impaired complement-mediated solubilization of ICs in glomeruli. Affected lambs are clinically normal at birth, but die at 1-3 months of age in renal failure. At autopsy, the kidneys are enlarged with pale cortices and glomeruli that are grossly visible as red spots. The glomerular lesion is characterized by mesangial proliferation, capillary wall thickening, and often by the formation of glomerular crescents. Subendothelial electron-dense deposits are present and consist of C3, smaller amounts of IgM and IgA and, with prolonged survival, progressively larger amounts of IgG. Glomerular changes begin in the lambs in utero and develop progressively after birth. Choroid plexus lesions also result from IC deposition, and lead to encephalopathy.

Maedi-visna viral infection has been associated with histologic evidence of MPGN in sheep, but investigative studies lack TEM and IF. Immunohistochemistry revealed viral antigen in tubular epithelial cells and interstitial cells. Glomerular staining was not reported. Bovine viral diarrhea viral antigen can be detected along the GBM and in the mesangium of persistently infected cattle. Glomeruli demonstrate mesangial hypercellularity and slight thickening of the GBM. Although IF has demonstrated viral antigen, IgG, and complement components in the glomerulus, it has been difficult to reproduce these results. Furthermore, similar histologic lesions with concomitant IgG and scattered C3 staining have been observed in bovine viral diarrhea virus (BVDV)-negative cattle.

Further reading

Angelopoulou K, et al. Detection of Maedi-visna virus in the kidneys of naturally infected sheep. J Comp Pathol 2006;134: 329-335.

Aresu L, et al. Membranoproliferative glomerulonephritis type III in a simultaneous infection of *Leishmania infantum* and *Dirofilaria immitis* in a dog. J Vet Diagn Invest 2007;19:569-572.

Aresu L, et al. Light and electron microscopic analysis of consecutive renal biopsy specimens from *Leishmania*-seropositive dogs. Vet Pathol 2013;50:753-760.

Cowgill LD, et al. Consensus recommendations for immunosuppressive treatment of dogs with glomerular disease based on pathology. J Vet Intern Med 2013;27:S44-S54.

De Loor J, et al. Urinary biomarkers for acute kidney injury in dogs. J Vet Intern Med 2013;27:998-1010.

Galav V, et al. Pathogenicity of an Indian isolate of bovine viral diarrhea virus 1b in experimentally infected calves. Res Vet Sci 2007;83:364-368.

Hegasy GA, et al. The molecular basis for hereditary porcine membranoproliferative glomerulonephritis type II: point mutations in the factor H coding sequence block protein secretion. Am J Pathol 2002;161:2027-2034.

Jennette JC. Rapidly progressive crescentic glomerulonephritis. Kidney Int 2003;63:1164-1177.

Klosterman ES, et al. Comparison of signalment, clinicopathologic findings, histologic diagnosis, and prognosis in dogs with glomerular disease with or without nephrotic syndrome. J Vet Intern Med 2011;25:206-214.

Littman MP. Lyme nephritis. J Vet Emerg Crit Care 2013;23:163-173.

Minkus G, et al. Familial nephropathy in Bernese mountain dogs. Vet Pathol 1994;31:421-428.

Nabity M, et al. Urinary biomarkers of renal disease in dogs with X-linked nephropathy. J Vet Intern Med 2012;26:282-293.

Ortloff A, et al. Membranoproliferative glomerulonephritis possibly associated with over-vaccination in a cocker spaniel. J Small Anim Pract 2010;51:499-502.

Paes-de-Almeida EC, et al. Kidney ultrastructural lesions in dogs experimentally infected with *Dirofilaria immitis*. Vet Parasitol 2003;168: 157-168.

Pickering MC, et al. C3 glomerulopathy: consensus report. Kidney Int 2013;84:1079-1089.

Sanchez-Cordon PJ, et al. Glomerulonephritis associated with simultaneous canine adenovirus-1 and *Dirofilaria immitis* infection in a dog. J Vet Med B Infect Dis Vet Public Health 2002;49:235-239.

Schneider SM, et al. Prevalence of immune-complex glomerulonephritides in dogs biopsied for suspected glomerular disease: 501 cases (2007-2012). J Vet Intern Med 2013;27(Suppl. 1):S60-S68.

Slade DJ, et al. Resolution of a proteinuric nephropathy associated with *Babesia gibsoni* infection in a dog. J Am Anim Hosp Assoc 2011; 47:e138-e144.

Steinbach S, et al. Plasma and urine neutrophil gelatinase-associated lipocalin (NGAL) in dogs with acute kidney injury or chronic kidney disease. J Vet Intern Med 2014;28:264-269.

Vezzali E, et al. Spontaneous glomerulonephritis in Göttingen minipigs. Toxicol Pathol 2011;39:700-705.

Wehner A, et al. Associations between proteinuria, systemic hypertension and glomerular filtration rate in dogs with renal and non-renal diseases. Vet Rec 2008;162:141-147.

Zhou Y, et al. Gene expression profiling of hepatic genes associated with lipid metabolism in nephrotic rats. Am J Physiol Renal Physiol 2008;295:662-671.

Glomerular diseases that are not immune-complex mediated

Amyloidosis

Amyloidosis is a group of disorders in which *amyloid—an eosinophilic, homogeneous, proteinaceous material—*is deposited in the walls of small blood vessels and extracellularly in a variety of sites, particularly in glomeruli. All amyloid fibrils have a β-pleated sheet structure, Deposition of amyloid causes pressure atrophy of adjacent cells, and, depending on the organs involved, can lead to chronic renal failure (CRF), nephrotic syndrome, thrombosis, hepatic failure, spontaneous hepatic hemorrhage and rupture, arthritis, or diabetes mellitus. Amyloidosis is seen in a number of presentations:

- **Reactive systemic amyloidosis** (secondary, or AA) is the most common form of amyloidosis in domestic animals (dogs, cattle, horses, cats; rare in swine and goats). **AA amyloid** is derived from *serum amyloid A* (SAA), an acute-phase lipoprotein made predominantly by hepatocytes. SAA is produced in excess as a result of chronic antigenic stimulation, such as occurs in persistent infectious, inflammatory or neoplastic conditions.
- **Immunoglobulin-derived amyloidosis** (primary, or AL) is the most common form in humans, but it is uncommon in domestic animals (dog, horse, cat). **AL amyloid** is produced from *immunoglobulin light chains* in plasma cell dyscrasias as a product of monoclonal B-cell proliferation. Either **λ** or **κ** light chains may predominate in this dysproteinemia. Systemic κAL amyloidosis has been described in a Holstein cow with bovine leukocyte adhesion deficiency.
- **Familial** amyloidosis occurs in a number of species and breeds. Systemic AA amyloidosis occurs in Beagles, Shar-Peis (likely autosomal recessive), gray Collies, English Foxhounds, Abyssinian cats (likely autosomal dominant with incomplete penetrance), and Siamese and Oriental cats.
- **Apolipoprotein A-I** (apoA-I)–derived amyloidosis affects the pulmonary vessels of old dogs.
- **Islet amyloid polypeptide** (IAPP)-derived amyloidosis is common in the pancreatic islets of cats with non–insulin-dependent diabetes mellitus.

Both AA and AL amyloidosis can occur in either systemic or localized forms. The *cause* of amyloid fibril formation and deposition is obscure, but the *nidus theory* postulates that amyloid fibrils serve as templates for fibril growth and as scaffolding for fibril polymerization; amyloid-enhancing factor may be involved. Macrophages appear to be important in the conversion of precursor proteins to amyloid fibrils. Other extracellular matrix components, including amyloid P component (a glycoprotein of the pentraxin family), glycosaminoglycans, and proteoglycans, are always associated with amyloid.

Most cases of amyloidosis in domestic animals are of the reactive systemic type. Deposits of AA amyloid may be found in many organs, but *the kidney is the organ most commonly involved in amyloidosis.* Localization of amyloid is usually *glomerular* in most breeds of dogs, but *medullary* localization predominates often in Shar-Pei dogs, cats, and occasionally cattle.

Amyloidosis is most common in older **dogs** and is usually idiopathic, although some cases occur in association with chronic suppurative and granulomatous lesions in other tissues. Canine glomerular amyloidosis has been associated with *Hepatozoon americanum* and *Ehrlichia canis* infections. Dogs with glomerular amyloidosis develop progressive renal insufficiency and proteinuria that may cause the *nephrotic syndrome.* Dogs with medullary amyloidosis without glomerular involvement may have little or no proteinuria. This presentation is most often seen in Shar-Pei dogs, because amyloid tends to be medullary as opposed to glomerular in this breed. Amyloidosis is less common in **cats** than dogs and is primarily medullary; hence marked proteinuria is an uncommon finding. Glomerular amyloidosis with concurrent IC-

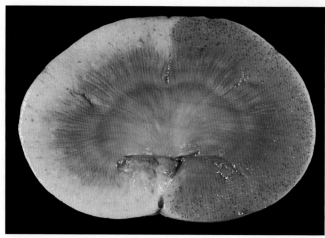

Figure 4-37 Renal amyloidosis in a cat. Right half of the kidney was treated with Lugol's iodine to demonstrate the amyloidotic glomeruli, resulting in red discoloration of the cortex. (Courtesy M.K. Keating.)

mediated glomerulonephritis with a membranous pattern has been reported in a cat, demonstrating that more than one glomerular disease can occur in the same patient. Recent research has suggested that amyloid may act as a prion, wherein exposure of naive animals to amyloid fibrils can induce them to produce more amyloid. In **cattle,** glomerular amyloidosis can cause severe proteinuria; medullary amyloidosis is reported as a common subclinical disease. Chronic inflammation is occasionally demonstrable in affected cattle. AA amyloidosis occurs systemically in **horses** used for antiserum production, whereas AL amyloidosis occurs in the skin and the upper respiratory system. **Sheep and goats** can develop glomerular and medullary amyloidosis in the course of chronic inflammatory processes. **Pigs** rarely develop amyloidosis.

Grossly, with small deposits of amyloid, the kidney may be only mildly increased in size. Characteristic renal changes include pallor, enlargement, and a waxy consistency. The capsule strips smoothly, and the cortical surface has a finely stippled appearance because of numerous fine yellow spots (glomeruli) and gray translucent points (dilated tubules). *Affected glomeruli stain brown-red when exposed to an iodine solution, and subsequent exposure to acetic acid changes the color to purple* (Fig. 4-37).

The **cat** (including Abyssinians, Siamese, domestic short-hairs, and captive tigers and cheetahs) differs somewhat from other species in that amyloid is deposited mainly in the papilla and outer medulla and usually spares glomeruli. Grossly, the kidneys may be indistinguishable from those with nonspecific chronic interstitial nephritis. The prevalence of amyloidosis in cats is much increased on diets providing excess vitamin A (see Vol. 1, Bones and joints).

Histologically, amyloid is first deposited in the mesangial area and in the subendothelial zones of glomerular capillaries. Nodules of amyloid gradually develop until the glomeruli are enlarged and converted to homogeneous spheres lacking endothelial and epithelial nuclei. Similarly, amyloid is deposited in tubular basement membranes, and eventually broad cuffs of amyloid appear around the tubules. The physical presence of amyloid causes ischemia and pressure atrophy of nephrons, and resultant scarring. Tubules may contain numerous pink hyaline casts of protein. Proteinuria is often severe.

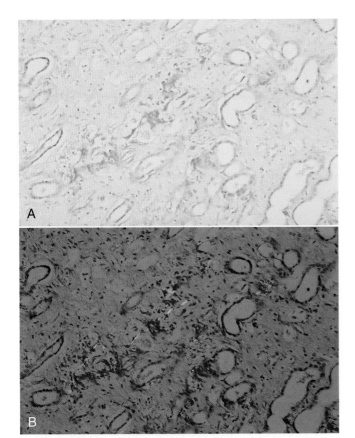

Figure 4-38 Medullary interstitial amyloidosis in a dog. **A.** Congo red staining of the medullary interstitium. **B.** Same field as **A**, with polarized light reveals apple green birefringence of a small portion of the orange material. Moving the polarizer will shift the apple green birefringence to other regions of the interstitium.

If medullary amyloidosis is present (Fig. 4-38), the animal may also be azotemic and have some degree of tubulointerstitial scarring.

Amyloid is eosinophilic in H&E sections, pale pink in PAS, a mix of pale blue to orange on trichrome, and does not take up silver on the JMS stain (Fig. 4-39; eFig. 4-20). *The histologic diagnosis must be confirmed with the Congo red (CR) stain*, with which it stains peach or orange-red, and exhibits green bire-fringence in polarized light. Importantly, to enhance the sen-sitivity of the CR stain, slides should be cut at 8-10 μm thickness. Elimination of the CR staining affinity by oxidation of tissue sections in potassium permanganate indicates it is AA amyloid. Retention of congophilia after pretreatment with potassium permanganate indicates the presence of AL amyloid; the potassium permanganate reaction may be unreliable in cats. Amyloid exhibits bright yellow fluorescence after stain-ing with *thioflavine-T*, which may be required in cats because of poor staining of amyloid with CR in this species. The above staining patterns of amyloid result from its characteristic β-pleated pattern, which also confers on it resistance to pro-teolysis and insolubility. Specific immunohistochemistry can be useful in identifying amyloid and in distinguishing amyloid types. Characteristic nonbranching 7-10 nm–diameter fibrils of amyloid may be seen by electron microscopy (see Fig. 4-39A, B). Definitive characterization of amyloid rests on isolation of the amyloid and amino acid sequencing; the amino acid sequences of feline SAA and AA amyloid vary slightly between Abyssinian and Siamese cats.

Of note, rare cases of nonamyloidotic fibrillary material have been observed in cats and dogs. Therefore birefringence on the CR stain is required for a definitive diagnosis of amy-loidosis. Ultrastructural analysis of nonamyloidotic fibrillary glomerulopathy cases usually demonstrates fibrils with a larger diameter than amyloid. In one such example in a cat, the material stained positive for IgM and IgG but negative for C3. The significance of the IF staining pattern in that particular cat is unknown. In humans, fibrillary glomerulonephritis and immunotactoid glomerulonephritis result from fibrillogenesis of immunoglobulin molecules. The presence of these immu-noglobulins activates complement, and there is usually strong C3 staining on IF. Fibrils that have a larger diameter than amyloid are identified via TEM. In immunotactoid glomeru-lonephritis, the fibrils have a microtubular structure with a central pore. Definitive, well-characterized examples of both of these diseases have not yet been reported in animals.

Further reading

Cavana P, et al. Noncongophilic fibrillary glomerulonephritis in a cat. Vet Pathol 2008;45:347-351.

Markowitz GS. Dysproteinemia and the kidney. Adv Anat Pathol 2004;11:49-63.

Mensua C, et al. Pathology of AA amyloidosis in domestic sheep and goats. Vet Pathol 2003;40:71-80.

Niewold TA, et al. Familial amyloidosis in cats: Siamese and Abyssinian AA proteins differ in primary sequence and pattern of deposition. Amyloid 1999;6:205-209.

Segev G, et al. Renal amyloidosis in dogs: a retrospective study of 91 cases with comparison of the disease between Shar-Pei and non-Shar-Pei dogs. J Vet Intern Med 2012;26:259-268.

Familial abnormalities of the glomerular basement membrane

There are multiple canine breed-related glomerulopathies that strongly resemble a hereditary glomerular disease in humans known as *Alport syndrome*. The basis of the disease is an abnormal, multilaminated GBM (seen on TEM) and results from various genetic mutations in type IV collagen alpha subunits. Clinically, young dogs are presented with protein-uria, hematuria, progressive azotemia, and juvenile-onset renal failure. Histology of late-stage disease reveals mesangial hyper-cellularity, numerous segmentally to globally sclerotic glom-eruli, and moderate to marked interstitial inflammation with fibrosis and tubular atrophy (Fig. 4-40A; eFig. 4-21A, B). Depending on the stage of the disease, there is global multi-lamination of the GBM and foot process effacement on TEM (Fig. 4-40B).

Type IV collagen is the main structural subunit of the GBM in adult dogs and humans. In humans, it is a heterotrimer, composed of 3 intertwined chains (α3, α4, and α5) encoded by the genes *COL4A3*, *COL4A4*, and *COL4A5*, respectively. *COL4A5* is located on the X chromosome in humans and dogs, and mutations in *COL4A5* can result in X-linked Alport syndrome in both species. Because of the extrarenal expres-sion of *COL4A5*, human patients also have hearing deficits and ocular abnormalities. There are 2 canine models of X-linked Alport syndrome: **Samoyed hereditary glomerulopa-thy** (the result of a mutation in exon 35 of the *COL4A5* gene) and a colony of **mixed-breed dogs** (the result of a 10–base pair deletion in exon 9 that causes a frame shift and a

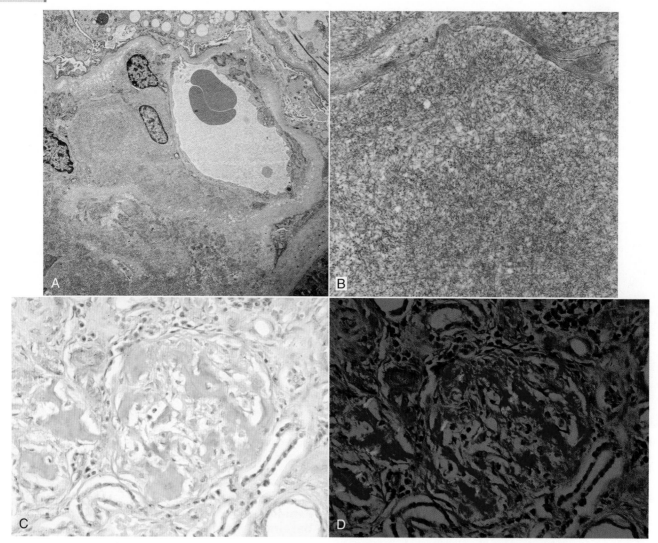

Figure 4-39 Glomerular amyloidosis in a dog. The material is pink and glassy to waxy with H&E and PAS, a mix of orange and blue on Masson trichrome, and does not take up silver with the Jones' methenamine silver method. **A.** TEM of the glomerulus demonstrates large accumulations of fibrillar material in the mesangium and smaller amounts in the GBM. Podocyte foot processes are globally effaced. **B.** Higher magnification of **A** reveals haphazardly arranged nonbranching fibrils, ranging from 9-11 nm in diameter. (**A** and **B** courtesy G. Lees, F. Clubb.) **C, D.** Congo red staining of glomerulus without (**C**) and with (**D**) polarized light.

premature stop codon in exon 10 in the *COLA5* gene). In both models, male dogs are more severely affected than females and have an earlier onset of clinical signs. Dogs do not have hearing loss or ocular disease; therefore the canine symptomatology does not entirely mimic that of humans. The clinical progression of Samoyed hereditary nephropathy is as follows: affected males develop proteinuria and wasting at 2-3 months of age, azotemia after 5 months, renal failure after 7 months, and death by 15 months of age. Mutations in both canine models result in decreased collagen expression in the GBM. Immunofluorescence tests to detect the alpha chains of type IV collagen are used to verify decreased (or lack of) protein expression. In Samoyeds, there is a 90% reduction in the amount of α5 chain in GBMs, probably leading to inadequate cross-linking of collagen type IV. The mixed-breed dogs with this disease have also been well characterized. Labeling of α3, α4, α5, and α6 collagen chains was absent

from GBMs in the affected mixed-breed dogs. As an aside, some normal adult dogs have expression of an α6 chain of type IV collagen in their GBM in addition to the α3-5 chains.

Both *COL4A3* and *COL4A4* reside on canine chromosome 25 and human chromosome 2, therefore mutations in these genes will result in an autosomal recessive disease. The canine model for autosomal recessive Alport syndrome is **English Cocker Spaniel hereditary nephritis**, which is the result of a single nucleotide substitution that causes a premature stop codon in exon 3. In affected dogs, α1-α2(IV) are increased, α3(IV) and α4(IV) chains are absent, α5(IV) chains are markedly decreased, whereas α6(IV) chains are present.

Last, there is also an autosomal dominant form of Alport syndrome in humans, and both **Bull Terriers** and **Dalmatians** have been proposed as animal models for this subtype. The ultrastructural appearance of the GBM is similar to that seen in autosomal recessive Alport, but there is a normal expression

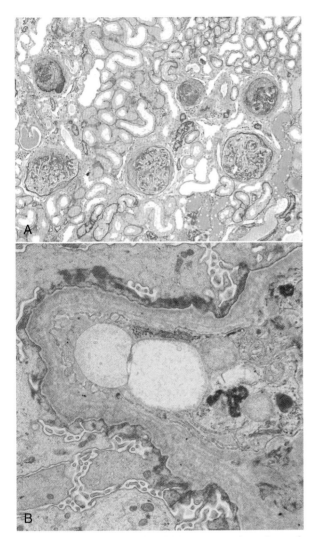

Figure 4-40 Hereditary nephritis (Alport syndrome) resulting from mutated type IV collagen in a severely azotemic and proteinuric 10-month-old dog. **A.** Glomeruli demonstrate sclerosis, mesangial hypercellularity and GBM thickening with accumulation of collagen and plasma in Bowman's space. Tubules are at various stages of degeneration and atrophy. Although this disease displays an MPGN pattern on light microscopy, it is not a true membranoproliferative glomerulonephritis because immune-complex deposition is not involved in the pathogenesis. PAS stain. **B.** TEM of a glomerular capillary loop reveals severe lamination of the GBM.

pattern of collagen chains α3(IV), α4(IV), and α5(IV) in humans and dogs. Although mutations in *COL4A3* and *COL4A4* genes have been documented in humans, the specific mutations have not been identified in either dog breed.

Other examples in which there is ultrastructural evidence of marked GBM lamination on TEM have been identified. These diseases and lesions are not yet well characterized, and more research into their pathogeneses is needed. There is a familial tendency in **Doberman Pinschers** to develop proteinuria and renal failure; the precise mode of inheritance is unknown. Grossly, the kidneys are light brown, slightly small, and have diffuse, fine, subcapsular pits that appear as radial streaks on cut surface. Females may have concomitant unilateral renal agenesis. The histologic renal lesion is mesangial hypercellularity with irregularly thickened GBM and various

degrees of tubulointerstitial disease. Ultrastructurally, GBMs display 2 distinct lesions: the lamina densa may be lamellated and contain intramembranous electron-dense material, or there may be diffuse attenuation of the lamina densa with thickening of the GBM by collagen fibers. Notably, the electron-dense material only stained positively for IgM in 1 of 9 dogs examined, and therefore this is not an example of familial ICGN. There is also a familial glomerulopathy of **Rottweilers** with multilaminated GBM; however, the disease phenotype and the pathogenesis are uncharacterized.

Familial glomerulopathies in other dog breeds

Familial renal diseases of uncertain inheritance occur in other breeds (see Table 4-1). Glomerular lesions (fetal and immature glomeruli and glomerulocystic atrophy) are prominent, but there are also significant tubulointerstitial lesions, making it difficult to definitively determine which compartment was primarily affected.

Familial renal disease in **Norwegian Elkhound** dogs is seen as rapidly progressive renal failure in juvenile dogs; the mode of inheritance is unknown. Glomerular changes begin as *periglomerular fibrosis* with hypertrophy and hyperplasia of parietal epithelium and progress to diffuse fibrosis of cortex and medulla and progressive loss of glomeruli. In contrast to the hereditary glomerulopathies discussed previously, the lesion in Norwegian Elkhounds may represent a primary tubular lesion with secondary prominent glomerular changes because microdissection of nephrons in early cases reveals saccular dilations of the distal segments. Genetic analysis has ruled out the possibility of an Alport-like syndrome.

Glomerulosclerosis

Glomerulosclerosis is the term used when the glomerulus is scarred, and *global glomerulosclerosis* is considered to be synonymous with glomerular obsolescence. Focal segmental glomerulosclerosis (FSGS) is a well-characterized cause of moderate to severe proteinuria in humans. In human nephropathology, this histologic pattern has such a close correlation with significant proteinuria that FSGS has become its own diagnostic entity. Affected patients have some glomeruli characterized by segmental glomerular scarring without evidence of IC deposition. The pathogenesis involves podocyte injury, followed by detachment and loss. Because podocytes cannot be replenished easily, the denuded GBM may be covered by cytoplasmic projections from neighboring podocytes. Alternatively, the GBM may adhere to Bowman's capsule (synechia). Eventually, the glomerular tuft may develop segmental effacement of peripheral capillary lumens by extracellular matrix (segmental sclerosis), although the relationship between podocyte injury and increased synthesis of extracellular matrix is not entirely understood. Often, insudation of hyaline material is also present in these segments. Segmental sclerosis can be due to innate podocyte defects (e.g., a mutation in a podocyte or slit diaphragm protein) or secondary to podocyte injury (e.g., from a toxic insult or hypertension).

As stated previously, ICGN can damage glomeruli such that podocytes are also injured and lost. Therefore chronic ICGN may have superimposed segmental sclerosis. This has led to the misconception in veterinary pathology that all cases with segmental GS have underlying IC disease. Although segmental sclerosis might suggest a previous episode of ICGN, TEM and IF evaluations of canine renal biopsies have revealed that ICs are not present in a considerable proportion of patients with segmental GS (see Fig. 4-26; eFig. 4-11). There-fore these cases fall into the diagnostic category of FSGS. In fact, 20% of North American dogs that underwent a renal biopsy for the clinical indication of proteinuria had FSGS-like disease.

In humans, the region of the kidney affected and the his-tomorphology of the sclerotic lesion within the glomerulus all have etiologic and prognostic implications; however, similar insights have rarely been established in domestic species. For example, in aging laboratory Beagles, the glomeruli in proxim-ity to medullary rays are predisposed to undergo segmental sclerosis, suggesting that these glomeruli (and podocytes) are exposed to injuries and stresses that do not affect other glomeruli.

There are 3 important points about segmental glomerulo-sclerosis:

1. It should be rare to absent in normal kidneys, and should not be considered as a step on the pathway to nephron senescence; when a nephron undergoes senescence, the entire glomerulus scars all at once.

2. Because the lesion is focal, an adequate number of glom-eruli need to be sampled in a renal biopsy. In humans, a biopsy core with 10 glomeruli has a 65% chance of detect-ing FSGS, even when only one tenth of the glomeruli are involved. The likelihood of detecting FSGS increases to 88% if the core contains 20 glomeruli. Although similar studies have not yet been done in veterinary species, it is assumed that a similar number of glomeruli should be evaluated to rule out FSGS in a biopsy core.

3. As mentioned previously, segmental sclerosis can be sec-ondary to a glomerular insult that damages podocytes. Therefore it can be seen in the setting of underlying ICGN. If ICs are not identified with additional modalities, then a diagnosis of FSGS should be rendered. Notably, the pres-ence of secondary segmental sclerosis superimposed on GN lesions should be mentioned in the morphologic diagnosis because it connotes irreversible glomerular scarring (e.g., membranous glomerulonephropathy with secondary seg-mental sclerosis).

In addition to its association with ICGN, some natural and experimental infections with *Dirofilaria immitis* led to fraying and thickening of the GBM with associated segmental GS. Immune complexes were not identified with TEM and IF studies. This suggests that some diseases can damage glomeruli through multiple pathways (both ICGN and non-ICGN). Focal segmental glomerulosclerosis has been reported in a colony of Maltese Beagle dogs with *glucose-6-phosphatase defi-ciency* (glycogen storage disease Ia); hepatomegaly and reno-megaly occur because of vacuolation of hepatocytes and proximal tubular epithelial cells, respectively. Nephrotic syn-drome secondary to FSGS has also been reported in a yearling Standardbred colt; TEM and IF studies did not reveal IC deposition.

The protein-losing nephropathy (PLN) in **Soft-coated Wheaten Terriers** is familial but of unknown inheritance. Affected dogs have a sclerosing phenotype and podocytes are often swollen with large cytoplasmic protein resorption drop-lets. Genome-wide association studies have revealed muta-tions in 2 podocyte genes, *NPHS1* and *KIRREL2*. Some of these dogs also have features of renal dysplasia. Food hyper-sensitivity was reported in a subset of dogs, suggesting mul-tiple abnormalities of the immune system in this breed. In the general pet population, PLN and FSGS in Soft-coated Wheaten

Terriers often occur in the absence of IC deposits, as demon-strated by TEM and IF.

A special type of GS is characterized by the primary depo-sition of collagen type III in glomeruli, whereas only collagen type IV should be present in normal adult glomeruli. This disease has been reported in dogs, pigs, and a cat (Fig. 4-41; eFig. 4-22). Proteinuria and renal failure result from sclerosis and obliteration of capillary lumina. This variant of GS resem-bles the human condition collagenofibrotic glomerulone-phropathy. One dog had both type III collagen as well as fibronectin deposition in the mesangium. Glomerulosclerosis resulting from fibrillar collagen deposition that was not subtyped was reported in Newfoundland dog littermates. *Col-lagenofibrotic glomerulonephropathy and fibronectin glomerulone-phropathy*, both of which are well characterized although poorly understood glomerular disease in humans, are differ-ential diagnoses for young animals with marked mesangial expansion and variable degrees of mesangial hypercellularity.

Minimal change disease

Histologic glomerular changes are slight, but clinical disease is marked, in **minimal change disease.** This disease is charac-terized by reversible global fusion of podocyte foot processes and is accompanied by significant proteinuria (Fig. 4-42; eFig. 4-23). Minimal change disease has been produced exper-imentally in dogs, by infection with *Ehrlichia canis*. Global foot process effacement with severe proteinuria has also been documented secondary to treatment with tyrosine kinase inhibitors in a cat and 2 dogs. One dog with severe proteinuria later developed acute renal failure (ARF), which was similar to minimal change disease with ARF, a well-known clinical entity in humans.

Glomerular lipidosis and miscellaneous glomerular lesions

Large *foam cells*, which contain sudanophilic (lipid) droplets, may be found in one or more lobules of glomerular tufts in many dogs. The cells are closely packed and finely vacuolated, and the cell boundaries are distinct (Fig. 4-43; eFig. 4-24). The source of these cells is unknown, but mesangial and endothe-lial cells have been proposed. Although glomerular lipidosis is thought to be an incidental finding, involvement of many glomeruli, aneurysmal dilation of capillary loops with associ-ated mesangiolysis suggests a more serious disease process. The original literature reported that most dogs with this lesion did not have renal dysfunction based solely on lack of azote-mia; UPC and urinalysis results were not provided. In rare renal biopsies taken from markedly proteinuric dogs, glomeru-lar lipidosis in many glomeruli was the sole lesion identified. Furthermore, experimental models of vascular injury in dogs via intravenous injection of biologic toxins (i.e., snake venom and diphtheria toxin) resulted in glomerular lipidosis.

Lipid embolization of renal arterioles and glomerular capillaries occurs occasionally in dogs with diabetes mellitus, dyslipidemia, or following trauma. The lipid emboli are intra-vascular rather than within foam cells (Fig. 4-44; eFig. 4-25). Cholesterol clefts may also be observed in glomerular capil-laries and interstitial vessels.

A syndrome of *idiopathic cutaneous and renal glomerular vasculopathy* has been documented in Greyhounds. Most dogs are diagnosed based on characteristic ulcers of the distal extremities, thrombocytopenia and ARF. Histologically, there is frequent necrosis of glomerular afferent arterioles with

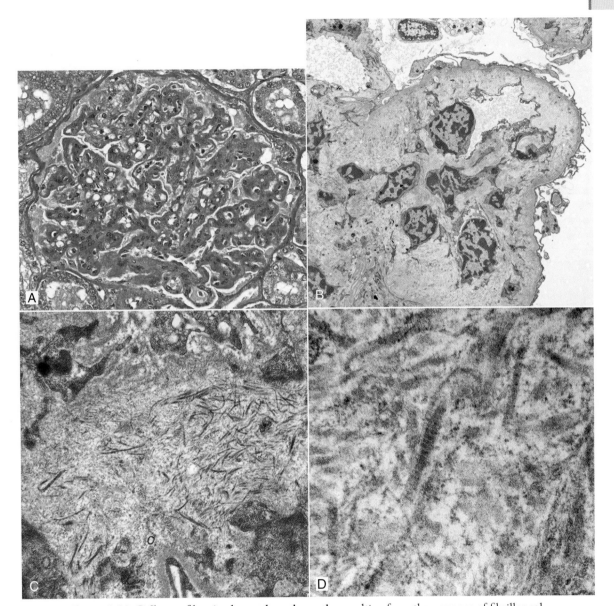

Figure 4-41 Collagenofibrotic glomerulonephropathy resulting from the presence of fibrillar collagen in the GBM in an azotemic, mildly proteinuric 9-month-old dog. **A.** Glomerular capillary loops are irregularly thickened, and there is marked mesangial hypercellularity. Although this disease displays an MPGN pattern on LM, it is not a true membranoproliferative glomerulonephritis because immune-complex deposition is not involved in the pathogenesis. Masson trichrome. (Courtesy G. Lees.) **B-D.**TEM of the glomerulus reveals the presence of haphazardly arranged collagen fibers. Periodicity of the fibers is observed in **D**. The fibrillar collagen is usually type III collagen, and its presence may be caused by overproduction or failure of the fetal glomerular type III collagen to switch to the adult glomerular type IV collagen during maturation. (B-D courtesy G. Lees, C. Brown.)

coagulation and necrosis of the tufts. Pulmonary and cutaneous vessels are sometimes similarly affected. Acutely, the ultrastructural lesions consist of endothelial cell injury and necrosis with aggregated platelets and fibrin. Over time, there is thickening of the glomerular capillary walls and associated narrowing of the lumens by cellular interpositioning and electron-densities that, based on IF, are not consistent with ICs. The clinical presentation and the glomerular ultrastructure are suggestive of primary endothelial cell injury (so-called thrombotic microangiopathy), which is not mediated by immune complexes. Thrombotic microangiopathy is well-

described in humans, but is only rarely documented in other species (Fig. 4-45; eFig. 4-26).

Experimentally-induced *pregnancy toxemia in sheep* led to significant proteinuria and azotemia. Glomerular abnormalities were characterized ultrastructurally by double contours of the GBM, occlusion of the capillary lumens by swollen endothelium, widespread fusion of podocyte foot processes, and absence of IC deposits. Affected sheep had significantly higher plasma levels of renin without a change in substrate concentration. Although comparisons to the glomerular thrombotic microangiopathy that can occur in human

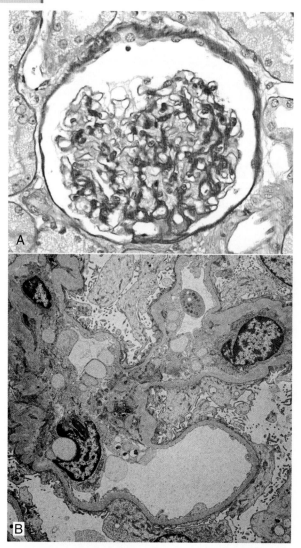

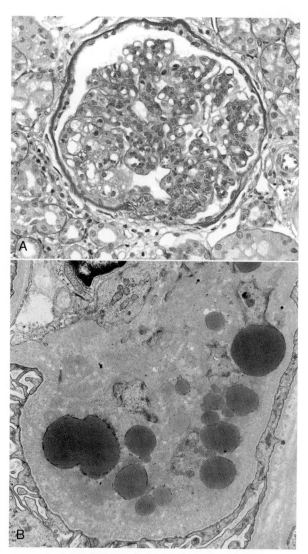

Figure 4-42 Minimal change disease in a severely proteinuric adult dog. **A.** Glomeruli are normocellular and the GBM is within normal limits. PAS stain. (Courtesy G. Lees.) **B.** TEM of the glomerulus reveals global effacement of podocyte foot processes. Neither immune complexes nor GBM abnormalities are present. (Courtesy G. Lees, F. Clubb.)

Figure 4-43 Glomerular lipidosis in a 1-year-old dog with marked proteinuria. **A.** PAS stain. **B.** TEM of a glomerular capillary reveals multiple osmiophilic lipid droplets. Immune complexes are not present. (Courtesy G. Lees, F. Clubb.)

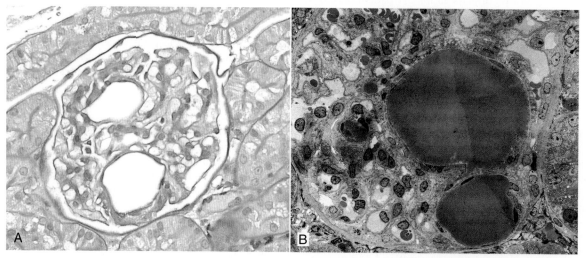

Figure 4-44 Glomerular lipid emboli in a severely proteinuric adult dog. **A.** PAS stain. **B.** TEM of the glomerulus reveals large osmiophilic lipid droplets distorting the capillary loops. (Courtesy G. Lees, F. Clubb.)

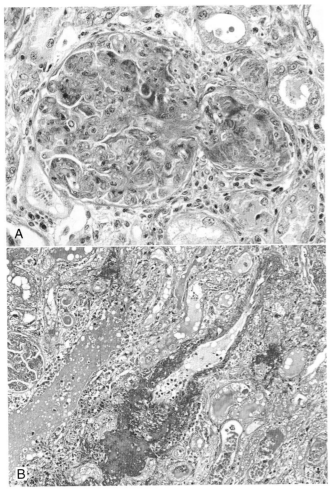

Figure 4-45 Thrombotic microangiopathy in a dog with acute renal failure and mild proteinuria. Masson trichrome stain. **A.** Fibrinoid necrosis of the afferent arteriole. **B.** Fibrinoid necrosis of an intralobular artery.

preeclampsia are understandable, the pathogenesis may be different. Specifically, the role of placental production of soluble vascular endothelial growth factor (VEGF) receptors in the pathogenesis of pre-eclampsia has been clearly demonstrated in humans, but similar research in sheep is lacking. Furthermore, hypertension is a key feature in human pre-eclampsia but was not reported in the sheep.

Mesangial hyaline droplets, of unknown pathogenesis and significance, were reported in 3 pigs; 2 of the pigs had concurrent mastocytosis and the third had mesangial cell proliferation. Droplets were assumed to be plasma constituents because IF demonstrated that they contained albumin, IgG, and fibrinogen, similar to protein droplets present in proximal tubules.

Further reading

Backlund B, et al. Minimal change glomerulopathy in a cat. J Feline Med Surg 2011;13:291-295.

Brown MR, et al. Mastinib-associated minimal change disease with acute tubular necrosis resulting in acute kidney injury in a dog. J Vet Intern Med 2013;27:1622-1626.

Davidson AG, et al. Genetic cause of autosomal recessive hereditary nephropathy in the English Cocker Spaniel. J Vet Intern Med 2007;21:394-401.

Kamie J, et al. Collagenofibrotic glomerulonephropathy with fibronectin deposition in a dog. Vet Pathol 2009;46:688-692.

Littman MP, et al. Glomerulopathy and mutations in NPHS1 and KIRREL2 in soft-coated wheaten terrier dogs. Mamm Genome 2013;24:119-126.

Pomeroy MJ, Robertson JL. The relationship of age, sex, and glomerular location to the development of spontaneous lesions in the canine kidney: analysis of a life-span study. Tox Pathol 2004;32:237-242.

Rortveit R, et al. A clinical study of canine collagen type III glomerulopathy. BMC Vet Res 2013;9:218.

Rule AD, et al. The association between age and nephrosclerosis on renal biopsy among healthy adults. Ann Intern Med 2010;152:561-567.

Sum SO, et al. Drug induced minimal change nephropathy in a dog. J Vet Intern Med 2010;24:431-435.

Wakamatsu N, et al. Histologic and ultrastructural studies of juvenile onset renal disease in four Rottweiler dogs. Vet Pathol 2007;44:96-100.

Wiersma AC, et al. Evaluation of canine COL4A3 and COL4A4 as candidates for familial renal disease in the Norwegian elkhound. J Hered 2005;96:739-744.

DISEASES OF TUBULES

Tubular diseases are primarily reflected in morphologic changes in the epithelial cells, although specific functional abnormalities that result from enzyme deletions may not be visible histologically. Patients are often azotemic or have abnormal urinary profiles. For example, glucosuria and amino aciduria in the setting of normal plasma levels can indicate proximal tubular defects, even when the serum creatinine is normal. Novel urinary biomarkers that have shown promise in identification of dogs with acute tubular injury (ATI) before the development of azotemia include retinol binding protein, neutrophil gelatinase-associated lipocalin, N-acetyl-β-D-glucosaminidase, β_2-microglobulin, cystatin C, and kidney injury molecule-1. As noted previously, *the tubules and interstitium are intimately associated, and damage to one affects the other.* Diseases that involve both compartments are discussed later under Tubulointerstitial diseases. Regeneration of tubular epithelium can occur, but postnatal development of entire nephrons is limited to a short period of time, depending upon species. The response of the kidney to destruction of tubules is limited to compensatory hypertrophy of remaining nephrons. Thus the tubules remaining in damaged kidneys are often large and dilated.

Degeneration and swelling of tubular cells cause the kidney to enlarge and bulge on cut surface. *Acute cellular swelling* results from damage to mitochondria and is visualized by the formation of clear spaces in the cytoplasm with some discrete vacuoles (Fig. 4-46A; eFig. 4-27). It is potentially reversible. *Necrotic tubular cells* are eosinophilic, have pyknotic nuclei, and slough into the lumen, where they form cellular or coarsely granular casts (Fig. 4-46B). Tubules filled with *proteinaceous fluid* usually indicate that there is increased glomerular permeability in that nephron. *Tamm-Horsfall mucoprotein*, which is produced in the ascending limb of the loop of Henle and the distal tubules, is bright magenta with the PAS stain and pale blue to pale peach with the Masson trichrome stain. *Hyaline droplets*, which are pink homogeneous globules of protein, appear in the cytoplasm of

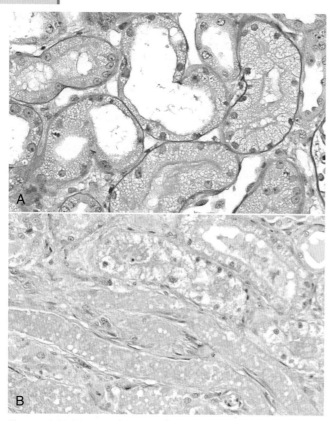

Figure 4-46 Various degrees of **acute tubular epithelial injury (ATI). A.** Tubulointerstitium from a dog with loss of the apical border (tubular simplification), attenuated epithelial cells, and marked isometric vesiculation. PAS stain. **B.** Tubulointerstitium from a cat with severely swollen proximal tubular epithelial cells (upper right) adjacent to denuded tubular basement membranes containing sloughed cellular debris (lower left). Interstitial inflammation is not a feature. H&E stain.

proximal tubular cells in nephrons with increased glomerular permeability. The hyaline droplets are lysosomes swollen by resorbed protein that is undergoing proteolysis and will be returned to the circulation as amino acids. Proteinaceous hyaline droplets are normal in proximal tubular epithelial cells of neonatal piglets. Protein resorption by proximal tubules is a physiologic process; hyaline droplets indicate that this mechanism is saturated. *Tubular lipidosis* is difficult to evaluate in swine, dogs, and cats, which normally have considerable quantities of fat in the renal epithelium. The lipid is usually found in the cells of the convoluted tubules.

Thickening of the tubular basement membrane is seen in a variety of situations involving chronic damage and is usually associated with atrophic tubular epithelium. In renal *amyloidosis*, amyloid is deposited on the tubular basement membrane, as well as in glomeruli. Disruption of the tubular basement membrane indicates severe or prolonged tubular injury, and may allow herniation of tubular epithelial cells, with some of these cells persisting as interstitial foam cells.

Acute tubular injury

There has been an evolution of terminology to describe and diagnose tubular injury, and these changes in terminology have been a response to our ever-increasing understanding of lesion pathogenesis. "**Nephrosis**" was the oldest term to describe an

acute injury to the tubular portion of the nephron. Next, the term acute tubular necrosis (**ATN**) was put forth as being more accurate. Unfortunately, this term implies that the functional disturbances in the kidney are the result of tubular epithelial cell death. This term can lead inexperienced pathologists astray by suggesting that overt necrosis is needed to make the diagnosis, when in fact the lesion may be limited to an increased number of pyknotic nuclei scattered amongst swollen, degenerative epithelial cells. Furthermore, recent research has revealed severe functional deficits resulting from cell degeneration, followed by sloughing of the apical portion of the cell into the lumen and maintaining the basal portion attached to the tubular basement membrane. This type of cell attenuation is sometimes misinterpreted by physician and veterinary pathologists as cell spreading over denuded tubular basement membranes as a part of the regenerative process. Examination of renal tissue over the time course of acute kidney injury has revealed that these attenuated cells are present early in the disease before any reparative phase. Therefore, acute tubular injury (**ATI**) is now the preferred term because it connotes a functional disturbance that can result in significant azotemia without implying the presence of coagulative or liquefactive necrosis. Even so, "ATN" is still often used by nephrologists and nephropathologists.

ATI is a reversible condition mediated by tubular degeneration and is an important cause of **ARF**. Affected animals are often *oliguric or anuric* and die within a few days unless given appropriate therapy. *The principal causes of ATI are ischemia and nephrotoxins.* The renal tubules, in particular the proximal straight tubule and the medullary thick ascending limb, are metabolically very active and are the components most susceptible to ischemia or nephrotoxins.

Ischemic or **tubulorrhectic ATI** follows a period of hypotension and/or marked renal ischemia. *Prolonged renal ischemia causes renal cortical necrosis*, that is, all cortical structures are affected (discussed previously). Massive hemolysis can cause ATI and produces a pattern known as *hemoglobinuria-associated ATI* (previously called hemoglobinuric or pigmentary nephrosis) (Fig. 4-47). The roles of hemoglobin and myoglobin as primary nephrotoxins are unclear, but renal failure is likely impacted by other factors, such as anemia. Ischemic ATI ranges in severity depending on length of the hypotensive episode. Mild ischemic ATI is characterized histologically by proximal tubular epithelial cell degeneration, and dilated, empty tubular lumens resulting from loss of the apical brush border. This apical portion is often rich in cytochrome pigments, and these cell portions can be identified as muddy brown casts in the urine if a specimen is collected soon after the insult. More severe cases of ischemia can affect distal tubules to some extent and may disrupt tubular basement membranes (tubulorrhexis). Eosinophilic hyaline and granular casts commonly occur in the distal tubules and collecting ducts. They consist of Tamm-Horsfall mucoproteins, dead epithelial cells, and other plasma proteins. Interstitial edema and accumulation of leukocytes in dilated vasa recta are common findings, especially acutely (Fig. 4-48). Glomeruli vary from normal to slightly wrinkled from poor perfusion. After about 1 week, *epithelial regeneration* may be seen as tubules lined by flattened, basophilic, karyomegalic epithelium, and frequent mitoses. The renewed cells are smaller than normal initially and may appear closely packed on the basement membrane. They tend to pile up in small clusters that will eventually disappear. If the initial injury is mild and/or supportive therapy

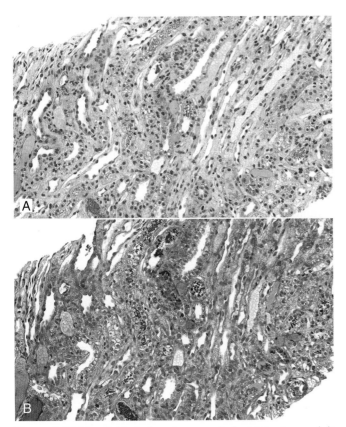

Figure 4-47 Myoglobin-induced acute tubular injury in an adult dog secondary to marked myonecrosis. **A.** H&E stain. **B.** Masson trichrome. Within the medulla, there are numerous intratubular granular to globular casts that are bright red-brown on both stains. There is associated vacuolar tubular degeneration. Of note, hemoglobin casts will have a histologically identical appearance.

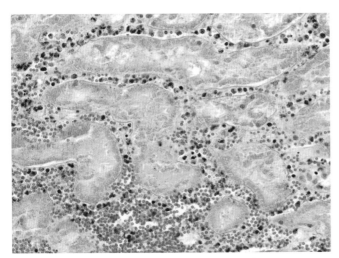

Figure 4-48 Ischemic tubular necrosis in a sheep with a **renal infarct.** Tubular outlines are preserved, and the interstitial acute inflammation provides evidence of reperfusion.

is adequate, *recovery* of architecture may be complete within about 2-3 weeks.

Nephrotoxic ATI differs in pathogenesis but often can overlap with ischemic ATI morphologically. Renal tubules, especially proximal tubules, are particularly susceptible to a wide variety of toxic agents as a consequence of their high metabolic activity and their exposure to agents in the ultrafiltrate that they contact during urine formation. Cellular enzyme systems are inactivated by toxic agents such as heavy metals, which bind to sulfhydryl groups. *Preservation of tubular basement membranes provides the framework for epithelial regeneration and is an important prognostic feature to evaluate in renal biopsies.* Ischemia, however, often complicates toxic ATI because edema compresses peritubular capillaries and decreases blood flow. The interaction between ischemia and nephrotoxicity is a prime example of why it is often difficult to discern the etiology of ATI in diagnostic cases. Given the interaction of ischemic and nephrotoxic ATI, the presence of a tubular basement membrane is not pathognomonic for either pathogenesis.

The *pathogenesis* of ARF and oliguria in either ischemic or toxic ATI remains controversial. Obstruction of tubular flow by cellular debris and casts and by interstitial edema appears to be an important factor. Other proposed mechanisms include preglomerular vasoconstriction, possibly because of activation of the renin-angiotensin system; leakage of tubular fluid into the interstitium (tubular backleak); and impaired glomerular permeability or vascular reactivity. Disruption of the actin cytoskeleton of proximal tubular cells and breakdown of apical microvilli occur because of ischemia. Redistribution of tubular cell membrane proteins causes loss of cell polarity, abnormal ion transport across tubular cells, and hence increased delivery of sodium to the distal tubule. The resulting tubuloglomerular feedback leads to vasoconstriction of afferent arterioles. *Oliguria* is the result of various combinations of these factors. At the oliguric stage of ARF, hyperkalemia can be life threatening. If the animal survives the oliguric phase, diuresis may occur, and electrolyte imbalances, such as hypokalemia, may contribute to death. As tubular regeneration proceeds, azotemia resolves and tubular function slowly returns.

Numerous toxic substances can cause ATI in domestic animals (Box 4-2). Some of these agents are no longer important as nephrotoxins. For example, organomercurials were commonly used as fungicides on grains that were occasionally inadvertently fed to animals and humans with disastrous results. This use of mercury has been banned. Similarly, highly chlorinated naphthalenes, which cause hyperkeratosis and ARF in cattle, have been excluded from the farm environment. Sulfonamides were formerly important nephrotoxins, but newer formulations are more soluble and less toxic. Some newly introduced agents have nephrotoxicity as a side-effect, for example, aminoglycosides. Numerous additional antibiotics that are toxic to humans (e.g., penicillin, semisynthetic penicillins, polymyxins) may also prove to be toxic to domestic animals. The toxicity of many of the exogenous agents is exacerbated by various systemic states, such as dehydration or shock, which concomitantly impair renal function in the affected animal. Discussion of specific examples of nephrotoxins follows.

Further reading

Haburjak JJ, Spangler WL. Isoniazid-induced seizures with secondary rhabdomyolysis and associated acute renal failure in a dog. J Small Anim Pract 2002;43:182-186.

Hsu WL, et al. Neutrophil gelatinase-associated lipocalin in dogs with naturally occurring renal diseases. J Vet Intern Med 2014;28: 437-442.

BOX • 4-2

Agents that are nephrotoxic in domestic animals

Exogenous
Animal venoms
Antimicrobials
    Aminoglycosides (neomycin, kanamycin, gentamicin, streptomycin, tobramycin, amikacin)
    Amphotericin B
    Cephalosporins
    Polymyxins
    Sulfonamides (sulfapyridine, sulfathiazole, sulfadiazine)
    Tetracyclines
Antineoplastic agents (cisplatin, doxorubicin, methotrexate)
Cantharidin (blister beetle)
Chlorinated hydrocarbons
Clostridium perfringens type D, epsilon toxin (pulpy kidney)
Contrast media
Ethylene glycol
Menadione (vitamin K_3)
Metals (arsenic, bismuth, cadmium, lead, mercury, thallium)
Methoxyflurane
Monensin
Mycotoxins (citrinin, ochratoxin A)
Paraquat
Plants
    Amaranthus retroflexus (pigweed)
    Isotropis
    Lantana camara
    Oxalates (various plants)
    Quercus spp. (oak; tannins)
    Terminalia oblongata (yellow-wood)
Sodium fluoride (superphosphate fertilizer)

Endogenous
Bile
Hemoglobin
Myoglobin

Maddens B, et al. Evaluation of kidney injury in dogs with pyometra based on proteinuria, renal histomorphology, and urinary biomarkers. J Vet Intern Med 2011;25:1075-1083.

Mene P, et al. Mechanisms of repair after kidney injury. J Nephrol 2003;16:186-195.

Vesely DL. Natriuretic peptides and acute renal failure. Am J Physiol Renal Physiol 2003;285:F167-F177.

Zhou X, et al. Evaluation of the usefulness of novel biomarkers for drug-induced acute kidney injury in beagle dogs. Toxicol Appl Pharmacol 2014;280:30-35.

Aminoglycosides

These antibiotics are widely used against gram-negative infections and include, in decreasing order of nephrotoxicity, **neomycin, kanamycin, gentamicin, streptomycin, tobramycin,** and **amikacin.** In cats, aminoglycosides are ototoxic as well as nephrotoxic. Foals are particularly prone to nephrotoxicosis. Aminoglycosides are not metabolized but instead are eliminated from the body primarily by glomerular filtration. They selectively accumulate in and damage proximal tubules. The *tubulotoxic effects* of aminoglycosides include loss of the brush border and formation of cytosegrosomes and myeloid bodies. Overloading of lysosomes with phospholipids (lysosomal phospholipidosis) results from aminoglycoside-induced inhibition of phospholipases. Lysosomal dysfunction and/or leakage may lead to tubular cell injury and death. Damage is dose related and is enhanced by pre-existing renal impairment. Toxicity is manifested clinically by an inability to concentrate urine, polyuria, enzymuria, proteinuria, hematuria and azotemia. ARF may ensue. Aminoglycoside nephrotoxicity is reversible, and recovery may occur in the face of continued therapy because the regenerating cells have increased resistance to aminoglycoside toxicity.

Tetracyclines

An overdose of oxytetracycline can produce ATI and renal failure in dogs. Tetracycline administration has been reported to cause ATI and death in calves because of the presence of tetracycline degradation products; high doses of oxytetracycline are nephrotoxic to cattle. *Use of tetracyclines is contraindicated in animals in renal failure.* Tetracyclines are excreted from the body primarily by the kidneys; thus renal dysfunction leads to increased serum drug concentrations and enhanced nephrotoxic potential. Doxycycline, a semisynthetic tetracycline, is not reported to be nephrotoxic.

Sulfonamides

Severe injury may follow ingestion of excessive doses of sulfonamides, especially if treated animals are dehydrated. Toxicity was more common previously when only less-soluble forms of the drug were available, for example, sulfapyridine, sulfathiazole, sulfadiazine. *Crystalline nephropathy is now rare because newer shorter-acting sulfonamides have greater solubility.* Affected kidneys are slightly enlarged and congested, and the sulfonamide crystals are grossly visible in the medulla, pelvis, and in some cases even in the bladder. The deposits are yellow and form pale radial lines in the medulla. Crystals are not observed in section because they are dissolved during processing. Epithelial cells of the proximal convoluted tubules and of Bowman's capsule undergo severe acute swelling. There is little evidence of necrosis in the distal and collecting tubules, but epithelial proliferation and swelling are prominent, and the tubules become densely populated with large basophilic cells. Some papillary formations into the lumen may be present, and there may be complete duplication of the epithelium lining the collecting ducts. The inner layer of epithelial cells surrounds faintly basophilic hyaline precipitate. There is a diffuse but mild interstitial reaction about the corticomedullary junction. It appears that the *renal lesions are the result of both local toxic and obstructive effects* and that hypersensitivity does not play a role in animals, as it apparently does in humans.

Amphotericin

Amphotericin B is an antifungal agent, a polyene antibiotic, whose most important toxic effect is renal dysfunction. It causes decreased renal blood flow and glomerular filtration because of *renal vasoconstriction*, and is also *directly toxic* to renal tubular epithelial cells. Necrosis of proximal and distal tubules occurs, and there is mineralization of intratubular casts. Nephrotoxicity of amphotericin B has been reduced by complexing the drug with lipids or entrapping it in liposomes.

Further reading

Ali BH, et al. Experimental gentamicin nephrotoxicity and agents that modify it: a mini-review of recent research. Basic Clin Pharmacol Toxicol 2011;109:225-232.

Deray G. Amphotericin B nephrotoxicity. J Antimicrob Chemother 2002;49(Suppl. 1):37-41.

Loo AS, et al. Toxicokinetic and mechanistic basis for the safety and tolerability of liposomal amphotericin B. Expert Opin Drug Saf 2013;12:881-895.

Lopez-Novoa JM, et al. New insights into the mechanism of aminoglycoside nephrotoxicity: an integrative point of view. Kidney Int 2011;79:33-45.

van der Harst MR, et al. Gentamicin nephrotoxicity—a comparison of in vitro findings with in vivo experiments in equines. Vet Res Commun 2005;29:247-261.

Ethylene glycol

Dogs and cats are commonly poisoned by ingestion of ethylene glycol. The seasonal incidence of this poisoning coincides with the changing of engine antifreeze solutions in the spring and autumn. Cattle are also occasionally poisoned. Ethylene glycol, which is present in a 95% concentration in antifreeze solutions, has a sweet taste and is usually ingested voluntarily, especially by young dogs. Cats are more susceptible, but less commonly affected, than dogs; the minimum lethal dose is 1.5 mL/kg for cats and 6.6 mL/kg for dogs.

Ethylene glycol, which itself is of low toxicity, is rapidly absorbed from the gastrointestinal tract. Most is excreted unchanged in the urine. A small percentage is oxidized by alcohol dehydrogenase in the liver to glycoaldehyde, which is in turn oxidized to glycolic acid, glyoxylate, and finally oxalate. *Glycoaldehyde and glyoxylate are the primary nephrotoxic metabolites;* they act by causing ATP depletion and damage to membrane phospholipids and enzymes. Other end products of metabolism are lactic acid, hippuric acid, and carbon dioxide.

Depression, ataxia, and osmotic diuresis develop within a few hours after ingestion of ethylene glycol. Although oxalate crystals are deposited around cerebral vessels and in perivascular spaces (Fig. 4-49), nervous signs are the result of the effect of aldehydes and possibly to the severe metabolic acidosis that develops as a result of accumulation of lactic acid, glycolate, and glyoxylate. Over the next 12 hours, pulmonary edema, tachypnea, and tachycardia occur. If the animal survives for 1-3 days after ingestion, ARF develops, primarily as the result of nephrotoxicity. Severe renal edema impairs intrarenal blood flow and contributes to injury. Soluble calcium oxalates in the blood precipitate in the ultrafiltrate of the renal tubules as the pH of the fluid decreases. Calcium oxalate crystals may be found in tubular lumens, in tubular cells, and in the interstitium; they are light yellow, arranged in sheaves, rosettes, or prisms, and are birefringent with polarized light (Fig. 4-50; eFig. 4-28). Tubular lesions, which are most severe in proximal tubules, range from acute cellular swelling to necrosis to regeneration.

In animals surviving the acute toxic insult, calcium oxalate crystals are thought to be of importance in causing renal failure. *Large numbers of crystals in tubules are virtually*

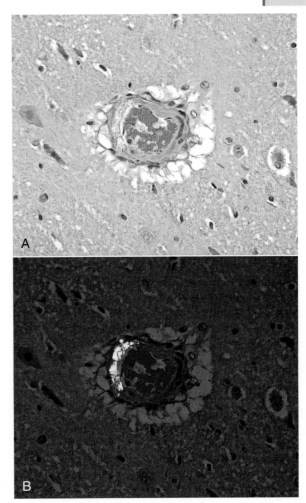

Figure 4-49 Ethylene glycol intoxication in a dog. **A.** Oxalate crystals in the wall of a vessel in the brain. **B.** As in A, with polarized light to demonstrate refractile calcium oxalate crystals. (**A, B.** Courtesy J. Davies.)

pathognomonic of ethylene glycol poisoning, whereas rare scattered oxalate crystals can be seen in many types of chronic kidney disease. Occasional calcium oxalate crystals are normally seen in urine sediment of dogs; large numbers of these crystals are highly suggestive of poisoning. Hypocalcemia resulting from the formation of crystals is usually mild in dogs. Animals that survive the acute exposure may develop tubulointerstitial scarring. Few crystals may be left in the tubules; they tend to be removed in the weeks following their deposition. The diagnosis may be confirmed by detection of ethylene glycol in stomach content or blood by gas chromatography early in the toxicosis, or by detection of glycolic acid in urine, serum, or ocular fluid by mass spectrometry later in the toxicosis. The renal calcium to phosphorus ratio may also be helpful in the diagnosis. In dogs dying from ethylene glycol intoxication, the ratio is often >2.5, whereas it is <0.1 in normal dogs.

Oxalate

Plants are the usual source of oxalate poisoning in sheep and cattle. Plants that can contain toxic amounts of oxalate are *Halogeton glomeratus,* halogeton; *Sarcobatus vermiculatus,* greasewood; *Rheum rhaponticum,* the common garden rhubarb; *Oxalis cernua,* soursob; and *Rumex* spp., sorrel, dock. Plants

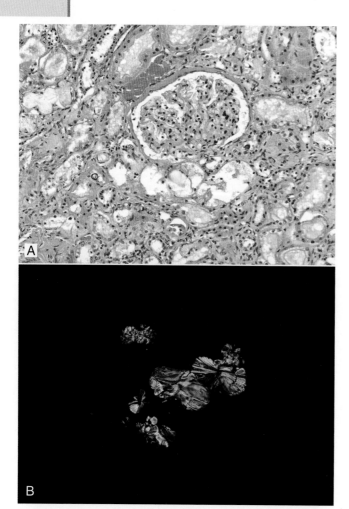

Figure 4-50 Acute tubular necrosis caused by ethylene glycol intoxication in a cat. **A.** Oxalate crystals are present within tubular epithelial cells and tubular lumens. **B.** As in A, with polarizer to demonstrate refractile oxalate crystals with the "sheaves of wheat" appearance.

of lesser importance are *Portulacca oleracea, Trianthema portulacastrum*, and *Threlkeldia proceriflora*, as well as some cultivated species such as mangels and sugar beet. Young plants may contain the equivalent of 7% or more of potassium oxalate; the amount decreases with maturity and drying of the plant. The above-listed plants are only eaten in unusual circumstances. Species of **grasses** in the genera *Cenchrus, Panicum*, and *Setaria*, which are widely cultivated in tropical and subtropical areas and accumulate large amounts of oxalate, have also been associated with renal oxalosis in cattle and sheep and with skeletal disease in horses, the latter the result of calcium deficiency (see Vol. 1, Bones and joints).

The **fungi** *Aspergillus niger* and *A. flavus* can produce large quantities of oxalates on feedstuffs. Large doses of **ascorbic acid** (vitamin C) have caused oxalate nephrotoxicosis in humans and in a goat; ascorbic acid is a metabolic precursor of oxalate. **Primary hyperoxaluria,** a rare inherited metabolic condition, occurs in humans, cats (inbred colony of domestic shorthairs), dogs (families of Tibetan Spaniels, and Shih Tzu), and in Beefmaster cattle (likely autosomal recessive). **Pyridoxine (vitamin B₆)** deficiency and **methoxyflurane** anesthesia can also cause renal oxalosis.

Mortality rates of 10% may occur in sheep when they graze on almost pure stands of halogeton or of soursob. It is more usual, however, for fatalities to be sporadic. Under natural conditions, sheep may ingest up to 75 g of oxalate a day; *the rumen degrades the salt efficiently by metabolism of oxalate to bicarbonate and carbonates.* Depending on the microbial composition of the rumen, some variation is expected in the ability of ruminal contents to degrade the salt. Cattle are less commonly affected under range conditions than are sheep, but cattle and sheep are equally susceptible to experimental poisoning. Horses are resistant to oxalate-induced nephrotoxicity and succumb to acute gastroenteritis only after receiving unnaturally large amounts of the chemical; they may develop osteodystrophia fibrosa with prolonged exposure.

Chelation of calcium by unmetabolized oxalate in the ingesta contributes to hypocalcemia. Following absorption, oxalates combine with calcium to form insoluble calcium oxalate; hypocalcemic tetany may result. Calcium oxalate may crystallize in vessel lumens or walls, causing vascular necrosis and hemorrhage, or in renal tubules, causing tubular obstruction and ARF. The nephrotoxicity of oxalates involves more than mechanical obstruction, and may be due in part to intracellular chelation of calcium and magnesium and hence interference with oxidative phosphorylation. Clinically, weakness, prostration, and death may follow within 12 hours of ingestion of oxalate-containing plants.

Endogenous oxalates are produced by the degradation of glycine, an important constituent amino acid of collagen and elastin. Uptake of normal dietary oxalate may increase in a variety of enteric diseases (enteric oxalosis). *Oxalosis can be prominent in the kidneys of aborted bovine fetuses,* and may reflect maternal intake of oxalate-containing plants or moldy feed. A few oxalate crystals can frequently be found in scarred tubules in any species; these crystals are usually without significance.

Melamine and cyanuric acid

Outbreaks of nephrotoxicity have been reported in dogs, cats, pigs, and human infants as the result of a combination of melamine and cyanuric acid in pet food, pig feed, and baby formula. The lesion involves the distal nephron, which contains prominent green to gold-brown circular crystals with radiating spokes (Fig. 4-51). Scattered oxalate crystals were also present and secondary to renal failure as opposed to being the cause. Interestingly, prolonged formalin fixation (>6 weeks) led to dissolution of crystals. Although many pets likely ingested the contaminated pet food, only some developed renal failure. The difference in response likely depended on underlying renal disease and urine pH.

Further reading

Cianciolo RE, et al. Clinicopathologic, histologic and toxicologic findings in 70 cats inadvertently exposed to pet food contaminated with melamine and cyanuric acid. J Am Vet Med Assoc 2008;233:729-737.

Dalal RP, et al. Melamine-related kidney stones and renal toxicity. Nat Rev Nephrol 2011;7:267-274.

Poldelski V, et al. Ethylene glycol-mediated tubular injury: identification of critical metabolites and injury pathways. Am J Kidney Dis 2001;38:339-348.

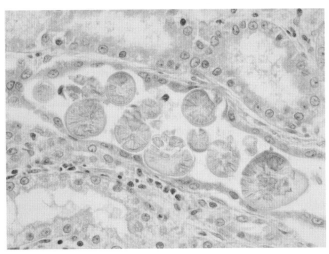

Figure 4-51 Acute tubular injury in a cat that consumed melamine and cyanuric acid in contaminated pet food. Crystals are often circular and gold-brown.

Rahman MM, et al. A review of oxalate poisoning in domestic animals: tolerance and performance aspects. J Anim Physiol Anim Nutr (Berl) 2013;97:605-614.

Mycotoxins

Aspergillus and *Penicillium* spp. produce a number of nephrotoxic mycotoxins, namely, **ochratoxins, citrinin, fumonisin, oxalate,** and **viridicatumtoxin,** which can contaminate feed grains. *Ochratoxin A (OTA)* is the most significant; the toxicity of OTA is enhanced by penicillic acid, which is coproduced by *Penicillium ochraceus*. In pigs, OTA and citrinin produce proximal tubular degeneration and atrophy with cortical interstitial fibrosis, but the renal insufficiency produced is usually subclinical. When ARF does occur, it is manifested by severe perirenal edema resembling that produced by redroot pigweed (*Amaranthus retroflexus*, see later). Ochratoxicosis also increases the susceptibility of pigs to secondary bacterial infections. Ochratoxins are normally degraded in the rumen; thus toxicity is unlikely to occur in ruminants.

Moldy feed also produces mycotoxic nephropathy in horses. *Fumonisins*, mycotoxins produced by *Fusarium* fungi, alter sphingolipid metabolism and cause leukoencephalomalacia in horses and pulmonary edema in pigs; they are hepatotoxic in all species. Fumonisins are nephrotoxic in sheep and cattle; renal lesions include vacuolar change, apoptosis, karyomegaly, and obstruction of proximal tubules.

Further reading

Milićević D, et al. Survey of slaughtered pigs for occurrence of ochratoxin A and porcine nephropathy in Serbia. Int J Mol Sci. 2008;9:2169-2183.
Stoev SD, et al. Experimental mycotoxic nephropathy in pigs provoked by a mouldy diet containing ochratoxin A and fumonisin B1. Exp Toxicol Pathol 2012;64:733-741.

Amaranthus

Ingestion of redroot pigweed, *Amaranthus retroflexus*, causes perirenal edema and ARF in swine and cattle, and uncommonly in horses. The nephrotoxic principle of *A. retroflexus*

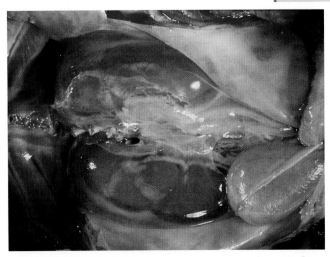

Figure 4-52 Perirenal edema caused by *Amaranthus retroflexus* toxicity in a pig. (Courtesy K. Potter.)

has not yet been identified; plants often contain high levels of nitrate and oxalate, but neither causes the toxic injury and they do not produce perirenal edema. Phenolic compounds have been identified in the leaves of *Amaranthus*, and may be of similar importance to those in *Quercus* spp. (oak, see later). Lush growth of pigweed occurs in early summer, and this plant often dominates the weed growth in disused lots to which animals are moved when other pasture is depleted. Weakness, recumbency, and often death follow 5-10 days after grazing begins.

Grossly, there is marked perirenal edema, which may be blood-stained and may be accompanied by edema of the mesentery, intestinal wall, and ventral abdominal wall, with moderate ascites and hydrothorax (Fig. 4-52). The kidneys are pale but not usually enlarged. Histologically, there is coagulative necrosis of both proximal and distal tubules and intratubular granular casts. There might also be mild glomerular epithelial injury and hypercellularity. The perirenal edema seen in acute cases is apparently the result of tubular backleak, with subsequent lymphatic drainage and leakage into perirenal connective tissue. The probable cause of death is heart failure resulting from hyperkalemia. Survivors may develop interstitial fibrosis and tubular atrophy.

Further reading

Kerr LA, Kelch WJ. Pigweed (*Amaranthus retroflexus*) toxicosis in cattle. Vet Hum Toxicol 1998;40:216-218.

Other plant toxicoses

Poisoning of ruminants and occasionally of horses by *blossoms, buds, leaves, stems, and acorns* of **oak shrubs and trees (*Quercus* spp.)** can occur. There are many species and varieties of oaks, but not all are palatable. They are all potentially poisonous by virtue of the *tannins* they contain, but toxicity is dose dependent. Ingestion of large amounts of the material can cause hydrothorax, ascites, perirenal edema, alimentary tract ulceration, ATI, microscopic hematuria, and death. The toxic substances are *gallotannins*; they are hydrolyzed to tannic acid, gallic acid, and pyrogallol, which appear to be the active toxic metabolites. Binding of tannins to endothelial cells results in *endothelial damage* and leads to perirenal edema, hydrothorax, and ascites. The alimentary lesions result from the binding of oak tannins to peptide bonds, which precipitates protein. The gastrointestinal ulcers are also partly the result of disseminated intravascular coagulation.

In acute oak poisoning, there is marked perirenal edema and hemorrhage. The kidneys are swollen and pale and, in cattle, have cortical hemorrhages of 2-3 mm diameter. Glomeruli are ischemic. After several days, dilation of Bowman's capsule may be present. Necrosis of the epithelium of the proximal tubules can be complete, producing homogeneous casts within the basement membranes. In less severe injury, adjacent groups of tubules may vary considerably in the extent of injury and necrosis. Animals may recover with or without scarring of the renal parenchyma. *The frank necrosis in groups of tubules with intratubular hemorrhage distinguishes the nephrotoxicity of acute oak poisoning from that of most other causes.*

Poisoning by the **yellow-wood tree,** *Terminalia oblongata,* in Australia is reputed to produce lesions similar to those of oak poisoning. Yellow-wood produces at least 2 toxic factors: punicalagin, a tannin that is hepatotoxic, and terminalin, a condensed tannin that is nephrotoxic. In acute yellow-wood poisoning of cattle and sheep, coagulative periacinar hepatic necrosis predominates over the nephrotoxic injury. Subacute and chronic intoxications are characterized by renal fibrosis and atrophy.

Several species of the genus *Isotropis* are toxic to ruminants. In both cattle and sheep, there is abomasitis, enteritis, perirenal edema, and accumulation of fluid in the body cavities and subcutis. Renal lesions are characterized by necrosis of proximal tubular epithelium. In many acute poisonings, there is abundant proteinaceous fluid in Bowman's space.

Various members of the **Liliaceae family** of plants are nephrotoxic in animal species, for example, *Narthecium ossifragum* (bog asphodel) in ruminants, and *Lilium* spp. in cats. Intoxicated cats are polyuric, polydipsic, glucosuric, proteinuric, isosthenuric, and azotemic. In addition to proximal tubular necrosis (eFig. 4-29), cats also have acute pancreatic necrosis and elevated creatine kinase. Ultrastructurally, renal tubules have swollen mitochondria, megamitochondria, and lipid accumulation.

Grapes and raisins contain an unknown toxin that causes proximal renal tubular degeneration and/or necrosis in dogs. Histology reveals the presence of intracellular gold-brown globular pigment that variably stains positively for iron with the Prussian blue stain. Dysregulation of calcium homeostasis might be involved in the pathogenesis because high calcium and high calcium:phosphorus products at the time of presentation are poor prognostic indicators.

Further reading

Eubig PA, et al. Acute renal failure in dogs after the ingestion of grapes or raisins: a retrospective evaluation of 43 dogs (1992-2002). J Vet Intern Med 2005;19:663-674.

Flaoyen A, et al. Tolerance to the nephrotoxic component of *Narthecium ossifragum* in sheep: the effects of repeated oral doses of plant extracts. Vet Res Commun 2001;25:127-136.

Rumbeiha WK, et al. A comprehensive study of easter lily poisoning in cats. J Vet Diagn Invest 2004;16:527-541.

Yoon SS, et al. Natural occurrence of grape poisoning in two dogs. J Vet Med Sci 2011;73:275-277.

Specific tubular dysfunctions

Renal tubular dysfunction may occur secondary to other systemic conditions. For example, glucosuria occurs when the tubular transport for glucose is exceeded in diabetes mellitus and acute enterotoxemia, whereas heavy-metal toxicity causes glucosuria and aminoaciduria because of tubular injury. The primary tubular transport defects identified in domestic animals are *hyperuricosuria in Dalmatian dogs, essential cystinuria, the syndrome of multiple resorptive defects in Basenji dogs, renal tubular acidosis,* and *primary renal glucosuria.* Hyperuricosuria and cystinuria predispose animals to urolithiasis and are discussed in that section.

Basenjis and several other breeds of dogs may develop a *proximal renal tubular disorder* similar to the **Fanconi syndrome** in humans; the condition is hereditary in Basenjis. The syndrome in dogs is characterized by polyuria, polydipsia, hyposthenuria, glucosuria with normoglycemia, hyperphosphaturia, proteinuria, and aminoaciduria. The aminoaciduria may be generalized or limited to cystinuria. Affected dogs have impaired renal tubular resorption of glucose, phosphate, sodium, potassium, uric acid, and amino acids. Research implicates abnormal fluidity of the proximal tubule brush border membrane resulting from significantly increased levels of cholesterol in affected Basenjis compared to normal dogs, and this likely affects the reabsorptive capacity of the proximal tubule. Polyuria results from the glucosuria and natriuresis. The syndrome develops in adult dogs and is usually slowly progressive. Dehydration and acidosis result in renal papillary necrosis, renal failure and death. Histologic renal lesions are nonspecific and include interstitial fibrosis and tubular atrophy. Affected dogs often have marked karyomegaly in scattered tubular cells. Ultrastructural abnormalities have not been noted in tubular cells. Acquired Fanconi syndrome has been reported in dogs in association with gentamicin nephrotoxicity, ethylene glycol nephrotoxicity, primary hypoparathyroidism, and copper storage hepatopathy (Fig. 4-53; eFig. 4-30).

Renal tubular acidosis that is part of the Fanconi syndrome is the most common example in dogs of **proximal, or type II, renal tubular acidosis,** in which proximal tubules fail to resorb filtered bicarbonate. Proximal renal tubular acidosis is usually

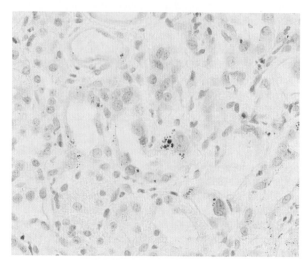

Figure 4-53 Acute tubular injury with karyomegaly in a dog with acquired **Fanconi syndrome.** Rhodanine stain. This case was associated with hepatic copper storage disease, and the rhodanine stain demonstrates small intracytoplasmic red-brown granules.

a self-limiting disease that is not evident clinically. **Distal, or type I, renal tubular acidosis** is caused by defective excretion of hydrogen ions by distal tubules and produces hyperchloremic metabolic acidosis that is more severe than that in the proximal form of renal tubular acidosis. It occurs in dogs, cats, and horses. Untreated distal renal tubular acidosis can result in osteomalacia, nephrocalcinosis, nephrolithiasis, and renal failure.

Primary renal glucosuria may occur as a singular transport abnormality without other defects. This defect is an inherited disorder in Norwegian Elkhounds.

The mannosidoses, hereditary **lysosomal storage diseases,** can cause vacuolation of neurons, renal tubular epithelial, and other cells in humans, cattle, goats, and cats. Salers calves affected with autosomal dominant β-mannosidosis have a variety of neurologic deficits and greatly enlarged kidneys, characterized by marked vacuolation of the cytoplasm of proximal tubular epithelial cells (eFig. 4-31). Although the renal lesion is marked, renal dysfunction is not reported (see Vol. 1, Nervous system). Importantly, similar tubular epithelial vacuolation can be caused by some plant intoxications, for example, *Swainsona, Astragalus, Oxytropis.*

Further reading

Aleman MR, et al. Renal tubular acidosis in horses (1980-1999). J Vet Intern Med 2001;15:136-143.

Appleman E, et al. Transient acquired Fanconi syndrome associated with copper storage of hepatopathy in 3 dogs. J Vet Intern Med 2008;22:1038-1042.

Thompson MF, et al. Acquired proximal renal tubulopathy in dogs exposed to a common dried chicken treat: retrospective study of 108 cases (2007-2009). Aust Vet J 2013;91:368-373.

Yearley JH, et al. Survival time, lifespan, and quality of life in dogs with idiopathic Fanconi syndrome. J Am Vet Med Assoc 2004;225: 377-383.

Pigmentary changes

Following acute hemolytic crises, *the kidneys may be very dark, almost black,* as a consequence of concentrated **hemoglobin** (Fig. 4-54). Initially, the discoloration is uniform, but shortly thereafter the kidneys have small foci of brown discoloration

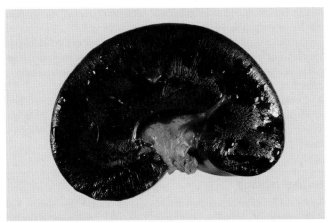

Figure 4-54 Marked discoloration (dark brown to black) of the renal parenchyma in a goat following a **hemolytic crisis in chronic copper poisoning.** (Courtesy E. Clark, D. Russell.)

as the result of retention of hemoglobin in scattered nephron units. The gross lesion is commonly observed in hemolytic crisis of chronic copper poisoning in sheep. Microscopically, the hemoglobin appears as fine red granules in the epithelial cells of the tubules and as red granular casts in the lower nephron, especially the loop of Henle and collecting tubules (see Fig. 4-48). Myoglobin casts are histologically indistinguishable from hemoglobin casts. The same histologic picture occurs following incompatible blood transfusions. In horses, hemoglobinuria resulting from *Acer rubrum* intoxication or neonatal isoerythrolysis should be differentiated from myoglobinuria, which can be seen in trauma, exertional rhabdomyolysis, polysaccharide storage myopathy, or intoxication with drugs (monensin) or plants (e.g., white snakeroot, coffee senna). Hemoglobin and myoglobin pigments persist in tubules after they are no longer detectable in urine samples. Heme proteins (hemoglobin and myoglobin) can reduce renal blood flow and are also cytotoxic. Other factors, such as anemia and dehydration, likely also contribute to renal failure. Tubular obstruction by myoglobin exacerbates ARF in horses with severe rhabdomyolysis.

Hemosiderosis results from chronic hemolytic anemia and from acute hemoglobinuric episodes. The pigment is found in epithelial cells of proximal tubules, where it is produced by the degradation of resorbed hemoglobin. It may be sufficient to produce brown discoloration of the cortex.

Lipofuscinosis of the kidneys of adult cattle is the result of *deposition of brown iron-free pigments* with staining characteristics of lipofuscin. On cut surface, the kidney has radiating dark lines in the cortex, but the medulla is spared. Microscopically, it is present as fine, brown granules in the epithelial cells of the convoluted tubules.

Cloisonné kidney is a nonclinical pigmentary condition in goats. The renal cortices are uniformly brown or black, because of thickening and *brown pigmentation of basement membranes* restricted to the convoluted portions of the proximal tubules. The basement membrane thickening is the result of the deposition of *ferritin and hemosiderin*, which is presumably the result of repeated episodes of intravascular hemolysis.

In congenital **porphyria** of cattle, swine, and cats, the renal cortices are discolored brown. Histologically, the pigment is present in the tubular epithelium and interstitium, and the pigment is excreted in the urine. When exposed to light, the urine develops a port-wine color because of photic activation of porphyrins. Urine and tissues fluoresce blue-green in ultraviolet light.

A *green-yellow pigmentation* of swollen kidneys is common in **icterus** of hepatic origin and less notable in hemolytic icterus unless there is concomitant hepatic injury. It is described in the section Hepatorenal syndromes. Olive-green coloration of the renal cortex is common in newborn lambs, calves, and foals. The pigment is bilirubin, and its presence is probably because of immaturity of hepatic conjugating mechanisms.

Light-green to green-yellow discoloration of renal and other abdominal lymph nodes is occasionally observed in cattle at slaughter. Histologically, numerous red-brown acicular crystals are present in the cytoplasm of renal tubular epithelial cells and hepatocytes. Crystals may be present in renal tubules, and renal calculi are rarely present. The crystals are **2,8-dihydroxyadenine (2,8-DHA)**, a metabolite of the purine adenine. The crystal deposition and pigmentation are of little significance, and the cause of this condition in cattle is unknown. In humans, these pigmented crystals are the result of adenine phosphoribosyltransferase deficiency and may result in urolithiasis. One case of 2,8-DHA urolithiasis has been reported in a dog; management for this disease is similar to that of urate urolithiasis.

Further reading

Agerholm JS, et al. Bovine renal lipofuscinosis: prevalence, genetics and impact on milk production and weight at slaughter in Danish cattle. Acta Vet Scand 2009;51:7.

Agrawal K, et al. Identification of protoxins and a microbial basis for red maple (*Acer rubrum*) toxicosis in equines. J Vet Diagn Invest 2013;25:112-119.

Furrow E, et al. An APRT mutation is strongly associated with and likely causative for 2,8-dihydroxyadenine urolithiasis in dogs. Mol Genet Metab 2014;111:399-403.

Herrera GA. Myoglobin and the kidney: an overview. Ultrastruct Pathol 1994;18:113-117.

Schumacher J. Hematuria and pigmenturia of horses. Vet Clin North Am Equine Pract 2007;23:655-675.

Miscellaneous tubular conditions

Hepatorenal syndrome

The term **hepatorenal syndrome** is applied to *functional renal failure that occurs in human patients with cirrhosis and ascites;* an exact parallel has not yet been identified in domestic animals. Marked renal hypoperfusion results from renal vasoconstriction, which is a manifestation of underfilling of the arterial circulation that occurs subsequent to splanchnic vasodilation. Cirrhosis also leads to an imbalance of vasodilators, for example, nitric oxide, and vasoconstrictors, for example, endothelin. Hypotension may result from the vasodepressor, cardiodepressor, and diuretic effects of cholemia; thus the azotemia in jaundiced patients may be of prerenal origin. Concentrations of bilirubin and bile acids are greatly elevated in the blood, especially in obstructive jaundice. Bile pigment accumulates in tubular epithelial cells, which are frequently swollen. In severe liver dysfunction, bile casts may form in tubules, resulting in so-called *"bile cast nephropathy."* Therefore the renal histology can range from normal, to ATI, to bile casts in tubules. In humans, resolution of the liver disease or liver transplantation will allow the kidneys to regain normal function.

Pseudohepatorenal syndromes include conditions in which liver and kidneys are both affected, but in which renal disease is not secondary to hepatic disease; included are a wide variety of infectious, circulatory, genetic, toxic, and other systemic disorders.

Glycogen accumulation in tubules

In diabetes mellitus in dogs and cats, glycogen accumulates in tubular epithelium, producing marked cytoplasmic clear spaces in the epithelium in the outer medulla and inner cortex. Glycogen can be readily demonstrated by appropriate techniques. The deposition occurs in the ascending limb of the loop of Henle, disappears following insulin administration, and has no effect on renal function.

Nephrogenic diabetes insipidus

This condition has been reported in dogs and foals with polyuria, polydipsia, and hyposthenuria. Affected animals are unresponsive to water deprivation, to exogenous administration of antidiuretic hormone (ADH), and to infusion of hypertonic saline. The basis of the defect is a *lack of responsiveness of the cells of the distal tubules and collecting ducts to ADH.* The defect may be *congenital* (possible X-linked disorder in 2 foals), or *acquired* as the result of tubulointerstitial diseases such as pyelonephritis or hypercalcemic nephropathy, or because of the effect of drugs such as tetracycline. If there is interference with production of ADH by the hypothalamus or ADH release from the posterior pituitary, the disease is referred to as *central or neurogenic diabetes insipidus.*

Hypokalemic nephropathy

Chronic potassium depletion can result in defects in urine concentration and polyuria. Hypokalemia may be caused by diarrhea, adrenal overactivity (hyperaldosteronism), and some renal diseases. Chronic potassium depletion can lead to lymphoplasmacytic tubulointerstitial nephritis and interstitial fibrosis, perhaps because of increased renal ammoniagenesis. Vacuolar change of proximal tubular cells has been reported in ewes deliberately given 11-17 times the recommended dose of *thiabendazole.* Many of the ewes developed hypokalemia, hypoproteinemia, uremia and death; potassium loss was thought to occur through the kidneys. *Corticosteroids* produce hypokalemia and reversible vacuolar change of tubular cells. Hypokalemia may be related to the tubular dilation commonly seen in piglets with *diarrhea* and is related to experimentally induced renal cysts.

Miscellaneous

There are several miscellaneous histologic changes that may be found in renal epithelium. *Some of the* **pyrrolizidine alkaloids** *cause megalocytosis in the proximal tubules.* The lesion is similar in type to that in hepatocytes but less conspicuous and does not cause functional disturbance. Some pyrrolizidine alkaloid-containing plants, particularly *Crotalaria* spp., cause significant glomerular megalocytosis (see Vol. 2, Liver and biliary system).

Occasional nuclei in tubules of old dogs may be polyploid. *In the proximal tubules, eosinophilic, crystalline, intranuclear inclusions* ("brick inclusions") *are commonly encountered in old dogs.* Similar inclusions occur in the liver. Their source is unknown, and they do not cause clinical disease. Their significance is the result of their similarity to certain heavy metal inclusions. *Subacute* **lead poisoning** *produces amorphous acid-fast inclusion material in proximal tubular epithelial nuclei that are large, pale, and vesicular.*

Large, eosinophilic, intranuclear inclusions occur in hepatocytes and renal collecting duct epithelial cells in goats. The pathogenesis of this **nuclear glycogenosis** is unknown, and it does not appear to be of functional significance.

Eosinophilic intracytoplasmic inclusion bodies have been reported in the renal collecting duct epithelial cells of dogs. The inclusions consisted of **iridovirus** particles, and the infection was not clinically significant.

Further reading

Betjes MG, Bajema I. The pathology of jaundice-related renal insufficiency: cholemic nephrosis revisited. J Nephrol 2006;19: 229-233.

Cohen M, Post GS. Water transport in the kidney and nephrogenic diabetes insipidus. J Vet Intern Med 2002;16:510-517.

Guevara M, Arroyo V. Hepatorenal syndrome. Expert Opin Pharmacother 2011;12:1405-1417.

Van Slambrouck CM, et al. Bile cast nephropathy is a common pathologic finding for kidney injury associated with severe liver dysfunction. Kid Int 2013;84:192-197.

TUBULOINTERSTITIAL DISEASES

This term comprises *diseases that involve primarily the interstitium and tubules,* and acknowledges that inflammatory and degenerative interstitial diseases almost always impair tubular function. Hence **interstitial nephritis** and **pyelonephritis** are classified as tubulointerstitial diseases. There is obviously overlap with the previous category of ATI, because animals often develop secondary interstitial inflammation and fibrosis. *Tubulointerstitial nephritis can be caused by a vast array of agents,* including infections, toxins, immunologic disorders, chemicals, and therapeutic drugs. Clinically, tubulointerstitial diseases usually result in impaired urine concentrating ability or specific tubular defects of resorption or secretion.

Histologic features of tubulointerstitial diseases include interstitial inflammation, interstitial fibrosis, and tubular dilation and atrophy. Pyelonephritis is usually caused by infectious agents, although they may not be identified, especially in chronic cases. Interstitial nephritis can be the result of infectious or noninfectious inflammatory conditions. Acute kidney injury, including glomerulonephritis, leads to release of a wide array of cytokines and growth factors from tubular epithelial cells and peritubular capillaries, resulting in interstitial inflammation and ongoing tubulointerstitial damage. Monocytes are recruited, interstitial fibroblasts are activated, interstitial myofibroblasts appear, and fibrosis ensues. Glomerular diseases can incite the above sequence of events through the action of filtered proteins on tubular epithelial cells. On the other hand, injury to glomeruli may occur secondarily in tubulointerstitial disease because of the interdependence of renal structures. In any case, *destructive fibrosis and nephron loss underlie progressive renal disease.*

The hallmark of glomerular disease is persistent proteinuria, whereas tubulointerstitial diseases are more likely to demonstrate defects of concentrating ability or specific tubular defects of resorption or secretion. However, the end point of both classes of renal disease is decompensated renal failure with isosthenuria and uremia.

Immunologically mediated tubulointerstitial disease has been identified in humans, and rarely in domestic animals. Hypersensitivity reactions occur to a variety of drugs, for example, methicillin. Tubular immune-complex disease occurs in some humans with lupus nephritis and glomerulonephritis, indicating that autoantibodies might cross-react with glomerular and tubular basement membranes; antitubular basement membrane autoantibody has been identified in a dog.

Nonsuppurative interstitial nephritis

Focal lymphohistiocytic inflammation with slight scarring is common in kidneys. The causes are seldom known and probably not specific; some lesions may be primarily inflammatory and some may be foci of antigen persistence. Nonsuppurative interstitial nephritis may be acute or chronic, and multifocal or generalized, depending upon the intensity of the insult and the efficiency of the host's responses. **Acute interstitial nephritis** is characterized by acute clinical onset, and histologically by *interstitial edema, leukocytic infiltration, and focal tubular necrosis.* In **chronic interstitial nephritis,** *there is mononuclear cell infiltration, interstitial fibrosis, and generalized tubular atrophy.* Many infectious agents are capable of causing nonsuppurative interstitial nephritis. Unfortunately, agents are often not identified, especially in chronic cases.

Interstitial nephritis is common in dogs and cats, both as a primary disease and secondary to glomerular diseases. In normal dogs, expression of major histocompatibility complex (MHC) class II molecules is usually limited to interstitial dendritic cells. In dogs with chronic tubulointerstitial nephritis, the tubular epithelial cells and peritubular capillary endothelial cells also expressed MHC class II molecules, and the expression correlates to the degree of proteinuria.

Leptospira interrogans serovars *canicola* and *icterohaemorrhagiae* have been associated with acute generalized interstitial nephritis in dogs, although their importance has declined because of the efficacy of vaccination. According to serologic evidence, leptospirosis is common in domestic animals and, in severe cases, interstitial nephritis occurs. In survivors of acute infections, there may be marked interstitial fibrosis and tubular atrophy. Diffuse interstitial nephritis is less common in large domestic animals than in dogs; the usual end result of leptospirosis in cattle and swine is multifocal interstitial nephritis. Leptospirosis is discussed in detail later.

Encephalitozoon cuniculi, an obligate intracellular microsporidian parasite, causes diffuse nonsuppurative to granulomatous interstitial nephritis and granulomatous encephalitis in immature dogs and rabbits. The renal lesion is characterized by heavy, almost pure, interstitial infiltrates of plasma cells. The gram-positive organisms occur in tubular epithelial cells, tubular lumens, and vessel walls. The disease is discussed in Vol. 1, Nervous system.

The best-known form of multifocal nonsuppurative interstitial nephritis is the *"white-spotted kidney"* of calves. It is common and is largely an incidental finding in young calves that can progress to scar tissue with advancing age. The cause is usually undetermined but is thought to be the result of bacteremia; *Escherichia coli* can occasionally be recovered from the lesions. *Salmonella* and *Brucella* are other suggested causes. Affected kidneys contain multiple small white nodules of up to 1 cm diameter throughout the cortex. Larger nodules may bulge from the capsular surface of the kidney and adhere to the capsule (Fig. 4-55; eFig. 4-32). Histologically, the initial

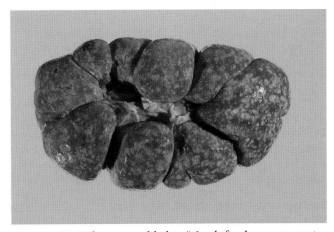

Figure 4-55 "White-spotted kidney" (multifocal nonsuppurative interstitial nephritis) from a calf. (Courtesy J.J. van der Lugt.)

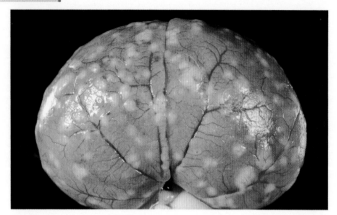

Figure 4-56 Perivascular pyogranulomatous nephritis in a cat with feline infectious peritonitis. (Courtesy R. Kohnken.)

lesion is a microabscess, which is soon replaced by numerous lymphocytes and occasional plasma cells and macrophages. Progressive fibrosis results in healing by scar tissue. The inflammation and scarring may cause tubular obstruction and/or atrophy.

Multifocal interstitial nephritis also occurs in cattle during the course of *malignant catarrhal fever, theileriosis, and lumpy-skin disease*. It can also be seen in a fatal *autosomal recessive disorder* in Japanese Black cattle (Wagyu) resulting from a null mutation of *claudin-16* gene (analogous to *paracellin-1* in humans), which is a tight junction protein expressed between tubular epithelial cells. Affected cattle are azotemic and proteinuric and have increased urinary magnesium excretion but normal serum magnesium levels. Homozygous animals usually die before 6 months of age, and there is marked interstitial inflammation and zonal fibrosis with cystically dilated tubules and Bowman's capsules. The relationship between the genetic mutation, abnormal magnesium dynamics, interstitial inflammation, and cystic tubules has not been clearly elucidated.

Interstitial nephritis is also seen in sheep infected with *sheep-pox* and *maedi-visna virus*, and the latter infection can also cause MPGN. In the horse, it has been associated with *equine infectious anemia*. The renal lesions do not contribute significantly to the course of these diseases, but are diagnostically important. Their gross and histologic features are given elsewhere. Multifocal pyogranulomatous lesions are a rather consistent finding in the kidneys of cats with *feline infectious peritonitis* (Fig. 4-56). *Canine herpesvirus* (Fig. 4-57) produces severe necrotizing nephritis as part of the systemic disease in puppies (see Vol. 3, Female genital system). Other causes of nonsuppurative interstitial nephritis in dogs include *Leishmania* spp., *Borrelia burgdorferi*, *Hepatozoon canis*, and *canine adenovirus 1*.

Cattle and horses grazing *vetch (Vicia* spp.) can develop dermatitis, diarrhea, and ill-thrift and develop lesions in skin, kidney, and other internal organs, characterized by multifocal eosinophilic granulomatous inflammation. Similar lymphocytic to lymphogranulomatous lesions are reported in cattle fed *citrus pulp*.

Suppurative interstitial nephritis

Bacterial infection of the kidneys may be either **hematogenous** or **ascending from the lower urinary tract**. The former causes embolic suppurative nephritis, whereas the latter

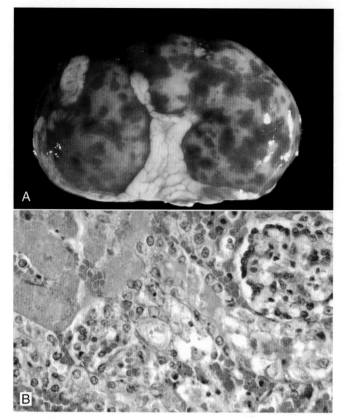

Figure 4-57 A. Multifocal renal cortical hemorrhages in a puppy infected with canid herpesvirus 1. **B.** Histology reveals **segmental tubular necrosis** and interstitial hemorrhage. (**A, B.** Courtesy L. Fry.)

causes pyelonephritis, with inflammation in both the pelvis and renal parenchyma.

Adenoviral infection of sheep primarily causes pneumonia, but also can cause mild, multifocal, suppurative interstitial nephritis, with characteristic large, basophilic, intranuclear inclusion bodies in endothelial and/or interstitial cells. Two young horses from the same farm succumbed to **equine polyomavirus infection** of the kidney. There was marked interstitial nephritis and tubulitis. Intranuclear inclusions were identified in tubular epithelial cells, with the distal nephron being primarily affected (Fig. 4-58). Immunohistochemistry revealed viral infection of most organs in one horse, whereas infection was limited to the kidney and a few cells of the gastrointestinal tract in the other. Immunosuppression in human renal transplant recipients puts them at risk of developing polyomaviral and adenoviral infections of the allograft kidney, indicating that immunocompromised states can predispose to these infections.

Embolic nephritis

This is analogous to abscess formation in any organ, and occurs when bacteria are seeded in the kidneys in the course of bacteremia or septic thromboembolism. Bacteria alone or in small septic emboli lodge mainly in glomerular and peritubular capillaries, and may produce variably sized abscesses. Larger emboli lodge in arteries, producing unilateral or bilateral septic infarcts.

Many bacteria undoubtedly pass through the glomerular capillary walls into the tubules, where they are probably

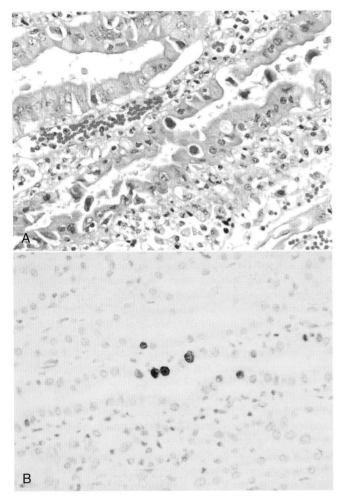

Figure 4-58 A. Acute tubular injury in a horse infected with **equine polyomavirus,** with intranuclear inclusions in epithelial cells of the distal nephron. **B.** As in **A,** immunostained with an antibody against polyomavirus antigens. (Courtesy S. Jennings, V. Nickeleit.)

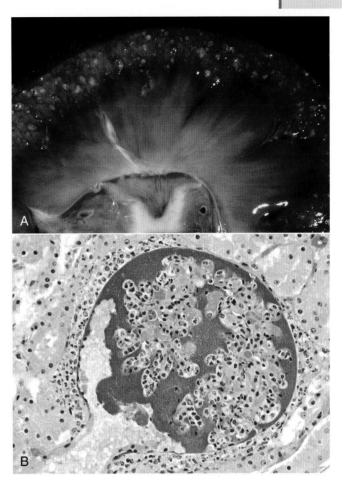

Figure 4-59 A. *Actinobacillus equuli* **embolic nephritis** in a foal. (Courtesy K. Potter.) **B.** Histopathology reveals myriad cocci in Bowman's space of glomerulus.

harmless unless there is stasis of urine. Abscesses are generally cortical rather than medullary; however, gram-negative enterobacteria can cause microscopic suppurative foci in the medulla. Healing of suppurative lesions occurs by scar formation.

In **horses,** the most common cause of embolic suppurative nephritis is *Actinobacillus equuli*, which is acquired *in utero*, during parturition, or shortly after birth as an umbilical infection. Death may occur because of fulminating septicemia. In foals that survive for several days, microabscesses are seen in the kidneys and other organs, and polyarthritis is present (Fig. 4-59; eFig. 4-33). The abscesses are usually green-yellow foci of up to 3 mm. The most common cause of embolic nephritis in **swine** is probably *Erysipelothrix rhusiopathiae*. Embolic glomerulonephritis may be seen grossly as glomerular hemorrhages. Microabscesses form in the interstitium. In adult **cattle,** most cases are caused by *Trueperella pyogenes* from valvular endocarditis, the septic emboli often producing large, randomly distributed abscesses and infarcts. In **sheep and goats,** renal abscesses caused by *Corynebacterium pseudotuberculosis* are common. In **dogs,** systemic protothecosis often involves the kidneys and is likely embolic. *Prototheca zopfii* organisms have been identified in glomerular capillaries, interstitial granulomas, and urine (eFig. 4-34).

Further reading

Angelopoulou K, et al. Detection of maedi-visna virus in the kidneys of naturally infected sheep. J Comp Pathol 2006;134:329-335.

Canaud G, Bonventre JV. Cell cycle arrest and the evolution of chronic kidney disease from acute kidney injury. Nephrol Dial Transplant 2014 Jul 12. pii: gfu230. [Epub ahead of print].

Drolet R, et al. Infectious agents identified in pigs with multifocal interstitial nephritis at slaughter. Vet Rec 2002;150:139-143.

Hirano T, et al. Null mutation of PCLN-1/Claudin-16 results in bovine chronic interstitial nephritis. Genome Res 2000;10:659-663.

Jennings S, et al. Polyomavirus-associated nephritis in 2 horses. Vet Pathol 2013;50:769-774.

Pressler BM, et al. Urinary tract manifestations of protothecosis in dogs. J Vet Intern Med 2005;19:115-119.

Uzal FA, et al. A study of "white spotted kidneys" in cattle. Vet Microbiol 2002;86:369-375.

Leptospirosis

Leptospirosis is an important, complex spirochetal infection of animals and humans caused by serovars of *Leptospira interrogans. It is particularly important as a cause of abortion and stillbirth in farm animals but also causes acute disease (septicemia, hepatitis, nephritis, meningitis) in these and other animals.* Many aspects of leptospirosis are poorly understood because of epidemiologic factors, difficulties in diagnosis, and the complexities of host-leptospiral relationships. Although generalizations are helpful, leptospirosis may best be understood in terms of the individual relationship between specific serovars and particular host species.

Leptospirosis can be caused by any of the ~250 serovars belonging to the 25 serogroups of what used to be recognized as one species, *Leptospira interrogans* (sensu lato), but which now contains 9 species of pathogenic, 5 intermediate, and 6 saprophytic species of *Leptospira*. Unfortunately, neither serogroup nor serovar reliably predicts the species of *Leptospira*, because the same serogroup (i.e., shares some common antigenic determinants) or serovar (i.e., antigenically indistinguishable isolate) may occur within 2 or more species. Thus some genetically unrelated leptospires can be antigenically identical. For example, serovar *hardjo* is found within *L. borgpetersenii*, *L. interrogans*, and *L. meyeri*. Serotyping is increasingly being replaced by restriction enzyme analysis of chromosomal DNA to identify "genotypes." Thus, using the same example, genotyping has divided serovar *hardjo* into 2 distinct types, hardjo-bovis and hardjoprajitno, (which correspond with the species *L. borgpetersenii and L. interrogans*, respectively) and they differ in geographic distribution and virulence. Restriction enzyme analysis has also assigned most North American serovar *pomona* isolates to genotype kennewicki, and further identified pig-associated and cattle-associated subtypes. The scheme used in this section is to use the species and serovar name with genetic type (e.g., *Leptospira borgpetersenii* serovar *hardjo*) where relevant.

Although many serovars are recognized globally, only a limited number are usually endemic to a particular region (Table 4-2). Geographic differences in the distribution of serovars are marked, but the true incidence and prevalence of leptospirosis are largely undetermined for most countries and regions. Serologic surveys tend to be flawed because antigens chosen may not represent serovars present in the country, because serologic prevalence does not necessarily indicate disease significance, because sampling is often done on the basis of convenience rather than in a carefully designed manner, and because titers designated as "significant" (usually ≥1:100 in the microscopic agglutination test [MAT]) may

underestimate the true seroprevalence of some host-adapted serovars.

Each serovar is adapted to and may cause disease in particular "maintenance" hosts, although they may cause disease in other species, the "incidental" hosts. The general distinctions between these types of host are shown in Table 4-3. *The natural reservoir of pathogenic leptospires is the proximal convoluted tubules of the kidney and, in certain maintenance hosts, the genital tract.*

In maintenance hosts particularly, transmission may be direct, that is, through contact with urine, postabortion discharges, milk, or through venereal or transplacental transmission. Infection of incidental hosts is often indirect, via environmental contamination by urine of carrier animals. Optimal conditions for survival of leptospires are moist, warm (optimal 28° C), and neutral or mildly alkalinized. Under ideal conditions, leptospires may survive weeks or months in waterlogged soil ("mud fever") or stagnant water. Under adverse conditions, survival is measured in minutes. *Leptospirosis thus occurs especially in the autumn in temperate climates ("fall fever"), and in the winter in tropical climates.*

Leptospires penetrate exposed mucosal surfaces or water-softened skin and disseminate throughout the body. Leptospiremia lasts up to 7 days. Organisms multiply especially well in the liver, kidneys, lungs, placenta, udder, and cerebrospinal fluid. Development of agglutinating and opsonizing antibody ~6 days after infection clears the organisms from most organs except immunologically privileged sites (i.e., proximal convoluted tubules of the kidney, cerebrospinal fluid, vitreous humor of the eye). Certain serovars can also survive in the genital tract of maintenance hosts.

Most leptospiral infections are supposedly subclinical, particularly in nonpregnant and nonlactating animals, and can only be detected by the presence of antibody or *minor lesions of interstitial nephritis at slaughter.* Infection may also cause *acute or subacute systemic disease* (i.e., nephritis, hepatitis, endotoxemia, hemoglobinuria) during the leptospiremic phase. After leptospiremia has ceased, *chronic disease* can manifest as abortion, stillbirth, infertility, or recurrent uveitis.

Acute and severe disease can occur in the leptospiremic phase, particularly in young animals. Clinical disease may be

Table • 4-2

Common leptospiral serovars of disease significance in domestic animals

Serovar	Maintenance host	Distribution	Species disease significance
autumnalis	Rodents	Global, tropics especially	+ ?Dogs
bratislava	Pigs, horses (dogs?)	Global	+ + + + Pigs + + + Horses, dogs
canicola	Dogs	Global	+ + + Dogs + All species
grippotyphosa	Raccoon, skunk, small rodents	Global	+ + Dogs + All species
hardjo type hardjo-bovis type hardjoprajitno	Cattle, sheep Cattle	Global Global? (some exceptions)	+ + Cattle, sheep + + + Cattle, sheep
icterohaemorrhagiae	Rats	Global? (some exceptions)	+ + + Dogs, humans
pomona type kennewicki	Pigs	Global? (some exceptions)	+ + + + Pigs + + + Cattle, all species
tarassovi	Wildlife, cattle, pigs	Europe, Australasia	+ + + Pigs

Kidney

Table • 4-3

General distinctions between maintenance and incidental hosts in leptospiral infection

Characteristic	Maintenance host	Incidental host
Susceptibility to infection by the serovar	+ + + +*	+ +
Endemic transmission within host species	+ + + +	+
Pathogenicity for the host	+ +	+ + +
Type of disease caused	Chronic, reproductive loss especially, nephritis	Acute or chronic
Persistence in kidney	+ + + +	+
Persistence in genital tract	+ + + (*bratislava, hardjo*)	-
Microscopic agglutinating antibody response	Low titer, sometimes nil	High titer
Efficacy of vaccination in controlling losses	± to + + + +	+ + + +
Examples:	Pig, *bratislava, pomona;* Dog, *canicola*	Pigs and cattle, *canicola, grippotyphosa;* Cattle, *pomona*

*Arbitrary scale for comparison.

characterized by fever, jaundice, hemolytic anemia, hemoglobinuria, pulmonary congestion, or occasionally meningitis. Capillary injury is caused by inflammatory cytokine release. *Jaundice* is a common manifestation of acute disease and might be the result of hemolysis from hemolysin production or because of toxic and/or ischemic hepatocellular injury. *Anemia* is initially the result of bacterial hemolysins but may later be the result of intravascular hemolysis caused by reaction of antibodies with leptospiral products coating red blood cells. Postsepticemic localization of leptospires in the kidneys is associated with focal or diffuse *interstitial nephritis and acute, transient tubular injury.*

Renal failure is a clinically recognized consequence of infection with *canicola* and other serovars in dogs, but is not often described in other animals, even though interstitial nephritis, especially in pigs, can be extensive. *Interstitial nephritis can be caused by all serovars.* Leptospires reach the kidney hematogenously and migrate randomly, persist briefly in the interstitium, and enter tubules at all levels of the nephron. Once antibody develops, the leptospires localize to the proximal convoluted tubules, where they may multiply. The physiologic changes to glomerular filtrate in the distal nephron damage leptospires. The *interstitial phase* is accompanied by marked vascular alterations that produce hyperemia, edema, and endothelial swelling. Tubular epithelial necrosis is likely the combined result of multiple factors, including hypoxia resulting from hypovolemia and hemolysis; bacterial toxins, including lipo-oligosaccharides and sphingomyelinases; free hemoglobin; and interstitial inflammation. Leptospiral antigen is demonstrable by immunoperoxidase staining in tubular epithelial cell phagosomes, and is the counterpart of minute, round, black spherical bodies seen with silver stains. By 2 weeks, the tubular changes are accompanied by *interstitial infiltration of plasma cells and lymphocytes,* which may be focal or diffuse. Leptospiral antigen is present in peritubular macrophages. The renal lesions may be clinically insignificant or might result in various degrees of renal insufficiency/failure.

Abortion, stillbirth, or the birth of congenitally infected young may occur weeks to months after maternal leptospiremia and is the most important form of the disease in ruminants and pigs. Serovar *bratislava* may also cause infertility in swine, as

may serovar *hardjo* infection in cattle. Horses are particularly likely to develop *recurrent uveitis* ("periodic ophthalmia") following serovar *pomona* infection, but uveitis can develop in other species following leptospirosis.

Leptospires are delicate, slender spirochetes (6-20 × 0.1 µm), with hooked ends like question marks, which led to the name *L. interrogans.* They do not stain with the usual aniline bacterial dyes but may be stained by Giemsa or, in tissue, by silver-impregnation techniques of Levaditi or Warthin-Starry. Dark-field microscopy of fluids is generally used in routine laboratory study. *Demonstration of leptospires by dark-field microscopy and silver staining of tissue sections are insensitive methods that give both false-negative and false-positive results. Immunofluorescence* of urine or of homogenates of tissues (e.g., fetal lung and kidney, or placenta) is an excellent diagnostic technique, almost equivalent in sensitivity to isolation in experienced laboratories. Difficulties may be experienced with serovar *bratislava* because of the small size of these organisms. *PCR-based diagnosis* will increasingly challenge IF as the diagnostic method of choice. A number of PCR procedures are available, which generally are more reliable for urine than for tissues. Leptospires die readily in tissues or body fluids unless kept at 4° C. Results may be improved if tissues are submitted to laboratories in leptospiral transport medium.

Culture is expensive and often time consuming, and usually restricted to highly specialized laboratories. *The microscopic agglutination test (MAT),* which is serovar specific and to some extent serogroup specific, has been a mainstay of diagnostic approaches to leptospirosis and is often made by comparison of acute to convalescent titers. In the diagnosis of abortion, the MAT suffers sometimes from the low titers that may occur with host-adapted serovars in their maintenance host, and also from difficulties in interpretation of titers. These may fail to rise between acute and convalescent phases because abortion may follow many weeks after infection in a maintenance host. In fetuses, MAT on fetal fluids is often a useful diagnostic approach, but dilutions should start at 1:10.

Cattle

Species and serovars of major importance are *L. borgpetersenii* serovar *hardjo* type hardjo-bovis and *pomona* type kennewicki in North America, and, in Europe, *L. interrogans* serovar *hardjo* type hardjoprajitno and *L. borgpetersenii* serovar *hardjo* type hardjo-bovis. There is serologic evidence of infection with other serovars, including *canicola, grippotyphosa,* and *icterohaemorrhagiae,* among others. These latter serovars are not often implicated in disease, although geographic variations will occur. Serovar *hardjo* has become increasingly recognized with a concomitant, apparent decline in importance of serovar *pomona.* Cattle and sheep are reservoir hosts for *hardjo.* Serovar *hardjo* type hardjoprajitno, which is recognized in Europe but not in North America or Australia and New Zealand, appears to be more virulent than type hardjo-bovis. In Northern Ireland, where serovar *hardjo* type hardjoprajitno occurs, *hardjo* was recognized in one study as responsible for nearly half of all abortions. This type was isolated from most aborted or stillborn fetuses, whereas type hardjo-bovis was mainly isolated from the kidney and genital tract of carrier cows. In one large study in Ontario, Canada, where only hardjo-bovis rather than hardjoprajitno is thought to occur, serovar *hardjo* was identified in about 6% of abortions; no serovar *pomona* was recognized.

The most severe (but uncommon) manifestation of acute infection occurs in calves infected with incidental serovars, especially *pomona.* Hemoglobinuria is usually the first sign and may be transient. In fatal cases, the urine is a port-wine color. Hematuria from hemorrhage into renal tubules may lead to blood clots in the urinary tract. There is fever, anemia, icterus, dyspnea because of pulmonary congestion, and occasionally meningitis. Albuminuria and bilirubinuria can be severe. In cows, agalactia with small quantities of discolored, viscous milk is also typical. Abortion may occur during the acute phase or several weeks later during convalescence. The fetus is frequently decomposed, indicating death some time before abortion.

The most common form of the disease is a less severe, "subacute" form characterized in dairy cows by a 2-10 day drop in milk production with transient pyrexia. In this "milk drop syndrome," the milk has the consistency of colostrum, with thick clots and yellow discoloration, and the udder is soft. This form is commonly associated with serovar *hardjo* type hardjoprajitno, but may be caused by all serovars. Hemoglobinuria is uncommon in milder infections.

The chronic form of the disease, most commonly associated with serovars *hardjo* and *pomona* in pregnant cows, is seen as abortion, stillbirth, or the birth of premature and weak infected calves as the result of infection of the fetus. The cow may have had an episode of illness up to 6 weeks *(pomona)* or 12 weeks *(hardjo)* earlier.

The postmortem appearance of an animal that dies of acute leptospirosis is characterized by mild icterus and severe anemia. Hemorrhages may be absent, or ecchymoses may be numerous on serous membranes and in the subcutis. The lungs are pale and edematous, and the liver is enlarged, friable, pale tan-yellow, with or without hemorrhages and small zones of necrosis around central veins. Massive hepatocellular necrosis is not typical. Hemoglobinuria may or may not be present. Kidneys are swollen. During a hemolytic crisis, they are diffusely dark red-brown, but later there is restriction of pigment to small groups of tubules, resembling numerous small hemorrhages grossly. Still later, the kidneys may have numerous small gray foci that are rather indistinct and more numerous in the cortex than in the medulla. It is doubtful that cattle die from chronic leptospiral interstitial nephritis. In animals that

have recovered from the acute disease, foci of renal inflammation might be the only morphologic traces remaining. Although leptospiral infection has been implicated in the pathogenesis of "white-spotted kidneys" in neonatal calves, various studies have implicated other pathogens or excluded leptospires as an etiology.

The histologic changes in most cases of bovine leptospirosis may be mild and nonspecific. There may be mild multifocal pulmonary edema and periacinar hepatocellular necrosis (from anemia). Kupffer cells are increased in number and contain excessive amounts of hemosiderin. There is diffuse but mild cellular infiltration in the portal triads. In the uncommon infections caused by *icterohaemorrhagiae,* necrosis in the liver and dissociation of hepatic cords may occur. Depending on the stage of the infection and degree of hemolysis, biliary canaliculi may contain bile plugs.

In acutely fatal disease, there are often marked degenerative changes in the epithelium of the cortical renal tubules. The changes vary in severity from acute cellular swelling to necrosis and desquamation. The desquamated epithelium forms granular and cellular casts, in addition to the protein, red blood cell, and pigment casts. There is also interstitial edema with mild diffuse infiltration of plasma cells, and lymphocytes (Fig. 4-60A). *In acute disease, organisms can often be demonstrated by appropriate stains in the liver,* in which they are partly intracellular, *and in the kidneys,* in which they occur in the tubular epithelium and frequently as clusters in the tubular lumen (Fig. 4-60B).

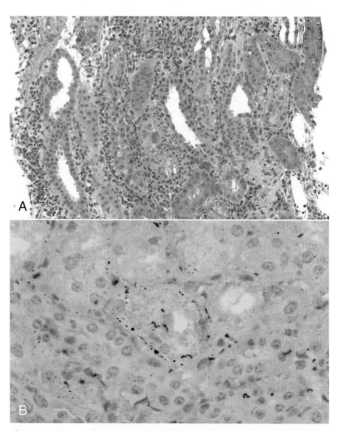

Figure 4-60 A. Severe neutrophilic and histiocytic tubulointerstitial nephritis in a dog with acute leptospirosis. **B. Leptospires** in a bovine kidney demonstrated by immunohistochemical staining. (Courtesy J. Ramsay.)

After recovery from acute disease and in subclinical illness, organisms localize in *microcolonies in the kidneys* and appear as intratubular aggregates; it is rare to find organisms in the interstitium. *There are widespread foci of interstitial nephritis.* The nonsuppurative inflammatory reaction is virtually confined to the cortex, and lymphocytes and plasma cells predominate. The reaction subsides slowly, and inflammatory cells decrease in number as the lesions scar. An odd feature of active lesions is an atypical regenerative pattern of tubular epithelium within the areas of inflammation wherein regenerating cells produce a few bizarre syncytia or a few giant cells.

Aborted fetuses show no specific changes, although the organism can often be demonstrated in fetal tissues (see Vol. 3, Female genital system). The fetuses are sometimes edematous, and in many cases, there is advanced autolysis or putrefaction by the time the fetus is aborted. The placenta may show mild placentitis; there is a tendency for it to be unduly retained.

Sheep, goats, and deer

Sheep, goats, and deer may be less susceptible than cattle to clinical leptospirosis. The major serovar in sheep is *hardjo*, which has a maintenance cycle independent of cattle. Acute disease in lambs resembles that of calves (eFig. 4-36). *Hardjo* infection of ewes may cause late-term abortion, stillbirth, weak lambs, and agalactia. Leptospirosis in goats is not often described, but clinical and pathologic changes are similar to those described for cattle. Fatal nephritis of farmed young red deer caused by serovar *pomona* has been described in New Zealand. Kidneys were markedly enlarged because of severe chronic active cortical interstitial nephritis.

Dogs

Dogs are susceptible to infection with a number of serovars, but those best recognized to cause severe diseases are *canicola* and *icterohaemorrhagiae*. *Canicola* is host maintained in the dog, but widespread use of vaccination has virtually eradicated this infection from dogs in many countries. *Icterohaemorrhagiae* is generally acquired from rats, and other serovars (*autumnalis, bratislava, pomona*) from their respective hosts (see Table 4-2). Serologic evidence of infection with serovar *bratislava* is increasingly recognized, and this organism may cause nephritis and abortion in dogs; it has been suggested that this serovar is host adapted to the dog, pig, and horse. Clinical infections with serovars *canicola* and *icterohaemorrhagiae* are now usually rare because of vaccination, but infection with other serovars may be under-reported. In recent years, leptospirosis in urban dogs has resurged in northeastern North America and elsewhere, associated with *grippotyphosa, pomona*, possibly *autumnalis*, and rarely other serovars acquired from urban wildlife. Clinically normal dogs can shed pathogenic leptospires in urine, which may pose a zoonotic risk. Serologic testing is a poor predictor of urinary shedding. Current *canicola*- and *icterohaemorrhagiae*-based vaccines provide only serovar-specific protection.

As a generalization, *icterohaemorrhagiae* exerts its effect predominantly on the liver, whereas *canicola* damages the kidney, although there may be overlap in the clinical presentations. Other serovars can affect both organs, although disease is usually less severe.

Hyperacute infection, which is usually seen in puppies and caused by *icterohaemorrhagiae*, causes fulminant septicemia; death occurs in a few hours to 2-3 days. There is fever, dehydration, hypersensitivity, hematemesis, melena, epistaxis, and petechiae on the mucous membranes. Icterus is usually absent in hyperacute infection, whereas it is prominent in *acute disease*, and may be the first abnormality observed. Fevers are usually mild.

Widespread hemorrhages characterize both the hyperacute and the acute disease. The most consistent gross lesions in acute cases consist of *subcapsular renal cortical hemorrhages*. With chronicity, these foci become pale tan, and the capsule adheres to the cortex. Lesions in dogs given viable *canicola* and killed 100 days later consisted of symmetrically enlarged kidneys with nodular and wedge-shaped lesions 4-8 mm in diameter at the corticomedullary junction. Lesions in the liver of dogs with spontaneous infections of *grippotyphosa* vary from gross enlargement to fibrosis with nodular hyperplasia to atrophy.

In animals dying acutely, focal hepatocellular necrosis is often, but not always, present. *The characteristic change is dissociation of the cells of the hepatic cords, but this is not pathognomonic.* Dissociated cells are discrete and rounded with eosinophilic, coarsely granular cytoplasm, and pyknotic or karyorrhectic nuclear debris. Regeneration is sometimes prominent and evidenced by cytomegaly, binucleation, and mitoses. Kupffer cells contain excess hemosiderin, and many canaliculi contain bile plugs. Organisms can be demonstrated by appropriate techniques in sinusoids and in hepatic epithelial cells. Serovar *grippotyphosa* may cause chronic active hepatitis, with peribiliary fibrosis, lobular disarray, and irregular fibrosis.

In dogs that survive the acute septicemia or fail to manifest a septicemic phase at all, the disease shifts from the liver to the kidneys. This is typical of infections by *canicola* and the incidental serovars (*grippotyphosa, pomona*). Clinical signs are those of *renal insufficiency* and vary in severity and progression. Death may occur rather rapidly from renal failure, but it also appears that initially inapparent infections, particularly with *canicola*, can smolder over the course of years, eventually leading to chronic renal failure from chronic interstitial nephritis (see Fig. 4-60). In these renal syndromes, the lesion caused directly by the leptospires is *acute diffuse interstitial nephritis*, from which the animal may recover or may progress to *subacute and chronic interstitial nephritis*.

In the acute phase, the renal changes are severe but largely characterized by tubular injury rather than inflammation. The brunt of the injury is borne by the convoluted tubules, with epithelial changes ranging from acute cellular swelling to necrosis. The latter may be extensive enough to denude considerable areas of tubular basement membrane. In the course of a couple of days, regeneration begins and atypical syncytial giant cells may form. This is accompanied by interstitial edema and a diffuse but sparse infiltration by lymphocytes and plasma cells. Leptospires are demonstrable in the tubular epithelium and in the lumens of tubules, frequently in clusters. Early on, organisms may be found in any part of the cortex, but later they are restricted to superficial, subcapsular areas. With chronicity, the interstitial inflammation decreases and fibrosis increases. Bowman's capsules may be thickened, and there may be periglomerular fibrosis, although both lesions are nonspecific. Likewise, lesions in the renal medulla are nonspecific and include fibrosis with mild inflammation. Lymph nodes and spleen may be enlarged and edematous or hemorrhagic, and microscopically, there is depletion of lymphocytes and increase of sinusoidal reticular cells. Erythrophagocytosis is prominent.

Although clinical disease is rarely reported in **cats**, there is a wide range of seroprevalence, and cats can shed leptospires in their urine. Furthermore, there was a significant difference in seropositivity between cats with kidney disease (15%) and healthy cats (7%), suggesting a role of exposure in the pathogenesis feline kidney disease. There was not a significant difference in PCR positivity, however. The most commonly detected serovars were *pomona* and *bratislava*.

Swine

Although any leptospiral serovar may cause disease in pigs, until recently the most important serovar recognized in North America was serovar *pomona* (type kennewicki), a subtype of which is host adapted to swine. In Australia and some European countries, *tarassovi* (formerly hyos), another pig-adapted serovar, causes losses as serious as those of *pomona*. More recently, *Leptospira fainei* has been isolated from pigs with reproductive problems in Australia, but its significance remains to be determined. Understanding of leptospirosis in swine is changing rapidly with the recognition of the widespread and dominant prevalence of antibodies to the Australis serogroup and the isolation of *bratislava* and *muenchen* from aborted and stillborn pigs. The role and importance of Australis serogroup leptospires are only partially understood, in part because of the difficulty of isolating these leptospires. Incidental infections with serovars *canicola, grippotyphosa, hardjo,* and other serovars have been locally important. Antibody to *icterohaemorrhagiae* is widespread, but the serovar is of rare disease significance.

Only a small proportion of infected animals develop clinical illness, usually an unrecognized transient episode of mild fever, anorexia, and depression. Hemoglobinuria and icterus may occur rarely in piglets. The principal aspect of the disease in pigs, apart from transmissibility to other species, *is abortion and the birth of small litters of weak piglets*, which may reach outbreak proportions. This is particularly liable to occur if pregnant sows with no acquired immunity are exposed during the second month of pregnancy. Abortion is associated with heavy leptospiral infection of the fetus.

The usual pattern of leptospirosis in pregnant sows, caused by serovars other than those of the Australis serogroup, is for the litter to be delivered 1-3 weeks prematurely, with some of the fetuses dead and some born alive, only to die shortly afterward. Not all aborted fetuses in the litter will yield leptospires. The organism can usually be recovered from the fresher ones, some of which in each litter are expected to have lesions. Straw-colored pleural effusion, somewhat viscid, may be accompanied by effusion of lesser volumes in the other serous cavities. Petechial hemorrhages may be present in the pleura, epicardium, renal cortex, and peripelvic tissue, and occasionally elsewhere. The liver and spleen are swollen and dark, with tan foci of necrosis, 2-5 mm in size, especially near the margins.

Histologic changes are also variable. Hepatitis is acute, consisting of neutrophils and lymphocytes in portal areas and surrounding the foci of coagulative necrosis. Focal nonsuppurative myocarditis with coagulative necrosis is less frequent than mild epicarditis and endocarditis. These latter mononuclear infiltrations can be quite diffuse. In addition to many minor foci of interstitial inflammation in the kidney, there may be large discrete infiltrates of mononuclear cells in the

peripelvic parenchyma, sometimes involving the papilla and encroaching on the adjacent cortex. The medulla may contain myriad organisms. The lesions are not specific for *pomona* infections, as they have also been observed with other serovars.

Infection with serovars belonging to the Australis serogroup produce subtler losses than those described for *pomona* or other serovars, and lesions have not been described. In Northern Ireland and the United States, late-term abortion is uncharacteristic, but stillbirths occur, characterized by the birth of live, dying, and dead piglets within a litter. Diagnosis is problematic because of the extreme difficulty of isolation of serovars *bratislava* and *muenchen*, but approaches include fetal and maternal serology, IF of fetal lung and kidney homogenates, and PCR-based diagnosis.

A distinct *infertility ("repeat breeder") syndrome* associated with Australis serogroup infection has been described in Northern Ireland. Disease is most noticeable in sows bred to infected boars for the first time or when susceptible animals are introduced into infected herds. Serovars *bratislava* and *muenchen* are commonly isolated from the genital tracts of sows and boars in infected herds. Venereal transmission is thought to be common.

The majority of instances of chronic interstitial nephritis in pigs, lesions of which are often observed at slaughter, are leptospiral in origin, particularly associated with serovar *pomona*.

Horses

There is widespread serologic evidence of leptospiral infection in horses, but acute disease is apparently rare. Clinical features include fever, anorexia, depression, and icterus in the acute disease, and abortion, premature foaling, and chronic uveitis ("periodic ophthalmia") in the chronic disease. Horses are maintenance hosts for *bratislava*. Leptospires are involved in fatal hepatic and renal disease in foals, may be important in abortion, and cause immune-mediated chronic uveitis in horses. Acute respiratory distress and failure has been reported in foals and adults, wherein bronchoscopy reveals pulmonary hemorrhages.

Leptospires of a variety of serovars have been isolated or identified by IF in neonatal foals or adults with fatal icterus. Different serovars, including *bratislava, canicola, grippotyphosa, hardjo, icterohaemorrhagiae* but particularly *pomona, may* also cause subacute disease characterized by fever, with or without icterus, in adults. Although of generally minor significance per se, these infections have important chronic sequelae in the form of abortion or chronic uveitis. In North America, serovars in leptospiral equine abortion are *pomona, grippotyphosa,* and *bratislava*. Abortion tends to occur in late gestation. *Giant cell hepatitis in aborted fetuses* has been associated with leptospiral infection; the lesions were characterized by dissociation of hepatocytes, disruption of hepatic cords, and numerous large, multinucleated hepatocytes. The placenta is edematous with necrotic, mineralized villi, and cystic adenomatous hyperplasia of the allantoic epithelium. Leptospires can be demonstrated in the placental villi and stroma.

Recurrent uveitis may develop several months after leptospiral infection, particularly with serovar *pomona*. There is a genetic predisposition for Appaloosas and horses, with the MHC-1 haplotype ELA-A9 being at higher risk, whereas Standardbreds are at lower risk. Following an acute infection, there may be recurrent ocular disease characterized by a thick hyaline membrane at the posterior iris, and the nonpigmented epithelial cells of the ciliary body can contain eosinophilic linear cytoplasmic inclusions. The inflammation can lead to cataracts, synechiae, lens luxation, and retinal detachment. Expression of the leptospiral proteins LruA and LruB in the eye, together with the presence of elevated antibodies against these proteins, has been demonstrated. Because the antibodies in the aqueous humor exceed serum antibody levels, local production is presumed. Furthermore, these antibodies can cross-react with normal ocular components. Specifically, LruA antibodies cross-react with α-crystalline B and vimentin, whereas LruB antibodies cross-react with β-crystalline B2.

Further reading

Azizi S, et al. Evaluation of "white-spotted kidneys" associated with leptospirosis by polymerase chain reaction based LipL32 gene in slaughtered cows. J S Afr Vet Assoc 2012;83:69.

Boutilier P, et al. Leptospirosis in dogs: a serologic survey and case series 1996 to 2001. Vet Ther 2003;4:178-187.

Cerri D, et al. Epidemiology of leptospirosis: observations on serological data obtained by a "diagnostic laboratory for leptospirosis" from 1995 to 2001. New Microbiol 2003;26:383-389.

Faber NA, et al. Detection of *Leptospira* spp. in the aqueous humor of horses with naturally acquired recurrent uveitis. J Clin Microbiol 2001;38:2731-2733.

Harkin KR, et al. Comparison of polymerase chain reaction assay, bacteriologic culture, and serologic testing in assessment of prevalence of urinary shedding of leptospires in dogs. J Am Vet Med Assoc 2003;222:1230-1233.

Prescott JF, et al. Resurgence of leptospirosis in dogs in Ontario: recent findings. Can Vet J 2002;43:955-961.

Rodriguez J, et al. Serologic and urinary PCR survey of leptospirosis in healthy cats and cats with kidney disease. J Vet Intern Med 2014;28:284-293.

Uzal FA, et al. A study of "white spotted kidneys" in cattle. Vet Microbiol 2002;86:369-375.

Verma A, et al. Leptospirosis in horses. Vet Microbiol 2013;167:61-66.

Ward MP, et al. Prevalence of and risk factors for leptospirosis among dogs in the United States and Canada: 677 cases, (1970-1998). J Am Vet Med Assoc 2002;220:53-58.

Pyelonephritis

Pyelonephritis is inflammation of the pelvis and renal parenchyma, usually resulting from infection ascending from the lower urinary tract. Hematogenous pyelonephritis is extremely uncommon. Ascending pyelonephritis is characterized by inflammation, necrosis, and eventually deformity of the calyces, in association with tubulointerstitial inflammation and necrosis. The location distinguishes it from other forms of nephritis. It is usually accompanied by ureteritis and cystitis. In *acute pyelonephritis*, inflammation and necrosis predominate, with the pelvis and medulla being more severely affected than the cortex. In *chronic pyelonephritis*, fibrosis replaces inflammation. In both cases, the disease can be asymmetrical, unilateral, or bilateral. Chronic pyelonephritis produces irregular contracture of the kidneys with pelvic deformities. **Pyonephrosis** denotes severe suppuration of the kidney in the presence of complete or nearly complete ureteral obstruction. The infected hydronephrotic kidney is converted to a sac of pus. Suppuration may extend through the renal capsule during the course of pyelonephritis to produce a **perinephric abscess.**

The pathogenesis of pyelonephritis begins with establishment of infection in the lower urinary tract. Organisms involved in urinary tract infection are usually endogenous bacteria of the bowel and skin, such as *Escherichia coli*, staphylococci, streptococci, *Enterobacter, Proteus,* and *Pseudomonas,* and more specific urinary pathogens, such as *Corynebacterium renale, C. cystitidis,* and *C. pilosum* in cattle, and *Actinobaculum (Eubacterium) suis* in pigs. Mycoplasmas are rarely involved in cattle. Infection can be mixed. *C. renale* is an obligate parasite of urinary mucosae. Fungal infections are rare causes of pyelonephritis in dogs.

Virulence of bacteria in the urinary tract is enhanced by the presence of pili on their surface. Pili assist in adhesion of *C. renale* to urinary epithelium in a pH-dependent manner. The type of pili expressed by the bacteria can also be important later in the course of pyelonephritis. Type 1 fimbriate *E. coli* induce greater activation of neutrophils and hence more renal scarring than do nonfimbriate or P-fimbriate *E. coli.*

One of the *urinary tract defenses* against bacterial infection and colonization is shedding of mature epithelial cells with attached bacteria. Normal voiding of urine helps maintain the sterility of the bladder. Once bacteria enter the bladder, they grow well in urine with low osmolality or alkaline pH. *Stasis of urine* is an important predisposing factor in the pathogenesis of cystitis and of pyelonephritis. Urinary obstruction can be caused by ureteral anomalies in young animals, kinked ureters in pigs, pregnancy, urolithiasis, and prostatic hypertrophy. *Females are predisposed to urinary tract infection* because of their short urethras, urethral trauma, and possibly because of hormonal effects. Clinically, urinary infection is indicated by bloody or cloudy urine, pyuria, and/or bacteriuria.

Once infection is established in the bladder, probably the most significant mechanism in causing renal infection is **vesicoureteral reflux**. This retrograde flow of urine up the ureters and into the kidney *(intrarenal reflux)* during micturition may carry bacteria as far as the urinary space of glomeruli, especially if there is urinary obstruction. It can also occur during manual compression of the bladder in dogs and cats for collection of urine samples. Swine have a long intravesical ureter—5 mm at birth, 36 mm at maturity—that should prevent reflux in mature animals. Transient vesicoureteral reflux is common in puppies and is related to the immaturity of the ureterovesical junction, wherein pressure in the bladder overcomes the vesicoureteral valve. Reflux should decrease with age because the intravesical portion of the ureter lengthens and has a more oblique entry through the bladder wall. Vesicoureteral reflux of sterile urine does little renal damage, but the ureteral muscular layers may hypertrophy. Cystitis and mucosal edema may impede the valve function, leading to reflux in adult dogs. Importantly, vesicoureteral reflux is a clinical diagnosis based on contrast radiographs or advanced imaging. Positioning of the patient, especially dogs, may affect the clinician's ability to detect this phenomenon, wherein dogs in lateral recumbency may have reflux that is not repeatable when they are in a supine position. Movement of the urinary bladder with kinking of the ureters is the likely cause of this discrepancy.

Cystitis can alter normal ureteral peristalsis, perhaps causing reversed peristaltic waves. Hence persistent pyelonephritis may result from vesicoureteral reflux, and possibly from reversed peristalsis in animals with cystitis. Progression of pyelonephritis probably depends upon persistence of bacterial infection or bacterial antigens.

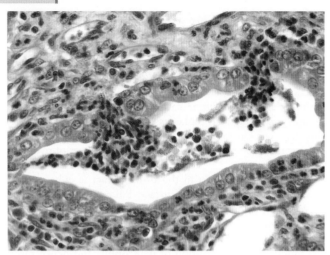

Figure 4-61 Acute pyelonephritis in a dog. Neutrophils cross the basement membrane of a collecting duct that contains cocci.

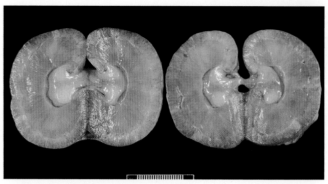

Figure 4-62 Chronic pyelonephritis in a dog. The renal parenchyma is scarred and atrophic. (Courtesy A. Koehne.)

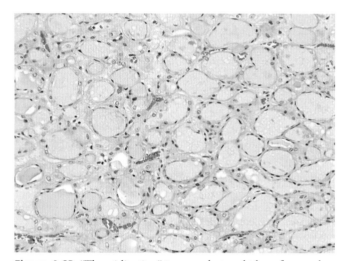

Figure 4-63 "Thyroidization" in an end-stage kidney from a dog.

For a number of reasons, *the medulla is the part of the kidney most susceptible to infection.* It is relatively hypoxic because of the low hematocrit in vasa recta. Hypertonicity depresses the phagocytic activity of leukocytes, and ammonia may interfere with activation of complement. In pigs, the renal poles are more susceptible to intrarenal reflux and infection because the collecting ducts serving those lobes do not collapse as readily as do those of the central lobes when exposed to the increased pelvic pressure. Invasion of the renal papilla probably progresses by way of the collecting ducts, as is suggested by the early development of lines of suppuration along the straight tubules and the presence of bacterial colonies within tubules. There can also be direct invasion across the eroded pelvic urothelium.

Pyelonephritis can be unilateral or bilateral; however, unilateral pyelonephritis can be clinically silent. A general description will be given of acute and chronic pyelonephritis before species differences are noted in more detail. **Acute disease** typically begins with necrosis and inflammation of papilla or renal crest ("necrotizing papillitis") in an irregular pattern. Bacteria may be abundant in the collecting ducts. Associated wedge-shaped areas of parenchyma are swollen, dark red, and firm. As the hyperemia subsides, *suppurative tubulointerstitial nephritis and tubular necrosis* develop in radially distributed wedges. Tubules are obliterated by the inflammation, and neutrophils cross the tubular basement membrane to enter the tubular lumen (tubulitis) (Fig. 4-61; eFig. 4-36). The leukocytic casts formed in the tubules may be found on urinalysis. Tubular dilation and obstruction are common. Glomeruli, although initially uninvolved, may eventually be obliterated. As the process becomes **chronic,** mononuclear cells replace neutrophils, and fibrosis develops. Contraction of the scars results in deep, flat cortical depressions (Fig. 4-62). The *scars in pyelonephritis* extend from capsule to pelvis. They can be distinguished from those of other nephritides and infarcts by the presence of fibrosis and deformation of the renal papilla. The calyces and pelves are dilated and often contain exudate and debris. Papillary defects may be subtle in mild cases. Generalized involvement of the kidney will produce a firm pale shrunken kidney with an irregular surface, and this will be difficult to differentiate from other end-stage kidneys of other etiologies.

In **dogs** and **cats,** acute pyelonephritis can go undetected, but scars attributed to chronic pyelonephritis are common. In dogs, accumulation of colloid-like material in tubules and glomerular capsules dilated from scarring produces a thyroid-like histologic appearance, called "thyroidization" (Fig. 4-63). Calculi can form in the pelvis on the nidi provided by cellular debris. Neither thyroidization nor pelvic calculi are pathognomonic for pyelonephritis, however. *Emphysematous pyelonephritis*, an uncommon variant caused by gas-forming organisms in dogs and cats with diabetes, is characterized by the presence of gas in the renal parenchyma, collecting system, or perinephric space.

In **swine,** acute pyelonephritis is seen occasionally, but chronic disease is rare. Shortening of the intravesical portion of the ureter and widening of the ureteric orifices occur in sows as a consequence of cystitis. This can facilitate vesicoureteral reflux and pyelonephritis. *Acute pyelonephritis occurs in sows postpartum or 3-4 weeks postbreeding.* Young males are occasionally affected, and some of these have urinary tract anomalies. Blood-stained urine or discharge can be seen, but it is not unusual for prostration and death to occur in 12 hours or so. Severe cystitis and ureteritis are usually present with yellow-brown or bloody mucoid tuxudate. The renal poles are preferentially involved, and the infection may be fulminant and erupt through the renal capsule to produce retroperitoneal hemorrhage and inflammation. Less severe disease is characterized by pale areas of leukocytic infiltration involving wedges or entire lobes.

In **cattle,** pyelonephritis is a significant sporadic disease. Unilateral pyelonephritis is as common as bilateral disease, which means that many animals are not azotemic. Suppurative destructive papillitis may predominate, whereas tubulointerstitial nephritis may be minimal. The medulla of each lobe is fairly uniformly destroyed. Eventually, the cortex remains as a narrow capsule surrounding large amounts of pus in the calyces. Alternatively, a pattern of radially distributed tubulointerstitial nephritis can be the main histologic pattern (eFig. 4-37). The kidney may have a granular surface because of interstitial inflammation and fibrosis. Rupture of the kidney occurs in males with obstructive urolithiasis, but it is less common in cattle than in swine. Pyelonephritis is uncommon in **sheep.** Pyelonephritis is also uncommon in **horses**; it can cause hematuria.

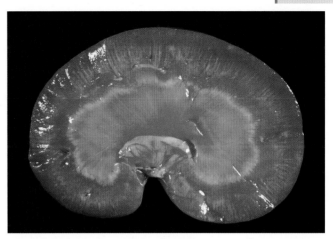

Figure 4-64 **Hypercalcemic nephropathy** in a dog. (Courtesy J. Grieves, P. Stromberg.)

Further reading

Braun U, et al. Clinical and ultrasonographic findings, diagnosis and treatment of pyelonephritis in 17 cows. Vet J 2008;175:240-248.

Coldrick O, et al. Fungal pyelonephritis due to *Cladrophialophora bantiana* in a cat. Vet Rec 2007;161:724-727.

Isling LK, et al. Pyelonephritis in slaughter pigs and sows: morphological characterization and aspects of pathogenesis and aetiology. Acta Vet Scand 2010;52:48.

Moon R, et al. Emphysematous cystitis and pyelonephritis in a nondiabetic dog and a diabetic cat. J Am Anim Hosp Assoc 2014;50:124-129.

Woldemeskel M, et al. Microscopic and ultrastructural lesions of the ureter and renal pelvis in sows with regard to *Actinobaculum suis* infection. J Vet Med A Physiol Pathol Clin Med 2002;49:348-352.

Hypercalcemic nephropathy

Hypercalcemia may be sufficiently severe to cause renal failure (hypercalcemic nephropathy) in dogs and cats.

- A common cause *is hypercalcemia of malignancy, or pseudohyperparathyroidism*, a paraneoplastic syndrome. A nonendocrine tumor, usually lymphosarcoma or adenocarcinoma of the apocrine glands of the anal sac, stimulates bone resorption via parathyroid hormone-related protein (PTHrp), a peptide that resembles parathyroid hormone (see Vol. 3, Endocrine glands and Vol. 3, Hematopoietic system). Hypercalcemia of malignancy is less commonly caused by osteolytic neoplasms.
- Poisoning by *rodenticides containing vitamin D* (0.075% cholecalciferol) has become an important cause of hypervitaminosis D and hypercalcemia in dogs and cats. The same syndrome follows ingestion of *human antipsoriatic preparations* that contain synthetic vitamin D analogues, for example, calcipotriol, tacalcitol. Diagnosis of cholecalciferol rodenticide poisoning may be aided by determination of the renal 25-hydroxyvitamin D ($25(OH)D_3$) concentration. The renal calcium to phosphorus ratio is <0.1 in normal dogs, but 0.4-0.9 in cholecalciferol-poisoned dogs.
- Hypercalcemia can also be seen in primary hyperparathyroidism, CRF with secondary hyperparathyroidism, and hypoadrenocorticism.

- Hypercalcemia resulting in nephrocalcinosis and mineralization of other soft tissues is well known in grazing animals that ingest plants containing vitamin D_3 sterol (e.g., *Solanum malacoxylon, Cestrum diurnum, Trisetum flavescens, Medicago sativa*).

Hypercalcemia results in inactivation of adenyl cyclase, and hence decreased cyclic adenosine monophosphate formation. Sodium transport is impaired in the ascending limb of the loop of Henle, the distal tubule, and collecting ducts, resulting in natriuresis. Hypercalcemia also interferes with ADH receptors in the collecting ducts, leading to nephrogenic diabetes insipidus. The resultant polyuria and compensatory polydipsia are reversible if the primary cause of the hypercalcemia is removed. If hypercalcemia persists, *progressive renal mineralization* occurs, beginning with basement membranes of tubules and Bowman's capsules, particularly in the outer zone of the medulla (Fig. 4-64) and eventually involving the interstitium, vessels, and glomeruli. Tubular epithelial mineralization and cast formation cause tubular obstruction and eventually loss of nephrons.

Other less significant examples of renal mineralization also occur. The deposition of calcium salts in the form of clumps of granules in the lumen and lining of collecting tubules and in the adjacent interstitium is rather common. They are associated with hypomagnesemia in some species and are not considered to be significant.

Mineralization is very common in dogs, but unusual in other species. Cellular casts, injured epithelium and basement membranes can mineralize quickly. In uremia, it may also involve the glomeruli and small blood vessels. Renal mineralization is a frequent result of *secondary hyperparathyroidism* induced by chronic renal insufficiency and coexists with similar deposits in the lungs, gastric mucosa, and other organs (see Renal disease, renal failure, and uremia). Dogs fed a high-phosphorus diet similarly develop diffuse renal mineralization.

Miscellaneous interstitial lesions

Extramedullary hematopoiesis occurs in the kidneys of dogs under a variety of circumstances, all of which probably have a common denominator of bone marrow depression or injury. When the kidneys are sites of hematopoiesis, the liver, lymph nodes, spleen, adrenals, and lungs are usually also involved. Pronounced hematopoiesis can occur in canine pyometra.

Bone occasionally develops in the urinary tract, for example, following urinary tract surgery or in hydronephrotic kidneys. Urothelium stimulates transformation of mesenchymal cells to osteoblasts.

Renal telangiectasia occurs in cattle, dogs, cats, mink, and ferrets; it is familial in Pembroke Welsh Corgis (eFig. 4-38). It is a rare cause of hematuria in dogs.

Further reading

Kruger JM, et al. Hypercalcemia and renal failure. Etiology, pathophysiology, diagnosis, and treatment. Vet Clin North Am Small Anim Pract 1996;26:1417-1445.

Peterson ME, Fluegeman K. Cholecalciferol. Top Companion Anim Med 2013;28:24-27.

Rumbeiha WK, et al. The postmortem diagnosis of cholecalciferol toxicosis: a novel approach and differentiation from ethylene glycol toxicosis. J Vet Diagn Invest 2000;12:426-432.

Parasitic lesions in the kidneys

Toxocara canis

The most common parasitic lesion in the kidneys is a focal scar secondary to *Toxocara canis* larval migration in canine kidneys. These small granulomas, 2-3 mm in diameter, are found in the cortical parenchyma. Early lesions are gray-yellow with soft centers; later, they become firm and white, and the superficial ones cause dimpling of the cortex. *Each granuloma surrounds an entrapped larva*, which may be hard to find in histologic sections (eFig. 4-39). Healing occurs after death and removal of the larvae. Residual scars typically consist of dense concentrically arranged fibrous tissue. Similar lesions are produced in calves by the migratory larvae of *T. cati* and *T. canis* acquired by fecal contamination of feed, and by *T. vitulorum*, especially in buffalo.

Stephanurus dentatus

Stephanurus dentatus is the kidney worm of swine. It is widely distributed in tropical and subtropical countries, and the prevalence in grazing swine can be very high. *The worms encyst in perirenal fat and adjacent tissues, and the cysts communicate with the renal pelvis.* The life cycle of *S. dentatus* can be direct or involve earthworms as transport hosts; the latter mechanism has not been shown to occur naturally. Eggs are passed in the urine of the pig, and the larvae hatch in 2-3 days. Infective stages are vulnerable to sunlight and drying. Infection may occur by penetration through the skin or by ingestion, and prenatal infections occur. Following oral infection, third-stage larvae migrate from the small and large intestine via the portal circulation and mesenteric lymphatics to the liver. A few migrate across the peritoneal cavity. After skin infection, most larvae migrate to the lungs and reach the intestines following tracheal migration. Deaths resulting from peritonitis and intestinal intussusception occur in some pigs 20-30 days after heavy infections. These are associated with larval migration from the mesenteric nodes to the liver. Infective larvae may migrate in the liver for several months. Hepatic migrations can cause severe hepatitis, with lesions similar to but often more severe than those produced by *Ascaris suum* larvae. *S. dentatus* also produces portal phlebitis with thrombosis in some pigs (see Vol. 2, Liver and biliary system). The liver is usually enlarged and may be very firm. The lobulation is enhanced by

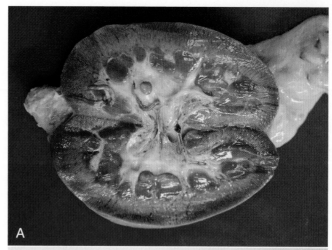

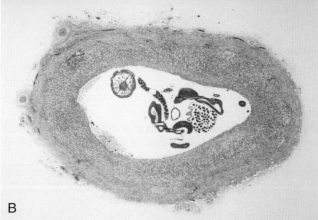

Figure 4-65 A. Encysted *Stephanurus dentatus* in hilus of a porcine kidney. **B.** Histopathology of *Stephanurus dentatus* in a dilated ureter. (Courtesy O. Illanes.)

perilobular fibrosis. Lobules may be obliterated by contracting and proliferating scar tissue in the portal areas.

Many larvae are destroyed in the liver by encapsulation in small abscesses. *From the liver, the larvae migrate across the peritoneal cavity to the perirenal region.* Many become encysted in abscesses in adjacent tissue, especially the pancreas. It is not unusual for some to invade the vertebral canal causing paraplegia. The definitive site is the tissue around the renal pelvis and ureter, wherein the adults encyst (Fig. 4-65). Occasionally, cysts may be found in the kidney itself. The cysts communicate with the lumen of the ureter, allowing escape of eggs. Developmental stages in the definitive host take a long time, and patent infections may not be established for 9 months or more. Mature females may lay eggs for 3 years or longer.

Dioctophyma renale

Dioctophyma renale is the *giant kidney worm*, the largest of parasitic nematodes. It has a worldwide distribution, but its incidence is unknown. The worm is red and cylindrical, and adult females measure 20-100 cm long and 4-12 mm in diameter. Males are 14-45 cm long and 4-6 mm in diameter. *D. renale* is usually found in dogs, mink, cats, and other fish-eating mammals, but has been reported in the pig, ox, and horse. Definitive hosts are wild fish-eating carnivores, especially mink, in which the worms are smaller and usually located in the kidney.

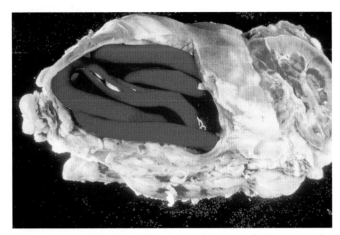

Figure 4-66 Adult ***Dioctophyma renale*** encysted adjacent to the kidney of a dog. (Courtesy University of Guelph.)

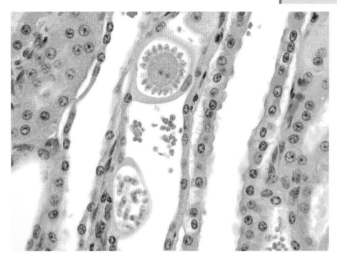

Figure 4-67 *Klossiella equi* in tubular epithelial cells of an equine kidney.

The life cycle involves 2 aquatic intermediate hosts. Eggs passed in the urine are resistant to the external environment and may survive for 2-5 years. Embryonation requires 1-7 months, depending on the climate. Embryonated eggs are ingested by the intermediate hosts, which are aquatic oligochaetes ("mud worms;" *Lumbriculus variegatus*), and develop through first and second larval stages. Third- and fourth-stage larvae can either develop directly in the worm, or within fish or frog intermediate hosts, for example, the northern black bullhead *(Ictalurus melas)*, green frog *(Rana clamitans)*. Following ingestion by mammals, infective third- or fourth-stage larvae penetrate the gut wall and migrate across the peritoneal cavity to the kidney. The life cycle from egg to adult requires 3.5-6 months, but may take up to 2 years.

Adult worms live in the renal pelvis but may also encyst in a body cavity, the uterus, mammary gland, or bladder (Fig. 4-66; eFig. 4-40). Adults are very destructive in the kidney, causing hemorrhagic pyelitis that becomes suppurative. The renal parenchyma is then progressively destroyed until the renal capsule only contains the worm and exudate.

Dogs are regarded as abnormal hosts because only one or a very small number of worms is present, worms of both sexes are found in only about one third of infections, and most infections are not patent. *Intrarenal parasites in dogs and mink are more common in the right kidney than the left.* In ~60% of infected dogs, parasites are only in the peritoneal cavity. *D. renale* may encircle a lobe of the liver, causing infarction or rupture with or without hemoperitoneum. Simultaneous renal and peritoneal infections occur in ~15% of dogs.

Pearsonema plica

Pearsonema (Capillaria) plica may be found in the lumen of the renal pelvis, ureter, or urinary bladder of dogs, foxes, and smaller carnivores. Although widely distributed, it is uncommon. The life cycle is not clearly known but is probably indirect, with earthworms as intermediate hosts. Ingestion of earthworms from infected premises causes patent infections in 61-68 days. Pathologic effects are not usually attributed to *P. plica* infection, but hematuria and dysuria are occasionally seen. Worms embedded in bladder, ureter, or pelvis may invoke mild submucosal inflammation.

Other species of *Pearsonema* occur in urinary bladder of other animals—*P. mucronata* in mink and *P. feliscati* in the cat; the latter may be the same as *P. plica*. Light infestations are common but harmless. At most, the rostral end of the worm embedded in the surface layer of epithelium may incite mild submucosal inflammation.

Klossiella equi

Klossiella equi is a *sporozoan parasite of the kidney of the horse and its relatives*, including the zebra, donkey, and burro. Infections are usually incidental. The life cycle is not fully known. It is thought that after infection with sporocysts from the environment, sporozoites are released and enter the circulation. One schizont generation develops in glomerular endothelium and another in proximal tubular epithelium. Sporogony occurs in the epithelium of the thick limb of Henle's loop (Fig. 4-67), and sporocysts may be passed in the urine. Heavy infections can result in rupture of tubules and lymphoplasmacytic interstitial nephritis.

Granulomas may be found in the renal pelvis in *schistosomiasis* of cattle and sheep (see Vol. 3, Cardiovascular system) and larvae of *Setaria digitata* may produce granulomas in the bladder of cattle in Asia (see Vol. 2, Alimentary system and peritoneum).

Halicephalobus gingivalis

Halicephalobus gingivalis (formerly *Micronema deletrix*) is a saprophagous nematode that produces granulomatous masses in the nasal cavity of horses and is occasionally responsible for cerebral vasculitis and granulomatous nephritis. Granulomas contain numerous larval and adult female rhabditiform nematodes and embryonated eggs. Urine and semen of infected horses may also contain multiple life stages of the parasites (Fig. 4-68).

Further reading

Basso W, et al. *Capillaria plica* (syn. *Pearsonema plica*) infection in a dog with chronic pollakiuria: challenges in the diagnosis and treatment. Parasitol Int 2014;63:140-142.

Ferreira VL, et al. *Dioctophyma renale* in a dog: clinical diagnosis and surgical treatment. Vet Parasitol 2010;168:151-155.

Kinde H, et al. *Halicephalobus gingivalis (H. deletrix)* infection in two horses in southern California. J Vet Diagn Invest 2000;12: 162-165.

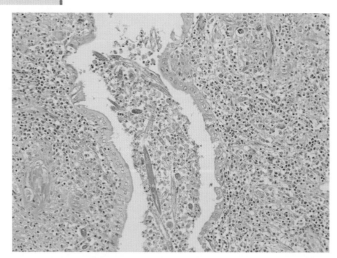

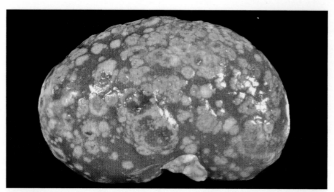

Figure 4-70 **Renal carcinoma** with intrarenal metastasis in a dog. (Courtesy E. Clark, P. Stromberg.)

Figure 4-68 *Halicephalobus gingivalis* nematodes in a tubule of an equine kidney with associated marked pyogranulomatous inflammation.

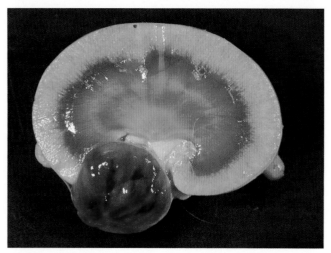

Figure 4-69 **Renal adenoma** in a cat. Incidental finding. (Courtesy N. Vapniarsky.)

RENAL NEOPLASIA

Primary renal tumors are uncommon. One abattoir survey in the United Kingdom found 8.5, 0.9, and 4.3 cases per million animals in cattle, sheep, and pigs, respectively. Renal tumors were found in ~0.15% of horses in 2 large surveys. Primary renal tumors comprise about 1% of all canine neoplasms and 1.5-2.5% of feline neoplasms. In one large retrospective study of primary canine renal neoplasms, most were of epithelial origin (85.2%), demonstrated metastatic disease, and had an associated poor prognosis (mean survival 6.8 months).

The vast majority of renal neoplasia is metastatic to the kidney, by hematogenous or lymphatic spread or by direct extension (eFig. 4-41).

Renal adenoma

Renal adenomas are rare; they are said to occur more often in cattle and horses than in other species. In dogs, they comprise about 15% of primary renal epithelial tumors. *Adenomas are usually incidental autopsy findings.* Renal adenomas arise from tubular epithelium. Grossly, they tend to be *solitary nodules* <2 cm across but occasionally are larger (Fig. 4-69).

Neoplastic cells are cuboidal with moderate to abundant acidophilic cytoplasm. They form solid sheets, papilliform or tubular structures, and stromal tissue is scant. Tumors with mixed architectural patterns occur. Histologic differentiation of adenoma and renal carcinoma is sometimes impossible; a few "adenomas" may be small, well-differentiated carcinomas. In cattle, adenocarcinomas are virtually always microscopically multiple.

Renal carcinoma

Carcinomas are the most common primary renal tumors of dogs, cattle, and horses. There are only sporadic reports in cats, sheep, and pigs. These tumors occur in mature and old animals; thus their incidence is relatively low in some species. The average age of affected dogs is ~8 years, although this tumor has been reported in dogs <2 years of age. Males are affected about twice as often as bitches. This is in contrast to the overwhelming higher occurrence in cows, likely because of a preponderance of females in the aged cattle population. Common presenting signs are hematuria, palpable abdominal mass, and weight loss. Polycythemia caused by excessive erythropoietin production is very rarely seen in animals, but paraneoplastic erythrocytosis occurs in 1-5% of humans with renal adenocarcinoma. Hypertrophic osteopathy may be seen in cases of renal carcinoma with pulmonary metastases. Disseminated intravascular coagulation, extreme neutrophilic leukocytosis, leukemoid blood response, and bone infarcts are additional rare paraneoplastic syndromes in dogs. Leukocytosis has been associated with synthesis of granulocyte-macrophage colony-stimulating factor by neoplastic cells.

Grossly, renal carcinomas are spherical or ovoid masses, typically located in one pole of the kidney. Usually, they are well demarcated from the remainder of the kidney, which is atrophic and compressed. The tumor may be much larger than the original size of the kidney but still has a discrete border. The tumor is usually gray or light yellow, often with darker areas of necrosis and hemorrhage (Fig. 4-70). Invasion of the renal pelvis, ureter, renal vein, and hilar lymphatics may be visible.

In humans, the types of renal carcinoma are recognized based on neoplastic cell morphology and organization and include clear cell and papillary renal cell carcinomas (RCC), both arising from the proximal tubule, and chromophobe RCC and oncytoma, both arising from the collecting duct, as well as other less common variants. Biallelic loss of the von Hippel-Lindau *(VHL)* gene has been documented in a majority of human clear cell RCC, but sequence analysis of *VHL* exons in canine RCC has not revealed mutations.

Immunohistochemistry and lectin staining can help distinguish cell origin because there are segment-specific patterns within the various levels of the nephron. Normal canine proximal tubules stain positively for CD10, whereas the distal tubules and collecting ducts stain with *Dichloros biflorus* agglutinin, peanut agglutinin, and *Ulex europaeus* agglutinin I. *Histologically*, there is a variety of cell types and architectures, and there is often a mix of clear cells, poorly stained chromophobe cells, and eosinophilic cells. They may be arranged in sheets, papillary or tubular structures (Fig. 4-71; eFig. 4-42), and occasionally, they line small cystic spaces. All of these patterns may occur in a single tumor, and the various patterns have not yet been associated with specific prognoses in veterinary species. However, the advent of immunohistochemical and lectin-based techniques mentioned previously may allow more accurate classification of tumor subtypes and improve prognostication. One study reported that all canine RCC expressed uromodulin. In addition, canine RCC often express vimentin, except for tumors with a papillary and cystic structure. This suggests that the vimentin-expressing tumors are derived from the metanephric mesenchyme. Likewise, papillary and tubulopapillary carcinomas express a few cytokeratins, whereas solid carcinomas (with sheet-like arrangements of neoplastic cells) may be cytokeratin negative. Expression of CD10, a marker for proximal tubules, is sporadic in canine RCC, but c-KIT is commonly expressed in most cases. This staining pattern is in contrast to that of human RCC, with frequent CD10 and absent c-KIT expression. Taken together, these data suggest that many canine RCC arise from a different segment of the nephron than that of human RCC. The stroma of renal carcinomas is scant but highly vascularized, which predisposes to the extensive hemorrhage often seen grossly.

Renal carcinomas tend to grow expansively, but satellite nodules can also develop. Invasion of the renal vein does not always lead to metastases. Peritoneal implantation may occur. Usually by the time a dog is presented for examination, widespread metastases are present, especially in lungs and liver, but also in brain, heart, and skin. In cases without metastases, unilateral nephrectomy might be curative. In contrast, **cattle** have a low rate of systemic metastasis, but bilateral renal involvement is common. This might be explained by multiple de novo development as opposed to intrarenal metastasis. Bovine RCCs often contain corpora amylacea. One study reported that they all stain positively for uromodulin via immunohistochemistry, indicating that they are derived from distal segments of the nephron. Reports of equine RCC are rare in the literature, but they are considered to be locally invasive with potential for metastasis. The oncocytic form of renal carcinoma has been reported infrequently in rats and

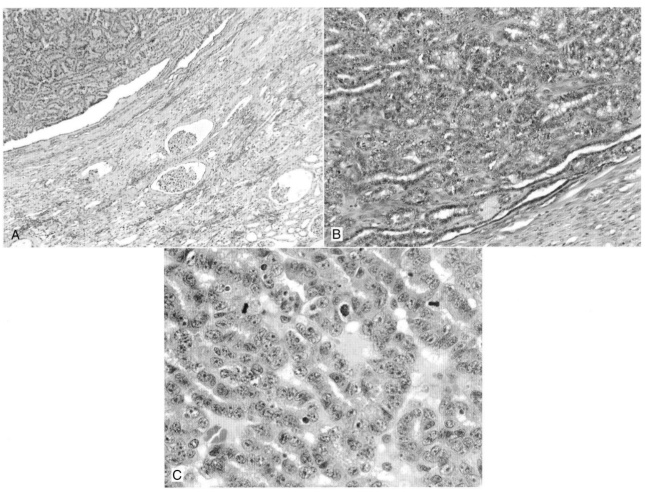

Figure 4-71 Renal cell carcinoma in a dog compressing adjacent parenchyma and consisting of tubules and ducts (**A-C**).

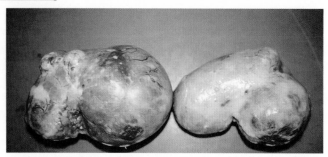

Figure 4-72 Renal cystadenocarcinoma from a German Shepherd dog.

dogs. Renal carcinomas are rarely diagnosed in **cats,** but typically occur unilaterally, in older cats (mean 9 years), with no sex or breed predilection and only sporadic metastases.

Middle-aged and older German Shepherd dogs with generalized *nodular dermatofibrosis* concurrently also have **renal cystadenocarcinomas** or cystadenomas, which are usually bilateral (Fig. 4-72; eFig. 4-43). The carcinomas will occasionally metastasize to regional lymph nodes, peritoneum, liver, spleen, lung, and bone. Affected bitches also often have multiple uterine leiomyomas. The syndrome may be the result of a paraneoplastic process in which renal tumor-derived growth factors stimulate accumulation of fibrous tissue in various sites. The syndrome is *inherited in an autosomal dominant mode in German Shepherd dogs,* and genetic mapping has linked the disease to mutations in the Birt-Hogg-Dubé locus located on chromosome 5. Mutations in this gene have previously been associated with a similar phenotype in humans. Because nodular dermatofibrosis with various cystic renal diseases has been reported in a variety of dog breeds, some postulate that there is concurrent initiation of fibrosis in both the skin and the kidney. Renal fibrosis can result in outflow obstruction of renal tubules with expansion and eventual cyst formation. There can be progression through a continuum of lesions, including renal epithelial cyst, cystic adenomatous hyperplasia, renal cystadenoma, and cystadenocarcinoma, with purebred dogs perhaps being prone to more rapid transformation to malignancy. Thus all dog breeds are potentially at risk.

Further reading

Gil da Costa RM, et al. Immunohistochemical characterization of 13 canine renal cell carcinomas. Vet Pathol 2011;48:427-432.

Kobayashi N, et al. Chromophobe renal cell carcinoma with sarcomatoid transformation in a dog. J Vet Diagn Invest 2010;22:983-987.

Lillakas K. Renal adenoma in a 5-year-old Labrador retriever: big is not always bad. Can Vet J 2013;54:179-181.

Merrick CH, et al. Hypercalcemia of malignancy associated with renal cell carcinoma in a dog. J Am Anim Hosp Assoc 2013;49:385-388.

Petterino C, et al. Paraneoplastic leukocytosis in a dog with a renal carcinoma. Vet Clin Pathol 2011;40:89-94.

Pressler BM, et al. Sequencing of the Von Hippel-Lindau gene in canine renal carcinoma. J Vet Intern Med 2009;23:592-597.

Wise LN, et al. A retrospective analysis of renal carcinoma in the horse. J Vet Intern Med 2009;23:913-918.

Nephroblastoma

Nephroblastoma (embryonal nephroma, Wilms' tumor) is the most common primary renal tumor of pigs and chickens. Abattoir

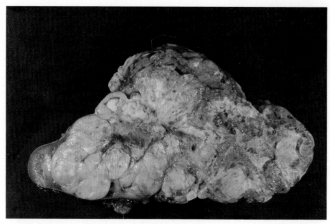

Figure 4-73 Nephroblastoma from a dog. (Courtesy J. Luff, P.A. Pesavento.)

surveys of pigs in the United Kingdom found 3.5 per million swine slaughtered, and in the United States, 43.5 per million, with a frequency of 197 cases per million in one area. Nephroblastomas occur far less often in calves and in dogs, and are uncommon in sheep, horses, and cats. They are usually seen in young animals and sometimes in fetuses. They may be seen in mature sows and are more common in adult dogs than in pups. In rats, various carcinogens, including dimethylnitrosamine, can induce formation of nephroblastomas, among other tumors.

Nephroblastomas are *true embryonal tumors* that arise in primitive nephrogenic blastema and in foci of renal dysplasia. The presence of tissues not typically associated with the kidney, such as cartilage and skeletal muscle, indicates an origin in pluripotential mesenchyme of the metanephron. These tumors establish the important principle that all component tissues of the kidney arise from a common blastema and that this neoplasm may represent a form of arrested development. Finding nephrogenic rests of nodular renal blastema in dogs suggests this species shares a similar pathogenesis and histogenesis to that seen in Wilms' tumors in humans.

Grossly, nephroblastomas can be large enough to cause abdominal distension. They can be multiple in the affected kidney, growing expansively and compressing the adjacent parenchyma (Fig. 4-73). They are usually unilateral, but a few are bilateral, and these sometimes unite across the midline to form a single large mass. Widespread metastases to lung and liver occur in more than half the canine cases, but are rare in pigs and calves. The cut surface of nephroblastomas is lobulated with myxomatous soft, gray-white or tan spongy tissue. Larger tumors have extensive hemorrhagic necrosis. Rarely, these tumors are seen as primary extramedullary and intradural spinal canal masses between T10 and L2 and are called *thoracolumbar spinal tumor* of young dogs. German Shepherd and male dogs seem to be over-represented with the spinal form, which may occur in the absence of renal involvement.

Histologically, the characteristic features are primitive glomeruli, abortive tubules, and a loose spindle-cell stroma that may show some differentiation to a variety of mesenchymal tissues, including striated muscle, collagen, cartilage, bone, and adipose tissue. The mesenchymal components may predominate over epithelial elements in certain tumors, especially in ruminants.

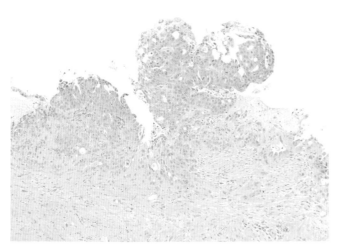

Figure 4-74 **Urothelial cell carcinoma** arising from the renal pelvis in a dog and producing frond-like proliferations into the pelvis.

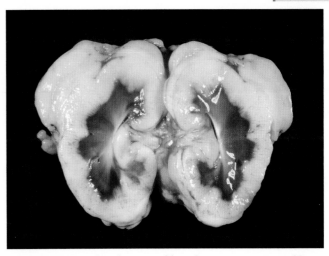

Figure 4-75 **Renal and perirenal lymphosarcoma** in a cat. (Courtesy E. Clark, D. Russell.)

When all 3 components (blastemal, epithelial, and stromal) exist in equal proportions, these forms are referred to as *triphasic (mixed)*. Commercially available antibody to the human Wilms' tumor gene product C-19 successfully binds with canine nephroblastomas. These tumors are also typically glial fibrillary acidic protein negative and variably vimentin and cytokeratin positive. Tubular and glomerular differentiation indicates a good prognosis, whereas anaplasia and sarcomatous stroma are associated with metastasis and poor prognosis. In pigs, the mesenchymal component can be immunolabeled with vimentin, whereas tubular structures can be labeled with various cytokeratins, with CK19 staining all tubules. Embryologically, this particular cytokeratin is transiently expressed as the epithelial cells of tubules undergo differentiation and then becomes limited to the parietal epithelium and distal tubules. This widespread presence of a transiently expressed protein in porcine nephroblastomas supports the embryonic origin of the neoplasm. Interestingly, glomeruloid structures did not contain factor VIII–positive cells, demonstrating a lack of capillary invasion. Rarely, polycythemia is seen as an associated paraneoplastic syndrome in nephroblastoma.

Other tumors

Urothelial papilloma and **carcinoma** of the renal pelvis are rare tumors, which occur in the dog, cat, cow, pig, and horse (Fig. 4-74; eFig. 4-44). Squamous and glandular metaplasia develops in the carcinomas. Primary pelvic **squamous cell carcinoma** is extremely uncommon, but in dogs, they have been noted in association with pelvic calculi. Urothelial cell tumors are discussed in Urinary bladder, later.

Primary **mesenchymal tumors** of the kidney occur, but may be diagnosed only after very careful examination to exclude a primary focus in some other tissue. The prognosis associated with renal mesenchymal neoplasms is usually grave. Fibrous and vascular tumors are the most common types. **Hemangioma** is the most frequently encountered benign mesenchymal renal neoplasm in dogs; hematuria is the most consistent accompanying sign. Renal **interstitial cell tumors** occur near the corticomedullary junction, arising from cells distinct from interstitial fibroblasts. **Benign cortical fibromas** also occur in older dogs. Other rare primary renal tumors include

neurofibroma, malignant fibrous histiocytoma, and oncocytoma. **Renal oncocytomas** are rare, usually unilateral, benign tumors composed of oncocytes, which are large polygonal cells with bright eosinophilic granular cytoplasm. PAS stain accentuates the cytoplasmic granules, which on electron microscopy are mitochondria. The cells are typically arranged as compact nests, cords, or tubules. The histogenesis is unclear, but it is thought that these tumors originate from intercalated cells of the collecting ducts; the cells express cytoplasmic keratin.

Metastatic tumors are common in the kidneys, and disseminated neoplasms of any type are likely to localize there, typically with bilateral involvement of the cortices. Many such metastases are microscopic and of hematogenous origin. Retrograde lymphatic invasion along the renal lymphatics may occur from carcinomas in adjacent organs.

In dogs, primary **pulmonary adenocarcinoma** with renal metastases may be difficult or impossible to distinguish from primary renal carcinoma with pulmonary metastases, because their microscopic appearance is quite similar.

Renal involvement in **lymphoma** is common in those species in which the neoplasm is common. This is the most common renal neoplasm in cats, but is more often a metastatic rather than a primary lesion (Fig. 4-75; eFig. 4-45). The involvement may be diffuse or nodular and possibly bilateral. When the nodular lesions are grossly visible, they are numerous, poorly defined, fatty in appearance, and project hemispherically above the surface. Diffuse lymphoma results in generalized enlargement with a uniform white fatty appearance. Metastases of other round cell tumors have similar gross appearances (Fig. 4-76). Differentiation of metastatic lymphoma from interstitial nephritis may require microscopic examination. Peripelvic and periureteral lymphoma, which can cause hydronephrosis, is seen in cattle.

Further reading

Dempster AG, et al. The histology and growth kinetics of canine renal oncocytoma. J Comp Pathol 2000;123:294-298.

Grieco V, et al. Immunohistochemical study of porcine nephroblastoma. J Comp Pathol 2006;134:143-151.

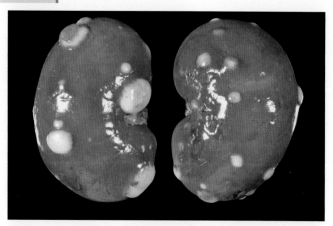

Figure 4-76 Multifocal metastatic **histiocytic sarcoma** in a dog. (Courtesy B. Harrington, P. Stromberg.)

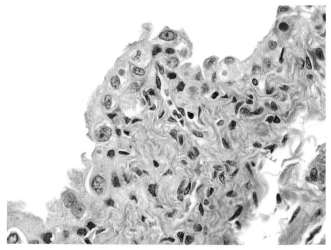

Figure 4-77 **Intracytoplasmic inclusion bodies** in the urothelium of a dog infected with canine distemper virus. (Courtesy E. Clark, P. Stromberg.)

Hanzlicek AS, et al. Renal transitional-cell carcinoma in two cats with chronic kidney disease. J Feline Med Surg 2012;14: 280-284.

Henry CJ, et al. Primary renal tumours in cats: 19 cases (1992-1998). J Fel Med Surg 1999;1:165-170.

Soldati S, et al. Congenital mesoblastic nephroma in a young basset hound dog. J Small Anim Pract 2012;53:709-713.

Yamamoto Y, et al. Nephroblastoma with transcoelomic metastasis in a Japanese black bull. J Vet Med Sci 2006;68:891-893.

LOWER URINARY TRACT

GENERAL CONSIDERATIONS

The lower urinary tract consists of **ureters, urinary bladder,** and **urethra.** The ureters and bladder, and also the renal pelvis, are lined by nonkeratinizing, stratified epithelium—the **urothelium.** The ureters are of uniform diameter throughout, and usually course directly to the bladder, although they may be tortuous and dilated distally in baby pigs. The ureters enter the bladder wall obliquely and are covered by a mucosal flap. Histologically, the ureteral mucosa is present in longitudinal folds; there are poorly defined internal and external longitudinal muscle layers, a prominent middle circular layer, and either adventitia or peritoneal serosa. Thus peritonitis may interfere with ureteric peristalsis. Ureters and the renal pelves of horses have simple branched tubuloalveolar mucous glands in the propria-submucosa. Histologically, the bladder is an expanded ureter, lined by stratified urothelium ranging from 3-14 cells thick, depending on the species and degree of distension. Superficial cells, which contain tubulovesicular compartments, supply additional membrane to allow for bladder distension. The basolateral plasma membrane of the superficial cells and the plasma membrane of the intermediate layer of urothelium interdigitate and are attached by desmosomes that provide structural stability and elasticity during distension and relaxation. Lymphoid nodules are commonly found in the lamina propria of all domestic animals. Eosinophilic intracytoplasmic inclusion bodies of canine distemper seen in urinary bladder epithelial cells (Fig. 4-77) must be differentiated from similar nonspecific inclusions.

The function of the ureter is to propel urine from the kidney to the bladder by peristalsis. Ureteral peristalsis is complex and influenced by the rate of urine production. The ureters pass obliquely through the muscular wall of the bladder at the ureterovesical junction. *The segment of ureter in the bladder wall, the intravesical ureter, forms the basis of the* **vesicoureteral valve,** *which prevents reflux of urine from bladder to ureter.* When the length of the intravesical ureter is short, as is often the case in puppies, reflux frequently occurs. Thus the angle of the ureteral entry and the thickness of the bladder wall influence the competence of the valve. The urinary bladder stores urine and, in concert with the urethra, expels it. During continence, the bladder is relatively flaccid, and the urethra acts as a valve. During micturition, contraction of the *detrusor muscle*—the urinary bladder musculature—pumps urine through the relaxed urethra. Sphincter mechanism incompetence or detrusor instability can lead to incontinence, seen most commonly in bitches.

Embryologically, the ureters are formed by buds from the mesonephric ducts, which develop craniad to their entrance into the cloaca. The cloaca is divided into a dorsal rectum and ventral urogenital sinus by the urorectal fold in such a way that the urogenital sinus is continuous with the allantois. The allantois originates as an evagination of the hindgut. At this stage of development, the mesonephric duct and ureteral bud form a Y shape; one arm of the Y is the ureteral bud, and the other arm plus the stem of the Y are formed by the mesonephric duct. As the allantois and urogenital sinus develop, the stem of the Y is absorbed, and the mesonephric duct and ureteral bud enter the urogenital sinus independently. In females, the entire urethra, plus the vaginal vestibule, is derived from the urogenital sinus, but in males, only the prostatic urethra is so derived. The penile urethra forms by closure of the urethral groove on the caudal face of the penis. The bladder, which is formed from the cranial part of the urogenital sinus and the caudal part of the allantoic diverticulum, communicates with the allantois via the urachus, a part of the intraembryonic allantoic diverticulum. The communication is severed at birth, and the urachus closes but remains as the umbilical ligament of the bladder.

Most ailments of the lower urinary tract are associated with obstruction and infection, which can be concomitant. Unlike the gastrointestinal tract, which has a normal microbial flora throughout its length, only the most distal part of the male urethra, and the female vagina, normally host microorganisms. The operation of sphincter-like mechanisms in the urethra and vesicoureteral valves, and the intermittent pulsatile flow of urine from the kidneys and bladder, normally prevents the movement of organisms higher up the tract. The susceptibility of the urinary bladder of the female to severe infections is undoubtedly related to its short distensible urethra and its proximity to the external environment and rectal flora. On the other hand, the anatomy of male urethras, with their flexures, ossa, and appendages, make them prone to obstruction, particularly by calculi. Specific factors concerned in the establishment and maintenance of infections in the urinary bladder and their spread to the kidney are discussed in the sections Cystitis and Pyelonephritis. The causes and effects of obstruction are considered in the sections Urolithiasis and Hydronephrosis.

The **urothelium** of the renal pelvis, ureter, and perhaps the trigone of the bladder originate from mesoderm, whereas, in the rest of the bladder, it has an endodermal origin. The urothelium responds to chronic irritation from infections, calculi, and excreted chemicals by proliferation and/or metaplasia, both of which are regarded as premalignant changes. Proliferation of urothelium, a common reactive change, results in groups of proliferating cells isolated in the submucosa, known as **Brunn nests.** If the center of the nest undergoes liquefaction, *cystitis cystica, ureteritis cystica,* or *pyelitis cystica* results. *Cystitis glandularis* develops if the epithelium lining the cyst undergoes mucous metaplasia. Metaplasia of squamous or mucous types is often superimposed on predominantly proliferative lesions. The male urethra has a thin lining of urothelium; that of the female is similar but has stratified squamous epithelium at its termination. Most adenomas and adenocarcinomas of the lower urinary tract develop in areas of mucous metaplasia. A few may arise in submucosal glands or mesonephric and urachal remnants. Urothelium that is not exposed to urine has a tendency to undergo metaplasia to an intestinal-type epithelium; such is the fate of some cystic urachal remnants.

Urine may be obtained for urinalysis or culture by cystocentesis at autopsy. The bladder may be distended in downer animals, even in states of dehydration, caused by either the absence of the correct posture needed for urination or decreased medullary tonicity resulting from hypoproteinemia (low urea production) that has led to polyuria. Dog bladders are often constricted at autopsy and hence have a thick wall. If the bladder can be dilated by pulling it between the fingers, the thickening is not pathologic. Horse urine normally contains mucus and crystals.

Further reading

Forsee KM, et al. Evaluation of the prevalence of urinary incontinence in spayed female dogs: 566 cases (2003-2008). J Am Vet Med Assoc 2013;242:959-962.

Silverman S, Long CD. The diagnosis of urinary incontinence and abnormal urination in dogs and cats. Vet Clin North Am Small Anim Pract 2000;30:427-448.

Verlander JW. Normal ultrastructure of the kidney and lower urinary tract. Tox Pathol 1998;26:1-17.

ANOMALIES OF THE LOWER URINARY TRACT

Ureters

Agenesis of the ureters is the result of failure of the ureteral bud to form, and may be unilateral or bilateral. In dogs, it is often accompanied by renal agenesis (see Anomalies of development). **Duplication** of a ureter is caused by the formation of 2 ureteral diverticula from the mesonephric duct. The caudal ureter drains the caudal part of the kidney and the cranial one drains the cranial part. Usually the caudal ureter empties normally, whereas the other is ectopic. Duplication is rare but occurs in dogs and pigs (eFig. 4-46). **Ureteral dysplasia** occurs in association with renal dysplasia. **Ureteral valves** are occasionally seen in dogs. **Retrocaval ureter** is a condition in which one ureter (often the right) traverses dorsal to the vena cava and then wraps around to run ventral to it (Fig. 4-78). Although it can be seen incidentally, it might predispose to unilateral obstruction in settings of urolithiasis.

Ectopic ureter *is the most important ureteral anomaly.* Rather than terminating at the trigone of the bladder, the affected ureter may empty into the vas deferens, vesicular gland, or urethra of the male, or the bladder neck, urethra, or vagina of the female (Fig. 4-79). In bitches, the ectopic ureter usually terminates in the vagina or urethra, whereas in cats urethral termination is most common. There are 2 possible causes: either the ureteral bud arises too far craniad to be

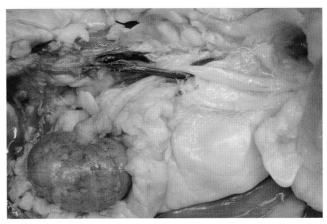

Figure 4-78 Retrocaval ureter from a cat. Incidental finding.

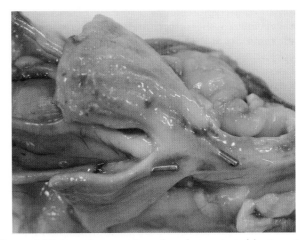

Figure 4-79 Ectopic ureter in a dog, demonstrated by insertion of probes through the ureters. (Courtesy J. Davies.)

incorporated into the urogenital sinus, or the differential growth of the sinus is abnormal and the ureter fails to migrate to its usual location. Ectopic ureters occasionally empty into the rectum because of anomalous cloacal division by the urorectal fold. Very rarely, they empty into the cervix, uterus, or uterine tube, possibly as a result of aberrant origin from the paramesonephric (Müllerian) duct. Even more rarely, an ectopic ureter may be blind ended cranially in cases with accompanying renal agenesis.

Ectopic ureter is most common in dogs and is diagnosed up to 20 times more frequently in females than in males. However, this sex difference may be exaggerated because affected females are usually incontinent from birth, whereas affected males may not be. Termination of the ectopic ureter proximal to the external urethral sphincter in males leads to retrograde filling of the bladder rather than to incontinence. Ectopia can be unilateral or bilateral and is often associated with other urinary tract abnormalities, including bladder agenesis or hypoplasia, renal agenesis or hypoplasia, ureteral or bladder duplication, and branching of the terminal ureter. In the United States, certain dog breeds have a high risk for the defect, including the Siberian Husky, Bulldog, Newfoundland, Labrador Retriever, West Highland White Terrier, Fox Terrier, and Miniature and Toy Poodles. The breed predilection in the United Kingdom includes the Golden Retriever, Labrador Retriever, Skye Terrier, Border Terrier, Briard, Bulldog, and the Griffon. The defect is familial in Siberian Huskies and Labrador Retrievers. Ectopic ureter also occurs in White Shorthorn bulls and tends to involve the region of the seminal vesicles. It is rare in horses.

A **ureterocele** is a congenital abnormality that is defined as *a focal submucosal dilation of the distal ureter*, especially involving that portion that lies within the urinary bladder wall. It may be associated with normal anatomic emptying (orthotopic or intravesical ureterocele), or an ectopic location (ectopic ureterocele). *Ureteral anomalies often predispose to hydronephrosis/hydroureter and urinary tract infection that may culminate in pyelonephritis.* **Ureteral diverticula** result from urothelial hyperplasia, mucinous metaplasia, and submucosal urothelial proliferation with the formation of small cysts. Neoplastic transformation may occur more readily in such sites.

Urinary bladder

Duplication of the urinary bladder occurs rarely in dogs and causes dysuria, incontinence, and, less frequently, abdominal distension and cryptorchidism. The extra bladder originates dorsally between the urinary tract and uterus or rectum. Cystic remnants of the urorectal fold may be responsible for this defect.

Patent or **pervious urachus** is the *most common malformation of the urinary bladder* and is seen more often in foals than in other animals. Animals with this defect dribble urine from the umbilicus because the urachal lumen fails to close and is a channel between the apex of the bladder and the umbilicus. A patent urachus is susceptible to infection. Rupture of the urachus causes uroperitoneum. The condition must be differentiated from perinatal rupture of the bladder. Occasionally, urachal obliteration is partial, and rests of epithelium remain intact to develop into **urachal cysts** at any point between the umbilicus and the bladder. Although these cysts may become quite large, they are usually small, multiple and attached to the midline of the bladder. Occasionally, they adhere to the intestinal serosa. The urachus is normally lined by urothelium, but metaplasia to squamous or mucus-secreting columnar epithelium is common in urachal cysts and sinuses. Urachal remnants in the bladder wall may give rise to neoplasms.

Diverticula of the bladder may be primary or acquired secondary to partial obstruction to urine outflow, or as the result of pressure changes exerted during normal contractions. Diverticula are usually seen at the apex, where they represent incomplete closure of the urachus (vesicourachal diverticulum) with an area of discontinuity in the muscle. They also occur less commonly in the trigone region in association with a malformation of the bladder muscle wall. Contraction of the bladder tends to distend the diverticulum, but rupture does not occur. Additionally, stasis of urine in the diverticulum eventually leads to persistent infection and inflammation. Calculi may form in the diverticulum. If the distal urachus remains patent to the exterior through the umbilical opening, a **urachal sinus** results.

Urethra

Urethral **agenesis, duplicated** urethra, **ectopic** urethra, and **imperforate** urethra occur rarely in dogs. A case of bovine urethral duplication was reported in a Swiss Braunvieh heifer with other urogenital malformations. This animal had cytogenetic confirmation of reciprocal autosomal translocation between chromosomes 20 and 22, suggesting that genetic anomalies could be responsible for this condition. Hypospadias is described with male genitalia. *The most common urethral anomaly is* **urethrorectal** or **rectovaginal fistula,** which is caused by incomplete division of the cloaca into rectum and urogenital sinus by the urorectal fold. In males, the communication involves the pelvic urethra, and affected dogs urinate from the rectum. In females, the opening is in the vagina and may be associated with imperforate anus. These defects are reported in dogs, cats, pigs, rabbits, alpacas, and foals, often as one of several congenital anomalies. These changes usually predispose to urogenital tract infections, but sometimes are incidental autopsy findings.

In male ruminants and swine, a **urethral recess** is normally present near the ischial arch and is an impediment to catheterization. Dilation of the urethral recess can cause midline perineal swelling in ruminants.

Urethral atresia and **urethral hypoplasia** have been noted in newborn freemartin intersex calves with uroperitoneum following rupture of the urethra or urinary bladder. **Urethral strictures** have been documented in intersex ruminants, a llama, and a Nubian goat.

Further reading

Agut A, et al. Unilateral renal agenesis associated with additional congenital abnormalities of the urinary tract in a Pekingese bitch. J Small Anim Pract 2002;43:32-35.

Chaney KP. Congenital anomalies of the equine urinary tract. Vet Clin North Am Equine Pract 2007;23:691-696.

Esterline ML, et al. Ureteral duplication in a dog. Vet Radiol Ultrasound 2005;46:485-489.

Holt PE, et al. Breed predisposition to ureteral ectopia in bitches in the UK. Vet Rec 2000;146:561.

Lautzenhiser SJ, Bjorling DE. Urinary incontinence in a dog with an ectopic ureterocele. J Am Anim Hosp Assoc 2002;38:29-32.

Reichler IM, et al. Ectopic ureters in dogs: clinical features, surgical techniques and outcome. Vet Surg 2012;41:515-522.

Stiffler KS, et al. Intravesical ureterocele with concurrent renal dysfunction in a dog: a case report and proposed classification system. J Am Anim Hosp Assoc 2002;38:33-39.

Acquired anatomic variations

Displacements of ureters and urethra can be caused by local inflammation and neoplasia. Their significance is related to obstruction of urine flow. Ureteral and urethral displacements may also occur with variations of position of the bladder.

Torsion of the bladder is uncommon; it may be partial or complete about the long axis of the organ. Presence of part of the bladder within the pelvis in dogs, so-called *"pelvic bladder,"* is a clinical diagnosis made via contrast urethrocystography; its clinical significance as a cause of urinary tract infection or incontinence is controversial. **Retroflexion** of the bladder can occur from vaginal prolapse in cows, sows, and bitches and occasionally in perineal hernia of older male dogs. In these cases, the retroflexed bladder may be present in the hernial sac with obstructive kinking of the neck of the bladder and sometimes of the urethra and ureters. If the ureters are patent, the accumulation of urine in the bladder contributes to the size of the hernia. Hydronephrosis or rupture of the bladder may occur if the condition is not corrected.

Eversion of the bladder *(invagination into and through the urethra)* occurs in females because the female urethra is short and wide. The bladder may arrive in the vagina. This is an issue in large animals and is perhaps most common in mares. Eversion occurs in circumstances in which increased intra-abdominal pressure or straining occurs, often after parturition. Hypocalcemia in periparturient dairy cows may contribute by resulting in decreased bladder tone before eversion. The everted bladder may allow for herniation of intestine. Rarely, *umbilical eversion* of the bladder can occur in foals that experience traumatic tearing of the umbilical cord and urachus during birthing. Eversion of the bladder should be distinguished from **prolapse** of the bladder. In eversion, the mucosal surface protrudes from the vulva, whereas *in prolapse the bladder is displaced through a rent in the vagina, and the serosal surface appears.*

Hydroureter, or *dilation of a ureter,* may be caused by obstruction by calculi, neoplasms, inflammation, scar tissue, or the result of accidental ligation during surgery, (e.g., ovariohysterectomy) (eFig. 4-47). It will lead to hydronephrosis. Dilation without physical obstruction occurs in association with peritonitis and may be because of loss of muscle tone. Dilation of ureters is often present in neonatal pigs with enteric infections. Congenital hydroureter and hydronephrosis often occur in piglets in association with epitheliogenesis imperfecta.

Ureters may **rupture** as a consequence of blunt physical trauma or rarely in association with parturition. Foals can have bilateral involvement after nonpenetrating, blunt trauma, which suggests a possible congenital predisposition. Ureters may also be accidentally **transected** during surgery, for example, ovariohysterectomy. Leakage of urine from a traumatized ureter is the most common cause of a **paraureteral or uriniferous pseudocyst,** which is basically a fibrous wall without an epithelial lining. Urethral obstruction and urine leakage from a rent in the renal capsule are also documented causes. **Perinephric pseudocysts** are similar but surround the kidney and may be associated with CRF in cats.

Dilation of the bladder may be the result of obstruction or neuromuscular disease. The wall is thin and almost transparent. Brief periods of distension may allow return of normal contractility. Severe or prolonged distension may result in loss of tone, which can be complicated by bacterial infection. *Causes of obstruction* include calculi, prostatic enlargement, inflammatory debris or blood clots in the urethra, urethral strictures, and tumors of the neck of the bladder or urethra. Detrusor atony of the bladder may follow prolonged dystocia in the dog. Distension of the bladder occurs when calves fed indigestible milk-replacer starve to death. Renal concentrating ability is depressed by starvation because of lack of urea and a partial insensitivity to ADH and mineralocorticoids. The bladder distension is possibly caused by overproduction of dilute urine.

Neurogenic disorders of micturition can arise from abnormalities of the sphincter or bladder, and also from failure to store and/or void urine. Neurogenic distension follows spinal injury, with loss of tonic parasympathetic outflow from the sacral plexus. In the dog, it most commonly follows herniation of intervertebral disks. Spinal myelitis can also cause paralysis of the bladder. Cystitis and ischemic necrosis, secondary to compression of vessels within the distended urinary bladder wall, are possible complications. In horses, bladder paralysis and distension may lead to sabulous urolithiasis, resembling sand (Fig. 4-80). Descriptions of *detrusor-urethral dyssynergia* in dogs have been rarely documented in young and middle-aged large-breed dogs. This condition is a functional disorder of the voiding phase of micturition, because of involuntary contraction of the external urethral sphincter in the postprostatic urethra, the smooth muscle of the neck of the bladder, or the prostatic urethra (internal sphincter). Typically, these animals have dysuria with interrupted spurting of urine and a large residual urine volume.

Sphincter mechanism incompetence *is the most common cause of urinary incontinence in middle-aged, spayed bitches,* but the prevalence is also higher those with body weights >30 kg, docked breeds (Doberman Pinschers, Old English Sheepdogs, Rottweilers, Weimaraners, and Setters). In females, an intrapelvic bladder neck, a short urethra, reduced urethral tone, and neutering before first estrus predispose to this condition. Restoration of normal anatomic location of urethra/urinary bladder by surgical procedures is often curative. Bladder neck

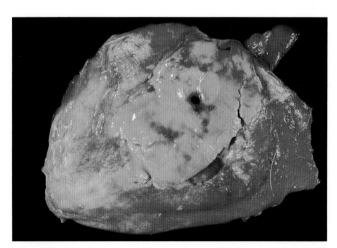

Figure 4-80 Sabulous cystitis in a horse. (Courtesy S. Siso, B.G. Murphy.)

position (i.e., intrapelvic), breed, prostate size, and castration status are significant risk factors for incontinence in male dogs. Congenital urethral sphincter mechanism incompetence in cats has been associated with genitourinary dysplasia (urethral hypoplasia and vaginal and/or uterine hypoplasia/aplasia).

Hypertrophy of the bladder wall is fairly common in dogs and less so in other species. It is a response to long-standing partial obstruction to the outflow of urine.

Rupture of the bladder (cystorrhexis) often occurs following urethral obstruction, such as occurs in urolithiasis. Rarely, it is secondary to pelvic trauma or dystocia. The interval between obstruction and rupture depends somewhat on the competence of the vesicoureteral valve and whether hydronephrosis develops. Rupture of the bladder occurs in newborn foals, with an incidence of 0.2–2.5%, affecting either the dorsal or ventral aspect of the organ. Males are most often affected. Some ruptures are congenital and are probably caused by birth trauma. Twists in the amniotic portion of the umbilical cord may compress the urachus, causing distension of both bladder and urachus and predisposing to rupture. Only rarely is the urinary bladder rupture secondary to atrophy of circular smooth muscle fibers in the dorsal bladder wall.

Urine in the peritoneal cavity, or **uroperitoneum,** follows leakage from the kidneys, ureter, bladder, or urethra. Diagnosis of uroperitoneum is supported by the finding of peritoneal-to-serum ratios for potassium, phosphate, and creatinine >2:1. Calcium carbonate crystals are occasionally seen in the peritoneal fluid. Uroperitoneum has been seen increasingly in foals in association with positive sepsis scores. It has been associated with a negative prognosis. *Escherichia coli, Actinobacillus equuli* and, less commonly, *Clostridium perfringens* are implicated in urosepsis or urachal infections. Abdominal trauma is the most common cause of urine leakage from the bladder in dogs and cats. Catheterization and bladder expression are the most common causes of urethral leakage in cats. Urinary calculi and obstruction by urothelial cell carcinoma are also causes.

Although uncommon in domestic swine, **urethral polyps** have been reported in Vietnamese pot-bellied pigs. It seems most likely that these lesions arise secondary to trauma to the mucosal folds of the urethral recess associated with repeated catheterization. **Urethral caruncles** have been described in humans and dogs and form as a result of chronic inflammation of the urethral mucosa. Glandular structures are intermixed with a granulomatous infiltrate, often producing an obstructive mass lesion.

Further reading

Braun U, et al. Ruptured urinary bladder attributable to urethral compression by a haematoma after vertebral fracture in a bull. Acta Vet Scand 2014;56:17.

Dunkel B, et al. Uroperitoneum in 32 foals: influence of intravenous fluid therapy, infection, and sepsis. J Vet Intern Med 2005;19:889-893.

Lores M, et al. Septic peritonitis and uroperitoneum secondary to subclinical omphalitis and concurrent necrotizing cystitis in a colt. Can Vet J 2011;52:888-892.

Moores AP, et al. Urinoma (para-ureteral pseudocyst) as a consequence of trauma in a cat. J Small Anim Pract 2002;43:213-216.

Morisset S, et al. Surgical management of a ureteral defect with ureterrhaphy and of ureteritis with ureteroneocystostomy in a foal. J Am Vet Med Assoc 2002;220:354-358.

Nwadike BS, et al. Use of bilateral temporary nephrostomy catheters for emergency treatment of bilateral ureter transection in a cat. J Am Vet Med Assoc 2000;217:1862-1865.

Textor JA, et al. Umbilical evagination of the urinary bladder in a neonatal filly. J Am Vet Med Assoc 2001;219:953-956.

Thieman KM, Pozzi A. Torsion of the urinary bladder after pelvic trauma and surgical fixation. Vet Comp Orthop Traumatol 2010;23:259-261.

Weisse C, et al. Traumatic rupture of the ureter: 10 cases. J Am Anim Hosp Assoc 2002;38:188-192.

Worth AJ, Tomlin SC. Post-traumatic paraureteral urinoma in a cat. J Small Anim Pract 2004;45:413-416.

CIRCULATORY DISTURBANCES

In the ureters and urethra, hemorrhages are associated with obstructive calculi or acute ascending infections. Urethral hematomas following pelvic trauma may predispose to urinary bladder rupture. In the bladder, hemorrhages are typically located in the propria mucosa and may occur in any septicemia. Small hemorrhages or hematomas are common and considered diagnostically significant in classical swine fever, African swine fever, porcine salmonellosis, and equine purpura hemorrhagica. Larger hemorrhages are seen in bracken fern poisoning of cattle. Hemorrhage occurs with acute cystitis and neoplasia, and following rupture of the bladder.

Further reading

Arnold CE, et al. Hematuria associated with cystic hematomas in three neonatal foals. J Am Vet Med Assoc 2005;227:778-780.

Braun U, et al. Ruptured urinary bladder attributable to urethral compression by a haematoma after vertebral fracture in a bull. Acta Vet Scand 2014;56:17.

UROLITHIASIS

Urolithiasis is the presence of calculi (uroliths or stones) in the urinary passages. Calculi are grossly visible aggregates of precipitated urinary solutes, urinary proteins, and proteinaceous debris. Minerals predominate in **calculi,** whereas matrix usually predominates in **urethral plugs.** *Calculi typically have a central nidus, surrounded by concentric laminae, an outer shell, and surface crystals.* Many calculi are hard spherical or ovoid structures with a small amount of organic matrix impregnated with inorganic salts. *Urethral plugs are masses of sandy sludge with a much higher organic component* whose form is largely determined by the shape of the cavity they fill. Even densely mineralized calculi of the same type may have quite a different appearance, depending on whether they are located in renal pelvis or urinary bladder. Many calculi contain significant quantities of "contaminants," such as calcium oxalates in "silica" calculi. A few calculi are relatively pure.

The diseases caused by uroliths are among the most important urinary tract problems of domesticated animals. Calculogenic material must occur in urine in quantities sufficient to be precipitated. Sometimes this concentration is achieved because a substance is metabolized in an unusual way, as is uric acid in Dalmatian dogs. Also a substance may be processed abnormally by the kidney, as is cystine in cystine stone–formers, or may be in abnormally high levels of a substance in the diet, such as silicic acid in native pastures. Regardless of the type of calculus, certain factors are more or less important; these are **urinary pH** and **reduced water intake,** in relation to the degree of urine concentration. Other predisposing conditions include **infection** (see Struvite calculi), obstruction, structural abnormalities, foreign bodies, and drug-induced changes in urine composition, for example, by sulfonamides. A foreign body, such as a suture, grass awn, catheter, or needle, can act as a nidus for urolith formation. Deficiency of vitamin A is frequently suggested as a factor predisposing to urolithiasis, but the evidence is equivocal; it may contribute in exceptional circumstances by producing metaplastic changes in the urinary epithelium.

Urine **supersaturation** is the essential precursor to initiation of urolith formation (nucleation). Supersaturation may be in the **unstable** region where spontaneous precipitation occurs (homogeneous nucleation, the precipitation-crystallization theory of urolith initiation), or in the **metastable** range, where precipitation occurs by epitaxy or heterogeneous nucleation (one type of crystal grows on the surface of another type). Although formerly it was thought that urinary proteins such as uromucoid, which make up 5-20% or more of some calculi, were pre-eminent initiators of crystal formation in the metastable range *(the matrix-nucleation theory of urolith initiation)*, it is now believed that in many cases either coprecipitation of proteins and minerals occurs or that proteins are adsorbed on to formed crystals. It is possible that crystals of one salt, for which urine is supersaturated in the unstable range, cause epitactic induction of crystals of another salt, for which supersaturation is metastable. Crystals are much more common in urine than are calculi. Even though equine urine, for example, is normally supersaturated with calcium carbonate and crystalluria is normal, horses experience a low prevalence of calculi. The factors that promote crystal growth and crystal aggregation or, more importantly, prevent them in some animals, are poorly understood. Experimentally, high levels of urinary inorganic pyrophosphate and magnesium are important inhibitors of calcium phosphate and calcium oxalate crystallization, and pyrophosphate also inhibits aggregation of calcium phosphate crystals. Certain urinary macromolecules, probably glycosaminoglycans, are also strong inhibitors of crystal aggregation in experimental systems. Deficiency of inhibitors of crystallization may be important in calcium oxalate and calcium phosphate calculogenesis *(crystallization-inhibition theory of urolith initiation)*. It is not known why calculi stay in the renal pelvis and urinary bladder until they are large enough to cause disease.

The important types of urinary calculi are listed according to species in Table 4-4. Although one mineral may predominate in a urolith, *many uroliths are of mixed composition.* Overlap in the gross appearance of uroliths usually precludes specific gross diagnosis of mineral type. *In general, calculi are important in cattle, sheep, dogs, and cats, less important in horses, and unimportant in pigs.* In pigs, uroliths are occasionally found in the renal pelvis of old animals and, more often, in the pelvis of dehydrated sucklings (see Renal disease, renal failure, and uremia; previously). In *horses,* they occur sometimes as single or several, spherical or faceted carbonate stones in the bladder; urethral obstructions are rare. In *dogs,* several breeds are predisposed to formation of calculi, namely, Dachshunds, Dalmatians, Cocker Spaniels, Pekingese, Basset Hounds, Poodles, Schnauzers, and small terriers.

Table • 4-4

Composition and importance of urinary calculi

Species	Common types	Uncommon types
Dog	Struvite Oxalate Purines (urate, uric acid, xanthine)	Silica Cystine Calcium phosphate
Cat	Struvite Oxalate	Urate Cystine
Ox	Silica Struvite Carbonate	Xanthine
Sheep	Silica Struvite Oxalate "Clover stones" Carbonate	Xanthine
Horse	Carbonate	
Pig		Urate

Calculi may form in any part of the urinary duct system, from the renal pelvis to the urethra. Some uroliths clearly originate in the lower urinary tract, but the point for development of most is not known. In experimental urolithiasis produced by oxalates or calcium phosphate in laboratory animals, the calculi, initially microscopic, form in the collecting ducts and encrust on the renal papilla. They may grow large enough to make voidance impossible (Fig. 4-81). It is not known whether this is a general phenomenon. Tubular microlithiasis may simply represent crystallization in the highly concentrated urine of the medulla, or, alternatively, it may indicate in situ production of an abnormal or excessive matricial substance. Obstructive nephroliths and ureteroliths occasionally develop in horses and cause secondary chronic tubulointerstitial nephritis; the suggested pathogenesis is renal medullary crest necrosis resulting from the use of nonsteroidal anti-inflammatory drugs in dehydrated horses, with subsequent mineralization of the sloughed necrotic renal crest material. Nephroliths are uncommon forms of uroliths in most species, representing only 1-4% of canine uroliths (Fig. 4-82).

Small calculi may be voided in the urine, but *impaction in the urethra is common in males.* The common sites of urethral impaction are the ischial arch, the sigmoid flexure of ruminants, the vermiform appendage of rams (Fig. 4-83), the proximal end of the os penis in dogs, and anywhere along the urethra of male cats. At the point of obstruction, there is pressure necrosis with ulceration of the mucosa. Because urinary stasis favors bacterial growth, acute hemorrhagic urethritis develops and can ascend to the bladder and kidney. Hydronephrosis is not common with completely obstructive urethral calculi because rupture of the urethra with associated infection and acute cellulitis terminates the condition fairly quickly.

Large numbers of companion animal uroliths have been studied, and knowledge is expanding on the prevalence of mineral composition, breed predilections, geographic region prevalence, and the association with urinary tract infections.

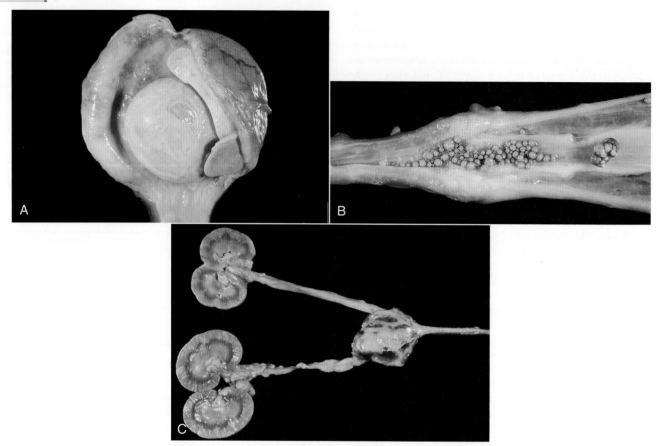

Figure 4-81 **A.** **Urolithiasis** in the urinary bladder of a dog. (Courtesy L. Himmel, C. Premanandan.) **B.** Multiple small uroliths in the urethra of a cat. (Courtesy C. Martin, C. Premanandan.) **C.** Granular uroliths in the urinary bladder and urethra of a cat with secondary hemorrhagic cystitis, unilateral hydroureter, and hydronephrosis. (Courtesy B. Harrington, D. Russell.)

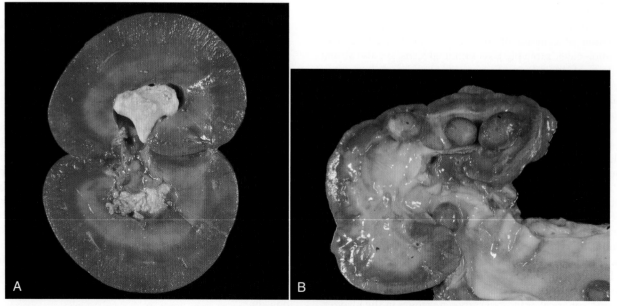

Figure 4-82 **A,** **Staghorn calculus in the renal pelvis** of a dog. (Courtesy L. Himmel, C. Premanandan.) **B.** **Multiple uroliths** in a hydronephrotic equine kidney. (Courtesy S. Jennings.)

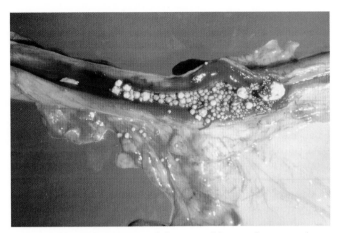

Figure 4-83 Obstructive urolithiasis and hemorrhagic urethritis resulting from impaction of multiple calculi at the sigmoid flexure of the penis of a steer. (Courtesy University of Guelph.)

Further reading

Adams LG. Nephroliths and ureteroliths: a new stone age. N Z Vet J 2013;61:212-216.

Duesterdieck-Zellmer KF. Equine urolithiasis. Vet Clin North Am Equine Pract 2007;23:613-629.

Houston DM, Moore AE. Canine and feline urolithiasis: examination of over 50,000 urolith submissions to the Canadian veterinary urolith centre from 1998 to 2008. Can Vet J 2009;50:1263-1268.

Low WW, et al. Evaluation of trends in urolith composition and characteristics of dogs with urolithiasis: 25,499 cases (1985-2006). J Am Vet Med Assoc 2010;236:193-200.

Osborne CA, et al. Analysis of 451,891 canine uroliths, feline uroliths, and feline urethral plugs from 1981 to 2007: perspectives from the Minnesota Urolith Center. Vet Clin North Am Small Anim Pract 2009;39:183-197.

Silica calculi

In **ruminants,** these calculi are hard, white to dark-brown, radiopaque, often laminated, and up to 1 cm across. They are spherical, ovoid, or mulberry shaped, and have smooth surfaces in the bladder of ruminants, but in the kidney, they are angular and irregular, having the shape of the minor calyces, where they are located almost exclusively.

"Pure silica" stones contain ~75% silica as silica dioxide. Mixed calculi contain some calcium oxalate or carbonate. Silica calculi contain about 20% organic matter. Most have a friable core, which is high in amorphous silica and low in organic matter. The core is surrounded by a layer of organic matter, which separates it from the outer concentric laminations that are rich in silica.

Silica calculi are very common in pastured ruminants and are a major cause of urinary tract obstruction. They occur with increasing prevalence in dogs and rarely in horses. Silica calculi are present in >50% of steers on native ranges in western Canada; <5% develop urethral obstruction. The singularity of adjacent laminae in the calculi is consistent with intermittent deposition as urine composition changes. Certain grasses contain 4-5% or more of silica; the level increases through the growing season. Most of it is relatively insoluble, but that in the cell sap is relatively soluble, unpolymerized silicic acid. Rumen fluid becomes saturated with silicic acid. After absorption, some is returned to the gut in digestive secretions; <1% of dietary silica is excreted in urine, and up to 60% is resorbed from the filtrate. However, when urine production is very low, either because of dehydration or because of high insensible fluid losses in hot climates, the concentration of silicic acid in urine may reach 5 times the saturation level. Even so, precipitation from solution requires other substances, probably proteins of renal or serum origin, in the urine. Calculus formation is reduced to subclinical levels by adding salt to the ration, thereby increasing water consumption. Acid-forming effects of the diet and a reduction in the dietary calcium-to-phosphorus ratio also reduce silica urolith formation.

In **dogs,** silica calculi are detected primarily in males, are located in the bladder and urethra, and often cause urinary obstruction. Male German Shepherd dogs and Old English Sheepdogs are at increased risk for formation of these calculi. Unlike cystic silica calculi in ruminants, bladder stones in dogs have very irregular shapes with surface protrusions. Silica uroliths in dogs may be multilayered or single-layered, and may contain calcium oxalate and struvite. Large quantities of plant-derived ingredients, particularly corn gluten feed, rice hulls, and soybean hulls, in dry dog food are implicated as risk factors for development of silica uroliths. Some cases are associated with lower urinary tract infections, often with *Staphylococcus* species. Silica uroliths are likely less soluble in acid than in alkaline urine.

Further reading

Kinsley MA, et al. Use of plain radiography in the diagnosis, surgical management, and postoperative treatment of obstructive urolithiasis in 25 goats and 2 sheep. Vet Surg 2013;42:663-668.

Lulich JP, et al. Recent shifts in the global proportions of canine uroliths. Vet Rec 2013;172:363.

Struvite calculi

Struvite is *magnesium ammonium phosphate hexahydrate* ($MgNH_4PO_4 \bullet 6H_2O$). Struvite stones are white or gray, radiopaque, chalky, usually smooth, and easily broken. They may be pure struvite but usually contain other compounds, such as calcium phosphate (which may form a shell around a struvite), ammonium urate, oxalate, or carbonate. They may be single and large, or numerous and sand-like. Single struvite calculi can form masses that mold to the shape of the cavity they occupy. They have also been referred to as "triple phosphate," a misnomer, and as "infection calculi" in recognition of their common association with infection.

Struvite calculi are important in dogs, cats, and ruminants. In **dogs,** they are the most common calculus, and females are particularly susceptible, perhaps because they develop bladder infections more often than males. Ureases from *Staphylococcus* and *Proteus* spp. induce supersaturation of urine with struvite by increasing urine pH and ammonium ions. Alkaline urine decreases struvite solubility and increases ionization of trivalent phosphate, both of which favor calculus formation. Factors other than urease production, which are associated with infection, are probably also important in the genesis of struvite stones. The reason for *sterile* struvite urolithiasis in 3 related English Cocker Spaniels and in an inbred line of Beagles is not known, but familial risk factors and dietary factors are postulated. Pugs are predisposed to developing both struvite uroliths and struvite urethral plugs, without evidence of underlying urinary tract infection. The somewhat refractory response of struvite calculi to medical or dietary manipulations in dogs is thought to be because of the presence of associated hydroxyl apatite and concentric laminations, which have low porosity.

In **cats,** most cases of the heterogeneous group of disorders referred to as **feline lower urinary tract disease** (FLUTD) are idiopathic, and are discussed in the section Cystitis. One manifestation of FLUTD is urolithiasis, in which discrete calculi develop in the urinary bladder of young to middle-aged cats (increased risk for cats between 4 and 10 years of age). Additional risk factors are associated with Russian Blue, Himalayan, or Persian breed, and castrated male or spayed female status. Intact females had a reduced risk. Struvite crystalluria is often seen in cats with and without calculi; the reasons for aggregation of crystals into sterile calculi are obscure. The prevalence of struvite uroliths and struvite urethral plugs has declined since the mid-1980s when cat foods were reformulated; there has been a concomitant increase in calcium oxalate urolithiasis in cats. Formation of struvite uroliths can be induced in previously normal cats fed calculogenic diets containing 0.15-1.0% dry weight magnesium. Primary pores in struvite calculi are an important feature and may allow dietary and medicinal manipulations to dissolve these uroliths. Coagulase-positive staphylococci and other bacteria may be cultured from the urine or calculi of some affected cats. Formation of infection-induced struvite calculi is similar to that seen in dogs, but these calculi are less common than sterile struvite uroliths.

Of considerably more importance than discrete calculi are the amorphous accumulations of protein, cellular debris, and struvite crystals that form *sabulous (matrix-crystalline) urethral plugs in male cats*, with castrated males being at a higher risk and spayed females at the lowest risk. Animals 2-7 years of age are predisposed. This condition was previously known as *feline urologic syndrome*, and it results from concomitant occurrence of urinary tract inflammation and the presence of various types of urine crystals. It is characterized by dysuria, hematuria, and urethral obstruction. If unrelieved, the obstruction can lead to bladder distension, hemorrhagic cystitis, azotemia, and death. *The obstructive material, which becomes molded to the shape of the urethra in male cats, may be either struvite "sand" or rubber-like protein matrix, or a mixture of the two;* the matrix contains Tamm-Horsfall mucoprotein, albumin, globulins, cells, and cellular debris. The inflammatory component of plugs may be caused by viral, bacterial, or fungal infections. Various viruses, including feline cell-associated herpesvirus (a strain of bovine herpesvirus 4), feline syncytia-forming virus, and feline calicivirus, have been implicated as potential urinary pathogens in cats; there is no concrete evidence for *Mycoplasma* or *Ureaplasma*. Addition of magnesium and phosphate to the diet causes disease in some cats and, conversely, reduction of dietary magnesium reduces the incidence. Alkaline urine pH is likely of more significance in the formation of struvite crystals than is magnesium intake. The increased incidence during cold winter months may be the result of decreased fluid consumption or increased intervals between urinations. The incidence of urethral plugs has decreased as more cats have been fed magnesium-restricted/pH-controlling diets.

In **ruminants,** struvite calculi usually occur in feedlot cattle or sheep on high grain rations, and obstruction may develop in up to 10% of steers. As in cats, *calculi usually form a gritty sludge with a high proportion of matrix.* Inhibition of urethral growth by early castration predisposes to obstruction, and increased water consumption tends to prevent obstruction. Animals with crystalluria often have crystals adhering to preputial hairs. Diets high in phosphate is associated with a high incidence of calculi in sheep, wherein a calcium-to-phosphorus ratio of 1:2 or greater appears to be the critical cutoff. The balance of other constituents, such as magnesium, sodium, and potassium, are probably also important. Additional potassium tends to promote phosphate urolithiasis. Magnesium deficiency leads to renal mineralization and tubular microlithiasis, at least in laboratory species. Both sodium and magnesium are competitive with calcium, and increase the solubility of calcium salts in urine. There may also be a genetic effect on urolithiasis in sheep, because it is more likely to develop in sheep that excrete phosphorus mainly in urine as opposed to fecal excretion.

Further reading

Houston DM, et al. Feline urethral plugs and bladder uroliths: a review of 5,484 submissions 1998-2003. Can Vet J 2003;44: 974-977.

Lekcharoensuk C, et al. Epidemiologic study of risk factors for lower urinary tract diseases in cats. J Am Vet Med Assoc 2001;218:1429-1435.

Okafor CC, et al. Risk factors associated with struvite urolithiasis in dogs evaluated at general care veterinary hospitals in the United States. J Am Vet Med Assoc 2013;243:1737-1745.

Palma D, et al. Feline struvite urolithiasis. Compend Contin Educ Vet 2009;31:E1-E7.

Stiller AT, et al. Urethral plugs in dogs. J Vet Intern Med 2014;28: 324-330.

Oxalate calculi

Oxalate calculi are hard, heavy, white, or yellow, and typically covered with jagged spines, although some are smooth. They tend to be large and solitary in the bladder.

Oxalate calculi occur as the calcium oxalates, *either calcium oxalate monohydrate* (whewellite) or *calcium oxalate dihydrate* (weddellite). Their development is not well understood, but *hypercalciuria and hyperoxaluria are involved.* There are several causes of hypercalciuria (see Hypercalcemic nephropathy; previously). Oxalic acid is synthesized from glyoxylic and ascorbic acid and may be ingested in certain foods. Hyperuricosuria may be involved in oxalate precipitation, because sodium hydrogen urate may act as a heterogeneous nucleator. Dietary magnesium and citrate inhibit the formation of calcium oxalate uroliths by forming soluble complexes with oxalate and calcium, respectively.

Oxalate (and silica) calculi may be important in **sheep** grazing grain stubble, but the source of the oxalate is not known. Oxalate-containing plants are not apparently a source because oxalate is metabolized in the rumen; nonetheless, occasional exceptions to this general rule do seem to occur. Feeding a low-calcium diet (0.3% Ca) has produced oxalate urolithiasis in steers, possibly because of increased bone resorption resulting in increased plasma concentrations of hydroxyproline, an oxalate precursor. High magnesium intake inhibits formation of oxalate calculi, whereas low levels induce formation in some species.

In **dogs,** oxalate calculi are second to struvite calculi in prevalence and are of increasing importance, but little is known of their origins. Calcium oxalate and calcium phosphate (hydroxyapatite or calcium apatite) calculi occur in dogs with primary hyperparathyroidism, hypercalcemia, hyperadrenocorticism, or following exogenous steroid administration. Canine dietary factors, such as high protein, fat, Ca, P, Mg, Na, K, Cl, and use of canned foods, are thought to decrease the risk of development of these stones. Males are more frequently affected than females, and they are seen more commonly in older animals. The Miniature Schnauzer, Bichon Frise, Lhasa Apso, Yorkshire Terrier, Shih Tzu, and Miniature Poodle are breeds at increased risk. In predisposed Miniature Schnauzers, hypercalciuria, decreased urinary oxalate, normal urinary citrate, increased brushite (calcium hydrogen phosphate dihydrate), urinary relative supersaturation, lower urine volume, and elevated excreted uric acid levels are consistent findings.

The prevalence of oxalate uroliths in **cats** has increased markedly from the early 1980s through the 1990s. This increase has been accompanied by a marked decline in the prevalence of struvite uroliths. The underlying cause for oxalate uroliths in cats is unknown, but likely related to diet. Several dietary factors can contribute to calciuria, including high animal-source protein, low magnesium, high sodium chloride, and diets formulated to acidify urine. Risk factors also include use of a single brand of cat food without additional supplementation, and maintaining cats in an indoor environment only. Persian, Himalayan, and several other breeds are at increased risk; cats with calcium oxalate uroliths tend to be older than cats with struvite uroliths. Additionally, male and neutered cats are at higher risk for the development of oxalate calculi. Oxalate uroliths in cats have been associated with parathyroid neoplasia, as in dogs.

Further reading

Dijcker JC, et al. Urinary oxalate and calcium excretion by dogs and cats diagnosed with calcium oxalate urolithiasis. Vet Rec 2012; 171:646.

Lekcharoensuk C, et al. Associations between dry dietary factors and canine calcium oxalate uroliths. Am J Vet Res 2002;63: 330-337.

Okafor CC, et al. Risk factors associated with calcium oxalate urolithiasis in dogs evaluated at general care veterinary hospitals in the United States. Prev Vet Med 2014;115:217-228.

Wisener LV, et al. Risk factors for the incidence of calcium oxalate uroliths or magnesium ammonium phosphate uroliths for dogs in Ontario, Canada, from 1998 to 2006. Am J Vet Res 2010;71: 1045-1054.

Uric acid and urate calculi

These *purine calculi* are usually multiple, hard, concentrically laminated and brown-green. In the bladder, they are frequently spherical and <5 mm across. Most contain ammonium urate with some uric acid and phosphate; in others, sodium urate is the predominant salt.

Urate stones are most common in dogs, especially Dalmatians, but also occur in pigs and rarely in cats. Neonatal piglets in a negative energy balance produce increased purine catabolites, which predispose to urate urolithiasis. Dalmatians excrete high levels of uric acid in their urine. This is the result of defective hepatocellular uptake of uric acid, leading to incomplete conversion of uric acid to allantoin, a more soluble product of purine metabolism. This defect is an inherited autosomal recessive trait and is linked to a mutation in *SLC2A9*, a glucose transporter that has been demonstrated to be involved in urate transport in humans and rodents and is believed to function similarly in dogs. Hepatic uricase levels are normal. Predisposing factors for urolith formation include male sex, hyperuricemia, hyperammonemia, hyperuricosuria, hyperammonuria, and aciduria. Other dog breeds with a higher incidence of urate urolithiasis include English Bulldogs, Miniature Schnauzers, Shih Tzu, and Yorkshire Terriers. Dogs with portosystemic shunts have ammonium biurate crystals in their urine, and may have urate-containing calculi in kidneys and bladder.

Urates exist in supersaturated urine as lyophobic colloids, which are flocculated (coalesced and precipitated), by high levels of ammonium ion and, to a lesser extent, by low pH. Urea-splitting organisms may be important in the development of urate calculi because production of ammonium ion favors calculus formation. Although higher pH inhibits precipitation of uric acid, it favors precipitation of ammonium urate and phosphates, which can be found in urate calculi.

Further reading

Dear JD, et al. Feline urate urolithiasis: a retrospective study of 159 cases. J Feline Med Surg 2011;13:725-732.

Karmi N, et al. Estimated frequency of the canine hyperuricosuria mutation in different dog breeds. J Vet Intern Med 2010;24:1337-1342.

McCue J, et al. Urate urolithiasis. Compend Contin Educ Vet. 2009; 31:468-475.

Xanthine calculi

Xanthine stones are yellow to brown-red, often concentrically laminated, friable, and irregularly shaped. They are radiolucent. *Xanthine is a metabolite of purines,* which seldom appears in urine because it is normally degraded by xanthine oxidase to uric acid.

Xanthine calculi occur occasionally in dogs and are reported in sheep, calves, and cats. A high incidence in sheep was circumstantially related to deficiency of molybdenum in unimproved pasture because molybdenum is a component of xanthine oxidase. Several cases in calves in Japan were also associated with deficiency of xanthine oxidase. Xanthine precipitates in acid urine. Calculi usually form in the collecting ducts and calyces of the kidney, and may cause hydronephrosis.

Two forms exist in dogs, as in humans. The *primary form* is inherited as an autosomal recessive and is caused by an inborn enzyme defect in xanthine oxidase. This hepatic enzyme catalyzes 2 sequential steps in degradation of purines, namely, conversion of hypoxanthine to xanthine, and then xanthine to uric acid. This form has been noted most often in Dachshunds and in a family of Cavalier King Charles Spaniels (CKCSs); examination of unrelated CKCSs did not reveal abnormal excretion or metabolism of uric acids and xanthines. The *secondary form* (iatrogenic) is the more common in dogs, especially Dalmatians, and is usually the result of previous treatment with allopurinol, which binds to and inhibits the action of xanthine oxidase.

Further reading

Jacinto AM, et al. Urine concentrations of xanthine, hypoxanthine and uric acid in UK Cavalier King Charles spaniels. J Small Anim Pract 2013;54:395-398.

Mestrinho LA, et al. Xanthine urolithiasis causing bilateral ureteral obstruction in a 10-month-old cat. J Feline Med Surg 2013;15: 911-916.

Cystine calculi

Cystine calculi are small and irregular, soft and friable, waxy, and light yellow to red-brown, turning to green on exposure to daylight. Many cystine calculi consist of pure cystine; others may also contain calcium oxalate, struvite, brushite (calcium hydrogen phosphate dihydrate), and complex urates.

Cystine stones occur in dogs, ferrets, and rarely in cats. They comprise about 1-3% of canine calculi in North America, but 20-30% in some European countries, being second to struvite calculi in incidence. Cystinuria occurs in both males and females, but cystine calculi and urinary obstruction occur almost exclusively in males. They are primarily found in the urinary bladder, but nephroliths are common in Irish Terriers, Scottish Terriers, and Newfoundlands. Other predisposed breeds include Dachshunds, Bulldogs, Mastiffs, Bassett Hounds, and Tibetan Spaniels. Although blood cystine levels are normal, an *inborn error of metabolism in affected dogs* results in high levels of urinary cystine because of defective proximal tubular resorption from glomerular filtrate. Many dogs with cystinuria also have high levels of other amino acids in their urine, but these are more soluble than cystine. Cystine precipitates in acid urine, but factors other than urinary pH are probably important in the genesis of cystine stones because dogs with crystalluria do not always form stones. The incidence of recurrent urolithiasis is enhanced in those dogs with higher excretions of urinary cystine. The mode of inheritance of cystinuria is either autosomal recessive or autosomal dominant in various breeds, the result of mutation in *SLC3A1* and *SLC7A9* genes. In some dogs, the severity of cystinuria may decrease with age.

Further reading

Brons AK, et al. SLC3A1 and SLC7A9 mutations in autosomal recessive or dominant canine cystinuria: a new classification system. J Vet Intern Med 2013;27:1400-1408.

Hoppe A, Denneberg T. Cystinuria in the dog: clinical studies during 14 years of medical treatment. J Vet Intern Med 2001;15:361-367.

Nwaokorie EE, et al. Epidemiological evaluation of cystine urolithiasis in domestic ferrets (*Mustela putorius furo):* 70 cases (1992-2009). J Am Vet Med Assoc 2013;242:1099-1103.

Clover stones

Sheep grazing estrogenic pastures, particularly subterranean clover, or those *injected or implanted with estrogens,* may have an incidence of fatal urinary obstruction as high as 10%. There are probably 3 *separate developmental patterns,* and in each, the obstructing material is soft or pulpy and scantily mineralized. Probably the most common pattern is urethral obstruction by desquamated cells and secretions of accessory glands originating in the pelvic urethra under the influence of estrogen. The second type, the so-called "clover stone," is usually found in the renal pelvis as a yellow, soft material, which eventually leads to scarring of the kidney. It affects both sexes equally. These calculi contain benzocoumarins, which may be metabolites of phytoestrogens. Third, sudden and serious mortalities may occur in male sheep grazing subterranean clover *(Trifolium subterraneum)* during its period of rapid maturation. The urethral process becomes impacted with soft white paste consisting mainly of calcium carbonate and an unidentified organic material probably related to isoflavones.

Further reading

Gardiner MR, et al. Urinary calculi associated with oestrogenic subterranean clover. Aust Vet J 1966;42:315-320.

Other types of calculi

Several other types of calculi develop in animals. They may be important locally, or iatrogenic and rare, such as **tetracycline, sulfonamide,** and **barium** stones. Other chemical compounds are more common but constitute a minor part of certain uroliths. Stones with high **carbonate** content are associated with very alkaline urines and are seen in ruminants consuming high-oxalate plants or clover-dominated pastures.

In horses, calcium carbonate crystals are seen commonly in normal urine. Calculi are much less frequent, but are most commonly composed of **calcium carbonate,** usually in the crystalline form of calcite, and substituted vaterite (the Ca of $CaCO_3$ is replaced in various amounts by Mg, K, and Mn); weddellite (calcium oxalate dihydrate) may also be present. Alkaline pH and dietary factors are implicated in their formation.

Less than 3% of canine uroliths are composed of **calcium phosphate.** Factors that decrease calcium phosphate solubility, predisposing to urolith formation include alkaline urine, hypercalciuria (hyperparathyroidism and other hypercalcemic disorders), reduced concentrations of crystallization inhibitors (inorganic pyrophosphates, citrate, magnesium ions, nephrocalcin), or increased concentrations of crystallization promoters (epitactic induction by calcium oxalate and monosodium urate crystals).

Further reading

Diaz-Espineira M, et al. Structure and composition of equine uroliths. J Eq Vet Sci 1995;15:27-34.

Lulich JP, et al. Recent shifts in the global proportions of canine uroliths. Vet Rec 2013;172:363.

INFLAMMATION OF THE LOWER URINARY TRACT

Inflammation of the lower urinary tract centers on involvement of the urinary bladder, that is, **cystitis. Ureteritis** is rare in the absence of cystitis, and clinical **urethritis** in animals is usually associated with obstruction by a calculus from the bladder. Under normal circumstances, the bladder is resistant to infection, and bacteria are quickly eliminated by the normal flow of normal urine. *Predisposition to urinary tract infection* (UTI) occurs when there is stagnation of urine because of obstruction, incomplete bladder emptying because of upper or lower motor neuron disease or dysautonomia, or urothelial trauma. *Other risk factors for UTI* include catheterization, vaginoscopy, urinary incontinence, vaginitis, or administration of antibiotics or corticosteroids. Of itself, normal voiding is not sufficient to prevent or eliminate bladder infection. Indeed, complete voidance does not occur, but residual urine is rapidly diluted or added to by continuing excretion. *Defense mechanisms* in the bladder and urethra, which prevent bacterial adhesion to mucosal surfaces, are essential if bacteria are to be removed by urine flow. Tamm-Horsfall mucoprotein, produced in the kidneys, may bind to bacterial adhesins and prevent adherence. Local production of IgA and a surface glycosaminoglycan layer is probably important in preventing attachment of organisms to the normal urothelium, and IgG may have similar activity in specific UTIs. Urinary oligosaccharides may be able to detach adherent bacteria. Voiding of sloughed urothelial cells with attached bacteria aids their clearance. Incomplete voiding at micturition may be a result of diverticula of the urinary bladder or vesicoureteral reflux. The presence of residual urine can maintain a bladder infection, allowing organisms to take advantage of any opportunity to invade the urothelium.

Unlike human urine, which tends to be a good medium for bacterial growth, animal urine usually has antibacterial activity. This activity is related to urine pH and particularly to urine osmolality. In general, the further the pH is from the optimum range of 6-7, the less likely it is to support bacterial growth. The antibacterial effect of acid urine is related to the concentration of undissociated organic acids. High urine osmolality also contributes to bacteriostasis.

To infect the urinary tract, uropathogens must compete with the normal bacterial flora of the distal urethra, vulva, or prepuce. *The usual causes of cystitis are* **bacteria** *from the urethra, the origin of which is almost always the rectal flora.* Cystitis is common in young animals with patent urachus, and the bacterial flora is mixed. When bacteria breach the surface defenses of the urothelium and attach to the epithelial cells, the cells are desquamated through a rapid apoptosis-like mechanism. When the urothelium is penetrated, clearance is prevented and neutrophils and macrophages in the submucosa respond.

A variety of bacteria may be involved in bladder infections and these include in all hosts *Escherichia coli, Proteus vulgaris,* streptococci, staphylococci, and enterococci. Other uropathogens include *Klebsiella, Pasteurella, Mycoplasma, Enterobacter,* and *Pseudomonas spp.* Coinfections with more than one bacterium are common. The *Corynebacterium renale* group *(C. renale, C. pilosum, C. cystitidis)* is important in cows, and less so in other species, where it is usually part of a mixed infection. *C. urealyticum* can cause "encrusted cystitis" in dogs and cats because of the deposition of struvite (magnesium ammonium phosphate) and calcium phosphate along the bladder mucosa secondary to ammonia release by these urease-producing bacteria. *Actinobaculum (Eubacterium) suis* is the primary cause of cystitis and pyelonephritis in swine and is an important cause of death in sows; *A. suis* infections typically produce gross hematuria and alkaline urine.

Mycoplasmas are uncommon causes of UTI in dogs and cattle. In the latter species, *M. bovirhinis* (a typical isolate from the respiratory tract) can also be isolated from semen and then may travel retrograde through the female reproductive tract to the bladder in recently bred cows and bulls with urethral obstruction. Urogenital infections causing prostatitis, orchitis, nephritis, and cystitis may occur in canine **blastomycosis.**

Aspergillus, Candida, and *Nocardia* are unusual causes of cystitis in dogs and cats. *Candida* infections can be seen more commonly with predisposing factors, such as diabetes mellitus, prolonged antibiotic or glucocorticoid usage, aciduria, indwelling catheters, or an immunocompromised state.

Bacterial pathogens of the urinary tract, such as *Escherichia coli,* can express a formidable array of *virulence factors,* including fimbriae or pili adhesins (P fimbriae, type 1 fimbriae), nonfimbrial adhesins, aerobactin (an iron chelator), hemolysin, capsular polysaccharide (K antigen), and anticomplementary serum resistance. The most urovirulent strains often express multiple virulence factors simultaneously to produce a synergistic or additive effect and are classified as uropathogenic *E. coli.* Certain virulence factors, such as adhesins, specifically favor the development of pyelonephritis, whereas others favor cystitis. In humans, *E. coli* with P fimbriae bind to renal pelvic urothelium and are thought to be responsible for pyelonephritis. Type 1 fimbriae (pili) are of most importance in bladder colonization. Type 1 pilus tips interact with membrane glycoproteins of urothelial cells, known as uroplakins. In contrast, gram-positive bacteria use extracellular polysaccharides for adhesion.

Once attached, *E. coli* can invade the urothelial cell and replicate to create small intracellular bacterial colonies. Interestingly, *E. coli* can replicate rapidly without increasing in length and change from a coliform morphology to a more coccoid shape. The clusters of bacteria have biofilm properties and will eventually distort the apical membrane of the superficial urothelial cell. Later, *E. coli* become motile and detach from the clusters to exit the cell. At this time, the bacteria attain a filamentous morphology, which helps them survive attacks by neutrophils. Urothelial cells will exfoliate as part of an innate host defense system.

Cystitis

Cystitis is a clinically significant disease in many species. There is a higher incidence in females, which is probably associated with the shorter urethra. Although glucosuria in diabetes mellitus promotes bacterial growth, other substances and mild proteinuria might also be significant in the development of cystitis with this disease. Decreased leukocyte efficiency may also be involved. Animals with diabetes mellitus, hyperadrenocorticism, or pyometra are at increased risk for developing urinary tract infections with *E. coli.* *Emphysematous cystitis* develops in some dogs and cats with diabetes mellitus and is thought to be a result of fermentation of sugar by glucose-fermenting bacteria. Emphysematous cystitis is less commonly detected in nondiabetic animals (Fig. 4-84). Hormone-induced changes, such as hyperestrogenism, can also affect the functional integrity of the urethral and vesicular epithelium. The role of hormones in the production of glycosaminoglycans in the urogenital tract might also change the susceptibility to UTIs. During estrus in sows, estrogen causes the urine pH to rise, producing an alkaline environment suitable for the growth of *Actinobaculum suis.*

As well as the opportunistic bacterial UTIs that develop in all species, other types of diseases also induce inflammation with or without hemorrhage of the lower urinary tract. Hemorrhagic cystitis sometimes occurs in *malignant catarrhal fever* in cattle and deer, and occasionally is the dominant gross lesion. In horses eating alfalfa hay, hematuria should raise the clinical suspicion of cantharidin intoxication. In *Schistosoma mattheei* infections in cattle, linear granulomas occur in the

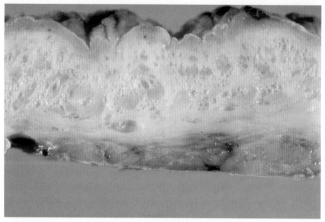

Figure 4-84 Emphysematous cystitis in a dog; not associated with diabetes mellitus. (Courtesy University of Guelph.)

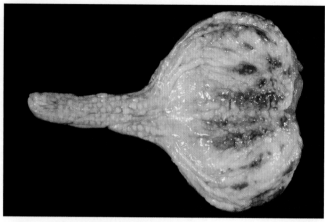

Figure 4-85 Follicular cystitis in a dog. (Courtesy D. Russell.)

renal pelvis, ureter, and bladder of. Urinary tract infection has been associated with recent calving, inadequate sanitation, and omphalitis in dairy cattle, but azotemia is uncommon. Cystitis in horses and cattle (but not sheep) grazing *Sorghum* sp. is associated with ataxia caused by degenerative encephalomy-elopathy; the bladder lesions are almost certainly neurogenic in origin.

Feline lower urinary tract disease (FLUTD) may result from UTI, uroliths, urethral plugs, congenital or acquired ana-tomic defects of the bladder or urethra, or iatrogenic causes. Abyssinian cats, cats >10 years of age, and spayed females are predisposed to bacterial UTI. Novel feline caliciviruses have been isolated from FLUTD cases; further studies are required to determine if these are uropathogens and/or causative agents. Although some studies report absence of infection in most cases of FLUTD, other studies have demonstrated bac-teriuria in up to one-third of cats presented with these clinical signs. Differences in prevalence may be the result of patient population, geographic location, and primary practice versus tertiary referral care centers. Even so, many cases of FLUTD are idiopathic and bear considerable resemblance to the some-what obscure condition in humans called "interstitial cystitis." **Feline interstitial cystitis** is characterized by chronic irritative voiding signs (dysuria, hematuria, pollakiuria, and/or inap-propriate urination), sterile and cytologically negative urine, and cystoscopically visible submucosal petechiae. This common feline condition may result from decreased urinary excretion of glycosaminoglycans, increased bladder permeabil-ity, and neurogenic inflammation. Increased sympathetic activity is confirmed in feline interstitial cystitis cases, and this affects bladder function locally. Nonspecific histologic changes in the bladders of affected cats include submucosal edema, dilated submucosal vessels with margination of neutrophils, and submucosal hemorrhage; there may also be increased numbers of submucosal mast cells. Cats 4-10 years of age are predisposed.

Sterile hemorrhagic cystitis may occur in dogs and cats treated for neoplastic or immunologic diseases with *cyclophos-phamide*. Activated metabolites of the drug cause mucosal ulceration, hemorrhage, and edema. Signs of cystitis occasion-ally follow an 8-week course of therapy, but have also been noted within 24 hours of administration of the first therapeu-tic dose. Concurrent treatment with other drugs, degree of diuresis, and pre-existing cystitis may influence the prevalence

of cyclophosphamide-induced lesions. Fibrosis and mineraliza-tion of the bladder may result in persistent hematuria and incontinence. Urothelial cell carcinoma may develop in the bladder of dogs in association with prolonged cyclophospha-mide therapy.

Eosinophilic cystitis is an uncommon form of cystitis in older dogs with a history of urolithiasis and characterized by the predominance of eosinophils in a proliferative fibroblastic mass.

Cystitis is differentiated into acute and chronic forms, but there is considerable overlap in both the lesions and the causes. In simple **acute** catarrhal inflammation, there is moder-ate hyperemia and submucosal edema, and the surface is covered with a layer of tenacious catarrhal exudate. The urine is cloudy. Histologically, there is necrosis and desquamation of the epithelium and prominent leukocytic infiltration. Submu-cosal vessels are dilated and cuffed by leukocytes. In more severe inflammation, leukocytes may infiltrate all layers of the bladder wall, the mucosa may ulcerate, and hemorrhage from the submucosal vessels may be severe enough to produce blood clots in the bladder lumen. These hemorrhagic compli-cations are common in cystitis following urethral obstruction, especially in cats and cattle. When the inflammatory process is severe, the cystitis may be of superficial fibrinous or deep diphtheritic type. In both, there is a thick, dirty-yellow friable surface encrustation, which may peel with difficulty. Ulcer-ations may penetrate the wall to the serosa or predispose to rupture.

Chronic cystitis may also have different patterns. The sim-plest occurs in association with vesical calculi. The mucosa is irregularly reddened and usually thickened. There is some urothelial desquamation, and the submucosa is infiltrated by mononuclear inflammatory cells; there are few neutrophils (eFig. 4-48). In addition, there is often submucosal fibrosis and hypertrophy of the muscularis. In **follicular cystitis,** which is common in dogs, the mucosa is studded with gray-white nodules ~1 mm across, which may be confluent or surrounded by a zone of hyperemia (Fig. 4-85). Histologically, the nodules are aggregates of proliferating lymphocytes. These are imme-diately beneath the epithelium, which may be normal or ulcerated. **Chronic polypoid cystitis** is common in any species. The mucosa is thrown into many folds or villus-like or sessile projections. The polyps are covered by epithelium over a core of proliferated connective tissue densely infiltrated with mononuclear leukocytes. The polyps often undergo mucoid degeneration in cattle, or the epithelium may undergo metaplasia to a mucus-secreting, glandular type, resembling colonic epithelium. Such polyps may break down, causing intermittent hematuria. Obstructive uropathy is another sequela. Biopsy is required to differentiate them from neoplasms.

Further reading

Briscoe KA, et al. Encrusting cystitis in a cat secondary to *Corynebacterium urealyticum* infection. J Fel Med Surg 2010;12:972-977.

Eggertsdóttir AV, et al. Bacteriuria in cats with feline lower urinary tract disease: a clinical study of 134 cases in Norway. J Fel Med Surg 2007;9:458-465.

Fuentealba IC, Illanes OG. Eosinophilic cystitis in 3 dogs. Can Vet J 2000;41:130-131.

Hung C, et al. A murine model of urinary tract infection. Nat Protoc 2009;4:1230-1243.

Lekcharoensuk C, et al. Epidemiologic study of risk factors for lower urinary tract diseases in cats. J Am Vet Med Assoc 2001;218:1429-1435.

Ling GV, et al. Interrelations of organism prevalence, specimen collection method, and host age, sex, and breed among 8,354 canine urinary tract infections (1969-1995). J Vet Intern Med 2001;15:341-347.

Rice CC, et al. Genetic characterization of 2 novel feline caliciviruses isolated from cats with idiopathic lower urinary tract disease. J Vet Intern Med 2002;16:293-302.

Smee N, et al. UTIs in small animal patients: part 1: etiology and pathogenesis. J Am Anim Hosp Assoc 2013;49:1-7.

Ulett GC, et al. Uropathogenic *Escherichia coli* virulence and host responses during urinary tract infection. Curr Opin Microbiol 2013;16:100-107.

Woldemeskel M, et al. Microscopic and ultrastructural lesions of the ureter and renal pelvis in sows with regard to *Actinobaculum suis* infection. J Vet Med A Physiol Pathol Clin Med 2002;49:348-352.

Yeruhaum I, et al. A herd level analysis of urinary tract infection in dairy cattle. Vet J 2006;171:172-176.

Enzootic hematuria

Enzootic hematuria is a syndrome in mature cattle characterized by persistent hematuria and anemia, and is associated with hemorrhages or neoplasms in the lower urinary tract. In >90% of cases, the hematuria originates from tumors of the urinary bladder. Outbreaks of the disease are reported in sheep.

Enzootic hematuria occurs on all continents, but is restricted to particular locations. In endemic areas, up to 90% of adult cattle may be affected. *The syndrome is attributed to chronic ingestion of* **bracken fern** and is reproducible experimentally. The extent and persistence with which toxic ferns are grazed probably influences the incidence of bladder lesions. There are 2 subspecies of bracken fern: *Pteridium aquilinum* subsp. *aquilinum* and *P. aquilinum* subsp. *caudatum*. It is not known whether all varieties are toxic. *P. revolutum*, a species of bracken fern common in South Asia, and *P. esculentum*, a bracken fern of Australia, also produce enzootic hematuria. In areas where bracken does not grow, other ferns, such as *Cheilanthes sieberi* (mulga or rock fern from Australia), are capable of producing enzootic hematuria.

Bracken fern is very common, and may be the only plant that causes naturally occurring tumors in animals. *It contains several toxic substances*, including a thiaminase, a variety of

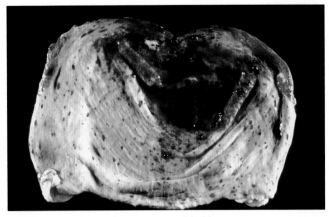

Figure 4-86 Hemorrhagic urinary bladder mucosa in **enzootic hematuria** in a cow. (Courtesy K. Potter.)

carcinogens (quercetin, shikimic acid, prunasin, ptaquiloside, ptaquiloside Z, aquilide A, and others), and a "bleeding factor" of unknown structure. Following administration of ptaquiloside to guinea pigs, hemorrhagic cystitis results, suggesting that this is one of the toxic principles in bracken fern hematuria. There is a strong link between bracken fern and bovine papillomavirus 2 (BPV-2) in the development of bladder neoplasms in animals with enzootic hematuria; the relationship of oncogenic viruses to bracken is discussed in Vol. 2, Alimentary system and peritoneum.

Cattle fed low levels of bracken fern develop microscopic, followed by macroscopic, hematuria. Microhematuria is usually associated with petechiae, ecchymoses, or suffusive hemorrhages in the urothelium of the renal calyces, pelvis, ureter, and bladder (Fig. 4-86). These lesions appear to be a manifestation of the hemorrhagic syndrome characteristic of acute bracken fern poisoning. In some cases, microscopic hematuria occurs before gross lesions are visible. Diffuse or patchy areas of pink discoloration develop in the bladder mucosa, and microscopically, ectatic and engorged capillaries are present. These altered vessels are prone to hemorrhage into the bladder wall or lumen, and nodular vascular lesions develop in affected areas. Macroscopic hematuria is usually, but not always, indicative of tumors, which ulcerate and bleed into the lumen. Occasionally, tumors also develop in the renal pelvis and ureter, and hepatic hemangiomas accompany bladder tumors in a few animals. Most neoplasms are located on the ventral and lateral walls of the bladder, where constant contact with urine occurs.

Several types of epithelial and mesenchymal neoplasms may develop, including urothelial cell and squamous cell carcinoma, papilloma, adenoma, hemangioma, hemangiosarcoma, leiomyosarcoma, fibroma, and fibrosarcoma. Multiple tumors of more than one type may be present, and in >50% of affected cattle mixed epithelial-mesenchymal neoplasms develop. *Papillomas, fibromas, and hemangiomas with carcinomas are the most common types.* Malignant types may invade locally, and about 10% of epithelial malignancies metastasize to iliac nodes or lungs. Chronic cystitis usually accompanies the neoplastic changes. Brunn nests may develop in the mucosa. Epithelial neoplasms appear to develop from the hyperplastic and metaplastic (squamous and mucous) changes in the urothelium that often accompany the vascular lesions. A pagetoid variant of urothelial carcinoma in situ has been reported in a cow that also had enzootic hematuria and concurrent BPV-2 infection; fragile histidine triad (Fhit) protein, expressed by the tumor suppressor gene *FHIT*, was found to be absent in some of the pagetoid cells, correlating with late-stage neoplastic progression. Uroplakins are urothelial cell differentiation products that are more consistently expressed in the superficial urothelium. In high-grade urothelial carcinomas that demonstrate muscle invasion, there is a decrease in the immunohistochemical uroplakin III staining of the neoplastic cells, whereas cytokeratin-7 expression is maintained. Research indicates that cyclin D1 may be dysregulated in all tumors (benign and malignant) from cattle with enzootic hematuria, whereas malignancies often have p53 mutations. Although it is not necessarily of use prognostically, staining for uroplakins may help identify metastatic urothelial cell clusters.

Further reading

Ambrosio V, et al. Uroplakin expression in the urothelial tumors of cows. Vet Pathol 2002;38:657-660.

Borzacchiello G, et al. The pagetoid variant of urothelial carcinoma in situ of urinary bladder in a cow. Vet Pathol 2001;38:113-116.

Cota JB, et al. Epithelial urinary bladder tumors from cows with enzootic hematuria: structural and cell cycle-related protein expression. Vet Pathol 2013;51:749-754.

NEOPLASMS OF THE LOWER URINARY TRACT

Neoplasia of the lower urinary tract is uncommon, but occurs most often in dogs, cats, and cattle (see Enzootic hematuria; previously). There are few data for other animals; thus the following discussion concerns mainly these species. Almost all bovine tumors are associated with enzootic hematuria. Tumors of the urinary bladder account for <1% of all canine neoplasms, and are even less prevalent in cats. Sex bias has not been definitively established. The Scottish Terrier, Shetland Sheepdog, Beagle, and Collie seem to be at greater risk than other breeds. The greater susceptibility of the urinary bladder than of other parts of the urinary tract may be the result of more prolonged exposure of the bladder mucosa to urinary carcinogens. *In general, urinary bladder tumors are slow growing and late to metastasize.* With the exception of rhabdomyosarcoma, neoplasia of the lower urinary tract usually occurs in old animals.

Bladder neoplasia may be caused by a variety of *industrial chemicals* (2-naphthylamine, benzidine), tryptophan metabolites (ortho-aminophenol), chronic irritation, foreign bodies (sutures), viruses, bracken fern, and cyclophosphamide. The greater concentration of *tryptophan* metabolites in dog urine than in cat urine may account for the higher prevalence of bladder tumors in dogs. *Grading of urinary tract neoplasms according to tumor invasiveness, lymph node involvement, and presence of metastases (the tumor-node-metastasis [TNM] system)* can assist with prognostication and selection of therapy.

Secondary tumors are rare, comprising ~5% of tumors of this organ. These originate in pelvic organs or as peritoneal implants.

Epithelial tumors

Epithelial tumors comprise ~80% of the lower urinary tract neoplasms. They occur as adenomas, papillomas, and carcinomas, and most of them develop in the bladder of old animals.

Adenomas are rare in all species; they originate from areas of mucous metaplasia of the urothelium and may be single or multiple with a papilliform or pedunculated appearance. Microscopically, they form glandular structures, some of which contain mucin. **Papillomas** constitute ~17% of primary tumors of the urinary bladder. They tend to be multiple and may be pedunculated or sessile, occasionally involving most of the mucosa. They are covered by well-differentiated transitional epithelium, which is demarcated by basement membrane from a delicate supporting stroma. Squamous metaplasia of the epithelium may develop. Papillomas are susceptible to superficial necrosis, which results in hematuria. In dogs, some papillomas undergo malignant transformation to form urothelial cell carcinoma (previously called *transitional cell carcinoma* or *TCC*) or adenocarcinomas. *Papillary hyperplasia*, to be differentiated from the rarer papilloma, occurs in the urinary bladder of cattle and can cause urinary obstruction and hydronephrosis.

Carcinomas of the lower urinary tract are of 4 histologic types: (1) urothelial cell; (2) squamous cell; (3) adenocarcinoma; and (4) undifferentiated carcinoma. Together they make up ~60% of primary bladder tumors in dogs and cats; the majority of these are of urothelial origin. Carcinomas may be solitary or multiple and usually do not reach a large size before they cause hematuria or death from urinary complications. Metaplastic changes to squamous or glandular epithelium are often adjacent to epithelial neoplasms. Brunn nests are most often found in association with adenocarcinomas.

Urothelial cell carcinomas may be papillary, polypoid, or sessile (Fig. 4-87). Occasionally, they are not visible on the vesical mucosa, even though the bladder wall is infiltrated diffusely; the tumors may be present in any part of the bladder, but are often in the bladder neck or trigone. Tumors originating in the prostatic urethra are easily overlooked at autopsy. Features of tumors that tend to be localized include papillary architecture, in situ tumor, low tumor grade, and a strong lymphoid response. Metastatic disease is seen with infiltrative and nonpapillary growths, increasing tumor grade, deeper invasion, vascular invasion, and peritumoral fibrosis. Occasionally, urothelium can induce fibroblasts from the desmoplastic areas surrounding metastases to produce heterotopic bone. A few urothelial cell carcinomas contain areas of squamous metaplasia. *About 50% of urothelial cell carcinomas metastasize.* The usual pattern is for metastasis to regional lymph nodes

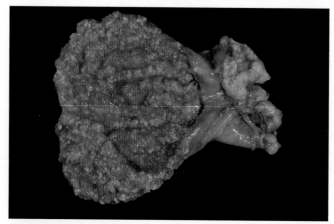

Figure 4-87 **Urothelial cell carcinoma** in the urinary bladder of a dog. (Courtesy E.E.B. LaDouceur.)

and lungs, but peritoneal implantation or retrograde lymphatic spread to the soft tissue and bones of the hindlimbs or vertebrae is common. Occasionally, solitary metastasis to bone occurs. Immunohistochemically, canine urothelial cell carcinomas often have antigens similar to tumor-associated glycoprotein 72 (TAG-72), a high-molecular-mass glycoprotein used in the diagnosis of carcinomas originating in numerous human tissues. Uroplakin III has been determined to be a specific and sensitive marker for canine urothelial cell neoplasms. The presence of uroplakin III was not noted to correlate with tumor grade. Expression of cyclooxygenase-2 in neoplastic urinary bladder epithelium, but not in normal epithelium, suggests this may be a useful marker for neoplastic transformation and growth and can be targeted for therapeutic effects. Furthermore, noninvasive biomarkers, such as urinary S100A8, A9, and A12, have shown promise as diagnostic tools in canine urothelial and prostatic carcinomas. *To assist clinical management of urothelial cell carcinoma pathology descriptions should include tumor architecture, tumor grade, and depth of invasion based on sampling of multiple sites.*

Squamous cell carcinomas and **adenocarcinomas** are usually nonpapillary infiltrative growths, which are grossly nodular or sessile and often ulcerated. They develop in areas of squamous or mucous metaplasia. Histologically, they are "pure," without urothelial cell areas. Squamous cell carcinomas and adenocarcinomas occur in dogs, cattle, and cats, and are the most common urinary bladder neoplasm in horses. Squamous cell carcinomas occur most often in bitches in the urethra, the distal two-thirds of which is lined by stratified squamous epithelium. Apparently, these are less likely to metastasize than are urothelial cell tumors. **Undifferentiated carcinomas** are rare primary neoplasms that do not conform to one of the histologic types mentioned previously.

Mesenchymal tumors

Mesenchymal tumors comprise <20% of tumors of the lower urinary tract. Neoplasms causing enzootic hematuria in cattle are ~10% mesenchymal and 55% mixed, with most of the nonepithelial tumors in these mixtures being hemangiomas. A few vascular tumors also occur in the bladder and about the urethra of dogs, but most mesenchymal tumors in dogs are leiomyomas or fibromas. **Leiomyomas** originate in the smooth muscle coats of the urinary bladder and form well-defined projecting spherical white nodules. The nodules may be multiple and seem to have a predilection for the neck of the bladder, where they may interfere with urine outflow. **Leiomyosarcomas** are very rare and generally do not metastasize; immunohistochemical staining for smooth muscle actin

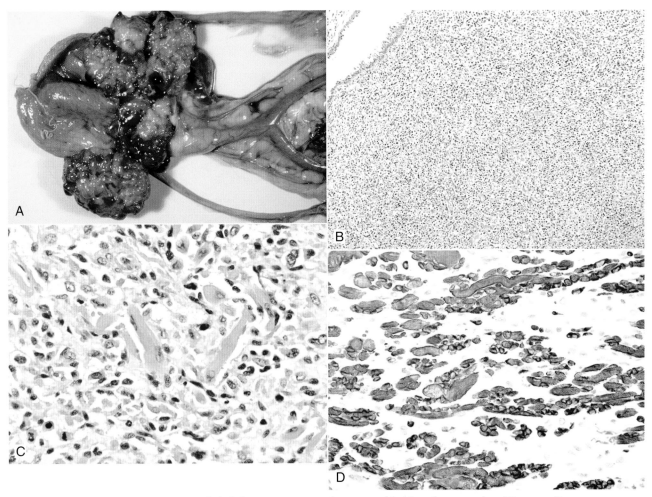

Figure 4-88 A. Botryoid rhabdomyosarcoma in the urinary bladder of a young dog. (Courtesy K. Potter and Kansas State University) **B, C.** Histopathology of a different dog reveals scattered strap cells with striations. **D.** Immunohistochemistry for desmin demonstrates diffuse cytoplasmic positivity in neoplastic cells.

and desmin are expected. **Fibromas** probably arise from sub-epithelial connective tissue, are usually solitary, and have a typical gross and microscopic appearance. **Fibrosarcomas** are rare; they are likely to metastasize widely.

Rhabdomyosarcoma is a rare tumor in any location (see Vol. 1, Muscle and tendon). **Botryoid** (shaped like a bunch of grapes) **rhabdomyosarcoma** occurs in the urinary bladder and occasionally the urethra of young dogs (Fig. 4-88). Large breeds, particularly the Saint Bernard, seem to be over-represented. This tumor has also been reported in a Maltese bitch, 2 Poodles, and a filly. The young age of the affected animals (<2 years of age in most cases) raises the possibility that these tumors arise in rests of embryonic myoblasts. Grossly, the tumors usually occur at the trigone and project into the bladder as botryoid masses. They may metastasize, but are usually identified because of urinary obstruction before this occurs. This tumor has been associated with hyper-trophic osteopathy in a dog. Microscopically, there is usually a mixture of fusiform and pleomorphic cells, with some strap cells and multinucleated cells. Cytoplasmic cross-striations are sometimes present. Immunoperoxidase staining of the inter-mediate filament desmin may aid in the diagnosis of this tumor.

Involvement of the urinary bladder in primary **lymphoma** has been reported only rarely in domestic animals; primary canine epitheliotropic T-cell lymphoma involving the urinary bladder is even more rare.

Further reading

Heilmann RM, et al. Measurement of urinary canine S100A8/A9 and S100A12 concentrations as candidate biomarkers of lower urinary tract neoplasia in dogs. J Vet Diagn Invest 2014;26:104-112.

Maiolino P, Devico G. Primary epitheliotropic T-cell lymphoma of the urinary bladder in a dog. Vet Pathol 2000;37:184-186.

Meuten DJ. Tumors of the urinary system. In: Meuten DJ, editor. Tumors in Domestic Animals. 4th ed. Ames, Iowa: Iowa State University Press; 2002. p. 509-546.

Patterson-Kane JC, et al. Transitional cell carcinoma of the urinary bladder in a Thoroughbred, with intra-abdominal dissemination. Vet Pathol 2000;37:692-695.

Reed LT, et al. Cutaneous metastasis of transitional cell carcinoma in 12 dogs. Vet Pathol 2013;50:676-681.

Sledge DG, et al. Differences in expression of uroplakin III, cytokeratin 7, and cyclooxygenase-2 in canine proliferative urothelial lesions of the urinary bladder. Vet Pathol 2015;52:74-82.

Takiguchi M, et al. Rhabdomyosarcoma (botryoid sarcoma) of the urinary bladder in a Maltese. J Small Anim Pract 2002;43: 269-271.

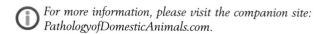 *For more information, please visit the companion site: PathologyofDomesticAnimals.com.*

CHAPTER 5

Respiratory System

Jeff L. Caswell • Kurt J. Williams

ACKNOWLEDGMENTS

We gratefully acknowledge the contributions to prior editions of this chapter by Drs. Ken Jubb, Peter Kennedy, Nigel Palmer, and Donald Dungworth.

GENERAL CONSIDERATIONS

Of all of the organ systems, *the respiratory tract may be unique in its vulnerability to injurious agents.* The involuntary nature of ventilation, necessitated by aerobic respiration and the need for oxygen, actively pulls large volumes of air into the lungs (estimated at 5,400 L/day in dogs and 11,400 L/day in horses). Along with this air, there is a variety of potentially injurious materials. In addition, the flow of the entire cardiac output through the extensive and delicate vascular bed of the gas exchange region of the lungs provides a separate avenue for the delivery of potentially harmful substances to the respiratory tract. These dual exposure routes are particularly important in determining the expression of disease in the lung, with *distinct patterns of lesions depending on whether the route of entry is airborne (aerogenous) or vascular (hematogenous)*. The array of potentially injurious agents includes airborne microorganisms, particulates, and toxic gases in ambient air, and a wide variety of infectious agents and extrinsic or intrinsic toxins delivered via the pulmonary circulation. Together, the injury, inflammation, and reparative responses to these insults compromise the gas exchange functions of the respiratory system.

The upper airway

Air flows through the *nares* into the *nasal vestibule*, past the *nasal valve*, and into the *nasal cavity*. There, the ventral, middle, and dorsal *meatuses* are demarcated by the osseous and cartilaginous *conchae* (turbinates). Air flows past the *ethmoid conchae* in the caudal nasal cavity, through the *choanae* and into the nasopharynx. The presence of respiratory turbinates is restricted to mammals and birds, and is assumed to be important in the evolution of endothermy and the high levels of oxygen consumption associated with metabolism in these species; similar structures are not present in ectothermic animals.

Functionally, the *respiratory turbinates warm and humidify the inspired air* to prevent desiccation of the lower respiratory tract, and reclaim moisture and heat from the saturated vapor leaving the lungs. The nasal submucosa is richly supplied with a complex vascular plexus, nerves, and mucosal glands. In addition to the air-warming functions, most species have vascular shunts between the respiratory turbinates and the brain vasculature, suggesting a role in *cooling the brain* during periods of intense activity in mammals and birds. Stimulation of the parasympathetic innervation in the nasal cavity leads to

increased vascular permeability and mucosal gland secretion, which may occlude the nasal airways and increase resistance to airflow. This is countered by the sympathetic nerve fibers, which favor vasoconstriction and decreased vascular permeability.

The mucosa of the nasal cavity has distinct epithelial types: (1) *stratified squamous*, (2) *transitional*, (3) *ciliated respiratory*, *and* (4) *olfactory*. The relative distribution and extent of each of these cell types vary among species. Stratified squamous epithelium is confined to the nasal vestibule at the entrance to the nasal cavity. Separating the squamous epithelium from the more caudal respiratory epithelium is a zone of nonciliated cuboidal to columnar cells, the transitional epithelium. Most of the epithelium lining the nasal mucosa is composed of *pseudostratified respiratory epithelium*. This is a complex epithelium that includes ciliated, mucous, nonciliated, and basal cells (Fig. 5-1). *Olfactory epithelium is located in the caudal and caudodorsal nasal cavity*, lining the ethmoid conchae. This is the most phylogenetically conserved of the nasal epithelium, reflecting the ancient origins of olfaction. The epithelium is composed of olfactory sensory neurons—bipolar neurons that have immotile cilia forming dendritic knobs bearing the olfactory receptors—as well as sustentacular cells and basal cells. Olfactory mucosa is readily recognized by a line of sustentacular cell nuclei at the mid-level of the epithelium, basal cells adjacent to basal lamina, and olfactory neurons scattered between these 2 layers, as well as Bowman's glands and prominent olfactory nerves in the lamina propria (see Fig. 5-1). *Olfactory epithelium is rich in cytochrome P450 monooxygenases*. These enzymes are essential for olfaction, and their biotransformation activity confers susceptibility to inhaled or ingested toxins, such as 3-methylindole in horses.

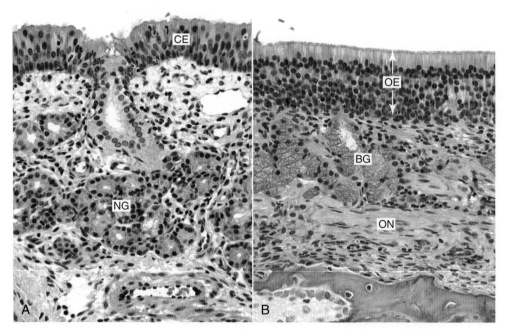

Figure 5-1 Microscopic anatomy of **nasal epithelium in a pig**. **A.** Respiratory epithelium is pseudostratified and contains ciliated epithelial cells (CE), with nasal glands (NG) in the lamina propria. **B.** Olfactory epithelium (OE) has dendritic knobs at the surface, apical cytoplasm, a mid-level layer of sustentacular cell nuclei, and nuclei of basal cells and bipolar neurons in the basal half of the epithelium. The lamina propria contains Bowman's glands (BG) and prominent olfactory nerves (ON).

The **nasopharynx** is lined by ciliated pseudostratified epithelium with zones of stratified squamous epithelium. *Lymphoid nodules* are abundant throughout the submucosa, and are one of the components of the pharyngeal lymphoid (Waldeyer's) ring, a collection of lymphoid tissues that encircle the oropharynx and nasopharynx. *The auditory (Eustachian) tubes* extend from the nasopharynx to the middle ears. In horses, diverticula of each auditory tube form the *guttural pouches*, which are located caudodorsal to the caudal pharynx. The function of the guttural pouches is not completely understood, but they may play a role in cooling blood destined for the brain during periods of intense activity and respiration. This respiratory-based cooling mechanism is facilitated by the anatomy of the internal carotid artery as it courses in a crease along the caudal wall up to the dorsal surface of the pouches. As with the pharynx and auditory tube, the mucosa of the guttural pouches is lined by pseudostratified ciliated epithelium.

The **larynx** is composed of a complex of cartilage plates lined by stratified squamous epithelium as well as pseudostratified ciliated respiratory epithelium. The larynx is at the boundary between the respiratory system and the pharynx, and communicates directly with the laryngopharynx. The cartilage of the larynx is important in vocalization in animals, and also resists deformation and obstruction from ingesta, external pressure, and the negative internal pressures experienced during inhalation.

The **trachea** extends from the terminus of the larynx to the *carina*, the branch point for the principal bronchi leading into the right and left lungs. With its relatively simple gross anatomy, and seemingly simple function serving as the conduit for air traveling to and from the lungs, the trachea is often overlooked in routine pathology examinations. The upper third of the trachea is arbitrarily considered to be the most distal part of the upper respiratory tract.

Organization of the lung

The organization and subdivision of the lower respiratory tract arise as a function of the development of the organ, and vary considerably by species (lung development is reviewed later in the chapter). Many of these gross features are important in the pathogenesis of disease and susceptibility of individual species to a variety of insults, including infectious agents and inhaled toxins and particulate matter. Additionally, proper usage of terminology is important in the gross description of lesions at the time of autopsy.

The divisions of the lungs, from largest to smallest, include lobe, bronchopulmonary segment, and terminal acinus. In all of the domestic species, the lung is divided into a right and left lung, each of which is served by a single **principal bronchus** (primary bronchi) arising at the tracheal bifurcation. Each of the 2 lungs is further subdivided into individual lobes. The **lung lobe** represents the largest subdivision of the right and left lungs. *The lobe is defined as the gas exchange region ventilated through the* **lobar (secondary) bronchus**. The numbers and distribution of lung lobes vary by species. All domestic species except the horse have 2 lobes in the left lung (cranial and caudal) and 4 lobes in the right lung (cranial, middle, caudal, and accessory); the horse lacks a right middle lung lobe. The cranial lobe of the left lung is subdivided into a cranial and caudal part in all species except the horse, and the right cranial lobe of domestic ruminants is similarly divided into a cranial and caudal part. The lobar bronchus **(tracheal bronchus)** of

the right cranial lung lobe of ruminants and pigs arises from the trachea before the primary bronchi bifurcate from the trachea to the right and left lungs.

Depending on the species, further subdivision into individual **lobules** by connective tissue septa may or may not be grossly visible; when present, these interlobular septa are contiguous with the pleura. *In humans, pigs, and cattle, lobulation is highly developed, with individual lobules readily seen on the pleural surface of the lung. Equine, ovine, and caprine lungs are intermediate in lobulation; canine and feline lung are essentially devoid of septation and lobule formation.* A **bronchopulmonary segment** is the area served by a tertiary bronchus that arises from the lobar (secondary) bronchi. Well-developed interlobular septa that nearly completely surround individual bronchopulmonary segments, as in the pig and cow, limit collateral ventilation as well as the movement of cells and molecules between adjacent segments. Functionally, this is important in these species in limiting the extension of inflammation between lobules. Well-developed connective tissue septa can effectively sequester inflammation in affected lobules, leading to the characteristic gross lesions especially common in bacterial bronchopneumonia, with severely affected lobules adjacent to those less affected. The lack of collateral ventilation is also largely responsible for the common, incidental, interlobular emphysema found in cattle lungs at the time of autopsy.

The **terminal acinus** *is composed of one terminal bronchiole and its associated gas exchange region.* The anatomy of the terminal acinus varies among domestic species, especially the length between the terminal bronchiole and the alveoli. This junction is composed of respiratory bronchioles and/or alveolar ducts, depending on the species. **Respiratory bronchioles** (prominent in dogs, cats, ferrets, and humans, but not in horses, cattle, sheep, or pigs) are lined by cuboidal epithelium that is interrupted by periodic alveolar outpocketings before transitioning into the gas exchange region. **Alveolar ducts** are cylindrical airways lined by a membranous epithelium and have multiple circumferential communications with alveoli; they may have smooth muscle in their wall.

Vascular supply to the lung

The vascular supply to the lung is dual, arriving through both the pulmonary and bronchial circulation. This unique system of perfusing the lung with blood has implications in the pathogenesis of pulmonary disease. The *pulmonary arterial circulation* receives the entire output of the right ventricle and is characterized as a high-flow, low-pressure system. In contrast, the *bronchial arterial circulation*, being a part of the systemic arterial blood vasculature, is a low-flow, high-pressure system. The bronchial circulation can arise from a variety of sites, including the aorta, intercostal arteries, and subclavian arteries. It delivers nutrition to the bronchi and bronchioles, and in some species also to the blood vessels, pleura, and much of the interstitium. Species vary in their vascular supply. The bronchial artery supplies the airways of dogs, and its obstruction causes bronchiolar necrosis, whereas this does not occur in rabbits because of contributions by the pulmonary artery. In cattle, sheep, pigs, and horses, the bronchial circulation also supplies the pleura, whereas in species with thin pleurae (dogs, cats, rodents), the pulmonary circulation serves this function. The pulmonary circulation nourishes the alveolar parenchyma and delivers blood to the site of alveolar gas exchange.

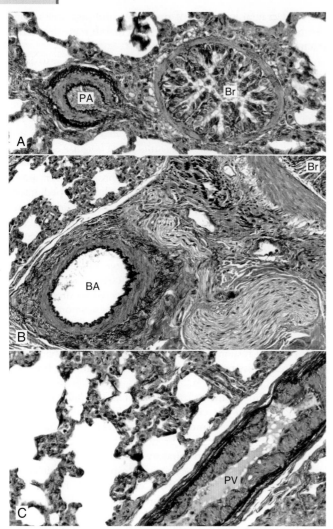

Figure 5-2 Microscopic anatomy of pulmonary vessels. Verhoeff–van Gieson elastic stain. **A.** The **pulmonary artery** (PA), located in the connective tissue ensheathing the bronchiole (Br), has both internal and external elastic laminae, and is about half the diameter of the bronchiole. **B.** The **bronchial artery** (BA) also follows the bronchiole (Br) but is smaller than the pulmonary artery, and has an internal but not an external elastic lamina. **C.** The **pulmonary veins** (PV) are most easily seen in the lung parenchyma, and may have an external but no internal elastic lamina. Pulmonary veins of cattle, shown here, have thick smooth muscle in the tunica media.

The morphology of the 2 vascular systems in most species can be discerned histologically, at least in their normal state (Fig. 5-2). Both arteries are adjacent to bronchi and bronchioles, but the pulmonary artery is much larger (at least half the diameter of the airway) than the bronchial artery. Further, the muscular pulmonary arteries have an internal and external elastic lamina of similar thickness, whereas bronchial arteries have an internal elastic lamina, but the external lamina is indistinct or absent. At the pulmonary trunk, the arteries of most species have considerable numbers of elastic fibers interspersed with the smooth muscle, whereas the more distal arteries and arterioles do not have elastic fibers. The smaller branches of pulmonary arteries vary considerably between species in their morphology, especially in the thickness of the

tunica media. *Cats, pigs, and cattle have the thickest pulmonary arteries of the domestic species,* and in domestic cats, the medial hypertrophy/hyperplasia can be quite pronounced, although usually incidental. Because of the presence of smooth muscle in the small pulmonary arterioles of many domestic species, care needs to be taken in diagnosing pulmonary arterial hypertension based simply on arteriolar histology.

Pulmonary veins drain the entire lung except the proximal trachea and lymph nodes. Cardiac muscle is present in the large proximal veins of rodents but not domestic species. The pulmonary veins follow the bronchial tree in most domestic species (in contrast to humans), and have a thin fibrous wall in all of the species except for cattle and pigs, where smooth muscle can be prominent and give a beaded appearance. Thus cattle >3 months of age have thick muscular veins next to airways and in the interstitium that resemble arteries (see Fig. 5-2C). In all species, the larger pulmonary veins are recognized by the presence of an external elastic lamina between the tunica media and the adventitia, but no internal elastic lamina.

The *lymphatic system* is the least well understood of the vascular systems in the lung. Lymphatic vessels are present within the visceral pleura and surround airways and blood vessels, but do not extend into the alveolar septa. The morphology of the pulmonary lymphatics varies by their location. Within the pleura and just below it, the interstitial space leading into proper lymphatics can be considered as prelymphatic space. This is a site of fluid accumulation during pulmonary edema and also, given that it collects fluids bathing the entirety of the surrounding tissue, is important in delivering antigens to regional lymph nodes. The prelymphatics in the pleura blend into reservoir lymphatics, which eventually connect with conduit lymphatics. Within the lung, saccular and tubulosaccular lymphatics surround all airways and non-capillary blood vessels (arteries and veins). These lymphatics are large (some >100 μm) and thin walled. Although they are histologically indistinct and are often overlooked, the lymphatics distend greatly with fluid as a result of pulmonary edema or pneumonia. Metastatic emboli filling lymphatics sometimes reveal the distribution of the pulmonary lymphatic system, and aggregates of inflammatory cells may accumulate around terminal airways and blood vessels in association with the local lymphatics. Thus the lung lymphatic system is important in fluid movement, regulating alveolar hydration, and acting as a conduit for movement of antigens, leukocytes, and metastasizing neoplasms.

Cellular architecture and cell biology of the lung

The cellular constituents of the respiratory system are functionally interdependent in relation to organ development, homeostasis, and response to injury. This interdependence is first evident in the close interactions between endodermal and mesodermal components in lung development (see Lung development and growth, later). In the adult lung, this anatomic and functional relationship has been termed the *epithelial-mesenchymal trophic unit* and includes the interactions among respiratory epithelial cells, smooth muscle cells, endothelial cells, extracellular matrix proteins, and leukocytes during development, health, and disease.

In all domestic species, the **trachea and bronchi** *are surrounded by rings of hyaline cartilage.* These rings resist physical deformation, thereby helping to maintain the patency of the upper airways. In spite of their greater diameter, relative to the bronchioles, ~80% of the resistance to pulmonary airflow resides within the first 4-7 generations of the conducting airways. Partly because of this, any process that results in significant narrowing of the bronchi can result in clinically detectable changes at an earlier stage than a similar process involving the bronchioles.

Bronchioles, in contrast to bronchi, *have no cartilage in their walls to prevent airway collapse.* Bronchiolar airway patency is dependent on the attachment of alveolar septa to the thin connective tissue layer in the bronchiolar wall. The one exception to this rule is marine mammals, both cetaceans and pinnipeds, which possess well-developed cartilage rings around even the smallest bronchioles that prevent airway collapse in the face of supra-atmospheric pressures found at depth within the oceans. In terrestrial mammals, the radially arranged alveolar septa are tethered to and pull on the bronchiolar wall to maximize the luminal diameter during peak lung volume during inspiration. During expiration, as the forces from the alveolar septa decrease, the bronchiolar lumen decreases in diameter. Because of their smaller diameter, collapsibility and thin-walled structure, bronchioles are much more susceptible to disease processes occurring in the surrounding alveolar parenchyma than are bronchi, and they individually have a higher resistance to airflow than individual bronchi. In spite of this, there is less resistance to airflow in the distal airways because of the higher number of bronchioles. Therefore a large percentage of bronchioles must be affected before clinical evidence of disease is detected.

Histologically, there is great cellular diversity within the mucosal epithelium of the conducting airways, the cell populations changing depending on the species and airway generation under consideration. The trachea, bronchi, and proximal bronchioles are lined by pseudostratified epithelium composed of a mix of ciliated, mucous, club (formerly Clara cells, see later), serous and chemosensory/brush cells. In general, the numbers of ciliated and mucous cells decrease within the distal airways, with a greater proportion of nonciliated cells present within the bronchioles (eFig. 5-1). These distribution factors can play an important role in the species- and region-specific susceptibility of the airway epithelium to specific forms of injury, especially infectious agents, particulate matter, and inhaled or systemic toxins.

The **ciliated cells** function mainly in clearance of airway-lining fluid and also have secretory functions. The **secretory cells** include mucous cells, serous cells, and club cells. The morphologic and functional differences among these secretory cells are not considered immutable, and microenvironmental conditions induce metaplasia from one type to the other. The contribution of these cells to the airway surface liquid includes not only mucus but also the innate defense molecules (see Lung defenses, later), immunoregulatory proteins such as club cell secretory protein and annexin A1, and cellular defense molecules, including antioxidants and trefoil factor. **Mucous cells** (goblet cells) are a source of mucins that form the mucus layer of the epithelial lining fluid. **Club cells** (formerly known as Clara cells) are nonciliated non–mucus-secreting cells that predominate in the distal airway of many species. The club cell functions as a *progenitor cell* for epithelial repair within the airway mucosa, as it has the capacity to divide and differentiate into other secretory cells or ciliated cells. Club cells of many species have abundant smooth endoplasmic reticulum that possesses high concentrations of cytochrome

P450-monooxygenase enzymes. Indeed, on a per-cell basis, club cells of some species have greater metabolic capacity than even hepatocytes. Therefore, *club cells are extremely sensitive to a variety of xenobiotics;* metabolism of these toxins can generate intermediate metabolites that form adducts with macromolecules and lead to cellular injury. Finally, club cell secretory protein (formerly Clara cell secretory protein, CC10, CC16), secreted by these cells in response to adrenergic stimuli, may dampen the inflammatory response by inhibition of phospholipase A_2. The **chemosensory or brush cells** are infrequent cells that are thought to detect irritants in the inhaled air. In addition to these cells lining the airway surface, **tracheobronchial glands** in the lamina propria and/or in the submucosa between the cartilage rings are the major source of mucus in these large airways.

Smooth muscle cells are located around the circumference of the bronchi and bronchioles, and extend to the ostia of alveolar outpocketings in the respiratory bronchioles, and into the alveolar ducts of some species. Historically, the *airway smooth muscle cell* was primarily seen as the transducer of bronchoconstriction and bronchodilation. However, smooth muscle cells can undergo hyperplasia in response to paracrine signals arising from the airway epithelium in inflammatory diseases, and this doubtless contributes to the accentuation of smooth muscle found histologically in chronic bronchitis and asthma. Further, smooth muscle cells *produce a wide array of cytokines, chemokines, growth factors, and extracellular matrix metalloproteases,* allowing them to modify the interstitial matrix directly around smooth muscle bundles. These cells also *secrete matrix proteins,* including fibronectin, elastin, and a variety of laminins and collagens, which then modulates the proliferation, migration, and apoptosis of the smooth muscle cells. For example, plasmin can stimulate release of active transforming growth factor-β from these cells, which in turn promotes collagen synthesis by the smooth muscle cells. This paradigm may partly explain the increased extracellular matrix found around smooth-muscle bundles in chronically inflamed airways.

The **alveolar parenchyma** is the site of the only essential function of the lung, that being *gas exchange to support cellular aerobic respiration.* Regardless of the media for gas exchange (water or air), the essential design of the gas exchange membrane in animals is remarkably similar, consisting of an epithelial layer exposed to the exchange media, in close apposition to blood-filled capillaries. This relatively simple arrangement belies the complexity of the biology of the region. In mammals, there are 5 major cell types associated with the alveolar parenchyma: *type I and type II pneumocytes, capillary endothelial cells, interstitial fibroblasts,* and *alveolar macrophages.*

Type I pneumocytes *are large, flat, membranous epithelial cells that line ~93% of the alveolar surface.* Type I pneumocytes are terminally differentiated and nonmitotic. They are particularly vulnerable to oxidant injury in part because of their large membrane surface area and low levels of important antioxidants, especially reduced glutathione. Irreversible injury to type I cells is quickly followed by sloughing of the cells from the alveolar basement membrane, which triggers a rapid regenerative response orchestrated by the type II pneumocytes. This description of type I cells suggests a passive role in the lung, facilitating gas exchange across the plasma membrane, and poised for injury and loss following any number of insults. Although this is true, they also play a critical part in maintaining normal lung fluid composition, providing a structural basis for preventing movement of fluid into the alveolus, and clearing fluid and protein from the alveolus during pulmonary edema.

Type II pneumocytes *are the main cuboidal cell lining the alveolus;* the brush cell or type III pneumocyte is also cuboidal, but much less numerous. Type II pneumocytes are found most commonly at the intersection of 2 alveolar septa, the so-called "corners" of the polygonal alveoli. Ultrastructurally, the type II pneumocyte has apical microvilli and characteristic cytoplasmic osmiophilic lamellar bodies, which are the site of surfactant storage. The primary functions of type II pneumocytes are to *synthesize pulmonary surfactant*, to serve as *progenitor cells* for replacement and turnover of alveolar epithelium, and to *metabolize xenobiotics.*

Pulmonary surfactant is a complex mixture that forms a film at the air-liquid interface of terminal bronchioles and alveoli. It consists of dipalmitoyl-phosphatidylcholine (DPPC, which is responsible for much of the surface-tension–lowering function) and other phospholipids, cholesterol, and surfactant proteins (SP-A, SP-B, SP-C, SP-D). Surfactant lipids are synthesized in type II pneumocytes; some are also produced by club cells. They are initially stored in lamellar bodies, then secreted onto the alveolar surface, where they arrange in a functional surface-active form known as *tubular myelin*, which adsorbs to the alveolar air-liquid interface. The main function of surfactant in the alveoli is to *lower surface tension in the alveolar space to prevent alveolar collapse during expiration.* The biology of the system is highly dynamic. With each breath, there is cycling between the subsurface surfactant reservoir and the bioactive surface film. Similarly, tubular myelin is constantly converted to a less functional vesicular form that must be recycled by type II pneumocytes or degraded by alveolar macrophages. SP-A, SP-B, and SP-C are important for secretion and recycling of the surfactant lipid, formation of tubular myelin, and the proper insertion of these lipids into the alveolar surface film. Beyond its role in regulating alveolar surface tension, SP-A and SP-D also have important immunoregulatory and pulmonary defense functions (see Lung defenses, later). The biology of this system is highly relevant to the pathogenesis of interstitial lung diseases.

The proliferative capacity of type II pneumocytes is important in alveolar development and postnatal lung growth; the lungs of most species are not fully developed, undergoing continued maturation after birth (see Lung development and growth, later). Type II cells can rapidly proliferate to repopulate denuded basement membrane following injury to type I pneumocytes. This process follows a general pattern, consisting of rapid migration to cover the basement membrane, followed by proliferation, and differentiation to the dominant alveolar epithelium. The process is dependent on the ability of the type II pneumocyte to modify the extracellular matrix to facilitate this process. Type II cells synthesize a variety of matrix components, including fibronectin, type IV collagen, and proteoglycans, as well as matrix-degrading enzymes such as metalloproteases.

Fibroblasts are found within the alveolar wall associated with a network of extracellular matrix proteins, including collagen and elastin. This network is not uniformly distributed within the membrane, leading to regions of the wall that are "thick" and "thin," with gas exchange only occurring in the latter. The fibroblasts of the lung are heterogeneous in terms of morphology, functionality, and expression of surface markers. This heterogeneity is particularly well documented

in experimental and human cases of pulmonary fibrosis. For example, the presence or absence of Thy-1 on lung fibroblasts is associated with variation in fibroblast adhesion to extracellular matrix, production of cytokines, and ability to produce extracellular matrix proteins including collagen. The array of matrix proteins potentially produced by lung fibroblasts is extensive, and includes collagen types I, III, IV, V, and VI; elastin; laminin; fibronectin; glycosaminoglycans; and proteoglycans.

Pulmonary macrophages are an important class of lung cells and are found in a variety of compartments within the organ. Five separate populations have been recognized: *alveolar macrophages, interstitial macrophages, pulmonary intravascular macrophages, dendritic cells,* and *pleural macrophages.*

Alveolar macrophages are resident cells in the lung that form a self-renewing pool derived from progenitors in the yolk sac and fetal liver; they are minimally supplemented by, but not dependent on, renewal from marrow-derived circulating monocytes. Inflammation induces massive proliferation of these resident cells as well as eliciting monocytes from the circulation, and it has become apparent that resident and elicited macrophages have considerable differences in function. Resident alveolar macrophages are integral to homeostasis of the alveolar parenchyma, and maintaining a noninflamed environment despite the presence of low numbers of bacteria. The role that pulmonary macrophages play in pulmonary defense is discussed subsequently (see Lung defenses). Less appreciated is the homeostatic role of alveolar macrophages in preventing the accumulation of native proteins, especially surfactant, within the alveolus. *Alveolar proteinosis,* a condition of alveolar accumulation of surfactant components, can be caused by local deficiency of granulocyte-macrophage colony-stimulating factor; this impairs the ability of the alveolar macrophage to clear surfactant, leading to its accumulation in the alveolus.

Alveolar macrophages function as *important regulatory cells* in the lung, controlling inflammatory, immune, and repair processes through the release of a wide array of cytokines and other regulatory molecules. Inflammation and immunity are promoted by macrophage synthesis and release of cytokines, such as interleukin-1 (IL-1), tumor necrosis factor-α, and interferon-γ, as well as by release of inflammatory mediators, such as leukotriene B$_4$ and C$_4$, platelet-activating factor, and thromboxane A$_2$. Repair processes are generally promoted or otherwise regulated by release of cytokines that include transforming growth factor-β and -α, fibroblast growth factor, insulin-like growth factor, and platelet-derived growth factor.

Dendritic cells are *ubiquitous immunoregulatory cells* found in all tissues. They are motile cells involved in surveillance for antigens at the epithelial and mesothelial surfaces of the respiratory tract. Various subpopulations can be distinguished by means of morphologic characteristics, primary location, and unique surface marker proteins. Morphologically, dendritic cells have numerous long processes and function as antigen-presenting cells, priming naïve T cells and driving the cells into T-helper type 1 (Th-1) or Th-2 effector cells. The ability to present antigen to T cells requires that the dendritic cells themselves mature; this occurs within regional lymph nodes under the influence of appropriate proinflammatory signals. The numbers of dendritic cells can increase markedly in the respiratory tract, given the proper stimuli, and they play an important role in allergic airway disease and asthma.

Interstitial macrophages are the least well-understood class of pulmonary macrophages. Because of their location within the interstitium of the conducting airways and alveolar parenchyma, they are more difficult to isolate and characterize than other macrophage populations. In mice, interstitial macrophages have less phagocytic activity than alveolar macrophages, and instead are primarily immunomodulatory cells, expressing more major histocompatibility complex class II molecules and producing more cytokines, such as IL-1 and IL-6, than the alveolar macrophage.

Pulmonary intravascular macrophages (PIMs) are unique mononuclear phagocytes found within the alveolar capillaries of select species, including cattle, sheep, goats, horses, pigs, cats, and cetaceans (eFig. 5-2). PIMs may be recruited into the lungs of rats and humans during inflammatory lung diseases, and this same process seems to occur in dogs. PIMs form membrane-adhesive complexes with the capillary endothelium, which *keeps them localized to the vascular bed*. These cells are highly phagocytic and play an important role in the clearance of circulating bacteria and particulates from the pulmonary circulation. PIMs release an array of proinflammatory mediators following interaction with particulates and bacterial endotoxin. Because of their proinflammatory properties, they can contribute to the lung injury coincident with acute lung inflammation. Depletion of PIMs can attenuate lung injury following experimental bacterial infections or exposure to endotoxin.

Further reading

Fahy JV, Dickey BF. Airway mucus function and dysfunction. N Engl J Med 2010;363:2233-2247.

Harkema JR, et al. The nose revisited: a brief review of the comparative structure, function, and toxicologic pathology of the nasal epithelium. Toxicol Pathol 2006;34:252-269.

Orgeig S, et al. Recent advances in alveolar biology: evolution and function of alveolar proteins. Respir Physiol Neurobiol 2010;173 (Suppl.):S43-S54.

Lung defenses

The necessary function of gas exchange requires that the lung remain exposed to the environment. Thus the lung is continuously challenged by immense quantities of microorganisms and foreign material in inhaled air, and by opportunistic pathogens within droplets that are aspirated from the nonsterile upper respiratory tract. Despite this constant bombardment, the lung must maintain the balance of normal microbiota now documented to reside in the lung and prevent increases in the numbers of noncommensal organisms in the alveoli, as such increases can induce inflammation that impedes gas exchange in the lung. Additionally, because of the tremendous blood flow through the lung, contamination of the lung by bacteria carries a significant risk of bacteremia. Thus *the lung requires a multilayered system of defense against infectious agents*. This is accomplished by the following:

- *Mucus* lines the airways, entrapping particles and microbes, and is propelled by coughing or by ciliary beating to the pharynx, where it is swallowed.
- *Antibody and innate defense proteins* kill microbes directly, prevent them from colonizing mucosal surfaces, and/or opsonize the microbes to make them more easily ingested by phagocytes.

- *Alveolar macrophages* recognize foreign invaders, particularly in the presence of opsonins, and engulf and kill these microbes without inducing inflammation.

If the infection cannot be contained by these mechanisms, inflammation is triggered in an attempt to control the threat. In these situations, macrophages and airway or alveolar epithelial cells produce cytokines and other mediators that recruit neutrophils and monocytes-macrophages. Inflammatory mediators also induce the production of antibacterial proteins by epithelial cells of the airway surface and tracheobronchial glands. But this response has the potential to do harm. *Inflammatory exudates impair gas exchange, leukocyte-derived enzymes and oxygen radicals cause injury to lung tissue, and repair processes may result in organization of alveolar exudates or fibrosis of alveolar septa that permanently decreases lung compliance and thickens the blood-gas barrier.* The significance of these sequelae depends on the extent of lung involvement. The tremendous reserve capacity of the lung means that many animals have localized areas of pneumonia that are of no clinical significance, yet mild changes present throughout the lung can seriously compromise pulmonary function.

Inspired air carries a variety of particulates, including infectious agents, allergens, and inert particles. *The site of* **particle deposition** *in the respiratory tract depends on their size, density, and charge.* Particles larger than ~10 μm are almost completely removed in the nasal cavity, mainly by impaction at sites in the nasal turbinates where the airflow changes direction. Particles that are 3-10 μm are more likely to impact the mucosa of the trachea and bronchi, where they can be cleared by the mucociliary apparatus. In general, particles <5 μm have the greatest potential to reach the deep lung (terminal bronchioles and alveoli), although this is most common with smaller particles (1-2 μm). The velocity of airflow declines precipitously in the terminal airways because the total cross-sectional area increases; as a result, particle deposition in the bronchioles and alveoli results from sedimentation, diffusion, and electrostatic charge.

Coughing and mucociliary clearance *are the major mechanisms for clearing particles that become entrapped in the airways.* Mucociliary clearance of particles from distal airways requires 2-6 hours, and the presence of innate defense proteins within the airway mucus, described in more detail later, probably serves to limit bacterial growth during this time. Mucociliary clearance may be as rapid as 10 mm per minute in the trachea, but the pace in the bronchioles is more languid. The airways are covered by a *periciliary liquid layer* (formerly known as the sol or hypophase) and a superficial mucous layer. The mucous layer contains abundant glycoproteins that are sticky and tend to trap a wide variety of particles that impact on the airway surfaces. The function of the periciliary liquid layer has long been considered to simply provide an aqueous medium in which the cilia can beat. However, recent evidence indicates that this layer forms a periciliary brush composed of mucins that transiently tether the cilia to the overlying mucus, trap water to maintain hydration, and prevent the mucus and other luminal substances from entering the periciliary layer. The quality of the periciliary liquid layer is also critical for clearance of entrapped particulates, because the low viscosity of this fluid permits the cilia of the epithelial cells to beat effectively. Additionally, clearance of sputum from the larger airways by coughing requires that the periciliary liquid layer be fluid and abundant, allowing the superficial mucous layer to be easily propelled. Finally, effective ciliary function is necessary for mucociliary clearance, and requires coordinated unidirectional ciliary beating at an adequate frequency of around 15 beats per second. The regulation of this system is not well known. However, shear stress on the epithelium both increases the ciliary beating frequency and promotes epithelial secretion to maintain the quality of the liquid and mucous layer. Nitric oxide, cyclic adenosine monophosphate, and cyclic guanosine monophosphate are other regulators of ciliary beat frequency.

When entrapped particles reach the nasopharynx, they have the opportunity to interact with the well-developed lymphoid tissue in the tonsils and nasopharyngeal mucosa before reaching the pharynx and being swallowed. Although this clearance of inhaled particles is normally beneficial, it is a method for the spread of agents such as *Mycobacterium bovis* and *Rhodococcus equi*, and is important in the migration of helminth eggs and larvae. Mucociliary clearance may be impaired by infection of the airway epithelium with viruses, mycoplasmas, or *Bordetella*; exposure to cold air or ammonia; squamous metaplasia resulting from chronic bacterial infection or toxin exposure (cigarette smoke and environmental pollutants being the best-characterized examples); inherited anomalies of ciliary structure or function; or abnormal mucus production in human cystic fibrosis.

The mucus covering the airway mucosa contains a rich spectrum of **antimicrobial factors,** which operate by several distinct mechanisms. Some cause *direct injury to pathogens,* such as the β-defensins, cathelicidins, lactoferrin, lysozyme, lactoperoxidase, the complement membrane attack complex, and anionic antimicrobial peptides. *Lactoferrin binds iron* and makes it unavailable for use by many bacteria, whereas neutrophil gelatinase-associated lipocalin—secreted by airway and alveolar epithelial cells and by neutrophils—binds the bacterial siderophores that otherwise allow pathogens to scavenge ferric iron. Other components, including immunoglobulin A and polysaccharides within the mucus, *block the attachment of bacteria to mucosal surfaces. Infectious agents may be opsonized* by immunoglobulin G, the complement component C3b, and surfactant proteins A and D. Two families of antimicrobial proteins, defensins and collectins, deserve particular mention. The *defensins* are a family of 3-5 kDa, cationic, arginine-rich peptides that are present in neutrophil granules, intestinal Paneth cells, and epithelial cells of the trachea and bronchi. Some defensins are constitutively expressed, whereas others are rapidly induced by proinflammatory cytokines, lipopolysaccharide and other Toll-like receptor agonists, or cytokines secreted by T-helper-17 cells. The defensins are able to kill bacteria, fungi, and enveloped viruses by forming pores within microbial membranes that are rich in anionic phospholipids, and they also have roles in leukocyte chemotaxis and wound healing. The *collectins* are a family of calcium-dependent carbohydrate-binding lectin proteins that include the surfactant proteins A and D. Both of these proteins are produced by type II pneumocytes; SP-A is also secreted by club cells in the bronchioles. These pulmonary collectins agglutinate and opsonize bacteria, viruses, and fungi, and also maintain surfactant homeostasis, have antioxidant activity, and bind lipopolysaccharide to regulate inflammatory responses.

Alveolar macrophages *are critical for defending the lung against particles that are deposited in alveoli, and also play a key role in recycling and removal of surfactant.* Alveolar macrophages are decorated with a variety of cell surface receptors that permit recognition of particles opsonized by antibody, complement, or collectins. In addition, CD14, Toll-like receptors, mannose receptors, and the scavenger receptor permit responses against bacteria that have not been previously encountered by the host. Alveolar macrophages phagocytose most opsonized particles within 2-4 hours, although the ingestion of inert particles such as carbon and silicates is much slower. Alveolar macrophages kill bacteria using reactive oxygen and nitrogen species and enzymes within their lysosomes. In addition, these cells promote an inflammatory response by *secreting cytokines, including chemokines* that recruit and activate neutrophils and macrophages. These newly recruited phagocytes are important in the clearance of more severe bacterial infections of the lung. Alveolar macrophages are integral to the immune response by presenting antigen, secreting cytokines that activate macrophages and modulate the immune response, and serving as effector cells in delayed hypersensitivity reactions. However, resident alveolar macrophages generally sequester or clear antigens and particulates from the alveoli without stimulating an immuno-inflammatory response and without migration to regional lymph nodes. In contrast, when blood monocytes are recruited to the lung during inflammation and differentiate into macrophages, their phlogistic nature further stimulates local inflammation and immune responses.

The actual physical removal of particulates from alveoli is inefficient, in contrast to their removal when deposited on the mucociliary blanket. Most particles phagocytosed by macrophages are either inactivated or sequestered. Alveolar macrophages are mainly cleared through the bronchioles on the mucociliary blanket. As the particulate load increases, as occurs in pneumoconioses, some particles penetrate into the pulmonary interstitium by endocytosis across the type I pneumocytes, where they are phagocytosed by interstitial macrophages. Particle-laden macrophages often cluster around bronchioles and blood vessels, associated with local lymphatics (well illustrated by the common finding in dogs of carbon-laden particles in the walls of terminal bronchioles), with some entering the lymphatics and eventually finding their way to local lymph nodes. In addition to the alveolar and interstitial macrophages, *intravascular macrophages* are present in the lung of cats, horses, ruminants, and pigs. These cells serve to remove infectious agents and other particles from the blood, and thus serve an analogous role to Kupffer cells in the liver and macrophages in splenic sinusoids.

Pulmonary immune responses are initiated when inhaled antigens are taken up by *dendritic cells* that inhabit the airway epithelium, and migrate to bronchial lymph nodes, where the antigen is presented to lymphocytes. Although *bronchus-associated lymphoid tissue* (BALT) is often visible histologically, this structure is not present in germ-free animals of most species and may represent a consequence of inflammation and antigenic stimulation. Homing of lymphocytes to BALT depends on $\alpha_4\beta_1$-integrin/vascular cell adhesion molecule 1 (VCAM-1), and chemokine receptor 10 (CCR10)/chemokine ligand 28 (CCL28). In contrast, migration of lymphocytes into alveolar tissue is exceptional because it occurs in capillaries rather than venules, and the homing receptors differ from those in the airways. These mechanisms allow *T lymphocytes and natural killer cells* to constantly survey the respiratory tissues, where they are most useful in defense against viruses, intracellular bacterial pathogens, and fungi.

Thus the lung is protected from inhaled bacteria by the filtering effect of the nasal cavity, innate and acquired humoral defenses, mucociliary clearance in the airways, resident alveolar macrophages, recruited neutrophils and elicited macrophages, and T lymphocytes and natural killer cells. These defenses can be considered in multiple layers, where most inhaled particles are removed in the nasal cavity or neutralized by innate defense proteins in the airway mucus prior to being cleared by the mucociliary apparatus. The small bronchioles seem to be a site of particular vulnerability, being poorly served by either mucociliary clearance or alveolar macrophages. Pathogens that reach the alveoli may be phagocytosed and killed by alveolar macrophages, particularly if the particles have been opsonized by complement or the surfactant proteins A and D, or by antibody if a previous encounter with the agent has resulted in an immune response. Still greater threats invoke a suppurative inflammatory response, which may be essential to clear bacteria from the lung but also carry the risk of compromised lung function and damage to the pulmonary tissue.

Further reading

Ackermann MR, et al. Innate immunology of bovine respiratory disease. Vet Clin North Am Food Anim Pract 2010;26:215-228.

Caswell JL. Failure of respiratory defenses in the pathogenesis of bacterial pneumonia of cattle. Vet Pathol 2014;51:393-409.

Parker D, Prince A. Innate immunity in the respiratory epithelium. Am J Respir Cell Mol Biol 2011;45:189-201.

NASAL CAVITY AND SINUSES
General considerations

The responses of the respiratory tract to injury, and the resulting patterns of disease, are largely determined by the structural and functional complexity of the system. Most of the diseases of the respiratory system are caused by agents arriving by either the airborne (aerogenous) or blood-borne (hematogenous) routes, each with its own special pathogenetic considerations.

The *upper respiratory tract* comprises the air-conducting structures from the external nares to the upper third of the trachea, including the specialized system of paranasal sinuses, the auditory tubes, and the guttural pouches of horses. The anatomy of the upper respiratory tract is described previously. Functionally, this system conducts and conditions the air moving into and out of the lower respiratory tract during respiration. The upper airways, constantly exposed to materials from the external environment, play an important role in surveying the inspired air for pathogens and are exposed to a variety of potentially toxic particulates and gases.

The upper respiratory tract accounts for >50% of the airway resistance in the entire respiratory tract. This resistance leads to negative pressure during inspiration, shown to be greatest in the nasal cavity overlying the rostral aspect of the soft palate, the larynx, and the trachea; and indeed these correspond to disease hotspots, such as for dorsal displacement of the soft palate in racehorses and tracheal edema and hemorrhage syndrome of cattle. The anatomy of the upper airways is also important in the generation of species-specific vocalization in animals, and abnormal vocal sounds (stertor, stridor), as well as inspiratory dyspnea, are clinical indicators of diseases involving the upper airways.

Further reading

Jeffrey AM, et al. Nasal cytotoxic and carcinogenic activities of systemically distributed organic chemicals. Toxicol Pathol 2006;34:827-852.

Congenital anomalies

Congenital anomalies of the nasal cavity and sinuses are rare but occur in all species. They are usually part of more extensive craniofacial defects accompanied by various malformations of the mouth and eyes. Animals with absent, underdeveloped, or severely distorted nasal regions are usually stillborn or die immediately after birth because of the severity of the craniofacial defects.

Choanal atresia *is a failure of formation of one or both of the communications between the nasal cavity and nasopharynx.* The condition is relatively common in llamas and alpacas, well recorded in foals, and has been described in dogs, sheep, and cats. The obstruction may be membranous or bony and unilateral or bilateral. Affected animals have partial or complete obstruction of airflow, exercise intolerance, or respiratory distress, or they develop aspiration pneumonia or malnutrition if mouth breathing interferes with suckling. The condition in llamas is often accompanied by other facial malformations.

Further reading

Reed KM, et al. Evaluation of CHD7 as a candidate gene for choanal atresia in alpacas *(Vicugna pacos)*. Vet J 2013;198:295-298.

Nasal amyloidosis

Deposits of amyloid sometimes occur in the nasal submucosa of horses. The deposition is not part of generalized amyloidosis, although there might be concurrent cutaneous amyloidosis. The amyloid usually forms one or more masses in the nasal vestibule and rostral portions of the nasal cavity and may obstruct air flow, but it can be located anywhere in the nasal cavity or form diffuse deposits. The amyloid forms multifocal deposits accompanied by numerous lymphocytes, macrophages and giant cells (Fig. 5-3). There may be ulceration of the mucosa, especially overlying large nodular masses. Nasal amyloidosis in horses is of the *AL type*, composed of immunoglobulin light chains or light-chain fragments. Although AL amyloid results from plasmacytic neoplasms in other species, no such association has been established in horses.

Further reading

Mould JR, et al. Conjunctival and nasal amyloidosis in a horse. Equine Vet J Suppl 1990;10:8-11.

Circulatory disturbances

Epistaxis *refers to hemorrhage from the nose, without regard to the source of the bleeding. Blood-stained foam* in the trachea and nasal cavity is often present in animals with pulmonary congestion and edema at autopsy, but should not be confused with epistaxis, in which larger amounts of blood are present. In epistaxis, the hemorrhage may arise from the nasopharynx, lungs, or elsewhere in the respiratory tract. Lesions within the nasal cavity often cause unilateral epistaxis; causes of such

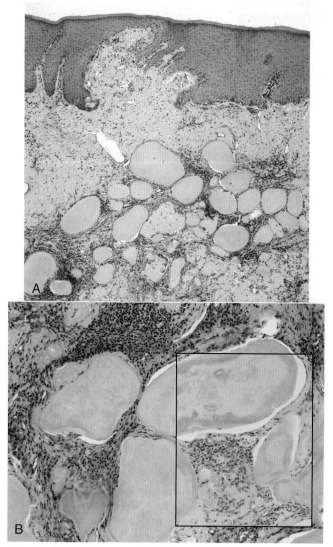

Figure 5-3 Amyloidosis of the nasal vestibule in a horse. **A.** The focal masses consist of amorphous eosinophilic aggregates of AL amyloid, separating a dense infiltrate of lymphocytes. **B.** Higher magnification. Inset: Congo red stain.

lesions include nasal trauma, severe rhinitis (lymphoplasmacytic, eosinophilic, or suppurative), mycotic infections of the nasal cavity or the guttural pouch, tooth root abscesses, and neoplasms. In contrast, bilateral epistaxis may indicate a severe manifestation of the above, hemorrhagic diatheses such as those causing thrombocytopenia, or lesions in or distal to the nasopharynx. The latter include pulmonary contusions, purpura hemorrhagica in horses, exercise-induced pulmonary hemorrhage in horses, rupture of embolic pulmonary abscesses in cattle, pulmonary neoplasia or granulomas, pulmonary hypertension, or vasculitis. Animals with epistaxis that swallow the blood may have considerable amounts in the stomach.

Further reading

Mylonakis ME, et al. A retrospective study of 61 cases of spontaneous canine epistaxis (1998 to 2001). J Small Anim Pract 2008;49: 191-196.

Immunology of the upper respiratory tract

As with other mucous membranes, the upper-airway mucosa has an indigenous immune system, the *nasal-associated lymphoid tissue* (NALT). NALT is considered to be a component of the broader mucosal-associated lymphoid system present in a variety of mucous membranes. The nasopharyngeal lymphoid (Waldeyer's) ring is a collection of lymphoid tissues that encircles the oropharynx and nasopharynx of animals. The degree of organization of this lymphoid tissue varies by species. In addition, there are lymphoid follicles and loose aggregates of mononuclear cells within the lamina propria. These lymphoid tissues induce a local immune response, and also stimulate a systemic immune reaction to nasally delivered antigens. This tissue is particularly prominent in foals, and gives a finely nodular appearance to the pharyngeal mucosa.

The organization of NALT is similar to mucosal lymphoid tissues at other sites. Specialized follicle-associated epithelium, with *microfold (M) cells,* covers the follicles and transfers antigen to the underlying lymphoid follicles. Within the follicles there are T-cell– and B-cell–rich regions, as well as dendritic cells and macrophages involved in antigen presentation. The formation of NALT is a postnatal event that is at least partly regulated by acquisition of commensal microbes in the nasopharynx. This resident microbial flora is often established by specific adherence of bacterial adhesins to carbohydrates on epithelial cells.

In addition to the role that nasopharyngeal commensals play in the formation of NALT, they can prevent colonization of the mucosa by more virulent organisms and modulate the immune response during infection. Injury to the nasal mucosa can allow infection of the underlying tissues by certain of the normal flora or, more importantly, affect surface binding sites so that adherence and colonization by pathogenic microorganisms can occur. Finally, disruption of the normal nasopharyngeal flora by prolonged antimicrobial therapy may result in fungal or opportunistic bacterial infections of the nasal cavity, further illustrating the role of these commensals in mucosal defense.

Further reading

Canessa C, et al. The immunity of upper airways. Int J Immunopathol Pharmacol 2010;23(1 Suppl.):8-12.

Rhinitis

Rhinitis, inflammation of nasal tissue, can be localized or a manifestation of systemic disease. The main causes include viral, bacterial, fungal, and parasitic infections; allergens; inhalation of irritant gases; and particulate dusts (Box 5-1). Most cases of significant acute rhinitis begin with serous exudation, which changes in the course of the disease to become catarrhal, purulent, or hemorrhagic. With **pseudomembranous rhinitis,** fibrinous membranes can be peeled off without leaving gross underlying defects. In contrast, **fibrinonecrotic (diphtheritic) membranes** adhere firmly to the underlying tissue, leave a raw ulcerated surface when removed, and are most commonly caused by inhalation of epitheliotoxic gases, alphaherpesviruses, or bacteria such as *Fusobacterium necrophorum*. Histologically, in acute rhinitis, the epithelial cells are normal or show hydropic degeneration, loss of cilia, or attenuation. Goblet cells may be inapparent from having secreted their contents, or may be hyperplastic. The lamina propria is

BOX • 5-1

Major causes of nasal and sinus disease in domestic animals

Dogs
- Foreign body
- Mycotic rhinitis
- Allergic rhinitis
- Idiopathic lymphoplasmacytic rhinitis
- Oronasal fistula
- Apical tooth infection
- Ciliary dyskinesia
- Adenocarcinoma
- Olfactory neuroblastoma
- Other considerations
  - *Bordetella bronchiseptica*
  - Canine adenovirus 2
  - Canine distemper virus
  - Canine parainfluenza virus
  - *Linguatula serrata*
  - *Pneumonyssoides caninum*
  - *Eucoleus boehmi*
  - *Rhinosporidium seeberi*

Cats
- Felid herpesvirus 1
- Feline calicivirus
- *Cryptococcus*
- Foreign body
- Nasopharyngeal stenosis
- Nasopharyngeal polyp
- Lymphoma
- Adenocarcinoma
- Other considerations
  - *Bordetella bronchiseptica*
  - *Chlamydophila* spp.
  - *Mycoplasma* spp.
  - Mycotic rhinitis
  - *Rhinosporidium*

Swine
- Inclusion body rhinitis
- Atrophic rhinitis

Horses
- Equid herpesvirus
- Influenza A virus
- Equine rhinitis virus
- *Streptococcus equi* ssp. *equi*
- *Streptococcus equi* ssp. *zooepidemicus*
- Bacterial sinusitis
- Ethmoid hematoma
- Sinonasal polyps
- Ethmoid and sinus cysts
- Squamous cell carcinoma
- Maxillary bone tumors (fibrous dysplasia, ossifying fibroma, osteoma, fibrosarcoma)
- Other considerations
  - Tooth root infection
  - Nasal amyloidosis
  - Glanders
  - Mycotic rhinitis or sinusitis
  - Phycomycosis
  - *Schistosoma* spp.

Cattle
- Bovine herpesvirus 1
- Bovine parainfluenza virus 3
- Mycotic nasal granuloma
- Allergic rhinitis
- Other considerations
  - *Limnatis* spp.
  - *Mammomonogamus* spp.

Sheep and goats
- *Salmonella enterica* ssp. *arizonae*
- *Oestrus ovis*
- Enzootic nasal tumor

edematous and contains inflammatory cells that often infiltrate the epithelium and may be visible in the surface exudate.

Chronic rhinitis may be classified by the nature of the leukocytic infiltrate, but caution should be exercised in equating this with a specific cause. For example, *suppurative rhinitis* can result from bacterial infection, aspergillosis, or an inhaled foreign body, but is a common nonspecific response to mucosal injury of other causes. Eosinophils predominate in the lesions of *allergic rhinitis* but may also be the dominant granulocyte in the tissue adjacent to fungal plaques or carcinomas. *Lymphoplasmacytic rhinitis* is a common reaction pattern in chronic nasal disease of diverse etiology. The nasal epithelium in chronic rhinitis is often attenuated because of necrosis or may develop squamous metaplasia or dysplasia. Other features of chronic inflammation include hyperplasia of lymphoid tissue, fibrosis of the lamina propria with atrophy of the glands, and

sessile or pedunculated *polyps* that may be mistaken clinically for neoplasms.

Nasal/nasopharyngeal stenosis or cicatrix formation occurs in cats and horses, probably as a result of previous erosive rhinitis with fibrous organization of exudates. *In horses*, the typical lesion is circumferential weblike scarring of the mucosa in the laryngopharynx rostral to the epiglottis, but may be elsewhere in the pharynx, nasal cavity, or trachea. *In cats*, nasopharyngeal stenosis appears as more uniform membranous narrowing of the opening between the nasopharynx and the caudal nasal cavity. The histologic findings are chronic nonspecific rhinitis and/or granulation tissue with chronic hemorrhage. Clinical signs often include upper respiratory noise or respiratory distress in the absence of much discharge. Rarely, the inspiratory efforts resulting from bilateral nasal obstruction can lead to hiatal hernia and megaesophagus.

Idiopathic lymphoplasmacytic rhinitis is an important condition in dogs, and to a lesser extent in cats. In dogs, the clinical disease may be either unilateral or bilateral, although histologic lesions are usually bilateral. Grossly, there is increased mucus production, mucosal inflammation, and turbinate destruction. Histologically, lymphocytes and plasma cells predominate, but neutrophils may be present. Chronic inflammation may lead to diffuse or polypoid thickening of the nasal mucosa and obstruction of nasal passages. The fibrotic stroma is heavily infiltrated by lymphocytes and plasma cells, and the surface epithelium may be hyperplastic, eroded, or undergo squamous metaplasia. The cause and pathogenesis of this disease remain unknown. It seems reasonable to consider that following an unknown initial insult, there develops a self-propagating cycle that involves dysregulation of the local immune system, resulting in mucosal damage and further infection by normally nonpathogenic commensal flora and self-sustaining inflammation. Nevertheless, *lymphoplasmacytic inflammation is a common reaction of the nasal mucosa to injury, and occult causes such as foreign body, bacterial or fungal infection, or neoplasia must be ruled out.*

Allergic rhinitis is observed sporadically in most domestic species. The disease in *dogs* is diagnosed on the basis of chronic and often seasonal oculonasal discharge, sneezing, nose-rubbing, head-shaking, and perhaps epistaxis, and the *presence of eosinophils in nasal exudate* (eFig. 5-3). There is no definitive information on either the pathologic or immunologic basis of the condition, but it is assumed to be a type I hypersensitivity. *Cattle,* and occasionally *sheep,* develop a seasonal rhinitis that available evidence suggests is an allergic response to pollen antigens. A familial predisposition has been reported, and the disease occurs chiefly in the summertime when pastures are in bloom. Affected animals have nasal discharge, lacrimation, sneezing, and evidence of nasal itching. The nasal mucosa is pale and thick from edema, and mucosal erosions may be visible in the rostral nares. Eosinophils and mucus are a prominent component of the exudate. Histologically, *the surviving nasal epithelium is hyperplastic or eroded and is infiltrated by eosinophils.* The glandular epithelium can be hypertrophied, and mucus is produced in excess. In more severe cases, in which there is extensive superficial diphtheresis, many of the small mucosal vessels show fibrinoid necrosis.

Nasal "granuloma" in cattle is generally considered to be a more chronic form of allergic rhinitis. The affected mucosa is mainly in the caudal portion of the nasal vestibule and the rostral region of the ventral nasal cavity but may extend caudally even to the larynx and proximal trachea. Grossly, *the hyperplastic epithelium is granular or has multiple nodular projections covered by intact epithelium,* and catarrhal exudate may be present. Histologically, the nodules typically consist of hyperplastic epithelium with areas of squamous metaplasia or ulceration, covering a superficial edematous lamina propria with a central core of inflamed granulation tissue. Goblet cell hyperplasia is more pronounced in the ducts of the nasal glands, at the lateral boundaries of the nodules. Eosinophils infiltrate the superficial lamina propria and epithelium, and lymphocytes, plasma cells, and mast cells are increased in number. Vascular proliferation, fibroplasia, and accumulation of mostly lymphocytes and plasma cells in the cores of nodules are features of chronicity. It is believed that the condition is an allergic reaction to plant pollens or fungal spores. Because

there appears to be a familial predisposition in Jersey cattle, and to a limited extent in other cattle, the existence of susceptible "atopic" animals has been proposed. The condition is therefore sometimes referred to as *atopic rhinitis.*

Specific infectious causes of suppurative rhinitis deserve mention. *Salmonella enterica* ssp. *diarizonae* (specifically, serovar 61:k:1,5,[7]) causes flock problems in sheep, with mucoid nasal discharge, nasal obstruction, and granular swelling or sessile polyp formation in the ventral conchae. Histologically, there is polypoid hyperplasia of the mucosa with intraepithelial bacteria and infiltration of neutrophils. *Streptococcus canis* and *Streptococcus equi* ssp. *zooepidemicus* cause outbreaks or sporadic cases of rhinitis and sinusitis in dogs and cats, with extension through the cribriform plate leading to fatal meningitis. *Aspergillus fumigatus* commonly causes nasal disease in dogs and cats, with ulceration and suppurative or eosinophilic rhinitis in which the fungal hyphae are found mainly in plaques on the mucosal surface. However, suppurative rhinitis is also a nonspecific reaction to foreign bodies, neoplasms, bacterial infection, tooth root infections, oronasal fistula, and other causes.

Infectious causes of granulomatous rhinitis, with or without eosinophils, are diverse and are discussed in detail later (see Infectious diseases of the respiratory system). *Cryptococcus neoformans* and *C. gatti* are readily recognized by the thick capsule; acapsular strains occur and incite more granulomatous inflammation but are recognized by the narrow-based budding. *Conidiobolus* spp. and *Basidiobolus haptosporus* cause granulomatous masses in the caudal nasal cavity of horses and ruminants that may invade surrounding tissues and disseminate to lung or brain. Histologically, granulomas contain macrophages, many giant cells, few eosinophils, central necrosis, and negatively stained fungal hyphae embedded in Splendore-Hoeppli material; silver stains reveal the hyphae to be 8-20 μm diameter, infrequently septate, with nonparallel walls and bulbous dilations. Although comparable, lesions caused by *Pythium insidiosum* occlude mainly the rostral nasal cavity, induce eosinophilic inflammation, and have smaller hypha-like oomycetes that are 2-7 μm diameter and infrequently septate with thick nonparallel walls. *Rhinosporidium seeberi* causes inflamed polyps with sporangia that are 15-75 μm or much larger and commonly have endosporulation. Granulomatous rhinitis caused by the yeast *Candida parapsilosis* is reported in an immunosuppressed cat. Nodular granulomatous rhinitis with eosinophils caused by *Pseudallescheria boydii* is described in dogs and cattle. *Besnoitia spp.* causes lesions in many organs, but the characteristic 150-450 μm diameter thick-walled protozoan cysts are often found in the nares, nasal cavity, nasopharynx, or larynx. Finally, *Prototheca wickerhamii* and *P. zopfii* affect the mucocutaneous junction of the nares in addition to the skin, with necrotizing pyogranulomatous lesions containing septated sporangia that are 3-15 μm and 7-30 μm diameter, respectively.

A variety of toxic agents cause necrosis of nasal respiratory or olfactory epithelium. These may be direct-acting irritants or toxins. Further, because of the cytochrome P450-dependent biotransformation activity of the nasal mucosa, systemic toxins such as acetaminophen, vincristine, coumarins, naphthalene, polychlorinated biphenyls, methimazole, and 3-methylindole target the nasal epithelium in some species. These are particularly well studied in rodents, but toxic nasal disease is not often investigated in domestic animals.

Further reading

Anon. AHVLA disease surveillance report: rhinitis associated with allergic nasal granuloma in Jersey cattle. Vet Rec 2012;171:468-471.

Barrs VR, et al. Sinonasal and sino-orbital aspergillosis in 23 cats: aetiology, clinicopathological features and treatment outcomes. Vet J 2012;191:58-64.

Lacasta D, et al. Chronic proliferative rhinitis associated with *Salmonella enterica* subspecies *diarizonae* serovar 61:k:1, 5, (7) in sheep in Spain. J Comp Pathol 2012;147:406-409.

Lobetti RG. A retrospective study of chronic nasal disease in 75 dogs. J S Afr Vet Assoc 2009;80:224-228.

Norman TE, et al. Association of clinical signs with endoscopic findings in horses with nasopharyngeal cicatrix syndrome: 118 cases (2003-2008). J Am Vet Med Assoc 2012;240:734-739.

Silva SMMS, et al. Conidiobolomycosis in sheep in Brazil. Vet Pathol 2007;44:314-319.

Diseases of the paranasal sinuses

Inflammation of the paranasal sinuses often goes undetected unless it has caused facial deformity or a fistula in the overlying skin. In acute catarrhal or purulent rhinitis, the mucosal swelling tends to occlude the orifices of the sinuses and impair drainage. The secretions and exudates then accumulate and predispose to bacterial infection and chronic purulent sinusitis. *The accumulation of seromucinous secretion is referred to as* **mucocele**, *and the accumulation of purulent exudate is known as* **empyema** *of the sinus* (eFig. 5-4). Sinusitis follows penetration of infection in dehorning wounds, fractures, and periodontitis. It is common in sheep infected with larvae of *Oestrus ovis*. Sinusitis is of most significance in the horse because of the size and complexity of its paranasal sinuses and the compounding effects of limited drainage and tendency for periodontitis to extend to the sinuses. In *horses*, primary sinusitis is most frequent in the maxillary sinus, but the exudates in the ventral conchal sinus are more likely to be inspissated and therefore respond more poorly to therapy. Other sinus diseases of horses include dental sinusitis from apical infection of a maxillary cheek tooth, oromaxillary fistula, mycosis, cysts, trauma, or progressive hematoma. Reported equine sinus neoplasms include cementoma, benign fibro-osseous tumor, myxoma, lymphoma, and carcinoma.

Further reading

Dixon PM, et al. Historical and clinical features of 200 cases of equine sinus disease. Vet Rec 2011;169:439.

Dixon PM, et al. Equine paranasal sinus disease: a long-term study of 200 cases (1997-2009): ancillary diagnostic findings and involvement of the various sinus compartments. Equine Vet J 2012;44:267-271.

Woodford NS, Lane JG. Long-term retrospective study of 52 horses with sinunasal cysts. Equine Vet J 2006;38:198-202.

Non-neoplastic proliferative disorders of the nasal cavity and sinuses

Sialoceles and nasal glandular mucoceles occasionally expand into the nasal cavity or nasopharynx with similar morphology to those found elsewhere (eFigs. 5-5, 5-6). *Polypoid thickening of the nasal mucosa* can occur in cases of chronic rhinitis and sinusitis. In these chronic inflammatory lesions, mucosal and submucosal hyperplasia may become florid enough to form a discernible mass within the nasal cavity or sinuses. Whereas this change is a nonspecific remodeling response in the nasal cavity, there are 2 specific types of polyps in domestic species, whose clinical features and pathology are distinctive.

Progressive ethmoid hematomas (PEH, hemorrhagic nasal polyp) **of horses** *arise from the ethmoid turbinate region of the equine nasal cavity*. These masses usually occur in older horses, and may be more common in the Thoroughbred and Arabian breeds. PEH are usually unilateral hemorrhagic growths arising from the submucosa of the ethmoid turbinates. The cause and pathogenesis of PEH remain to be determined, although it is assumed that it represents an aberrant vasoproliferative response to submucosal hemorrhage. The lesions are progressive and may continue to enlarge until the cylindrical mass extends to the external nares. Grossly, PEH is a mottled, hemorrhagic fibrovascular mass that can fill the ipsilateral nasal meatus, or occasionally grow into the maxillary sinus. Histologically, PEH mostly consists of organizing hemorrhages of various ages with extensive siderosis and mineralization of connective tissue fibers and vessel walls. The inflammatory response is variable, but multinucleated giant cells are usually present within the stroma. The surface is often covered by attenuated epithelium with underlying glands, or squamous metaplasia may occur. Ulceration of the surface epithelium is common.

Nasopharyngeal polyps of cats *are non-neoplastic inflammatory masses arising within the middle ear or auditory tube* (Fig. 5-4). Clinical disease is seen primarily in young cats 1-3 years of age. The clinical signs are dependent on the location of the polyp. Extension of the mass into the pharynx is associated with dyspnea, dysphagia, and gagging; involvement of the nasal cavity may cause sneezing, nasal discharge, and protrusion through the nares, whereas involvement of the middle ear may result in ataxia, Horner's syndrome, and/or facial nerve paralysis. The cause and pathogenesis are not known, although the appearance of the lesions suggests progressive expansion of the mucosa in response to localized chronic inflammation. Histologically, feline nasopharyngeal polyps

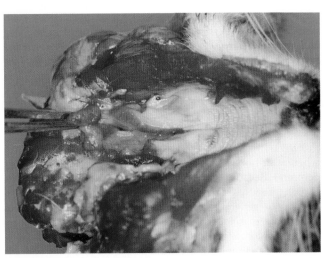

Figure 5-4 Nasopharyngeal polyp in a cat. Forceps grasp the polyp, which has a stalk extending from the nasopharynx into the auditory tube. The soft palate has been incised.

consist of a loose fibrovascular core covered by ciliated respiratory or squamous epithelium. Even when the surface epithelium has undergone squamous metaplasia, ciliated cells are usually visible within nests of epithelial cells buried in the stroma. The stroma is infiltrated by a mixed chronic inflammatory infiltrate of lymphocytes, plasma cells, and macrophages; surface erosions, when present, elicit neutrophil infiltration of the stroma. Recurrence of the polyps is relatively common when removed by simple traction, if the base of the mass is not excised. A *second form of feline nasal polyps* arises from nasal turbinate; consists of fibrous tissue, woven bone, and blood-filled spaces; and is covered by columnar ciliated epithelium. *These have been termed* **inflammatory polyps of the nasal turbinates of cats** *or feline mesenchymal nasal hamartoma.*

Paranasal sinus cysts in foals or young adult horses are within a maxillary or frontal sinus, and have a thin bony wall lined by respiratory epithelium and filled with fluid. The masses can distort the profile of the maxillary bone sufficiently to cause obstruction of the ipsilateral nasal passage, destruction of the nasal turbinates, distortion of the teeth, and deviation of the nasal septum. **Cystic nasal conchae** are congenital lesions that cause progressive nasal obstruction with inspiratory and expiratory noise in cattle. They are bilateral or unilateral, and otherwise similar to those of horses. **Epidermal inclusion cysts** lined by stratified squamous epithelium are described in the nasal diverticulum (false nostril) of horses and have been seen in dogs.

Further reading

Conti MB, et al. Diagnosis and treatment of progressive ethmoidal haematoma (PEH) in horses. Vet Res Commun 2003;27(Suppl. 1):739-743.

Greci V, et al. Inflammatory polyps of the nasal turbinates of cats: an argument for designation as feline mesenchymal nasal hamartoma. J Feline Med Surg 2011;13:213-219.

Neoplasms of the nasal cavity and sinuses

Although primary neoplastic disease of the nasal cavity and sinuses of domestic animals is not common, pathologists frequently examine nasal biopsy specimens to rule out such disease. Primary nasal neoplasia is most frequent in the dog and cat, with fewer reports in horses. Most nasal epithelial neoplasms in sheep and goats are of retroviral etiology (see Infectious respiratory diseases of sheep and goats, later). Interestingly, there is some epidemiologic evidence of a link between exposure to environmental tobacco smoke and coal-burning and kerosene heat sources, and the development of nasal neoplasms in dogs.

Origin from the nasal cavity is usual in dogs and cats, whereas in horses, tumors of the paranasal sinuses are most common. Because of the inflexible osseous encasement, even benign growths can be associated with significant clinical disease. In general, *most neoplasms of the nasal cavity and sinuses are carcinomas,* followed in decreasing frequency by chondrosarcoma, fibrosarcoma, and osteosarcoma.

Nasal carcinomas are common in dogs and cats, and are classified as adenocarcinoma, adenoid cystic carcinoma, transitional carcinoma, adenosquamous carcinoma, squamous cell carcinoma, acinic cell carcinoma, neuroendocrine carcinoma, oncocytoma, and undifferentiated (solid) carcinoma. Regard-

less of the type, locally invasive growth is the usual reason for euthanasia. *Stage I neoplasms* have unilateral growth resulting in nasal discharge with or without blood. *Stage II neoplasms* are bilateral and may cause dyspnea from obstruction of the nasal cavity. *Stage III neoplasms* invade adjacent tissues, such as nasal, palatine, or facial bones to cause facial distortion or ocular discharge, the retro-orbital space to cause exophthalmos, or the cribriform plate and brain to cause seizures or depression. These consequences of invasive growth are the usual reason for euthanasia, and metastasis occurs relatively late in the course of disease. Median survival time in dogs is ~3 months, and the presence of epistaxis confers a worse prognosis.

Adenocarcinoma is the most common type, and the diagnosis is based on identifying an invasive carcinoma, with formation of many or few acini, tubules, or papillary structures (Fig. 5-5). Occasional cases have prominent mucin production. **Adenoid cystic carcinomas** are formed by nests and cords of neoplastic basal-like cells with scant cytoplasm and hyperchromatic nuclei; these cellular nests have a cribriform pattern with sharply demarcated "punched out" centers containing

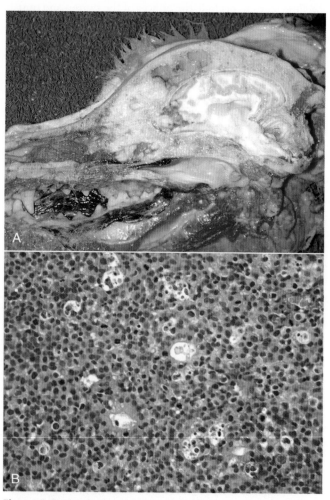

Figure 5-5 **Nasal adenocarcinoma** in a dog. **A.** Adenocarcinoma arising from the ethmoid conchae, with invasion of paranasal sinus and through cribriform plate into brain. **B.** The cells have a nearly solid arrangement, with a few acini lined completely by a ring of neoplastic cells. Focal cellular necrosis is present but should not be interpreted as acini.

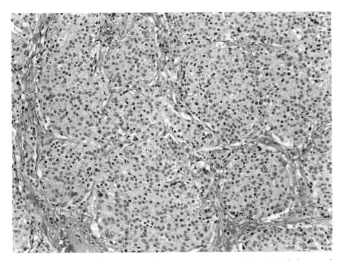

Figure 5-6 Nasal transitional carcinoma in a dog. Nodules and nests of neoplastic cells, without acinus formation or squamous differentiation. (Courtesy S. Youssef.)

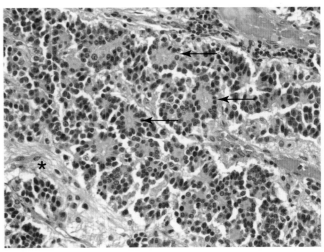

Figure 5-7 Olfactory neuroblastoma in a dog. The epithelioid cells form rosettes (arrows), with finely fibrillar material in the stroma (asterisk).

basophilic mucus. Lakes of this same material are present between the nests of cells. **Transitional carcinomas** (nonkeratinizing squamous cell carcinomas) form nodules or nests of stratified cuboidal epithelium that lack keratinization (Fig. 5-6); microcysts are sometimes present within the epithelial layers and must be distinguished from the acini seen in adenocarcinomas. **Adenosquamous (mucoepidermoid) carcinomas** have mucin-filled acinar components and foci with squamous differentiation, and are reported to be more aggressive tumors. **Squamous cell carcinomas** are similar to those seen in other organs, with nodules or nests of epithelial cells that keratinize to form abundant glassy eosinophilic cytoplasm and occasional central aggregates of keratin. These are frequent tumors in the cat, where most originate from the nasal vestibule, and in the horse, where the maxillary sinus is a common site. **Acinic cell carcinomas** have a faintly packeted or acinar arrangement of cells that resemble salivary serous cells, with abundant pale cytoplasm containing fine basophilic periodic acid–Schiff (PAS)-positive diastase-resistant granules; this type is invasive, but metastases are not expected. **Oncocytomas** form cords or nests of large epithelioid cytokeratin-positive cells with angular borders, with abundant eosinophilic cytoplasm containing numerous mitochondria that appear as fine phosphotungstic acid–hematoxylin (PTAH)-positive granules; the few cases reported had either noninvasive or invasive growth habits. **Neuroendocrine carcinomas** have delicate septa of fibrous stroma separating nests or packets of neoplastic epithelial cells and express synaptophysin, chromogranin A, and other markers of neuroendocrine differentiation. Because these markers are also expressed by some adenocarcinomas, the morphologic features are essential for the diagnosis. **Undifferentiated carcinomas** are solid epithelial neoplasms that lack the patterns of differentiation mentioned previously. Differential diagnoses for nasal carcinomas in general include lymphoma, olfactory neuroblastoma, and amelanotic malignant melanoma. The distinction between carcinoma and lymphoma can be particularly difficult in cats, and immunohistochemistry may be needed to resolve uncertainty. **Benign epithelial neoplasms** are rare but include papilloma (eFig. 5-7), adenoma, and basal cell tumor (of the vestibule).

Olfactory neuroblastoma (esthesioneuroblastoma, esthesioneuroepithelioma) is a rare neoplasm derived from olfactory neuroepithelium and arising in the ethmoid conchae. The neoplastic cells form indistinct serpiginous ribbons, nests, or lobules with delicate fibrovascular stroma, and are epithelioid but have indistinct borders and scant cytoplasm. *Rosette formation* is a characteristic feature (Fig. 5-7), more frequent in cats than dogs, and includes pseudorosettes (neoplastic cells palisading around a blood vessel), Homer-Wright rosettes (neoplastic cells arranged around neurofibrillary material), and infrequent Flexner-Wintersteiner rosettes (neoplastic cells arranged around an empty space). *Neurofibrillary material* often separates the cells, mineralization may be present, and necrosis is usually extensive in dogs and cats. Immunohistochemistry for chromogranin and neuron-specific enolase (NSE) may be helpful, although nonspecific background staining can be problematic with NSE, and synaptophysin is often negative. Neuron-specific markers such as microtubule-associated protein 2 (MAP-2) and NeuN are more specific but less widely available. Because some are cytokeratin positive, this is not useful in distinguishing olfactory neuroblastoma from adenocarcinoma. A grading scheme is proposed, with higher-grade tumors having lack of lobular architecture, fibrillary matrix or mineralization, few or no rosettes, and a greater degree of nuclear pleomorphism, necrosis, and mitotic activity. Penetration through the cribriform plate and into the cerebral cortex is commonly observed.

Of the round-cell neoplasms, **lymphoma** is most frequent, particularly in cats. Nasal lymphoma in cats is usually primary, arising from the nasal cavity or uncommonly the nasopharynx, and is not associated with retroviral infection. Less often, nasal tissues can be secondarily affected in cases of multiorgan lymphoma. Feline nasal lymphoma is easily confused with carcinoma, because the large neoplastic cells are often arranged as dense sheets, and faint packeting can result from the presence of delicate bands of stroma. The vast majority are of diffuse large B-cell phenotype, but low-grade follicular B-cell lymphoma as well T-cell lymphoma do occur. Epitheliotropism suggests a T-cell phenotype, yet nasal epitheliotropic B-cell lymphoma is reported. Diffuse large B-cell nasal lymphoma can develop in other organs as the disease progresses

(22-67% of cases, depending on the study), but invasion of local tissues, including brain, is the more common clinical problem. Other round cell tumors of the nasal cavity include mast cell tumor, melanoma, and transmissible venereal tumor.

Of the mesenchymal neoplasms, **chondrosarcoma** is most frequent followed by **osteosarcoma** and **fibrosarcoma**. The appearance is typical of that in other tissues (eFig. 5-8). **Paranasal meningioma** occurs in dogs and horses, and in dogs appears similar to intracranial meningioma but has a more invasive behavior. **Nasopharyngeal angiofibroma** in dogs forms a papillary mass composed of loose proliferative fibrous tissue with numerous tiny branching capillaries, with infiltration of neutrophils and lymphocytes. Despite the benign histologic appearance, these masses have an aggressive, locally invasive growth habit. **Nasomaxillary tumors of young horses,** including fibrosarcoma, ossifying fibroma, and fibrous dysplasia, are described elsewhere (see Vol. 1, Bones and joints). Other mesenchymal tumors of the nasal cavity include melanoma, hemangiosarcoma, and fibroma.

Further reading

Brosinski K, et al. Olfactory neuroblastoma in dogs and cats—a histological and immunohistochemical analysis. J Comp Pathol 2012;146:152-159.

Day MJ, et al. An immunohistochemical investigation of 18 cases of feline nasal lymphoma. J Comp Pathol 2004;130:152-161.

Little L, et al. Nasal and nasopharyngeal lymphoma in cats: 50 cases (1989-2005). Vet Pathol 2007;44:885-892.

Mukaratirwa S, et al. Feline nasal and paranasal sinus tumours: clinicopathological study, histomorphological description and diagnostic immunohistochemistry of 123 cases. J Feline Med Surg 2001;3:235-245.

Ninomiya F, et al. Nasal and paranasal adenocarcinomas with neuroendocrine differentiation in dogs. Vet Pathol 2008;45:181-187.

Rassnick KM, et al. Evaluation of factors associated with survival in dogs with untreated nasal carcinomas: 139 cases (1993-2003). J Am Vet Med Assoc 2006;229:401-406.

PHARYNX, LARYNX, AND TRACHEA
Pharynx and guttural pouch

The pharynx, as the site where the respiratory and alimentary systems conjoin, is exposed to both inhaled and ingested materials, some of which may have deleterious effects on the animal. In **pigs**, a *caudal diverticulum of the pharynx lies immediately dorsal to the esophagus.* In young pigs, plant awns and similar foreign materials occasionally lodge in this diverticulum, causing pharyngitis and cellulitis that may lead to dysphagia and death from starvation. Iatrogenic pharyngitis, even with perforation of the caudodorsal wall of the pharynx, may occur in **cattle** during incorrect oral administration of boluses or esophageal intubation.

In young **horses,** it is common to find prominent lymphoid follicles within the pharyngeal mucosa. This is usually an incidental finding, as these follicles are part of the normal mucosal immune system in the horse (eFig. 5-9).

The **guttural pouches** of equids are ventral diverticula of the auditory tubes. Suppurative inflammation leading to guttural pouch empyema occurs mostly after upper respiratory infections, particularly with *Streptococcus equi* or other streptococci. Guttural pouch mycosis, generally caused by *Aspergillus* spp., causes fibrinonecrotic inflammation that extends deeply to invade vessels and other structures (Fig. 5-8). Thus severe complications are much more likely than for guttural pouch empyema. Guttural pouch inflammation can extend to involve nearby vessels, cranial nerves (VII, IX, X, XI, XII), and the cranial sympathetic trunk, or even spread to adjacent bones, middle ear, brain, or atlanto-occipital joint. Thus erosion of the internal or external carotid artery or the maxillary artery causes epistaxis, damage to the glossopharyngeal or vagus nerves causes dysphagia, damage to the cranial sympathetic trunk or cranial cervical ganglion causes Horner's syndrome, or damage to the facial nerve causes facial paralysis. Other complications include laryngeal hemiparesis, or permanent dorsal displacement of the soft palate. Guttural pouch hemorrhage may also result from fracture of the basisphenoid bone. A less common condition is *guttural pouch tympany.* This

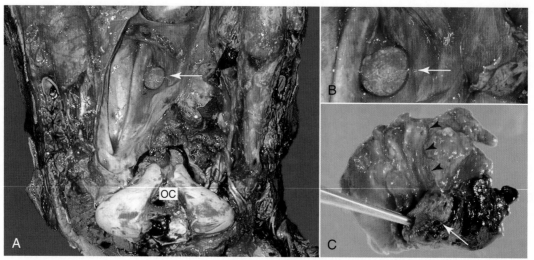

Figure 5-8 Guttural pouch mycosis in a horse. **A, B.** The fungal plaque (arrow) is adjacent to the stylohyoid bone. Ventral view of the head, with occipital condyles (OC) labeled for orientation. **C.** Within the guttural pouch, the carotid artery (blue arrowheads) is focally invaded by a fungal plaque (arrow). The pouch was filled with blood at the time of autopsy (different case from **A** and **B**).

is seen mostly in young animals, and the accumulation of air is presumed to be due to valvular action of the nasopharyngeal orifice of the auditory tube. *Tumors of the guttural pouches are rare, but squamous cell carcinoma is most likely.* Pharyngeal tumors are discussed with neoplasia of the mouth (see Vol. 2, Alimentary system and peritoneum).

Further reading

Borges AS, Watanabe MJ. Guttural pouch diseases causing neurologic dysfunction in the horse. Vet Clin North Am Equine Pract 2011;27: 545-572.

Larynx

In the **horse,** *subepiglottic cysts* are believed to arise from thyroglossal duct remnants. *Entrapment of the epiglottis* below the aryepiglottic fold is usually associated with congenital hypoplasia or acquired shortening or distortion of the epiglottis. A short epiglottis also predisposes to *dorsal displacement of the soft palate,* and these conditions sometimes occur together. *Persistent frenulum of the epiglottis* has been reported in newborn foals, predisposing to oronasal reflux of milk after nursing and aspiration pneumonia. The persistent frenulum of the epiglottis leads to dorsal displacement of the soft palate, which can be assessed endoscopically.

Laryngeal paralysis in horses is frequently subclinical but may cause abnormal respiratory noise *(roaring)* and poor performance. *The condition is almost always a left-sided hemiplegia caused by idiopathic degeneration of the left recurrent laryngeal nerve.* The resulting denervation atrophy affects the intrinsic laryngeal muscles supplied by this nerve, but the atrophy is not uniform; the lateral cricoarytenoid muscle is affected first and most severely, followed by the dorsal cricoarytenoid. Grossly, the affected muscles are pale and atrophic (Fig. 5-9). The cricothyroid muscle, which is supplied by the cranial laryngeal nerve, is the only intrinsic muscle not affected. Because the dorsal cricoarytenoid muscle is the main abductor of the larynx, denervation atrophy and dysfunction of this muscle allows the left arytenoid cartilage to sag into the lumen and obstruct airflow during inspiration.

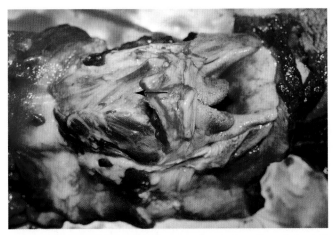

Figure 5-9 Equine laryngeal neuropathy, with pallor of the left dorsal cricoarytenoid muscle (arrow) resulting from severe neurogenic atrophy. Dorsal view, tongue to the right. The transverse incision was made at autopsy.

Microscopic examination of affected nerve fibers reveals *severe loss of myelinated fibers in middle and distal portions of the left recurrent laryngeal nerve.* Ultrastructural features indicate progressive loss of fibers in the left recurrent nerve accompanied by chronic demyelination, remyelination, and abortive regenerative attempts. Similar but milder changes can be detected ultrastructurally in the distal right recurrent nerve. The axons in the left recurrent laryngeal nerve are much longer than those in the right recurrent nerve, and this presumably makes them more susceptible to degeneration. *Idiopathic laryngeal paralysis in horses*—the most common form encountered—is unilateral, whereas bilateral paralysis is more typical of cases caused by hepatic encephalopathy and general anesthesia.

Laryngeal paralysis in dogs occurs most commonly in older males of large or giant breeds as well as Labrador retrievers. The condition is less common in cats. The disease is usually bilateral, in contrast to that in horses. Although the cause is often not identified, the relationship between recurrent laryngeal axonopathy and denervation atrophy of the laryngeal muscles is usually as described in horses. In dogs, unlike horses, laryngeal paralysis may be a single manifestation of generalized neuromuscular disease. Some breeds of dogs are predisposed to developing laryngeal paralysis, including Bouvier des Flandres and mixed Husky-Malamute puppies, where it is associated with apparent hereditary degeneration of the nucleus ambiguus; Rottweilers, as a manifestation of a polyneuropathy; and white-coated German Shepherd dogs. Occasionally, laryngeal paralysis occurs secondary to hypothyroidism or following general anesthesia. In dogs, laryngeal paralysis predisposes to aspiration pneumonia.

Laryngeal edema may be part of a local or systemic inflammatory process, and can be caused by infections of the laryngeal mucosa or surrounding connective tissues, inhalation of irritant materials, local trauma, anaphylaxis, or hyperthermia. The amount of edema varies, but is most severe in the region of the epiglottis, the aryepiglottic folds, and the ventricles. Mild laryngeal edema is a common incidental finding in many species at autopsy.

Laryngitis accompanies inflammatory diseases of either the upper or lower respiratory tract, or can occur without involvement of other tissues. Laryngitis can occur as a part of *oral necrobacillosis* (calf diphtheria) caused by *Fusobacterium necrophorum* in calves and swine. *Laryngeal erosions* can develop in response to exposure to noxious agents, such as anhydrous ammonia (eFig. 5-10). *Laryngeal ulcers* occur in feedlot cattle with bronchopneumonia, and probably represent mucosal damage by the repeated trauma of laryngeal closure in dyspneic animals. *Laryngeal infarcts* with ulceration may overlie lesions of septic phlebitis in calves with *Histophilus somni* septicemia and pneumonia. Inhalation or aspiration of toxicants is a rare cause of laryngeal and epithelial necrosis (see eFig. 5-4). The nematode parasite *Mammomonogamus laryngeus* can inhabit the laryngeal surface of cattle.

Laryngeal lesions in racing horses occur commonly. The simplest form is small mucosal ulcers in a variety of locations. *Laryngeal chondritis (arytenoid chondropathy)* is characterized by ulceration of mucosa at the rostral margin of the arytenoid cartilage, immediately caudal to the attachment of the vocal fold, resulting in deformation of the laryngeal cartilage (eFig. 5-11). The histologic lesions include variable combinations of chronic suppurative inflammation, granulomatous inflammation, granulation tissue, and necrosis of cartilage. The

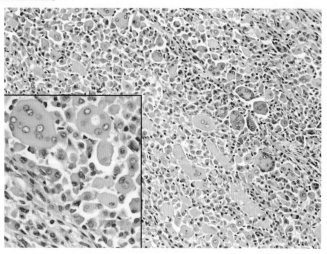

Figure 5-10 Laryngeal rhabdomyoma in a dog. The neoplastic cells are round or spindle-shaped, occasionally strap-like, pleomorphic, with abundant eosinophilic cytoplasm, and often multinucleated. Inset: higher magnification.

pathogenesis is not known, but may involve mucosal trauma as the larynx closes forcefully in rapidly breathing animals, with introduction of bacteria that stimulate inflammation and cartilage degradation.

Primary neoplasms of the larynx are rare in domestic species. **Papillomas** involving the larynx are usually part of widespread papillomatosis, as may be seen in immunocompromised animals. **Squamous cell carcinoma** is the most common malignant tumor. The laryngeal epithelium has a florid hyperplastic response to underlying inflammation, so care should be taken in differentiating (non-neoplastic) pseudoepitheliomatous hyperplasia from laryngeal squamous cell carcinoma. **Plasmacytoma** is a round cell tumor with eccentric nuclei, abundant glassy cytoplasm, and occasional karyomegaly or multinucleation. As for alimentary plasmacytoma, laryngeal plasmacytoma has a more aggressive course than those arising in skin. Laryngeal neoplasms consisting of cells with abundant granular cytoplasm include rhabdomyoma, oncocytoma, and granular cell tumor. **Laryngeal rhabdomyoma** occurs in young dogs as a solitary benign raised nodule in or near the lateral ventricle of the larynx (eFig. 5-12). It consists of lobular masses of angular pleomorphic cells with abundant deeply eosinophilic granular or foamy cytoplasm (Fig. 5-10). Although this appearance has been interpreted as an oncocytoma, the diagnosis of rhabdomyoma is confirmed by demonstrating *myosin and muscle-specific actin* by using immunohistochemistry. **Granular cell tumor**, probably of Schwann cell origin, is less common in the larynx than in the tongue of dogs. The neoplastic cells have abundant cytoplasm with fine PAS-positive diastase-resistant granules (lysosomes and phagosomes), and are positive for S100 and vimentin. A miscellany of other neoplasms is described in the larynx (eFig. 5-13).

Further reading

Aitken MR, Parente EJ. Epiglottic abnormalities in mature nonrace-horses: 23 cases (1990-2009). J Am Vet Med Assoc 2011;238:1634-1638.
Diab S, et al. Study of laryngopharyngeal pathology in Thoroughbred horses in southern California. Equine Vet J 2009;41:903-907.

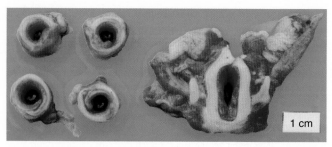

Figure 5-11 Brachycephalic airway syndrome in a Bulldog. The larynx is hypoplastic, with thickening of the mucosa and a narrow lumen. The trachea could be stretched to normal diameter, but is collapsed from excessively negative inspiratory pressure, causing overlap of the ends of the cartilage rings.

Dixon PM, et al. Laryngeal paralysis: a study of 375 cases in a mixed-breed population of horses. Equine Vet J 2001;33:452-458.
Thieman KM, et al. Histopathological confirmation of polyneuropathy in 11 dogs with laryngeal paralysis. J Am Anim Hosp Assoc 2010;46:161-167.

Trachea

Brachycephalic airway syndrome is a constellation of lesions occurring in brachycephalic dogs and to a lesser extent in cats. It may include stenotic nares, insufficient pharyngeal space for the soft palate ("elongation" and thickening of the soft palate), and tracheal hypoplasia. In this syndrome, **tracheal hypoplasia** appears as reduced diameter of the lumen resulting from small tracheal rings, with an inapparent dorsal tracheal ligament. Greater negative intraluminal pressures during forced inspiration secondarily cause eversion of laryngeal saccules, hypertrophied and folded pharyngeal mucosa, everted tonsils, laryngeal edema, collapse of the larynx, and/or collapse of the trachea with overlapping of the ends of the cartilage rings (Fig. 5-11). These factors aggravate the problem by further obstructing airflow, as does mucosal thickening or exudates resulting from tracheitis or pneumonia. Aspiration pneumonia is often present in fatal cases. A comparable condition resulting from narrowing of the larynx occurs in *Norwich Terriers*.

Tracheal collapse refers to *dorsoventral narrowing of the trachea* resulting in coughing and exercise intolerance. The disease is most common in middle-aged miniature breeds of dogs and is described in miniature horses. The cartilage rings are abnormally shaped and form shallow arcs, and the dorsal tracheal muscle (tracheal membrane) is widened and flaccid (Fig. 5-12). The condition is not limited to the trachea; bronchoscopy reveals bronchomalacia and collapse in many affected dogs. Earlier descriptions of the histologic and histochemical features associated with tracheal collapse describe foci of hypocellularity of the hyaline cartilage and areas where cartilage is replaced by fibrous and/or fibrocartilaginous tissue. It remains to be determined if these changes are causative or the result of biomechanical changes resulting from the tracheal collapse.

Tracheal edema and hemorrhage syndrome of feedlot cattle, in which the lumen is partially obstructed by severe mucosal and submucosal edema and hemorrhage of the dorsal region of the distal half of the trachea, occasionally causes death by asphyxiation in feedlot cattle (Fig. 5-13). The loud inspiratory noise made by severely affected animals has given rise to the clinical term "honker syndrome." The cause is not

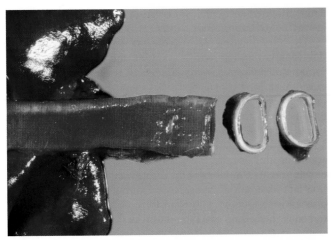

Figure 5-12 Tracheal collapse in a dog. The dorsal tracheal ligament is stretched and lax, with oblong flattening of the malacic cartilage rings. (Courtesy University of Guelph.)

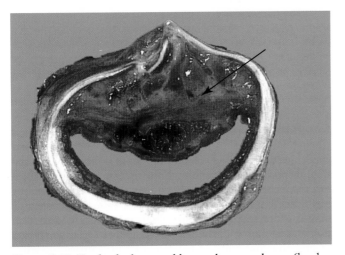

Figure 5-13 Tracheal edema and hemorrhage syndrome (honker syndrome) in a feedlot calf. Edema and focal hemorrhage asymmetrically thickens the dorsal tracheal mucosa (arrow) and partially occlude air flow. (Courtesy E.G. Clark.)

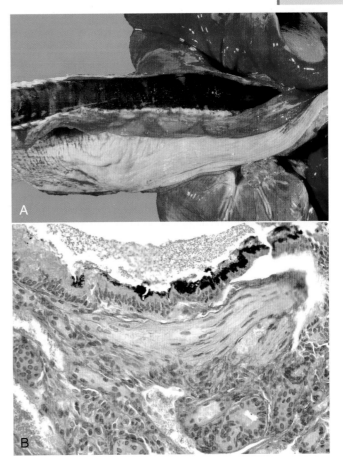

Figure 5-14 Smoke inhalation. A. Black discoloration of the tracheal mucosa confirms the dog was alive at the time of the fire. **B.** Histologic appearance (a different case), with black soot on the mucosal surface, and heat-induced coagulation of the tracheal tissue. (Courtesy University of Guelph.)

known, but the increased prevalence during hot weather and the frequent presence of concurrent bronchopneumonia suggest that hyperpnea with negative intratracheal pressures during inspiration may cause mechanical injury to the tracheal mucosa.

Miscellaneous lesions occur uncommonly in the trachea. *Tracheal froth* is normally present (eFig. 5-14), may increase as a result of pulmonary edema, but is abundant in normal sheep and horses at autopsy. *Malformations of the cross-sectional shape of the trachea* can be found as an incidental finding, especially in cattle. *Tracheal trauma*, such as during dystocia, causes fracture or collapse of the cartilage. Necrosis of tracheal epithelium occurs after *endotracheal intubation* if the cuff is inflated with excessive pressure. *Squamous metaplasia* of tracheal epithelium is a feature of vitamin A deficiency and severe iodide toxicosis. Black discoloration of the tracheobronchial mucosa is seen with smoke inhalation (Fig. 5-14). Foci of chronic polypoid tracheitis, probably as a result of chronic inflammation, are occasionally observed in dogs and cats and may cause stenosis and dyspnea. *Pox viruses* (lumpy skin disease and sheep pox) cause hyperplastic nodules in the

trachea. Tracheitis frequently accompanies bronchitis and bronchopneumonia. Small foci of *mineralization*, often with accompanying granulomatous inflammation, occur in the lamina propria of the dorsal trachea and ventral turbinates of adult pigs. The cause is not known. *Parasitic diseases* of the trachea of dogs, discussed later in the chapter, include *Eucoleus aerophilus*, *Oslerus osleri*, and *Spirocerca lupi*.

Tracheal carcinoma is recognized in cats and rarely in dogs. *Tracheal chondroma and osteochondroma* is an uncommon condition of young dogs, and may represent a dysplastic cartilaginous mass rather than a true neoplasm. It forms an expansile mass of disorganized cartilage, with ossification of the central core of some lesions.

Further reading

Adamama-Moraitou KK, et al. Canine bronchomalacia: a clinicopathological study of 18 cases diagnosed by endoscopy. Vet J 2012;191:261-266.

Clarke DL, et al. Partial resolution of hypoplastic trachea in six English Bulldog puppies with bronchopneumonia. J Am Anim Hosp Assoc 2011;47:329-335.

Fasanella FJ, et al. Brachycephalic airway obstructive syndrome in dogs: 90 cases (1991-2008). J Am Vet Med Assoc 2010;237:1048-1051.

Johnson LR, et al. Upper airway obstruction in Norwich terriers: 16 cases. J Vet Intern Med 2013;27:1409-1415.

LUNGS

Lung development and growth

The lungs develop early in gestation, forming from a ventral diverticulum in the foregut endoderm. The 6 stages of lung development and growth are the embryonic, pseudoglandular, canalicular, saccular, alveolar, and vascular maturation stages. Important development continues postnatally in most mammalian species.

During the **embryonic** stage of lung growth (30-50 days of gestation in a bovine fetus), the primordial trachea and right and left primary bronchi develop, growing into the surrounding mesenchyme. The growth of the conducting airways occurs primarily in the **pseudoglandular** stage; in most species, the airways develop through a series of asymmetrical dichotomous branching. Differentiation of conducting airway epithelial cells begins proximally and extends distally at this stage, with development of ciliated cells, mucous cells, basal cells, and bronchial cartilage. At the end of the pseudoglandular period, all branches of conducting airways have developed and are embedded in mesenchymal stroma. Distal airway branches are lined by cuboidal to columnar epithelial cells that contain abundant cytoplasmic glycogen. During the **canalicular** stage of growth (120-180 days of gestation), vascular "canalization" of the interstitium occurs, with capillaries growing in apposition to the airway epithelium to form the developing air-blood interface. Also during the canalicular stage, there is development of type II pneumocytes and type I pneumocytes within the newly formed terminal airspaces. Fetal lung development to the **saccular** stage (180-240 days gestation in the bovine fetus) is important for survival outside of the uterus. Lung volume and gas exchange surface increase markedly, and there is further reduction in mesenchyme between airspaces. The terminal branches of the conducting airways extend through the nascent parenchyma, and conditions are set for alveolar development. Small accumulations of elastic fibers, the site of secondary alveolar septal development, are deposited during this stage. During the **alveolar** stage of lung growth (240-260 days), true alveoli form by ingrowth of septa from intersaccular crests at the sites of elastic fiber deposition. These secondary septa have a doubled capillary layer separated by mesenchymal tissue (eFig. 5-15). The acquisition of a mature air-blood interface, with a single capillary layer, occurs after birth in the final stage of lung development, the stage of **microvascular maturation.** The end result is a reduction of the interstitium and maturation of the interalveolar wall. Further subdivision of alveolar septa results in continued increases in alveoli and alveolar surface area during a period of rapid postnatal growth. Airways increase in diameter and length through coordinated growth as overall lung volume and weight increase.

Movement of fetal lung fluid is important in directing normal lung development. Fetal respiration and spontaneous contraction of fetal conducting airways facilitate the movement of the fluid. Contraction of fetal airways occurs even in lung explants without central neurologic control because of the phasic contraction of the airway smooth muscle. Neural innervation of the developing lung occurs early in development, arising from neural tissue migrating through the fetal mesenchyme. Studies in the fetal pig show that both developing nerves and ganglia are present within the fetal bronchial tree as early as the pseudoglandular stage of development.

This cholinergic neural innervation coordinates the fetal airway contractions mentioned previously.

The coordination of intrauterine and extrauterine lung development and growth is complex and influenced by both local tissue factors as well as influences originating beyond the developing lung. Local epithelial-mesenchymal interactions, outlined previously, are necessary for directing the distal expansion of the lungs; indeed, the formation of the diverticula from the foregut endoderm, branching morphogenesis, and cell differentiation are specifically coordinated by the adjacent lung-specific mesenchyme. In each stage of lung development, a number of diffusible mediators and transcription factors direct organogenesis. Examples include the fibroblast growth factor family, transforming growth factor-β, and the sonic hedgehog signaling pathway.

Further reading

Castleman WL, Lay JC. A morphometric and ultrastructural study of postnatal lung growth and development in calves. Am J Vet Res 1990;51:789-795.

Maritz GS, et al. Fetal growth restriction has long-term effects on postnatal lung structure in sheep. Pediatr Res 2004;55: 287-295.

Shannon JM, Hyatt BA. Epithelial-mesenchymal interactions in the developing lung. Annu Rev Physiol 2004;66:625-645.

Congenital anomalies

Congenital anomalies of the lung are rare and may reflect abnormal development of the lung bud, pulmonary circulation, or both. Major malformations such as pulmonary agenesis are incompatible with life and are often accompanied by malformations in other organs. When investigating congenital masses of lung-like tissue, key observations include the location of the lesion and whether it is contained within the pleura or not, the continuity of the trachea and primary bronchus with the bronchi within the mass, and the nature of the pulmonary and systemic arterial supplies.

Pulmonary hypoplasia *is defined as reduced lung weight; hypoplastic lungs usually also have reduced numbers of alveoli* (eFig. 5-16). In contrast, the airways generally develop normally. Pulmonary hypoplasia may accompany malformations in other organs, and may include anasarca. Its development is closely linked to the presence of lung liquid that is secreted by the pulmonary epithelium, fills the airspaces, and is required for growth of the lung mass. *Pulmonary hyperplasia* is the result of overdistension of the lung, resulting from tracheal obstruction or laryngeal paralysis. In contrast, pulmonary hypoplasia ensues if the lung volume is not maintained. Pulmonary hypoplasia is caused by conditions that compress the lung, including congenital diaphragmatic hernia, intrathoracic masses, pleural effusions, or malformations of the thoracic cage; by oligohydramnios, in which the reduced uterine volume causes abnormal fetal positioning that compresses the chest and lungs; by impaired fetal breathing movements from abnormalities of the fetal nervous or musculoskeletal systems; by a tracheal fistula; and perhaps by reduced fluid secretion as a result of fetal hypoxemia or high levels of epinephrine.

Bronchogenic cysts and accessory lungs probably arise from aberrant (ectopic) outpouchings of the foregut. **Bronchogenic** cysts are single unilocular cystic masses that do not communicate with the airways. They may be located anywhere in the thorax but are most frequent near the hilus of the lung or in the mediastinum. Their walls contain cartilage plates, and the cystic cavity is lined by bronchial epithelium. **Accessory lung (extralobar sequestration,** choristoma) *is a mass of pulmonary tissue completely separated from the lung* (with a separate pleural covering) and found in the pleural space, mediastinum, or abdominal cavity. The term *sequestration* refers to the lack of connection to the normal airways. Bronchi are absent or rarely connect to the upper alimentary system (bronchopulmonary foregut malformations), and the mass is supplied by systemic but not pulmonary arteries.

Various sequelae of bronchial obstruction probably underlie the following malformations, and indeed, several of these can occur together. **Bronchial atresia** or complete obstruction results in accumulation of secreted mucus in the isolated lung tissue distal to the defect. This excessive lung fluid induces hyperplasia of bronchial tissue (adenomatoid malformation) or alveolar tissue (polyalveolar lobe). Conversely, partial obstruction of a bronchus, such as from maldevelopment of the cartilage or compression by external masses, leads to air trapping within the distal areas of lung after birth (**congenital lobar emphysema,** described later in Pulmonary emphysema). **Congenital cystic adenomatoid malformation** (adenomatoid hamartoma) is characterized by one or more intrapulmonary masses that are swollen, spongy or cystic, fluid- or air-filled, and lobulated (eFig. 5-17). The masses are formed by cysts varying from microscopic to several centimeters in diameter, which are lined by pseudostratified columnar or cuboidal epithelium. In the microcystic form, these give the lung an adenoma-like appearance. Microcystic spaces are separated by loose connective tissue, whereas the larger cysts may have walls of fibromuscular tissue. Bronchi, if present, are hypoplastic and lack cartilage and smooth muscle in their walls.

Pulmonary hamartoma (intralobar bronchopulmonary sequestration) *is a tumor-like mass of pulmonary tissue within the lung,* enveloped by the normal pleura but cut off or sequestered from the normal airways. It may be supplied by anomalous branches of the aorta and drained by pulmonary veins, but lacks communication with the bronchi or with the pulmonary arteries. Histologically, the development of bronchi, bronchioles, alveoli, and blood vessels is variable; those formed by excessive amounts of alveolar tissue relative to bronchioles and vessels are termed **polyalveolar lobe.** These are thought to result from bronchial atresia, with pulmonary hyperplasia in response to trapped secretions. The differential diagnosis includes pleuropulmonary or pulmonary blastoma.

In **anomalous pulmonary venous drainage,** the pulmonary veins drain into the right rather than the left atrium. Completely (total) or partially anomalous forms differ in whether all of the pulmonary veins are abnormal or not.

Further reading

Agerholm JS, Arnbjerg J. Pulmonary hypoplasia and anasarca syndrome in a belted Galloway calf. Vet Rec 2011;19(168):190.

Deutsch GH, et al. Diffuse lung disease in young children: application of a novel classification scheme. Am J Respir Crit Care Med 2007;176:1120-1128.

Lee JY, et al. Congenital cervical bronchogenic cyst in a calf. J Vet Diagn Invest 2010;22:479-481.

Leroith T, et al. Respiratory epithelial adenomatoid hamartoma in a dog. J Vet Diagn Invest 2009;21:918-920.

Wright C. Congenital malformations of the lung. Curr Diagn Pathol 2006;12:191-201.

Lung lobe torsion

Lung lobe torsion most often affects the right middle lobe of large deep-chested breeds of dogs as well as cats, presumably because of the narrow waist at the hilus, whereas the left cranial lobe is more commonly affected in small-breed dogs. Underlying causes are not apparent in most cases, but a minority have neoplasia, pneumonia, or atelectasis of the affected lobe, congenital dysplasia or hypoplasia of the bronchial cartilage, previous thoracic surgery, or pneumothorax. The clinical signs are variable and include respiratory distress, coughing, and hemoptysis. The affected lobe is twisted at the hilus and deeply congested (Fig. 5-15). Pleural effusion is consistently present and may be transudative, chylous, exudative, or bloody. Histologic lesions vary from simple congestion in acute or partial torsions, to diffuse alveolar damage with fibrinous alveolar exudates, to pulmonary infarction with coagulative necrosis of all tissue elements.

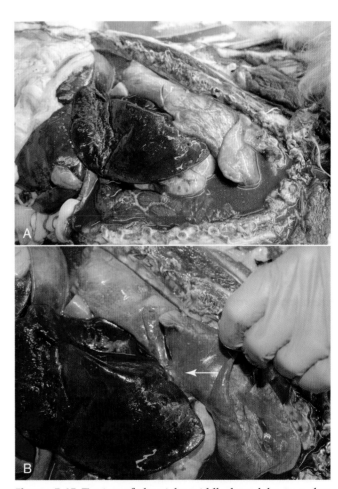

Figure 5-15 Torsion of the right middle lung lobe in a dog. **A.** The affected lobe is purple-red because of venous obstruction; there is abundant bloody thoracic fluid. **B.** The torsion is palpable and barely visible at the hilus of the lobe (arrow).

Further reading

Neath PJ, et al. Lung lobe torsion in dogs: 22 cases (1981-1999). J Am Vet Med Assoc 2000;217:1041-1044.

Atelectasis

Atelectasis *refers to incomplete expansion of the lung.* Atelectatic lung is homogeneously dark red and sunken relative to aerated lung, and the texture is fleshy or firmer and nonspongy. Microscopically, simple atelectasis appears as slightly congested alveolar walls lying in close apposition with slit-like residual lumina having sharp angular ends (eFig. 5-18). Atelectasis is a common artifact in immersion-fixed lung tissue. In **congenital atelectasis,** the lungs appear as in the fetus, but dark red-blue because of dilation of alveolar capillaries, of fleshy consistency and do not float (eFig. 5-19). **Obstructive atelectasis** *is caused by complete airway obstruction.* Whether atelectasis follows obstruction depends on the size of airway obstructed and the degree of collateral ventilation. *A lobular pattern of atelectasis suggests bronchial obstruction as the cause,* prompting a search for the offending exudates or tumors.

Compressive atelectasis *is caused by pleural or intrapulmonary space-occupying lesions.* Examples are hydrothorax, hemothorax, exudative pleuritis, and tumors. In large animals, the atelectasis caused by pleural effusions often occurs below a sharply demarcated fluid line. Abdominal distension, as in severe ascites and ruminal tympany, may cause partial atelectasis, typically in the cranial regions where ventilatory movements are most easily compromised by intra-abdominal pressure. Large animals with prolonged recumbency, such as anesthesia, may develop atelectasis of the down side. Generalized and severe atelectasis is mostly seen as a *sequel to pneumothorax.*

What appears to be total atelectasis is seen in animals that die while breathing 80-100% oxygen during anesthesia or intensive care. Because of the speed with which the oxygen is resorbed into tissues and the lack of nonabsorbable gas (especially nitrogen, as is present within atmospheric air), *the lungs are usually completely devoid of gas by the time they are examined after death.* Grossly, the lungs are markedly reduced in size, so the heart is especially prominent when the pluck is examined.

Pulmonary emphysema

Emphysema in its widest sense refers to tissue expansion by air or other gas. In the lung, there are 2 major forms:
1. **Alveolar (vesicular) emphysema,** which is rare in animals, refers to abnormal and permanent enlargement of alveoli resulting from destruction of alveolar septa, and an absence of obvious fibrosis. Emphysema thus differs from **overinflation of alveoli** caused by air trapping, which is a reversible lesion that is commonly encountered.
2. **Interstitial emphysema** is the presence of air within interlobular, subpleural, and other major interstitial zones of the lung. *"Emphysema," unless otherwise qualified, should only be used for alveolar emphysema.*

Emphysematous areas of lung are grossly voluminous, pale, and puffy. The enlarged airspaces are often visible as small vesicles, and in severe cases, coalescence of airspaces can produce large air-filled bullae. Emphysematous bullae occasionally rupture to cause fatal pneumothorax.

Enlargement and coalescence of airspaces are apparent histologically, and are most reliably assessed on lungs that have been infused with fixative to a volume approximating the in vivo state. *In true emphysema, fragments of alveolar wall may be apparent histologically,* in contrast to the more frequent lesion of alveolar overinflation. However, emphysema and overinflation are often difficult to distinguish. Emphysema may affect the terminal bronchioles and adjacent alveoli (centrilobular or centriacinar emphysema), or more uniformly involve the entire lobule (panlobular or panacinar).

Current knowledge of the **pathogenesis of emphysema** is based on investigations of the human disease and of animal models. Emphysema is an important condition in humans, where it frequently coexists with chronic obstructive pulmonary disease attributable to cigarette smoking and is the result of an imbalance between proteases and antiproteases. *Neutrophil-derived serine proteases, particularly elastase, and matrix metalloproteinases from a variety of sources are the likely culprits,* and their concentrations are enhanced by the neutrophil and macrophage activation induced by chronic bronchitis. Although antiproteases—α_1-antitrypsin, secretory leukoprotease inhibitor, and tissue inhibitors of matrix metalloproteinases—protect normal lung from proteolytic damage, their function may be reduced by genetic deficiency or by oxidative stress from cigarette smoke and the resulting inflammation. Unchecked proteases degrade elastin and other matrix proteins in the interstitium, and the weakened alveolar septa are vulnerable to stress-induced failure with the tensions generated by each ventilatory cycle.

The emphysematous lung is dysfunctional because the loss of alveolar septa reduces the alveolar surface area; although the affected portion of lung may be larger than normal, gas exchange is reduced. Loss of elastic recoil caused by degradation of elastin further compromises lung function. These factors make hyperpnea necessary to maintain lung function, which may exacerbate the disease by placing additional ventilatory stresses on the damaged lung.

Overinflation of alveoli is commonly encountered, although this does not qualify as alveolar emphysema unless it leads to destruction of alveolar septa. Overinflation is mostly the result of airway obstruction or spasm, with air trapping in alveoli and failure of the lung to deflate normally. Distended airspaces can be found at in the apices of the lungs of dogs, cats, and horses with underlying causes of respiratory distress, or along the margin of a consolidated lung (secondary to bronchiolar obstruction by exudate). Lobar overinflation may result from bronchial mucus plugs or lung lobe torsion. Overinflated lobules are a common finding in horses with bronchiolar mucus plugging associated with recurrent airway obstruction ("heaves").

Congenital lobar overinflation (congenital lobar emphysema) is rare in dogs, and results from collapse or obstruction of a lobar bronchus, such as by hypoplasia of the cartilage, leading to air trapping in the affected lobe. The right middle or cranial lung lobes are greatly enlarged by alveolar overinflation and/or bullous emphysema, sometimes with bronchiectasis. Pneumomediastinum, subcutaneous edema, or pneumothorax may occur. Affected dogs typically have slowly progressive dyspnea and coughing, and surgical excision is usually curative.

Interstitial emphysema is distinguished from alveolar emphysema by the presence of air in the connective tissues and lymphatics of the lung, including the interlobular septa,

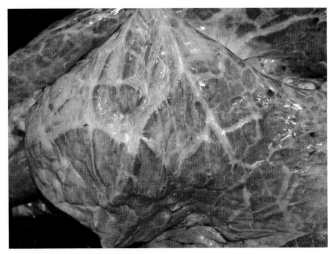

Figure 5-16 Interlobular emphysema in a "downer" dairy cow, with no respiratory distress and no other evidence of pulmonary disease. Pale bubbles of air distend the interlobular septa.

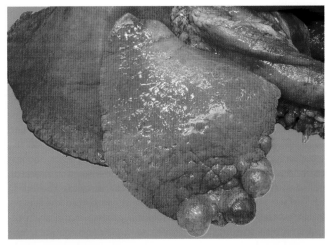

Figure 5-17 Bullae at the apices of the lung in a dog. Rupture of such bullae causes spontaneous pneumothorax.

beneath the pleura, and around vessels and airways. Positive-pressure ventilation with excessively high tidal volume is an occasional cause in all species. Interstitial emphysema without alveolar emphysema occurs frequently in cattle, presumably because of their well-developed interlobular septa and lack of collateral ventilation of the alveoli (Fig. 5-16; eFig. 5-20). It is an incidental finding in cattle at slaughter, and is common in recumbent ("downer") cows with periparturient paresis or toxic mastitis, where it may develop as cows forcibly exhale or grunt against a closed glottis. Thus *the finding of interstitial emphysema in cattle does not necessarily imply primary lung disease.* Dramatic interstitial emphysema occurs in cattle with respiratory distress caused by 3-methylindole toxicity, other toxins, or pneumonia caused by bovine respiratory syncytial virus. Interstitial emphysema in such cases may result from abnormally high intra-alveolar pressures caused by increased expiratory effort or bronchiolar obstruction, or perhaps from altered permeability or strength of the barrier between air-spaces and interstitium. In animals surviving a sufficient length of time with severe interstitial emphysema, the air can extend along lymphatics to the bronchial and mediastinal lymph nodes or along fascial planes of the mediastinum to beneath the skin of the back.

Blebs and bullae are common causes of spontaneous pneumothorax in dogs. They occur mainly in large-breed or deep-chested dogs. The respiratory distress may be acute or worsen over a period of weeks, and be continuous or intermittent. Surgical removal of the affected lobe is usually curative. These lesions appear as air-filled "bubbles" at the apices of the lung, usually in cranial or middle lobes, with more than one lobe affected in about half of cases (Fig. 5-17). Ruptured blebs and bullae are notoriously inconspicuous at autopsy, but holding the lungs under water and distending the lung by infusing air into the trachea or bronchus usually identifies the pleural leak. This should be done routinely in cases of anesthesia-associated death.

Histopathology distinguishes the 2 lesions: *air-filled spaces within the pleural connective tissue are termed blebs* (see eFig. 5-20), *whereas those arising in the lung parenchyma (by distention of alveoli or rupture of alveolar septa) and bulging into the pleura are bullae* (eFig. 5-21). Patchy subpleural areas of alveolar distention are often present within lobectomy samples, and

some cases have prominent smooth muscle hypertrophy in alveolar ducts or bronchioles, or chronic bronchitis. Whether these airway lesions cause the air trapping, and thereby bulla formation, is uncertain. A differential diagnosis is congenital lobar overinflation caused by hypoplasia of bronchial cartilage.

Further reading

Lipscomb VJ, et al. Spontaneous pneumothorax caused by pulmonary blebs and bullae in 12 dogs. J Am Anim Hosp Assoc 2003;39:435-445.

Wright JL, Churg A. Current concepts in mechanisms of emphysema. Toxicol Pathol 2007;35:111-115.

Circulatory disturbances of the lung

The lung is a vascular organ comprised of hundreds of billions of capillaries organized into hundreds of millions of alveoli whose surface area is estimated, in humans, to be 50-100 m². The entire output of the right ventricle is delivered to the lung with each contraction, delivering mixed venous blood from the peripheral tissues through the alveoli for reoxygenation. Given the anatomy and physiology of the lung, it is not surprising that circulatory disturbances are important in many lung diseases.

The color of the lungs at the time of postmortem examination is highly variable, but may or may not reflect any underlying disease. The lungs of animals that die from exsanguination will often be nearly white. Active **hyperemia**, as part of the acute inflammatory response, is a feature of acute pulmonary injury. Pulmonary **congestion** may be caused by left heart failure or inflammation. However, pulmonary congestion is a common incidental finding at autopsy, and therefore *the color of the lung is often deceptive. Changes in lung texture are a more reliable indicator of underlying disease.*

Pulmonary edema

Pulmonary edema is a frequent complication of many diseases and is therefore one of the most commonly encountered pulmonary abnormalities. If severe, pulmonary edema has a catastrophic effect on lung function by reducing pulmonary compliance, blocking ventilation of the alveoli, obstructing gas exchange across the alveolar septa, and reducing the surface area of the air-liquid interface in the alveoli. In addition, proteins present in the edema fluid interfere with surfactant function, further reducing compliance and contributing to pulmonary dysfunction. Edema of the lung is, in many respects, similar to edema of other tissues, and is governed by the permeability of the vascular wall and by Starling forces—the balance of hydrostatic and osmotic pressures between the intravascular and interstitial compartments. Distinctive aspects of edema in the lung include the importance of type I pneumocytes as barriers to fluid movement, the role of type II pneumocytes and club cells in active transport of water from the alveolus, the effect of surface tension on fluid movement, and fluid exchanges between the alveolar and bronchiolar airspaces and the pulmonary interstitium. It is useful to consider separately the means by which the alveoli are kept dry, and the ways in which excessive fluid is removed from the alveoli.

Alveoli are kept "dry" by several related mechanisms. Tight junctions between type I pneumocytes are relatively impermeable to fluid and proteins and confer >90% of the barrier to albumin flux across the blood-air barrier. In contrast, in the lung, capillary endothelium is relatively permeable to movement of fluid and small molecules into the interstitium. Complementing the barrier function of the type I pneumocyte are Na^+-K^+–ATPase channels (sodium pumps) on the basolateral surface and passive sodium channels on the apical surface of type II pneumocytes. The net effect is to actively transport sodium out of the distal airspaces into the interstitium, drawing water along the same pathways by osmosis, thus resulting in a slow but steady flow of liquid from the alveoli to the interstitium. Drainage of interstitial fluid from the interstitium to the lymphatics is facilitated by negative pressure in the lymphatic vessels. In addition, the surface tension in airways may draw fluid out of alveoli into distal bronchioles, where fluid resorption by club cells is driven by a variety of ion channels. The rate at which fluid is cleared from the distal airspaces varies by species, being slowest in dogs, intermediate in sheep, and fastest in rodents and rabbits.

Active transport of alveolar fluid is enhanced by catecholamines (through β_2-adrenergic receptors) and glucocorticoids; this is probably important in clearance of fluid from the lungs of neonates, and is also used to advantage in the therapy of pulmonary edema. Conversely, active transport mechanisms are impaired by hypoxia, for example, as a result of high altitude, reactive oxygen and nitrogen species (as a result of inflammation), halogenated anesthetics, oleic acid, and perhaps lidocaine, suggesting that these factors, in addition to damage to type II pneumocytes or club cells, are additional contributors to development of pulmonary edema.

Causes of pulmonary edema *include elevated hydrostatic pressure, increased permeability of the alveolar wall, impaired lymphatic drainage, and several miscellaneous causes* (Box 5-2). *Elevated hydrostatic pressure* (increased pulmonary venous pressure) is commonly caused by left-sided heart failure (*cardiogenic edema*, see Pulmonary hypertension, later), or less often from hypervolemia caused by excessive fluid administration. In these situations, fluid loss into the alveoli may occur from either the alveolar septa or the peribronchiolar or perivascular connective tissue.

Increased permeability of the blood-alveolar barrier (noncardiogenic edema) is the second major mechanism of pulmonary edema, and is typified by a rapid onset of high-protein edema.

BOX • 5-2

Causes of, and contributors to, pulmonary edema

Increased venous hydrostatic pressure
- Left heart failure
- Increased blood volume
- Pulmonary venous occlusion

Increased permeability of the alveolar barrier
- Pneumonia
- Diffuse alveolar damage
- Endotoxemia/septicemia
- Anaphylaxis

Impairment of active transport of fluid from distal airspaces
- Damage to type II pneumocytes or club cells
- Hypoxia (high altitude)
- Oxygen and nitrogen radicals (increased by inflammation)
- Halogenated anesthetics
- Possibly lidocaine
- Malnutrition
- High alveolar protein content

Reduced oncotic pressure
- Hypoproteinemia (uncommon)

Lymphatic obstruction
- Neoplastic emboli in lymphatics or lymph nodes (rare)

Neurogenic pulmonary edema, secondary to brain trauma

Acute upper-airway obstruction
- Strangulation, hanging

Hypoglycemia

This form of edema develops in pneumonia of various causes, diffuse alveolar damage (see Interstitial and bronchointerstitial lung disease, later), sepsis or endotoxemia, anaphylaxis or drug-induced histamine release, and mechanical ventilation causing barotrauma or rapid re-expansion of collapsed alveoli. In the case of diffuse alveolar damage, edema may result from more minor injury than is needed to cause formation of hyaline membranes. Fumonisin toxicity in swine, African horsesickness virus and Hendra virus infection in horses, and bluetongue are specific causes of spectacular pulmonary edema.

Several *additional causes of pulmonary edema* are uncommonly encountered. Hypoproteinemia from glomerular, intestinal, or liver disease, or severe endoparasitism, may cause pulmonary edema, but edema in other tissues is usually more prominent. Obstruction of lymphatic vessels or lymph nodes by neoplastic cells is a rare cause of pulmonary edema. Increased intracranial pressure from trauma to the central nervous system causes *"neurogenic pulmonary edema,"* probably related to catecholamine-induced pulmonary hypertension and increased vascular permeability. Hypoxia resulting from high altitude induces pulmonary edema, an effect of both impaired alveolar active sodium transport and pulmonary hypertension. Postanesthetic pulmonary edema seems to involve multiple mechanisms. Acute upper-airway obstruction from asphyxiation can cause pulmonary edema, likely resulting from the drop in intra-alveolar pressure that leads to a net increase in transmural pressure across the alveolar wall, increasing fluid movement into the interstitium.

On **gross examination,** edematous lungs are wet, heavy, and do not completely collapse when the thorax is opened; fluid oozes from the cut surface. The ratio of lung weight to body weight (or to heart weight in ruminants) is a useful measure of pulmonary edema. Edema is prominent in the pleura and the pulmonary interstitium, and may form shallow pools in the hilus of the lung or the mediastinum. In cattle and swine, the interlobular septa are obviously distended by clear fluid (eFig. 5-22). Foam often fills the trachea and bronchi and flows from the nostrils, although this is a common and nonspecific finding in horses and sheep (see eFig. 5-14). The thoracic cavity may contain excess fluid. It is important to understand that the above features occur in severe cases, but pulmonary edema may be functionally significant yet grossly unremarkable.

Histologically, edema is first detected within the perivascular and peribronchial/bronchiolar interstitium, interlobular septa, and pleura, where it is cleared by the lymphatic system. At this stage, the fluid has little impact on lung function. If fluid accumulation exceeds clearance by the lymphatics, then it will accumulate within alveoli, where it can reduce surfactant function, decrease surface tension, and facilitate alveolar collapse; at this stage, decrements in lung function can be expected. Microscopically, edema fluid is often colorless and manifests simply as expansion and separation of constituents of the interstitial extracellular matrix, especially surrounding blood vessels and the bronchovascular bundle. With increased protein content, edema appears acidophilic, especially within alveoli, where it is homogeneous or finely granular except for occasional discrete holes that represent trapped air bubbles.

Chronic edema is accompanied by a diffuse increase in the number of alveolar macrophages, and in left-sided heart failure, these may contain phagocytosed erythrocytes or hemosiderin, the so-called "heart failure" cells (see Pulmonary hypertension, later). Histopathology is neither sensitive nor specific for detection of pulmonary edema. Low-protein edema must be abundant before it is detected histologically, the protein in edema fluid can leach from sections during processing and be quite inconspicuous, and conversely, pink material often fills the alveoli in autolysed carcasses or those euthanized with barbiturates. Therefore radiographs, measurement of lung weight, and the gross appearance are usually more accurate indicators of the presence and severity of edema.

Further reading

Kaartinen MJ, et al. Post-anesthetic pulmonary edema in two horses. Vet Anaesth Analg 2010;37:136-143.

Martin GS, Brigham KL. Fluid flux and clearance in acute lung injury. Compr Physiol 2012;2:2471-2480.

Matthay MA, et al. Lung epithelial fluid transport and the resolution of pulmonary edema. Physiol Rev 2002;82:569-600.

Thrombosis, embolism, and infarction

Pulmonary thromboembolism may result from in situ thrombus formation within pulmonary veins or arteries, or embolism to the pulmonary arteries of a thrombus, bacteria, parasites, hair, or foreign material. Clinically, pulmonary thromboembolism often goes undetected, particularly in horses. Reported clinical signs are not specific and include dyspnea, tachypnea, coughing, lethargy, hemoptysis, cyanosis, or sudden death. Because the clinical features may be vague, the branches of the pulmonary arteries must be opened at autopsy in all animals with clinical evidence of respiratory disease.

In situ development of pulmonary thrombi involves Virchow's triad of underlying mechanisms: increased blood coagulability, damage to endothelial cells or the vessel wall, or stasis of blood flow. The major causes are listed in Box 5-3. Hypercoagulability is of prime importance in most cases. Thrombi that develop in situ within the lung are usually microscopic (eFig. 5-23), whereas grossly visible thrombi are usually emboli from a distant site (Fig. 5-18); exceptions to this rule do occur. Microvascular thrombi dissolve rapidly after death if the fibrinolytic system has been activated, as is expected in disseminated intravascular coagulation; thus the absence of thrombi does not rule out this condition.

The lungs are strategically situated to catch **emboli** carried in venous blood; the most common sources are listed in Box 5-3.

The significance and sequelae of pulmonary thromboembolism depends on the extent of vascular obstruction, the rapidity of its development, and the presence of sepsis. Because the lung is supplied by both pulmonary and bronchial arteries and has extensive collateral vessels, thromboembolism does not often cause infarction. Ischemia and infarction are more likely if thrombosis or embolism occurs at the periphery of the lung (rather than affecting the large central vessels), or if the

---

BOX • 5-3

Causes of pulmonary thrombosis and embolism

Pulmonary thrombosis
- Glomerulonephritis, glomerular amyloidosis: loss of antithrombin
- Immune-mediated hemolytic anemia
- Hyperadrenocorticism or corticosteroid therapy
- *Dirofilaria immitis, Angiostrongylus vasorum*
- Disseminated intravascular coagulation: sepsis, neoplasia, pancreatitis, peritonitis, burns, massive trauma, bacterial pneumonia
- Heart disease
- Atherosclerosis, pulmonary vasculitis

Sources of emboli
- Valvular endocarditis
- Jugular thrombosis associated with catheterization
- Hepatic abscess with thrombosis of the caudal vena cava (cattle)
- Thrombosis of uterine and pelvic veins (cattle)
- Thrombi in deep veins of the legs, in recumbent (downer) cows

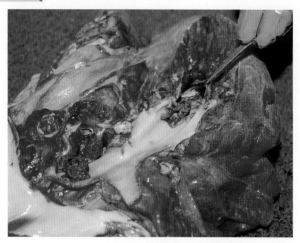

Figure 5-18 Pulmonary embolus in a caudal branch of a pulmonary artery (forceps) from a calf with endocarditis of the right atrioventricular valve. The affected lung tissue is grossly normal, and the embolus would have been overlooked had the pulmonary artery not been fully opened.

bronchial or systemic circulation is also impaired, such as by concurrent heart failure. When infarcts occur, they form sharply demarcated, wedge-shaped, or polygonal raised, firm, red-blue hemorrhagic lesions at the periphery of the lung lobes (eFig. 5-24); fibrin may give the pleural surface a dull granular appearance. Pulmonary hemorrhage and pleural effusion are frequent gross findings, even when infarcts are absent. Sublethal ischemia causes histologic lesions of diffuse alveolar damage, whereas infarcts manifest as foci of coagulative necrosis, sometimes delineated by macrophages, fibroplasia, and inflammation of vessel walls. Emboli that obstruct large branches of the pulmonary artery may cause sudden death, or over time lead to cor pulmonale and right heart failure; right ventricular dilation may or may not be present. Large thrombi are detected by dissection of the terminal branches of the pulmonary arteries; these lesions are easily missed if only cross-sections of lung are examined.

Septic embolism with massive numbers of bacteria, as occurs when an abscess ruptures into a vein, induces acute pulmonary edema or interstitial lung disease. Septic emboli that are less fulminant result in multifocal infarcts, abscesses, or suppurative embolic pneumonia. **Fat embolism** is rarely important in animals. The fat can originate from bone marrow at sites of fracture, from severe hepatic lipidosis when the hepatocytes rupture, or from subcutaneous fat necrosis caused by pancreatitis, diabetes mellitus, or vitamin E deficiency. The emboli lodge in alveolar capillaries and produce sausage-shaped distensions that are empty in routine paraffin sections, but special stains of frozen sections reveal the presence of fat. Small numbers of **megakaryocytes** are frequently found in pulmonary capillaries, particularly in dogs, and are usually of no diagnostic significance. **Emboli of brain or spinal cord** occur in cattle when improper use of captive bolt guns induce marked increases in intracranial pressure.

Further reading

Goggs R, et al. Pulmonary thromboembolism. J Vet Emerg Crit Care 2009;19:30-52.

Johnson LR, et al. Pulmonary thromboembolism in 29 dogs: 1985-1995. J Vet Intern Med 1999;13:338-345.

Yousem SA. The surgical pathology of pulmonary infarcts: diagnostic confusion with granulomatous disease, vasculitis, and neoplasia. Mod Pathol 2009;22:679-685.

Pulmonary hemorrhage

Pulmonary hemorrhage varies from petechiae to extensive filling of large regions by blood. It is usually possible to distinguish hemorrhage from congestion based on gross appearance. *Hemorrhages are usually multifocal or patchy splashes of blood, whereas congestion is diffuse within the affected region of the lung.* Pulmonary hemorrhages occur frequently in hemorrhagic diatheses, including thrombocytopenia and anticoagulant rodenticide toxicity, sepsis, disseminated intravascular coagulation, and with severe congestion. They can also be caused by vasculitis, pulmonary hypertension, infarction, ruptured aneurysms, trauma, migrating foreign bodies (eFig. 5-25), hemangiosarcoma, tumors that have undergone necrosis, bronchopneumonia, leptospirosis, or drug reactions. Aspiration of blood is frequent at slaughter, and has a characteristic pattern of multiple, small, bright red foci with feathery borders (eFig. 5-26). In lung biopsies, distention of alveoli with blood suggests pre-existing hemorrhage, whereas the hemorrhage of surgical trauma is more likely accompanied by alveolar collapse.

Abscesses *that erode large blood vessels cause massive hemorrhage.* Affected animals may develop hemoptysis or be found dead with blood flowing from the nares, and expectorated blood is often detected in the stomach. Liver abscesses in cattle may extend into hepatic veins, spreading to the lungs via the caudal vena cava to cause pulmonary thromboembolism, acute interstitial lung disease, or chronic lung abscesses. Such abscesses occasionally erode pulmonary vessels, leading to epistaxis and sudden death from exsanguination.

Equine exercise-induced pulmonary hemorrhage (EIPH). Equine exercise-induced pulmonary hemorrhage is a common occurrence in strenuously exercising horses. Approximately 75% of racehorses have endoscopically detectable blood in their airways following a single post-race examination, and this increases to 95% following a second examination. The severity of hemorrhage in EIPH-affected horses varies from mild to severe, and may lead to epistaxis. *Severe bleeding negatively impacts race performance and length of racing career, but beyond that, there are few reported clinical signs in horses that experience EIPH.*

Because EIPH does not typically lead to the death of the animal, and affected horses can be retired and used for other purposes, for many years, there had been few studies of the pathology. Recent studies have expanded our understanding of the pathology and pathogenesis of EIPH. *Most EIPH lesions occur in the caudodorsal lung* (Fig. 5-19; eFig. 5-27). *The most widely reported gross lesion associated with EIPH is dark brown to blue-black discoloration of the caudodorsal pleura.* Pleural and interlobular septal fibrosis may be present, as well as patchy interstitial fibrosis and brown foci in the parenchyma, reflecting hemosiderophage accumulation. In severe cases, discrete mass-like and curvilinear foci are noted in the caudodorsal lung (see Fig. 5-19B) and histologically consist of edema and fibrosis. These lesions may be found months after racing, indicating that the changes persist for considerable periods of time.

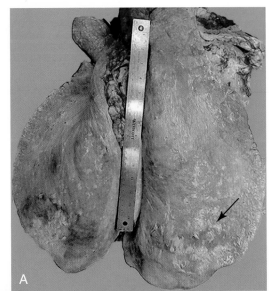

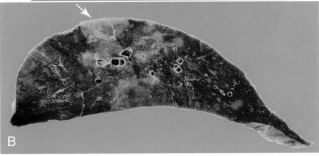

Figure 5-19 Equine exercise-induced pulmonary hemorrhage in a horse. **A.** Bilateral, primarily caudodorsal, regions of pleural discoloration (arrow). **B.** Discrete focus of edema and fibrosis (arrow).

Histologically, EIPH is characterized by the following constellation of lesions: pleural and interlobular septal fibrosis, pulmonary vein fibrosis, hemosiderophage accumulation, and interstitial fibrosis. The venous fibrosis especially affects the adventitia of small (100-200 μm) veins; in some veins, fibrosis also involves the intima and can narrow the vein lumen. In severe EIPH, discrete foci of interstitial edema and fibrosis may accompany the aforementioned lesions.

The pathogenesis of EIPH has been debated for years, leading to diverse hypotheses, from bleeding occurring as a result of preexisting airway inflammation to shock waves being transmitted into the lung from the forefeet striking the ground. The bleeding in EIPH has been postulated to arise from rupture of the alveolar capillary bed as a result of the high vascular pressures achieved within the lung during strenuous exercise. However, the distribution and features of the gross and histologic pathology of EIPH are not explained by simple pressure-induced capillary rupture. The most recent data suggests that *the cause of EIPH is regional venous remodeling. This remodeling likely occurs as a result of the high vascular pressures and flow experienced by veins in the caudodorsal lung.* It is known that blood flow is preferentially distributed to the caudodorsal lung of horses at rest and increases further to this lung region during exercise, which could explain the regional distribution of the venous lesions in the EIPH lung. Further, data have shown that the other lesions in the EIPH lung,

namely, hemosiderin accumulation and interstitial fibrosis, do not occur without venous remodeling being present, *suggesting that venous remodeling is central to the pathogenesis of EIPH.* The proposed pathogenesis of EIPH can be summarized as follows. Strenuous exercise in horses leads to extremely high vascular pressures and flow preferentially in the caudodorsal lung, leading to the characteristic remodeling of small veins of this region of lung; the venous remodeling reduces wall compliance, resulting in supraphysiologic upstream capillary pressures, during exercise, that cause capillary rupture and bleeding.

Equine exercise-associated fatal pulmonary hemorrhage. Massive diffuse pulmonary hemorrhage and edema are among the most common causes of sudden death in racing horses. Because these animals die during or shortly after strenuous exercise, often in the warmer months, there is often considerable autolysis by the time they are examined by the pathologist. Blood may be noted at the nares and often pours forth from the nose when the carcass is shifted. The *gross pathology* of exercise-associated fatal pulmonary hemorrhage (EAFPH) consists of widespread hemorrhage and edema in both lungs (eFig. 5-28). Raised hemorrhagic foci, suggestive of acute infarcts, are occasionally found along the margins of the lung lobes. The degree of hemorrhage is usually more prominent within the caudodorsal regions but also extends into more cranial regions.

Histologically, hemorrhage is present throughout the alveoli, interlobular septa, and subpleural tissue, and also surrounds airways and vasculature. In addition to the hemorrhage, vasculature is markedly congested throughout the lung. Because of hemorrhage and autolysis, it is difficult to evaluate the integrity of the blood vessels and alveolar septa. Horses affected by EAFPH may or may not have obvious histologic lesions of antecedent EIPH.

The pathogenesis of EAFPH is not well understood. Acute cardiac failure has been suggested, but this seems unlikely, as clinically apparent or fatal pulmonary edema would be expected before vascular pressures increased sufficiently to cause such widespread vascular rupture and hemorrhage. Because hemorrhage is the dominant feature of EAFPH, some refer to it as "fatal EIPH." Based on the limited descriptions and personal experiences, it is not clear that EIPH is consistently present in horses that die suddenly from EAFPH. Further, the lung involvement in horses dying from EAFPH is much greater than for EIPH, which is mostly a disease of the caudodorsal lung. It is speculated that if, during exercise, horses developed sudden widespread spasm of small postcapillary venules within the lungs, this could lead to a rapid rise in capillary pressures that might be sufficient to cause widespread acute rupture and hemorrhage, as is seen in EAFPH. In rodents, there are smooth muscle sphincters in postcapillary veins that are capable of constricting and regulating local vascular perfusion and pressures through adrenergic receptors. If such structures are present in the equine lung, this might provide a mechanism for the sudden global edema and hemorrhage that occurs in EAFPH. This hypothesis remains to be tested.

Further reading

Derksen FJ, et al. Regional distribution of collagen and haemosiderin in the lungs of horses with exercise-induced pulmonary haemorrhage. Equine Vet J 2009;41:586-591.

BOX • 5-4

Causes of pulmonary hypertension

- Idiopathic (primary) pulmonary arterial hypertension
- Familial pulmonary arterial hypertension (humans)
- Systemic-to-pulmonary vascular shunts: ventricular septal defect, patent ductus arteriosus
- Chronic pulmonary thromboembolic disease
- Disorders of pulmonary blood vessels: *Dirofilaria immitis,* pulmonary veno-occlusive disease, pulmonary vasculitis
- Hypoxic vasoconstriction of pulmonary arterioles: high altitude (brisket disease), bronchiolitis obliterans, chronic bronchitis or bronchiolitis (equine heaves)
- Chronic interstitial lung disease with fibrosis and occlusion of pulmonary vessels
- Left-sided heart failure causing pulmonary venous hypertension: mitral insufficiency or stenosis, subaortic stenosis, cardiomyopathy

Lyle CH, et al. Sudden death in racing Thoroughbred horses: an international muticentre study of post mortem findings. Equine Vet J 2001;43:324-331.

Williams KJ, et al. Regional pulmonary veno-occlusion: a newly identified lesion of equine exercise-induced pulmonary hemorrhage. Vet Pathol 2008;45:313-326.

Williams KJ, et al. Distribution of venous remodeling in exercise-induced pulmonary hemorrhage of horses follows reported blood flow distribution in the equine lung. J Appl Physiol 2013;114: 869-878.

Pulmonary hypertension

The clinical diagnosis of pulmonary arterial hypertension (PAH) is based on documenting pulmonary arterial pressure >30 mm Hg. In veterinary medicine, this is usually measured using echocardiography rather than direct catheterization of the right heart. Pulmonary hypertension is often classified by the underlying cause (Box 5-4). The *pathogenesis* of PAH historically had been considered to involve excessive vasoconstriction and thrombosis leading to vascular remodeling. PAH is now understood to be a vasculopathy, characterized by dysregulation of vascular tone, abnormal vascular cell growth, and apoptosis, along with inflammation. The vascular remodeling characteristic of PAH is a cause rather than a result of the disease. The dysregulation of vessel tone in PAH is caused by an imbalance in vasodilatory (e.g., prostacyclin, nitric oxide, cyclic guanosine monophosphate) and vasocontricting (e.g., endothelin, thromboxane A_2, serotonin) molecules, whereas a number of growth factors and cytokines, such as TGF-β, bone morphogenetic protein 2, platelet-derived growth factor, and fibroblast growth factors are implicated in the vascular lesions of PAH.

Gross lesions in cases of primary idiopathic PAH are often not present within the lungs. In secondary PAH, the gross lesions reflect the precipitating disease, such as interstitial lung disease, canine heartworm disease, or pulmonary thromboembolism. Severe PAH leads to right ventricular and sometimes atrial dilation, and hypertrophy develops with time. Lesions of right heart failure may be present. Irrespective of the cause, *PAH has a spectrum of characteristic histologic lesions that*

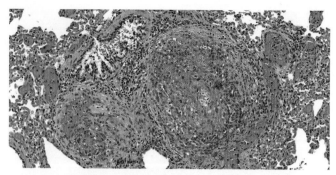

Figure 5-20 Intimal proliferation in 2 pulmonary arteries, as a consequence of pulmonary hypertension in a dog with patent ductus arteriosus.

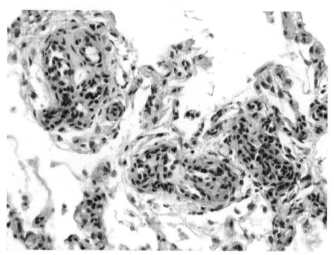

Figure 5-21 Plexiform arteriopathy in a dog with pulmonary hypertension.

mainly reflect chronic remodeling of pulmonary arterioles. These include thickening of the tunica intima by endothelial cell proliferation and later by fibrosis, hypertrophy of smooth muscle in the tunica media, and more variable fibrosis or edema of the adventitia (Fig. 5-20). Small arterioles at the level of the terminal airway that normally have a thin tunica muscularis may become muscularized. A *range of morphologic variants* in cases of PAH in humans are recognized: intimal proliferation that may be concentric (in familial PAH), eccentric (as a result of thromboembolism and other causes), or obliterative; thrombosis and recanalization of the lumen; and plexiform lesions. The latter are web-like plexuses of vascular lumens, each surrounded by concentric rings of endothelial cells and matrix, which appear as a branching or outpouching of a larger artery, and are thought to represent chronic attempts to repair damage to the parent vessel wall (Fig. 5-21). *Severe acute PAH results in endothelial degeneration, vasoconstriction, fibrinoid necrosis of the vessel wall, vasculitis, and "onion skin" fibrosis and proliferation of smooth muscle cells* (eFig. 5-29).

Pulmonary venous hypertension is commonly caused by left-sided heart failure, and may lead to pulmonary arterial hypertension. Left heart failure causes pulmonary edema as a result of elevated pressure in the lung vascular bed, and varies with the rapidity of onset of venous and capillary hypertension. In animals with long-standing left-sided failure (e.g., mitral valve insufficiency in small-breed dogs), the edema may

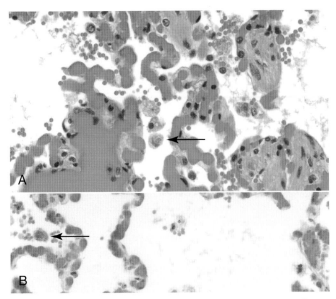

Figure 5-22 Heart failure cells. A, B. Alveolar macrophages contain brown pigment (**A,** top, arrow) that stains blue with Perls' Prussian blue (**B,** bottom, arrow) and is in the typically scant amount seen in animals with heart failure, in a cat with hypertrophic cardiomyopathy.

be relatively modest compared to that occurring in an animal experiencing acute heart failure. This difference reflects the ability of the lymphatic system to clear the fluid. Thoracic effusion is also common in acute heart failure, again reflecting the inability of pleural lymphatics to clear the sudden increase in pressure-driven pleural fluid formation.

Histologically, chronic left-sided heart failure results in pulmonary edema, increased numbers of lung macrophages, and remodeling of pulmonary veins. The edema initially forms around airways and blood vessels (see Pulmonary edema, previously), reflecting the location of the lymphatics that expand to clear the edema fluid. As fluid production increases and exceeds lymphatic clearance, fluid is more apparent within the alveolar interstitium and the alveoli. Alveolar macrophages are increased in number and usually have abundant cytoplasm with ruffled cell borders, a feature that is characteristic of chronic alveolar edema. *Hemosiderin-laden alveolar macrophages,* the so-called "heart failure cells," are inconsistently present in chronic left heart failure and absent in acute heart failure (eFig. 5-30; Fig. 5-22). Histochemical stains for iron are helpful for subtle lesions. This lesion affects alveolar macrophages more or less uniformly throughout the section; single or focally intense accumulations of hemosiderin-laden alveolar macrophages, or pigment-laden macrophages in the bronchiolar interstitium, are not indicative of heart failure. Conversely, the presence of hemosiderin-laden alveolar macrophages is not pathognomonic of heart failure, as pulmonary hemorrhage causes the same lesion. Careful evaluation of pulmonary veins, especially small- to medium-sized vessels, often reveals increased amounts of collagen within the adventitia. In acute heart failure, there is greater and more widespread edema, without "heart failure cells" or the aforementioned increases in adventitial collagen around pulmonary veins.

Pulmonary veno-occlusive disease (PVOD) is a rare and serious cause of pulmonary hypertension in humans that

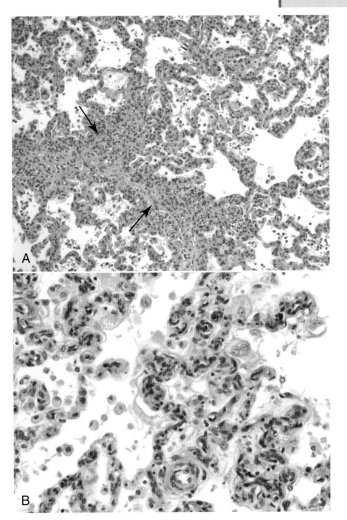

Figure 5-23 Canine pulmonary veno-occlusive disease. A. Two branches of remodeled pulmonary veins (arrows) are evident along with segmental alveolar capillary engorgement and hemosiderophages. **B.** The histologic lesion is patchy, with areas in which alveolar septal capillaries have proliferation of endothelial cell nuclei. Alveolar macrophages are hypertrophied, and alveoli contain hemorrhage. (Case courtesy S. Priestnall, Royal Veterinary College.)

results from progressive remodeling of pulmonary veins. We have reviewed the lungs from a series of adult dogs with similar lesions. Clinically, affected dogs experience rapidly progressive respiratory signs that include coughing, tachypnea, dyspnea, and hypoxia; epistaxis and hemoptysis may be reported. The *gross pathology* of canine PVOD is striking. The lungs are diffusely firm and have widespread, relatively well-demarcated, foci of hemorrhage or congestion (eFig. 5-31). *Histologically,* the lesions are patchy rather than diffuse, with extensive remodeling of small- to medium-sized pulmonary veins located in the alveolar interstitium (Fig. 5-23). The lumen of the most severely affected veins is obscured by plump spindle cells and collagen. Within the alveolar parenchyma, alveolar capillaries have segmental lesions of marked congestion and often extensive hypercellularity caused by endothelial proliferation. This lesion is similar to "capillary hemangiomatosis" reported in humans with PVOD. The cause of the remarkable venous remodeling in dogs is not known.

Further reading

Malherbe CR, et al. Right ventricular hypertrophy with heart failure in Holstein heifers at elevation of 1,600 meters. J Vet Diagn Invest 2012;24:867-877.

Mandel J, et al. Pulmonary veno-occlusive disease. Am J Respir Crit Care Med 2000;162:1964-1973.

Simonneau G, et al. Updated clinical classification of pulmonary hypertension. J Am Coll Cardiol 2013;62(Suppl. 25):D34-D41.

Stacher E, et al. Modern age pathology of pulmonary arterial hypertension. Am J Respir Crit Care Med 2012;186:261-272.

Zabka TS, et al. Pulmonary arteriopathy and idiopathic pulmonary arterial hypertension in six dogs. Vet Pathol 2006;43:510-522.

Pulmonary vasculitis

Pulmonary vasculitis is uncommon in domestic animals. *Septic pulmonary vasculitis* may be hematogenous or arise within lesions of bronchopneumonia, and results in numerous necrotic neutrophils in vessel walls, often with thrombi occluding the lumen, and necrosis of vessel walls (eFig. 5-32). Specific infectious causes include feline infectious peritonitis virus; *Dirofilaria immitis* in dogs; acute bovine viral diarrhea virus infection, malignant catarrhal fever, *Histophilus somni*, and *Aspergillus* in cattle; equine arteritis virus, equid herpesvirus 1, African horse sickness virus, and Hendra virus in horses; and porcine circovirus 2 and Nipah virus in swine. Oral selenium supplementation of lambs causes subtle vasculitis affecting pulmonary alveolar septa, leading to edema and hemorrhage in addition to myocardial necrosis. Immune complex vasculitis, other mechanisms of immune-mediated vascular injury, and drug-induced pulmonary vasculitis are well recognized in humans and probably occur in dogs.

Further reading

Brown PJ, et al. Pulmonary haemorrhage and fibrillary glomerulonephritis (pulmonary-renal syndrome) in a dog. Vet Rec 2008;162:486-488.

Tiwary AK, et al. Comparative toxicosis of sodium selenite and selenomethionine in lambs. J Vet Diagn Invest 2006;18:61-70.

Pulmonary mineralization

Mineralization of the pulmonary interstitium is a feature of *uremic pneumonopathy* in dogs with acute or chronic renal failure, and similar lesions may result from hypercalcemia, hyperphosphatemia, vitamin D toxicosis, alkalosis, or hyperadrenocorticism. Dogs with uremic pneumonopathy may have tachypnea and dyspnea. The magnitude of respiratory signs and lesions is not related to the severity of renal dysfunction nor to the clinical outcome. There are often no gross lesions, or the lung may be gritty and porous. Mineralization occurs within the smooth muscle and connective tissue fibers in alveolar septa, pulmonary veins, and the walls of bronchioles (Fig. 5-24). Alveoli are edematous and contain increased numbers of macrophages, and giant cells occasionally engulf the mineralized material. Hemorrhage, thin strands of fibrin, and edema may be prominent in acute exacerbations (see Fig. 5-24). Alveolar septa and pulmonary veins, such as the gastric mucosa, may be predisposed to mineralization because of the *alkaline microenvironment* resulting from carbon dioxide excretion. Mineral deposits in the lung undergo ossification with time.

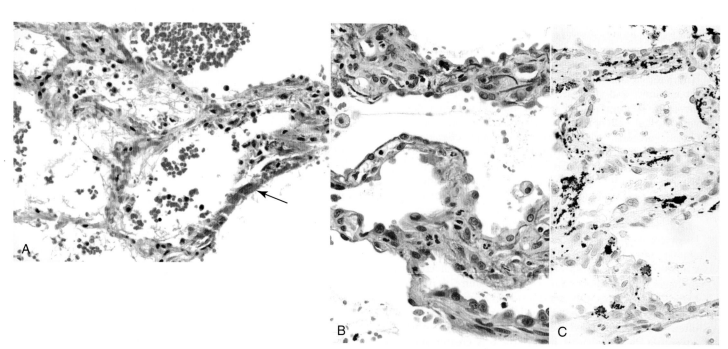

Figure 5-24 Uremic pneumonopathy caused by chronic renal failure. **A.** Acute exacerbation in a dog. In addition to mineralization of alveolar septa (arrow), alveoli contain lacy fibrin and hemorrhage. **B.** Subacute lesions in a cat. Alveolar septa have basophilic mineralization of fibers, are thickened by fibrous tissue, and covered by type II pneumocytes. **C.** Black staining (von Kossa) of mineral within the alveolar septa.

Further reading

Le Boedec K, et al. Pulmonary abnormalities in dogs with renal azotemia. J Vet Intern Med 2012;26:1099-1106.

Pulmonary neoplasia

Primary pulmonary neoplasms are encountered most often in dogs and cats, and are rare in other domestic animals. A variety of mechanisms explains the clinical effects of lung tumors. Respiratory failure is rare but may ensue if tumors occupy a large proportion of lung parenchyma. More commonly, effects on specific anatomic structures explain the clinical signs: coughing caused by compression of a bronchus, pleural effusion and dyspnea caused by invasion of pleural lymphatics and regional lymph nodes, hemoptysis from erosion of blood vessels, or rarely regurgitation caused by esophageal obstruction. Other sequelae include cytokine production, leading to malaise, anorexia, and cachexia; the distant effects of metastasis; and paraneoplastic syndromes, including hypertrophic osteopathy, hypercalcemia, fever, or adrenocorticotropic hormone secretion.

Epithelial tumors are the most frequently encountered type. For primary epithelial lung tumors, hilar or central neoplasms are more likely of bronchial origin, whereas peripheral tumors, which are far more common, are more likely to have arisen from distal bronchiolar or alveolar epithelium. Because the lung is a frequent site for metastatic neoplasms, it is essential to differentiate metastases of a distant tumor from primary lung neoplasms. *Features supporting the diagnosis of a primary lung neoplasm* include the absence of a primary tumor in a distant organ, the presence of a single large lung mass with or without smaller metastases (eFig. 5-33), detection of thyroid transcription factor-1 (TTF-1), or mucus production or ciliated cells (neither of which are commonly present even in primary tumors). Because pulmonary carcinomas often form intrapulmonary metastases, the presence of tumor emboli within vessels is not helpful in distinguishing primary from metastatic tumors. Expression of TTF-1 is detected in most (64-95%, depending on the study) primary pulmonary adenocarcinomas and adenosquamous carcinomas, but is usually absent in pulmonary squamous cell carcinoma, mucinous pulmonary adenocarcinoma, mesothelioma, or nonpulmonary nonthyroid metastatic tumors. Thus peripheral neoplasms of bronchioloalveolar origin are generally TTF-1 positive, whereas central neoplasms arising from large airways are negative. Pulmonary adenocarcinomas are consistently labeled for pancytokeratins (AE1/AE3), and vimentin is co-expressed in the less-differentiated tumors.

The classification of pulmonary carcinomas in humans has undergone 2 major revisions since the last consensus on classification of these tumors in domestic animals (Box 5-5), and the revised system has a much-improved relationship to clinical behavior. Lung tumors of animals follow similar patterns, so this scheme seems highly relevant, but the existing literature on tumors of animals cannot be directly translated into this current system. Caution is necessary because this scheme has not yet been formally studied in animals, and the prognostic relevance for dogs and cats is unknown. Important changes include abandoning the term bronchioloalveolar carcinoma, highlighting the concept of lepidic growth, and a different definition of invasive growth than what has been used in veterinary pathology (Table 5-1).

BOX • 5-5

Classification of epithelial lung tumors in domestic mammals

Benign epithelial lung tumors
- Papilloma
- Adenoma

Malignant epithelial lung tumors
- Adenocarcinoma: see Table 5-1
- Squamous cell carcinoma
- Adenosquamous carcinoma
- Bronchial gland carcinoma
- Large cell carcinoma
- Small cell carcinoma
- Neuroendocrine tumor
- Pulmonary blastoma
- Combined carcinoma
- Carcinosarcoma

From Dungworth DL, et al. Histological Classification of Tumors of the Respiratory System of Domestic Animals. 2nd series. Vol. VI. Washington, DC: Armed Forces Institute of Pathology, 1999.

Papillary adenomas are solitary circumscribed tumors of the bronchi or lung parenchyma, characterized by papillary growth of well-differentiated epithelial cells; these occur in dogs but are rare. **Peribronchiolar metaplasia** (Lambertosis) is a non-neoplastic condition thought to result from bronchiolar injury, which involves hyperplasia but not dysplasia of the terminal bronchiolar epithelium, and extension of club cells, goblet cells, or squamous cells into adjacent alveoli (eFig. 5-34). The bronchiolar origin of the alveolar cells can be confirmed by detection of specific cytokeratins. **Atypical adenomatous hyperplasia** and **adenocarcinoma in situ** (see Table 5-1) do not cause clinical disease in humans; its occurrence in dogs has not been defined. **Minimally invasive, lepidic-predominant, and papillary predominant adenocarcinomas** (see Table 5-1; Fig. 5-25; eFigs. 5-35, 5-36) are the most frequent lung tumors in dogs, forming pale moderately firm masses, usually arising in subpleural or peripheral areas of lung. Some neoplasms have accumulations of eosinophilic secretion within the lumen of the tumor, or mucus secretion is occasionally prominent. Minimally invasive and lepidic tumors in dogs are associated with prolonged survival, whereas papillary predominant tumors behave similarly but occasionally invade adjacent tissues or metastasize. In contrast, **acinar-predominant or solid-predominant adenocarcinoma**, although less frequent in dogs, carry a higher risk of invasive growth and metastasis. **Micropapillary adenocarcinoma** seems to occur as an aggressive neoplasm in dogs and cats but has not been formally described.

Grading of adenocarcinoma in dogs (McNiel et al., 1997) has been based on overall differentiation, degree of nuclear pleomorphism, mitotic rate, nucleolar size, tumor necrosis, fibrosis, and demarcation of the mass. Grades were assigned from the sums of the above scores. Of these criteria, degree of differentiation, mitotic rate (with cutpoints of >1 and >3 mitoses per high-power field), necrosis of >50% of the tumor, and nucleolar size were most predictive of outcome. Unpublished data indicate more aggressive neoplasms include histologic pattern (solid or acinar pattern), disordered or

Table • 5-1

Classification of human pulmonary adenocarcinoma

General points
1. The term "bronchoalveolar carcinoma" has been abandoned.
2. The *lepidic pattern of growth* is an important feature of several neoplasms described later, and is characterized by pre-existing alveoli whose septa are covered by a single layer of neoplastic epithelial cells that do not invade the connective tissue (see eFigs. 5-30, 5-35). Simple finger-like ingrowths may occur, but secondary or tertiary branching indicates a papillary rather than lepidic pattern. Identifying elastic fibers in the walls of alveoli (lepidic pattern) may be useful, as these are absent in papillae. The name lepidic refers to the resemblance to a row of butterflies perched on a branch. In addition to lepidic, other patterns of growth are papillary (see Fig. 5-25B; see also eFig. 5-36), acinar, micropapillary, and solid.
3. *Invasion* does *not* refer to extension of neoplastic cells into lung tissue adjacent to the neoplasm, but instead indicates invasion of neoplastic cells into the tumor stroma (see Fig. 5-35C, eFig. 5-37), blood or lymphatic vessels, or pleura. Invasion of stroma is recognized by areas of fibroblastic or myofibroblastic stroma (desmoplastic reaction) containing neoplastic cells. In addition, any papillary, acinar, micropapillary, or solid growth pattern is considered invasive growth.
4. Invasive adenocarcinomas often have more than one morphologic pattern in a single mass, and the classification is based on the predominant pattern across the entire tumor. It is recommended to state the percentage of the mass comprising each of the various patterns, in 5% increments.

Atypical adenomatous hyperplasia	Small (≤0.5 cm) solitary lesions in which alveoli are lined by scattered cuboidal bronchioloalveolar epithelial cells with gaps between the peg-like cells (lepidic noninvasive). In contrast to carcinoma in situ, crowding or stratification of cells is not present, and there is gradual transition with normal adjacent alveoli. In contrast to alveolar injury, stromal thickening is present only in areas of epithelial proliferation.
Adenocarcinoma in situ	Small lesion (≤3 cm) with neoplastic cells continuously lining the surface of pre-existing alveoli; anisokaryosis or nuclear atypia are absent. There is no necrosis, papillary or acinar growth, neoplastic cells growing in alveolar lumens, or invasion into the tumor stroma, blood or lymphatic vessels or pleura (any of these features indicate invasive adenocarcinoma). These tumors do not cause clinical disease in humans.
Minimally invasive adenocarcinoma	Small (≤3 cm) solitary lesion, similar to adenocarcinoma in situ, but with small foci (≤0.5-cm diameter in humans) of invasion into the tumor stroma or pleura.
Lepidic-predominant adenocarcinoma	Similar to adenocarcinoma in situ, with lepidic growth along pre-existing alveoli (see Fig. 5-25A, eFig. 5-35), but has evidence of invasive growth forming an area >0.5-cm diameter.
Papillary predominant adenocarcinoma	Growth of neoplastic cells on stalks containing fibrovascular connective tissue, that project into spaces within the tumor. Note that the aforementioned patterns involve growth of neoplastic cells along pre-existing alveoli, whereas the alveolar architecture is lost in papillary adenocarcinoma, and the cells grow upon stroma of newly formed papillae (see Fig. 5-25B, eFig. 5-36).
Acinar-predominant adenocarcinoma	Neoplastic cells arranged around clearly visible glandular spaces.
Solid adenocarcinoma	Sheets of neoplastic cells lacking papillary or acinar growth.
Micropapillary predominant adenocarcinoma	Neoplastic cells form tiny finger-like protrusions into spaces within the mass but, unlike true papillae, these protrusions lack fibrovascular cores. The micropapillae often have clear cystic centers surrounded by rings of neoplastic cells. This pattern has a highly aggressive growth habit in humans.
Other patterns	Mucinous variants of each subtype (cells contain abundant mucin in the cytoplasm, correlating with molecular changes and neoplastic behavior in humans), as well as colloid adenocarcinoma (abundant mucin distends the air spaces within the tumor).

Data from Travis WD, et al. International association for the study of lung cancer/American Thoracic Society/European Respiratory Society international multidisciplinary classification of lung adenocarcinoma. J Thorac Oncol 2011;6:244-285.

multilayered arrangement of neoplastic cells lining papillae, invasion of neoplastic cells into intratumoral stroma, poor demarcation of tumors, and filling of alveolar lumens adjacent to the tumor by clusters of neoplastic cells. Tumor grading is not widely used for human pulmonary adenocarcinomas, but mitotic rate and abnormal mitotic figures in addition to tumor subtype provides prognostic information.

Staging of adenocarcinoma, in addition to tumor type, is predictive of outcome in dogs. The presence of more than one tumor (stage T2 in animals), significant invasion of adjacent

tissues (T3), or the presence of lymph node (N1) or distant (M1) metastases correlate with progressively shorter survival times. In humans, key elements of staging include the size of the mass, invasion along a bronchus (rare in animals), careful examination of pleural puckers to detect invasion through the elastic layer of the pleura or through the pleural surface, invasion across an interlobar fissure into a different lobe, formation of physically separate additional tumor nodules (only those recognized grossly, not incidental microscopic nodules) of the same histologic subtype in the same or different lobes, and

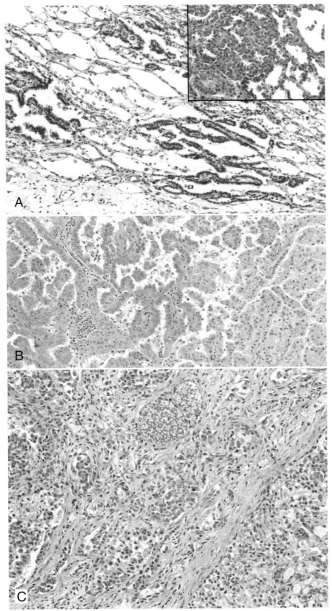

Figure 5-25 Pulmonary adenocarcinoma. A. Lepidic growth of neoplastic cells in pulmonary adenocarcinoma. Pre-existing alveoli adjacent to the main mass are lined by a continuous layer of cuboidal neoplastic epithelial cells that do not invade the stroma. Inset: ovine pulmonary adenocarcinoma (jaagsiekte) showing detail of the lepidic growth pattern along pre-existing alveolar septa. **B. Papillary-predominant** pulmonary adenocarcinoma in a cat. A stalk of fibrovascular tissue lined by neoplastic epithelial cells protrudes into a space within the tumor. Lack of the stromal core at the tips of the papillae could be confused with a micropapillary pattern. **C.** Invasive growth of pulmonary adenocarcinoma into fibroblastic stroma within the tumor, in a dog. Invasion is defined by growth of neoplastic cells into tumor stroma, blood vessels, or pleura. The invasive focus shown is bordered above and below by a papillary pattern of tumor growth (not visible).

micrometastases of neoplastic cells in lymph nodes (cell clusters, but not isolated neoplastic cells).

Pulmonary adenocarcinoma is a relatively common neoplasm of older **cats.** The tumors may be single, multiple, or lobar (eFigs. 5-37, 5-38), and follow the above-mentioned lepidic, papillary, acinar, and adenosquamous patterns (see Box 5-5 and Table 5-1). Tumors ≥1 cm diameter are more likely to metastasize, but the histologic pattern has not been shown to correlate with clinical outcome; in fact, frequent metastasis is reported for large lepidic tumors. Affected cats develop progressive dyspnea and coughing from the expansile tumor, or there may be intrapulmonary metastasis, or pleural invasion with effusion arising from the intrapleural metastases (eFig. 5-39). However, affected cats often exhibit no evidence of respiratory disease, and the clinical signs result from metastasis to other viscera, brain, muscle, eye, bone, or skin. *A peculiar feature of this tumor is the propensity to cause lameness by metastasizing to the digits*, especially to the dermis on the dorsum of a distal phalanx and beneath the footpad epidermis (eFig. 5-40). Occasionally, the epithelial hyperplasia associated with *feline idiopathic pulmonary fibrosis* (IPF) is mistaken for an adenocarcinoma. Unlike true epithelial neoplasms, which have features consistent with their clonal origin, feline IPF is a heterogeneous lesion with evidence of smooth muscle proliferation, fibrosis, and honeycomb lung formation. Conversely, cats with feline IPF can have coincident primary lung carcinomas, so it is important for the pathologist to inspect the pulmonary parenchyma far from the lung neoplasm to identify changes typical of feline IPF.

Carcinoma in situ and lepidic-predominant adenocarcinoma are characteristic of ovine pulmonary adenocarcinoma (jaagsiekte), the retroviral lung tumor discussed in the section Infectious respiratory diseases of sheep and goats (see Figs. 5-25A, 5-62; see also eFig. 5-35).

Non-adenocarcinomatous epithelial neoplasms are less frequent in animals. **Bronchial gland carcinoma** is a rare low-grade malignancy that shows clear evidence of arising from the wall of a bronchus. The neoplastic cells form acini composed of well-differentiated epithelial cells with prominent mucus production. **Squamous cell carcinoma** is common in the lung and is histologically similar to that in other tissues, with a usual mix of small basaloid cells and larger differentiated cells that are polygonal, with abundant glassy eosinophilic cytoplasm. **Adenosquamous carcinoma** forms both acinar/tubular and squamous patterns of differentiation (each forming ≥10% of the tumor), with prominent atypia of neoplastic cells, higher grade, and a particularly aggressive growth habit (Fig. 5-26). Squamous and adenosquamous patterns reflect the pattern of differentiation, and do not imply an origin from squamous epithelium. **Large cell carcinoma** is a rare and anaplastic variant of pulmonary carcinoma, in which the individual neoplastic cells are large, polyhedral, sometimes separated from one another, and have abundant often-vacuolated cytoplasm, pleomorphic nuclei with anisokaryosis and multinucleation, but lack keratinization, intercellular bridges, acini, or mucin. Histiocytic sarcoma and large cell neuroendocrine tumor are important differential diagnoses in cases of large cell carcinoma. **Carcinosarcoma** is a primary pulmonary tumor with both adenocarcinomatous and sarcomatous components, rarely seen in animals, which is thought to represent epithelial-mesenchymal transition of carcinomatous cells.

Neuroendocrine tumors in humans are classified as low-grade carcinoid, intermediate-grade atypical carcinoid, high-grade small cell carcinoma, and high-grade large cell neuroendocrine carcinoma. All are rare in domestic animals and mainly affect the young. *Pulmonary neuroendocrine tumor is the preferred term because the validity of subclassifying these*

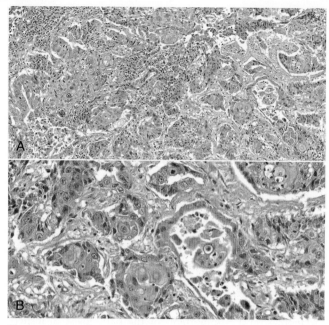

Figure 5-26 **Adenosquamous pulmonary carcinoma** in a cat. Acinar differentiation with formation of lumens is clearly evident (**A, B**), along with obvious squamous differentiation of cells containing abundant glassy eosinophilic cytoplasm (**B**), with each component forming at least 10% of the mass.

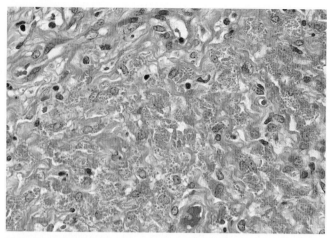

Figure 5-27 **Pulmonary granular cell tumor** in a horse. The neoplastic cells have indistinct borders and innumerable eosinophilic granules in the cytoplasm, and abundant collagenous matrix is present.

tumors in animals is unknown. **Carcinoids** in humans are thought to arise from bronchial neuroendocrine tissue and exhibit the characteristic features of neuroendocrine tumors: arrangement in nests, palisades, or pseudorosettes; expression of chromogranin and serotonin (synaptophysin is weak; neuron-specific enolase [NSE]) is considered nonspecific); and the presence of dense-core granules visible by electron microscopy. The few cases of pulmonary neoplasms in dogs that resemble carcinoids have developed adjacent to a bronchus and have a neuroendocrine pattern of nests or ribbons of cells separated by delicate vascularized stroma. The cells are uniform, round to polygonal, with abundant pale eosinophilic cytoplasm and relatively small nuclei. Features in humans indicative of an intermediate grade (i.e., atypical rather than typical carcinoid) are mitotic rate >2 per 10 high-power fields and punctate coagulative necrosis of the tumor. *Large cell neuroendocrine carcinoma* has >1 mitosis per high-power field with comedo-like necrosis. In the few cases of neuroendocrine tumors reported in dogs, increasing tumor grade correlates with progression from well-demarcated nodules to infiltrative or metastatic neoplasms. The diagnosis is based firmly in morphology, and immunohistochemical findings alone do not justify the diagnosis. **Small cell carcinoma** is a rare and poorly characterized neuroendocrine tumor described in dogs and cows. It has a hilar location and consists of loosely arranged packets of small cells (~10 μm diameter) separated by a thin stroma. The neoplastic cells have scant cytoplasm, and may be round (resembling lymphocytes), fusiform ("oat cells") or polygonal. The immunohistochemical staining patterns in domestic animals are not characterized.

Pulmonary blastoma, rarely described in animals, is a multinodular lesion that implants in the pleural cavity, metastasizes to lymph nodes, and invades extrapulmonary structures. Blastoma consists, by definition, of *malignant epithelial and*

mesenchymal components, although there is much variation in the relative amount of each component between tumors and within different areas of the same neoplasm. The cuboidal epithelial cells are arranged in nests or branching tubules. The mesenchymal component appears embryonal, with loose matrix separating spindle-shaped, stellate, or angular cells with vesicular or hyperchromatic nuclei. Pleuropulmonary blastoma is of similar morphology and is located in pleura, lung, or mediastinum, but the epithelial component is well differentiated rather than atypical. The differential diagnoses include pulmonary hamartoma and mesothelioma.

Granular cell tumor *is the most common primary lung tumor in horses, and is thought to originate from Schwann cells in the peribronchial tissue.* It is often discovered as an incidental finding in older horses, but can cause coughing or, rarely, dyspnea. Metastasis is not described. Grossly, the mass is white to beige, usually multinodular, and unilateral. Granular cell tumors are associated with large bronchi, and often bulge into the bronchial lumen to cause variable degrees of obstruction. Histologically, the neoplasm is composed of sheets or lobular aggregates of large, round, or angular cells with abundant cytoplasm containing innumerable tiny acidophilic granules (Fig. 5-27). There is minimal variation in cell size, and few mitotic figures are found. The granules usually stain with Luxol fast blue and more variably with periodic acid–Schiff. Immunohistochemical markers for pulmonary granular cell tumors in horses are widely expressed in a variety of other cell types, and so are not pathognomonic for this neoplasm; S100 and vimentin are consistently present, with inconsistent expression of NSE and glial fibrillary acidic protein (GFAP).

Histiocytic sarcoma *is a malignant neoplasm of myeloid interstitial dendritic cell phenotype* (see Vol. 3, Hematopoietic system). Histiocytic sarcoma arises in the lung and spreads to thoracic lymph nodes, or histiocytic sarcoma of splenic origin may secondarily involve lung and other organs. The infiltrate may replace an entire lung lobe, or form multifocal infiltrates throughout the lung. The morphology varies from individualized round cells with scant to abundant eosinophilic cytoplasm, to spindle-shaped or dendritic cells with indistinct borders (Fig. 5-28). The nuclei are round or cleaved with marked anisokaryosis. Most cases have significant numbers of

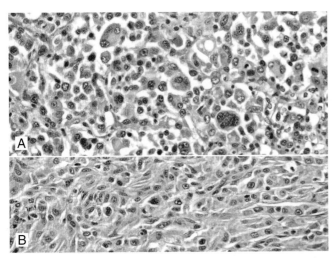

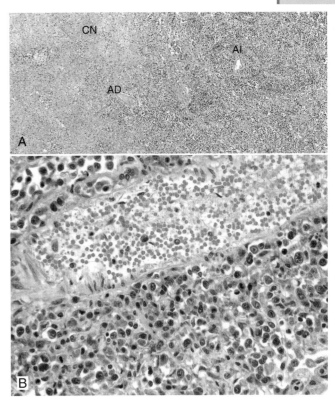

Figure 5-28 Pulmonary histiocytic sarcoma in a dog. Within the same mass, the phenotype varies from pleomorphic round cells with abundant cytoplasm and frequent multinucleation (**A**), to spindle-shaped cells with less obvious histiocytic differentiation (**B**).

Figure 5-29 Angioinvasive lymphoma in a dog resembling lymphomatoid granulomatosis. **A.** At low magnification, there is angioinvasive growth of neoplastic cells (AI), angiodestructive behavior with effacement of a vessel wall (AD), and coagulative necrosis (CN) caused by infarction of adjacent neoplastic tissue. **B.** High magnification shows the pleomorphic nature of the large neoplastic round cells and small non-neoplastic lymphocytes, with infiltration of a vessel wall.

multinucleated cells, lymphocytes, and plasma cells intermingled with the neoplastic cells. Definitive diagnosis requires immunohistochemistry on frozen sections to demonstrate expression of CD1, CD11c, major histocompatibility complex class II, and intercellular adhesion molecule 1 (ICAM)-1. However, in formalin-fixed specimens, demonstration of a typical morphology along with expression of CD18 but absence of CD3, CD20, and CD79a provides tentative confirmation of the diagnosis. Dogs with splenic hemophagic histiocytic sarcoma (of macrophage phenotype) may have neoplastic cells within pulmonary blood vessels.

Feline pulmonary Langerhans cell histiocytosis is a rare condition of old cats, causing multifocal coalescing masses or diffuse infiltrates within the lung, and may affect pancreas, kidney, liver, and local or distant lymph nodes. The infiltrate targets the bronchioles and extends to adjacent alveoli. The histiocytic cells are pleomorphic, with a moderate amount of homogeneous or finely vacuolated eosinophilic cytoplasm, anisokaryosis, poikilokaryosis, and nuclear hyperchromasia. These cells express CD18 and E-cadherin and have ultrastructurally visible Birbeck granules, consistent with a Langerhans cell phenotype. In addition to this disease, cats with **progressive histiocytosis** and dogs with **cutaneous Langerhans cell histiocytosis** or **systemic histiocytosis**, described elsewhere, may have involvement of the lungs.

Angiocentric lymphoma (also known as **lymphomatoid granulomatosis**) is a rare and poorly understood disease of dogs, and very rarely of cats. In humans, lymphomatoid granulomatosis is a B-cell proliferation associated with Epstein-Barr virus infection. Although the disease is discussed here as a pulmonary neoplasm, there is considerable debate as to whether the analogous condition in humans represents a neoplasm or a non-neoplastic lymphoproliferative disorder. No data are available in veterinary medicine addressing the clonality of the lymphoid cells, so the biology of this disease remains enigmatic. Most cases affect young dogs (4-9 years of age), with cases as young as 9 weeks of age recorded. The masses are multiple and usually found within the caudal lung lobes. They are poorly demarcated and pale, or can occur as a diffuse

infiltrate within the affected lobes. Histologically, angiocentric lymphoma *is an angioinvasive, angiodestructive, pleocellular infiltrate* (Fig. 5-29). A requirement for the diagnosis is a mixed infiltrate of small lymphocytes (mainly T cells) as well as large atypical cells, along with a variable infiltrate of plasma cells and eosinophils. The atypical cells are round with distinct borders, large but variably sized, occasionally binucleate, and often have a high mitotic rate. Characterization of the condition in dogs is limited but suggests that the atypical cells include both T and B cells. *Destructive invasion of the pleomorphic cells into the walls of blood vessels is the characteristic feature of the disease*, and infarction of adjacent tissue may be present. The infiltrates frequently involve the bronchial lymph nodes and occasionally the liver and other viscera, but it is the progressive involvement of the lung that causes death in most cases. The differential diagnosis includes eosinophilic granulomatosis, anaplastic carcinoma, and pulmonary round cell tumors, such as histiocytic sarcoma, lymphoma, and mast cell tumor.

Metastatic tumors commonly arise within the lung because of the organ's rich capillary and lymphatic network. Criteria for differentiating metastases of nonpulmonary neoplasms from intrapulmonary spread of a primary lung neoplasm are described previously. An important part of the diagnosis of a primary lung tumor is thorough examination of the body to exclude possible nonpulmonary sites of primary neoplasia.

Metastatic carcinomas may form acini, solid sheets, lepidic growth along pre-existing alveolar septa, and/or clusters within blood vessels. Some of the most common metastatic neoplasms include lymphoma in all species; uterine adenocarcinoma in cows and sows; malignant melanoma in horses; and osteosarcoma, hemangiosarcoma, oral melanoma, mast cell tumor, transitional cell carcinoma, and adenocarcinomas of mammary, biliary, pancreatic, intestinal, anal sac, or thyroid origin in dogs and cats (eFigs. 5-41, 5-42).

Further reading

Affolter VK, Moore PF. Localized and disseminated histiocytic sarcoma of dendritic cell origin in dogs. Vet Pathol 2002;39:74-83.

Busch MD, et al. Feline pulmonary Langerhans cell histiocytosis with multiorgan involvement. Vet Pathol 2008;45:816-824.

D'Costa S, et al. Morphologic and molecular analysis of 39 spontaneous feline pulmonary carcinomas. Vet Pathol 2012;49:971-978.

Goldstraw P. International Association for the Study of Lung Cancer, Staging Manual in Thoracic Oncology. Orange Park, Fla: Editorial Rx Press, 2009. Available at umfiasi2015.files.wordpress.com/2013/03/pulmon-iaslc-manual.pdf.

Park HM, et al. Pulmonary lymphomatoid granulomatosis in a dog: evidence of immunophenotypic diversity and relationship to human pulmonary lymphomatoid granulomatosis and pulmonary Hodgkin's disease. Vet Pathol 2007;44:921-923.

Ramos-Vara JA, et al. Usefulness of thyroid transcription factor-1 immunohistochemical staining in the differential diagnosis of primary pulmonary tumors of dogs. Vet Pathol 2005;42:315-320.

Travis WD, et al. International Association for the Study of Lung Cancer/American Thoracic Society/European Respiratory Society international multidisciplinary classification of lung adenocarcinoma. J Thorac Oncol 2011;6:244-285.

Anatomic patterns of lung injury

Damage to lung tissue varies according to the nature of the causative agents, their distribution (particularly the route by which they reach the lung), and their persistence. Pulmonary diseases can be classified in several ways:

- *Morphologic pattern,* according to initial site of involvement and the pattern of spread of the lesion: bronchopneumonia, interstitial lung disease, airway disease, bronchointerstitial lung disease, and embolic pneumonia (Fig. 5-30)
- *Histologic character:* fibrinous, suppurative, granulomatous, necrotizing, proliferative, fibrosing
- *Etiology:* viral, bacterial, parasitic, toxic, allergic
- *Duration:* acute, subacute, chronic
- *Functional abnormality:* obstructive versus restrictive
- *Epidemiologic patterns:* shipping-fever pneumonia, enzootic pneumonia

The approach described here emphasizes morphologic patterns of pneumonia, for 2 reasons. First, gross and histologic examination is usually sufficient to classify a condition by this scheme, even if the etiology cannot be identified. Second, knowledge of the pattern of pneumonia provides important clues as to the probable etiology, route of exposure to the causative agent, pathogenesis of the lesions, effect on pulmonary function, and the sequelae and complications. Emphasizing the similarities between specific diseases, by grouping them based on morphologic patterns, often enhances our ability to recognize the sometimes subtle differences among these conditions.

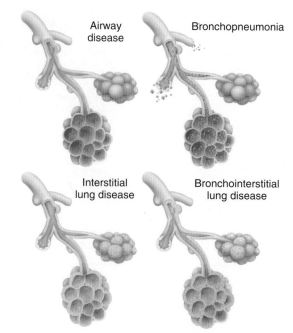

Figure 5-30 The 4 morphologic patterns of lung disease. *Airway disease* involves necrosis and/or inflammation targeting bronchi or bronchioles. In *bronchopneumonia,* leukocytes and edema fill airspaces (alveoli and bronchioles) because of airborne spread of bacteria. *Interstitial lung disease* arises from the non-airway tissues of the lung, mainly the alveolar and interlobular septa. *Bronchointerstitial lung disease* is a combination of airway and interstitial lung disease. (Courtesy M. Danko.)

Airway disease

Lesions that specifically target the airways include those that primarily cause epithelial necrosis and those that induce airway inflammation; often, a combination of necrosis and inflammation is present. Diseases may affect the bronchi, bronchioles, or both, and the diagnosis of bronchointerstitial pneumonia, described later, is appropriate when both airway and alveolar epithelial cells are damaged. *The major consequences of these diseases are coughing, airway obstruction, and impairment of lung defenses.* The flow of air can be obstructed by bronchoconstriction resulting from contraction of airway smooth muscle, by leukocytes or mucus within the lumen of the airway, and by thickening of the airway wall by edema and leukocytes. The consequence is failure of alveolar ventilation that may cause hypoxemia and hypercapnia. As a result of alveolar hypoxia inducing reflex vasoconstriction, there is reduced perfusion of hypoventilated areas of lung that, if widespread, may lead to pulmonary hypertension. Pulmonary compliance is reduced because of the increased pressure needed to ventilate the alveoli. Clinically important airway obstruction is particularly notable with bronchiolar disease, where it manifests as expiratory dyspnea because the airway obstruction is exacerbated from the slight collapse that occurs during exhalation.

Bronchitis is relatively common in domestic animals but receives inadequate attention by pathologists because it is not usually fatal. Bronchitis and/or bronchial necrosis may be caused by viral or bacterial infection, parasitism, allergic disease, or exposure to irritants or toxins.

Morphologic manifestations of acute bronchitis include the same range of inflammation described for upper airways. The

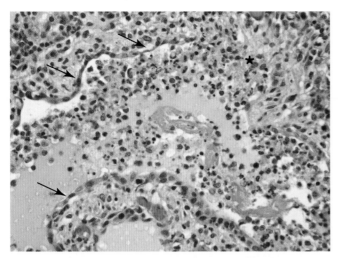

Figure 5-31 Acute bronchiolar necrosis caused by **Nipah virus** infection in a pig. There is complete loss of bronchiolar epithelium (asterisk) with exudation of fibrin, leukocytes, and necrotic cells. The adjacent epithelium is attenuated (arrows) in an attempt to cover the denuded basement membrane. Epithelial attenuation is a more reliable criterion for necrosis, as sloughed cells are a common artifact of autolysis.

exudates may be catarrhal, mucopurulent, fibrinous, fibrinopurulent, or purulent. Ciliated epithelial cells are most sensitive to a wide array of injurious agents and are often the first to undergo necrosis and slough (Fig. 5-31). *Catarrhal bronchitis* represents a relatively mild reaction in which the irritation induces both a mild neutrophil-dominated inflammatory response and secretion of mucus by goblet cells and bronchial glands. In *purulent bronchitis*, the exudate is yellow or white and viscid. *Fibrinonecrotic bronchitis* resulting from viral or occasionally mycotic infection is characterized by areas of epithelial necrosis with loosely adherent fibrinous exudate. In such cases, gentle removal of the exudate reveals a granular lesion of epithelial necrosis, which differentiates the lesion from the expectorated mucus that is often present in the large airways of animals with chronic bronchopneumonia. Animals with aspiration pneumonia often have extensive necrosis of the bronchial epithelium, with green-brown foul-smelling exudate.

Bronchial necrosis can resolve by epithelial regeneration if the offending stimulus is removed or neutralized. More severe or prolonged injury to epithelium results in fibrosis of the lamina propria, as well as accumulation of lymphocytes, macrophages, and plasma cells. Epithelial hyperplasia, mucous hyperplasia, and/or squamous metaplasia may also become prominent following mucosal injury of any cause (eFig. 5-43). Chronic infection with damage to the airway wall may result in bronchiectasis, discussed later. Fibrous polyps are a rare response to bronchial mucosal injury.

Common airway diseases in domestic animals include acute tracheobronchitis ("kennel cough") of dogs (discussed in the section Infectious respiratory diseases of dogs, later), chronic bronchitis and eosinophilic bronchopneumopathy of dogs, feline asthma, recurrent airway obstruction ("heaves") in horses, and *Dictyocaulus* spp. in cattle, sheep, goats, and horses. Bronchitis also results from inhalation of bacteria from the upper respiratory tract and, rarely, when the focal lesions of tuberculosis or caseous lymphadenitis erode into a large

airway. Bronchitis causes coughing that may be paroxysmal, and airway obstruction manifests in wheezing. However, it is not expected to be fatal unless the lesion induces widespread bronchoconstriction, obstructs a large airway, or leads to secondary bronchopneumonia as a result of aspiration of infected material or impaired mucociliary clearance.

Chronic bronchitis in dogs. Chronic bronchitis is a common condition in older, small- and medium-sized dogs, and manifests as chronic productive or nonproductive cough, exercise intolerance, expiratory or inspiratory wheezes, reduced expiratory airflow, and hypoxemia. The etiology is rarely identified. Proposed causes include dry air; airborne pollutants, including sulfur dioxide and particulates; environmental tobacco smoke; chronic gingivitis with aspiration of debris; immune-mediated inflammation; and viral infection. Opportunistic bacterial pathogens are occasionally isolated, but their significance as a primary cause is questionable; similarly, viral and bacterial infections are well recognized to induce acute exacerbations in human patients with chronic bronchitis in which infection is not the primary cause. Many dogs with chronic bronchitis also have chronic left heart failure, suggesting that cardiogenic pulmonary edema may result in chronic coughing that generates airway inflammation and mucus hypersecretion.

The major gross finding in chronic bronchitis is excessive mucus or mucopurulent exudate in the trachea and bronchi. The bronchial mucosa in severe cases is hyperemic, thickened, edematous, and granular rather than glistening, and lymphoid nodules or hyperplastic polyps may project into the lumen. Microscopically, the bronchial mucosa is edematous and contains many lymphocytes, plasma cells, and occasional macrophages and neutrophils. Eosinophils may or may not be present. There is hyperplasia and hypertrophy of bronchial glands, hyperplasia of goblet cells, and variable hyperplasia, ulceration, or squamous metaplasia of the surface epithelium. Intraluminal mucus is commonly mixed with abundant neutrophils. Many cases of uncomplicated bronchitis persist for years, but *sequelae* in severe cases include bronchiectasis; bronchopneumonia; or alveolar atelectasis, leading to pulmonary hypertension, cor pulmonale, and medial hypertrophy of pulmonary arteries. Collapsing trachea and chronic bronchitis are frequent companions. Chronic inflammation is thought to progress to malacia of the tracheobronchial cartilage in some cases and contribute to development of tracheal collapse. Emphysema is not an important sequel to chronic bronchitis in dogs.

Eosinophilic bronchopneumopathy is an uncommon, usually steroid-responsive condition of young dogs. It causes chronic gagging, cough, dyspnea, nasal discharge, and variable blood eosinophilia and neutrophilia. The nodular or diffuse lung lesions are not completely described, but include chronic eosinophilic bronchitis with epithelial hyperplasia, ulceration, or squamous metaplasia, which destroys the airway walls and leads to bronchiectasis in ~25% of cases. In addition to bronchial lesions, most cases have extensive involvement of lung parenchyma with diffuse eosinophilic and granulomatous infiltrates, focal eosinophilic granulomas centered on necrotic tissue and densely eosinophilic material (probably masses of eosinophil secretions), and large areas of necrosis and fibrosis (Fig. 5-32). Eosinophilic bronchopneumopathy is perhaps the most common cause of bronchiectasis in dogs (eFig. 5-44). Cases with involvement of the lung parenchyma overlap with eosinophilic pulmonary granulomatosis, which is discussed

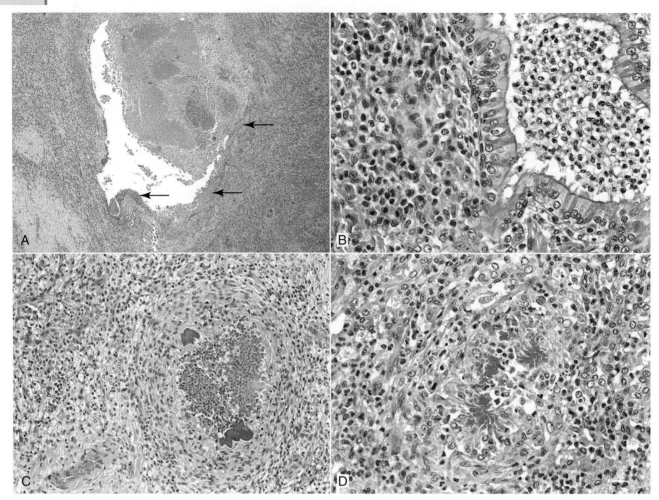

Figure 5-32 Eosinophilic bronchopneumopathy in a dog. **A.** A dense infiltrate of eosinophils, lymphocytes, and macrophages targets and effaces a bronchus. Remnants of bronchial epithelium (arrows) remain visible and have undergone squamous metaplasia. **B.** Higher magnification of a more mildly affected bronchiole. **C, D.** Pulmonary parenchyma contains a diffuse leukocyte infiltrate with formation of granulomas around necrotic eosinophils (**C**) or deposits of brightly eosinophilic material (**D**).

later. Eosinophilic bronchopneumopathy is thought to be immune mediated, but specific causes should be ruled out: the tracheobronchial parasites *Crenosoma vulpis*, *Eucoleus aerophilus (Capillaria aerophila)*, and *Oslerus osleri*; the lungworms *Angiostrongylus vasorum* and *Filaroides hirthi*; occult *Dirofilaria immitis* infection (causing eosinophilic granulomas in lung); as well as pulmonary carcinoma, histiocytic sarcoma, lymphoma, and lymphomatoid granulomatosis. Allergic bronchopulmonary aspergillosis and drug reaction cause similar lesions in humans but have not been identified in dogs.

Aspergillus fumigatus and *A. flavus* rarely cause chronic destructive bronchitis in German Shepherd dogs, with erosion of epithelium, neutrophil infiltration, and formation of granulation tissue in the wall of small and large airways. The lesion can progress to form an aspergilloma or fungus ball, a cavitated mass in the lung composed mainly of fungal hyphae (eFig. 5-45). However, hyphae may be difficult to detect in the chronic bronchial lesions. Progression to invasive systemic aspergillosis is not described in dogs, and excision with antifungal therapy has been curative.

Further reading

Clercx C, Peeters D. Canine eosinophilic bronchopneumopathy. Vet Clin North Am Small Anim Pract 2007;37:917-935.

Kulendra E, et al. Cavitary pulmonary lesion associated with *Aspergillus fumigatus* infection in a German shepherd dog. J Small Anim Pract 2010;51:271-274.

Padrid PA, et al. Canine chronic bronchitis. A pathophysiologic evaluation of 18 cases. J Vet Intern Med 1990;4:172-180.

Acute and chronic bronchitis in cats. **Feline asthma** *is relatively common, and is defined by the clinical findings of reversible airway obstruction with inflammation.* Most cases have an acute onset or recurrent bouts of cough, dyspnea, or wheezing that respond to treatment with bronchodilators and corticosteroids, and are *mainly the result of bronchial inflammation, airway smooth muscle hyper-reactivity,* and bronchoconstriction. Thickening of the bronchial wall may be noted radiographically, and eosinophils are usually numerous in bronchoalveolar lavage fluid. Neutrophils or macrophages predominate in bronchoalveolar lavage fluid in some cases that are otherwise typical of feline asthma (eFig. 5-46). Other cats have chronic rather than episodic coughing or wheezing; chronic bronchitis is a more accurate diagnosis in these cases if it cannot be demonstrated that the signs are readily reversible. Cats parenterally sensitized then challenged with Bermuda grass allergens develop allergen-specific immunoglobulin E (IgE), IgG, and IgA; airway hyper-reactivity; and the following histologic lesions in the bronchi: narrowing of the lumen, smooth muscle hypertrophy, infiltrates of eosinophils in the wall and lumen, hypertrophy and hyperplasia of goblet cells and bronchial glands, and hyperplasia and exfoliation of the surface epithelium. The histologic findings in natural cases are not as well characterized because mortality is uncommon. In addition to smooth muscle hyperplasia and eosinophil infiltration, lymphoplasmacytic infiltrates with lymphoid follicles may develop in the adventitia of the bronchi, and bronchioles may contain similar lesions.

Chronic bronchitis in cats may be a manifestation of ongoing low-grade allergic reactions, although these do not fulfill the criteria of acute onset of reversible airway obstruction, as is necessary for the diagnosis of asthma. The exudate in airways is dominated by neutrophils, but the histologic lesions have not been defined. The role of infectious agents, including *Mycoplasma* spp., as causes of chronic bronchitis in cats is controversial. Bronchial parasites are rare in cats.

Further reading

Padrid P. Feline asthma. Diagnosis and treatment. Vet Clin North Am Small Anim Pract 2000;30:1279-1293.

Venema CM, et al. Histopathologic and morphometric evaluation of the nasal and pulmonary airways of cats with experimentally induced asthma. Int Arch Allergy Immunol 2013;160:365-376.

Bronchiectasis. *Bronchiectasis is defined as permanent dilation of bronchi as a result of chronic bronchial obstruction and infection.* Such bronchi become unable to clear the inflammatory exudate and will no longer perform their normal functions. Although most cases are a complication of bronchopneumonia or bacterial bronchitis, bronchiectasis may occur with immune-mediated bronchitis, or rarely as a congenital malformation. Bronchiectasis is relatively common in **cattle** with chronic bronchopneumonia, because complete lobular septation and lack of collateral ventilation both impair resolution of bronchopneumonia and lead to more extensive atelectasis because of airway blockage. Bronchiectasis is common in **dogs.** The lesions commonly affect the right cranial or middle lung lobes, and are usually the result of eosinophilic bronchopneumopathy, bacterial infection or occasionally tumors, bronchial foreign bodies, or ciliary dyskinesia. The condition in **cats** usually affects the caudal or middle lobes, and is often a sequel to chronic bronchitis, bronchopneumonia, or pulmonary neoplasia. Endogenous lipid pneumonia and emphysema are concurrent findings in some cases. Bronchiectasis infrequently develops in **pigs, sheep,** and **goats** with severe parasitic bronchitis. There are 3 anatomic forms of bronchiectasis: (1) *cylindrical bronchiectasis* causes relatively uniform dilation of the bronchus; (2) *saccular bronchiectasis* is probably a more advanced stage, where there are circumscribed or fusiform cyst-like lesions at the end of

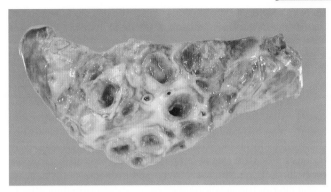

Figure 5-33 Bronchiectasis in a cow with chronic bronchopneumonia. The seemingly increased numbers of large airways simply results from dilation of smaller airways, because of degradation of their walls by the purulent exudate that had pooled within.

progressively dilated airways; (3) *varicose bronchiectasis—* rarely identified in animals—forms focal constrictions along dilated airways. The smaller distal bronchi are usually affected by bronchiectasis, and a similar lesion may involve the bronchioles.

Destruction of bronchial walls with luminal obstruction by exudate is the key to development of bronchiectasis, and leads to their permanent dilation. In these situations, neutrophil- or eosinophil-derived proteases and oxygen radicals are thought to damage the bronchial wall. This results not only in weakening of the bronchial wall, but also failure of mucociliary clearance that perpetuates the infection and pooling of exudates in the lumen. The exudates cause obstruction; as a result, the weakened airways can be pulled outward with each inspiration and thus dilate over time.

Grossly, the dilated bronchi are filled with viscid yellow-green creamy exudate (Fig. 5-33), which may eventually form caseous or inspissated masses in the lumen. The intervening parenchyma may be atelectatic and fibrotic. The bronchi may be so dilated as to be visible from the pleural surface, but are best appreciated when sectioned transversely. *They may be confused with abscesses, but form cylindrical tracts, have remnants of cartilage, and are eventually continuous with recognizable bronchi* (eFig. 5-47). In severe cases, the dilated bronchi give a honeycombed or cystic appearance to the lobe (see Fig. 5-33). Microscopically, the lumen is filled with mucus, cellular debris, leukocytes, and occasionally blood. The epithelium often has some combination of attenuation, ulceration, mucous or squamous metaplasia, and hyperplasia. The bronchial wall is infiltrated with leukocytes and may be obscured by granulation tissue, and this destructive and fibrotic lesion may extend to the deeper tissues and destroy cartilage and bronchial glands. Normal bronchi are dynamic structures that actively regulate airflow and defend the lung through mucociliary clearance; those crippled by bronchiectasis are forever dilated and unable to clear their burden of harmful pus and pathogens.

Further reading

Hawkins EC, et al. Demographic, clinical, and radiographic features of bronchiectasis in dogs: 316 cases (1988-2000). J Am Vet Med Assoc 2003;223:1628-1635.

Norris CR, Samii VF. Clinical, radiographic, and pathologic features of bronchiectasis in cats: 12 cases (1987-1999). J Am Vet Med Assoc 2000;216:530-534.

Primary ciliary dyskinesia. Cilia are complex structures. The "9 + 2" or "9 + 0" arrangement of microtubular doublets forms the basic structure, inner and outer dynein arms are the motors that forces the cilium to bend, and nexin links and radial arms provide support. These structures contain hundreds of proteins, so it is not surprising that *primary ciliary dyskinesia is a diverse collection of disorders* involving mucus-propelling cilia in the nasal cavity and bronchi, sperm flagella, nodal cilia in the developing embryo, water-propelling cilia in the ependyma and epididymis, and cilia in the middle ear and retina. Primary ciliary dyskinesia, or *immotile cilia syndrome*, is an inherited condition reported infrequently in many dog breeds, which manifests as recurrent or persistent rhinitis and sinusitis, bronchiectasis, bacterial pneumonia, and/or male infertility caused by reduced spermatozoal motility with abnormal tails. About half of affected humans and dogs have *Kartagener's syndrome*, defined as the combination of sinusitis, bronchiectasis, and situs inversus. The latter is a left-right reversal of the thoracic and/or abdominal viscera resulting from dysfunction of cilia in the embryologic node. Otitis media or hydrocephalus may occasionally be present.

The *diagnosis* of ciliary dyskinesia is based on abnormal ciliary motility in short-term cell cultures, in vivo imaging studies to measure movement of mucus, and/or detection of ultrastructural abnormalities in cilia. Because bacterial toxins or adhesion of *Bordetella* or perhaps *Mycoplasma* cause ciliary dysfunction, detection of dysfunction in cilia from more than one tissue is necessary. Ultrastructural studies are also useful in differentiating primary from acquired ciliary dyskinesia. Absence or reduced number of inner and/or outer dynein arms, of the radial spokes that extend from these arms, and/or of the central microtubules are common ultrastructural lesions in primary ciliary dyskinesia, and other primary and secondary changes are described. The ultrastructural diagnosis depends heavily on the quality of the preparation, and some dogs with the syndrome do not have ultrastructural changes in cilia.

Further reading

Cavrenne R, et al. Primary ciliary dyskinesia and situs inversus in a young dog. Vet Rec 2008;163:54-55.

Leigh MW, et al. The challenges of diagnosing primary ciliary dyskinesia. Proc Am Thorac Soc 2011;8:434-437.

Bronchiolar necrosis and inflammation

Bronchiolitis and/or bronchiolar necrosis are *caused by* viral infection, inhalation of toxic gases, toxins that are metabolized by cytochrome P450 in nonciliated club (Clara) cells, hypersensitivity reactions, or inflammatory reactions to inhaled irritants. Autoimmune disorders, drug reactions, and reactions to mineral dusts are further causes of bronchiolar injury in humans. In addition, bronchiolar lesions are frequently an extension of bronchitis, bronchiectasis, or bacterial bronchopneumonia. The designation of *bronchointerstitial pneumonia* is appropriate when necrosis targets both the bronchiolar and the alveolar epithelium, as occurs particularly in viral infections and toxic injury (see Fig. 5-30). Bronchiolar epithelial

hyperplasia and lymphocytic bronchitis are common sequelae to viral infections (eFig. 5-48).

Airway obstruction occurs more readily in bronchioles than in bronchi because their lack of cartilage rings and small luminal size readily permits collapse and occlusion by exudate. According to Poiseuille's law of frictional resistance, resistance to airflow varies with the fourth power of the radius, so narrowing of the airway by half will increase airway resistance 16-fold. Thus, if it is of diffuse distribution, even minor airway obstruction by bronchoconstriction, intraluminal exudates or mucus, or edema of the wall has profound effects on the work of breathing and on alveolar ventilation. These functional changes manifest as forced expiratory effort, hypoxemia, and hypercapnia in the later stages. *Complete airway obstruction causes atelectasis, whereas partial obstruction leads to air trapping and overdistension of alveoli* (see Fig. 5-17). Both of these situations lead either to shunting of non-oxygenated blood past the perfused but hypoventilated alveoli, or arteriolar constriction that reduces perfusion of these hypoventilated alveoli but causes pulmonary hypertension if the airway obstruction is widespread.

Bronchiolitis obliterans (also known as *bronchiolitis fibrosa obliterans, obliterative bronchiolitis,* or *organizing bronchiolitis*) is a sequel to chronic bronchiolar damage. The term is used here to describe the presence of fibrous polyps occluding the bronchiolar lumen (Fig. 5-34); bronchiolitis obliterans is occasionally used elsewhere to describe acute lesions in which intraluminal aggregates of neutrophils obstruct airflow. The lesion is distinct from **constrictive bronchiolitis**, a lesion not commonly identified in animals, in which fibrosis of the bronchiolar wall causes external compression that reduces the diameter of the lumen. **Hyaline scars** are described in lambs with chronic viral or mycoplasmal pneumonia, and appear as nodular masses of fibrillar eosinophilic matrix and fibroblasts within the wall of bronchioles that bluntly compress the lumen, but do not form the intrabronchiolar polyps seen in bronchiolitis obliterans (eFig. 5-49).

Bronchiolitis obliterans is wound healing gone awry. Any agent that severely damages the bronchiolar epithelium—viral

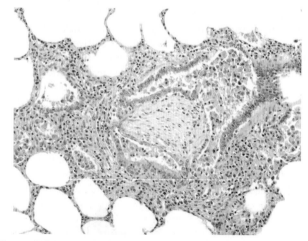

Figure 5-34 Bronchiolitis obliterans in a feedlot calf. A polyp of fibrous tissue, covered by epithelium, protrudes into and partially occludes the lumen of a bronchiole. Peribronchiolar leukocyte infiltration may reflect the presumed viral infection that initiated the lesion. This calf had cor pulmonale with arterial medial hypertrophy, subcutaneous edema, and ascites.

infection, neutrophil-mediated injury caused by bacterial pneumonia, toxic gases, toxins metabolized by club cells, lungworms, and rejection of transplanted lung—may lead to fibrin formation in the bronchiolar lumen (see Fig. 5-28). As in any wound, fibrinous exudates that are not rapidly removed heal by fibroblast infiltration, neovascularization, and migration and proliferation of epithelial cells across their surface. Organization of exudate into granulation tissue can take place in as little as 7-10 days after injury, and regeneration of epithelium over its surface can occur in a similar time period. The presence of *fibrous polyps occluding the airways has disastrous and permanent effects on airflow and alveolar ventilation.*

Bronchiolitis obliterans is commonly identified within lesions of chronic bronchopneumonia in cattle, as a consequence of viral or neutrophil-mediated epithelial damage. Calves with a prior history of viral pneumonia occasionally develop right heart failure with right ventricular dilation, subcutaneous edema, hepatomegaly, and ascites. These lungs may be grossly normal, but histologic examination reveals epithelium-covered fibrous polyps that occlude the lumen of most bronchioles (see Fig. 5-31) as well as medial hypertrophy of pulmonary arterioles. The latter is a histologic indicator that widespread alveolar hypoventilation has incited pulmonary hypertension, in turn causing cor pulmonale with right heart failure.

Scattered subpleural foci of **bronchioloalveolar hyperplasia** are a common incidental finding in dogs (see Fig. 5-34). The lesions can be difficult to distinguish from early bronchioloalveolar carcinoma, but the hyperplastic lesions are usually multifocal, line terminal bronchioles, do not enlarge to form masses, are usually associated with fibrosis and lymphocytic inflammation of the adjacent tissue, and have no features of cellular atypia.

Further reading

Fulton RW, et al. Lung pathology and infectious agents in fatal feedlot pneumonias and relationship with mortality, disease onset, and treatments. J Vet Diagn Invest 2009;21:464-477.

Li X, et al. Oleic acid-associated bronchiolitis obliterans-organizing pneumonia in beagle dogs. Vet Pathol 2006;43:183-185.

Recurrent airway obstruction in horses. Recurrent airway obstruction (RAO, or "heaves") is a common condition of mature horses. *The term chronic obstructive pulmonary disease is not appropriate for the equine disease,* as the condition is more similar to human asthma. RAO is usually induced or exacerbated by exposure to organic dusts (particularly dusty, poor-quality hay) that may contain allergens, endotoxins, fungi, actinomycetes, and particulate irritants. *RAO is a nonseptic, inflammatory airway disease of adult horses, characterized by airway hyper-responsiveness and episodes of reversible airway obstruction resulting from bronchospasm.* Other factors contributing to the airway obstruction include accumulation of mucus and neutrophils in bronchiolar lumina and thickening of the bronchiolar wall (Fig. 5-35).

Although RAO is undoubtedly an inflammatory disease, it remains controversial whether allergy (IgE- and mast cell–mediated type I hypersensitivity) is important to the pathogenesis. Evidence supporting a mast cell–dependent or allergic basis includes elevated levels of IgE and histamine in bronchoalveolar lavage fluid, and enhanced histamine release from pulmonary mast cells of horses with heaves. However, skin

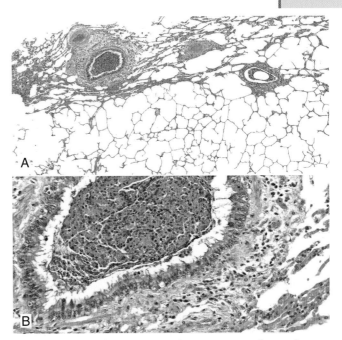

Figure 5-35 Recurrent airway obstruction in a horse. Lesions target the bronchioles (**A**), with mucus, neutrophils and sloughed epithelial cells filling the lumen, goblet cell metaplasia of the epithelium, and thickening of the adventitia by mononuclear cells and edema (**B**). The alveoli are overinflated because of air trapping but, in contrast to true emphysema, fragments of alveolar walls are not observed (**A**).

tests induce delayed rather than immediate reactions and do not correlate with airway reactivity, antigen-specific IgE levels are similar to controls, and stimulated bronchoalveolar lavage cells in horses with RAO produce both interleukin-4 (IL-4) and interferon-γ (in addition to tumor necrosis factor-α, IL-1β, and IL-8) mRNA, suggesting that a pure type 2 immune response is not characteristic of this disease. Alternatively, dysregulation of the normal anti-inflammatory functions of club cells may promote airway inflammation in affected horses. Challenge with molds, mold extracts, or endotoxin-containing dusts has induced airway neutrophilia and obstruction in heaves-susceptible but not normal horses, implying that all of these factors contribute to the airway responses.

The disease occurs in stabled horses in northern regions and as a summer pasture-associated form in warm wet climates. *Affected horses have chronic cough, increased expiratory effort, wheezing, variable nasal discharge, and exercise intolerance.* Increased pulmonary resistance and reduced dynamic compliance are typical functional changes, and the bronchioles are hyper-responsive to agonists. The signs wax and wane depending on exposure to dusts, and a seasonal effect is common, but many cases are slowly progressive over the course of months or years.

The lesions specifically target the small bronchioles, and alveolar changes are usually minor. Bronchioles contain mucus, neutrophils, and sloughed epithelial cells in their lumens; increased numbers of goblet cells in the epithelium; hyperplasia and/or sloughing of club cells; lymphocytes, plasma cells, and mast cells in the lamina propria and adventitia; hyperplasia of smooth muscle; and inconsistent peribronchiolar fibrosis (see Fig. 5-35). Of these, the presence of mucus and neutrophils in bronchiolar lumens and hyperplasia of goblet cells are most characteristic, whereas leukocyte infiltrates in the airway wall and smooth muscle hyperplasia are seen in horses without RAO. Lesions are more severe in the caudodorsal lung. Eosinophils are usually infrequent but numerous in some cases; their presence perhaps reflects a different stage of the disease. Mucus spills into the adjacent alveoli in severe cases. Overinflation of alveoli may result from trapping of air distal to the obstructed bronchioles, but true emphysema with destruction of alveolar septa is not expected.

Inflammatory airway disease is a term used to describe an RAO-like condition in younger horses. It occurs in 2- to 4-year-old horses, causes no clinical signs at rest, but exercise induces excessive airway mucus production and coughing, leading to exercise intolerance and poor racing performance. Bronchoalveolar lavage cytology reveals mild neutrophilia in some cases, eosinophilia in others, and some with increased numbers of mast cells. The histologic features are not described. Prior viral infection and exposure to airborne environmental allergens, dusts, and/or endotoxins are proposed causes.

Further reading

Couëtil LL, et al. Inflammatory airway disease of horses. J Vet Intern Med 2007;21:356-361.

Katavolos P, et al. Clara cell secretory protein is reduced in equine recurrent airway obstruction. Vet Pathol 2009;46:604-613.

Pirie RS. Recurrent airway obstruction: a review. Equine Vet J 2014;46:276-288.

Bronchopneumonia

The hallmark of bronchopneumonia is an exudative lesion originating at the bronchiolar-alveolar junction, and an airborne route of entry of the causative agents. The lesions of bronchopneumonia most often affect the cranioventral regions of the lungs, with neutrophils and sometimes fibrin or macrophages filling the air spaces of the bronchioles and alveoli (eFig. 5-50, Fig. 5-36; see Fig. 5-30).

The terminal bronchioles are the major site of deposition of 0.5-3.0 μm diameter particles, yet they seem to be particularly vulnerable to bacterial infection. In particular, the terminal bronchioles receive limited protection from the mucociliary clearance that is more active in the larger airways, or from the alveolar macrophages that protect the more distal airspaces. This situation is worsened by the fact that clearance of large volumes of debris from the alveoli requires that this material transits the narrow lumen of the bronchiole, so inflammation of the bronchiole readily obstructs clearance of bacteria and exudates from the alveoli, especially in species that lack collateral alveolar ventilation.

The characteristic cranioventral distribution of bacterial bronchopneumonia in animals is probably explained by gravitational influences, which result in both increased deposition of inhaled particles and pooling of aspirated secretions in these regions. There is also evidence that intravenous administration of *Mannheimia haemolytica* also causes pneumonia in cranioventral regions, perhaps suggesting that defenses might be less effective in this area of the lung.

Causes and predisposing factors. *Bronchopneumonia is, in most cases, caused by opportunistic bacterial pathogens* (Table 5-2), and development of disease requires increased exposure of the lung to bacteria, impairment of the pulmonary defenses, or both. The bacteria found in the lungs are generally similar

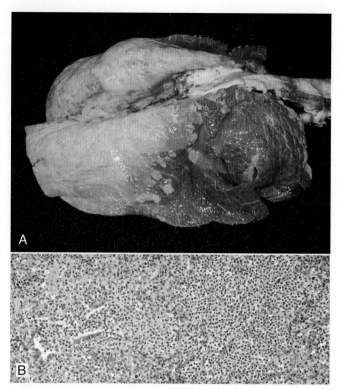

Figure 5-36 Lesions of bronchopneumonia. **A.** Typical gross appearance of subacute bronchopneumonia with red-tan discoloration and firmness of cranioventral areas of the lung, in a dairy calf. The lobular distribution is visible at the leading edge of the lesion, where completely consolidated lobules contrast with neighboring lobules that are unaffected. **B.** Histologic appearance of bronchopneumonia, in a dog with *Bordetella bronchiseptica* infection, with neutrophils filling the airspaces of alveoli (right) and a bronchiole (left), but no damage to the epithelium.

to those in the upper respiratory tract of the same individual, but at 2-4 logs lower number. *Aspiration pneumonia* (described later) is an obvious situation where pulmonary challenge with massive numbers of bacteria overcomes the lung defenses. Similarly, in cattle, *stress* leads to increased numbers of *Mannheimia haemolytica* bacteria colonizing the nasal cavity, with increased numbers of bacteria in inhaled droplets challenging the lung defenses. The *causes of impaired lung defenses* include stress, viral and mycoplasmal infection, unadapted exposure to cold, toxic gases, and inherited conditions. Agents or conditions that impair mucociliary clearance include exposure to cold, bovine herpesvirus 1, bovine respiratory syncytial virus, bovine parainfluenza virus 3, *Mycoplasma hyopneumoniae*, a variety of toxic gases, and ciliary dyskinesia. Corticosteroids (stress) and bovine viral diarrhea virus dampen the ability of airway epithelial cells to produce antimicrobial peptides. Alveolar macrophage function is reduced by bovine herpesvirus 1, porcine reproductive and respiratory syndrome virus, stress, aflatoxin, and T-2 mycotoxin. Conditions that reduce the number or function of circulating neutrophils may also predispose to opportunistic bacterial pneumonia, including parvoviral enteritis, acute bovine viral diarrhea virus infection, chemotherapy, stress, acidosis, uremia, and several mycotoxins. *Bovine leukocyte adhesion deficiency* (BLAD) is an autosomal recessive disease present in Holstein cattle. Neutrophils in affected animals have abnormal expression of the

Table • 5-2

Major causes of bacterial bronchopneumonia in domestic animal species

Cattle and sheep	Swine	Horses	Dogs and cats
Mannheimia haemolytica	Actinobacillus pleuropneumoniae	Streptococcus spp.	Bordetella bronchiseptica
Histophilus somni	P. multocida	Rhodococcus equi (Rhodococcus hoagii, Prescotella equi)	Streptococcus spp.
Pasteurella multocida	Streptococcus suis	Actinobacillus spp.	Pasteurella spp.
	Haemophilus parasuis	Klebsiella spp.	Staphylococcus spp.
	Actinobacillus suis		Escherichia coli
	Bordetella bronchiseptica		Anaerobic bacteria

β_2 integrin leukocyte adhesion molecule CD11a,b,c/CD18. Affected cattle have persistent marked neutrophilia and develop a variety of chronic bacterial infections, including severe chronic bronchopneumonia with bronchiectasis as a result of ineffective neutrophil function.

Morphology. *The typical gross appearance of bronchopneumonia is irregular, somewhat symmetrical consolidation in cranioventral regions* (see Fig. 5-36A), and most cranioventral lung lesions in domestic animals represent bronchopneumonia. There are, however, several exceptions to this rule. First, some viral infections, including bovine respiratory syncytial virus and influenza A virus in swine, typically induce a cranioventral pattern of bronchointerstitial pneumonia that can easily be mistaken for bronchopneumonia. Second, the lesions of bronchopneumonia in swine caused by *Actinobacillus pleuropneumoniae* and *Actinobacillus suis* usually affect the caudal lung lobes. Third, whereas the lesions of bronchopneumonia in dogs and cats may be cranioventral, it is not unusual to find a patchy distribution throughout the lung.

Consolidation—an increase in texture or induration—is best detected on a cut section to avoid the pleura, with deep and purposeful palpation of individual lobules. The lesions are dark red-purple, maroon, or pink-gray depending on the age and nature of the process, but a color change without altered texture often represents congestion or hemorrhage rather than bronchopneumonia. The cut surface is usually edematous, and catarrhal or purulent material can be expressed from small airways in subacute cases. In contrast, there is no exudate in fulminant cases because leukocytes are enmeshed in a tangle of fibrin, and the affected lung is discolored, dry, or edematous, and cuts crisply. Lesions of bronchopneumonia have a lobular or lobar distribution.

- **Lobular bronchopneumonia** *involves some lobules in their entirety, whereas adjacent lobules are unaffected,* most notably at the border of the lesions. It reflects the slow expansion of such lesions, and is most apparent in species with well-developed interlobular septa, such as cattle and swine.
- **Lobar pneumonia** *is characterized by consolidation of an entire pulmonary lobe.* This is usually a fulminating bronchopneumonia, and typical causes are *M. haemolytica* in cattle, *Actinobacillus pleuropneumoniae* in swine, and aspiration pneumonia. In many such cases, the pulmonary parenchymal lesions are accompanied by *pleuritis*, which may vary from a dull granular appearance to a spectacular coating of fibrin with large pockets of edema.

Histologically, the nidus of inflammation in bronchopneumonia is in the bronchiolar-alveolar junction. Neutrophils begin to infiltrate these air spaces about 30 minutes after experimental infection. In early bronchopneumonia, bronchioles and adjacent alveoli are filled with neutrophils and sometimes cell debris, mucus, fibrin, and macrophages, and the wall of the bronchiole is edematous and infiltrated by neutrophils. By the time the bronchopneumonia is clinically apparent, the exudate has usually filled bronchioles and alveoli throughout the lobule (see Fig. 5-36B). The bronchiolar epithelium is usually normal; extensive bronchiolar necrosis suggests an underlying viral infection. However, bronchiolar necrosis can develop during experimental infection with *M. haemolytica* and probably with other bacteria, and is thought to represent neutrophil-mediated damage to the epithelium. Suppurative or lymphoplasmacytic inflammation may be visible in the bronchi but, despite the term "*broncho*pneumonia," this is not always apparent and not a requirement of the diagnosis. Alveoli in mild or early lesions are atelectatic and edematous, but this is obscured by neutrophils in severe lesions.

Resolution and sequelae. Resolution of bronchopneumonia is possible if the infectious agent is destroyed by the immune response or antimicrobial therapy. Neutrophils undergo apoptosis within a day or 2, and fibrin may be removed by plasmin and/or phagocytosed by macrophages. Macrophages and extracellular debris are mostly cleared through the airways with the aid of coughing and collateral ventilation. If there is minimal damage to the alveolar septa and blood vessels, catarrhal or mild purulent bronchopneumonia can begin to resolve within 7-10 days and return to normal within 3-4 weeks. In ruminants and swine, the lack of collateral ventilation impedes clearance of alveolar exudates, and these species have a greater propensity to develop chronic suppurative bronchopneumonia.

Death from fulminant lobar bronchopneumonia may occur with only 20-40% of the lung affected. In such cases, the cause of death is not respiratory failure but rather *sepsis*, with or without bacteremia, and these animals are profoundly depressed and have grossly apparent petechiae on serosal surfaces and muscles throughout the body. *Bacteremia* is frequent in animals with severe peracute bronchopneumonia. In mouse models, both the bacterial pathogen and the genetic background of the mouse dictate the frequency of bacteremia and subsequent mortality. The extent of lung involvement in animals with chronic bronchopneumonia—up to 80% of the lung in some calves with chronic *Mycoplasma bovis* pneumonia—highlights the tremendous reserve capacity of the lung that must be consumed before bronchopneumonia causes death by simple filling of alveoli with exudate, and emphasizes sepsis as the major mechanism of death in acute disease.

Reduced lung function does occur in bronchopneumonia. The obvious reason is the edema and neutrophils that fill alveoli and bronchioles, which impede ventilation of affected alveoli and block gas exchange in the alveolus. Further, filling of air spaces and disruption of the surfactant system reduces the compliance of the lung and increases the work of breathing. Finally, pulmonary arterial vasoconstriction is the natural response to hypoxia in hypoventilated alveoli. However, prostaglandins and other inflammatory mediators cause vasodilation and thus maintain perfusion of the pneumonic tissue, resulting in shunting of non-oxygenated blood past the hypoventilated alveoli into the systemic circulation; this ventilation-perfusion mismatching worsens the hypoxemia.

Chronic suppurative bronchopneumonia *develops if the infection remains active.* In many such cases, the lesions are colonized by secondary pathogens, such as *Trueperella (Arcanobacterium) pyogenes* in cattle, and the primary cause can no longer be identified. Chronic bronchopneumonia may manifest simply as filling of bronchioles and alveoli with neutrophils, caused by persistent bacterial infection and ongoing recruitment of neutrophils. In other cases, the chronic infection results in *pulmonary fibrosis, bronchiectasis, abscess formation, or sequestration.* Extensive fibrinous exudate or injury to alveolar septa may heal by fibroplasia, which causes thickening of alveolar septa or locally extensive areas of fibrosis. Organization of fibrinous pleural exudate produces *pleural adhesions. Abscesses* develop within areas of chronic bacterial infection (eFig. 5-51; see eFig. 5-50).

A **sequestrum** *is a mass of necrotic lung parenchyma, often separated from viable lung tissue by purulent exudate, and usually encased in a fibrous capsule.* Sequestra commonly develop from the infarcted lung tissue in contagious bovine pleuropneumonia, and in pneumonia caused by *M. haemolytica* or *M. bovis* in cattle or *Actinobacillus pleuropneumoniae* in swine. The lesions vary in size from several centimeters to large masses that occupy much of one lung (eFig. 5-52), and are firm, gray or red, and may be friable or have a foul odor. *Sequestra are permanent and nonfunctional, and act as a nidus of persistent bacterial infection.* "Pulmonary sequestration" describes quite a different condition in human pathology, wherein a congenitally anomalous mass of pulmonary tissue is not connected to the bronchial tree (see Congenital anomalies, later).

Aspiration pneumonia. *Aspiration pneumonia refers to pneumonia caused by aspiration of foreign material, often in liquid form, reaching the lungs through the airways.* This distinguishes it from most bronchopneumonias that are caused by inhalation of tiny droplets or particles. The response to the aspirated material depends on 3 factors: (1) the nature of the material; (2) the bacteria that are carried with it; and (3) the distribution of the material in the lungs.

Conditions that cause septic aspiration pneumonia in animals include force-feeding or inadvertent passing of a nasogastric tube into the lungs; vomiting and regurgitation (e.g., megaesophagus, myasthenia gravis, laryngeal paralysis, and parvoviral enteritis in dogs, recumbency or white muscle disease in cattle); anesthesia; cleft palate; neurologic or laryngeal disease; mouth breathing, including choanal atresia; and bronchoesophageal fistula.

The lesions of septic aspiration pneumonia are similar to those described for other forms of bronchopneumonia, with

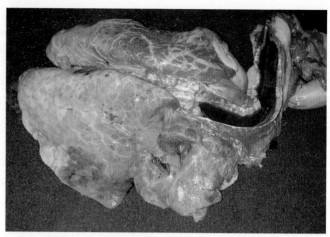

Figure 5-37 **Aspiration pneumonia** in a dairy cow. The unilateral distribution, green discoloration and necrosis, and foul smell are characteristic of pneumonia from aspiration of rumen content. Interlobular emphysema is extensive in the left lung.

some characteristic features (Fig. 5-37). First, they are usually localized or unilateral rather than bilaterally symmetrical. Second, aspiration, especially of anaerobes, incites extensive necrosis, liquefaction, foul smell, and rapid green discoloration of the affected tissue. Third, in herbivores, plant material may be visible microscopically along with an associated inflammatory reaction. In contrast, grossly visible plant material is often absent, and when present is of little diagnostic significance. Ruminants frequently aspirate rumen content at the time of death, but this has no associated inflammatory reaction and is irrelevant to the cause of death. Finally, in cases of septic aspiration pneumonia, bacterial culture yields mixed flora of relatively low pathogenicity, whereas one or a few recognizable pathogens are isolated from cases of opportunistic bronchopneumonia.

The above conditions introduce large numbers of bacteria into the lung, in contrast to the aspiration of mostly sterile material, such as milk, mineral oil, radiographic contrast material, (eFig. 5-53) or drugs. These sterile reactions are referred to as aspiration pneumonitis in human medicine.

Widespread distribution of inhaled milk is occasionally observed in *pail-fed or tube-fed calves.* The course of the disease in these cases can be as short as 1 day. The gross appearance is not characteristic. The lungs remain inflated; they are hyperemic, and excessive fluid may be present in the small bronchi. Histologically, there is acute bronchiolitis with various degrees of acute alveolitis, and the air spaces are filled with deep-staining amphophilic material containing variably sized clear lipid droplets (Fig. 5-38).

The aspiration of vomitus in a simple-stomached animal may be rapidly fatal as a result of laryngeal spasm or acute pulmonary edema, before there is time for much inflammation to develop. Alternatively, acid-induced lung injury can lead to infiltration of neutrophils and diffuse alveolar damage. Disease resulting from aspiration of oil is discussed later (see Lipid pneumonia and alveolar filling disorders, later).

Further reading

Caswell JL. Failure of respiratory defenses in the pathogenesis of bacterial pneumonia of cattle. Vet Pathol 2014;51:393-409.

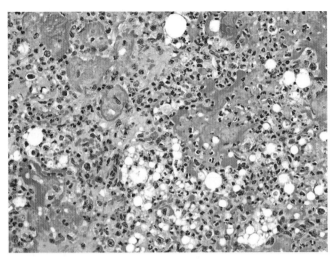

Figure 5-38 Milk aspiration in a dairy calf. Alveoli are filled with densely amphophilic fluid (protein-rich milk), extracellular lipid droplets, and neutrophils.

Dagleish MP, et al. Characterization and time course of pulmonary lesions in calves after intratracheal infection with *Pasteurella multocida* A:3. J Comp Pathol 2010;142:157-169.

Kogan DA, et al. Clinical, clinicopathologic, and radiographic findings in dogs with aspiration pneumonia: 88 cases (2004-2006). J Am Vet Med Assoc 2008;233:1742-1747.

Interstitial and bronchointerstitial lung disease

Interstitial lung disease *is a broad term that describes damage to, or inflammation involving, the alveolar or interlobular septa, which represent the interstitium of the lung.* This contrasts with bronchitis and bronchiolitis, which involve the airways, and bronchopneumonia, which forms exudate in the airspaces of the alveoli and distal airways (see Fig. 5-30). The terminology used to classify the interstitial lung diseases suffers from a lack of consensus in veterinary pathology. We use the term interstitial lung disease to define a broad range of conditions affecting or arising from the pulmonary interstitium. In addition to diffuse alveolar damage, other forms of interstitial lung disease in animals include granulomatous and eosinophilic pneumonia; mononuclear cell infiltrates targeting alveolar septa and vascular adventitia (e.g., porcine reproductive and respiratory syndrome, maedi, and metastrongylid nematode infections such as *Muellerius* and *Aelurostrongylus*), multifocal lesions dominated by necrosis (e.g., toxoplasmosis or canine herpesvirus infection) or epithelial proliferation and fibrosis (e.g., equine multinodular pulmonary fibrosis), and most pneumoconioses. There are many histologic patterns of interstitial lung disease identified in humans, including diffuse alveolar damage, usual interstitial pneumonia, nonspecific interstitial pneumonia, organizing pneumonia, respiratory bronchiolitis, desquamative interstitial pneumonia, and lymphocytic interstitial pneumonia; most of these have little relevance to diseases of domestic animals.

The term "**interstitial pneumonia**" is used in 2 different ways in veterinary medicine: as a synonym for interstitial lung disease to describe a broad range of inflammatory (e.g., viral) or noninflammatory (e.g., toxic) diseases affecting the interstitium, or more narrowly to describe increased numbers of leukocytes, usually lymphocytes and macrophages, within the alveolar septa (such as in porcine reproductive and respiratory syndrome). The term "**atypical pneumonia**" has been used in the past to describe interstitial pneumonias; we suggest that its use be abandoned because it also denotes unusual forms of bronchopneumonia.

Diffuse alveolar damage. *The most commonly identified form of interstitial lung disease is diffuse alveolar damage (DAD),* which represents diffuse injury to type I pneumocytes or endothelial cells in the alveolar septa, and results in pulmonary edema, formation of hyaline membranes, proliferation of type II pneumocytes, and interstitial fibrosis (Fig. 5-39). *Acute respiratory distress syndrome* is a clinically defined condition with an acute onset of bilateral pulmonary disease characterized by hypoxemia but no evidence of left atrial hypertension; diffuse alveolar damage is the histologic lesion in many cases.

Gross lesions *of DAD are widely distributed throughout the lungs, often with greater involvement of caudodorsal regions* (see Fig. 5-39A). This pattern is in sharp contrast to the cranioventral distribution in most cases of bronchopneumonia. The lesions can either be uniformly diffuse, or lobular with a resulting checkerboard appearance throughout the lung. Histologically, most causes of diffuse alveolar damage follow a stereotyped pattern of response, with an *acute exudative phase, subacute proliferative phase, and chronic fibrosing phase.* Because of the similar histologic appearance irrespective of etiology, identifying the specific cause is often based on clinical investigations and identifying lesions in other organs.

In the **acute exudative phase,** alveolar septa are congested, and alveoli contain protein-rich edema fluid with flocculent material or delicate interlacing fibrin strands and variable numbers of neutrophils and macrophages. Although it may be histologically indistinct, alveolar edema is highly detrimental to lung function, and more readily revealed by diagnostic imaging than by histopathology. *The characteristic pathologic finding is the presence of hyaline membranes,* which are aggregates of fibrin, other serum proteins, and cell debris (see Fig. 5-39B). These appear in alveoli and/or alveolar ducts as linear masses of discrete, densely eosinophilic material lining the junction between the airspace and the septum. Because type I pneumocytes are 10 times less permeable than endothelial cells, injury to type I pneumocytes causes loss of interstitial fluid into the alveolus. Alveolar type I and type II pneumocytes reabsorb alveolar fluid by active transport, so injury to these cells further promotes alveolar edema. Although type II pneumocytes cover only 10% of the alveolar surface, they are critical in production and recycling of surfactant lipids and proteins, and their damage leads to abnormal intra-alveolar surface tensions that further damage the epithelium. Similarly, production of secretory phospholipase A_2 in the early stages of diffuse alveolar damage degrades phosphatidylglycerol and results in surfactant dysfunction.

Type II pneumocytes *repair the alveolar epithelium by spreading along the alveolar surface, proliferating to repopulate the epithelium, secreting new basement membrane, and differentiating into membranous type I pneumocytes.* Type II pneumocytes rapidly spread to cover the denuded alveolar surface prior to undergoing mitosis. Single type II pneumocytes are impossible to distinguish from alveolar macrophages on hematoxylin and eosin–stained (H&E) sections; however, type II pneumocytes are more easily recognized when they form a single layer of cuboidal cells lining the alveolus (see Fig. 5-39C), and cytokeratin immunohistochemistry can be used to confirm subtle lesions. Proliferation of type II pneumocytes

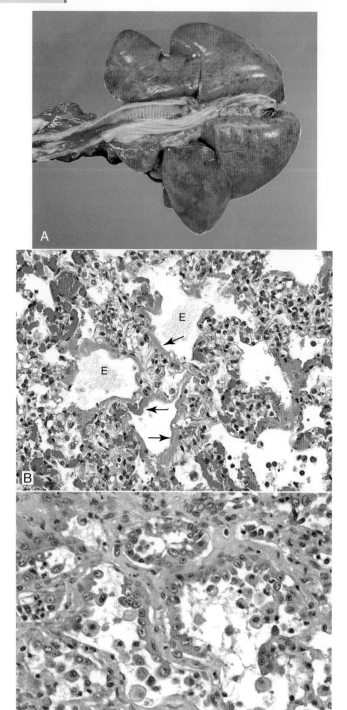

Figure 5-39 Interstitial lung disease. A. The lung is uniformly firmer than normal, with rubbery texture that lacks the sponginess of normal lung. The cause in this dog was not identified. **B.** Hyaline membranes (arrows) line the alveoli, and there is protein-rich edema that appears as flocculent material in the alveoli (E). From a 5-month-old foal with severe bronchointerstitial pneumonia and minor lesions of *Rhodococcus* pneumonia. **C.** Alveolar septa have marked diffuse thickening by fibrous tissue, with extensive type II pneumocyte proliferation with increased numbers of foamy alveolar macrophages. Chronic interstitial lung disease in a West Highland White Terrier.

is initially observed at 2-3 days and is extensive by 6 days after insult. It is a dysfunctional stage of epithelial repair because these cuboidal cells block effective gas exchange. Type II pneumocytes are the major source of basement membrane if this structure has been previously damaged. If the injurious stimulus has been removed, then the type II cells differentiate into type I pneumocytes, and surplus cells undergo apoptosis. The cuboidal type II cells may no longer be visible histologically by 5-7 days after a single mild insult, but may remain for prolonged periods if the injurious stimulus persists or in the presence of interstitial fibrosis. In some cases, the remarkable proliferation of type II pneumocytes may be mistaken for carcinoma.

Interstitial fibrosis develops in 2 ways. Fibrinous alveolar exudates may be invaded by fibroblasts and organized into fibrous tissue that resembles granulation tissue in a skin wound; this fibrous tissue is later incorporated into the alveolar wall and covered by type II pneumocytes. Alternatively, fibrous tissue may develop within the alveolar septum itself as a consequence of repetitive, persistent, or severe damage to epithelial or endothelial cells, or induced by fibrogenic cytokines produced by alveolar macrophages (see Fig. 5-39C). Fibroblasts can appear within alveoli by 3-5 days after fibrin exudation, collagen fibers can be detected histologically by 5-7 days, and fibrosis may be well developed by 14 days. Myofibroblasts or smooth muscle cells are a prominent feature of some interstitial lung diseases, particularly in sheep (maedi) and cats (feline idiopathic pulmonary fibrosis).

The intimate encounters shared by alveolar epithelial cells, fibroblasts, and macrophages are crucial to understanding the chronic sequelae of diffuse alveolar damage. Normal type II pneumocytes limit fibroblast proliferation and the development of fibrosis; conversely, repetitively injured type II pneumocytes and macrophages (or those experiencing endoplasmic reticulum stress) secrete transforming growth factor-β and other growth factors that stimulate interstitial fibrosis. On the other hand, growth factors secreted by fibroblasts and macrophages promote type II pneumocyte proliferation and may preclude their differentiation to type I pneumocytes, and this possibly accounts for the observation that fibrotic alveolar septa are often lined by cuboidal epithelial cells. Alveolar fibrosis is not necessarily permanent, as fibrous tissue is remodeled and may be removed by matrix metalloproteases. However, because this process occurs over many months, and because the cause of chronic injury to the alveolar septa is often not identified or eliminated, *the finding of marked interstitial fibrosis confers a guarded prognosis.*

Diffuse alveolar damage causes hypoxemia that is refractory to oxygen supplementation, the difference between alveolar and arterial oxygen tension resulting from the barrier to diffusion of oxygen across the alveolar wall. Carbon dioxide diffuses more readily than oxygen, so hypercapnia is less frequent than hypoxemia in interstitial lung disease. Pulmonary compliance is reduced, which increases the work of breathing and may reduce the functional lung volume. Cardiac function is expected to be normal.

The causes of diffuse alveolar damage are legion (Box 5-6), and most induce direct injury to alveolar epithelial cells or capillary endothelial cells in the alveolar septa. Many **infectious agents** infect type I pneumocytes, including respiratory syncytial viruses, parainfluenza viruses, herpesviruses, feline calicivirus, adenoviruses, and *Toxoplasma gondii*. Many viruses also infect airway epithelial cells and cause bronchiolar

BOX • 5-6

Causes of acute or chronic diffuse alveolar damage, a form of interstitial lung disease

- Pulmonary infections: many viruses, *Toxoplasma gondii*, feline infectious peritonitis virus, ascarid larval migration, *Dictyocaulus*
- Thermal injury: inhalation of steam or smoke in barn or house fires
- Acid-induced injury from aspiration of sterile vomitus in monogastric animals
- Toxic gases: nitrogen dioxide, sulfur dioxide, chlorine, 100% oxygen, ammonia, phosgene, ozone
- Ingested toxins: paraquat, kerosene, 3-methylindole, ipomeanol, perilla mint ketone, *Brassica*, Crofton weed
- Septicemia and endotoxemia, disseminated intravascular coagulation, possibly shock
- Massive trauma, strangulation, near drowning, pulmonary contusion
- Ischemic lung injury: lung lobe torsion, reperfusion injury
- Chronic left heart failure
- Pancreatitis, uremia, parvoviral enteritis, irradiation
- Surfactant dysfunction: prematurity (hyaline membrane disease), inherited defects in surfactant proteins B or C
- Ventilator-induced lung injury
- Adverse drug reactions
- Acute hypersensitivity pneumonitis

necrosis; this pattern of damage to bronchioles and alveoli represents bronchointerstitial pneumonia and is discussed later.

Noninfectious causes of direct injury to type I pneumocytes include *physical forces* (as in surface tension in neonatal hyaline membrane disease, or ventilator-induced lung injury); *thermal and chemical injury* from inhalation of steam or smoke, as occurs in barn or house fires; *acid-induced injury* from aspiration of sterile vomitus in monogastric animals (associated with vomiting, anesthesia, or seizures); and inhalation of *toxic gases*, such as chlorine, nitrogen dioxide, sulfur dioxide, phosgene gas, and high concentrations of oxygen. Other xenobiotics must be *metabolized* by type II pneumocytes to reactive intermediates that damage the alveolar epithelium. These include 3-methylindole, ipomeanol, perilla mint, Crofton weed, and chemotherapeutic nitrosourea, and are considered in the section Toxic lung injury.

Ventilator-induced lung injury occurs when high tidal volumes cause injury to the alveolar septa and/or the small bronchioles. The most intuitive mechanism is overdistension of alveoli with damage to the septa, leading to interlobular emphysema, pneumomediastinum, or pneumothorax. Less obvious is the repetitive trauma suffered by alveoli and small bronchioles as they collapse at the end of expiration and are subjected to the high pressures required for reinflation. This mechanical strain and shear stress damages the type I pneumocytes and endothelial cells, and thus results in alveolar edema, formation of hyaline membranes, and infiltration of neutrophils in the alveoli or terminal bronchioles. Finally, ventilator-induced injury may result in neutrophil influx and increased levels of proinflammatory cytokines in the alveolar lining fluid, and this inflammatory response may be stimulated by abnormal stretch or strain pressures on macrophages or

epithelial cells. The histologic lesions include hyaline membranes, bronchiolar necrosis, and/or neutrophil infiltration into alveoli, but it is often impossible to determine if these lesions are caused by mechanical ventilation or pre-existing lung disease. Pneumothorax, if present, is more suggestive of ventilator-induced injury, if the clinical history is supportive.

Sepsis and endotoxemia *are well-recognized causes of interstitial lung lesions.* Sepsis induces an inflammatory cascade that affects the function of endothelial cells in the alveolar septa, by cytokine-induced retraction of endothelial cells leading to increased permeability, neutrophil-mediated damage to the endothelium or matrix proteins, and/or by promoting capillary thrombosis. Sepsis also causes surfactant dysfunction; in addition to direct injury to surfactant-producing type II pneumocytes, the serum proteins that flood the alveoli inhibit surfactant function. This in turn provokes atelectasis and abnormal surface tensions in the alveoli that physically damage the type I pneumocytes.

Septicemic lung injury has various histologic manifestations (Fig. 5-40). One is a pulmonary interstitial reaction (interstitial pneumonia), in which the alveolar septa appear hypercellular resulting from hypertrophy of pulmonary intravascular macrophages and/or aggregation of neutrophils and mononuclear cells. A second manifestation is marked congestion and serofibrinous exudation into the alveoli, which appears histologically as flocculent or loosely fibrillar material in the alveoli. Third, some cases have hyaline membranes and type II pneumocyte proliferation typical of diffuse alveolar damage. Finally, thrombi may be identified in small venules and capillaries in some cases of septicemia. Apart from severity and chronicity, the reasons for these differing manifestations are not apparent.

Additional causes of diffuse alveolar damage *include massive trauma, shock, disseminated intravascular coagulation, pancreatitis, multi-organ failure, postvaccinal reactions, and uremia.* Although these associations are established, the exact mechanisms are poorly described. Neutrophil-induced lung injury contributes to diffuse alveolar damage in several experimental models, but the importance of this effect in natural disease is controversial.

Bronchointerstitial pneumonia. Bronchointerstitial pneumonia has 2 meanings in veterinary pathology. *Usually, it denotes the presence of both bronchiolar necrosis and diffuse alveolar damage, and is thus a manifestation of injury to both the bronchiolar and the alveolar epithelium* (see Fig. 5-30). In this context, bronchointerstitial pneumonia can be caused by aerogenous viral infections or inhaled or ingested toxins that affect both of these cell types. *Alternatively, bronchointerstitial pneumonia has been used to describe diseases in which mononuclear cells encircle airways and infiltrate alveolar septa,* such as in *Mycoplasma hyopneumoniae* infections of swine or in mild or subacute viral infections. These patterns are not to be confused with bronchopneumonia, which in a sense is the opposite of bronchointerstitial pneumonia. In bronchopneumonia, bronchioles and alveoli are filled with leukocytes as a result of bacterial infection of the airspace, but necrosis of the bronchiolar or alveolar epithelium is not usually present.

Further reading

American Thoracic Society/European Respiratory Society. International Multidisciplinary Consensus Classification of the Idiopathic Interstitial Pneumonias. Am J Respir Crit Care Med 2002;165:277-304.

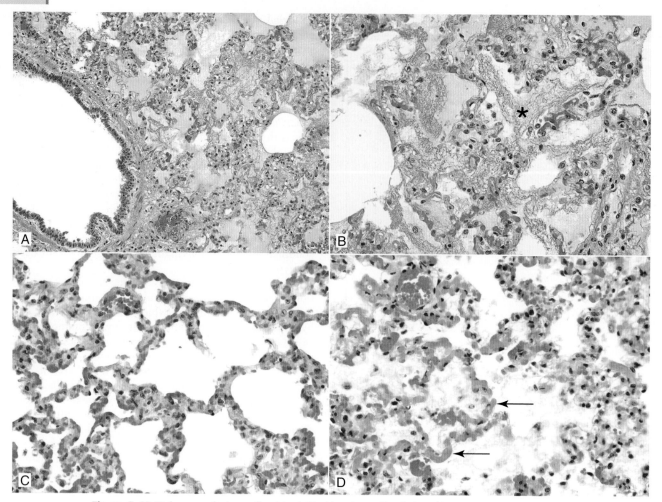

Figure 5-40 Pulmonary lesions of sepsis. A, B. Alveoli are flooded with protein-rich edema fluid, which appears as lightly eosinophilic material containing delicate strands of fibrin (asterisk), in a heifer, with sepsis caused by necrotizing colitis. **C.** An alternative appearance is hypercellularity of alveolar septa, probably corresponding to hypertrophied pulmonary intravascular macrophages, in a cow, with sepsis caused by acute mastitis. **D.** A third manifestation of sepsis is thrombosis (arrows) of capillaries in the alveolar septa, in a cow, with sepsis caused by periparturient acute mastitis.

Orgeig S, et al. Recent advances in alveolar biology: evolution and function of alveolar proteins. Respir Physiol Neurobiol 2010; 173(Suppl.):S43-S54.

Specific noninfectious interstitial lung diseases

Anaphylaxis and hypersensitivity pneumonitis. Anaphylaxis affects the lungs in cattle, causing bronchoconstriction, pulmonary hypertension, and systemic hypotension. The lungs are congested and contain alveolar and interlobular edema, the trachea and bronchi contain froth, and emphysema may result from the marked dyspnea. Congestion or edema of the larynx is prominent and potentially fatal in some cases. Bronchoconstriction without marked alveolar changes is more typical of anaphylaxis in cats and horses.

Other reactions to injected materials result from administration of products contaminated by bacteria or their toxins, or inadvertent intravenous administration of vaccines or other drugs. These are not mediated by IgE, and may result from activation of complement, coagulation, or pulmonary macrophages. Whether such reactions should be termed anaphylac-

tic or anaphylactoid is a matter of debate. The onset of disease is typically 2-8 hours after vaccination, whereas IgE-mediated anaphylaxis usually occurs within 5-30 minutes. Histologic lesions include alveolar edema containing macrophages and neutrophils, congested alveolar septa with infiltrates of mononuclear cells and neutrophils, and periarterial hemorrhages. In diagnostic cases, additional testing may be necessary to distinguish anaphylaxis, sepsis, and other mechanisms of postvaccinal reaction.

Hypersensitivity pneumonitis in animals occurs mainly in adult cattle reared in confinement, and rarely in horses, and often affects multiple animals in the group. It results from chronic inhalation of spores of thermophilic actinomycetes (especially *Saccharopolyspora rectivirgula*, formerly *Micropolyspora faeni*) in moldy hay, leading to inflammatory reactions that occur through several mechanisms concurrently. The bacteria directly activate complement by the alternative pathway, and there is solid evidence for immune-complex (type III) reactions, even though the morphology suggests a delayed (type IV) hypersensitivity reaction. In cattle, tiny gray foci may be grossly visible throughout the lung.

Lymphoplasmacytic or granulomatous infiltrates are consistently present in alveolar septa, often around the bronchi and bronchioles, and multinucleated macrophages are occasionally seen. During acute exacerbations, noncaseating granulomas are accompanied by edema and infiltration of eosinophils, neutrophils, and lymphocytes. Proliferation of alveolar type II pneumocytes, fibrosis of the alveolar septa and peribronchiolar tissue, and bronchiolitis obliterans occurs in chronic cases. Hyaline membranes are uncommon but may follow acute challenge. Similarly, the characteristic lesions in humans and in experimentally challenged dogs are airway-centered, with non-necrotizing poorly formed granulomas in the bronchiolar adventitia and extending into alveolar septa, mononuclear cell infiltrates in bronchioles and centrilobular alveolar septa, peribronchiolar fibrosis, and bronchiolar epithelial hyperplasia. *The airway-centered distribution is a major diagnostic clue.*

Further reading

Ramsay JD, et al. Fatal adverse pulmonary reaction in calves after inadvertent intravenous vaccination. Vet Pathol 2005;42:492-495.

Shmuel DL, Cortes Y. Anaphylaxis in dogs and cats. J Vet Emerg Crit Care 2013;23:377-394.

Granulomatous interstitial pneumonia. Granulomatous pneumonia has diverse infectious causes, including *Mycobacterium*, *Rhodococcus*, *Actinobacillus*, *Actinomyces*, and *Nocardia*; the fungal pathogens *Blastomyces*, *Cryptococcus*, *Coccidioides*, *Histoplasma*, and *Pneumocystis*; a wide variety of parasites, including *Angiostrongylus* in dogs and *Dictyocaulus* in cattle; occasional viruses, such as porcine circovirus 2, equine herpesvirus 5, and feline infectious peritonitis virus; and rarely protozoa, such as *Balamuthia* or *Acanthamoeba*. Noninfectious conditions include silicosis and other pneumoconioses, hypersensitivity pneumonitis, inadvertent inhalation of barium-containing contrast materials, intravenous injection in horses of Freund's complete adjuvant or immunostimulants containing mycobacterial cell-wall extracts, porcine dermatosis vegetans, endogenous lipid pneumonia, and alveolar histiocytosis.

Eosinophilic interstitial pneumonia. The eosinophilic interstitial pneumonias are a compilation of pulmonary diseases united by the presence of eosinophils in the alveoli or alveolar septa. The best described are those caused by parasites, which are discussed more fully in later sections but include both adult parasites residing in the lung and migrating larva. Other conditions probably represent hypersensitivity reactions. Those primarily affecting the airways (including **eosinophilic bronchopneumopathy**) are discussed above. **Eosinophilic pulmonary granulomatosis** is a rare condition in dogs, characterized by chronic cough, variable dyspnea, and blood eosinophilia. The lungs contain nodular necrotizing lesions formed by eosinophils, epithelioid macrophages, and fibrosis, with type II pneumocyte proliferation and eosinophil infiltrates in the surrounding alveoli. Many dogs with eosinophilic pulmonary granulomatosis have heartworm disease, although microfilariae are not detected in the granulomas. **Less severe eosinophilic pneumonias** are poorly described in dogs and cats, in part because the steroid responsiveness of many cases precludes their examination at autopsy. The alveoli contain eosinophils, lymphocytes, and macrophages, and the degree of fibrosis is variable. A similar condition occurs in horses, and should be distinguished from the eosinophilic granulomas of multisystemic eosinophilic epitheliotropic disease. **Other causes** of eosinophilic lung disease in dogs and cats include angiotropic lymphoma (lymphomatoid granulomatosis), eosinophil infiltrates associated with carcinomas and lymphomas, other parasitisms, and fungal infections. Drug reactions cause eosinophil-rich lesions in humans, but are not described in animals.

Further reading

Bell SA, et al. Idiopathic chronic eosinophilic pneumonia in 7 horses. J Vet Intern Med 2008;22:648-653.

Katajavuori P, et al. Eosinophilic pulmonary granulomatosis in a young dog with prolonged remission after treatment. J Small Anim Pract 2013;54:40-43.

Acute interstitial lung disease in feedlot cattle. Interstitial lung disease commonly causes an acute onset of dyspnea and open-mouth breathing in feedlot beef cattle, particularly those approaching slaughter weights, and is most prevalent in the summer and autumn. Heifers are disproportionately affected in many reports, and the case fatality rate is high. The gross lesions are often variegated as a result of a lobular distribution, and are most prominent in the caudodorsal lung. The red, rubbery, edematous, heavy lungs fail to collapse when the chest is opened, and interlobular and subpleural emphysema is frequent (Fig. 5-41). Many cases have concurrent gross lesions of acute or chronic bacterial bronchopneumonia in the cranioventral lung, but these cases may represent a separate disease. *Hyaline membranes* are the characteristic histologic feature of the acute lesions, and *type II pneumocyte proliferation* is often present. More variable lesions include bronchiolitis obliterans, infiltration of neutrophils and eosinophils, and patchy alveolar hemorrhages that possibly arise from emphysematous rupture of alveolar septa.

The cause is uncertain. Epidemiologic evidence suggests 3-methylindole, melengestrol acetate (fed to feedlot heifers to suppress estrus), high-energy diets, dusty environment, hot weather, and concurrent bacterial infection as possible causes or contributing factors. Although bovine respiratory syncytial

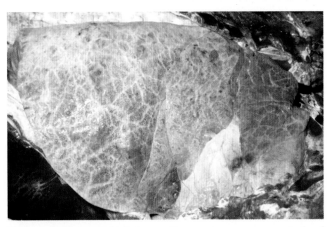

Figure 5-41 Interstitial lung disease in a cow, typical of 3-methyindole toxicity. Palpation reveals crepitus caused by interlobular emphysema, but individual lobules are firmer than normal and edematous. (Courtesy of the University of Guelph.)

virus occasionally causes acute bronchointerstitial pneumonia soon after arrival in feedlots, it seems not to cause the form of interstitial lung disease occurring late in the feeding period. Some more chronic cases, in which eosinophils and granulomas are present, may represent a hypersensitivity reaction.

Further reading

Stanford K, et al. Effect of dietary melengestrol acetate on the incidence of acute interstitial pneumonia in feedlot heifers. Can J Vet Res 2006;70:218-225.

Interstitial and bronchointerstitial pneumonia in foals. Bronchointerstitial pneumonia in 1- to 4-month-old foals has been recognized as a sporadic disease for many years, yet the etiology remains mysterious. Affected foals may be found dead without premonitory signs or develop acute onset of severe dyspnea, tachypnea, and pyrexia, with profound hypoxemia and variable hypercapnia. Case fatality rates are high and the foals respond poorly to therapy. It remains possible that there is not a single etiology for this disease, but that the reaction pattern may result from any of several infectious and noninfectious insults.

At autopsy, lesions are present throughout the lungs in a diffuse or lobular pattern. The lungs are firm, heavy, edematous, reddened, and fail to collapse (eFig. 5-54). Concurrent lesions of *Rhodococcus equi* pneumonia are present in up to 40% of cases, with cranioventral bronchopneumonia or scattered foci of liquefactive pyogranulomatous pneumonia. *Histologic lesions* reflect the bronchointerstitial pneumonia, and include necrosis of the epithelium lining terminal bronchioles, alveolar hyaline membranes, exudation of fibrin and a few neutrophils in alveoli, and syncytial cells in the bronchi or alveoli (see Fig. 5-39B). The prevalence of syncytial cells and the extent of bronchiolar versus alveolar lesions are variable.

A viral etiology is possible, as the age of affected foals correlates with waning maternal passive immunity. A respiratory syncytial virus and equid herpesvirus 2 (EHV-2) have been identified in some cases, but attempts to identify viral agents in the vast majority of cases have been unsuccessful. Other proposed causes include an aberrant response to *R. equi* or other bacterial pathogens, surfactant dysfunction resulting from production of secretory phospholipase A_2 by infected macrophages, a complication of hyperthermia resulting from bacterial pneumonia or treatment with erythromycin; endotoxemia; and xenobiotics, including 3-methylindole, pyrrolizidine alkaloids, and pentachlorophenol, that are metabolized by club cells and type II pneumocytes. *Pneumocystis carinii* infection (see Infectious respiratory diseases of horses) is a differential diagnosis for subacute lesions with extensive type II pneumocyte hyperplasia and foamy macrophages in alveoli.

Further reading

Britton AP, Robinson JH. Isolation of influenza A virus from a 7-day-old foal with bronchointerstitial pneumonia. Can Vet J 2002;43:55-56.

Donkey pulmonary fibrosis. Donkey pulmonary fibrosis (DPF) is a common finding, having been documented in the lungs of 35% of aged donkeys (mean age 30 years). DPF may be discovered as an incidental finding at autopsy or, when there is more extensive lung involvement, may result in chronic respiratory disease and debilitation. *Grossly*, DPF appears as *multifocal and coalescing large foci of visceral pleural fibrosis* (without parietal pleural fibrosis) over the dorsal lungs (eFig. 5-55). *Histologically*, there is *pleural and subpleural fibrosis with subpleural intra-alveolar fibrosis* and occasional foci of septal and peribronchiolar fibrosis, as well as arterial and venous intimal fibrosis. In the most severely affected regions, fibrosis extends to the ventral lung. Elastin staining of affected tissue reveals abundant elastin fibers within the regions of fibrosis and disruption of the normal pleural elastic fiber architecture. The pathology of DPF shares features with pleuroparenchymal pulmonary fibrosis in humans, a rare form of idiopathic interstitial pneumonia. The cause of DPF remains unknown. There is no evidence that the development of DPF is related to lung infection with asinine herpesviruses (AHV) as has been reported with AHV-4 and AHV-5 and the development of chronic interstitial pneumonia in donkeys (see Infectious respiratory diseases of horses, later).

Further reading

Miele A, et al. Chronic pleuropulmonary fibrosis and elastosis of aged donkeys—similarities to human pleuroparenchymal fibroelastosis (PPFE). Chest 2014;145:1325-1332.

Interstitial lung disease in dogs. Diffuse alveolar damage manifesting clinically as **acute respiratory distress syndrome** is occasionally encountered in dogs of various ages. Affected animals develop acute onset of dyspnea with tachypnea, and variable coughing and lethargy, which is usually rapidly progressive and fatal within 3 days. Findings considered secondary to dyspnea include pneumothorax and subcutaneous emphysema, and gastroesophageal intussusception. At autopsy, the lungs are diffusely firm with a liver-like texture, edematous and heavy, and mottled (eFig. 5-56; see Fig. 5-39A). *Hyaline membranes* are a nearly consistent feature and often affect alveolar ducts, with proliferation of type II pneumocytes in the less fulminant cases. Epithelial necrosis or attenuation is often present in terminal bronchioles. Diffuse alveolar damage may be considered to result from either direct injury to alveolar epithelium or as a result of *multiple organ dysfunction syndrome*. Specific inciting causes include massive trauma, shock, disseminated intravascular coagulation, septicemia, bacterial pneumonia in other areas of lung, aspiration of sterile gastric acid, smoke inhalation, oxygen toxicity, other toxins, viral infection, near drowning, and strangulation. Many cases are idiopathic. Similar findings, but localized, may be identified in lung lobes that have undergone torsion, or in areas of ischemia resulting from thromboembolism.

West Highland White Terrier dogs, *6-12 years old, develop a syndrome of interstitial fibrosis* with chronic dyspnea, exercise intolerance, or coughing. Histologic lesions include deposition of collagenous matrix in the alveolar septa and around small blood vessels (Fig. 5-42; see Fig. 5-39C). The interstitial fibrosis is diffuse or patchy in distribution but may be more severe near the pleura or bronchioles, and is quite variable in severity between animals. Mildly affected cases have discontinuous deposition of matrix in alveolar septa that is most obvious when it forms concentric rings around alveolar capillaries. Severe cases have distortion of alveoli with honeycombing.

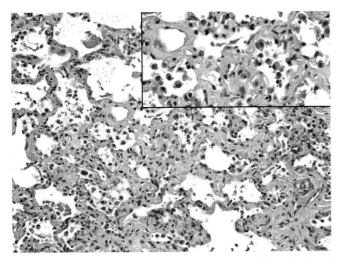

Figure 5-42 Chronic interstitial lung disease in a West Highland White Terrier. There is an irregular distribution within the sections, of marked interstitial fibrosis, hyperplasia of type II pneumocytes, increased numbers of reactive alveolar macrophages, and a light infiltrate of lymphocytes. Inset: higher magnification of alveolar lesion.

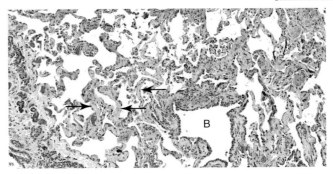

Figure 5-43 Idiopathic pulmonary fibrosis in a cat, with a characteristically irregular distribution of lesions in the lung. In this case, lesions are dominated by interstitial fibrosis (arrows), with mild proliferation of type II pneumocytes and subtle attenuation of bronchiolar (B) epithelium. Other cases display smooth muscle metaplasia of alveolar septa, or more extensive type II pneumocyte proliferation.

interstitial pneumonia and usual interstitial pneumonia in man. J Comp Pathol 2013;149:303-313.

Some cases have proliferation of alveolar type II pneumocytes with atypia, cytomegaly, and occasional multinucleation. Other findings may include proteinaceous material in alveoli, increased number of alveolar macrophages, diffuse alveolar damage with hyaline membranes, or interstitial infiltrates of lymphocytes, plasma cells, and macrophages.

Progressive fibrosing interstitial lung disease of unknown cause also occurs sporadically in adult dogs of a variety of other breeds. Histologically, the disease differs from what is seen in West Highland White Terriers. In these dogs, the fibrosis is not uniformly dense collagen as in usually seen in Westies, but rather consists of a mix of plump fibroblasts, immature collagen, and mild inflammation. The alveolar epithelial cells overlying the regions of fibrosis vary from plump and cuboidal in some cases, to markedly attenuated with features of atypia in others.

Dalmatian dogs, 4-10 months-old, develop an apparently inherited condition characterized by *bronchiolar epithelial hyperplasia and dysplasia*. Affected dogs have a short course of tachypnea, increased respiratory noise, and dyspnea. The lungs are diffusely wet, heavy, firm, and purple-red with scattered hemorrhages. The microscopic findings are multifocal, peribronchiolar, or subpleural, with bronchiolar epithelial cells affected by hyperplasia, atypia, and sometimes squamous metaplasia, as well as alveolar type II pneumocyte proliferation, fibrosis of alveolar septa, and mild infiltrates of mononuclear leukocytes. The adjacent lung tissue is edematous with hyaline membranes.

Further reading

Campbell VL. Respiratory complications in critical illness of small animals. Vet Clin North Am Small Anim Pract 2011;41:709-716.

Syrjä P, et al. Pulmonary histopathology in dalmatians with familial acute respiratory distress syndrome (ARDS). J Comp Pathol 2009;141:254-259.

Syrjä P, et al. The histopathology of idiopathic pulmonary fibrosis in West Highland white terriers shares features of both non-specific

Idiopathic pulmonary fibrosis in cats. Chronic interstitial lung disease is uncommon but not rare in cats, and is usually seen as *chronic progressive tachypnea, respiratory distress, and cough in middle-aged to older cats*. The disease has been likened to idiopathic pulmonary fibrosis (cryptogenic fibrosing alveolitis) in humans. Lesions are often present throughout the lung, but tend to be patchy or multinodular rather than diffuse (eFig. 5-57). The histologic lesions include multifocal or irregular areas in which alveolar septa are remarkably thickened by smooth muscle, fibrosis, and focal clusters of fibroblasts, and myofibroblasts. Alveoli are lined by prominent cuboidal or columnar epithelial cells, which often contain mucus or occasionally undergo squamous metaplasia. There is variation in the relative prominence of the epithelial proliferation and matrix deposition (Fig. 5-43). Interstitial infiltration of lymphocytes is a variable finding, and concurrent bronchioloalveolar carcinomas are identified in some affected cats. The cause of idiopathic pulmonary fibrosis in cats and humans is unknown. Emerging evidence in humans and animal models suggests that apoptosis of type II pneumocytes, resulting from shortened telomere length or from endoplasmic reticulum stress, leads to a failure to maintain and repair the alveolar epithelium. Subsequently, epithelial cell apoptosis is known to stimulate fibrosis in the underlying connective tissue. Thus dysregulation of type II pneumocyte survival and function is a possible mechanism for development of idiopathic pulmonary fibrosis.

Further reading

Williams K, et al. Identification of spontaneous feline idiopathic pulmonary fibrosis: morphology and ultrastructural evidence for a type II pneumocyte defect. Chest 2004;125:2278-2288.

Neonatal respiratory distress syndrome. *Interstitial and bronchointerstitial lung disease is common in neonatal foals and is occasionally encountered in other species. In foals, the*

causes include equid herpesvirus 1, septicemia, hyaline membrane disease, and meconium aspiration. Other causes of respiratory disease in neonates include bronchopneumonia secondary to placentitis or aspiration of ingesta, and persistent pulmonary hypertension. *The biology of pulmonary surfactant* (see Cellular architecture and cell biology of the lung, previously) is central to the pathogenesis of hyaline membrane disease.

Neonatal hyaline membrane disease is well recognized in premature or full-term foals, and is occasionally seen in premature puppies, calves, lambs, and piglets. A similar condition is prevalent in cloned calves. The pathogenesis in domestic species is assumed to result from *a failure of the immature type II pneumocytes to secrete functional surfactant*, leading to elevations in surface tension that cause alveoli and small bronchioles to collapse with each exhalation. The tension and shear stress imparted on the lung during reinflation of these collapsed airspaces injures type I pneumocytes and club cells. Abnormalities of surfactant have been documented in premature calves with hyaline membrane disease, but have not been adequately investigated in other species of domestic animals. Fetal hypothyroidism and possibly hypoadrenocorticism are causes of the condition in piglets, because thyroid hormone is necessary for maturation of type II pneumocytes. Other contributing factors in all species are fetal asphyxia, aspiration of meconium in amniotic fluid, reduction in pulmonary arteriolar blood flow, and inhibition of surfactant by fibrinogen, other serum constituents in edema fluid, or by components in aspirated amniotic fluid.

Affected foals have respiratory distress from the time of birth, an expiratory grunt or "bark," hypoxemia, and in some cases heart failure and/or convulsions and opisthotonos. The lungs are diffusely atelectatic, plum-red, rubbery, and sink or become partially submerged in formalin. Histologically, in addition to the thickened hypercellular alveolar septa expected in immature lung (see eFig. 5-15), hyaline membranes line the collapsed alveoli and sometimes the small bronchioles (eFig. 5-58). Alveoli are edematous, and cellular debris is occasionally noted.

Pulmonary hypertension results from pulmonary arterial vasoconstriction that may develop in neonatal hypoxia. The elevations in pulmonary arterial pressure can maintain patency of the ductus arteriosus and foramen ovale, with right-to-left shunting exacerbating the hypoxemia. **Bronchopulmonary dysplasia,** a chronic complication of prematurity, mechanical ventilation, and oxygen therapy in human infants, is characterized by alveolar hypoplasia, thickening of alveolar septa by type II pneumocyte proliferation and fibrosis, bronchiolar damage, and medial hypertrophy of pulmonary arteries; this complication is rare in domestic animals.

Meconium aspiration syndrome is described in human infants, neonatal calves, and rarely in other species. Affected lungs contain variable but usually low amounts of amorphous yellow-orange meconium, keratin, and/or squamous epithelial cells, associated with atelectasis, hemorrhage, and a mild but diffuse alveolar infiltrate of neutrophils, macrophages, and occasional multinucleated cells. When bacterial placentitis is present, pneumonia caused by aspiration of fluids before or during delivery can induce similar lesions and should be ruled out by bacterial culture. Aspirated meconium immediately obstructs airways, thereby inducing hypoxic pulmonary vasoconstriction, which leads to pulmonary hypertension and right-to-left shunting across the ductus arteriosus or foramen

ovale. After a few hours, meconium compromises lung function by eliciting an inflammatory response and by interfering with surfactant activity. In contrast, aspiration of squamous epithelial cells elicits little reaction and is a common incidental finding (eFig. 5-59).

Familial forms of neonatal respiratory distress seem to occur but are not documented in domestic species. Interstitial lung disease caused by mutation of genes involved in surfactant function are described in humans and rodents, and their manifestations vary between genotypes and species: Deficiency of the phospholipid transporter ABCA3 causes lymphocytic interstitial infiltrates and alveolar proteinosis; SP-A deficiency is associated with bronchopulmonary dysplasia and/or increased susceptibility to bacterial infection; SP-B mutations result in alveolar proteinosis, failure of formation of tubular myelin, and/or diffuse alveolar damage; SP-C mutations in humans cause fibrosis of the alveolar septa with infiltration of mononuclear cells, similar to that seen in idiopathic pulmonary fibrosis; and SP-D–deficient mice develop alveolar lipidosis with type II pneumocyte proliferation. A familial form of neonatal respiratory distress is described in pigs, and may result from pulmonary dysmaturity caused by congenital hypothyroidism. Affected piglets have diffuse alveolar damage with hyaline membranes and bronchiolar necrosis, and features suggesting hypothyroidism, including mildly prolonged gestation, fine hair coat, generalized edema, and thyroid follicular hyperplasia with lack of colloid.

Further reading

Lopez A, Bildfell R. Pulmonary inflammation associated with aspirated meconium and epithelial cells in calves. Vet Pathol 1992;29:104-111.

Peek SF, et al. Acute respiratory distress syndrome and fatal interstitial pneumonia associated with equine influenza in a neonatal foal. J Vet Intern Med 2004;18:132-134.

Wert SE, et al. Genetic disorders of surfactant dysfunction. Pediatr Dev Pathol 2009;12:253-274.

Lipid pneumonia and alveolar filling disorders. *Lipid pneumonia is a special form of aspiration pneumonia in which droplets of oil are aspirated into the lung.* Spectacular flooding of the lungs occurs when mineral oil is drenched through a stomach tube accidentally placed into the lung, or lesser amounts are aspirated if the oil is carelessly given per os. Oily droplets are noticed in the trachea and bronchi, or when sections of lung are immersed in formalin (eFig. 5-60). The reaction is typically dominated by macrophages, but the appearance depends on the nature of the oil. In general, *vegetable oils* such as olive oil are not irritating and eventually resorbed with little reaction or fibrosis. *Oils of animal origin* are irritants and provoke early exudation of serofibrinous fluid and leukocytes. This is later replaced by foamy macrophages and giant cells that fill the alveoli; the alveolar septa are thickened by mononuclear cells and fibrosis. The oil is ultimately resorbed. The purest cellular response occurs to *mineral oil*, which is the usual offender in animals. Mineral oil can be identified by its permanence and by its failure to stain with osmic acid. The alveolar lipid is both extracellular and intracellular within macrophages. In time, lipid-laden macrophages accumulate in peribronchial and interlobular septal lymphatics, and there is fibrosis of these tissues and of alveolar septa. *Pneumonias* caused by aspiration of exogenous lipid must be differentiated from the so-called endogenous lipid pneumonias described later. The most important distinguishing feature is that, in lipid aspiration pneumonias, there are extracellular globules of lipid. In paraffin-embedded sections, these appear as clear spherical spaces with distinct borders formed by the compressed cytoplasm of macrophages and giant cells. Lipoid pneumonia caused by mycobacteria is a differential diagnosis.

Alveolar filling disorders *are a group of conditions characterized by accumulation of abnormal material within alveoli.* They are usually incidental findings but are occasionally responsible for clinical disease. In general, material accumulates in alveoli because its clearance is impeded by obstructed airways, it is produced in excess, or its removal is impaired. These conditions are often overlapping, and include alveolar histiocytosis, endogenous lipid pneumonia, alveolar proteinosis, alveolar phospholipidosis, pulmonary hyalinosis, and alveolar microlithiasis.

Alveolar histiocytosis and endogenous lipid pneumonia (foam cell pneumonia, cholesterol pneumonia) *are opposite ends of a spectrum characterized by focal accumulations of foamy macrophages in alveoli.* The condition is most frequently encountered in laboratory rodents and mustelids but is also seen in cats. Minor lesions of alveolar histiocytosis are common in dogs. Many cases are idiopathic, but some are sequelae to obstruction of airways by exudates, bronchoconstriction, tumors, or anomalous bronchi, with the result that lipids such as surfactant accumulate within alveoli. Drug-induced alveolar phospholipidosis in laboratory rodents is a well-described sequel to administration of a group of cationic amphophilic drugs, and is also seen with mutations in the surfactant protein D. Lipid storage diseases and injury to type II pneumocytes by particulates and irritant gases are additional causes described in humans. The lesions should be distinguished from the foamy macrophages encountered in *Pneumocystis, Histoplasma, Leishmania,* or environmental mycobacterial infections.

Grossly, the lungs have irregularly distributed, often subpleural, yellow-white, firm foci that appear as sharply defined flecks or bulging nodules that rarely exceed 1-cm diameter (eFig. 5-61). Histologically, *lesions of alveolar histiocytosis are often subpleural and multifocal, consisting of alveoli filled with foamy macrophages,* with only small amounts of interstitial fibrosis and accumulation of lymphocytes and plasma cells (eFig. 5-62). The lesion is considered *endogenous lipid pneumonia* if lipids can be demonstrated within the macrophages by oil red O or Sudan black stains on frozen sections. In severe cases, there are intracellular and extracellular cholesterol crystals (but no extracellular lipid droplets), more severe interstitial fibrosis, accumulation of neutrophils and mononuclear cells, and type II pneumocyte proliferation. The large cholesterol crystals stimulate development of giant cells and intra-alveolar fibroplasia.

Alveolar proteinosis *(and lipoproteinosis) is a rare but clinically significant disorder characterized by accumulation within alveoli of acellular granular eosinophilic or amphophilic material consisting of surfactant proteins and phospholipids.* The material is strongly PAS-positive and diastase-resistant, particularly at the periphery, and ultrastructurally consists of lamellar and tubular myelin-like arrays. Alveoli may be lined by type II pneumocytes, and foamy macrophages are present, but inflammation and fibrosis are usually minimal. The accumulation of

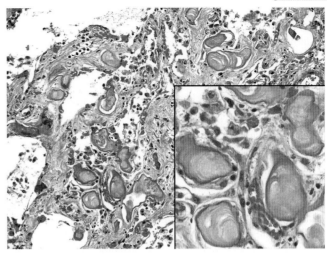

Figure 5-44 Alveolar microlithiasis. Eosinophilic concretions arise in alveoli as well as within septa and have a characteristic laminated appearance. This dog had progressive respiratory distress for 9 months. The central (hilar) area of lung was hard, gritty, and could not be incised without demineralization; peripheral areas were more normal. Inset: higher magnification. (Courtesy B. Stevens.)

surfactant lipids and proteins may result when they are produced in excess by type II pneumocytes, as occurs in rabbits and rats following inhalation of silica dust, surfactant protein (SP)-B deficient humans, or SP-D knockout mice. Alternatively, impaired degradation of these lipids and proteins by alveolar macrophages induces a similar lesion, as occurs in granulocyte-macrophage colony-stimulating factor (GM-CSF) knockout mice, humans with autoantibodies to GM-CSF, interleukin-10–induced inhibition of GM-CSF function, or inherited absence of the receptor. A similar lesion occurs in goats with pneumonia caused by caprine arthritis encephalitis virus.

Pulmonary hyalinosis, *which consists of multifocal accumulations of macrophages and giant cells containing hyaline or laminated material,* is seen as an incidental finding in the lungs of old dogs. Histologically, the cytoplasm of macrophages and giant cells is greatly distended by amorphous or laminated, amphophilic, strongly PAS-positive material. This finding is in contrast to the extracellular deposits seen in pulmonary alveolar microlithiasis.

Pulmonary alveolar microlithiasis is characterized by *concentrically laminated PAS-positive concretions* that form extracellular deposits in the alveoli and may be incorporated into the alveolar septa (Fig. 5-44). This condition is rare in animals, but may be associated with clinical signs of respiratory disease if the lesions are extensive. An analogous condition in humans has an apparently familial basis in some cases, whereas others are sequelae to heart failure. X-ray energy-dispersive spectroscopy of the microliths reveals phosphorus and calcium, reflecting their composition of calcium phosphate, calcium hydroxyapatite, or carboxyapatite.

Multifocal osseous metaplasia (ectopic ossification, "osteoma") of the pulmonary interstitium is frequently encountered as an incidental finding in dogs and other species (eFig. 5-63). Histologically, this appears as well-demarcated tiny nodules of bone within the lung parenchyma.

Further reading

de Brot S, Hilbe M. Pulmonary alveolar microlithiasis with concurrent pleural mesothelioma in a dog. J Vet Diagn Invest 2013;25:798-802.

Michaud CR, et al. Spontaneous pulmonary alveolar proteinosis in captive "moustached tamarins" (*Saguinus mystax*). Vet Pathol 2012;49:629-635.

Pneumoconiosis. *Pneumoconiosis—lung disease ensuing from inhalation and retention of inorganic dusts—is* uncommon in animals because they lack occupational exposures that are the basis for most human cases. In general, inorganic dusts are engulfed by and persist within macrophages, which secrete mediators that induce the *characteristic fibrosis and granulomatous inflammation.* Mild pulmonary **anthracosis** is a common incidental finding in city-dwelling animals or those cohabiting with cigarette smokers, in which carbon particles accrue within macrophages adjacent to airway bifurcations, including the wall of terminal bronchioles. **Asbestosis** is characterized by *asbestos (ferruginous) bodies*—asbestos fibers coated with ferritin and hemosiderin that are linear with a beaded appearance and globose ends—within granulomatous and fibrosing lung lesions. The ability to form ferruginous bodies varies by species, thus asbestos-related lung disease in some animals can be difficult to diagnose. Sheep have been used as an experimental model of the disease, but natural cases are rare. Asbestos-associated mesothelioma seems not to occur in domestic animals.

Silicate pneumoconiosis in horses, and rarely dogs, is the only reported clinically important pneumoconiosis in animals. In horses, this disease is occasionally erroneously referred to as "silicosis". *Silicosis* is a disease caused by inhalation of crystalline silica—a 3-dimensional arrangement of silicon dioxide (SiO_2) tetrahedra—particles that are largely derived from quartz, and thus most common in people who work with quartz-bearing stone or rocks. **Silicates**, on the other hand, are common crustal minerals formed when SiO_2 combines with a variety of cations, especially magnesium, calcium, and aluminum. Asbestos is a fibrous silicate whose inhalation may result in asbestosis (described previously), whereas non-asbestos silicate pneumoconioses refers to disease associated with inhalation of a variety of non-asbestos, that is, nonfibrous, silicates. The clinical signs associated with silicate pneumoconiosis in horses include weight loss, exercise intolerance, and dyspnea, and the condition in horses has been associated with osteoporosis. Miliary firm or gritty lesions are distributed throughout the lung. Microscopically, the lesions are mainly centered on bronchioles or, less frequently, target the interlobular septa and consist of multifocal fibrosis with granulomatous inflammation, often with necrosis and mineralization in the centers. Clear, brown, or black crystals are indistinctly visible in the cytoplasm of the macrophages. These are sometimes birefringent, can usually be highlighted by acid-fast stains, and are identified by X-ray spectroscopy. Although the cause of this severe pulmonary disease is reported to be the result of inhalation of silicate particles, based on finding such particles associated with the characteristic granulomatous inflammation, no studies have been performed to confirm the pathogenicity of silicates in horses. Histologically, silicates are commonly detected in the lungs of many species as an incidental finding unrelated to progressive fibrosing lung disease, and pulmonary lesions similar to silicate pneumoconiosis have been documented in horses beyond California. Thus the pathogenesis may be more complex than is currently assumed, and may not be the result of silicate inhalation.

Further reading

Arens AM, et al. Osteoporosis associated with pulmonary silicosis in an equine bone fragility syndrome. Vet Pathol 2011;48:593-615.

Khalil N, et al. Environmental, inhaled and ingested causes of pulmonary fibrosis. Toxicol Pathol 2007;35:86-96.

Matros L, et al. Silicate pneumoconiosis in a dog: case report and current concepts of pathogenesis. J Am Anim Hosp Assoc 2005;30:375-381.

Toxic lung injury. *The lung is the target of toxic injury by several mechanisms:* inhalation of gases or fumes that are directly toxic to epithelial or endothelial cells, ingestion or inhalation of toxins that are metabolized to reactive intermediates mainly by club cells or type II pneumocytes, hypersensitivity reactions, effects of inhaled persistent material such as asbestos or fiberglass, and xenobiotic-induced carcinogenicity. Typical lesions include epithelial cell necrosis, hyperplasia, dysplasia, squamous metaplasia, or neoplastic transformation; alveolar histiocytosis; or fibrosis. Inhaled or ingested xenobiotics causing nasal lesions are well studied in animal models, but are rarely encountered in diagnostic veterinary pathology.

Severe lung injury from **inhalation of toxic gases** is rarely encountered in domestic animals because they do not have the occupational exposures that are usually responsible in humans. The anatomic location of injury by inhaled toxins depends on the dose, chemical reactivity, aqueous solubility, and particle size. Water-soluble gases, such as sulfur dioxide and ammonia, usually cause upper respiratory injury, whereas less soluble gases, such as nitrogen dioxide, are more widely distributed and may cause bronchiolar or alveolar injury. Poisoning of cattle, pigs, and chickens by **nitrogen dioxide (silo gas)** can cause massive mortality, with lesions of pulmonary edema and congestion, necrosis of bronchial and bronchiolar epithelium, and alveolar hemorrhage and/or fibrin exudation. Acute pulmonary injury caused by **smoke inhalation** is seen in animals trapped in burning buildings (see Fig. 5-14). When asphyxiation is not immediate, the combined chemical and heat effects of smoke can cause widespread epithelial necrosis and exudation, and death within a few days. Exposure to **copper-containing drenches**, perhaps by aspiration, causes bronchiolar necrosis in sheep, with elevated copper levels in lung but not liver. **Hydrocarbon waterproofing sprays** are reported to cause lung disease in dogs, but the lesions or mechanisms are not defined.

Exposure to 85-100% **oxygen** (or perhaps lower levels, in animals with pre-existing lung disease) damages capillary endothelium and type I pneumocytes, and causes serofibrinous exudation in alveoli or diffuse alveolar damage. In intensive care patients, it may be impossible to determine if diffuse alveolar damage was caused by the underlying disease, or hyperoxic or ventilator-induced lung injury. *Reactive oxygen species* (superoxide, hydroxyl radicals, and hydrogen peroxide) are currently favored as the injurious metabolites, causing cellular injury by lipid peroxidation, protein oxidation, and DNA strand breaks. Neutrophil-dependent lung injury and dysfunction of surfactant are additional proposed mechanisms of hyperoxic lung injury.

The toxicity of other compounds depends on their **conversion to reactive intermediate metabolites by phase I enzymes** that include several cytochrome P450 (CYP) isozymes. The CYP isozymes have a species-dependent distribution in nasal tissue, club cells, type II pneumocytes, and to a lesser extent in ciliated epithelial cells, type I pneumocytes, endothelial cells, and pulmonary macrophages. Reactive intermediates generated by CYP isozymes are further detoxified by phase II enzymes, including glutathione-S-transferases and glucuronyltransferases, to form water-soluble metabolites that are excreted. However, toxicity may develop when the phase II systems are inadequate (e.g., when glutathione is depleted or glutathione-S-transferase activity is impaired or absent) or overwhelmed by high concentrations of the reactive metabolite. In these situations, the electrophilic metabolite binds to essential proteins or nucleic acids, or leads to formation of oxygen radicals that damage cell membrane lipids. Thus *the cellular susceptibility to toxic injury depends not only on cell-specific expression of the appropriate cytochrome P450 isozymes, but also on the adequacy of the antioxidants (glutathione, vitamin E, superoxide dismutase, and others) and phase II enzymes that protect the cell from injury.* Inherited polymorphisms in CYP genes and induction of CYP by glucocorticoids or other drugs may also influence the susceptibility of individual animals to pulmonary toxins.

3-Methylindole (3-MI) toxicity *causes acute bovine pulmonary emphysema and edema, or fog fever, in cattle.* L-tryptophan in grazed pastures is metabolized in the rumen (or the large colon of nonruminants) to 3-MI, and this is converted primarily by CYP to an electrophilic intermediate that alkylates cellular macromolecules, resulting in lipid peroxidation and membrane damage. The early ultrastructural changes are necrosis of nonciliated and ciliated bronchiolar epithelial cells and type I pneumocytes, and transient swelling of endothelial cells. Although type II pneumocytes have high CYP activity, the high levels of glutathione and phase II enzymes are thought to spare these cells from injury.

3-MI toxicity affects adult cattle in the autumn, within 4-10 days after they are moved from dry to lush pastures; younger animals are resistant to the toxic effects of 3-MI. Affected animals have acute onset of dyspnea with expiratory effort, tachypnea, open-mouth breathing, and froth in the mouth. The trachea is filled with foam, and the lungs contain striking alveolar and interlobular edema, resulting in heavy wet lungs that fail to collapse. Interlobular or bullous emphysema is prominent in the caudal lobes in less fulminant cases (see Fig. 5-41). Histologically, hyaline membranes line the edematous alveoli and alveolar ducts, and type II pneumocyte proliferation is extensive in the subacute stages. The alveolar septa are distended by edema, and may contain eosinophils and/or neutrophils in natural cases. Although bronchiolar lesions are often absent in natural cases, bronchiolar necrosis is described following intentional administration of 3-MI. The *differential diagnoses* for this histologic picture includes other toxins listed later as well as post-patent forms of *Dictyocaulus viviparus* infection, for which the histologic lesions are very similar, but recent access to lush pasture would favor fog fever; acute infection with *Ascaris suum* or *Dictyocaulus* larvae, which generally occur in younger calves and have many eosinophils with at least a few histologically visible larvae; viral pneumonia, which may be difficult to distinguish without laboratory testing unless viral syncytia or inclusion bodies are present; anaphylaxis, which causes pulmonary edema,

congestion, emphysema, and rarely eosinophil infiltration, but not hyaline membranes; and extrinsic allergic alveolitis, in which lymphocytes and granulomas form beside bronchioles and within alveolar septa. In contrast to the predominantly alveolar damage in ruminants, experimental 3-MI toxicity in horses causes necrosis of club cells in the bronchioles, probably reflecting the species-dependent distribution of cytochrome P450.

4-Ipomeanol from moldy sweet potatoes induces a comparable condition in calves, of diffuse alveolar damage with or without bronchiolar injury following CYP-induced formation of a reactive intermediate. **Perilla ketone** toxicity (from perilla mint, *Perilla frutescens*) in cattle and horses follows a similar pattern, ascribed to the toxin 1-(3-furyl)4-methylpentatone. Other toxins causing diffuse alveolar damage in cattle include stinkwood (*Zieria arborescens*, a small tree in southeastern Australia), moldy garden beans, *Brassica* (turnip tops or kale), and rape. **Crofton weed** (*Eupatorium adenophorum, Ageratina adenophora*)—specifically, the flowering plant—causes multifocal or diffuse chronic interstitial lung disease in horses, in which proliferation of alveolar epithelial cells and fibroplasia are the prominent features. Similarly, horses chronically ingesting *Crotalaria* spp. containing **pyrrolizidine alkaloids** develop interstitial fibrosis with hyperplasia and dysplasia of bronchiolar and alveolar duct epithelium, with or without alveolar type II pneumocyte proliferation. **Carbolic dips** used to prepare sheep for showing is also reported to cause fatal pulmonary disease 1-3 days later, probably by absorption through the skin, with pulmonary lesions of hyperemia, edema, and type II pneumocyte proliferation.

Paraquat *is a highly toxic herbicide that can cause acute diffuse alveolar damage* if inhaled or ingested. Acute lung injury has been reported in cattle, sheep, pigs, and dogs following ingestion of foodstuffs contaminated with the herbicide. Paraquat is taken up by type I pneumocytes and induces alveolar injury through reduction-oxidation (redox) cycling, depleting the cells of NADPH and glutathione, which results in uncontrolled generation of superoxide anion and oxidant injury. Cases of malicious poisoning are more likely to cause fulminating pulmonary edema and hemorrhage because of the high dosage, whereas in accidental poisonings, there is more often time for hyperplasia of alveolar type II cells and fibroplasia to be superimposed on the earlier exudative changes. In the acute intoxication with survival up to 2-3 days, the lungs are heavy, dark, and rubbery, and alveolar spaces are filled with fluid and blood, with much fluid in the hilar connective tissue. Hyaline membranes are present in alveolar ducts. With longer survival, profuse fibroplasia and type II pneumocyte proliferation thicken the alveolar septa. Extrapulmonary lesions are often present and include patchy necrosis of the adrenal zona glomerulosa and of renal tubular epithelium.

Other toxins cause pulmonary vascular disease. **Fumonisin B1**, a mycotoxin usually associated with corn, causes massive interlobular pulmonary edema and hydrothorax as well as pancreatic necrosis in pigs. The toxin causes damage to alveolar endothelial cells associated with altered sphingolipid metabolism. Similarly, poisoning by the rodenticide α-**naphthylthiourea (ANTU)** causes respiratory distress resulting from pulmonary edema and pleural effusion. Pulmonary vascular lesions are also produced in horses, pigs, sheep, and cattle by **pyrrolizidine alkaloids** (*Crotalaria, Trichodesma, Senecio*); the resulting vascular lesions are described in the sections Pulmonary vasculitis and Pulmonary hypertension, previously. *Pimelea* spp. (St. George disease), which contains simplexin and dihydroxycoumarin glycoside toxins, is another toxic cause of pulmonary hypertension in cattle and horses in Australia. Sodium selenite and selenomethionine, found in **selenium-accumulator plants** ingested by lambs, causes mainly myocardial necrosis but also pulmonary edema and hemorrhage resulting from vasculitis of the alveolar septa.

Drug reactions are important causes of acute or chronic pulmonary injury in humans, manifesting as pulmonary edema, asthma-like disease, bronchiolar necrosis, diffuse alveolar damage, eosinophilic pneumonia, pulmonary vascular disease with hemorrhage, or pleural effusion. Pulmonary drug reactions are poorly described and apparently rare in domestic animals. *CCNU, a nitrosourea chemotherapeutic* used for treatment of lymphoma, causes chronic lung injury with interstitial fibrosis and smooth muscle hyperplasia as well as type II pneumocyte hyperplasia.

Further reading

Botha CJ, et al. Crotalariosis equorum ("jaagsiekte") in horses in southern Mozambique, a rare form of pyrrolizidine alkaloid poisoning. J Vet Diagn Invest 2012;24:1099-1104.

Medeiros RM, et al. Bovine atypical interstitial pneumonia associated with the ingestion of damaged sweet potatoes *(Ipomoea batatas)* in northeastern Brazil. Vet Hum Toxicol 2001;43:205-207.

Sells DM, et al. Respiratory tract lesions in noninhalation studies. Toxicol Pathol 2007;35:170-177.

Shuler CM, et al. Retrospective case series of suspected intentional paraquat poisonings: diagnostic findings and risk factors for death. Vet Hum Toxicol 2004;46:313-314.

Skorupski KA, et al. Pulmonary fibrosis after high cumulative dose nitrosourea chemotherapy in a cat. Vet Comp Oncol 2008;6:120-125.

Embolic pneumonia and lung abscesses

Embolic pneumonia results from hematogenous distribution of infectious and/or inflammatory processes within the lung. The pattern of embolic pneumonia is multifocal, and grossly appears as discrete, variably sized, rounded foci of necrosis and inflammation leading to abscess formation (eFig. 5-64). Few forms of embolic pneumonia have characteristic clinical presentations or pathology. An exception is embolic aspergillosis in horses with colic. These animals develop severe hemorrhagic and necrotizing embolic pneumonia associated with disseminated *Aspergillus* spp. infection in association with a history of antecedent colitis. *Pulmonary abscesses may reflect an embolic process but can also arise from chronic bronchopneumonia.* A cranioventral location and associated bronchiectasis are evidence of the abscess originating from bronchopneumonia. Multiple widely distributed abscesses usually indicate hematogenous origin, and are often associated with an obvious source of septic emboli elsewhere in the body, such as endocarditis, or hepatic abscesses with phlebitis of the hepatic vein in cattle. The occurrence of abscesses in other tissues supports a hematogenous route of infection. *Other causes* of pulmonary abscess include aspirated foreign bodies such as plant awns, direct traumatic penetration of the lung, or multisystem diseases such as caseous lymphadenitis and melioidosis. It is often impossible to determine the pathogenesis of isolated abscesses if lesions are not identified in other tissues. Abscesses may erode through the pleura to cause empyema, through blood vessels and into airways to cause massive blood loss, or into a bronchus to cause suppurative bronchopneumonia.

PLEURA

The relatively simple anatomy of the pleura belies the underlying complexity of the tissue. Mesothelial cells form a thin continuous layer and produce an underlying basal lamina. Although the thoracic mesothelial lining is contiguous, it is subdivided into *parietal pleura*, covering thoracic wall, diaphragm, and mediastinum; and *visceral pleura*, covering the lungs.

Mesothelial cells are flat cells with surface microvilli on their apex; tight junctions between the cells have an important role in maintaining proper thoracic fluid balance. Mesothelial cells sample materials within the thoracic cavity, using both pinocytosis to take in pleural fluid as well as phagocytosis to engulf particles such as bacteria. The cells participate in inflammation through production of cytokines and deposition of extracellular matrix, and are capable of synthesizing large amounts of collagen and other extracellular matrix proteins. Both procoagulant and anticoagulant proteins are produced by the mesothelium, and an imbalance in these proteins, especially plasminogen-activator inhibitor, can promote pleural fibrin deposition.

Mesothelial cells normally have little baseline mitotic activity, and their ability to replace themselves following injury is not well understood. In response to pleural injury, mesothelial cells become cuboidal, and during long-standing stimulation often form villus projections into the pleural cavity covering a core of mesothelial-derived extracellular matrix and small capillaries.

The pleura has limited local defenses. *Kampmeier's foci*, found within the parietal pleura of the costal surface and mediastinum, are aggregates of lymphocytes and macrophages and are covered by a layer of modified mesothelial cells that are assumed to function similarly to mucosal-associated lymphoid tissues in the surveillance of the pleural fluid. Grossly, these aggregates may be seen as small white foci within the costal parietal pleura.

Pleural fluid is present in very small amounts (1-2 mL) in health. It provides for mechanical coupling between the lung and the chest wall in the negative-pressure environment of the thoracic cavity, and acts as a lubricant during respiration. Fluid enters the pleural cavity through stomata in the parietal pleura, following a hydrostatic gradient, and is pulled into the pleural space with the recoil of the lung during respiration. Pleural fluid is removed through stoma in the visceral and parietal pleura, and to a lesser extent by transcellular means through mesothelial cells. **Pleural effusion** *occurs when filtration of fluid exceeds reabsorption.* Less commonly, pleuroperitoneal migration of fluid may result in fluid accumulation in the thoracic cavity through microscopic portals in the diaphragm when ascites is present.

Congenital anomalies of the pleura and mediastinum are of little significance. *Congenital cysts of branchial pouch origin* are rarely encountered, most often in brachycephalic dogs. They are found in the cranial mediastinum, often in close association with thymic tissues, and are lined by a single layer of cuboidal epithelium. *Bronchogenic cysts* are occasionally identified in the mediastinum. **Degenerative** changes in the pleura occur in uremia in dogs, with mineralization of elastic and collagen fibers in the parietal pleura of the intercostal spaces; this change is grossly most consistently evident in the first 3-4 cranial intercostal spaces. *Pleural cysts* lined by keratinizing squamous epithelium are described in horses, but their cause is uncertain. Tetrathyridia of the cestode *Mesocestoides* spp. cause cystic lesions on the pleural surface.

Further reading

Baum B, et al. Multifocal pleural cystic squamous metaplasia in a horse with chronic obstructive bronchopneumonia. Vet Pathol 2004;41: 532-534.

Pneumothorax

Pneumothorax *refers to the presence of air or gas in the pleural cavities, and results in atelectasis because negative intrapleural pressure cannot be maintained.* In normal animals at the time of autopsy, the diaphragm billows caudally with an in-rush of air reflecting the loss of negative intrathoracic pressure when the diaphragm is pierced; these features are absent in cases of pneumothorax (but may also be lost with significant autolysis of the body). In small animals, where detection of this diaphragmatic movement and in-rush of air in normal animals may be challenging, pneumothorax could be detected by opening the chest under water and observing the escape of air bubbles. Pneumothorax results in atelectasis, but in chronic cases, there may also be hyperplasia or metaplasia of the pleural mesothelium as well as type II pneumocyte proliferation in the adjacent alveoli.

Pneumothorax can be spontaneous or traumatic. *Primary spontaneous pneumothorax* refers to rupture of blebs or bullae in the absence of apparent lung disease. Blebs and bullae are common causes of pneumothorax in dogs (see section Pulmonary emphysema, previously). *Secondary spontaneous pneumothorax* refers to those cases resulting from an underlying lung disease. The causes include rupture of lesions that form a communication between the airway and pleural space, such as parasitic cysts (e.g., paragonimiasis), abscesses, pyogranulomas, neoplasms, migrating foreign bodies, or infarcts. Other causes lead to emphysematous bulla formation: barotrauma (from forced ventilation during anesthesia), bronchopneumonia, asthma, chronic bronchitis, and thromboembolism. *Traumatic pneumothorax* is usually the result of accidental puncture of the thoracic wall and/or visceral pleura. Traumatic pneumothorax can also be a complication of cardiac resuscitation or biopsy of the lung. Air that tracks through the pulmonary interstitium to the mediastinum *(pneumomediastinum)* does not usually escape into the pleural cavities unless there is traumatic rupture of the mediastinum.

Further reading

Mooney ET, et al. Spontaneous pneumothorax in 35 cats (2001-2010). J Feline Med Surg 2012;14:384-391.

Pawloski DR, Broaddus KD. Pneumothorax: a review. J Am Anim Hosp Assoc 2010;46:385-397.

Noninflammatory pleural effusions

Hydrothorax *is the accumulation in the pleural space of transudate, which is clear, watery, colorless or light yellow, and has a low protein and cell content* (eFig. 5-65). Chronic hydrothorax causes pleural opacity because of reactive hyperplasia of mesothelial cells, which produce fibrous thickening of the underlying pleural connective tissue. Hydrothorax is caused by increased venous pressure, lymphatic obstruction, rarely hypoproteinemia, or by extension from a peritoneal effusion. It is particularly common in cats with cardiomyopathy (with either left- or right-sided heart failure), and occasionally develops from heart failure in other species. Hydrothorax is also a feature of specific diseases such as lung lobe torsion, "mulberry heart disease" in swine, black disease in sheep, African horsesickness, and **α-naphthylthiourea** poisoning.

Chylothorax *is the accumulation in the pleural space of lymph, which appears milky and has a high triglyceride and lymphocyte content* (eFig. 5-66). The diagnosis is confirmed by measurement of a higher triglyceride concentration in the fluid than in serum, or a reduced cholesterol-to-triglyceride ratio. Chylothorax is seen in cats and occasionally dogs, and *most cases are idiopathic.* Recognized causes include cardiomyopathy and right-sided heart failure, where increased central venous pressure prevents emptying of lymph from the thoracic duct into the vena cava; vena caval thrombosis; thoracic masses, such as lymphoma, thymoma, or granulomas that cause thoracic duct obstruction; or infrequently dirofilariasis, lung lobe torsion, diaphragmatic hernia, or congenital anomalies in Afghan Hounds. Traumatic rupture of the thoracic duct is a well-known but rarely identified cause. *Chylous effusion causes atelectasis and stimulates noninflammatory pleural fibrosis.* Repeated removal of the effusion may induce dehydration, electrolyte disturbance, depletion of lipids and fat-soluble vitamins, hypoproteinemia, and lymphopenia.

Hemothorax *is the presence of blood in the pleural cavity.* It is most often the result of traumatic rupture of blood vessels, but it can also be caused by coagulopathies, such as anticoagulant rodenticide toxicity; rupture of highly vascularized tumors, such as hemangiosarcoma; lung lobe torsion; or erosion of a vessel by an inflammatory or neoplastic process (eFigs. 5-67, 5-68). Chronic hydrothorax or chylothorax may lead to the development of well-vascularized papillae on the pleura, and rupture of these may result in a blood-stained effusion.

Further reading

Singh A, et al. Idiopathic chylothorax: pathophysiology, diagnosis, and thoracic duct imaging. Compend Contin Educ Vet 2012; 34:E2.

Pleuritis

Infectious agents most often reach the pleura from the blood or from lesions of bronchopneumonia, aspiration pneumonia, or abscesses in the underlying lung. Other routes of infection include perforation of the chest wall or diaphragm, penetrating foreign bodies from the esophagus or reticulum, perforating esophageal ulcers, lymphatic permeation from the peritoneal cavity, or direct extension from a mediastinal abscess. *Pleural defenses against microorganisms are much weaker than those of the lung*, and even a few organisms reaching the pleural surfaces are apt to have serious consequences. The appearance varies depending on the species affected, cause, magnitude of infection, and chronicity. Fibrinous exudates often form loosely adherent strands or veils of elastic material on the pleural surface (eFig. 5-69). In more florid

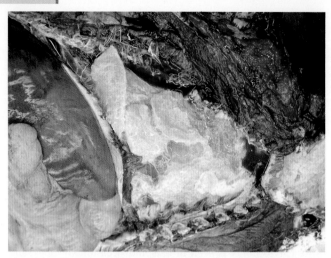

Figure 5-45 *Histophilus somni* **pleuritis** in a feedlot calf, with abundant yellow pleural fluid and thick mats of fibrin covering the pleural surface. The underlying lung tissue is otherwise normal.

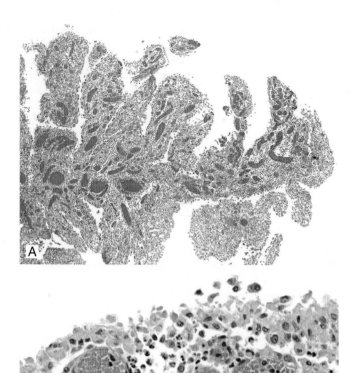

Figure 5-46 Chronic pleuritis in a dog. **A.** Papillary hyperplasia of the pleural tissue. **B.** Hyperplastic tissue is covered by loosely arranged mesothelial cells and infiltrated by neutrophils and macrophages.

fibrinous lesions, the prosector may find voluminous serofibrinous exudate when the chest is opened, and lakes of watery clear yellow fluid alternate with pockets of turbid and foul-smelling exudate (Fig. 5-45). Creamy white suppurative exudate fills the pleural space in cases of **pyothorax** or **thoracic empyema** (eFig. 5-70). Chronic lesions readily form adhesions between the parietal and visceral pleura, yet the functional impact of adhesions on lung function is usually minimal.

Pleuritis in **swine** may be an extension from obvious lesions of bronchopneumonia caused by *Actinobacillus pleuropneumoniae* or *A. suis*. *Streptococcus suis*, *Haemophilus parasuis*, and *Mycoplasma hyorhinis* are common causes of septicemia in swine, and the fibrinous or fibrinopurulent pleuritis caused by these agents is usually accompanied by exudates on other serosal surfaces, joints, or meninges. The causes in **cattle** include bronchopneumonia, especially from *Mannheimia haemolytica* or *Histophilus somni*, direct extension from lesions of traumatic reticuloperitonitis, septicemic *H. somni* infection (see Fig. 5-45), and *Pasteurella multocida* type B.

Pleuritis in mature **horses** often occurs with a recent history of travel, and is described later (see Infectious respiratory diseases of horses). The pleural exudate is unilateral or bilateral, and usually so florid that it masks the causative underlying lung lesion, but nearly all cases have either a focal area of consolidated lung that suggests aspiration pneumonia (eFig. 5-71), or a bilateral lesion of necrotizing bronchopneumonia. *Mycoplasma felis* is an uncommon cause of pleuritis in horses without underlying lung lesions. Pleuritis occurs in neonatal foals with septicemia caused by *Actinobacillus equuli* or other gram-negative bacteria.

In **dogs,** pyothorax occurs mostly in hunting dogs or those with access to rural environments. The lesions are bilateral or occasionally unilateral, and pneumonia is absent or minor. The exudate is often bloody and opaque, resembling tomato soup, or creamy or darkly serofibrinous (eFig. 5-72). The pleural surfaces are usually thickened and velvety, red or gray-yellow, and fibrotic. *Actinomyces*, *Nocardia*, and *Bacteroides* spp. are the most frequently recovered organisms, and these are commonly associated with the presence of yellow "sulfur" granules amid the pus. Histologically, the characteristic pyogranuloma-

tous pleuritis and mediastinitis contain infrequent aggregates of filamentous bacteria (Fig. 5-46). Inhaled or ingested grass awns or florets that migrate into the pleural space are thought to be the source of infection in most cases, although they are usually impossible to find in the copious pleural exudate.

Other causes of pleuritis in dogs include bite wounds, esophageal perforation, or bacteremia. *Sparganosis*, caused by larval cestodes of the genus *Spirometra*, result in pleural thickening caused by chronic inflammation, with the presence of 6-mm long rice-grain–like structures (plerocercoids or spargana). The latter have multiple invaginations of the tegument, subtegmental muscle, loose stroma of low cellularity that contains clear "osmoregulatory canals," no coelomic cavity, and no reproductive or digestive tracts.

In **cats,** feline infectious peritonitis is a common cause of pleuritis, and multifocal pyogranulomas are visible on the pleural surface. Pyothorax is fairly common in cats, and *Pasteurella multocida*, various gram-negative enteric bacteria, streptococci, and staphylococci are commonly isolated, often in mixed infection. Although most cases are idiopathic, penetrating bite wounds, extension from bacterial pneumonia, migrating awns, or penetration of a foreign body from the esophagus are likely causes.

Further reading

Barrs VR, Beatty JA. Feline pyothorax—new insights into an old problem: part 1. Aetiopathogenesis and diagnostic investigation. Vet J 2009;179:163-170.

Epstein SE. Exudative pleural diseases in small animals. Vet Clin North Am Small Anim Pract 2014;44:161-180.

McFadden AM, et al. Outbreaks of pleuritis and peritonitis in calves associated with *Pasteurella multocida* capsular type B strain. N Z Vet J 2011;59:40-45.

Simpson C, et al. Molecular diagnosis of sparganosis associated with pneumothorax in a dog. Mol Cell Probes 2012;26:60-62.

Neoplastic conditions of the pleura

Mesothelioma arises from the pleura, as well as from the pericardium or peritoneum (eFig. 5-73). Histologically, *epithelioid, sarcomatous, and biphasic patterns* are described. The epithelioid cells form nests, ribbons, acini, or papillary protrusions that resemble carcinoma, and the mesenchymal component may resemble fibrosarcoma. Distinguishing mesothelial hyperplasia from mesothelioma can be a diagnostic challenge. The latter is expected to fully invade collagenous connective tissue within the pleura and usually extends into underlying lung tissue along interlobular or alveolar septa. In contrast, in humans, features suggesting a reactive lesion include abundant pleural fibrin, multinucleated mesothelial cells in the fibrin, capillaries growing perpendicular to the pleural surface into the fibrin, and parallel rather than storiform arrangement of collagen. *Immunohistochemical detection of both vimentin and cytokeratin, and detection of acid mucins by Alcian blue stain, are useful in distinguishing mesothelioma from other epithelial or nonepithelial neoplasms.* However, pulmonary adenocarcinomas also frequently co-express cytokeratin and vimentin; positive thyroid transcription factor-1 (TTF-1) labeling may be useful for differentiation from epithelioid mesothelioma. Calretinin and HBME-1 are used as markers of mesothelioma in humans but have been inconsistent or negative in animals. Pleural mesothelioma spreads and implants within the pleural cavity to cause persistent thoracic effusion, invades the underlying tissue, and may reach the abdominal cavity via lymphatics.

Metastatic neoplasms localizing to the pleura are more common than mesothelioma. Transpleural dissemination of carcinomas and sarcomas may occur by extension from the lungs, chest wall, or mediastinum, and carcinomas from the abdominal cavity can reach the pleura by pleuroperitoneal migration of fluid through the diaphragm.

Further reading

Sato T, et al. Peritoneal biphasic mesothelioma in a dog. J Vet Med A Physiol Pathol Clin Med 2005;52:22-25.

INFECTIOUS DISEASES OF THE RESPIRATORY SYSTEM

Infectious respiratory diseases of swine

Viral diseases

Porcine reproductive and respiratory syndrome. Porcine reproductive and respiratory syndrome (PRRS) was first identified in the late 1980s and is now worldwide in distribution, with the notable exceptions of Australia and Sweden. It is an *important cause of reproductive failure and interstitial pneumonia*, and a predisposing factor for bacterial pneumonia and septicemia. The disease varies greatly in severity and clinico-pathologic presentation, depending on the strain of the PRRS virus (PRRSV), the age of pigs affected, the level and distribution of immunity within the herd, and the presence of other pathogens.

On initial exposure, infection spreads slowly through the naive herd and causes a variety of clinical presentations: anorexia and lethargy of all age groups; reproductive failure characterized by late-term abortion, stillbirth, mummified fetuses, and weak-born piglets; and interstitial pneumonia causing fatal hyperpnea, dyspnea, and lethargy in suckling pigs infected in utero or in the neonatal period; respiratory disease is also common in weaned and grower-finisher pigs. "Sow abortion and mortality syndrome" describes a devastating disease resulting from PRRSV infection of naive herds, in which up to half of the sows may abort and sow mortality may reach 10%.

Viral infection often persists and circulates within the herd indefinitely, the result of prolonged viral shedding from individual animals and continuous entry of naïve animals. The disease in endemically infected herds is highly variable. Many herds have stable infections in which virus continues to circulate but does not cause clinical disease; others have endemic respiratory disease or a failure to thrive in nursery and grower-finisher pigs, or a PRRSV-induced increase in susceptibility to bacterial pneumonia and septicemia, and some herds have continuing losses because of abortion in gilts or dyspnea in neonatal or weaned pigs.

The PRRS virus is an enveloped, 50-65 nm diameter, positive-sense, single-stranded RNA virus in the family *Arteriviridae*. The viral genome includes 8 open reading frames (ORFs): ORF 1a and 1b encode proteins necessary for replication and transcription, ORFs 2-4 encode structural glycoproteins of uncertain function, ORF 5 encodes an envelope glycoprotein, ORF 6 encodes the integral membrane protein M, and ORF 7 encodes the nucleocapsid protein N. PRRSV isolates are divided into type 1 (European-like) and type 2 (North American–like) genotypes.

Genomic variability is an important feature of PRRSV, and may be attributed to the high mutation rate associated with the error-prone RNA polymerase and perhaps recombination between viral strains in coinfections. As a result, PRRSV isolates vary in terms of the severity of respiratory disease, reactivity in antigen- and nucleic acid–based diagnostic assays, and possibly in patterns of lesions in other organs, including brain and heart. These differences in virulence have not been shown to correlate with simple alterations in specific genes; rather, the virulence of particular strains is apparently determined by a combined effect of many genetic differences. Highly virulent strains have been associated with greater replication of virus within tissues; higher levels of inflammatory cytokines, including interferon-γ (which may lead to systemic disease resulting from "macrophage activation syndrome"); more severe lesions within tissues; and greater susceptibility to septicemia from secondary bacterial pathogens.

Modified live vaccine strains may rarely cause disease. Vaccine strains of the virus can infect in-contact animals and persist in herds, but do not commonly cause clinical disease. However, as these vaccine strains circulate in swine herds, *mutation to a less attenuated form of the virus may result in disease caused by vaccine-derived strains.* Extra-label intranasal administration of modified live PRRSV vaccine has induced clinical signs and lesions typical of PRRS.

The common mode of *transmission* of PRRSV is direct nasal, oral, or coital contact with saliva, oropharyngeal mucus, urine, semen, serum, mammary secretions, or perhaps feces of infected pigs. Transmission of PRRSV by artificial insemination has been documented, and transmission by contamination of pharmaceutical preparations or needles with infected serum is a potential risk. Transmission by fomites may occur, but because the enveloped virus is rapidly inactivated in most environmental conditions, disinfection procedures should be effective. Aerosol transmission is apparently of limited importance, but can occur at low frequency over short distances.

The pathogenesis of PRRS centers on infection of macrophages at the site of nasal, tonsillar, or pulmonary infection, extension to associated lymphoid tissue, rapid viremia, and infection of macrophages throughout the body. Following experimental intranasal challenge, viral antigen is expressed within 12 hours of infection in nasal and tonsillar macrophages and epithelium; pulmonary alveolar, intravascular, and interstitial macrophages; bronchiolar epithelium, and endothelial cells of pulmonary arterioles. Viremia occurs rapidly, in some cases within 12 hours of infection, and leads to widespread infection of monocytes and tissue macrophages. Viral antigen may be detected in myocardial macrophages and endothelium, follicular macrophages and dendritic cells in lymph node, interdigitating cells in the thymus, macrophages and dendritic cells in the spleen and Peyer's patches, and macrophages in hepatic sinusoids, adrenal gland, interstitium of the kidney, and choroid plexus.

Persistent infection is a key feature of PRRSV. Virus has been detected in serum for 3 weeks; in nasal mucosa, pulmonary macrophages, and spleen for 4 weeks; and in oropharyngeal mucosa for up to 22 weeks after infection. Animals remain infectious for in-contact naive pigs for at least 22 weeks after infection. Persistent infections are of epidemiologic importance in the maintenance of PRRSV infection in endemically infected herds; yet the reasons for failure of the immune response to clear the infection and the role of cell-mediated immunity in protection and viral clearance are unknown. Following experimental PRRSV infection, serum antibody detectable by ELISA and virus-neutralizing tests are first detectable at 7-14 days and 9-28 days after infection, peak at 5 weeks and 10 weeks, and remain detectable for 46 weeks and >1 year, respectively. Antibody responses are directed against all proteins encoded by ORFs 2-7; the products of ORF 3, 4, and 5 may represent protective epitopes.

Infection with PRRSV impairs host defenses, and increases susceptibility to infection with *Streptococcus suis*, *Haemophilus parasuis*, *Salmonella enterica* serovar Choleraesuis, and other opportunistic pathogens. Experiments to investigate this effect have been conflicting, and the ability of PRRSV to predispose to other agents is probably dependent on the viral and bacterial strains examined and on the specific experimental conditions. The ability of PRRSV to infect and reduce the function of pulmonary intravascular macrophages is one mechanism whereby PRRSV predisposes to septicemia; a similar impairment of alveolar macrophage functions, including phagocytosis, oxidative burst, and cytokine secretion, may reduce lung defenses against bacterial bronchopneumonia. Subclinical or clinical infection with *Mycoplasma hyopneu-*

moniae exacerbates the clinical signs and lesions of PRRS, possibly because mycoplasma-induced proliferation and activation of macrophages enhance the replication or persistence of PRRSV. In contrast, infection with PRRSV has little effect on the severity of mycoplasmal lesions. This finding is of clinical importance, as control of *M. hyopneumoniae* is one strategy for minimizing the effect of PRRSV in endemically infected herds. The effect of PRRSV infection on immune responses to other pathogens has not been fully addressed, but a state of generalized immunosuppression is not a likely feature of PRRS.

Animals infected with PRRSV develop apoptosis of alveolar and pulmonary intravascular macrophages, and of mononuclear cells in alveolar septa. Because apoptotic cells are more numerous than virus-infected cells, the mechanism of apoptosis may not represent a direct effect of viral infection. Similarly, although interstitial pneumonia is extensive in swine with PRRS, virus-infected cells are relatively infrequent, suggesting a role for host-derived factors such as cytokines in development of lesions.

The major **lesions** *of the postnatal form of PRRS include interstitial pneumonia, generalized lymphadenopathy, and lymphocytic infiltrates in multiple organs.* Gross lung lesions vary from undetectable to affecting the entire lung, and tend to be most striking in younger age groups. The lungs fail to collapse when the diaphragm is incised, occasionally retain impressions of the ribs, and have generalized, patchy, lobular, or diffuse distributions of lesions. Affected areas of lung are discolored tan or red, and have a firm texture reminiscent of thymus, which contrasts with the crisp hard texture of bacterial pneumonia (Fig. 5-47). A cut section reveals separation of lobules and oozing of edema fluid. In pigs that develop bacterial bronchopneumonia secondary to PRRS, lesions of cranioventral consolidation may be superimposed on the diffuse interstitial pneumonia. In these cases, the lesions of PRRS may be subtle, yet play a critical role in the development of pneumonia in the herd. Lymph nodes throughout the body—most notably the bronchial, mediastinal, cervical, and inguinal nodes—are enlarged, white or tan, solid, and rarely contain multiple clear cavitations on cut section. Periocular and subcutaneous edema, pulmonary infarcts, myocardial necrosis, renal petechiae, and serous effusions into body cavities are variable findings.

Histologic *lung lesions are of interstitial pneumonia.* Alveolar septa are thickened because of infiltration of lymphocytes and macrophages (see Fig. 5-47B). This feature is easily obscured by atelectasis in routinely prepared samples, but can usually be confirmed by searching for areas of lung in which alveoli are not collapsed. Alveoli contain a cellular infiltrate of macrophages, lymphocytes, and fewer neutrophils, and scattered clusters of alveoli are filled with necrotic cells with pyknotic nuclei or free chromatin. *The finding of necrotic alveolar macrophages and aggregates of free chromatin is highly suggestive of PRRS.* Type II pneumocytes are increased in number, but may or may not form a continuous layer of cuboidal epithelium lining the alveolus. Bronchiolar epithelium is not affected by PRRSV, and a finding of bronchiolar necrosis should incite a search for an alternative or additional diagnosis.

Histologic examination of lymph nodes, tonsils, and spleens of pigs with PRRS may reveal *follicular and paracortical hyperplasia, and apoptosis of follicular lymphocytes.* Multinucleated cells, probably of histiocytic origin, may be present. Although this lesion is also common in porcine circovirus 2 (PCV-2)

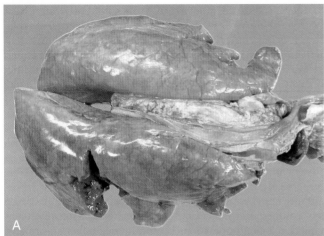

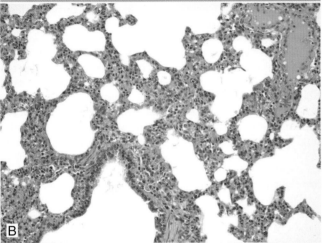

Figure 5-47 Porcine reproductive and respiratory syndrome. **A.** Grossly, the lungs show failure to collapse, diffuse firmness and rubbery texture, increased weight resulting from alveolar edema, and interlobular edema visible on the pleural surface. **B.** Diffuse thickening of alveolar septa by mononuclear cells. Lesions caused by circovirus or septicemia could appear similar.

infection, it has been described in PRRSV-infected pigs that have no evidence of PCV-2 infection.

Perivascular infiltrates of lymphocytes, macrophages, and plasma cells occur in many organs in PRRS. Commonly affected sites include the nasal mucosa, heart, kidney, and brain. Severe neurologic disease occasionally occurs in association with other manifestations of PRRS, possibly related to the infecting viral strain, and lesions of the central nervous system include lymphocytic meningoencephalitis, lymphocytic perivascular cuffs, and focal gliosis. PRRSV may cause *vasculitis* in the lung and other organs, manifesting as necrosis of the walls of large and small blood vessels in addition to perivascular and mural infiltrates of lymphocytes and plasma cells.

Aborted fetuses usually lack gross or histologic lesions, and, when present, the lesions are often not specific for PRRSV. Infection may progress from one fetus to another, resulting in live, stillborn, and mummified fetuses in the same litter. Fetal lesions that suggest PRRS include segmental or diffuse hemorrhage of the umbilical cord resulting from fibrinoid necrosis and suppurative inflammation of the umbilical artery, mild

interstitial pneumonia, pulmonary arteritis, lymphocytic myocarditis and encephalitis, and retroperitoneal and mesocolonic edema.

Diffusely firm lungs and histologic lesions of interstitial pneumonia are common findings at autopsy. In addition to PRRS, *a major differential diagnosis is septicemia.* Lesions of lymphadenopathy and mild proliferation of type II pneumocytes favor a diagnosis of PRRS, but differentiation requires ancillary testing. PCV-2 may cause a similar pattern of bronchointerstitial pneumonia, but granulomatous infiltrates and inclusion bodies are often present in lymph nodes and Peyer's patches. Proliferative and necrotizing pneumonia causes a similar alveolar lesion to PRRS, but bronchiolar necrosis is a feature of this disease that is absent in PRRS.

Polymerase chain reaction (PCR) and immunohistochemistry have become mainstays for the **diagnosis** of PRRS in tissue specimens although other assays may be of value: virus isolation, fluorescent antibody tests, and in situ hybridization. Detection of viral nucleic acid by PCR is a rapid technique that is as sensitive as virus isolation and has become widely used. In addition to tissue samples, PCR assays are performed on serum, oral fluids obtained with cotton ropes, or semen. Serology is useful on a herd level to identify prior exposure to PRRSV in unvaccinated herds. Immunohistochemistry on formalin-fixed paraffin-embedded sections of lung and tonsil is an economical approach to diagnosis, but because these assays are less sensitive than PCR, multiple sections should be examined. Virus isolation on chilled or frozen samples of lung, lymphoid tissues, serum, EDTA-treated blood, or pulmonary alveolar macrophages is a highly sensitive but slow method of diagnosis, but is necessary for further sequence analysis.

Results of diagnostic assays must be interpreted with caution in herds vaccinated with modified live viruses, as vaccine strains of PRRSV may circulate and persist in these herds and cause positive tests. An advantage of using PCR or virus isolation is the use of subsequent molecular analyses that assist in differentiating field and vaccine strains of virus in vaccinated herds. Identification of patterns of restriction fragment length polymorphisms (RFLP) in ORF 5 is commonly used to monitor patterns of PRRSV infection in large herds, and to differentiate vaccine strains from some field strains. However, the RFLP pattern of vaccine strains may change to an intermediate pattern as they circulate in herds. A second strategy distinguishes vaccine and field strains by identifying glycine and arginine, respectively, in residue 151 of ORF 5.

Obtaining a diagnosis of PRRS in aborted fetuses can be frustrating, because lesions are usually absent or nonspecific, and the agent often cannot be identified. Two techniques—the use of PCR assays on fetal lung and lymphoid tissue, and identification of antibody to PRRSV in precolostral sera—are currently recommended, but the low diagnostic rate remains a problem considering the importance of reproductive failure in infected swine herds.

Further reading

Gauger PC, et al. Genetic and phenotypic characterization of a 2006 United States porcine reproductive and respiratory virus isolate associated with high morbidity and mortality in the field. Virus Res 2012;163:98-107.

Li Y, et al. Emergence of a highly pathogenic porcine reproductive and respiratory syndrome virus in the Mid-Eastern region of China. Vet J 2007;174:577-584.

Mateu E, Diaz I. The challenge of PRRS immunology. Vet J 2007;177: 345-351.

Swine influenza. Orthomyxoviruses are pleomorphic, spherical to filamentous, 80-120 nm viruses containing negative-sense single-stranded RNA. Transcription of viral genes occurs in the nucleus, viral proteins are produced in the cytoplasm, and virions bud from the plasma membrane. Three genera of orthomyxoviruses are described based on variation of the nucleocapsid proteins: (1) *influenza A viruses* cause influenza in swine, horses, humans, and other species; (2) *influenza B viruses* represent human isolates only; and (3) *influenza C viruses* are rare and cause mild or subclinical infections in humans and swine. Orthomyxoviruses readily develop genomic variants, because of *genetic drift* caused by point mutations and *genetic shift* caused by recombination of genomic segments. *Identification of viral strains is based on antigenic variation of the 15 hemagglutinin (H) and 9 neuraminidase (N) envelope glycoproteins*, which mediate virus entry into cells and release of virus from infected cells, respectively. Analysis of viral strains is of practical importance in epidemiologic tracking of outbreaks and changing disease patterns, and to ensure that vaccine strains are representative of those in the field to ensure protective immunity.

Influenza viruses are usually host specific, and although several strains are known to cross species barriers, transmission rates are generally low, and most foreign strains are not maintained in the population. Although the direct zoonotic potential is of only moderate consequence, this phenomenon is important in the evolution of new viral strains. *Because swine possess cell-surface receptors for both avian and human viral strains, swine may act as hosts for reassortment among avian, porcine, and human strains of influenza viruses, with the potential for human pandemics resulting from the introduction of novel pathogenic strains into immunologically naive human populations.* However, it is now recognized that such reassortment can also occur in other species.

Influenza viruses are transmitted by aerosol or by contact with secretions. Infection is usually restricted to the respiratory tract, although myocarditis, myositis, and encephalitis are more frequent in carnivores and occasionally seen in horses and humans. Such non-respiratory lesions may be a consequence of viremia, or an effect of "cytokine storm" with dysregulation of cytokine production in the respiratory tissues.

Swine influenza is an important form of respiratory disease, manifesting as rapidly spreading outbreaks of severe nonfatal disease or as endemic disease as part of the porcine respiratory disease complex. Disease outbreaks are most common in the winter in cool climates, or late summer in warm climates. Disease severity may be enhanced by stresses, seasonal change in climate, PRRSV infection, or concurrent disease. Vaccination may enhance the disease that results from subsequent challenge with heterologous strains of the virus. Outbreaks of disease have a characteristic clinical presentation: The disease appears acutely and spreads rapidly to affect all ages of pigs, and despite severe clinical signs of coughing, fever, and stiffness, most pigs recover in 5-14 days, and the mortality rate is low. An endemic form of disease is also common, in which pigs develop bacterial bronchopneumonia secondary to subclinical infection with influenza virus. In this form of disease, the clinical picture is not specific for influenza and differentiation from other causes of porcine respiratory disease complex requires laboratory testing.

Identification of influenza A virus subtypes is important because there is limited cross-protection between subtypes; thus it is imperative that vaccines in current use are representative of circulating field strains. Subtypes H1N1, H3N2 and H1N2 are common in swine in North America, but infection of swine is documented with many other subtypes, including reassortants of swine, avian, and human viruses. Influenza virus is transmitted by infected droplets, aerosol, or contact with infected secretions. After experimental infection, serum antibody titers are detectable in many pigs by 7 days and peak 2-3 weeks after infection, and mucosal immunoglobulin A (IgA) and IgG are maximal at 1 and 4 weeks after infection, respectively. Pigs shed virus for 5-7 days after infection, although viral antigen is often cleared from the lung in as little as 72 hours after infection. Virus infection is probably maintained in swine populations by continuous infection of naive swine, as there is no evidence of a long-term carrier state or significant wildlife vector.

The **gross lesions** of swine influenza include a *cranioventral lobular distribution of atelectasis*, which is often sharply demarcated from normal lung tissue (eFig. 5-74, Fig. 5-48). Affected lobules are red, firm, and collapsed. Adjacent lobules are occasionally emphysematous. Generalized pulmonary edema may occur. Mediastinal and bronchial lymph nodes are enlarged and edematous, but usually not congested. The mucosa of the trachea and bronchi is often hyperemic and edematous. The development of secondary bacterial bronchopneumonia may obscure the gross lesions of swine influenza and cause red, firm, raised, lobular lesions in the cranioventral lung.

The **histologic lesions** reflect *necrosis of airway epithelium* and, to a lesser extent, alveolar epithelium, and include attenuation of bronchiolar epithelial cells; necrotic debris and neutrophils in bronchiolar lumens; atelectasis; and peribronchiolar, perivascular, and interstitial infiltrates of lymphocytes and plasma cells (see eFig. 5-74, Fig. 5-48). Vacuolation of bronchial and bronchiolar epithelial cells with loss of cilia occurs by 8 hours after experimental infection. By 24 hours, there is necrosis of bronchiolar and bronchial epithelial cells, and accumulation of sloughed necrotic cells in the lumen. Airway

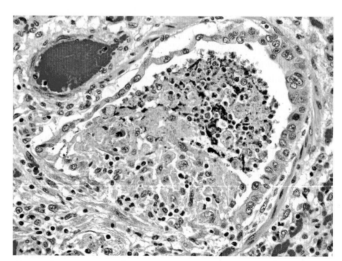

Figure 5-48 Swine influenza. Natural disease with focal erosion of bronchiolar epithelium, attenuation of adjacent epithelium, and early hyperplasia, giving a jumbled appearance of epithelial cell nuclei. The lumen is filled with cellular debris and leukocytes.

lumens and, to a lesser extent, alveoli contain neutrophils, and alveoli are atelectatic and edematous. Mononuclear cell infiltration occurs by 48 hours after infection. Alveolar injury, manifesting as exudation of neutrophils and scant fibrin with thickening of alveolar septa, is described in experimental cases at 48 hours after infection, but is often inapparent in pigs experiencing natural disease, or obscured by bacterial pneumonia. Later lesions include hyperplasia of airway epithelium as regeneration occurs, and peribronchiolar and perivascular aggregation of lymphocytes and plasma cells as immune responses develop. Infection is, in most cases, restricted to the respiratory tract and associated lymph nodes, although viremia has been infrequently described in neonates.

The **diagnosis** of swine influenza is suggested by the characteristic clinical signs of severe rapidly spreading disease with high morbidity and low mortality, and by the characteristic histologic lesions of bronchiolar necrosis or bronchiolar targeting of the neutrophil infiltrate (eFig. 5-75). *Differential diagnoses* for bronchiolar necrosis include porcine circovirus 2 infection, proliferative and necrotizing pneumonia, pseudorabies, Nipah virus infection, and airway injury caused by inhaled toxic gases. The diagnosis is confirmed by PCR testing of fresh lung tissue, antigen-detection ELISA on nasal or bronchial swabs, or immunohistochemistry on fixed tissues using monoclonal antibodies to conserved type A nucleoproteins. Initial PCR testing can target the conserved matrix gene, followed by subtype-specific testing or sequencing of the hemagglutinin gene. Virus isolation using embryonated eggs or cell lines is advantageous for subtyping, characterization of isolates, and partial sequencing to compare current and past isolates in a herd. Sample selection is critical for the diagnosis of swine influenza. Viral titers are highest 24 hours after infection, before gross lesions are obvious, and virus often cannot be identified by 72 hours after infection. Consequently, *selecting tissue from the cranioventral areas of the lung, from pigs early in the course of the disease, is critical for both histologic and virologic diagnosis.* Pigs with a high fever are the most suitable subjects for diagnostic investigation. The transient nature of the infection may complicate an investigation of the role of swine influenza in herds with endemic respiratory disease. In these cases, herd-level serology may be useful. Herd-level PCR testing is also of value, using nasal swabs or oral fluids collected with cotton ropes.

Further reading

Detmer S, et al. Diagnostics and surveillance for swine influenza. Curr Top Microbiol Immunol 2013;370:85-112.

Gauger PC, et al. Kinetics of lung lesion development and pro-inflammatory cytokine response in pigs with vaccine-associated enhanced respiratory disease induced by challenge with pandemic (2009) A/H1N1 influenza virus. Vet Pathol 2012;49:900-912.

Janke BH. Influenza A virus infections in swine: pathogenesis and diagnosis. Vet Pathol 2014;51:410-426.

Jung K, et al. Pathogenesis of swine influenza virus subtype H1N2 infection in pigs. J Comp Pathol 2005;132:179-184.

Yassine HM, et al. Interspecies and intraspecies transmission of influenza A viruses: viral, host and environmental factors. Animal Health Res Rev 2010;11:53-72.

Porcine circovirus and postweaning multisystemic wasting syndrome. Porcine circoviruses (genus *Circovirus*, family *Circoviridae*) are 17-nm, non-enveloped viruses that contain circular single-stranded DNA. Porcine circovirus 1 (PCV-1) is a nonpathogenic virus that was discovered as a cell culture contaminant. **Porcine circovirus 2** (PCV-2) is pathogenic and was first isolated in 1997 from pigs with a novel disease, *postweaning multisystemic wasting syndrome* (PMWS). Three genogroups—2a, 2b, and 2c—are recognized. Since its original identification in 2004, PCV-2b has become the predominant genogroup, but the associated spectrum of lesions appears comparable among the 3 genogroups.

PMWS was originally described in high-health herds, but many herds with PMWS are infected with PRRSV or other pathogens. *Serum antibody to PCV-2 is widespread in swine herds, and PCV-2 infection is common in herds with no clinical evidence of PMWS.* PMWS usually progresses slowly within the herd, with most cases developing in 5- to 12-week-old pigs. Morbidity is typically 5-10% but may be up to 20%, and most affected animals die or are euthanized. Pigs with PMWS lose weight or gain poorly, and have a variable combination of tachypnea, respiratory distress, diarrhea, pallor, and jaundice. Although uncommon, the finding of jaundice in swine should suggest a diagnosis of PMWS.

Porcine circoviral antigen and nucleic acid are most consistently present in the cytoplasm of monocytes, macrophages, and dendritic cells throughout the body, and less often in the nuclei and cytoplasm of epithelial cells in bronchioles, pulmonary alveoli, liver, renal tubules, stomach and intestine, and pancreas. Vascular smooth muscle and endothelial cells occasionally express circoviral antigen. Transmission is poorly characterized.

PCV-2 is sufficient to cause PMWS, as experimental infection of gnotobiotic or cesarean-derived colostrum-deprived pigs induces mild clinical signs and lesions of PMWS in the absence of other demonstrable pathogens. However, coinfection with PCV-2 and other pathogens, including parvovirus or PRRSV, results in more severe disease. Immunostimulation itself, either as a consequence of viral infection or vaccination, precipitates more severe disease. Thus *activation of the immune response may encourage replication of PCV-2, resulting in more severe manifestations of PMWS.* The role of PCV-2 in other swine diseases, termed PCV-associated diseases (PCVAD), remains controversial, in part because the virus can be isolated from many healthy pigs. In particular, although many pigs with dermatitis-nephropathy syndrome, proliferative and necrotizing pneumonia, sow abortion and mortality syndrome, congenital hypomyelination, and abortion with fetal myocarditis have evidence of PCV-2 infection, definitive proof of their causal association is lacking.

The spectrum of **gross lesions** and their severity are highly variable. Swine with PMWS are often thin, pale, and may be jaundiced. Lymph nodes throughout the body—particularly the inguinal, mesenteric, and bronchial nodes—are enlarged, soft, and white or gray-tan, and *this lymphadenopathy is the most consistent feature of PMWS.* Lung lesions, which are common, consist of interstitial pneumonia with generalized firm or rubbery texture, failure to collapse, and mottled color (see Fig. 5-47A). Cranioventral bronchopneumonia is a frequent concurrent lesion. The liver may be atrophic and discolored yellow-orange. Kidneys may contain patchy pallor or obvious white foci. Lesions resembling dermatitis-nephropathy syndrome may also occur, including swelling and edema of the kidneys, and cutaneous hemorrhages and necrosis. Infrequent lesions include splenic and cutaneous infarcts, cerebellar hemorrhages, renomegaly and pallor, or necrotizing colitis.

The **histologic lesions** of PMWS include *lymphoid depletion and granulomatous lymphadenitis, bronchointerstitial pneumonia, enteritis, interstitial nephritis, myocarditis, meningoencephalitis, and vasculitis*. Inclusion bodies were commonly observed when the disease initially emerged in the 1990s but are less common in contemporary cases. The inclusions are in macrophages, intracytoplasmic, usually multiple in a single cell, and basophilic. Inclusion bodies are most numerous and obvious in lymphoid tissues, including lymph nodes, Peyer's patch, tonsil, splenic periarteriolar lymphoid sheaths, and thymus (Fig. 5-49). In these tissues, there is depletion of lymphocytes from B-cell follicles, with striking infiltration of macrophages into follicles and, to a lesser extent, T-cell–rich paracortical areas. Multinucleated histiocytes may be present amid the granulomatous infiltrates. Widespread necrosis of lymphocytes in follicles is described but rare.

Histologic examination of the lungs of pigs with PMWS reveals diffuse or patchy *granulomatous interstitial pneumonia*. Epithelioid macrophages, multinucleated macrophages, lymphocytes, and fewer eosinophils or neutrophils infiltrate alveolar septa and may fill the alveoli. Lymphocytes and macrophages often encircle bronchioles and blood vessels. Bronchiolar necrosis is a variable finding, and may progress to bronchiolitis

obliterans in chronically affected pigs. Peribronchiolar fibroplasia with relatively mild lymphocytic inflammation is suggestive of PCV-2 infection. Liver lesions are highly variable, progressing from mild aggregates of lymphocytes in portal tracts, to single-cell necrosis of hepatocytes, periacinar necrosis, or widespread hepatocellular loss with condensation of hepatic stroma. Granulomatous enteritis with multinucleated cells may be prominent in the ileum, or infrequently in the colon. Perivascular infiltrates of lymphocytes and macrophages may be present in other organs, including kidney, myocardium, leptomeninges, pancreas, adrenal, stomach, and intestine. These lesions may be associated with renal tubular necrosis, interstitial nephritis, or necrosis of cardiac myocytes. Vasculitis, with necrosis of tunica muscularis accompanied by lymphohistiocytic infiltrates, and exudative glomerulonephritis are less common lesions. Lymphohistiocytic meningoencephalitis with or without vasculitis are reported.

Infection with PCV-2 is usually identified using *immunohistochemistry or PCR*. Assessing the viral load by PCR may be of value, as this is higher in wasting than in subclinically infected pigs. The virus may be isolated in PK15 cells or identified by in situ hybridization, but these find more use in research than as diagnostic techniques. Serologic assays, including indirect immunofluorescence and immunoperoxidase tests, have been developed, but the high prevalence of antibodies to PCV-2 in healthy pigs limits the diagnostic usefulness of these tests.

It is critical to recognize that demonstrating PCV-2 infection does not in itself indicate a diagnosis of PMWS. A **diagnosis** of PMWS is mainly based on the demonstration of consistent clinical findings and gross and histologic lesions, and is supported by the demonstration of active PCV-2 infection by immunohistochemistry or PCR. PRRS is the major differential diagnosis for lesions of interstitial pneumonia and lymphadenopathy in pigs. The following are helpful differentiating features, but *the lesions of PMWS and PRRS may be difficult to distinguish, and many pigs are coinfected with PCV-2 and PRRSV*:

- Multiple basophilic inclusion bodies in macrophages are a diagnostic feature of PCV-2 infection, and support the diagnosis of PMWS.
- Bronchiolar necrosis is present in some cases of PMWS (and swine influenza), but is not a lesion of PRRS.
- Lung lesions of PMWS tend to be dominated by macrophages, whereas lesions in PRRS are more lymphocytic, although there is much overlap in the morphology of these diseases.
- Granulomatous infiltrates and multinucleated macrophages in lymphoid organs are more typical of PMWS than of PRRS, although both lesions may be present in PRRS.

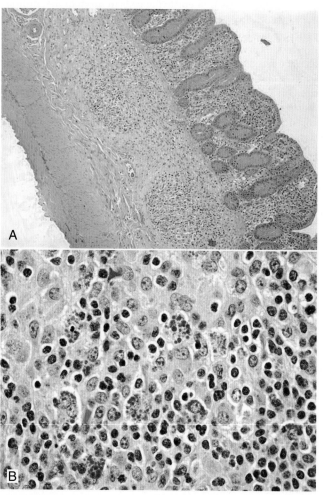

Figure 5-49 Postweaning multisystemic wasting syndrome caused by porcine circovirus 2. **A.** Peyer's patches in the ileum are depleted of lymphocytes and contain inclusion bodies visible even at low magnification. **B.** Multiple basophilic inclusion bodies in the cytoplasm of macrophages.

Further reading

Carman S, et al. The emergence of a new strain of porcine circovirus-2 in Ontario and Quebec swine and its association with severe porcine circovirus associated disease—2004-2006. Can J Vet Res 2008; 72:259-268.

Ellis J. Porcine circovirus: a historical perspective. Vet Pathol 2014;51: 315-327.

Langohr IM, et al. Vascular lesions in pigs experimentally infected with porcine circovirus type 2 serogroup B. Vet Pathol 2010;47:140-147.

Opriessnig T, Langohr I. Current state of knowledge on porcine circovirus type 2-associated lesions. Vet Pathol 2013;50:23-38.

Szeredi L, et al. Association of porcine circovirus type 2 with vascular lesions in porcine pneumonia. Vet Pathol 2012;49: 264-270.

Proliferative and necrotizing pneumonia. *Proliferative and necrotizing pneumonia is a severe acute disease of weaner and grower pigs.* Affected animals have acute onset of severe dyspnea, tachypnea, and fever. Gross lesions usually affect the entire lung, but may be restricted to the cranial and middle lobes. Lung lesions include remarkably increased firmness, failure to collapse, reddening, and edema. Generalized lymphadenopathy is usually present. Histologically, alveoli are edematous, contain macrophages and abundant necrotic cellular debris, and are lined by cuboidal type II pneumocytes. Alveolar septa are thickened by mononuclear cell infiltration (eFig. 5-76). Although many of these lesions may be present in severe cases of PRRS, *bronchiolar necrosis is often present in proliferative and necrotizing pneumonia but absent in PRRS.*

The understanding of the cause of this lesion is made difficult by the presence of multiple viruses. When the lesion was first reported in the early 1990s, it was associated with an H1N1 influenza virus that was genetically and antigenically distinct from common North American swine influenza virus isolates. Later publications associated proliferative and necrotizing pneumonia with PRRSV infection, PCV-2, and H3N2 influenza virus. It remains uncertain whether this lesion is caused by particular strains of PRRSV or by combined infection with several agents, or if it represents a pattern of reaction shared by more than one pathogen.

Further reading

Drolet R, et al. Detection rates of porcine reproductive and respiratory syndrome virus, porcine circovirus type 2, and swine influenza virus in porcine proliferative and necrotizing pneumonia. Vet Pathol 2003;40:143-148.

Grau-Roma L, Segales J. Detection of porcine reproductive and respiratory syndrome virus, porcine circovirus type 2, swine influenza virus and Aujeszky's disease virus in cases of porcine proliferative and necrotizing pneumonia (PNP) in Spain. Vet Microbiol 2007;119: 144-151.

Porcine respiratory coronavirus. Porcine respiratory coronavirus (PRCoV) is a minimally pathogenic virus that arose in the mid-1980s by deletion and point mutation of the transmissible gastroenteritis virus (TGEV) genome. European and American isolates of PRCoV differ, and apparently developed independently from TGEV. Following experimental challenge, neonatal pigs develop viremia and respiratory infection, whereas in 5-week-old pigs, viral antigen is limited to the respiratory tract, particularly alveolar and bronchiolar epithelial cells and alveolar macrophages. Lesions of naturally infected pigs are not described. In experimental cases, there is necrosis of bronchiolar epithelium, mild proliferation of type II pneumocytes, mononuclear cell infiltrates in alveolar septa, and lymphocytes and macrophages in alveoli. Most field cases are subclinical, although coinfection with *Bordetella* or PRRSV appears to exacerbate the disease. The major importance is that *antibodies to PRCoV cross-react with those to TGEV, leading to false-positive serologic tests in swine herds that are expected to be free of TGEV.* Diagnosis is based on isolation of the virus or indirect fluorescent antibody tests. Newer blocking ELISAs differentiate these coronaviruses.

Further reading

Brockmeier SL, et al. Coinfection of pigs with porcine respiratory coronavirus and *Bordetella bronchiseptica.* Vet Microbiol 2008;128: 36-47.

Halbur PG, et al. Pathogenicity of three isolates of porcine respiratory coronavirus in the USA. Vet Rec 2003;152:358-361.

Inclusion body rhinitis. Suid herpesvirus 2 (SuHV-2; cytomegalovirus) infections are ubiquitous and occur throughout the world, but clinical disease is much less frequent. *Inclusion body rhinitis, which is caused by SuHV-2, is typically an acute to subacute disease of 3- to 5-week-old suckling piglets.* Piglets exhibit fever, sneezing, catarrhal nasal exudate, shivering, and occasional dyspnea. Morbidity is high and mortality is low unless secondary bacterial infections develop. Systemic cytomegalovirus infections usually affect piglets <3 weeks of age. Such animals may be found dead without premonitory signs, or exhibit sneezing, lethargy, and anorexia, subcutaneous edema of the jaw and tarsal joints, and dyspnea. Infection of naive pregnant sows induces mild lethargy, anorexia, and delivery of stillborn or weak piglets.

Piglets commonly shed the virus soon after weaning at 3 weeks of age, suggesting that infection is usually acquired by contact with nasal secretions of infected cohorts. Other pigs, particularly those that develop generalized disease, are probably infected from the sow in the neonatal period. The virus replicates in nasal submucosal and lacrimal glands. Viremia develops 5-14 days after infection, depending on the age of the pig, and leads to infection of epithelial cells in renal tubules, liver, duodenum, and elsewhere. Pulmonary alveolar and splenic macrophages may be additional sites of viral replication. Virus is shed in nasal and ocular secretions, in the urine, and in vaginal secretions of sows.

Gross lesions in pigs infected with cytomegalovirus are usually only seen in piglets <3 weeks of age with generalized disease, and may include catarrhal rhinitis, hydrothorax, hydropericardium, pulmonary and subcutaneous edema, and renal petechiae. **Histologically,** *large 8-12 μm basophilic intranuclear inclusion bodies* are numerous in the epithelial cells of the nasal mucosal glands and their ducts (Fig. 5-50). Affected glands are not diffusely distributed but tend to occur in irregular clusters. As the inclusion forms, cytomegaly and karyomegaly develop. The nuclear membrane becomes indistinct, the inclusions appear as blue-gray smears, and the necrotic epithelium sloughs into the lumen. The developing immune response incites a lymphocytic infiltrate in the lamina propria, macrophages and lymphocytes cluster within degenerating glands, and there is squamous metaplasia of the surface epithelium.

Systemic lesions develop following viremia, with intranuclear inclusion bodies in epithelial cells of renal tubules and glomeruli; lacrimal, Harderian, and salivary glands; and less commonly in hepatocytes and sinusoidal lining cells, adrenal gland, esophageal glands, lymph nodes, spleen, renal medulla, lung, and elsewhere. *Inclusions are most numerous in epithelium but also occur in macrophages and endothelial cells;* this vascular disease accounts for the petechiation and edema. Inclusion bodies are often accompanied by cytomegaly, lymphocytic infiltrates, and occasionally focal necrosis. Focal gliosis with intranuclear inclusions in scattered glial cells occurs throughout the central nervous system. The viremic phase may last

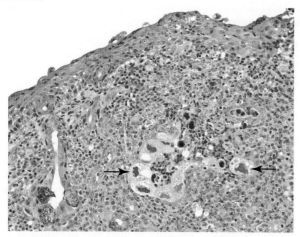

Figure 5-50 Inclusion body rhinitis in a pig. Cytomegaly of affected epithelial cells in nasal glands with large, homogeneous, smudgy, basophilic inclusions (arrows) that completely fill the nucleus. The lamina propria is diffusely infiltrated by lymphocytes.

for 2-3 weeks and is followed by persistent infection in pulmonary macrophages.

Inclusion bodies, cytomegaly, and karyomegaly are pathognomonic when present. Adenovirus is the only viral agent likely to cause similarly large basophilic intranuclear inclusion bodies, but adenovirus does not induce cytomegaly and is usually restricted to intestinal epithelium in swine. The intranuclear inclusions of pseudorabies are eosinophilic, less obvious than those of cytomegalovirus, focal necrosis is more prominent, and lesions are most prominent in brain, respiratory tract, and lymphoid tissue. Confirmation of cytomegalovirus infection may be achieved by electron microscopy to search for herpesviral particles, or by virus isolation, immunofluorescence, or PCR on nasal scrapings, lung wash cells, or kidney homogenates.

Further reading

Edington N, et al. Generalized porcine cytomegalic inclusion disease: distribution of cytomegalic cells and virus. J Comp Pathol 1976;86:191-202.

Pseudorabies. Pseudorabies (Aujeszky's disease), caused by **suid herpesvirus 1**, is described in more detail in Vol. 1, Nervous system, for neurologic signs predominate in most cases of pseudorabies in young swine. However, *certain strains of pseudorabies virus tend to cause respiratory disease*, particularly following aerosol exposure of older pigs. The respiratory form is typified by high morbidity and low mortality, unless secondary bacterial pneumonia develops. Affected pigs are depressed, febrile, and display episodes of sneezing, coughing, and dyspnea. Gross lesions in the upper respiratory tract are most common, and include necrotizing rhinitis and laryngotracheitis, with foci of necrosis in the tonsils. Lung lesions are less consistent, but patchy areas of reddening and consolidation may be scattered throughout the lung, or target the cranioventral lung. Histologically, *bronchointerstitial pneumonia* is characterized by necrosis and sloughing of bronchial and bronchiolar epithelium, *with frequent intranuclear eosinophilic or faintly basophilic inclusions* in the early stages of disease.

Alveolar lesions include multifocal necrosis; sloughing of necrotic alveolar epithelium; fibrinous exudate in alveoli; hemorrhage; infrequent inclusion bodies; and infiltration of lymphocytes, macrophages, and fewer plasma cells and neutrophils. Experimentally, necrotizing lesions develop within 3-6 days of infection, infiltration of lymphocytes is prominent by days 5-8, and repair occurs during days 6-10.

Further reading

Segales J, et al. Immunohistochemical demonstration of the spread of pneumotropic strain 4892 of Aujeszky's disease virus in conventional pigs. J Comp Pathol 1997;116:387-395.

Nipah virus. *Nipah virus* emerged as an epidemic cause of nervous and respiratory disease in pigs and humans in Malaysia in 1998 and 1999 and in humans in Bangladesh in 2004. The disease also affects dogs and cats, and horses and goats develop an antibody response. Nipah and Hendra viruses are the lone members of the genus *Henipavirus* (family *Paramyxoviridae*). *Pteropus* fruit bats (flying foxes) are the reservoir and major source of infection; pigs are considered a major source of infection for humans and other pigs, whereas human-to-human transmission appears to be rare.

Gross lesions are nonspecific, but *the characteristic histologic findings are lymphocytic and/or fibrinoid vasculitis; lymphoid necrosis; syncytial cells within lymphoid tissues, endothelium, and perivascular cells; and intracytoplasmic eosinophilic inclusion bodies.* The lesions include lymphocytic meningitis and, to a lesser extent, encephalitis that is present throughout the brain but most severe in the olfactory bulb; necrotizing, lymphocytic, and/or hyperplastic rhinitis, tracheitis, bronchitis, and bronchiolitis (see Fig. 5-31); lymphohistiocytic bronchointerstitial pneumonia; necrosis of lymphoid tissues, particularly tonsil and submandibular and bronchial lymph node; and lymphocytic infiltrates in multiple organs.

Nipah virus is readily isolated from blood, tonsil, nasal mucosa, lung, and other lymphoid tissues. Viral antigen is demonstrated by immunohistochemistry in epithelial cells in tonsil, trachea, bronchioles, and alveoli; alveolar macrophages; meningeal connective tissue and possibly astrocytes; endothelium and muscularis of inflamed blood vessels; and areas of lymphoid necrosis.

Further reading

Hooper P, et al. Comparative pathology of the diseases caused by Hendra and Nipah viruses. Microbes Infect 2001;3:315-322.

Other viral respiratory diseases of swine. Porcine rubulavirus (family *Paramyxoviridae*) causes "blue-eye disease," an important condition of pigs in Mexico. Clinical manifestations include neurologic disease, respiratory disease, and less frequently, corneal opacity or reproductive failure. Lesions in experimentally infected pigs are of lymphocytic interstitial pneumonia with cuffs around bronchioles. Porcine genogroup 1 torque teno virus (family *Anelloviridae*) is not considered important as a primary pathogen, but it may exacerbate other infections, such as with PCV-2. Challenge of gnotobiotic pigs induced interstitial pneumonia, thymic atrophy, glomerulopathy, and lymphocytic hepatitis.

Further reading

Krakowka S, Ellis JA. Evaluation of the effects of porcine genogroup 1 torque teno virus in gnotobiotic swine. Am J Vet Res 2008;69:1623-1629.

Rivera-Benitez JF, et al. Respiratory disease in growing pigs after Porcine rubulavirus experimental infection. Virus Res 2013;176:137-143.

Bacterial diseases

Actinobacillus pleuropneumoniae. *Actinobacillus pleuropneumoniae (APP) causes contagious pleuropneumonia, an important cause of severe, often fatal, pneumonia in growing pigs.* The disease is most common in 6-week-old to 6-month-old hogs. Disease severity is highly variable, but case fatality rates of 20-80% are common in acute outbreaks. Clinical signs in severely affected swine include fever, lethargy, severe dyspnea, cyanosis, bloody discharge from the nose, and occasionally vomiting or diarrhea. Convalescent pigs with chronic pneumonia may fail to thrive and display exercise intolerance and coughing.

APP is a gram-negative coccobacillus of the family *Pasteurellaceae*. Twelve serotypes are defined by antigenic variation in capsular polysaccharide and cell-wall lipopolysaccharide. Serotypes 1, 5, and 7 are most common in North America; serotypes 2 and 9 are prevalent in Europe; and serotypes 1, 7, and 12 are frequent in Australia. Serotypes 1, 5, 9, and 11 secrete both Apx I and II toxins and tend to cause more severe disease than other serotypes. Immunity to heterologous serotypes is only partially protective.

APP has a rich spectrum of *virulence factors* important in pathogenesis. Three cytotoxins, named Apx I, II, and III, are members of the RTX (repeats in toxin) family of secreted toxins that includes *Mannheimia haemolytica* leukotoxin and *Escherichia coli* hemolysin. A fourth Apx toxin gene expressed in vivo but not in vitro is of uncertain significance. The Apx toxins are potent inducers of cytolysis in porcine neutrophils, alveolar macrophages, erythrocytes, and epithelial cells. Low concentrations induce an oxidative burst in porcine neutrophils. These toxins appear critical to development of disease, as Apx toxin–deficient mutants have reduced virulence that is restored when the toxin genes are reintroduced. Lipopolysaccharide induces macrophage activation and secretion of neutrophil chemoattractants, procoagulant activity, and complement activation, similar to that described for *M. haemolytica*. The capsule impairs phagocytosis by macrophages and may prevent complement activation. Isolates with thin capsules may be less pathogenic. APP produces superoxide dismutase, catalase, and hydroperoxide reductase, which may protect against oxidative killing by neutrophils and macrophages. Other virulence factors include fimbrial adhesins, outer-membrane proteins, iron-binding proteins, metalloproteinase, and urease.

Infection is acquired by direct contact with infected pigs or by spread of aerosol droplets over short distances. The bacteria may be carried in the nasopharynx of apparently healthy animals, and these carriers are the principal method of introduction onto a naive farm. In contrast to *Pasteurella multocida* and *Bordetella bronchiseptica* in pigs and *M. haemolytica* of cattle, APP often causes disease in the absence of predisposing factors. Nevertheless, disease severity is enhanced by *Mycoplasma hyopneumoniae* or pseudorabies infections, and

by factors that cause ciliary stasis. The interaction between PRRSV and APP infections is controversial.

Following inhalation, APP rapidly binds to the epithelium lining terminal bronchioles and alveoli. Neutrophil infiltration and alveolar exudate develop as early as 90 minutes after infection. Neutrophil recruitment is primarily due to secretion of neutrophil chemoattractants by macrophages in response to infection, for bacterial products themselves do not directly induce neutrophil chemotaxis. *Leukocyte necrosis is a prominent feature of the histologic lesions*, and is presumably mediated by the Apx cytotoxins.

Immunity to APP is conferred by mucosal IgA and serum IgG antibody responses, particularly to the Apx cytotoxins. However, heterologous infections impart only partial immunity, and this effect is not dependent on patterns of Apx toxin expression, implying that antibody against other bacterial antigens also contributes to protection. Antibody against surface components, such as capsular polysaccharide, greatly enhances phagocytosis of APP by neutrophils and macrophages, and neutrophils but not macrophages effectively kill these opsonized bacteria in vitro. In endemically infected herds, maternal antibody declines over the first 12 weeks of life, and active immune responses contribute to increasing titers thereafter. In experimental infections, serum antibody titers are detectable at 2 weeks and maximal at about 5 weeks after infection.

Gross findings in pigs that die of contagious pleuropneumonia are typified by *fibrinosuppurative, hemorrhagic, and necrotizing lobar pneumonia or pleuropneumonia*. Identical gross lesions may be caused by *Actinobacillus suis* and, less frequently, by *Salmonella enterica* serovar Choleraesuis; these are important differential diagnoses in minimal-disease herds expected to be free of APP. The lesions commonly affect the *middle or caudal lung lobes*, and may be unilateral or bilateral (Fig. 5-51). Lesions are deep red, firm to hard, protrude above the surrounding lung, and cut crisply. The cut surface often exhibits sharply demarcated, irregularly shaped, 1-10 cm foci of coagulative necrosis that are friable and pale. In peracute cases, interlobular septa are expanded by fibrin and edema, and fibrinous exudate on the pleural surface ranges in appearance from a haze resembling ground glass to mats of fibrin.

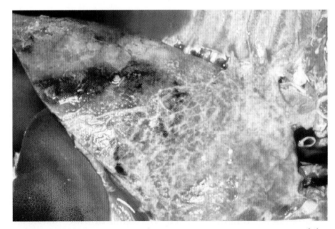

Figure 5-51 Contagious pleuropneumonia in a pig caused by *Actinobacillus pleuropneumoniae*. The primary lesion of hemorrhage and fibrinosuppurative pneumonia is characteristically located in the caudal lobe, and a mat of fibrin covers the pleural surface. (Courtesy University of Guelph.)

The bronchi may contain frothy or bloody fluid, and blood may ooze from the nostrils. Bronchial and mediastinal lymph nodes are enlarged, edematous, and congested. The pericardial and peritoneal cavities may contain scant serosanguineous fluid. Lesions in chronically affected pigs include fibrous pleural adhesions, sequestra, and locally extensive pulmonary fibrosis or abscess formation. Acutely affected pigs occasionally develop hyaline thrombi and fibrinoid necrosis of glomerular capillaries, afferent arterioles, and interlobular renal arteries, perhaps mediated by endotoxemia.

Microscopic investigation of these lesions reveals filling of alveoli and terminal bronchioles by fibrin, neutrophils, fewer macrophages, and many necrotic leukocytes that are probably neutrophils. The foci of necrosis, which are often centered on alveolar septa, are delineated by a basophilic band of intense neutrophil infiltration and extensive neutrophil necrosis. In the center of the necrotic areas, the exudate varies from protein-rich edema, to fibrin, to leukocytes. Many leukocytes contain streaming, lightly basophilic, homogeneous chromatin similar to the "oat cells" of bovine shipping fever pneumonia. These neutrophils are in an apparent state of activation, and express tumor necrosis factor-α, IL-1, and IL-8 mRNA at high levels.

The mucosa of bronchi and bronchioles may be infiltrated by neutrophils with fewer macrophages, and bronchiolar epithelium may be necrotic or sloughed. In this regard, the lesions can resemble those of swine influenza. Thrombi may develop in small venules and capillaries in the alveolar and interlobular septa, and fibrinoid vasculitis has been infrequently described. Lymphatics in the alveolar septa are distended by serofibrinous exudate with variable numbers of neutrophils. Extrapulmonary lesions are uncommon, but include renal glomerular thrombosis, renal vasculitis, or osteomyelitis.

Lesions of localized or locally extensive fibrinous and necrotizing pneumonia suggest APP, *A. suis* or, less commonly, *S. enterica* serovar Choleraesuis, as likely causes. *Definitive* **diagnosis** *depends on isolation of the agent, and microscopic identification of suppurative bronchopneumonia with neutrophil necrosis.* Isolation on blood agar requires a *Staphylococcus* streak or supplemented medium containing a source of nicotinamide adenine dinucleotide. Alternatively, bacteria in lung smears or primary cultures can be identified using antigen detection techniques such as ELISA or latex agglutination. Serologic identification of APP is particularly useful in the maintenance of minimal-disease herds.

Further reading

Merialdi G, et al. Survey of pleuritis and pulmonary lesions in pigs at abattoir with a focus on the extent of the condition and herd risk factors. Vet J 2012;193:234-239.

Sibila M, et al. Comparison of four lung scoring systems for the assessment of the pathological outcomes derived from *Actinobacillus pleuropneumoniae* experimental infections. BMC Vet Res 2014; 10:165.

Bronchopneumonia caused by opportunistic bacterial pathogens. *The porcine respiratory disease complex is an exemplar of multifactorial disease causation.* Although bacterial pneumonia is the final cause of death in many cases of porcine respiratory disease, its development is highly dependent on host factors, environmental influences, and other infectious agents. Important contributing environmental factors include elevated levels of dust and ammonia, temperature fluctuations, and extremes of temperature and humidity. In temperate climates, the incidence of swine pneumonia is maximal in the autumn and early winter, in part caused by fluctuating temperatures and the impact of cold weather on barn ventilation and air quality. Immunity to respiratory pathogens is dependent on patterns of pig flow through production units, vaccination practices, and alterations in innate resistance caused by social and environmental stresses, nutrition, and management practices. Against this background of host and environmental factors, interactions between multiple pathogens are commonly identified in swine pneumonia. Thus *effective control of disease requires that diagnostic investigations identify not only the immediate causes of fatal disease, but also the underlying infectious and noninfectious factors.*

Porcine reproductive and respiratory syndrome virus, *Mycoplasma hyopneumoniae*, influenza A virus, and porcine circovirus 2 all cause primary lung disease. In addition, each of these agents impair the normal pulmonary defenses against inhaled bacterial pathogens by, among other mechanisms, impairing mucociliary clearance and suppressing alveolar macrophage function. Swine are commonly exposed to the **opportunistic pathogens** *Pasteurella multocida, Streptococcus suis, Bordetella bronchiseptica*, and *Haemophilus parasuis*, and failure of lung defenses caused by viral or mycoplasmal infection, poor air quality, and stresses are key factors in development of disease caused by these bacterial pathogens.

P. multocida serotypes A and D are important causes of fatal pneumonia in weaner and grower-finisher pigs. The massive doses of *P. multocida* needed for experimental induction of disease suggest that the predisposing causes listed above are necessary components of the natural disease. *Bordetella* is particularly noteworthy as a cause of fatal pneumonia in piglets <3 weeks of age, but may also cause bronchopneumonia in older swine. The pathogenesis of bordetellosis is described in the section Infectious respiratory diseases of dogs, later.

Gross lesions of bronchopneumonia, in which cranioventral areas of lung are swollen, consolidated, reddened, and sharply demarcated from more normal lung, are typical of infection with these opportunistic bacterial pathogens. In many cases, but not all, mucopurulent exudate may be expressed from airways on cut section. Fibrinous pleuritis may be present but is usually minor. Bronchial lymph nodes are often enlarged and mottled red and white. The predominant **histologic findings** are numerous neutrophils and macrophages filling alveoli and bronchioles. Fibrin exudation may occur but is usually minor. These lesions contrast with those of *A. pleuropneumoniae* and *A. suis*, where fibrinous exudate in airspaces and on the pleural surface is often prominent, most of the neutrophils are necrotic and have streaming basophilic chromatin, and focally extensive coagulative necrosis is often present. In cases of bronchopneumonia, the bronchiolar epithelium is generally normal or mildly hyperplastic, but bronchiolar necrosis is usually absent unless there is underlying swine influenza virus or PCV-2 infection. *M. hyopneumoniae* also causes a cranioventral pattern of bronchopneumonia, but in contrast to the red swollen lung of bacterial bronchopneumonia, the acute lesions of mycoplasmosis are red and atelectatic, whereas the subacute lesions are gray to tan and only mildly swollen to firm. Cranioventral bronchopneumonia superimposed on generalized or patchy lesions of interstitial pneumonia suggests underlying PRRSV or PCV-2 infection, or septicemia.

Although bacterial bronchopneumonia may be the immediate cause of death, viral or mycoplasmal pathogens should be considered as underlying causes. Microbiologic testing is commonly used to identify the spectrum of pathogens causing pneumonia, but the plethora of currently available tests does not diminish the importance of morphologic examination of the lung. Determining the patterns of gross and histologic lesions allows the pathologist to narrow the list of differential diagnoses to select a panel of ancillary tests efficiently, to provide a tentative diagnosis when rapid therapeutic intervention is required or when ancillary microbiologic tests are negative, and to evaluate critically the contribution of particular pathogens, many of which are commonly present in healthy swine, to the case being investigated.

Further reading

Hansen MS, et al. An investigation of the pathology and pathogens associated with porcine respiratory disease complex in Denmark. J Comp Pathol 2010;143:120-131.

Hillen S, et al. Occurrence and severity of lung lesions in slaughter pigs vaccinated against *Mycoplasma hyopneumoniae* with different strategies. Prev Vet Med 2014;113:580-588.

Pors SE, et al. Occurrence and associated lesions of *Pasteurella multocida* in porcine bronchopneumonia. Vet Microbiol 2011;150:160-166.

Atrophic rhinitis. Nonprogressive atrophic rhinitis (NPAR), caused by *Bordetella bronchiseptica* and other factors, causes mild transient sneezing and nasal discharge, and is *not usually of herd significance.* In contrast, **progressive atrophic rhinitis (PAR)** is caused by toxin-producing strains of *Pasteurella multocida*, often in concert with other bacterial pathogens, and *causes production loss.* PAR affects pigs of at least 6-12 weeks of age, causing sneezing, mucopurulent nasal discharge, unilateral epistaxis, nasal deformity, failure to thrive, and secondary bacterial bronchopneumonia. Freedom from PAR is a frequent requirement in minimal-disease herds, so *differentiation of PAR and NPAR is of substantial significance.* Toxigenic *P. multocida* infects rodents, cats, dogs, and ruminants, and may be of zoonotic concern.

Both NPAR and PAR are multifactorial conditions for which air quality and the presence of other pathogens influence the severity of disease. NPAR is primarily caused by strains of *B. bronchiseptica* that adhere to nasal cilia and tonsillar epithelium, and produce a toxin that causes mucosal edema, loss of cilia, and resorption of turbinate bone. Infection is acquired by inhalation of infected aerosol droplets.

Progressive atrophic rhinitis is caused by cytotoxin-producing strains of **P. multocida type D** *or, less commonly, type A.* Infection is acquired by inhalation following direct contact with infected pigs. Colonization of the nasal mucosa and tonsil is inefficient, but augmented by factors that harm the nasal mucosa, including *B. bronchiseptica* infection, ammonia, and dusts. The *cytotoxin*, also referred to as *dermonecrotic toxin*, is a secreted, heat-labile toxin encoded by the *toxA* gene. Intranasal or intramuscular administration of *P. multocida* cytotoxin has similar effects on the nasal turbinates, including epithelial hyperplasia, glandular atrophy, resorption of turbinate bone by osteoclasts, reduced formation of bone by osteoblasts, and fibroblast proliferation. The cytotoxin does not directly affect

osteoclast function; rather, hyperplasia and increased function of these cells are apparently stimulated by soluble mediators secreted from nearby stromal cells in response to the cytotoxin.

Distortion of the snout is a prominent external finding in pigs with chronic atrophic rhinitis. Brachygnathia superior occurs when the maxillary bones of the snout fail to grow. Lateral deviation toward the most severely affected side is common.

Atrophy and malformation of the nasal turbinates are the principal lesions of atrophic rhinitis, and are more severe in the ventral than the dorsal conchae. To assess the integrity of the nasal turbinates, cross-sections of the snout should be made at the level of the first or second upper premolar teeth; in affected pigs, the normally scroll-like turbinates are misshapen and blunted. Turbinate atrophy may be partial or complete, leaving a hollow nasal cavity with an often-deformed nasal septum. Regeneration of atrophic turbinates has been demonstrated in a longitudinal computed tomography study.

Histologic lesions in the nasal turbinates include osteoclast hyperplasia, *osteoclast-mediated resorption of bone, and replacement with fibrous tissue containing many plump fibroblasts.* Lymphocytes and fewer neutrophils infiltrate the nasal mucosa, and there may be squamous metaplasia of the ciliated epithelium.

The gross lesions of NPAR and PAR are qualitatively similar, although those of NPAR are generally less severe. Nevertheless, given the significance of a diagnosis of progressive atrophic rhinitis caused by toxigenic *P. multocida*, definitive identification is usually warranted. *B. bronchiseptica* and *P. multocida* can be readily isolated from swabs of nasal mucosa or tonsil, but *definitive diagnosis of PAR depends on demonstrating P. multocida cytotoxin production using PCR or an ELISA.* Various grading systems have been described to assess the severity of nasal turbinate atrophy. These grading systems are not intended to differentiate NPAR from PAR, but are useful in monitoring the herd response to management or therapeutic interventions.

Further reading

Davies RL, et al. Characterization and comparison of *Pasteurella multocida* strains associated with porcine pneumonia and atrophic rhinitis. J Med Microbiol 2003;52:59-67.

Magyar T, et al. Regeneration of toxigenic *Pasteurella multocida* induced severe turbinate atrophy in pigs detected by computed tomography. BMC Vet Res 2013;9:222.

Mycoplasmal diseases

General features of mycoplasmas. Mycoplasmas, which are members of the class Mollicutes, are the smallest self-replicating organisms, lack a cell wall, and have a protein- and lipid-rich plasma membrane. They are obligate parasites, and several species lack the ability to synthesize required amino acids, cholesterol, and fatty acids. The success of culturing mycoplasmas in vitro is highly dependent on the particular species. Some mycoplasmas grow so readily that they commonly contaminate cell cultures, yet many of the pathogenic mycoplasmas grow slowly, have frustratingly fastidious growth requirements, and are easily overgrown by other agents. Mycoplasmas have a relatively small genome, 580-1,380 kb, which contains many repetitive elements and a propensity for genomic rearrangement through homologous recombination. Many mycoplasmas have highly specific host and tissue tropism, and are commonly commensals on mucosal surfaces. Nevertheless, spread of infection through the blood with subsequent localization in joints or serosal surfaces is a feature of some mycoplasmoses. *Most mycoplasmal pathogens of the respiratory tract adhere to ciliated epithelium*, mediated in some species by a specialized attachment organelle. A few mycoplasmas invade host cells, but this has not been demonstrated for mycoplasmal pathogens of animals.

High-frequency variation of surface antigens allows several mycoplasmas to evade the humoral immune response by changing their surface lipoprotein antigens as antibodies against these structures are formed. The mechanisms by which *Mycoplasma* infections result in disease remain poorly characterized. Mycoplasmas have not been shown to secrete exotoxins. *Pathogenic mechanisms* of respiratory disease include ciliostasis resulting from membrane alterations, alteration of host prostaglandin synthesis, biofilm formation, induction of apoptosis in lymphocytes or other host cells, non–antigen-specific stimulation of immune responses as a consequence of superantigens in the mycoplasmal plasma membrane.

Further reading

Citti C, Blanchard A. Mycoplasmas and their host: emerging and re-emerging minimal pathogens. Trends Microbiol 2013;21:196-203.

Mycoplasma hyopneumoniae. *Mycoplasma hyopneumoniae* is the cause of *mycoplasmal pneumonia of swine*, often known as *enzootic pneumonia*. It is a common, chronic, usually nonfatal disease of young pigs. The disease may be endemic, or spread slowly but progressively through a facility over the course of weeks, and the morbidity rate may be as high as 70-100%. Although pigs as young as 5 weeks of age may develop disease, it is *most important in grower-finisher pigs* and may be a key component of fatal multifactorial pneumonia in 4- to 6-month-old hogs. Clinical expressions of the uncomplicated disease are coughing, unthriftiness, poor weight gain, and reduced feed conversion. Because there is usually low mortality associated with mycoplasmal pneumonia, the lesions are generally seen in slaughtered animals or those dying from other diseases. When deaths do occur, they are mainly due to superimposed infections with other bacteria.

Like other mycoplasmal pathogens, *M. hyopneumoniae* is a tiny bacterium that lacks a cell wall. The agent adheres to ciliated epithelium of the large airways and, in lower number, of the bronchioles, using 97- and 145-kDa outer membrane proteins. Adherent organisms are closely associated with the cilia, and there is often extensive ciliary loss. In chronic infections, mycoplasmal antigen and nucleic acid are also present in alveolar and interstitial macrophages. The cell membranes of many mycoplasmas, presumably including *M. hyopneumoniae*, contain superantigens that induce polyclonal proliferation of lymphocytes and result in the characteristic aggregates of lymphocytes around airways and blood vessels. Infection with *M. hyopneumoniae* is mainly transmitted by direct contact with nasal secretions from infected pigs, although aerosol transmission over short distances may occur. A common clinical scenario involves infection of a few young pigs by contact with an infected sow, followed by slow spread

to in-contact pigs when groups are assembled in weaner or grower-finisher units.

Clinical disease is not an inevitable consequence of infection with *M. hyopneumoniae*. Rather, its development is highly dependent on other predisposing factors, including crowding, poor air quality, fluctuations in temperature or humidity, and the presence of other pathogens. Many infections are subclinical, and carrier animals are important sources of infection of naive herds. Primary *M. hyopneumoniae* infection is not expected to be fatal, but reduced mucociliary clearance and possibly impaired macrophage function may lead to fatal bacterial pneumonia caused by opportunistic pathogens such as *Pasteurella multocida*, *Streptococcus suis*, *Bordetella bronchiseptica*, or *Haemophilus* spp. The interaction of PRRSV with *M. hyopneumoniae* is particularly noteworthy. Mycoplasmal infection exacerbates the severity and the duration of PRRS, although the effect of PRRSV infection on mycoplasmal pneumonia is apparently minor. As a result, new infections with *M. hyopneumoniae* may cause outbreaks of PRRS in herds with previously subclinical PRSSV infections.

The characteristic **gross feature** *of mycoplasmal pneumonia is red-tan-gray discoloration, collapse, and rubbery firmness affecting cranioventral regions of the lungs in a lobular pattern* (Fig. 5-52). Lesions often affect cranial and middle lung lobes, accessory lobe, and cranioventral portions of the caudal lobes. The mildest lesions resemble atelectasis, with a lobular pattern of reddening and collapse. More severe lesions evolve from dark red through gray-pink to more homogeneous gray as the lesion ages. The rubbery or thymus-like texture of the lung contrasts with the more firm or hard consistency of *Pasteurella* pneumonia, although this is often present concurrently. The cut surface of affected lung is edematous, and catarrhal exudate can be squeezed from bronchi. The bronchiolar orientation of the inflammation often results in a regular pattern of tiny gray foci against a red background. *M. hyopneumoniae* rarely causes serofibrinous pleuritis or polyserositis, but this is more commonly due to opportunistic bacteria or *M. hyorhinis*. Pulmonary lymph nodes are enlarged and on cut surface are moist, usually bulging, and sometimes hyperemic.

Histologically, subacute to chronic mycoplasmal pneumonia in swine is typified by lymphocytic infiltrates around airways, increased numbers of alveolar macrophages, and alveolar edema. In the fully developed mycoplasmal pneumonia, there is *extensive lymphoid hyperplasia* around bronchi, bronchioles, and their associated vessels; and lymphocytes infiltrate the lamina propria of the airway mucosa (see Fig. 5-52). The epithelium is often histologically normal or mildly hyperplastic. Although ciliary loss and exfoliation of ciliated epithelium may occur, this is difficult to detect by light microscopy. Goblet cells in the airway mucosa are increased in number, and the bronchial glands are hyperplastic, reflecting the excessive mucus secretions seen grossly. The alveolar exudate consists predominantly of macrophages and protein-rich edema, but variable numbers of plasma cells, lymphocytes, and neutrophils are present. The alveolar septa are mildly thickened by lymphocytes and a few plasma cells.

Experimental studies of the pathogenesis of mycoplasmal pneumonia indicate that typical gross lesions do not occur until 2-4 weeks after infection. The rate of development of lesions is dependent on the dose and strain of *M. hyopneumoniae*, method of administration, and susceptibility of the pigs exposed. Young pigs naturally exposed to infectious aerosols soon after birth can develop lesions by the time they are

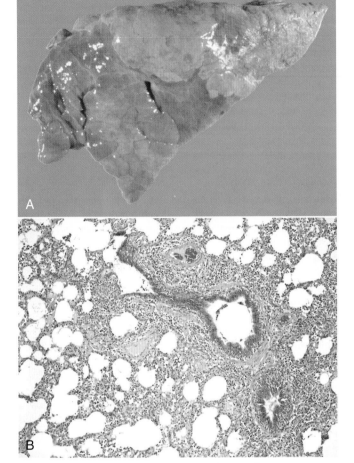

Figure 5-52 *Mycoplasma hyopneumoniae* **infection** in a pig. **A.** Cranioventral lung (to the left) is collapsed, grey-brown, with firm-rubbery or fleshy texture. **B.** Thick cuffs of lymphocytes encircle bronchioles as well as blood vessels, and alveoli contain increased numbers of mononuclear cells. (Courtesy University of Guelph.)

3-5 weeks of age. In the first week after experimental infection, neutrophils are present in airway lumens and, to a lesser extent, in alveoli. The numbers of neutrophils diminish and lymphoid cells increase over the subsequent several weeks to reach the fully developed stage of consolidation. After it has reached its peak some 5-6 weeks after infection, lesions of uncomplicated mycoplasmal pneumonia may either persist or completely resolve within 2 months.

The gross lesions of gray-tan discoloration and thymus-like texture are quite characteristic. However, many fatal cases are secondarily infected by opportunistic bacteria, resulting in red, firm or hard, cranioventral consolidation that appears identical to the bacterial pneumonia that complicates PRRSV, PCV-2, or influenza. Similarly, the well-developed histologic lesions with thick peribronchial cuffs of lymphocytes are highly suggestive, yet lymphoplasmacytic peribronchiolitis—usually milder—is also often present in chronic PRRSV, influenza, or PCV-2 pneumonia. In these cases, other histologic features can suggest a *tentative diagnosis: M. hyopneumoniae* also induces alveolar edema and increased numbers of plump alveolar macrophages, PRRSV results in diffuse lymphocytic infiltrates in alveolar septa, influenza virus and some PCV-2 infections are accompanied in the acute stages by bronchiolar necrosis and

neutrophils, and granulomatous infiltrates in lymph nodes suggest PCV-2 infection.

Establishing a definitive **diagnosis** in swine herds with pneumonia often requires laboratory support. *M. hyopneumoniae* is fastidious in its growth requirements, and isolation in culture is not a useful method of diagnosis. More sensitive confirmation of a morphologic diagnosis can be obtained by identifying antigen in lesional lung tissue by immunohistochemistry, or detection of *M. hyopneumoniae* DNA by PCR using lung tissue, nasal swabs, or transtracheal washes. Detection of serum antibody by ELISA is a useful method of confirming prior exposure, or validating the *M. hyopneumoniae*–free status of minimal-disease herds.

Further reading

Kwon D, et al. Chronologic localization of *Mycoplasma hyopneumoniae* in experimentally infected pigs. Vet Pathol 2002;39:584-587.

Thacker EL. Diagnosis of *Mycoplasma hyopneumoniae*. Anim Health Res Rev 2004;5:317-320.

Woolley LK, et al. Evaluation of clinical, histological and immunological changes and qPCR detection of *Mycoplasma hyopneumoniae* in tissues during the early stages of mycoplasmal pneumonia in pigs after experimental challenge with two field isolates. Vet Microbiol 2012;161:186-195.

Fungal diseases

Pneumocystis carinii. *Pneumocystis carinii* is a sporadic cause of acute or chronic dyspnea, usually without fever, in pigs, foals, dogs, and other domestic animals. Outbreaks of respiratory disease in pigs have been associated with *Pneumocystis* infection, but it is uncertain whether *Pneumocystis* was the primary cause of respiratory disease. *Clinical disease caused by Pneumocystis is thought to be unlikely without underlying immunosuppression;* identified causes include corticosteroid or other immunosuppressive therapy; severe combined immunodeficiency in foals, sometimes in association with adenovirus or *Rhodococcus* infection; common variable immunodeficiency of Miniature Dachshunds, demodicosis, or canine distemper in dogs; and perhaps PRRSV or PCV-2 infection in pigs. Nonetheless, the recent finding that *Pneumocystis* causes transient disease in immunocompetent rats, and persistent infection in immunodeficient rats, should motivate its reconsideration as a primary pathogen.

Pneumocystis is a fungus, in the class Pneumocystidomycetes. Isolates from different host species should be considered distinct species or subspecies; *P. jiroveci* causes disease in humans, but there is little evidence that isolates from animals (*P. carinii*) are of zoonotic importance. The life cycle is based only on morphologic evaluation, but involves a 1-4 μm diameter, thin-walled, *uninucleate, trophic form* that replicates by binary fission; and a 5-8 μm diameter, *thick-walled, multinucleate cyst form* that develops 8 intracystic bodies, which may be daughter forms that are products of sexual replication. The latter are released, attach to type I pneumocytes, and presumably develop into trophic forms. The cell wall is composed of mannose-rich polysaccharides and the major surface glycoprotein. This glycoprotein A is the immunodominant antigen and mediates binding of *Pneumocystis* to type I pneumocytes and macrophages, surfactant proteins, and fibronectin. Both macrophages and cell-mediated immune responses are essential for controlling *Pneumocystis;* hence clinical disease implies that there has been impairment of macrophage function or cell-mediated immune responses. In addition to the space-occupying effect of the fungus, *Pneumocystis* may alter lung function by interfering with surfactant homeostasis.

Gross lesions of *Pneumocystis* pneumonia are diffuse or patchy, red to yellow-brown regions of rubbery firmness or consolidation. The characteristic histologic finding is *foamy or "honeycomb" material filling alveoli*, caused by the presence of numerous intracellular and extracellular, 8-μm diameter, round or crescent-shaped, clear fungal bodies, each containing one or more 0.5-μm diameter, lightly basophilic bodies (Fig. 5-53). Foamy macrophages are present and contain the organisms, but the presence of lymphocytes, plasma cells, type II pneumocytes, and interstitial fibrosis is variable. *The diagnosis is made by identifying the fungi in histologic sections.* They are easily overlooked on H&E-stained sections, but the wall of the cyst forms stains with methenamine silver or PAS. It is notable that immunocompetent rats develop lymphohistiocytic interstitial pneumonia with perivascular cuffs of lymphocytes but few *Pneumocystis* cysts, whereas immunodeficient rats develop a similar lesion with many cysts. *Pneumocystis* cannot be cul-

tured using conventional techniques. PCR assays are a more sensitive method of detection than histopathology, in rats.

Further reading

Henderson KS, et al. *Pneumocystis carinii* causes a distinctive interstitial pneumonia in immunocompetent laboratory rats that had been attributed to "rat respiratory virus. Vet Pathol 2012;49:440-452.

Kim KS, et al. Epidemiological characteristics of pulmonary pneumocystosis and concurrent infections in pigs in Jeju Island, Korea. J Vet Sci 2011;12:15-19.

Parasitic diseases

Metastrongylus *apri (elongatus), M. pudendotectus,* and *M. salmi* (family *Protostrongylidae*) are all parasitic in the bronchi and bronchioles of pigs. Because the intermediate host is the earthworm, pulmonary metastrongylosis is now rare in housed swine, but it is common in wild boar. They are believed to be responsible for the occasional transmission of influenza A virus. The adult worms are white, threadlike, and 14-60 mm in length (eFigs. 5-77, 5-78). In heavy infections, which are mostly in young pigs, they may be found in all lobes of the lung. When there are fewer worms, particularly as occurs in older animals, the worms may be restricted to airways along the caudoventral borders of the caudal lobes. In histologic sections, the adults have polymyarian-coelomyarian musculature, cuboidal multinucleated intestinal epithelium with an indistinct microvillus layer, and thick-shelled eggs or embryonated eggs in the uterus (see eFigs. 5-77, 5-78). Eggs are laid in the bronchi, and a few of them hatch there, but most hatch after passing to the exterior in the feces. First-stage larvae are inactive and are capable of prolonged survival in moist conditions. Their further development depends on ingestion by earthworms, which are the intermediate hosts. The larvae develop to the third, infective stage in about 10 days, and then remain quiescent unless the earthworm is eaten by a pig. The larvae may survive for as long as 18 months in the earthworms and, by that time, thousands may be accumulated by a single worm. Migration within the pig is through the lymphatics from the intestine to the lungs. Some larvae pass through the liver and produce focal hepatitis.

Even with heavy adult infestations, gross lesions are inconspicuous. The worms live in the smallest airways, and on superficial examination of the lungs, the presence of the parasites is frequently only indicated by gray-pink nodules l-3 mm in diameter and by hyperinflated lobules along the caudoventral margins of the caudal lobes. Histologically, the lesions are similar to those produced by *Dictyocaulus* spp. The initial lesions are multiple foci of intense accumulations of eosinophils surrounding larvae in alveoli. Subsequently, when reproduction is active, an eosinophilic and granulomatous response occurs to the eggs and larvae in the alveoli. The prepatent period for *Metastrongylus* spp. is about 25 days, after which the rate of egg production rapidly reaches a peak and then subsides to a low level. At this later stage, the adults persist mainly in the bronchioles, and small bronchi and provoke goblet cell hyperplasia and exudation of mucus, eosinophils, neutrophils, and mononuclear cells. The bronchiolar epithelium is mildly hyperplastic, and eosinophils, lymphocytes, and plasma cells permeate the lamina propria.

Ascaris suum is an intestinal nematode in swine. The female worms have tremendous biotic potential, producing

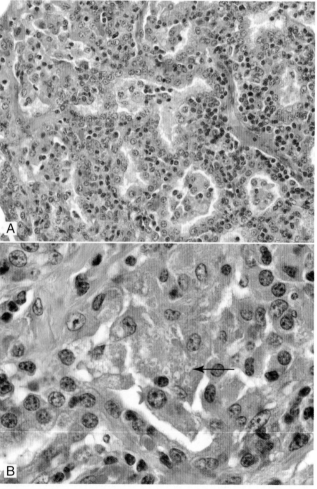

Figure 5-53 *Pneumocystis carinii* in a foal with no evidence of immunosuppression. **A.** Extensive proliferation of type II pneumocytes line alveoli, with interstitial infiltrates of lymphocytes. **B.** In a few areas, alveoli contain foamy material containing fungal cysts (arrow). Note the type II pneumocyte hyperplasia (bottom center).

numerous eggs that are passed in the feces. Consumption of large numbers of embryonated eggs or ingestion of infected paratenic hosts (usually earthworms) may result in the synchronous migration of huge numbers of larvae, which can occasionally be fatal. The lesion is *acute, diffuse, eosinophilic, interstitial lung disease* associated with the presence of large numbers of larvae. Characteristic morphologic features of the larvae are the lateral alae, prominent lateral chords, and uninucleate intestinal epithelial cells (eFigs. 5-79, 5-80).

Rare parasitisms of the respiratory tract of pigs include *Paragonimus* spp. and **hydatid disease.**

Further reading

Gassó D, et al. An identification key for the five most common species of *Metastrongylus*. Parasitol Res 2014;113:3495-3500.

Infectious respiratory diseases of cattle

Viral diseases

General features of herpesviruses. Herpesviruses are 120-200 nm diameter, and composed of an icosahedral nucleocapsid surrounded by a proteinaceous tegument and an outer envelope. Herpesviruses have large genomes composed of double-stranded DNA. Viral infection of cells induces a highly regulated cascade of viral gene expression: preformed tegument proteins and the products of immediate-early and early genes regulate the host transcriptional machinery and viral gene expression, and late genes encode structural proteins of the virus. Viral glycoproteins often form peplomers that project from the surface of the envelope; in addition to being key targets of protective immune responses, these envelope glycoproteins mediate viral entry into target cells, cellular fusion to form syncytia, and spread of virus between cells without exposure to extracellular antibody. Some envelope glycoproteins act as complement C3b or immunoglobulin Fc receptors, and several herpesviruses encode chemokine or chemokine receptor homologues that modulate the immunoinflammatory response. Viral replication occurs in the nucleus, and virions acquire an envelope by budding through the nuclear membrane. Lysis of the cell releases the mature virions to the extracellular space.

Herpesviruses are classified into *Alpha-, Beta-, and Gammaherpesvirinae subfamilies. The **alphaherpesviruses** are characterized by rapid growth in cell culture, lytic infection of cells, necrotizing lesions, the formation of syncytia in some instances, eosinophilic intranuclear inclusion bodies, latent infections, and narrow or broad host ranges.* Most alphaherpesviruses establish latent infections in neurons of the trigeminal ganglia and other sensory ganglia, as well as other sites, such as olfactory bulb, optic nerve, nasal turbinate, and cornea. During latent infection, the so-called latency-associated transcripts are the only evidence of viral gene expression; these have been used as markers of latent infection. Alphaherpesviruses affecting the lung of domestic mammals include bovine herpesvirus 1 (infectious bovine rhinotracheitis), caprine herpesvirus 1, suid herpesvirus 1 (pseudorabies), equid herpesviruses 1 and 4 (equine abortion, equine viral rhinopneumonitis), canid herpesvirus 1, and felid herpesvirus 1 (feline viral rhinotracheitis).

The **betaherpesviruses,** including suid herpesvirus 2 (porcine cytomegalovirus), have a limited host range, and these cytomegaloviruses induce pathologic enlargement of infected cells and prominent basophilic intranuclear inclusion bodies. Replication of cytomegaloviruses is slower than that of alphaherpesviruses, and disease is more chronic. As the immune response is generally effective, disease caused by cytomegalovirus occurs principally in immunodeficient or immunosuppressed animals.

Infectious bovine rhinotracheitis. Infection with **bovine herpesvirus 1** (BoHV-1, infectious bovine rhinotracheitis virus) is widespread in cattle populations, but the disease infectious bovine rhinotracheitis (IBR) is uncommon in areas where vaccination is practiced. IBR in feedlot calves causes an abrupt onset of fever, anorexia, tachypnea, mucopurulent nasal discharge, and dyspnea or open-mouth breathing. The nasal mucosa and muzzle are often hyperemic, suggesting the epithet "red nose," and white, loosely adherent plaques may peel from the surface. The mortality rate is low unless secondary bacterial pneumonia develops.

Bovine alphaherpesvirus infections cause infectious bovine rhinotracheitis, keratoconjunctivitis, bronchointerstitial pneumonia, abortion, encephalitis, systemic herpesvirus infection in young calves, and pustular vulvovaginitis or balanoposthitis. The factors that determine the manifestation are not fully understood, but include the following: route of infection (genital infection usually manifests as vulvovaginitis or balanoposthitis), strain of the virus (a distinct virus type, BoHV-5, is the usual cause of herpesviral encephalitis in calves), and degree of immunity (systemic herpesviral infection develops in young calves with low serum antibody titers to the virus).

BoHV-1 has a large 136-kb genome encoding 67 proteins; 12 envelope glycoproteins have been described. The glycoproteins gC and gD bind cell surface receptors, allowing virus entry into the cell by gB, gH, and gL. Fusion of cells, mediated by gB and gD, allows intercellular spread of virus and evasion of the immune response, and is the molecular basis of the epithelial syncytia that are occasionally noted histologically. The gC glycoprotein binds C3 component of complement and prevents complement activation, whereas gI and gE are Fc receptors for immunoglobulin that impair antibody-mediated neutralization of the virus.

BoHV-1 infects a wide range of animals, including cattle, sheep, goats, llamas, swine, water buffalo, mustelids, and rabbits, but *primary viral respiratory disease is only described in cattle.* Sources of BoHV-1 infection include clinically or subclinically infected cattle, and reactivation of latent infections. Wild ruminants may be subclinical reservoirs. Infection is transmitted by aerosol; direct contact with nasal, ocular, or vaginal secretions; or by indirect contact with fomites, semen, feed, or water. Systemic spread of the virus is a feature of the syndromes of systemic infection, abortion, and encephalitis. Viremia is not usually evident in cases of IBR, keratoconjunctivitis, vulvovaginitis, or balanoposthitis, although monocyte- or lymphocyte-associated viremia may occur at low level. In the latter conditions, virus spreads along mucosal epithelium, nerves, and lymphatics. *Latent infection of trigeminal or other sensory ganglia is common,* and follows axonal spread of infection rather than viremia. In latently infected neurons, viral DNA is present but, with the exception of a few "latency-associated transcripts," viral RNA or protein cannot be detected. Stress, administration of glucocorticoids or epinephrine, hyperthermia, or hypothermia trigger reactivation of the latent infection, and virus reaches the mucosal surface by anterograde axonal transport, where mucosal replication leads to shedding of infectious virus. Reactivated infections are usually subclinical, but may act as a source of contagion to naive, in-contact animals.

Infection of the respiratory tract induces *clinical disease* after an incubation period of 2-6 days, and virus is shed in nasal secretions for at least 10-16 days. Clinical IBR results from lytic infection of nasal and airway epithelial cells. Functional abnormalities such as serotonin- or dopamine-induced bronchoconstriction may also contribute to clinical signs. Secondary bacterial pneumonia in calves with IBR is a consequence of the destruction of ciliated epithelium by lytic viral infection, and impairment of the ability of alveolar macrophages to phagocytose bacteria and secrete neutrophil chemotactic factors. These impairments of lung defenses are maximal at 4-5 days after viral infection.

Interferon-α and -β secretion is detectable within 5 hours of BoHV-1 infections, and peaks at 36-72 hours. These interferons mediate innate resistance to spread of the infection, in part by recruiting macrophages and natural killer cells to the sites of viral infection. Cell-mediated immune responses are detectable in the respiratory tract within 5 days of infection, and mediate lysis of virus-infected cells. Neutralizing IgG is first detected at 10 days after infection, and IgA responses develop later. Antibody prevents disease in calves exposed to the virus. In infected calves, antibody neutralizes free virus and may prevent mucosal shedding of virus following reactivation of latent infection. However, because the virus evades the humoral immune response by spreading locally from cell to cell, a combination of cellular and humoral immunity is probably necessary for recovery from infection.

Gross lesions of IBR are usually restricted to the *nasal cavity, larynx, and trachea*. Pustules erupt early after infection, but are fragile and rarely observed. Petechiae, a granular appearance of the mucosa, and serous exudate may be present in acute lesions. More commonly, there is intense hyperemia of the mucosal tissue, multifocal to coalescing erosions with loosely adherent plaques of white debris, or diffuse ulceration covered by a fibrinonecrotic membrane (Fig. 5-54). When the exudate is peeled from the surface of the trachea or nasal cavity, dull granular eroded tissue remains. In contrast, in cases of bacterial pneumonia in which expectorated material accumulates on the tracheal or nasal mucosa, gentle removal of

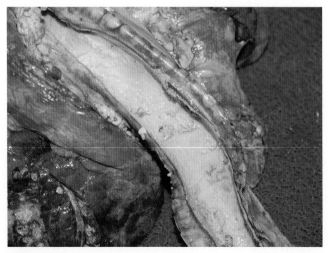

Figure 5-54 Infectious bovine rhinotracheitis, with necrosis of tracheal epithelium leading to formation of a fibrinonecrotic membrane.

the exudate reveals a shiny intact mucosal surface. In severe cases, obstruction of the laryngeal or tracheal lumen by abundant exudate may prove fatal. Emphysema is a sequel to dyspnea in severely affected calves.

The earliest **histologic lesions,** in the first 2 days after infection, include cytoplasmic vacuolation and pallor, and nuclear pyknosis or karyolysis. Eosinophilic intranuclear inclusion bodies are present in the epithelium of the nasal turbinates, tracheobronchial glands, and bronchial epithelium, but are rare in the tracheal surface epithelium. *Inclusions are absent in most diagnostic cases,* and the lesions at these later times include erosion or ulceration of nasal and tracheal mucosa, with necrosis and exfoliation of infected epithelial cells and exudation of neutrophils and fibrin. Neutrophils and mononuclear cells infiltrate the lamina propria. Mild perivascular infiltrates of lymphocytes may be detected in the trigeminal ganglion and brainstem.

Bronchointerstitial pneumonia may develop, with erosion of bronchiolar epithelium and proliferation of type II pneumocytes. *Primary viral pneumonia occurs in young calves* without significant upper respiratory lesions and without evidence of bacterial pneumonia. These calves may have epithelial syncytia in alveoli, and eosinophilic intranuclear inclusion bodies are more common than is seen in IBR.

Systemic lesions of BoHV-1 infection in young calves <2 months of age include multiple, coalescing, 1-7 mm diameter, sharply demarcated foci of necrosis in the upper digestive tract, including the oral cavity, esophagus, and rumen. Necrotic foci are often covered by adherent debris and ingesta, which appears as caseous clumps of curdled milk. Multifocal, pinpoint to 1-mm diameter, white foci of necrosis are often present in the liver, and occasionally in kidney and spleen. The nasopharynx and larynx may contain erosive and exudative lesions, but tracheal and pulmonary lesions are not typical. Histologically, eosinophilic intranuclear inclusion bodies are usually apparent at the margins of the necrotic lesions. The lesions of herpesviral abortion are described in Vol. 3, Female genital system.

The gross appearance of IBR is highly suggestive of the causative agent. A casual observer may mistake loosely adherent expectorated material for the tracheal ulceration of IBR. Bovine parainfluenza virus 3 can cause nasal erosions, but aspiration or inhalation of chemical irritants, which is rarely encountered, is the only process likely to be confused with florid lesions of IBR. However, as subclinical BoHV-1 infection impairs pulmonary defenses, laboratory investigation to demonstrate this pathogen is often warranted in calves with bacterial pneumonia. The virus grows readily in cell culture and produces characteristic cytopathic effects. Thus *virus isolation* from nasal swabs, nasal mucosa, trachea, or lung is an excellent means of definitive diagnosis, and has the advantage that novel strains may be identified and archived. PCR tests and immunohistochemistry are advantageous when a rapid diagnosis is needed. An important caveat is warranted when identifying BoHV-1 infection in the absence of characteristic lesions. *Cattle with other diseases experience stress-induced reactivation of latent herpesviral infections, leading to identification of the reactivated virus in any of these diagnostic assays.* Samples should be obtained early in the course of disease, as antibody in the exudate of subacute lesions may preclude isolation of the virus and block antigen-antibody interactions in antigen-based assays. Detection of seroconversion is useful to associate BoHV-1 infection with clinical disease.

Further reading

Levings RL, Roth JA. Immunity to bovine herpesvirus 1: I. Viral lifecycle and innate immunity. Anim Health Res Rev 2013;14:88-102.

Bovine respiratory syncytial virus. Infection with bovine respiratory syncytial virus (BRSV) is common in North American and European beef and dairy herds. Seroprevalence studies suggest that about half of range calves in North America are exposed to BRSV, and most non-exposed calves seroconvert within a month of entering feedlots. The seroprevalence of BRSV in adult cattle varies from 40-95%. *BRSV is an important cause of both acute outbreaks of respiratory disease and "enzootic pneumonia"* in 2-week-old to 5-month-old dairy and beef calves, with a peak incidence at 1-3 months of age. BRSV certainly causes *fatal bronchointerstitial pneumonia* soon after arrival in beef feedlots, but rarely causes acute interstitial lung disease in the late feeding period. Finally, *BRSV predisposes to bacterial pneumonia* in feedlot beef cattle by impairing lung defenses, and occasionally causes respiratory disease in naive adult dairy cows.

The disease is most prevalent in the autumn or early winter. *Clinical signs* in calves and cows are similar and include high fever, coughing, tachypnea, and variable nasal discharge and conjunctivitis. Some animals develop dyspnea with open-mouth breathing and increased abdominal effort. Calves often maintain a reasonable appetite in the face of severe respiratory distress, in contrast to the consistent depression of cattle with bacterial pneumonia. A biphasic clinical course is not present in all cases; when present, it is characterized by transient pyrexia and mild respiratory disease, temporary improvement for days to weeks, then rapid onset of severe respiratory distress.

BRSV, a member of the genus *Pneumovirus* in the family *Paramyxoviridae*, is pleomorphic, spherical or irregularly shaped, enveloped, 80-450 nm diameter, and contains negative-sense single-stranded RNA. The viral genome encodes 10 proteins, including the G glycoprotein, which mediates attachment of viral particles to host cells; the F protein, which induces fusion of infected cells; matrix proteins (M, M2, or 22 K); nucleocapsid protein (N); phosphoprotein (P); polymerase (L); small hydrophobic protein (SH); and nonstructural proteins (NS1[1C] and NS2[1B]). Subgroups of BRSV have been defined by antigenic and nucleotide differences of the G and F proteins, but their clinical significance is uncertain.

An understanding of the **pathogenesis** of BRSV pneumonia has been hindered by the difficulty of establishing experimental infections that are representative of naturally occurring disease. In general, experimentally infected calves develop less severe clinical disease and less extensive lesions than natural cases, in part because in vitro passage of the virus in cell culture rapidly attenuates virulence. As a result, descriptions of the pathogenesis of experimental infections are not necessarily representative of natural disease. *Airborne spread, probably by aerosol, is the common route of infection.* Clinical signs are observed from 2-7 days after experimental infection. In natural cases, viral infection is restricted to the respiratory tract, and viral antigen is most abundant in bronchiolar epithelium of the cranioventral areas of lung. Alveolar type II pneumocytes and macrophages express lesser amounts of viral antigen, and infrequent virus-infected cells are present in nasal, tracheal, and bronchial epithelium. The virus infects but does not replicate in lymphocytes in vitro. Following experimental infection of naive calves, viral shedding was first detected on the second day after infection, was maximal at about 4 days, and was absent by 7-10 days after infection. This transient infection is consistent with the difficulty experienced in demonstrating virus in naturally occurring subacute or chronic cases.

Interactions with other agents contribute to the severity of disease. Experimental BRSV infections result in more severe disease if calves are also infected with bovine viral diarrhea virus or exposed to 3-methylindole. BRSV is an important predisposing factor in the development of bacterial bronchopneumonia in cattle, because the virus impairs alveolar macrophage function, reduces mucociliary clearance, and may enhance proteolysis to facilitate bacterial invasion of the blood.

Calves with BRSV develop specific serum and mucosal antibody responses; however, most antibody is directed to the F and N proteins and is non-neutralizing, and serum titers are poorly correlated with protection from disease. Similarly, passively acquired colostral antibodies do not prevent disease. Although virus-neutralizing antibody is produced during infection, the role of humoral immunity in protection from disease requires further investigation. As for many viral infections, CD8+ T-lymphocyte responses may be important in recovery of calves following BRSV infection.

The role of the immune response in enhancing disease is controversial. It has been proposed that vaccination with inactive virus promotes a type 2 immune response in which antiviral IgE exacerbates the disease. Further, the biphasic clinical course, noted in some but not all natural cases, has been interpreted to represent a worsening of the disease as an immune response develops. Such comparisons have been used as a model to study human RSV infection, where children vaccinated with a formalin-inactivated vaccine developed more severe and prolonged disease course than nonvaccinates. However, attempts to reproduce this phenomenon in cattle have given conflicting results, and vaccinated calves developed milder disease than nonvaccinates in several studies. Similarly, it has been proposed that virus- or immune-complex–induced activation of complement or production of IgE may contribute to bronchoconstriction or pulmonary lesions in calves infected with BRSV, but the significance of complement activation and IgE responses in infected calves remains uncertain.

Gross lesions *in lungs of calves with naturally occurring BRSV pneumonia often differ in cranioventral and caudodorsal areas of lung.* The cranioventral lung is atelectatic, deep red or mottled, and rubbery (Fig. 5-55). In contrast, the caudodorsal areas are voluminous because they fail to collapse, and are edematous, heavy, and firmer than normal. *Variations in these gross lesions occur commonly:* First, occasional cases have a generalized rubbery texture and red discoloration, with no difference between cranial and caudal lung; second, calves that die in respiratory distress may develop marked subpleural and interlobular emphysema with formation of bullae; and third, the raised, consolidated, firm to hard lesions of bronchopneumonia may obscure the aforementioned viral lesions in cases with secondary bacterial infection. Apart from hypertrophy and edema of bronchial and mediastinal lymph nodes, lesions in other organs are usually not noted. Chronic cases of viral pneumonia with bronchiolitis obliterans, including those caused by BRSV, may die of heart failure caused by pulmonary

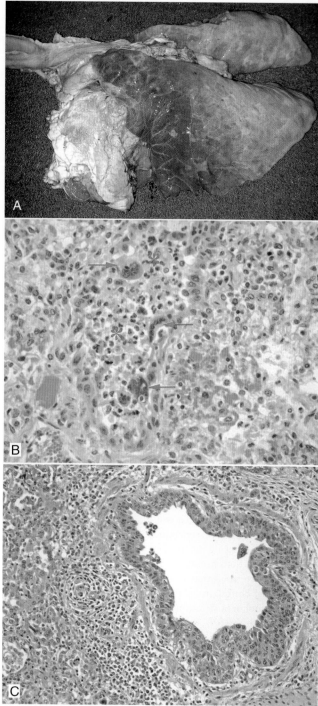

Figure 5-55 Bovine respiratory syncytial virus infection.
A. Grossly, individual lobules throughout the lung have firm-rubbery texture. Cranioventral areas are reddened and collapsed because of atelectasis; caudodorsal areas are expanded by overin-flation or emphysema. The white opacity of the caudal pleura is normal in cattle. **B.** Soon after infection, a bronchiole contains multinucleated syncytial cells (arrows), attenuation of remaining epithelium, and cellular debris and leukocytes in the lumen (asterisk). **C.** At a later stage, syncytial cells are absent, but hyperplasia gives the bronchiolar epithelium a multilayered appearance, and lymphocytes and plasma cells accumulate around bronchioles and blood vessels. Alveoli (at the left) are lined by a continuous layer of cuboidal type II pneumocytes, justifying the diagnosis of bronchointerstitial lung disease.

hypertension, as a result of hypoxic vasoconstriction. Lesions in these animals include hypertrophy of the right ventricle of the heart, subcutaneous edema, and ascites.

The **histologic hallmarks** of pneumonia caused by BRSV are *bronchointerstitial pneumonia with formation of bronchiolar and alveolar epithelial syncytia*. The lesions and the presence of viral antigen are most obvious in the cranioventral areas of lung. In the acute lesions, from 1-8 days after infection, bronchioles are lined by flattened epithelium, bronchiolar lumens contain necrotic epithelial cells and modest numbers of neutrophils, and lymphocytes infiltrate around bronchioles. Alveoli contain neutrophils and macrophages, and alveolar septa may be mildly thickened by mononuclear cells, but hyaline membranes are infrequent. Syncytia are prominent in the early stage, and appear as multinucleated cells closely associated with the bronchiolar or alveoli epithelium (see Fig. 5-55). Sloughed multinucleated cells with pyknotic nuclei are often more numerous than those within the epithelial layer. Alveolar syncytia may closely resemble the multinucleated macrophages that clear fibrin from alveoli in cases of fibrinous pneumonia, so the presence of bronchiolar syncytia is a more reliable indicator of viral infection. *Intracytoplasmic eosino-philic inclusion bodies* are occasionally present in syncytial cells and uncommonly in bronchiolar and alveolar epithelium (eFig. 5-81).

The *subacute lesions* of BRSV infection, beginning at about 8 days after infection, represent *early repair of the above lesions following lymphocyte-mediated lysis of virus-infected cells*. The bronchiolar epithelium becomes hyperplastic (see Fig. 5-55, eFig. 5-81), and there is disappearance of syncytial cells as viral antigen is cleared. Proliferation of type II pneumocytes appears as scattered "tombstone-like" cells or complete cuboidal epithelialization of the alveoli. Lymphocytes and plasma cells encircle bronchioles and blood vessels and thicken alveolar septa, and are most numerous 10 days after infection. Bronchiolitis obliterans may occur as early as 10 days after infection, forming polyps of fibrous tissue covered by epithelium that partially occlude bronchiolar lumens. Medial hypertrophy of pulmonary arterioles may be prominent in calves that develop pulmonary hypertension secondary to bronchiolitis obliterans.

The histologic lesions of necrotizing bronchiolitis with syncytial cells should be highly suggestive of BRSV infection, but 2 caveats should be considered. First, bovine parainfluenza virus 3 infection may also induce the formation of syncytia with intracytoplasmic inclusion bodies. Second, alveolar multinucleated macrophages are a common finding in fibrinous bronchopneumonia, and probably represent an attempt to remove the fibrinous alveolar exudate (eFig. 5-82). This can present a diagnostic dilemma, because many calves with BRSV develop secondary bacterial pneumonia. Thus if alveolar but not bronchiolar multinucleated cells are present, a diagnosis of BRSV infection is not indicated unless ancillary laboratory tests support the diagnosis. Finally, when syncytia are absent, the lesions resemble those caused by other viruses, and laboratory testing is needed for diagnosis.

Various assays are available to confirm BRSV infection. Lesional cranioventral areas of lung are the most profitable sites to detect virus; viral antigen or nucleic acid is less frequent in caudodorsal lung tissue. Virus isolation is not recommended for routine diagnostic use, because the development of an immune response interferes with virus isolation, and the virus is easily inactivated by transport conditions. Quantitative

RT-PCR assays are ideal and more sensitive than immunohistochemistry. Nevertheless, *identification of viral antigen by immunohistochemistry or antigen detection by ELISA is also useful and cost effective.* Cattle vaccinated with intranasal modified live-virus vaccines have detectable viral nucleic acid for 10 days, and up to 20 days in some calves. Thus positive RT-PCR tests in this time interval may not indicate the true cause of the respiratory disease.

Further reading

Gershwin LJ. Immunology of bovine respiratory syncytial virus infection of cattle. Comp Immunol Microbiol Infect Dis 2012;35:253-257.

Sacco RE, et al. Respiratory syncytial virus infection in cattle. Vet Pathol 2014;51:427-436.

Timsit E, et al. Detection by real-time RT-PCR of a bovine respiratory syncytial virus vaccine in calves vaccinated intranasally. Vet Rec 2009;165:230-233.

Bovine parainfluenza virus 3. Infection with bovine parainfluenza virus 3 (BPIV-3) is widespread in 2- to 8-month-old beef and dairy cattle, but *clinically significant disease caused by primary BPIV-3 infection is rare.* Clinical findings in uncomplicated primary BPIV-3 infection include transient fever, nasal discharge, sporadic coughing, mild depression, and increased respiratory rate. The virus causes occasional outbreaks of nasal disease in mature cows, with nasal erosions, fibrinous casts, epistaxis, and submandibular edema. Seroconversion to BPIV-3 commonly occurs during periods of temperature fluctuations in the autumn, in association with shipping fever of feedlot calves, and with enzootic pneumonia of dairy calves. The prevalence of positive serum titers to BPIV-3 varies from 2-67% on arrival in feedlots, but 23-91% of animals seroconvert within a month after arrival. There is a variable association between seroconversion to BPIV-3 and development of pneumonia, and BPIV-3 is one of the viruses that predisposes to shipping fever.

BPIV-3 is a member of the genus *Respirovirus* in the family *Paramyxoviridae*. Paramyxoviruses are pleomorphic, 150-200 nm diameter, and contain negative-sense single-stranded RNA. Structural proteins include hemagglutinin-neuraminidase glycoprotein (HN), fusion glycoprotein (F), high-molecular-weight protein (L), a phosphoprotein (P), nucleocapsid protein (NP), and matrix protein (M). The HN protein mediates viral attachment to and release from infected cells, and the F protein allows penetration and spread of the virus between infected cells. Both the HN and F proteins are necessary for formation of syncytia and virulence. Two distinct BPIV-3 genotypes occur: BPIV-3a and BPIV-3b.

BPIV-3 infects ciliated and nonciliated epithelial cells of the upper and lower respiratory tract, alveolar macrophages, type II pneumocytes, and lymphocytes. The *virus reduces pulmonary defenses* by several mechanisms. Injury to ciliated epithelium results in functional and structural impairment of mucociliary clearance, alveolar macrophages from infected calves have reduced capacity for phagocytosis and oxidative killing of bacteria, and infected alveolar macrophages induce contact-mediated suppression of lymphocyte responses.

The HN and F proteins are immunodominant antigens, and serum antibody titers to these antigens correlate with disease resistance. Serum antibody responses develop at 8 days after experimental infection and peak at ~12 days, and a strong anamnestic response occurs after later infections. Cytotoxic cell–mediated immune responses, which are probably important for clearance of virus-infected cells, are maximal at 6-9 days after infection.

The **gross lesions** in natural cases of primary BPIV-3 pneumonia are usually mild, and consist of a *cranioventral or generalized, lobular pattern of gray-red discoloration, firm, or rubbery texture, and mild swelling or atelectasis of lung tissue.* In calves that die in respiratory distress, there may be emphysema of the caudal lung lobes. *Bronchiolitis and mild bronchitis are the major* **histologic lesions** in natural cases of primary uncomplicated BPIV-3 pneumonia. Epithelial cells lining small bronchioles are rounded, occasionally vacuolated, and slough into the lumen, and the epithelial layer may be discontinuous, attenuated, or hyperplastic. In the acute stages, many bronchial, bronchiolar, and alveolar epithelial cells and alveolar macrophages contain prominent *eosinophilic intracytoplasmic inclusion bodies.* In experimentally infected calves, inclusions are most numerous from 2 to 4 days after infection, and less common from 5 to 12 days. *Epithelial syncytial cells may be present in alveoli,* but are fewer than in bovine respiratory syncytial virus infection. Airways contain low numbers of neutrophils, and lymphocytes infiltrate the mildly edematous bronchiolar walls. Alveoli are atelectatic, edematous, and contain increased numbers of macrophages and neutrophils, and may have proliferation of type II pneumocytes. Fibroblasts and macrophages begin to organize the bronchiolar exudate at 7-12 days after experimental infections, and bronchiolitis obliterans may develop thereafter.

BPIV-3 infection should be considered in calves with necrotizing bronchiolitis. Confirmation of the **diagnosis** is based on *virus isolation, or detection of viral antigen by immunohistochemistry or nucleic acid by RT-PCR testing.* These diagnostic methods are effective in acute cases (<9-12 days after infection), but may be unrewarding in the more common presentation of chronic bacterial pneumonia with concurrent bronchiolar necrosis or bronchiolitis obliterans. *Definitive diagnosis in these cases may be impossible,* because viral antigen may be cleared long before the bacterial pneumonia proves fatal. If acute and convalescent sera are available, then demonstration of a *rising antibody titer* by using the hemagglutination inhibition assay supports the histologic diagnosis.

Further reading

Ellis JA. Bovine parainfluenza-3 virus. Vet Clin North Am Food Anim Pract 2010;26:575-593.

Horwood PF, et al. Identification of two distinct bovine parainfluenza virus type 3 genotypes. J Gen Virol 2008;89:1643-1648.

Bovine coronavirus. *Bovine coronavirus (BCoV) is an important cause of enteric disease in young calves, and the same strains occasionally induce respiratory disease in calves 2-16 weeks of age.* BCoV is a less frequent but nonetheless important cause of respiratory disease in calves, and deserves more attention than it has received in the past. Isolates from occurrences of respiratory and diarrheic diseases have similar genotypes, and a single outbreak may include both forms of disease. Respiratory signs include fever, serous nasal discharge, sneezing, and coughing. The virus replicates primarily in the nasal and tracheal epithelium, and occasionally in the lung.

Many calves shed BCoV in their nasal secretions and/or seroconvert to BCoV in the first month after arrival in feedlots, but the association between seroconversion or virus shedding and increased risk of respiratory disease has been variable in the studies reported. Bronchiolar necrosis is the typical *lesion* seen in BCoV-infected calves (eFig. 5-83). Bronchiolar syncytia have been described in feedlot calves with concurrent BCoV infection and bacterial pneumonia, but the contribution of other viruses, such as bovine respiratory syncytial virus, to these lesions is uncertain. BCoV may be demonstrated using immunohistochemistry or RT-PCR, or isolated using specific rectal tumor cell lines.

Further reading

Bidokhti MR, et al. Tracing the transmission of bovine coronavirus infections in cattle herds based on S gene diversity. Vet J 2012;193:386-390.

Fulton RW, et al. Bovine coronavirus (BCV) infections in transported commingled beef cattle and sole-source ranch calves. Can J Vet Res 2011;75:191-199.

Park SJ, et al. Dual enteric and respiratory tropisms of winter dysentery bovine coronavirus in calves. Arch Virol 2007;152:1885-1900.

Bovine viral diarrhea virus. *The contribution of bovine viral diarrhea virus (BVDV) to pneumonia in cattle is a long-standing source of controversy.* Virus can be isolated from the lung in primary (acute) infections and in persistently infected calves. *Epidemiologic and experimental studies show that BVDV-infected calves do indeed have a heightened susceptibility to bacterial pneumonia,* and respiratory signs may be the chief clinical complaint resulting from acute BVDV infections. Mechanisms by which BVDV predisposes to bacterial pneumonia include reduced antimicrobial protein production by virus-infected airway epithelial cells, reduced function of alveolar macrophages, and virus-induced neutropenia. BVDV has also been shown to exacerbate bovine respiratory syncytial virus and bovine herpesvirus 1 infections in experimental situations.

It has been proposed that some isolates of BVDV induce primary respiratory disease, independent of opportunistic bacterial pathogens. During primary BVDV infection, viral antigen is present in pulmonary alveolar macrophages and in airway epithelium (eFig. 5-84). In addition, viral antigen may be demonstrated in the tunica muscularis of arterioles in the lung, heart, and occasionally in other tissues, often in association with lesions of lymphocytic arteritis. Calves or lambs challenged with certain isolates of BVDV develop fever and hyperpnea or, in other studies, nasal discharge and coughing. The lesions described are mild, consisting of peribronchiolar, perivascular, or interstitial aggregates of lymphocytes and macrophages, and/or mild suppurative exudate in bronchioles. However, other studies have found no lung lesions in calves infected with BVDV, and *the importance of BVDV as a cause of primary lung disease is probably minimal.*

Further reading

Al-Haddawi M, et al. Impairment of innate immune responses of airway epithelium by infection with bovine viral diarrhea virus. Vet Immunol Immunopathol 2007;116:153-162.

Confer AW, et al. Viral antigen distribution in the respiratory tract of cattle persistently infected with bovine viral diarrhea virus subtype 2a. Vet Pathol 2005;42:192-199.

Bovine adenovirus. *Bovine adenoviruses are a recognized cause of hemorrhagic colitis, but their role in respiratory disease*

is more controversial. Epitheliotropic bovine adenoviruses are occasionally isolated from feedlot calves with bacterial pneumonia, and many calves seroconvert to a range of bovine adenovirus (BAdV) serotypes within 5 weeks of entering feedlots. Adenoviruses may predispose to bacterial pneumonia by injuring ciliated epithelium and, for some strains, by impairing alveolar macrophages. However, compared to the roles of stress and other viral infections, *adenoviruses are probably minor contributors to bacterial pneumonia in feedlot cattle.*

Calves experimentally infected with BAdV generally develop only mild respiratory disease; the severity of primary adenoviral pneumonia is probably dependent on both the strain of the BAdV and the immune status of the calf. Experimentally infected calves developed lobular or patchy areas of atelectasis and reddening. *Histologic lesions* include proliferation of bronchial and bronchiolar epithelium, lymphocytic infiltration of airway epithelium, formation of *large basophilic intranuclear inclusions* in airway epithelial cells, and exfoliation or necrosis of virus-infected cells. In well-developed cases, there is extensive bronchiolar necrosis, occlusion of bronchiolar lumens by sloughed epithelium, and inclusions in intact or sloughed epithelial cells. Thickening of alveolar septa by mononuclear cells may occur, but proliferation of type II pneumocytes is uncommon.

Further reading

Narita M, et al. Bovine adenovirus type 3 pneumonia in dexamethasone-treated calves. Vet Pathol 2003;40:128-135.

Bovine rhinitis virus. Two bovine rhinitis viruses (BRAV, BRBV) are widespread in cattle populations, but are *generally believed to be of little importance as a cause of respiratory disease in cattle.* Virus isolation and serologic responses occasionally provide circumstantial evidence that it is involved in causing upper respiratory disease. Experimental infection has inconsistently induced bronchointerstitial pneumonia.

Further reading

Rai DK, Rieder E. Homology modeling and analysis of structure predictions of the bovine rhinitis B virus RNA dependent RNA polymerase (RdRp). Int J Mol Sci 2012;13:8998-9013.

Bacterial diseases

Bacterial bronchopneumonia caused by *Pasteurellaceae: Mannheimia haemolytica, Histophilus somni, Pasteurella multocida.* *Bacterial bronchopneumonia is a common and economically important disease of cattle,* particularly in temperate climates, and is mainly caused by bacteria of the family *Pasteurellaceae. The most important clinical entities are enzootic pneumonia of young calves and shipping fever of feedlot cattle,* but bacterial pneumonia may occur in any age group, often as a complication of stress, viral infection, or inclement weather.

Shipping-fever pneumonia has long been considered the most economically important disease of beef cattle in temperate climates. Recent years have seen considerable advances in understanding of pathogenesis and preventive strategies, with the result that, although the disease remains prevalent, mortality rates are lower than in the past. The *classic presentation* of shipping fever is of pneumonia affecting multiple calves, 3 days to 3 weeks after being shipped from their farm of origin to a feedlot. Affected animals exhibit acute onset of depression, pyrexia, anorexia, rapid and shallow respiration, and mucopurulent nasal discharge. Coughing is variably present, and dyspnea develops in later stages. Most cattle respond rapidly to appropriate antibiotic therapy if given early in the course of disease, but relapses are common. Most reports of shipping fever describe 15-45% morbidity, 1-5% mortality, and case fatality rates of 5-10%, depending on the rapidity with which treatment is initiated. *Risk factors* for shipping fever include those associated with (1) increased exposure of naive calves to animals shedding viral pathogens, such as mixing of calves from various sources; (2) stress, such as weaning, transport, crowding, disruption of social groups, deprivation of feed and water, handling, vaccination, dehorning, and pregnancy checking; (3) metabolic acidosis, such as rapid introduction to grain or corn silage; and (4) exposure of calves to adverse environmental conditions, such as changes in temperature and humidity, cool weather in the autumn months, snow or rain, or dusty environment.

Bacterial pneumonia is also common in 1- to 4-month-old dairy and veal calves, and less common in suckling beef calves. Although commonly referred to as *"enzootic pneumonia,"* cases may be sporadic, enzootic, or occur in outbreaks. Affected calves are febrile, hyperpneic, variably dyspneic, depressed, and anorexic. *Risk factors* include those that (1) affect air quality, such as indoor housing, poor ventilation, high stocking density, high levels of airborne droplets or dust, and humid conditions; (2) reduce lung defenses, such as failure of passive transfer of immunoglobulin and high environmental ammonia concentrations; (3) expose calves to viral or mycoplasmal pathogens, such as housing calves and adults together; and (4) cause stress, such as concurrent diseases.

Pasteurellaceae are gram-negative coccobacilli; several members of the family are common causes of pneumonia or septicemia in domestic animals. *Many species of Pasteurellaceae inhabit the upper respiratory tract of healthy animals,* but cause pneumonia when pulmonary defenses are impaired, or cause septicemia in naive animals or those with reduced systemic defenses. In general, the defense against many *Pasteurellaceae* depends on a combination of innate resistance mechanisms and acquired humoral immunity. The most common pathogenic *Pasteurellaceae* of domestic animals include *Pasteurella multocida* of swine, ruminants, and cats; *Mannheimia haemolytica* and *Bibersteinia trehalosi* of ruminants; *Actinobacillus pleuropneumoniae* and *A. suis* of swine; *A. equuli* of horses; *Histophilus somni* of cattle and sheep; and *Haemophilus parasuis* of swine.

***Mannheimia haemolytica* and *Bibersteinia trehalosi*:** 12 serotypes of *M. haemolytica* are discerned based on soluble capsular polysaccharide antigens. Serotype names were maintained when the species *P. haemolytica* biotypes A and T were reclassified as *M. haemolytica* and *B. trehalosi*, respectively; as a result, serotypes 3, 4, 10, and 15 are represented only by *B. trehalosi* (discussed in Infectious respiratory diseases of sheep and goats). Serotype 2, and, to a lesser extent, serotype 1, is a sporadic isolate from the nasopharynx of healthy calves. Serotype 1 is the most common isolate from pneumonic lung, but other serotypes in addition to many untypable isolates regularly cause bovine pneumonia.

Virulence factors of *M. haemolytica* include leukotoxin, lipopolysaccharide, a polysaccharide capsule, transferrin-binding proteins A and B, O-sialoglycoprotease, neuraminidase, IgG1-specific protease, outer membrane proteins, adhesins, and fimbriae. All serotypes secrete *leukotoxin,* a member of the RTX (repeats in toxin) family of gram-negative bacterial toxins, during the logarithmic phase of growth. The gene products of *lktA* and *lktC* represent the active leukotoxin, whereas *lktB* and *lktD* are necessary for toxin secretion. At high concentrations, leukotoxin induces lysis of ruminant leukocytes and platelets, mediated by binding to CD18 on the leukocyte surface and formation of pores in the cell membrane. At lower concentrations, leukotoxin activates leukocytes and platelets. Although leukotoxin clearly plays a role in the pathogenesis of pneumonia, disease does develop in calves vaccinated against leukotoxin and in those challenged with *M. haemolytica* constructs that do not secrete leukotoxin.

Lipopolysaccharide is a major component of the cell wall, and the presence of O-polysaccharide side chains confers a smooth phenotype to most serotypes. Lipopolysaccharide from *M. haemolytica* stimulates alveolar macrophages to secrete inflammatory mediators, including tumor necrosis factor-α (TNF-α), interleukin-1 (IL-1), and the chemokines IL-8, epithelial neutrophil-activating peptide (ENA), and growth-regulated oncogene-α (GRO-α). Other effects of *M. haemolytica* lipopolysaccharide on alveolar macrophages include triggering of oxidative burst, an important bactericidal mechanism that may also lead to oxidative tissue injury; expression of tissue factor, a mediator of the thrombosis characteristic of the disease; and secretion of nitric oxide, which may augment lung defenses but is also a potent mediator of vasodilation and hypotension. Other effects of lipopolysaccharide include activation of the extrinsic coagulation pathway, and complement activation. The mannose-rich polysaccharide capsule confers resistance of *M. haemolytica* to phagocytosis by macrophages and neutrophils, and may also block complement-dependent killing. Neuraminidase enhances adhesion of bacteria to mucosal epithelium by cleaving sialic acid from the surface of epithelial cells, and may reduce mucus viscosity to prevent mucociliary clearance.

Low numbers of M. haemolytica colonize the nasopharynx of normal calves, and there are several potential explanations for the shift from a commensal to a pathogenic relationship. First, stress or exposure to cold results in greater numbers of nasopharyngeal bacteria, so inhalation of droplets containing increased numbers of bacteria may overwhelm pulmonary defenses. The mechanisms whereby stress or exposure to cold induces expansion of the bacterial population, and whether these factors also alter expression of bacterial virulence factors, have not been defined. Second, some studies indicate that stress and cold exposure induce a shift from serotype 2 to the more pathogenic serotype 1. Third, viral infections or stress impair lung defenses. The lung is normally exposed to low numbers of aspirated *M. haemolytica,* but a combination of mucociliary clearance, antimicrobial function of secreted mucosal proteins, and phagocytosis by alveolar macrophages controls this infection without inciting an inflammatory response. Bovine herpesvirus 1 (BoHV-1), bovine respiratory syncytial virus (BRSV), and bovine parainfluenza virus 3 infect ciliated epithelium and reduce mucociliary clearance, and BoHV-1 and BRSV infect and impair the function of alveolar macrophages. In addition, BoHV-1 infection upregulates CD18 on the surface of bovine neutrophils, which, because CD18 is a receptor of *M. haemolytica* leukotoxin, makes these cells more susceptible to the leukotoxin. Viral infections may also impair secretion of antimicrobial proteins by airway or alveolar epithelium. The mechanisms whereby stress impairs innate pulmonary defenses are poorly defined. As a result of one or more of these processes, exposure of the lung to increased numbers of virulent *M. haemolytica* coincides with a reduction in pulmonary defenses, leading to increased colonization of the cranial lung lobes. The finding that outbreaks are often polymicrobial (with isolates of multiple *Pasteurellaceae* bacteria, including diverse genotypes of *M. haemolytica*) supports the notion that this disease results from failure of lung defenses, with colonization by opportunistic pathogens that are well equipped to evade the remaining defenses and incite disease.

Clinical disease is principally a consequence of the host response to infection of the lung with *M. haemolytica*, rather than a direct effect of bacterial toxins on lung tissue. Massive exudation of fibrin into alveoli is a prominent feature of severe pneumonia in cattle, and is mediated in part by a direct effect of lipopolysaccharide on endothelial cells, but also by macrophage-derived inflammatory mediators, such as TNF-α. Phagocytosis of *M. haemolytica* by alveolar macrophages is limited unless the bacteria are opsonized by antibody or complement; the significance of other opsonins, such as the collectins, remains speculative. Alveolar macrophages that have ingested *M. haemolytica* or been exposed to bacterial products secrete an array of neutrophil chemoattractants, including IL-8, ENA, GRO, platelet-activating factor, and leukotriene B$_4$. Neutrophils migrate to the alveoli and terminal bronchioles within 3 hours of experimental challenge with *M. haemolytica*. Neutrophil migration to alveoli uses a β_2 integrin–independent mechanism, whereas neutrophil recruitment to airways is dependent on interactions between β_2 integrin and intercellular adhesion molecule 1 ICAM-1. In contrast to most bacterial infections, in which neutrophils phagocytose and kill the offending bacteria, neutrophils recruited to the sites of established infection with *M. haemolytica* are probably lysed by the effects of leukotoxin. Thus *this disease is characterized by massive recruitment of neutrophils that are ineffective in killing bacteria, but nonetheless exacerbate the severity of clinical disease.* Infiltration of neutrophils and additional macrophages into alveoli is harmful in several ways. The physical presence of these cells precludes normal ventilation and gas exchange; oxygen radicals, nitric oxide derivatives, and proteinases secreted by leukocytes may injure pulmonary cells and the interstitial stroma; expression of tissue factor by activated alveolar or intravascular macrophages promotes fibrin formation in the alveolus and thrombosis of blood vessels in the alveolar septa; and both macrophages and neutrophils secrete chemoattractants that perpetuate the recruitment of additional leukocytes.

Focal areas of coagulative necrosis are a characteristic feature of infection with M. haemolytica. Some represent infarcts caused by thrombosis of intralobular blood vessels, but leukocyte secretions might also cause direct lung injury. These foci of necrosis are encircled by a dense band of leukocytes, many of which are necrotic, and these leukocytes are in a state of intense activation featuring prominent gene expression of IL-8 and inducible nitric oxide synthetase. Profound depression and "toxemia" or sepsis are constant features of acute infection with *M. haemolytica*; although the basis for this systemic illness is unknown, TNF-α in the plasma of some cases may be responsible.

Immune responses to *M. haemolytica* occur rapidly following exposure, with alveolar IgM detectable by 48 hours after experimental infection, detectable serum IgM by 5 days, and IgG by 7 days after infection. Animals that recover from disease or are vaccinated with live bacteria are immune to subsequent challenge, and serum antibody titers to leukotoxin, outer- membrane proteins, and capsule all correlate with resistance to naturally occurring disease. However, it is likely that an immune response to several antigens is necessary for protection, for the presence of antibody to individual antigens, including leukotoxin, capsular polysaccharide, lipopolysaccharide, or outer-membrane proteins, does not confer complete protection.

Histophilus somni causes bronchopneumonia, pleuritis (see Fig. 5-45) or pericarditis, polyarthritis, and infectious thrombotic meningoencephalitis, although an individual animal is usually affected by only one of these conditions. The importance of *H. somni* as a cause of bovine pneumonia varies considerably between geographic regions. As with *M. haemolytica*, this pathogen uses a broad array of virulence factors. Resistance to serum- and complement-mediated killing is mediated by proteins that bind the Fc component of immunoglobulin, making these Fc receptors unavailable for complement activation. Lipo-oligosaccharide has many proinflammatory effects, analogous to lipopolysaccharide in other gram-negative bacteria. The lipo-oligosaccharide of disease-associated, but not commensal, isolates of *H. somni* undergoes structural and antigenic variation during the course of an experimental infection, and this variation may serve as a mechanism of immune evasion and resistance to complement-mediated killing. Transferrin- and hemoglobin-binding proteins enable the bacteria to acquire iron for growth. *H. somni* binds to and induces apoptosis in endothelial cells in vitro, and although this effect may contribute to the vasculitis that is characteristic of *H. somni* septicemia, these processes are as yet poorly characterized. Immune-complex deposition is apparently not the cause of vasculitis. *H. somni* is considered a facultative intracellular pathogen as it survives within monocytes, yet both intracellular and extracellular bacteria are numerous in acute pneumonia, and biofilm formation is described. Finally, *H. somni* impairs the phagocytic function of neutrophils and macrophages, and induces degeneration of macrophages and apoptosis of neutrophils. Vasculitis in *H. somni* infection occurs by diverse mechanisms, including induction of an inflammatory response, apoptosis of endothelial cells, activation of platelets, and histamine production by the bacteria.

Pasteurella multocida is an important but less-studied cause of pneumonia in cattle. Capsular serotype A:3 is most commonly isolated from cases of pneumonia. As for *M. haemolytica*, the bacteria are carried in the nasopharynx of many clinically normal calves. Adhesins, an antiphagocytic capsule, neuraminidase, iron-binding proteins, and lipopolysaccharide are among the described virulence factors.

The **gross lesions** of acute fulminant shipping-fever pneumonia caused by *M. haemolytica*, *H. somni*, or *P. multocida* are not reliably distinguished and include *cranioventral lobar or lobular fibrinous bronchopneumonia, foci of coagulative necrosis, and variable fibrinous pleuritis* (Fig. 5-56). Lesions are most severe in the cranial and middle lung lobes, but may also affect the caudal lung. Acute fulminant cases often exhibit lobar fibrinous pneumonia and pleuritis and may die with as little as 30% of the lung affected, because of systemic effects of the infection rather than failure of lung function. Lesions are often sharply demarcated from less affected areas of lung, are

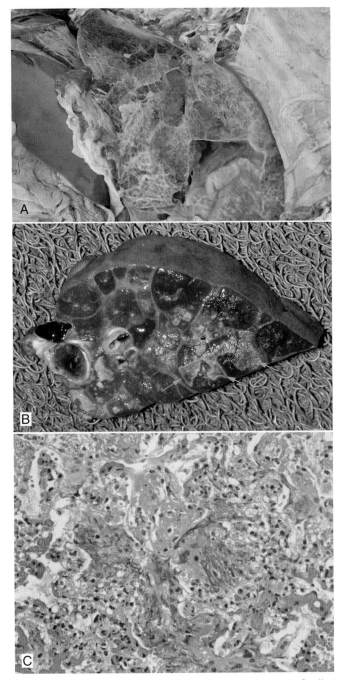

Figure 5-56 Peracute fibrinous bronchopneumonia in a feedlot calf. **A.** Characteristic lesions of a peracute bronchopneumonia: mats of loosely adherent fibrin on both visceral and parietal pleura (see the reflected ribs at the right), and red-purple discoloration and hard texture of affected lung tissue that cuts crisply with a knife. A thin line of ventilated pink tissue remains visible along the dorsal border of the lung. **B.** The cut section reveals irregularly shaped foci of coagulative necrosis typical of *Mannheimia haemolytica* infection, outlined by a white rim of leukocytes (arrows). **C.** Histologically, alveoli are filled with eosinophilic fibrin, and the necrotic leukocytes have streaming chromatin characteristic of "oat cells."

discolored purple-red and later tan-gray, and the filling of alveoli with fibrin bestows a firm or hard texture to the affected lung.

The cut section of the lung is purple-red, firm or hard, and moist. It is often not possible to express exudate from the transected airway, for the leukocytes are enmeshed in polymerized fibrin. Sharply demarcated, irregularly shaped, 0.5-5 cm diameter, pale, dry foci of coagulative necrosis are frequent in fulminant cases of *M. haemolytica* or *H. somni* infection, but are not expected with *P. multocida* (see Fig. 5-56). Bronchi may contain catarrhal or suppurative material or hemorrhage, or may be free of exudate. Interlobular septa are distended with fibrinous or serofibrinous exudate, and this lends a marbled appearance to the cut surface. In the most severe cases, fibrin forms a lattice or mat over the pleural surface of affected lung lobes, and the pleural cavity may contain serofibrinous yellow fluid that clots when the chest is opened. Fibrinous pericarditis may accompany the pleuritis.

Necrosis of laryngeal epithelium at the point of contact of the vocal folds is commonly identified in cattle with severe pneumonia, resulting from mucosal trauma induced by abrupt laryngeal closure in a dyspneic animal. Vasculitis resulting from *H. somni* bacteremia can cause a similar lesion.

Differentiation of acute from subacute lesions is challenging but important to determine whether early clinical recognition of ill animals was adequate. Indicators of peracute pneumonia include red-purple hemorrhagic and infarcted lobules, crisp texture of the cut section, abundant and loosely adherent pleural fibrin, and systemic petechiae (see Fig. 5-56). Characteristics of subacute bronchopneumonia may include a lobular distribution of lesions (see Fig. 5-36, eFig. 5-50), mottled tan-grey as well as red appearance, suppurative exudate that oozes from small bronchi when a cut section is compressed, purulent or catarrhal exudate on the mucosal surface of the large airways, and pleural adhesions. Mild subacute cases with atelectasis and rubbery consolidation may be difficult to distinguish from lesions of viral pneumonia.

Sequelae indicative of chronic disease include *sequestra, bronchiectasis, abscesses, and fibrous pleural adhesions*. Sequestra consist of a necrotic core of firm but friable tissue, sometimes surrounded by fluid or caseous exudate, enveloped in a capsule of fibrous tissue. Bronchiectasis manifests as dilated airways that are filled with purulent exudate and thickened by fibrous tissue (see Fig. 5-33). The surrounding lung tissue is invariably atelectatic, and may be swollen because of persistent bronchopneumonia. Ectatic bronchi appear similar to abscesses, but bronchiectasis is typified by cylindrical tracts filled with pus, the occasional presence of cartilage remnants on gross or histologic examination, and communication with a bronchus. Lesions of bronchiectasis and abscesses are often secondarily colonized by *Trueperella pyogenes* or other opportunistic pathogens.

The **histologic lesions** of *acute fulminant shipping-fever pneumonia caused by M. haemolytica or H. somni are characterized by fibrinous and suppurative bronchopneumonia with necrosis of leukocytes*. Alveoli and small bronchioles are filled with variable proportions of neutrophils and macrophages, fibrin, edema fluid, erythrocytes, necrotic cellular debris, and aggregates of bacteria. Necrosis of intra-alveolar leukocytes with a fusiform streaming pattern of pale basophilic chromatin (termed "oat cells" for their resemblance to grains of oats) is a characteristic feature of infection with *M. haemolytica* (see Fig. 5-56), where leukotoxin is the likely cause of the neutrophil cell death. Leukocyte necrosis may also be present in *H. somni* infection, and this agent is capable of inducing apoptosis in neutrophils in vitro. The nature of the necrotic leukocytes has long evaded definitive identification, but *it is likely that both neutrophils and macrophages are affected*. Larger airways may contain suppurative exudate, but neutrophil infiltration of the mucosa is often absent.

Necrosis and attenuation of bronchiolar epithelium, when present, should prompt a search for underlying viral infection. However, this lesion is present in some calves experimentally infected with *H. somni* or *M. haemolytica*, and may represent neutrophil-induced damage to the epithelium or a direct effect of *H. somni*. Thrombi commonly occlude arterioles, venules, and alveolar septal capillaries. Interlobular septa are distended with serofibrinous exudate, and septal lymphatics are often filled with fibrin. Sharply demarcated, irregularly shaped areas of coagulative necrosis are often apparent. In these, alveolar and bronchiolar lesions are as described above, but all cells within the lesions are necrotic, and karyolysis or karyorrhexis is prominent. A dense band of necrotic leukocytes encircles these foci of necrosis, and thrombi occasionally fill blood vessels at the edge of or within the lesions. Suppurative phlebitis with fibrinoid necrosis may occur in pneumonia caused by *H. somni*, but is only common in acute fulminant cases (eFig. 5-85).

The appearance of these lesions changes in later stages. Macrophages and multinucleated histiocytic cells encompass the alveolar masses of polymerized fibrin; removal of fibrin by these macrophages and by fibrinolysis presumably occurs in some nonfatal cases. Otherwise, alveolar fibrin is infiltrated by fibroblasts and replaced by connective tissue, visible by 5 days after infection, with 2 possible sequelae: incorporation of the re-epithelialized alveolar fibrous tissue into the alveolar septum to form a thickened alveolar septum and a "recanalized" alveolar lumen, or large expanses of pulmonary fibrosis. Chronic suppurative or lymphoplasmacytic bronchitis occurs regularly in calves with chronic pneumonia.

Less fulminant cases tend to lack the fibrinous alveolar exudate, thrombosis, and interlobular fibrin that are typical of fulminant shipping-fever pneumonia. Rather, these lesions are dominated by exudation of neutrophils in alveoli and bronchioles, congestion of pulmonary vessels, but little other morphologic change in lung tissue.

The gross lesions of cranioventral bronchopneumonia are usually **diagnostic**. The swollen and hard nature of bacterial pneumonia aids in the differentiation from the atelectatic cranioventral lesions of bovine respiratory syncytial virus pneumonia. A histologic finding of suppurative bronchopneumonia implies a diagnosis of bacterial pneumonia; the important challenge is to identify the underlying causes. Lesions of aspiration pneumonia may closely resemble bacterial pneumonia; however, necrosis of alveolar leukocytes is not expected, and focal or unilateral, necrotizing, and foul-smelling lesions containing histologically recognizable foreign material are more typical of aspiration. Differentiation of the foci of necrosis from those seen in *Mycoplasma bovis* pneumonia is discussed in the section on bovine mycoplasmal disease.

The use of *aerobic and microaerophilic culture* to identify the specific etiology is commonly successful unless animals have been medicated with antimicrobials. Subacute or chronic cases are often colonized by opportunistic bacteria, and the primary bacterial cause may no longer be present. Immunohistochemistry to identify *M. haemolytica* and *H. somni* has

been described, and may be of use in antimicrobial-treated, autolysed, or archival tissues, or if fresh tissue is not available. Detection of serum antibody to *M. haemolytica* by using a bacterial agglutination assay, leukotoxin neutralization assay, or leukotoxin ELISA is a common research tool, but finds limited use in field investigations.

Further reading

Agnes JT, et al. Bovine respiratory syncytial virus and *Histophilus somni* interaction at the alveolar barrier. Infect Immun 2013;81:2592-2597.

Aulik NA, et al. *Mannheimia haemolytica* and its leukotoxin cause macrophage extracellular trap formation by bovine macrophages. Infect Immun 2012;80:1923-1933.

Booker CW, et al. Microbiological and histopathological findings in cases of fatal bovine respiratory disease of feedlot cattle in Western Canada. Can Vet J 2008;49:473-481.

Caswell JL. Failure of respiratory defenses in the pathogenesis of bacterial pneumonia of cattle. Vet Pathol 2014;51:393-409.

Confer AW. Update on bacterial pathogenesis in BRD. Anim Health Res Rev 2009;10:145-148.

Dagleish MP, et al. Characterization and time course of pulmonary lesions in calves after intratracheal infection with *Pasteurella multocida* A:3. J Comp Pathol 2010;142:157-169.

Fulton RW, et al. Lung pathology and infectious agents in fatal feedlot pneumonias and relationship with mortality, disease onset, and treatments. J Vet Diagn Invest 2009;21:464-477.

Sandal I, Inzana TJA. A genomic window into the virulence of *Histophilus somni*. Trends Microbiol 2010;18:90-99.

Singh K, et al. *Mannheimia haemolytica*: bacterial-host interactions in bovine pneumonia. Vet Pathol 2011;48:338-348.

Timsit E, et al. Transmission dynamics of *Mannheimia haemolytica* in newly-received beef bulls at fattening operations. Vet Microbiol 2013;161:295-304.

Hemorrhagic septicemia of cattle. *Hemorrhagic septicemia of cattle is caused by Pasteurella multocida, and usually serotypes B:2 or E:2.* Hemorrhagic septicemia is now limited largely to tropical countries of Asia and Africa, and in these regions is primarily a disease of buffalo and, to a lesser extent, cattle. Outbreaks in tropical climates occur particularly during the rainy season. In intervening periods, the organism is apparently maintained in the nasopharyngeal regions of carrier cattle or buffalo. The start of an outbreak depends on some stress disturbing the balance in a carrier animal. This results in extensive proliferation and dissemination of the organisms to susceptible contact animals.

Approximately 10% of animals survive subclinical infections and become immune, but once clinical signs are apparent, the mortality is almost 100%, even with appropriate antimicrobial therapy. This, together with the immense proliferation of organisms in the clinical disease, suggests that bacterial toxins (particularly endotoxin) are important in causing death.

Hemorrhagic septicemia is a peracute disease, and many animals die without clinical signs. Less fulminant cases exhibit high fever and rapid prostration, with profuse drooling. The saliva and feces contain large numbers of bacteria. Petechial hemorrhages are present on the serous membranes and in various organs, especially the lungs and muscles. Severe endotoxemia may cause *acute, fibrinohemorrhagic interstitial lung disease*. Lymph nodes are swollen and hemorrhagic, and there may be blood-stained fluid in the serous cavities. Acute gastroenteritis, which can be hemorrhagic, is often present. The spleen is not greatly enlarged, which is a point of differentiation from anthrax.

There is a *subacute edematous form of hemorrhagic septicemia*, in which edema of the throat is unusually pronounced. The whole head, tongue, brisket, or a limb may also be affected. The swellings are produced by copious, clotted, straw-colored exudate. Although these lesions are caused by hemorrhagic septicemia, death is caused by asphyxiation.

Further reading

Shivachandra SB, et al. A review of hemorrhagic septicemia in cattle and buffalo. Anim Health Res Rev 2011;12:67-82.

Cilia-associated respiratory bacillus. Cilia-associated respiratory (CAR) bacillus (*Helicobacter* sp.) is a recognized cause of chronic respiratory disease in rats, mice, and rabbits. The bacilli interdigitate between cilia and induce lymphocytic bronchitis and bronchiolitis, bronchiectasis, and lung abscesses. Morphologically similar bacteria have been observed in the tracheal epithelium of cattle, deer, swine, and cats. The bacteria are of similar length and diameter as the cilia, but are visualized with Warthin-Starry silver stains (Fig. 5-57). In *calves*, there is an association between the presence of CAR bacilli and the presence of lymphoid follicles in the airway wall, but it remains unknown if this is a causal relationship. *Porcine* CAR bacilli are apparently nonpathogenic, for they are present in pigs with and without respiratory disease, and experimentally infected pigs have not developed clinical signs or lesions. The major differential diagnosis is *Bordetella bronchiseptica*.

Further reading

Pravettoni D, et al. Cilia-associated respiratory (CAR) bacillus infection in veal calves and adult cattle. Dtsch Tierarztl Wochenschr 2001; 108:386-389.

Tuberculosis. *Bovine tuberculosis, caused by* **Mycobacterium bovis**, *is a chronic disease characterized by caseating granulomas in lung, lymph nodes, and other organs.* Control programs have minimized the occurrence of bovine tuberculosis in many developed countries. The disease is rare in Canada, the United States, and Australia, although infected wildlife reservoirs remain and cases continue to occur in domestic livestock. Most recent reports of bovine tuberculosis in the United States and Canada have occurred in farmed cervids or in localized geographic areas. In much of Europe, <0.4% of cattle herds are infected, but the prevalence is higher in Ireland, United Kingdom, Spain, and Italy. In contrast, bovine tuberculosis is endemic in New Zealand and many countries in Africa, Asia, Central and South America; 10-35% of herds are infected in many of these endemic areas.

The success of tuberculosis eradication schemes is complicated by *wildlife reservoirs*, which maintain infection and transmit disease to cattle. Wildlife reservoirs of *M. bovis* infection include European badgers *(Meles meles)* in Ireland and the United Kingdom, brush-tailed possum *(Trichosurus vulpecula)* in New Zealand, feral pigs in Spain, swamp buffalo *(Bubalus bubalis)* in Australia's Northern Territory, Cape buffalo *(Syncerus caffer)* and lechwe antelope *(Kobus leche)* in southern Africa, bison *(Bison bison)* in Wood Buffalo National Park in western Canada, and various species of deer in the United States and New Zealand. In contrast, dead-end or spill-over hosts, including goats, wart hogs, cats, mustelids, and humans, may be infected with *M. bovis* but do not maintain infection in an area and rarely transmit infection to cattle.

Many mycobacteria persist in soil for prolonged periods, and the infectivity of *M. bovis* is likely maintained for several weeks in the environment. However, because oral infections require high doses of bacilli, the importance of environmental survival in the epidemiology of disease is likely limited.

The classic tubercle bacilli are *M. tuberculosis* (human) and *M. bovis* (bovine). Related species are *M. avium, M. microti,* and *M. africanum.* To avoid confusion, the term **tuberculosis** is limited to diseases caused by *M. tuberculosis* or *M. bovis.* Disease conditions caused by other "nontuberculous" mycobacteria are referred to as **mycobacteriosis** or atypical

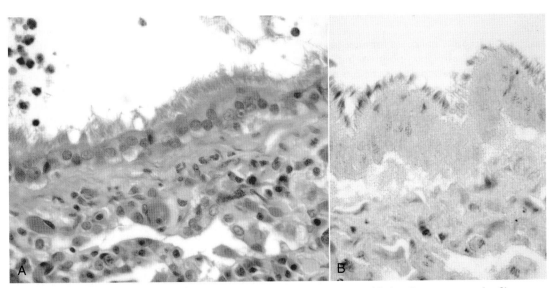

Figure 5-57 Cilia-associated respiratory bacillus in a rat. Innumerable bacilli accentuate the filamentous appearance of the cilia in a bronchus stained with H&E (**A**), and are more readily identified in the Warthin-Starry silver-stained section (**B**).

mycobacteriosis. Nontuberculous mycobacteria are widespread in soil and water. Examples include members of the *M. avium* complex as well as *M. fortuitum* and *M. smegmatis*. The >160 species of nontuberculous mycobacteria were once classified by the Runyon system, but this has been replaced by 16S rRNA gene sequencing. These organisms typically cause disease in immunocompromised hosts, and the manifestations are cervical lymphadenitis, pulmonary lesions similar to tuberculosis, or cutaneous lesions associated with local penetration of organisms through wounds.

The 3 main species of tubercle bacilli, *M. tuberculosis*, *M. bovis*, and *M. avium*, occur most frequently in their respective hosts, but cross-infections do occur, and various other species of animals are affected.

- **Bovine tuberculosis** refers mainly to disease in cattle caused by *M. bovis*, but the term is also used to describe the pathogenic effects of this bacterium in other hosts. The host range of *M. bovis* is broad, including cattle, deer, elk, bison, buffalo, goats, camels, llamas, swine, elephants, rhinoceros, dogs, foxes, cats, mink, badgers, and nonhuman and human primates. Natural disease is most common in cattle, cervids, humans, and swine.
- **M. avium** causes mycobacteriosis chiefly in birds and is occasionally found in cattle, swine, horses, sheep, and monkeys.
- **M. tuberculosis** is chiefly responsible for tuberculosis in humans, and occasionally infects pigs, captive monkeys, dogs, cats, cattle, and psittacine birds.
- **Human infections** with *M. bovis* are well documented, but are much less common than *M. tuberculosis*. Immunosuppressed individuals, such as those with the acquired immunodeficiency syndrome (AIDS), are at particular risk. Ingestion of milk from cows with mammary tuberculosis is a major route of infection in humans, typically inducing cervical lymphadenitis or other nonpulmonary forms of disease. This pattern of disease is of great historical importance as the impetus for identification of the tubercle bacillus and the subsequent *pasteurization of milk*, but infection from raw milk continues to occur in regions where bovine tuberculosis is common. Transmission from cattle to humans by aerosol or by contamination of cutaneous wounds also occurs, mainly in those in close contact with infected cattle.
- Mycobacteria are nonmotile, nonspore-forming pleomorphic coccobacilli. They are gram-positive but almost unstainable by the simpler bacterial stains because of their high content of lipids. They are routinely stained with carbol-fuchsin, and then resist decoloration by inorganic acids. This property of acid-fastness of the stained bacilli depends on the amount and spatial arrangement of mycolic acids and their esters in the bacterial wall. They are also demonstrable by fluorescent dyes such as auramine. Sometimes, in cultures or in old lesions, the organisms have a beaded or granulated appearance. This beading is partly caused by the presence of lipid droplets within the bacteria and is an indication of an unfavorable environment for organisms in the postexponential growth phase.

In addition to the cell membrane and peptidoglycan layers found in other bacteria, *the mycobacterial cell wall contains a large hydrophobic layer of mycolic acids, which bestows hydrophobicity on the cell wall, conferring environmental and antimicrobial resistance.* The waxes and cell-wall glycolipids are important inducers of the initial macrophage response and,

together with peptidoglycan (muramyl dipeptide), are responsible for most of the adjuvant activity of mycobacteria that facilitates recruitment of antigen-presenting cells. Increased glycolipid content of mycobacterial cell walls, acid-fastness, and the amount of trehalose dimycolate (cord factor) in the cell wall are associated with increased virulence. Other glycolipids (mycosides) form a barrier against lysosomal digestion and partly explain the ability of the organisms to survive after phagocytosis by macrophages; intracellular survival is also facilitated by preventing fusion of phagosomes and lysosomes. The differing effectiveness of such mechanisms determines the relative ability of various mycobacteria to resist intracellular degradation.

Tuberculoproteins are the other major category of immunoreactive substances in mycobacteria. They provide most of the antigenic determinants, but the adjuvant activity of the lipids and polysaccharides in the mycobacterial cell wall is needed for an animal to produce an immunologic response to these tuberculoproteins. *Purified protein derivatives* (PPD) from mycobacteria are capable of eliciting delayed-type hypersensitivity once the animal is sensitized, however, and this is the basis of *intradermal skin testing*. Both tuberculoproteins and the adjuvant lipids are present in infection, and the result is the development of both humoral and cell-mediated immune responses. Humoral antibodies can be demonstrated by serologic techniques, but do not participate in the development of lesions or in the production of immunity. Cell-mediated responses are responsible for both aspects of the disease.

The *method of transmission* influences the spectrum of lesions of bovine tuberculosis. Inhalation of droplet nuclei or dust particles containing *M. bovis* is the most common route of infection and leads to infection of the upper and lower airways. Oral infection requires a greater dose of bacilli than airborne infection to cause disease, and elicits lesions in the gut and associated lymph nodes. Transplacental transmission is a sequel of endometrial tuberculosis, and leads to fetal lesions in hepatic and portal lymph nodes. Less common routes of infection include percutaneous inoculation and genital transmission.

Important concepts in the pathogenesis of tuberculosis include the ability of mycobacteria to survive within macrophages, and the role of cellular immune responses in inciting granulomatous inflammation and enhancing the ability of macrophages to kill bacilli. Most animals that are infected with *M. bovis* do not develop clinical disease. The outcome of infection depends on bacterial factors, including the dose and virulence of infecting bacteria, but also on host factors, including the state of immune competence and heritable resistance to tuberculosis. Heritable variation in disease susceptibility has been identified in cattle and in deer. In humans and mice, mycobacterial resistance is partly related to allelic variation in the natural resistance–associated macrophage protein *(Nramp)* genes 1 and 2, which affect intracellular survival of pathogens by modifying lysosomal transport of divalent cations, including iron and manganese. Other forms of heritable resistance to *M. bovis* are unrelated to variation in *Nramp* genes.

There are several facets to immune-mediated control of tuberculosis, and most of this understanding is based on the study of *M. tuberculosis* infections in humans and laboratory animals. In the early phases of infection, bacilli are phagocytosed by macrophages and may be eliminated. Alternatively, infected macrophages may remain at the site of primary infection for prolonged periods before the disease progresses. An initial innate immune response develops at this site of primary infection, as macrophages secrete cytokines—particularly tumor necrosis factor-α (TNF-α) and the C-C chemokines—that recruit additional macrophages and lymphocytes to the site. Macrophages stimulated by exposure to mycobacteria secrete interleukin (IL-12), which skews the immune response to favor secretion of interferon-γ (IFN-γ) and IL-2 by CD4+ T-helper-1 lymphocytes. These IFN-γ–producing T-helper lymphocytes signal the development of **cell-mediated immunity,** first detected at 14-28 days after infection by positive tuberculin skin test reactions. The arrival of these antigen-specific lymphocytes is crucial for host defense, activating macrophages and thus allowing them to overcome the block in phagosome maturation, and upregulate production of bactericidal products, including reactive nitrogen and oxygen intermediates and lysosomal enzymes that kill intracellular bacilli. Activated macrophages appear epithelioid, with abundant cytoplasm and indistinct cell borders, or form multinucleated giant cells.

The cytokines TNF-α and IFN-γ act synergistically to promote formation of the **tuberculoid granuloma,** a dynamic structure that prevents spread of infection to other sites in the lung, as well as animal-to-animal transmission, and represents a localized target for the immune response. An excessive tissue-damaging cell-mediated immune response is thought to kill heavily infected macrophages and form the caseous center of the granuloma. Matrix metalloproteinases released from activated macrophages are a likely cause of the characteristic cell necrosis and liquefaction of tissues in some lesions of tuberculosis. Bacilli within the caseous center may remain dormant for years, until immunosuppression caused by diseases, drugs, hormones, or malnutrition, or other unidentified factors disturb the balance between host and agent, allowing proliferation of the pathogen and reactivation of the disease.

Whether the delayed-type hypersensitivity reaction is beneficial or harmful to the host depends on the circumstances. On the one hand, the reaction to relatively small numbers of bacilli causes accelerated tubercle formation that enhances the killing of the organisms, and helps prevent reinfection or dissemination from the initial site of infection. On the other hand, the delayed-type hypersensitivity response to large amounts of mycobacterial antigen causes extensive cell necrosis and tissue destruction, which is seriously detrimental. Liquefaction, brought about by hydrolytic enzymes of macrophages and possibly neutrophils, is the most harmful response. The bacilli multiply extracellularly in the liquefied material and are available in large numbers for dissemination through cavities, vessels, and airways. In summary, *the final determinants of the nature and intensity of lesions are the magnitude of the bacterial infection, the intensity and appropriateness of the immune response, and the modifying influences of the structure of the tissue involved.*

Gross or histologic lesions are absent in the majority of cattle that react to tuberculin skin tests, and although *M. bovis* cannot be isolated from many of these cases, they are generally considered to be infected for the purposes of epidemiology and control. Thorough examination of lymph nodes throughout the body is necessary before declaring a carcass free of visible lesions, as *gross lesions may be absent, few, or multiple.* The distribution of lesions of bovine tuberculosis depends on the mode of transmission. In most cases, gross lesions are restricted to the respiratory tract and associated lymphoid tissues and suggest inhalation as the route of infection.

Tubercles or craterous ulcers in gut or mesenteric lymph nodes suggest an oral route of infection, or ingestion of infected sputum that has been coughed up from the lung. Generalized disease is less common but well described.

In **respiratory infections,** *lesions are most common in retropharyngeal, tracheobronchial, and mediastinal lymph nodes,* and less frequent in palatine tonsils and mandibular, parotid, and mesenteric lymph nodes. Lung lesions are detected in only 10-30% of cattle with gross lesions, and often affect the caudal lobes. Thus secondary lesions in lymph nodes may be easier to detect than primary lesions in the lung. *The classic gross lesion is the tubercle: a circumscribed, often encapsulated, pale-yellow or white focus of granulomatous inflammation, often with central caseous necrosis and/or mineralization* (Fig. 5-58). Larger lesions may contain liquefied or suppurative exudate and be mistaken for abscesses caused by pyogenic bacteria.

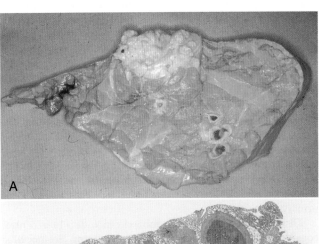

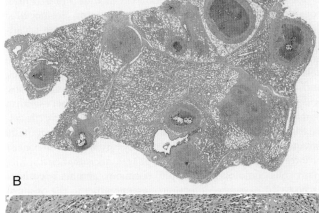

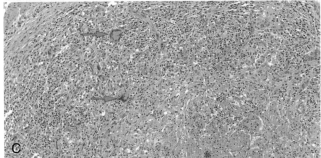

Figure 5-58 Bovine tuberculosis. A. Granuloma in the lung of a cow appears as a pale homogeneous bulging mass. **B.** Lung from an elk, with multiple granulomas containing central areas of caseous necrosis and mineralization. **C.** Lung from the same elk, showing central caseous necrosis (asterisk), a wall of macrophages, giant cells (arrows) and lymphocytes, and a peripheral fibrous capsule (top left).

Bacilli are released from expanding tubercles into the airways, and coughing up of infected sputum may spread the infection by ingestion to cause lesions in intestine or mesenteric lymph nodes, by adhesion to laryngeal or tracheal mucosa to incite ulcers or ulcerating tubercles, or by aspiration to seed secondary sites in the lung. Multiple, raised, yellow, 1-3 mm plaques on the mucosal surface of the nasal cavity and nasopharynx are early lesions following experimental intranasal infection. Erosion of pulmonary tubercles through the pleura may result in implantation of bacilli throughout the pleural cavity, with development of multiple granulomas on pleural surfaces. Lymphatic spread has been suggested as an alternative route of pleural infection.

Generalized lesions are reported in about 1% of animals with gross lesions of tuberculosis, and probably result from hematogenous dissemination of bacilli following erosion of the wall of a blood vessel by an expanding tubercle. Embolic lesions are most common in lung, and may involve lymph nodes, bone, liver, kidney, mammary gland, uterus, pleura, peritoneum, pericardium, and meninges. Lesions are rare in salivary gland, pancreas, spleen, brain, myocardium, or muscle. In some instances, presumably following substantial release of bacilli into the blood, the presence of innumerable tiny white foci justifies the term *"miliary tuberculosis."* In contrast, other carcasses display generalized lesions that are variable in size and degree of caseation or fibrosis, and imply a less catastrophic but more prolonged bacteremia. Erosion through serosal or mucosal surfaces by expanding tubercles spreads the infection by implantation on pleural, peritoneal, pericardial, or meningeal surfaces, or along the airways, intestine, or urinary tract.

Histologic features of the tubercle include (1) a central coagulum of caseous necrosis, consisting of eosinophilic homogeneous material with scant nuclear debris and a variable degree of mineralization; (2) a mantle of macrophages and Langhans-type multinucleated giant cells; (3) a capsule containing lymphocytes, clusters of neutrophils in some cases, and a rim of collagenous connective tissue in chronic lesions; and (4) acid-fast bacteria—often in very low number—within macrophages and giant cells of the mantle zone or extracellularly in the caseous core (see Fig. 5-58). In experimentally infected cattle, the early lesions at 7 days after infection consist of intra-alveolar clusters of macrophages, necrotic neutrophils, giant cells containing neutrophil remnants, and acid-fast bacteria. At 14 days after infection, corresponding to the onset of lymphocyte proliferative responses, tubercles contain central aggregates of neutrophils surrounded by epithelioid macrophages. Necrosis in the center of the tubercles develops later, at 21-42 days after infection, and the first mineralized lesions are at 35-60 days. However, this progression is variable among granulomas, with significant heterogeneity in a single animal. The amount of fibrosis increases with time, and tends to be more prominent in individuals and species with greater resistance. The presence of neutrophils is highly variable, and their presence in large numbers is most common in cases with rapid multiplication of bacteria, numerous reactive lymphocytes, and easily distensible tissues.

In **cervids**, *M. bovis* causes a similar spectrum of lesions as in cattle, but several unique features are of note. As in cattle, lesions are most common in retropharyngeal lymph nodes, lungs, thoracic lymph nodes, and mesenteric lymph nodes. However, deer may develop superficial lymphadenitis and abscesses that drain to the skin surface. Disease progression

may be more rapid in cervids than cattle; deer shed larger numbers of bacilli, and the disease may be more likely to remain subclinical. These features suggest that deer are less able to contain *M. bovis* infections than cattle, although limited evidence indicates they are not more susceptible to infection.

In elk *(Cervus elaphus nelsoni)*, red deer *(C. elaphus elaphus)*, and fallow deer *(Dama dama)*, fibrosis and giant cells are less evident than in cattle, the presence of mineralization is more variable, and importantly, *suppurative inflammation may be prominent.* Multifocal lesions of caseous necrosis or suppurative inflammation in the lungs and lymph nodes of cervids are commonly caused by *Fusobacterium necrophorum* infection, and it has been recommended that these lesions be carefully examined for acid-fast bacteria as a routine procedure. Occasional cases of tuberculosis in these species may have concentrically laminated caseous abscesses reminiscent of caseous lymphadenitis in sheep and goats. The lesions of tuberculosis in sika deer *(C. nippon)* are distinctive, consisting of nonencapsulated invasive accumulations of epithelioid macrophages and numerous irregularly shaped giant cells, few neutrophils, and minimal necrosis or mineralization.

Tuberculosis in **horses** is often *alimentary*, with lesions in *retropharyngeal and mesenteric lymph nodes and intestine.* Intestinal infection may cause localized ulcers or thickened mucosal lesions reminiscent of Johne's disease in cattle. Tubercles in horses are usually uniform, gray, smooth (lardaceous), with little caseation or mineralization but abundant fibrosis, and may resemble sarcomas. Tuberculosis in **small ruminants** is uncommon, and many cases have cavitary lesions with numerous bacilli. Tuberculosis in **swine** is often *systemic*, and the morphology depends on the infecting pathogen. *Mycoplasma bovis* produces caseous and mineralized tubercles similar to those that occur in cattle, and the lesions are often surrounded by a fibrous capsule. In the liver, there is a tendency for the caseous centers to liquefy. *M. avium* produces lesions that are proliferative in nature and consist of tuberculous granulation tissue resembling the lardaceous or sarcomatous lesions described in equine tuberculosis. The histologic appearance is of diffuse infiltration of macrophages, epithelioid cells, and Langhans' giant cells accompanied by extensive fibroplasia and numerous bacilli.

Tuberculosis in **dogs and cats** often appears as *granulation tissue* in which macrophages are scattered at random and giant cells are rare. *Discrete tuberculous granulomas are uncommon,* and composed principally of epithelioid cells surrounded by narrow zones of fibrous tissue in which there are scattered small collections of lymphocytes and plasma cells. Necrosis is often present in the centers of larger granulomas. Giant cells are rare. In cats, the presence of central necrosis and fairly small numbers of acid-fast bacilli helps to distinguish lesions of tuberculosis from those of feline leprosy. In dogs, intrabronchial dissemination within the lungs occurs quite rapidly and can lead to tuberculous bronchitis and bronchiolitis. Pleuritis or peritonitis often accompanies primary infections in the lungs or intestine, respectively, with diffuse or finely nodular pleural thickening by granulation tissue containing few macrophages and bacilli. Dogs are susceptible to *M. tuberculosis*, by contact with infected humans, and the lesions affect lung and cervicothoracic lymph nodes or may be disseminated.

A thorough examination is the most sensitive method of detecting tuberculosis after death, as the likelihood of isolating M. bovis in culture is low if gross lesions are not detected. The differential diagnosis for granulomas of lung or lymph nodes includes cestode cysts; pyogranulomas caused by fungi, bacteria, or inhaled foreign material; bacterial abscesses; and neoplasms. Thus the presence of many eosinophils, lymphoid hyperplasia, or bacterial colonies should prompt a search for alternative causes.

Gross lesions of focal caseous lesions in lymph nodes or lung, or histologic detection of granulomas, particularly with central areas of necrosis and/or mineralization, should prompt an extensive and thorough search for the low numbers of acid-fast bacilli that are typically present. Finding few bacilli is more suggestive of bovine tuberculosis than of mycobacteriosis caused by *M. avium*. However, *bacterial culture and PCR-based assays are necessary for definitive diagnosis of bovine tuberculosis*, particularly if the diagnosis is likely to have a serious impact. Immunohistochemical identification of *M. bovis* has been described. This procedure is more sensitive than examining acid-fast-stained sections, in terms of number of animals detected, staining intensity, and ease of detection, but the antibodies in current use cross-react with other mycobacteria as well as some gram-positive bacteria and fungi.

Further reading

Cassidy JP. The pathology of bovine tuberculosis: time for an audit. Vet J 2008;176:263-264.

Fitzgerald SD, Kaneene JB. Wildlife reservoirs of bovine tuberculosis worldwide: hosts, pathology, surveillance, and control. Vet Pathol 2013;50:488-499.

Johnson IK, et al. Histological observations of bovine tuberculosis in lung and lymph node tissues from British deer. Vet J 2008;175:409-412.

Liebana E, et al. Pathology of naturally occurring bovine tuberculosis in England and Wales. Vet J 2008;176:354-360.

Palmer MV, et al. Lesion development and immunohistochemical changes in granulomas from cattle experimentally infected with *Mycobacterium bovis*. Vet Pathol 2007;44:863-874.

Sakamoto K. The pathology of *Mycobacterium tuberculosis* infection. Vet Pathol 2012;49:423-439.

Chlamydial diseases

Chlamydophila psittaci infections, usually subclinical, have occasionally been identified in cattle. In a recent study, experimentally challenged calves had *C. psittaci* DNA detected in exhaled breath, blood, and lung tissue. The challenged calves had fever, tachypnea, cough, conjunctival hyperemia, and blood neutrophilia. Histologic lesions were of fibrinous and suppurative bronchopneumonia with multifocal necrosis, and chlamydial inclusion bodies in alveolar epithelial cells, neutrophils, and macrophages. It is unknown whether *Chlamydophila* infection in cattle is a zoonotic threat to humans.

Further reading

Ostermann C, et al. Infection, disease, and transmission dynamics in calves after experimental and natural challenge with a bovine *Chlamydia psittaci* isolate. PLoS ONE 2013;8:e64066.

Mycoplasmal diseases

Contagious bovine pleuropneumonia. Contagious bovine pleuropneumonia (CBPP), an OIE (World Organization for Animal Health) listed disease, is an important barrier to global trade, and a production-limiting disease in Africa. The disease is present in much of Africa except the Mediterranean and southeast African countries, and has recently occurred in southern Europe, central and eastern Asia, and the Middle East. CBPP caused devastating epidemics in cattle populations in the 19th century, but *sporadic disease is now more common in endemically infected countries practicing vaccination*. When the agent is introduced into naive populations, the effects vary from insidiously spreading disease to spectacular mortality affecting up to 50% of the animals.

The clinical signs and mortality rates are highly variable, depending on the strain of the pathogen, the age of the animal (adults are more susceptible than young), and the presence of other diseases, crowding, or stressors. Peracute cases die without premonitory signs. Acutely ill animals are febrile, anorexic, and depressed, with profound loss of milk production, open-mouth rapid breathing, mucoid nasal discharge, and occasional coughing. Chronically affected animals may be clinically normal or have an intermittent cough and fever, yet shed the organism intermittently. Calves <6 months of age commonly develop polyarthritis affecting carpal and tarsal joints, rather than pneumonia.

CBPP is caused by **Mycoplasma mycoides ssp. mycoides small colony type**, which is different from the large colony type that causes pleuritis and pneumonia in goats in many countries throughout the world. There is marked strain-dependent variation in virulence, and the pathogenicity apparently declines as in vivo passage of the organism occurs during an outbreak. Galactan in the mucus capsule is correlated with virulence, and induces necrosis, thrombosis, and inflammation. The host range includes cattle (*Bos taurus*), zebu (*B. indicus*), water buffalo (*Bubalus bubalis*), bison, and yak, although *cattle are most commonly affected by clinical disease*. *M. mycoides* is an obligate pathogen that survives poorly in the environment, so transmission usually depends on close contact with animals shedding the bacteria. Transplacental infection may occur. *The respiratory tract is the site of primary infection*, and bacteremia develops secondarily. The incubation period varies from 5-200 days, but is typically 20-40 days.

Gross lesions are often unilateral and restricted to the *caudal lung lobes*. In the acute stages, there are mats of fibrin and fluid exudate covering the pleural surface. Interlobular septa are remarkably distended with serous fluid, and the lobules vary from normal to consolidated and red or yellow-gray. The pattern of interlobular edema and lobular consolidation lends a *characteristic marbled appearance* to the lung. Focal areas of necrosis increase in size over time, and eventually develop into sequestra. *Sequestrum formation and fibrous thickening of the pleura with adhesions to the ribs are typical of chronic CBPP.* Pericarditis, peritonitis, and polysynovitis occur infrequently in adult cattle.

Histologic examination of bronchioles and alveoli reveals serofibrinous or suppurative exudates with necrosis of neutrophils, and multifocal areas of coagulative necrosis in the lung parenchyma. Interlobular septa are expanded by edema and fibrin, and interlobular lymphatics contain fibrin. Thrombosis of arteries, veins, and lymphatics is common, and nonsuppurative arteritis may be evident. *Vasculitis is central to the development of the necrotic lesions and sequestration of lung tissue.*

The **differential diagnosis** includes *Mannheimia haemolytica* and *Mycoplasma bovis*. The unilateral lesions, caudal lobe involvement, prominent inflammation in interlobular septa, and frequent development of sequestra should suggest a diagnosis of CBPP, although the latter 2 features do occur in shipping fever caused by *M. haemolytica*. The lesions of *M. bovis* lack the extensive fibrinous exudates in interlobular septa and on the pleural surface seen in CBPP.

Definitive **diagnosis** is based on *culture on special media*, which may take several weeks. *Frozen samples of lesional lung, pleural fluids, and lymph nodes are optimal for isolation of the agent.* Immunohistochemistry and the PCR assay are more rapid methods of diagnosis. Various serologic assays are useful for screening of herds, but not for individual diagnosis. Development of improved methods to detect subclinical carriers is an area of intensive research, as current serologic assays lack sensitivity.

Further reading

Pilo P, et al. Molecular mechanisms of pathogenicity of *Mycoplasma mycoides* subsp. *mycoides* SC. Vet J 2007;174:513-521.

Mycoplasma bovis. The role of *M. bovis* as a cause of mastitis and of infertility of dairy cows is discussed elsewhere. The 2 principal manifestations of *M. bovis* in the respiratory system are as a component of *enzootic pneumonia of young dairy and veal calves,* and *chronic pneumonia and polyarthritis in feedlot beef cattle.* In contrast to the appearance of shipping fever, calves with lesions of *M. bovis* pneumonia or polyarthritis usually die or are euthanized in the second or third month after arrival. These calves have often had prolonged antimicrobial therapy for nonresponsive or relapsing respiratory disease, which is indistinguishable from shipping fever in the early stages. Calves may be lame and have swelling of one or more joints, and many calves exhibit both respiratory disease and lameness.

The prevalence of chronic pneumonia and polyarthritis is often low, although up to 30% of calves may be affected in exceptional cases. Nevertheless, because the diagnosis is only made on fatal cases, the true prevalence of the disease is unknown. In contrast, the prevalence of infection with *M. bovis* has been reported to vary from 20-70%, and most calves seroconvert to *M. bovis* during the first month in the feedlot. Bovine herpesvirus and bovine viral diarrhea virus are suggested to predispose to severe mycoplasmal disease, but this remains controversial.

M. bovis may be carried and shed in the secretions of the respiratory tract, the genital tract, and the mammary gland. Infection of the respiratory tract probably occurs by direct contact with nasal secretions, or perhaps by inhalation of infected droplets. Contact with genital secretions or ingestion of infected milk may cause infection in neonatal calves. Infection may remain confined to the respiratory tract, or extend from the lung to cause bacteremia with subsequent infection of joints and other tissues.

M. bovis is seemingly well equipped to evade the immune response. The bacterium induces apoptosis of bovine lymphocytes, suppresses the proliferative response of lymphocytes to mitogens, and impairs neutrophil activation. The bacterial surface is decorated with a family of highly immunogenic variable-surface lipoproteins, encoded by at least 13 *vsp* genes containing multiple repeat sequences, which undergo high-frequency phase variation (turning expression on and off) and

size variation. *M. bovis* seems to alter surface lipoprotein expression in response to binding of specific antibody, suggesting that rapid changes in surface antigen expression is a mechanism of evading the humoral immune response. In support of this hypothesis, although antibody titers develop 2-3 weeks after experimental infections, the cellular and humoral immune responses are not protective.

Assessing the antimicrobial susceptibility patterns of *Mycoplasma* spp. is problematic, but several reports indicate that many isolates of *M. bovis* are resistant to antimicrobials commonly used in feedlot medicine, including β-lactam antibiotics, florfenicol, tilmicosin, oxytetracycline, and spectinomycin. The pathogenetic implications of this antimicrobial resistance are uncertain. However, one theory suggests that *M. bovis* may be one of several pathogens infecting calves as they enter the feedlot, but the ability of this bacterium to resist antimicrobials and evade the immune response leads to chronic disease that fails to respond to therapy.

Many calves with lesions of *M. bovis* pneumonia are also infected with *Mannheimia haemolytica*, and there is epidemiologic and morphologic evidence that the lesions of *M. bovis* may evolve out of those of *M. haemolytica*. Most cases have concurrent infection with *Mycoplasma arginini*, suggesting possible synergy. The role of *M. bovis* in predisposing to bacterial pneumonia is uncertain, as *M. bovis* is reportedly less effective than *Mycoplasma dispar* at impairing ciliary function.

The **gross appearance** of *M. bovis* pneumonia may be indistinguishable from suppurative bronchopneumonia of other causes. There is cranioventral reddening and consolidation, scant fibrin may cover pleural surfaces, and bronchial lymph nodes are enlarged and diffusely white. However, *the characteristic lesion is of caseonecrotic bronchopneumonia, in which the consolidated cranioventral lung contains raised, white, sharply demarcated, friable foci of caseous necrosis* (Fig. 5-59). These foci of necrosis are often 2-10 mm in diameter, but occasionally enlarge to many-centimeters diameter. The largest lesions may contain fluid pus rather than caseous exudate, presumably caused by secondary or concurrent bacterial infection. These foci of necrosis form sequestra in some cases (eFig. 5-86). Uncommonly, foci of necrosis and inflammation may be present in bronchial lymph nodes, and similar nodular masses are rarely encountered in the tracheal submucosa, along the dorsal tracheal ligament, or in other tissues.

Joint lesions are present in ~50% of calves with *M. bovis* pneumonia, and the lesions may vary considerably within the same animal. *Pneumonia is found in nearly all calves with M. bovis arthritis.* Acute lesions consist of serofibrinous exudate within joint cavities and tendon sheaths, and the synovium is reddened and hyperplastic. Cartilage erosion is reported in experimental cases but is often absent in clinical material. Purulent or fibrinopurulent exudate is often florid in more established lesions. Foci of caseous necrosis, similar to those described in the lung, may be present in the synovium or joint capsule. Other joints have minimal lesions in the articular cavity, but extensive edema and foci of caseous necrosis in the tendon sheaths or the periarticular soft tissues.

Other manifestations of *M. bovis* infection include fibrinous, purulent, or caseating *otitis media* in young calves, which may be associated with feeding of mastitic milk; *decubital abscesses*; and a proposed association with *necrotizing myocarditis* of the papillary muscle that resembles *Histophilus somni* myocarditis.

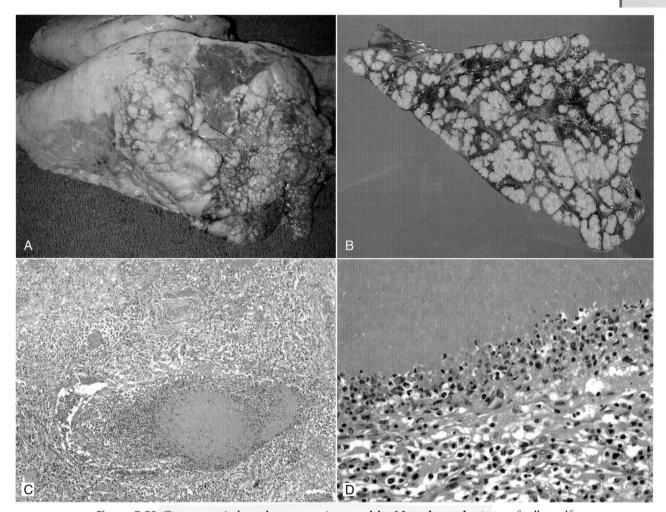

Figure 5-59 Caseonecrotic bronchopneumonia caused by *Mycoplasma bovis* in a feedlot calf. **A.** Cranioventral consolidation containing pale raised nodules. **B.** On cut section, the nodules are pale, round, dry, and friable. **C.** A focus of caseous necrosis arising in a bronchiole, with remnants of bronchiolar epithelium remaining at the right. **D.** The caseonecrotic lesion has an eosinophilic core with ghostlike remnants of leukocytes (top), a thin layer of viable macrophages and a few neutrophils, and a periphery of fibrous tissue with mononuclear cells.

The **histologic lesions** of suppurative bronchopneumonia are nonspecific, but the characteristic appearance of the foci of caseous necrosis suggests a diagnosis of *M. bovis*. The lesions originate in small bronchioles, alveoli, and alveolar septa. The mildest, and probably earliest, lesion consists of suppurative exudate within small bronchioles, in which leukocytes have a characteristic appearance. They are necrotic but retain their cellular outlines, and have hypereosinophilic cytoplasm and inapparent or fragmented nuclei (see Fig. 5-59). As the lesion progresses, there is erosion of bronchiolar epithelium, with expansion of the necrotic foci to incorporate peribronchiolar alveoli. Macrophages and lymphocytes infiltrate the margins, infrequent giant cells may be present, and immature fibrous tissue develops at the outermost edge of the lesion. Large lesions may contain coagulative necrosis in their centers, with retention of the alveolar and bronchiolar architecture of the dead parenchyma. Mineralization of the necrotic tissue is frequent. Lesions affecting bronchi may progress to bronchiectasis.

Using immunohistochemistry, mycoplasmal antigen is most abundant at the periphery of the foci of necrosis and within the bronchiolar exudate. Lesser amounts of antigen are present at the apical surfaces of bronchiolar and bronchial epithelial cells, and within alveolar macrophages and neutrophils. Foci of necrosis or lymphoplasmacytic inflammation may be present in the liver, kidney, or other viscera.

The gross and histologic appearance of caseonecrotic bronchopneumonia is distinctive. The foci of necrosis caused by *M. haemolytica* or *H. somni* are irregular in shape, nonfriable, delineated by a white rim (see Fig. 5-56B), retain the histologically visible tissue architecture (coagulative necrosis), and contain streaming necrotic leukocytes. In contrast, the lesions of *M. bovis* are usually circular and white throughout, and appear histologically as an eosinophilic coagulum exhibiting the ghostlike outlines of necrotic leukocytes (see Fig. 5-59B). Larger foci with fluid pus rather than crumbly content may be appropriately termed abscesses if a fibrous capsule can be demonstrated, and *M. bovis* may be isolated along with other bacterial pathogens such as *Trueperella pyogenes*. Sequestra caused by *M. bovis* are indistinguishable from those caused by *M. haemolytica* or *H. somni*, unless typical foci of caseous necrosis are detected in the adjacent consolidated lung tissue.

Various techniques are available to confirm the tentative **diagnosis** of *Mycoplasma bovis*. It grows readily on *Mycoplasma* enrichment media, and is occasionally isolated on blood agar. However, many calves without apparent pneumonia are infected with *M. bovis*. Thus *the diagnosis rests on identifying both infection with this agent and the presence of the characteristic lesions;* immunohistochemistry is advantageous for correlating the location of mycoplasmal antigen with the characteristic lesions. Seroconversion occurs in many healthy calves in the first month after entering feedlots, making this assay of no value for diagnosis of disease.

Mycoplasma bovis causes particularly severe disease in farmed **bison,** with high morbidity and mortality. The lesions are of caseonecrotic bronchopneumonia, which may be unilateral, pleuropneumonia, polyarthritis, necrotic pharyngitis, endometritis and placentitis with vasculitis, or disseminated abscesses in multiple viscera and lymphoid tissues.

Further reading

Arcangioli MA, et al. The role of *Mycoplasma bovis* in bovine respiratory disease outbreaks in veal calf feedlots. Vet J 2008;177:89-93.

Castillo-Alcala F, et al. Prevalence and genotype of *Mycoplasma bovis* in beef cattle after arrival at a feedlot. Am J Vet Res 2012;73:1932-1943.

Hermeyer K, et al. Chronic pneumonia in calves after experimental infection with *Mycoplasma bovis* strain 1067: characterization of lung pathology, persistence of variable surface protein antigens and local immune response. Acta Vet Scand 2012;54:9.

Register KB, et al. Systemic mycoplasmosis with dystocia and abortion in a North American bison *(Bison bison)* herd. J Vet Diagn Invest 2013;25:541-545.

Miscellaneous *Mycoplasma* spp. of calves. *Mycoplasma* spp. are regularly isolated from the lungs of calves with pneumonia, but their importance in disease is often difficult to interpret. Only *M. bovis* is likely to cause severe primary disease. Infection with *M. dispar, Ureaplasma diversum,* and perhaps *M. bovirhinis* and *M. alkalescens* causes bronchiolitis and may contribute to development of acute or chronic enzootic pneumonia in young calves by predisposing to bacterial pneumonia. Experimental infections with *M. bovigenitalium, M. arginini,* and *M. canis* induce mild lesions and no clinical signs.

Mycoplasma spp. attach to ciliated epithelial cells, on and between microvilli and covering the base of the cilia. *The typical lesion is chronic catarrhal bronchitis and bronchiolitis with prominent lymphocytic cuffs around airways.* Affected lungs contain patchy, cranioventral, purple-red foci of atelectasis. When secondarily infected by opportunistic bacterial pathogens, more confluent, meaty consolidation may also occur. Microscopically, accumulations of neutrophils and mucus are present in airway lumens, and there is increased prominence of goblet cells. Moderate infiltrates of lymphocytes and fewer plasma cells encircle the airways and accompanying blood vessels. Inflammation of alveoli adjacent to terminal bronchioles occurs in experimental infections in colostrum-deprived, specific–pathogen-free calves and can probably occur in heavy natural infection. Alveolar lesions are not specific, and include atelectasis, accumulation of neutrophils and alveolar macrophages with occasional lymphocytes and plasma cells, and mild hypercellularity of alveolar septa. As the infection becomes chronic, lymphocytic peribronchiolar cuffs thicken, develop germinal centers, and extend to the lamina propria of the bronchiole. At this stage, the epithelium may be hyperplastic with goblet cell hyperplasia and hypertrophy of bronchial glands.

Further reading

Ayling RD, et al. *Mycoplasma* species and related organisms isolated from ruminants in Britain between 1990 and 2000. Vet Rec 2004;155:413-416.

Kokotovic B, et al. *Mycoplasma alkalescens* demonstrated in bronchoalveolar lavage of cattle in Denmark. Acta Vet Scand 2007;49:2.

Fungal diseases

Mortierellosis. *Acute fatal mycotic pneumonia* is a sequel to placental infection with *Mortierella wolfii, the most important cause of mycotic abortion of cattle in New Zealand.* This condition has rarely been reported elsewhere. Acute fibrinonecrotic pneumonia occurs in infected cows within a few days of abortion or parturition, resulting from extensive hematogenous dissemination of fungi when the placenta detaches. In the acute disease, the lung is diffusely firm, edematous, and red-yellow. Histologic lesions include serofibrinous and suppurative exudate in alveoli, with vascular necrosis, thrombosis, and coagulative ischemic necrosis of lung parenchyma. In the subacute and chronic disease, there is an embolic pattern of multifocal fibrinous and suppurative inflammation. Similar lesions may occur in the spleen. Fungal hyphae are present within the lesions, but may be inconspicuous in chronic lesions. The hyphae are periodic acid–Schiff positive, nonseptate, branching, and are 2-12 μm in diameter.

Other fungi such as *Aspergillus, Mucor,* and *Rhizopus* are occasional opportunistic invaders of lung, and cause nodules of caseous necrosis or granulomatous inflammation.

Further reading

Gabor LJ. Mycotic pneumonia in a dairy cow caused by *Mortierella wolfii.* Aust Vet J 2003;81:409-410.

Parasitic diseases

Dictyocaulus viviparus. *Dictyocaulus viviparus* is a common and important cause of respiratory disease in cool, wet, seasonal climates. **Primary infections,** sometimes known as "husk" or "hoose," cause disease in calves during their first grazing season, and occasionally affect mature animals that have not had sufficient exposure to develop immunity. Although clinical disease may develop within 3 weeks of access to infected pastures, it is most common late in the grazing season when calves have been at pasture for 3-5 months. Affected herds usually have high disease prevalence, and mortality rates are variable, depending on the degree of pasture contamination. A second manifestation, **reinfection syndrome,** occurs when partially immune adult cattle on endemically infected farms have access to pastures that are contaminated with large numbers of infective larvae. In these herds, there is a high prevalence of coughing, tachypnea, and depression about 2 weeks after exposure. Some animals develop fatal dyspnea without coughing.

D. viviparus, the only adult nematode known to infect the lung of cattle, is a member of the superfamily

Trichostrongyloidea, family *Dictyocaulidae. Adult lungworms inhabit the large bronchi.* The eggs are embryonated when laid, and hatch rapidly. First-stage larvae are expelled from the lung by coughing, are swallowed, and then passed in the feces. Further development to infective third-stage larvae occurs on the ground over the next 5-7 days. Larval development is optimal in moist cool conditions; the larvae can develop at temperatures as low as 5° C, and their viability is prolonged at these temperatures. The third-stage larvae are ingested by cattle, penetrate the wall of the intestine, and migrate via the lymphatics to the mesenteric lymph nodes. In the lymph nodes, they molt to form fourth-stage larvae, and then go by way of lymph and blood to enter the lungs about 7 days after infection. Some larvae accidentally take the portal route and are destroyed in the liver, or rarely enter the systemic circulation to cause intrauterine infections in the fetus. The final molt to the fifth-stage larvae occurs in the bronchioles, and adults develop in the larger airways. Eggs are first detectable in feces at 21-30 days after infection; the infection is usually patent for another 1-3 months. However, a few egg-laying adults may persist in some animals over the winter months, and serve as a source of pasture contamination in the following grazing season.

The clinical and pathologic manifestations of *Dictyocaulus* infestation are dependent on the stage of infection, the level of immunity of the host, and the number of invading larvae. *The following description pertains to primary infections of naive animals;* reinfection of partially immune cattle is discussed subsequently. *Lesions differ in the prepatent period, the patent period, and the period of recovery.* During the **prepatent period,** from 7-25 days after infection, the principal lesions are eosinophilic bronchiolitis and/or alveolitis with fibrin or hyaline membranes, in response to the presence of larvae in the alveoli and bronchioles. Clinical signs include coughing and tachypnea, and calves infected with many larvae may die at this stage. Where the larvae emerge from pulmonary capillaries, they cause microscopic foci of necrosis and fibrin exudation, with an alveolar infiltrate of eosinophils and fewer neutrophils, macrophages, and giant cells. Mononuclear cells thicken the alveolar walls, and hyaline membranes or hyperplasia of type II pneumocytes may occur. The larvae, some of them dead, can be found in the alveoli. When the number of larvae is large, the foci of acute interstitial pneumonia may be visible grossly as lobular or smaller foci that are slightly depressed, purple, and widely distributed throughout the lungs.

By about day 10, many of the larvae have reached the terminal bronchioles. Frothy fluid is present in the bronchi and, in very heavy infestations, there is edema, atelectasis, and/or emphysema. Eosinophils invade the septal tissues in large numbers and pursue the larvae into the bronchioles. Most of the bronchioles contain plugs of exudate composed largely of eosinophils. Neutrophils, lymphocytes, and macrophages are present in smaller numbers in both the lumens and walls of the bronchioles. The early bronchiolar epithelial response is of necrosis, sloughing and flattening of remaining cells, but subsequently hyperplasia and metaplasia occur. At this stage, adult worms are not present in the airways, but larvae are detectable histologically or in a smear of exudate harvested from the smallest airways.

During the **patent period,** beginning 25 days after infection, the inflammatory response targets adult worms in the bronchi, and eggs and recently hatched first-stage larvae that have been aspirated into the alveoli. At this stage, calves may exhibit chronic coughing, increased respiratory rate, and weight loss, or develop severe dyspnea and death. Adult worms, which are slender, white, and up to 8 cm long, are most numerous in the caudodorsal bronchi of the caudal lobes (Fig. 5-60). Infections may be missed if only the trachea and large cranial bronchi are examined, as *many infestations are restricted to the small branches of the caudal bronchi.* Patchy lobular atelectasis may be the only other gross finding in mild infestations. In more severe cases, there are wedge-shaped, red-gray, firm, depressed areas of consolidation at the caudal border of the caudal lung. Examination of a cut section may reveal similar areas of consolidation in much of the pulmonary tissue surrounding larger bronchi.

Histologic lesions in patent infections include eosinophilic catarrhal bronchitis and bronchiolitis, and eosinophilic granulomatous alveolitis (see Fig. 5-60). The bronchi and large bronchioles contain adult worms, eggs, and larvae mixed with mucus and numerous eosinophils. In histologic sections, adult worms have thick intestinal epithelium composed of a few multinucleated cells with indistinct microvilli, prominent lateral chords, and coelomyarian-polymyarian musculature, and the uterus may contain larvae or embryonated eggs. The airway mucosa contains infiltrates of eosinophils and mononuclear cells, the epithelium is necrotic or hyperplastic and contains increased numbers of goblet cells, and the peribronchial lymphoid tissue is expanded (eFig. 5-87). The accompanying alveolar lesions consist of atelectasis secondary to the obstructive bronchiolitis, and macrophages, giant cells, and lymphocytes encircling fragments of cuticle, aspirated eggs, or newly hatched larvae. It is complicated in some cases by bacterial bronchopneumonia. Alveolar septa are thickened by cellular infiltration, slight fibroplasia, and inconsistent proliferation of type II pneumocytes. At this stage, the infection may be diagnosed by gross observation of adult worms in the bronchi, examination of histologic sections of bronchi and alveoli, identification of all stages in wet mounts of airway mucus, identifying larvae in feces by the Baermann technique, and/or detection of antibodies in serum or milk by ELISA.

During the **period of recovery,** *adult worms are eliminated.* However, gross lesions of consolidation may persist, and there is bronchiolitis obliterans, lymphocytic cuffs around bronchi, hyperplasia of type II pneumocytes, and fibrosis of peribronchiolar alveoli. Establishing a firm diagnosis at this stage may be impossible, as adults are not present and the feces no longer contain larvae. The distribution of lesions in the caudal lung helps to differentiate chronic parasitism from mycoplasmosis, which usually affects the cranioventral areas of lung. Acutely fatal exacerbations of the disease during the period of recovery, when larvae and adults are no longer present, have been described. These cases may be impossible to differentiate from toxic interstitial lung disease, but acute exacerbation of a chronic illness is not typical of pulmonary toxicity.

Emphysema may be a prominent gross lesion in severe cases of *Dictyocaulus* infection, and is probably a consequence of forced expiration, caused by severe dyspnea, in the presence of bronchiolar obstruction by exudate and bronchoconstriction. Cases in which emphysema is the major lesion may be mistaken for acute interstitial lung disease of toxic cause. This is particularly likely when the pulmonary damage is caused by massive invasion of larvae, and mature worms are not yet present for gross detection. Microscopic detection of larvae and immature worms usually provides the diagnosis.

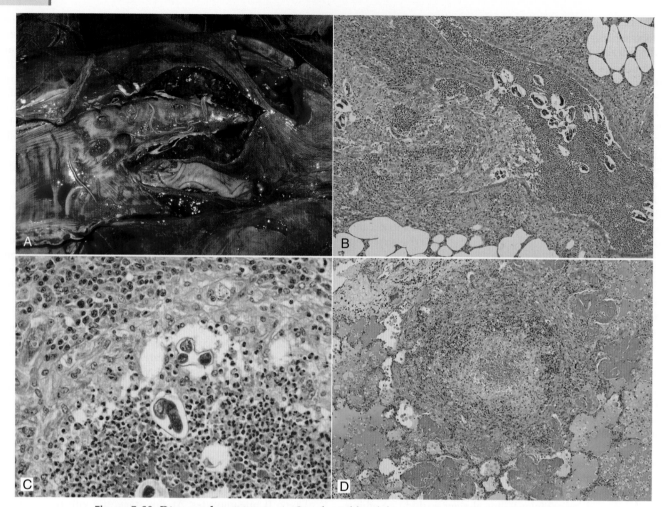

Figure 5-60 *Dictyocaulus viviparus.* **A.** Grossly visible adult nematodes in the caudal bronchi of an elk, accompanied by mild frothy exudate. (Courtesy D.G. Campbell, Canadian Wildlife Health Cooperative.) **B.** In a cow, effacement of a bronchus with attenuation of remaining epithelium (arrows), fibrosis, an intense infiltrate of eosinophils and mononuclear cells, and numerous nematode larvae and ova. **C.** Detail of embryonated ova and associated granulomatous inflammation in a bronchiole. **D.** Granuloma formation in the lung parenchyma in response to aspirated ova and larvae.

The typical lesions in the **reinfection syndrome,** in which partially immune adult cattle are infected with numerous larvae, are scattered, 2-4 mm diameter, gray nodules that often contain a green caseous center. The nodules represent dense accumulations of lymphocytes and plasma cells, encircling an eosinophilic and granulomatous response to a degenerating larva. As a result of this robust immunoinflammatory response, the larvae do not reach the large airways or develop into adults, and the infection does not usually achieve patency.

Further reading

Mangiola S, et al. Analysis of the transcriptome of adult *Dictyocaulus filaria* and comparison with *Dictyocaulus viviparus*, with a focus on molecules involved in host-parasite interactions. Int J Parasitol 2014;44:251-261.

Panciera RJ, Confer AW. Pathogenesis and pathology of bovine pneumonia. Vet Clin North Am Food Anim Pract 2010;26:191-214.

Miscellaneous parasites. *Ascaris suum* larvae occasionally cause severe interstitial lung disease in calves housed where

pigs were previously kept. In these situations, infective eggs are ingested, larvae hatch within 18 hours, and migrate to the lungs 5-13 days after infection. The lesions are of *severe acute interstitial lung disease*, in which the lungs are diffusely rubbery, wet, and heavy, and interlobular septa are distended with clear fluid. Migration of larvae through the liver may cause white streaks. Histologically, there is alveolar edema and hyaline membranes or type II pneumocyte proliferation, and numerous eosinophils infiltrate alveolar septa and exude into the alveoli (Fig. 5-61). Larvae are readily identified in cases that die about a week after infection, but a diligent search may be required in calves that survive for 2-3 weeks after infection. Larvae cannot be consistently recovered from lung digests. The histologic appearance of the larvae is characteristic: They have lateral alae, large lateral chords, and an intestine (the only internal organ present) composed of few uninucleate cells.

The trematodes *Fasciola gigantica* and *F. hepatica* occasionally invade the lungs accidentally from the liver. Because they are large parasites that wander extensively, a small number in the lungs can produce extensive cavitations. *Schistosoma nasalis* causes nasal granulomas in India. In cattle,

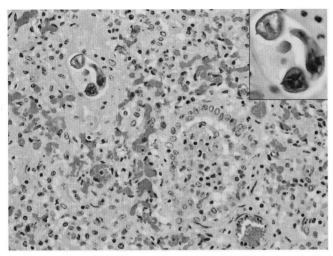

Figure 5-61 *Ascaris suum* **larval migration** in a dairy calf housed in a shed formerly used for pigs. Alveoli and bronchioles contain fibrin and eosinophils, and there are a few nematode larvae with characteristic lateral alae. Inset: higher magnification of the larva.

lung is less common than liver as a site of hydatid cysts caused by *Echinococcus granulosus.*

The leeches *Limnatis nilotica* and *L. africana* are taken in while drinking and attach to the mucosa of the pharynx and nasopharynx. They suck large quantities of blood, and their presence induces localized edema that leads to dyspnea or asphyxiation. The nematodes *Mammomonogamus (Syngamus) nasicola* and *M. ierei* are found in the nasal passages of ruminants in tropical countries, and *M. laryngeus* causes lymphocytic polypoid hyperplasia in the pharynx and larynx of cattle in tropical Asia and South America.

Further reading

Marques SMT, et al. *Mammomonogamus laryngeus* (Railliet, 1899) infection in buffaloes in Rio Grande do Sul, Brazil. Vet Parasitol 2005;130:241-243.

Infectious respiratory diseases of sheep and goats

Viral diseases

Ovine respiratory syncytial and parainfluenza viruses. Many aspects of the pathogenesis, lesions, and role of these viruses in predisposing to bacterial pneumonia are similar to those described for the bovine viruses. Ruminant respiratory syncytial viruses have been divided into bovine and ovine subgroups based on nucleotide and antigenic differences in the G protein. Sheep are susceptible to infection and disease with both ovine and bovine subgroups, and ovine strains infect cattle and deer.

Further reading

Sow FB, et al. Respiratory syncytial virus infection is associated with an altered innate immunity and a heightened pro-inflammatory response in the lungs of preterm lambs. Respir Res 2011;12:106.

Adenovirus. Adenoviral infections are common in sheep, but primary adenoviral pneumonia is rare. Ovine adenovirus (OAdV) serotype 6 exacerbates disease caused by experimen-

tally inoculated *Mannheimia haemolytica*, and adenoviruses are occasionally isolated from outbreaks of bacterial pneumonia in lambs. These findings suggest that adenoviral infection may predispose to development of bacterial pneumonia in some groups of lambs. Lesions in experimentally infected lambs are similar to those described for calves. A noteworthy feature of the lesions caused by at least one strain of OAdV is the enlargement of both nucleus and cytoplasm of inclusion-bearing bronchiolar and alveolar epithelial cells, which could be mistaken for cytomegalovirus infection. Adenoviruses have been isolated from goats, but their role in causing disease appears minor.

Further reading

Cutlip RC, et al. Lesions in lambs experimentally infected with ovine adenovirus serotype 6 and *Pasteurella haemolytica*. J Vet Diagn Invest 1996;8:296-303.

Peste des petits ruminants. Peste-des-petits-ruminants virus (PPRV) (see Vol. 2, Alimentary system and peritoneum) is closely related to rinderpest virus in the genus *Morbillivirus*. Sheep and goats with PPR ("ovine rinderpest") commonly have clinical signs and lesions affecting the respiratory system, in addition to enteric lesions that resemble those of rinderpest. The gross lesions usually affect the cranioventral lobes of the lung, which are firm, reddened, and may have fibrinous exudate on the pleural surface. Nasal and tracheal erosions with a fibrinonecrotic membrane may be present. Histologic lesions are of *bronchointerstitial pneumonia*, and resemble the lesions of canine distemper, another morbillivirus. There is necrosis and attenuation of epithelial cells lining the trachea, bronchi, and bronchioles; proliferation of type II pneumocytes; and formation of epithelial syncytia in the alveoli. Infected epithelial cells often contain eosinophilic inclusion bodies in the cytoplasm or the nucleus. As the virus is difficult to isolate in culture, definitive diagnosis depends on immunohistochemistry, PCR, or serology.

Further reading

Kul O, et al. Natural peste des petits ruminants virus infection: novel pathologic findings resembling other morbillivirus infections. Vet Pathol 2007;44:479-486.

Kumar N, et al. Peste des petits ruminants virus infection of small ruminants: a comprehensive review. Viruses 2014;6:2287-2327.

Sheep pox and goat pox. Sheep and goat pox (see Vol. 1, Integumentary system), OIE (World Organization for Animal Health) listed diseases, cause disseminated white nodules in the lung in addition to the cutaneous lesions. Histologically, these appear as hyperplasia of virus-containing type II pneumocytes and bronchiolar epithelial cells, variable numbers of neutrophils and lymphocytes, flocculent eosinophilic extracellular material, and foci of caseous necrosis. "Sheep pox cells" in these lesions are enlarged angular or stellate cells with vacuolated nuclei and intracytoplasmic inclusion bodies.

Further reading

Beytut E. Sheep pox virus induces proliferation of type II pneumocytes in the lungs. J Comp Pathol 2010;143:132-141.

Small ruminant lentiviruses: maedi (ovine progressive pneumonia) and caprine arthritis-encephalitis. Small ruminant lentiviral infections are common in sheep and goats worldwide, with the exceptions of Iceland, where the disease was eradicated in 1965, and Australia and New Zealand, where ovine lentiviral disease has not been recorded. The seroprevalence varies greatly, for example, from 1-70% in various areas of the United States. Most infected animals are not clinically ill, and infection may become widespread before diseased animals are noticed. *Lentiviruses cause slowly progressive pneumonia, encephalomyelitis, arthritis, and mastitis; the various syndromes may occur independently or concurrently.*

The descriptive terminology of the ovine disease is a colorful consequence of the history of the disease. The respiratory form in sheep, which is termed **maedi** ("dyspnea" in Icelandic) in much of the world and **ovine progressive pneumonia** in the United States, is the most common presentation, and manifests as inexorably progressive dyspnea, hyperpnea, and weight loss in sheep >3 years of age. Other outcomes in sheep are less frequent and include encephalitis, arthritis, and mastitis. Encephalitis—**visna** ("fading away" in Icelandic)—was common in the original Icelandic description but is now less common, and results in ataxia, weakness, tremors, hypermetria, and profound weight loss. Mastitis and arthritis are uncommon in sheep, and manifest as agalactia and a hard udder, or lameness and swollen joints (particularly carpal joints), respectively.

Goats with caprine arthritis-encephalitis (CAE) develop one or more of arthritis, encephalitis, and pneumonia. *Arthritis affects adult goats,* resulting in acute or chronic lameness and swelling of carpal or tarsal joints. *Neurologic disease,* occurring in 2- to 4-month-old kids, or less commonly in older animals, is characterized by progressive ataxia and weakness beginning in the hindlimbs. *Pneumonia* may occasionally be the major presenting complaint in kids or adults, or occur concurrently with arthritis or neurologic disease.

Maedi-visna and CAE are caused by closely related lentiviruses in the family *Retroviridae,* genus *Lentivirus.* The extreme genetic diversity created by replicative infidelity of the lentiviruses has blurred the concept of distinct viral species: Some strains infect only sheep or only goats, whereas others are capable of cross-species infection, so the term *small ruminant lentiviruses* is generally more appropriate than maedi-visna virus or caprine arthritis-encephalitis virus (CAEV). These viruses are enveloped, 100-nm diameter, and contain a dense nucleoid and a positive-sense single-stranded RNA genome. Viral genes include *gag,* which encodes group-specific nucleocapsid and matrix glycoproteins that are detected by antibody-based diagnostic tests; *pol,* which encodes reverse transcriptase and other enzymes; *env,* encoding the surface glycoprotein that mediates receptor binding and virus entry into cells, and is the target for neutralizing antibody; and the regulatory proteins encoded by *vif, rev,* and *vpr-like.* Long terminal repeats that flank the encoding regions of the genome bind transcription factors and are necessary for replication.

Lentiviral diseases in sheep and goats are marked by their variability. Viral strains or quasispecies may differ in their rapidity of replication, cytopathic effects, tropism for particular cell types, and their propensity to cause pulmonary, nervous, joint, or mammary disease. Disease manifestation is also influenced by host genetics, as certain breeds of sheep

are more susceptible than others. Finally, the local tissue microenvironment affects viral replication and development of disease; for example, proinflammatory cytokines generated in response to concurrent infection with other pathogens augment lentiviral replication and hasten disease onset.

Transmission of small ruminant lentiviruses through colostrum or milk is the major method of disease spread. Inhalation of nasal secretions following prolonged close contact, as occurs in confined animals in the winter months, is a recognized mode of horizontal transmission. In utero transmission occurs infrequently in sheep. The virus is shed in semen, but infection by coitus or artificial insemination has not been documented. Mucosal dendritic cells are thought to deliver virus to lymph nodes, where the mannose receptor is the likely route of entry into macrophages. Ovine lentivirus infects a variety of cell types, including choroid plexus and mammary epithelium, fibroblasts, endothelial cells, and monocytes. However, viral replication is restricted in these cells, and complete viral replication and assembly occur in mature macrophages. Viral antigen is widespread, having been detected in lung, bone marrow, mammary gland, lymph node, spleen, synovium, brain, and spinal cord of sheep with maedi, and is most abundant in areas of lymphocytic inflammation. Similarly, viral nucleic acid is demonstrable in lung, liver, spleen, lymph nodes, brain, synovium, intestine, kidney, and thyroid gland of goats with CAE. Infected alveolar macrophages produce cytokines that recruit and activate leukocytes in the area of infection, and may also incite fibrosis and smooth muscle metaplasia. Cytokine-dependent activation of macrophages stimulates lentiviral replication, which may in turn stimulate additional leukocyte recruitment. Altered organ function is a result of the immunoinflammatory response, rather than a direct effect of the lentiviral infection.

In contrast to primate and feline lentiviruses, *immunosuppression is not a feature of small ruminant lentiviral infection. Infection and shedding of the virus persist for life,* but the disease in sheep develops slowly, and the incubation period usually exceeds 2 years. The mechanisms of persistent lentiviral infection are not clear, but may include proviral integration, lack of avidity of neutralizing antibody, or decoy viral antigens that are immunodominant but non-neutralizing. Integration of provirus into the host genome is necessary for viral replication, occurs increasingly as the disease progresses, and may facilitate persistence of the virus. The development of serum neutralizing antibody responses during persistent infection is perplexing; the higher affinity of virus for macrophage receptors than for antibody has been suggested as a reason for failure of these antibodies to prevent cell-to-cell spread of infection in vivo.

The lungs of **sheep** with maedi are remarkably heavy, pale gray or tan, and fail to collapse when the chest is opened (Fig. 5-62). The lesions are generalized but most obvious in the caudal lobes, and vary from a diffusely firm or rubbery texture, to multiple coalescing gray and firm foci. Mediastinal and bronchial lymph nodes are enlarged, white, and edematous. Lesions of cranioventral bronchopneumonia caused by *Pasteurella multocida* or *Trueperella pyogenes* are commonly superimposed on the lesions of maedi. Lungworms, *Dictyocaulus* or *Protostrongylus,* are common in sheep with maedi, and an association between maedi and retroviral pulmonary adenomatosis has been described.

The histologic pulmonary lesions are of interstitial pneumonia (eFig. 5-88; see Fig. 5-62). Infiltrates of lymphocytes, plasma

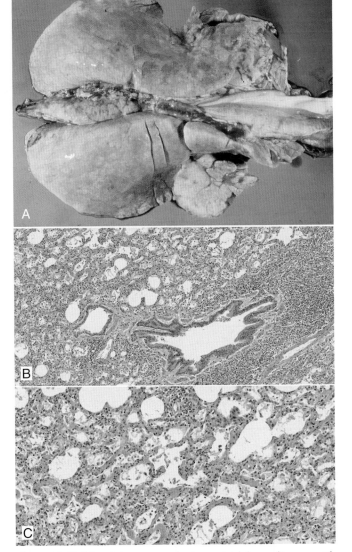

Figure 5-62 Maedi in a ewe. A. Interstitial lung disease with diffuse pallor, failure to collapse, and firm-rubbery texture. (Courtesy University of Guelph.) **B.** Low magnification reveals a dense cuff of lymphocytes around a bronchiole. **C.** At higher magnification, alveolar septa are thickened by metaplasia of smooth muscle, scant fibrosis, prominent infiltration of lymphocytes in the interstitium, and increased numbers of hypertrophied alveolar macrophages.

cells, and macrophages thicken alveolar septa and form cuffs around blood vessels and airways. The tendency for these cellular infiltrates to form *lymphoid nodules with germinal centers* is a characteristic feature of maedi. In addition to the cellular infiltrate, alveolar septa are thickened by *hypertrophy of smooth muscle* and by *mild interstitial fibrosis*. Hyperplasia of type II pneumocytes is not prominent, in contrast to pulmonary adenomatosis and CAE viral pneumonia. Mild hyperplasia of bronchiolar epithelium is occasionally present.

Brain and spinal cord lesions of sheep with maedi-visna are mainly periventricular in the brain and affect white matter of spinal cord, and may be perivascular or infiltrative. The lesions consist of lymphocytic and/or histiocytic leukoencephalomyelitis, gliosis, demyelination leading to malacia, and meningitis,

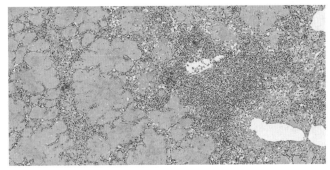

Figure 5-63 Pneumonia caused by caprine arthritis encephalitis virus in a goat kid. Dense infiltrates of lymphocytes are present diffusely and aggregate around blood vessels. Densely eosinophilic fluid fills alveoli in affected areas, and there is hyperplasia of type II pneumocytes.

with mononuclear infiltrates forming lymphoid follicles in choroid plexus. *Mastitis* is an uncommon clinical presentation of maedi-visna, but is a frequent subclinical lesion. There is diffuse firmness and pallor of the mammary gland, and histologic lesions include follicular aggregates of lymphocytes, plasma cells, and macrophages in the mammary interstitium. Mesangial or proliferative glomerulonephritis is an uncommon lesion in lentivirus-infected sheep.

In **goats**, the *lung lesions* of CAEV are distinctive. The gross appearance is of diffuse or multifocal pale firm lesions throughout the lung. Histologically, these foci are abruptly demarcated from relatively unaffected areas of lung. In the lesional areas, alveoli are filled with densely eosinophilic fluid containing foamy macrophages and lined by a continuous or patchy layer of cuboidal type II pneumocytes, and alveolar septa are thickened by lymphocytes and fibrosis (Fig. 5-63, eFig. 5-89).

Arthritis caused by CAEV is unilateral or bilateral, and affects the carpal joints or less commonly the tarsal, fetlock, stifle, and atlanto-occipital joints. Histologic lesions include striking villus hyperplasia of the synovium, and synovial infiltrates of lymphocytes, plasma cells, and macrophages. Fibrosis, mineralization, and necrosis of synovium and joint capsule develop in chronically affected animals. The brain and mammary lesions of CAE are similar to those of sheep with maedi.

Serology (agar gel immunodiffusion [AGID] or ELISA) is useful to detect infected flocks but of less value for individual-animal diagnosis. For both serologic and molecular diagnostic tests, false positives can occur in preweaned lambs because of uptake of antibody and provirus from infected colostrum and milk. False-negative serologic tests can result from the delayed development of antibodies after infection, or transient periods of seronegativity. *Quantitative PCR assays* to detect proviral DNA or viral RNA in blood mononuclear cells or lung tissue may be positive earlier in the disease course than serologic assays. PCR assays are considered less sensitive than serology, but may be positive before development of an antibody titer. Depending on the specific PCR assay, genetic variability of the virus can cause false-negative tests. *Immunohistochemistry*, such as for detection of the p27 or gp130 viral proteins, has the advantage of associating the presence of viral antigen with the histologic lesion. Antigen is usually in macrophages within the inflammatory lesions.

Further reading

Blacklaws BA. Small ruminant lentiviruses: immunopathogenesis of visna-maedi and caprine arthritis and encephalitis virus. Comp Immunol Microbiol Infect Dis 2012;35:259-269.

Glaria I, et al. Visna/maedi virus genetic characterization and serological diagnosis of infection in sheep from a neurological outbreak. Vet Microbiol 2012;155:137-146.

Herrmann-Hoesing LM. Diagnostic assays used to control small ruminant lentiviruses. J Vet Diagn Invest 2010;22:843-855.

Polledo L, et al. Patterns of lesion and local host cellular immune response in natural cases of ovine maedi-visna. J Comp Pathol 2012;147:1-10.

Ramírez H, et al. Small ruminant lentiviruses: genetic variability, tropism and diagnosis. Viruses 2013;5:1175-1207.

Enzootic nasal tumor. Viral adenomas and carcinomas of the nasal cavity of sheep and goats are geographically widespread, but absent from Australia and New Zealand. The prevalence is geographically variable, and many flocks have multiple animals affected over long periods of time. Clinical disease typically arises in adults, but lambs as young as 6 months have been affected. Clinical signs are insidious, progressive, and include stertor, inspiratory dyspnea, open-mouth breathing, nasal discharge, nasal deformity, and weight loss.

Enzootic nasal tumor virus (ENTV) includes 2 types, ENTV-1 from sheep and ENTV-2 from goats, which are related to jaagsiekte sheep retrovirus (JSRV). The viral envelope glycoprotein, which is responsible for tumor development (at least in mice), is detectable within neoplastic epithelial cells but not in the adjacent normal tissue. The disease has been transmitted to sheep and goats by using cell-free nasal fluids or tumor filtrates. Incubation periods after experimental infection are as little as 3 months, although those in the natural disease are thought to be 1-3 years. Transmission is thought to be by contact with nasal secretions. However, subclinical infection is common, and most experimentally challenged animals do not develop tumors.

Tumors may be unilateral or bilateral and *usually originate from the ethmoid turbinates*, but fill much of the caudal nasal cavity before severe clinical signs develop (Fig. 5-64). In protracted unilateral cases, the entire nasal cavity is occluded by tumor, there is deviation of the nasal septum, and tumor may

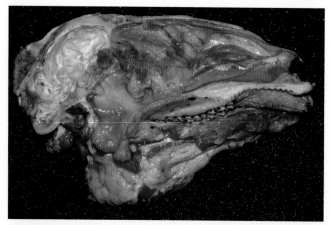

Figure 5-64 Enzootic nasal tumor in a ewe, with a mass arising from the ethmoid conchae, filling the right nasal cavity, and protruding into the nasopharynx.

protrude from the nostril. Most cases are adenomas that expand into sinuses, contralateral nasal cavity, or pharynx; the term adenocarcinoma may be justified in those cases with demonstrable invasion of bone, but metastasis is not reported. The neoplastic tissue is white, firm, and multinodular, or may contain brown-red areas of hemorrhage and necrosis.

The histologic appearance is of adenoma or low-grade adenocarcinoma. The cuboidal or pseudostratified nonciliated epithelial cells form orderly tubular, papillary, or acinar arrangements; squamous differentiation is described but rare. Neoplastic cells have basal round nuclei and a variable mitotic rate. Mucus secretion is occasionally abundant, and the fibrovascular stroma is usually scant. Neoplastic tissue and adjacent non-neoplastic tissues often contain numerous lymphocytes, and glandular hyperplasia or polyps may be present.

The *diagnosis* is usually based on gross and histologic findings. However, morphologic features do not differentiate viral neoplasms from the sporadic (nonviral) nasal tumors that occasionally develop in small ruminants. Immunohistochemistry, PCR, or electron microscopy are useful to detect the virus in tumors. An ELISA may be of value for identifying infected animals in flocks.

Further reading

Santry LA, et al. Genetic characterization of small ruminant lentiviruses circulating in naturally infected sheep and goats in Ontario, Canada. Virus Res 2013;175:30-44.

Walsh SR, et al. Experimental transmission of enzootic nasal adenocarcinoma in sheep. Vet Res 2013;44:66.

Ovine pulmonary adenocarcinoma (jaagsiekte). *Ovine pulmonary adenocarcinoma (OPA), also known as jaagsiekte or ovine pulmonary adenomatosis, is a contagious retroviral pulmonary carcinoma of sheep, and rarely of goats.* The disease is common in South America, South Africa, and Scotland, where 5-20% of infected animals contain pulmonary tumors. OPA occurs regularly in the rest of Europe, Africa, and Asia, but is rare in North America and not reported in Australia. Mortality rates tend to increase gradually for several years following introduction of infection, and subsequently decline gradually. Clinical disease is most common in 2-4 year-old sheep, but 3-month-old lambs have been affected. Clinical signs include progressive dyspnea, tachypnea, exercise intolerance, nasal discharge, coughing, and weight loss; fever and anorexia are unusual unless secondary infections occur. Drainage of lung fluids from the nose following elevation of the hindlimbs is a characteristic clinical sign seen in some sheep.

Jaagsiekte sheep retrovirus (JSRV), the agent of OPA, is a 100-nm diameter, enveloped, betaretrovirus. The following arguments support the role of JSRV as the etiology: JSRV is consistently present in neoplastic cells but minimally in non-neoplastic epithelium or stroma, the disease can be reproduced with cell-free JSRV-containing filtrates of tumor tissue, and the incubation period is dependent on the amount of retroviral reverse transcriptase in the experimental inoculum. However, defining the exact role of JSRV in disease development is complicated by the presence of endogenous retroviral proviral sequences that are common in neoplastic and non-neoplastic tissue of affected and normal sheep.

OPA is thought to be acquired by direct contact of young animals with nasal secretions of infected animals. Most naturally infected animals do not have tumors. In those that do, the typical incubation period has been estimated to be 2 years, but is age and dose dependent; tumors may develop in 10-20 days if high doses are administered experimentally to neonatal lambs. The increased propensity for tumor development in neonatally infected lambs may relate to the greater frequency of proliferating type II pneumocytes during post-natal lung development. In contrast, lung cells from adult sheep or goat kids are restrictive for JRSV replication. Disease is more common in certain breeds of sheep, but the reasons for this familial predisposition are unknown.

The envelope glycoprotein is sufficient to induce similar tumors in immunodeficient mice, and is the likely mechanism of tumor formation in sheep. It is exceptional that a retroviral structural protein should induce neoplasia, but oncogenes have not been identified in JSRV. Weak cellular and humoral immune responses in infected sheep, probably resulting from the continued presence of related endogenous retroviruses, may permit the persistent infection that typifies the disease.

Lungs of sheep with OPA contain multifocal or locally extensive lesions that are firm, gray, and exude fluid from the cut section (Fig. 5-65, eFig. 5-90). Affected lungs are heavy, up to 3 times their normal weight, and airways are filled with foamy secretion from the neoplastic cells. The tumors are expansile, and metastases to regional lymph nodes are present in about 10% of cases. Metastases to other tissues are reported but rare. Maedi and/or bacterial pneumonia are often present in sheep with OPA, and the diffuse lymphocytic interstitial pneumonia or cranioventral suppurative bronchopneumonia induced by these diseases may complicate the gross and histologic appearance of the tumors.

The histologic appearance is of a well-differentiated pulmonary carcinoma (see Figs. 5-25A, 5-65; see also eFig. 5-35). The neoplastic masses usually have a lepidic pattern in which alveoli are lined by cuboidal or columnar neoplastic epithelial cells. Other tumors have papillary or acinar patterns, a myxomatous variant is described, and polypoid lesions arising from bronchioles may be seen. The neoplastic cells variably express immunohistochemical markers of type II pneumocytes and bronchiolar club cells, suggesting an origin from multipotent lung epithelial progenitor cells. Alveoli adjacent to the tumors are atelectatic and contain many macrophages, and interstitial fibrosis may be present in advanced cases.

In the most frequent or classic form, tumors are poorly demarcated and extend into adjacent alveoli or form locally extensive lesions within affected lobes. An atypical form of the disease is subclinical and probably nonprogressive, and the tumors are isolated or well demarcated, dry, and firmer than the classic form, and surrounded by a more prominent infiltrate of lymphocytes and plasma cells. It is suggested that the classic progressive form reflects abundant JSRV replication in proliferating alveolar epithelial cells, promoting infection of the surrounding lung tissue, with ensuing expansion of the tumors. In contrast, the atypical form may reflect infection of lungs that have less alveolar epithelial cell proliferation, with well-demarcated nonprogressive tumors resulting from expression of the tumor-causing envelope glycoprotein but minimal viral replication.

The pulmonary lesions of OPA are characteristic, but cannot be distinguished from the rare nonviral pulmonary carcinomas of sheep without further testing. Immunohistochemistry for the JSRV envelope glycoprotein is useful for confirmation of the viral origin of the tumors. A PCR assay is able to

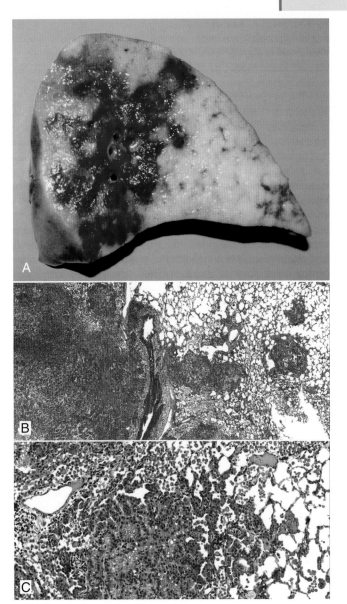

Figure 5-65 Ovine pulmonary adenocarcinoma caused by jaagsiekte sheep retrovirus. **A.** Coalescing white nodules within the lung. **B.** Multiple nodules coalesce to form a mass (at left), and satellite tumors pepper the adjacent lung tissue (right). **C.** Detail, showing lepidic and papillary patterns, and increased number of reactive alveolar macrophages. (Courtesy B. Cloak, J. Cassidy, University College Dublin.)

differentiate JSRV from endogenous sheep retroviral sequences and enzootic nasal tumor virus, although the low JSRV loads in blood leukocytes limit its sensitivity for analysis of blood samples.

Further reading

Caporale M, et al. Host species barriers to jaagsiekte sheep retrovirus replication and carcinogenesis. J Virol 2013;87:10752-10762.

De Las Heras M, et al. Solitary tumours associated with jaagsiekte retrovirus in sheep are heterogeneous and contain cells expressing markers identifying progenitor cells in lung repair. J Comp Pathol 2014;150:138-147.

Griffiths DJ. Pathology and pathogenesis of ovine pulmonary adenocarcinoma. J Comp Pathol 2010;142:260-283.

Wootton SK, et al. Envelope proteins of Jaagsiekte sheep retrovirus and enzootic nasal tumor virus induce similar bronchioalveolar tumors in lungs of mice. J Virol 2006;80:9322-9325.

Bacterial pneumonia

The bacteria causing pneumonia in sheep include *Mannheimia haemolytica*, *Pasteurella multocida*, *Histophilus somni*, hemolytic streptococci, and *Helcococcus ovis*. The important role of mycoplasmas is discussed later. Caseous lymphadenitis (eFig. 5-91) is described elsewhere (see Vol. 3, Hematopoietic system). *M. haemolytica* can also cause septicemia in the absence of pneumonia in lambs <2 months of age. The causative agents, predisposing factors, and pathogenesis are in many respects similar to those described in cattle. Sudden climatic changes, gathering and handling, and infection with *Mycoplasma* spp., ovine or bovine respiratory syncytial virus, bovine parainfluenza virus 3, or adenovirus are the most commonly recognized predisposing causes. The *Pasteurellaceae* bacteria listed above cause hemorrhagic or fibrinonecrotic, lobar or lobular bronchopneumonia and serofibrinous pleuritis in acute cases, and fibrinopurulent bronchopneumonia leading to abscess formation and fibrous pleural adhesions in subacute to chronic cases. *M. haemolytica* causes sporadic cases and small outbreaks of acute pneumonia and pleuritis in goat kids. The disease usually occurs as a peracute disease in late autumn and winter. At autopsy, a sheet of yellow fibrin adheres loosely to the pleural surfaces. The cranial lobes of the lungs are firm and dark red, with a transition to less-firm tissue with mottled gray-pink discoloration in the caudal lobes. Acute diffuse bronchopneumonia is characterized microscopically by neutrophils, protein-rich exudate, and numerous bacteria filling bronchioles and alveoli. There is usually little evidence of necrosis. In the caudal lobes, neutrophils fill the bronchioles and extend into the alveoli.

Helcococcus ovis has been recently associated with chronic suppurative bronchopneumonia, lung abscesses, and pleuritis in a sheep and a goat. The gram-positive bacterial cocci are visible histologically amid necrotic debris in the abscesses or on the pleural surface.

Further reading

García A, et al. *Helcococcus ovis* isolated from a goat with purulent bronchopneumonia and pulmonary abscesses. J Vet Diagn Invest 2012;24:235-237.

Sheehan M, et al. An aetiopathological study of chronic bronchopneumonia in lambs in Ireland. Vet J 2007;173:630-637.

Zhang Y, et al. Isolation of *Helcococcus ovis* from sheep with pleuritis and bronchopneumonia. J Vet Diagn Invest 2009;21:164-166.

Septicemic pasteurellosis. Septicemia caused by *Bibersteinia trehalosi* occurs mainly in weaned lambs during the fall months, but it can occur in other age groups and at other times of the year. Deaths, which seldom exceed 5% of the sheep at risk, usually follow within a few days of changes in pasture, feed, or other management practices.

Signs of illness are vague, and the usual course is short, or lambs may be found dead with no opportunity to exhibit clinical signs. At autopsy, *petechial and ecchymotic hemorrhages* are usually present in subcutaneous tissues, particularly of the neck and thorax, in intermuscular fascia, and in the pleura, epicardium, and mesentery (Fig. 5-66). Retropharyngeal and

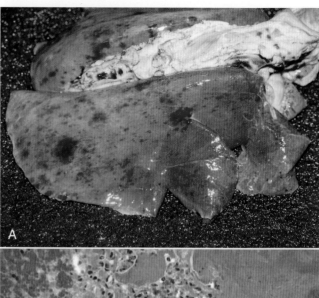

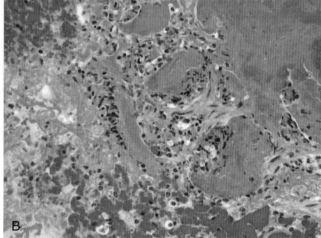

Figure 5-66 *Bibersteinia trehalosi* **septicemia** in a weaned lamb. **A.** Petechiae and ecchymoses throughout the lung, and also present in other tissues. **B.** Histologically, the lung is deeply congested and edematous, and myriad tiny bacteria fill blood vessels with only a minimal reaction of leukocytes. (Courtesy M.J. Hazlett, University of Guelph.)

mesenteric lymph nodes are hemorrhagic and edematous. *Ulcerative lesions* covered by yellow plaques of fibrin and necrotic debris are common on the tongue, pharynx in the area of tonsillar crypts, larynx, and esophagus. The abomasal, intestinal and colonic mucosae occasionally have shallow ulcers. The lungs are diffusely congested and edematous. *Multiple foci of hemorrhagic necrosis may be scattered throughout the lungs*, and the liver may contain pinpoint to 1-cm diameter yellow necrotic foci. There is occasionally inflammation of joints, pericardium, meninges, and choroid plexus, but these lesions are absent in peracute cases.

Microscopic examination of tissues reveals *widespread bacterial embolism* (see Fig. 5-66). The pulmonary lesions consist of multifocal masses of bacteria filling capillaries, accompanied by hemorrhagic and fibrinous exudate into alveoli. A peripheral zone of necrotic leukocytes may be present. The pale hepatic foci consist of colonies of bacteria with a surrounding zone of ischemic necrosis. There may be thrombosis of the adjacent tributaries of the portal vein and small amounts of parenchymal necrosis, but the leukocyte response is generally slight. This is probably related to the short course of the disease and perhaps to the effects of bacterial toxin on leukocytes. Bacterial emboli are regularly found in the spleen and adrenals, occasionally in the kidney, but are rare in other organs. Masses of bacteria adhere to the surface of the pharyngeal ulcers and occlude underlying blood vessels and lymphatics, and probably represent the *principal site of bacterial proliferation and systemic invasion.*

Further reading

Miller DS, et al. Domestic sheep *(Ovis aries) Pasteurellaceae* isolates from diagnostic submissions to the Caine Veterinary Teaching Center (1990-2004). Vet Microbiol 2011;150:284-288.

Melioidosis. Melioidosis is a systemic infectious disease affecting a wide range of animal species in tropical climates. The disease is endemic in Southeast Asia and northern Australia, is probably common in the Indian subcontinent and the Caribbean, and also occurs in southern Africa and the Middle East. The prevalence is highest in wet seasons, and causes acute outbreaks or chronic endemic disease. Clinical signs are variable and reflect the range of organs affected, and case fatality rates are high. Melioidosis is most common in goats, sheep, pigs, and rodents, and is an emerging tropical disease of humans. Horses, deer, camels, and laboratory animals are less commonly affected, whereas dogs, cats, cattle, water buffalo, and fowl are resistant to the disease unless they are immunosuppressed.

Melioidosis is caused by **Burkholderia pseudomallei**, a facultatively anaerobic gram-negative bipolar-staining bacillus. Infection is acquired from contaminated soil or water, by inhalation, ingestion, or inoculation of cutaneous wounds. *Acute disease,* most common in young animals, may initially affect the lungs, with later spread to other organs, or be primarily septicemic from the site of inoculation. *Chronic disease* is the more frequent manifestation, in which abscesses in multiple organs cause chronic nonspecific illness or are an incidental finding of public health importance at slaughter.

Virulence factors of *B. pseudomallei* include the iron-scavenging protein malleobactin, secreted proteases that degrade host tissues, a polysaccharide capsule that confers resistance to killing by phagocytes, lipopolysaccharides, and *Burkholderia* lethal factor 1, a protein toxin that inhibits translation and causes cell death. The bacterium survives within macrophage phagolysosomes and in epithelial cells, and elicits a granulomatous and suppurative tissue reaction.

Melioidosis causes abscesses in multiple organs. The lungs are most consistently affected, with disseminated coalescing nodules, or locally extensive areas of consolidation. Abscesses also affect the spleen, liver, lymph nodes, subcutis, kidney, or joints, and may occur in any visceral tissue. Lesions are particularly widespread in goats, and may include mastitis or aortic aneurysm. Neurologic disease is most common in goats; gross lesions are rare, but multifocal aggregates of neutrophils and lymphocytic perivascular cuffs are present in the brainstem and spinal cord. Nodular lesions in the nasal mucosa may be mistaken for glanders. Endometritis and placentitis are important manifestations in cattle.

The abscesses of melioidosis are not distinctive in their appearance. *The chronic lesions are encapsulated nodular masses, up to 5-cm diameter, with creamy or caseous yellow centers.* Multifocal aggregates of neutrophils form within 12 hours of infection. Granulomas, present by 3 days, form nodular aggregates of epithelioid macrophages and lymphocytes, and these develop central areas of caseous necrosis and neutrophil infiltration.

The gross and histologic appearance of melioidosis is not pathognomonic. Caseous lymphadenitis, glanders, and abscesses caused by other bacteria may have a similar appearance, and the brain lesions may be mistaken for listeriosis. A tentative diagnosis may be based on identifying gram-negative bipolar-staining bacilli in sections or tissue smears, but *definitive diagnosis requires culture.* Because of its zoonotic potential, great care should be taken when dealing with suspect cases during autopsy and subsequent tissue handling and testing.

Further reading

Galyov EE, et al. Molecular insights into *Burkholderia pseudomallei* and *Burkholderia mallei* pathogenesis. Annu Rev Microbiol 2010; 64:495-517.

Sprague LD, Neubauer H. Melioidosis in animals: a review on epizootiology, diagnosis and clinical presentation. J Vet Med B Infect Dis Vet Public Health 2004;51:305-320.

Chlamydial diseases

Intratracheal challenge of lambs with *Chlamydophila abortus (psittaci)* induces mild infiltration of neutrophils and macrophages into alveoli and alveolar septa, and mild proliferative alveolitis. Lesions are most prominent adjacent to terminal bronchioles. Moderately sized cuffs of lymphocytes are present around bronchioles and small blood vessels at the height of the lesion. The chlamydiae are mostly destroyed during the acute phase of inflammation, which then subsides. Resolution can be complete within 3-4 weeks of experimental infection. Chlamydiae may contribute to some cases of enzootic pneumonia in lambs and calves, in combination with other agents, but are probably of *limited importance as primary pulmonary pathogens.*

Further reading

Dungworth DL, Cordy DR. The pathogenesis of ovine pneumonia. J Comp Pathol 1962;72:49-79.

Mycoplasmal diseases

Contagious caprine pleuropneumonia. Contagious caprine pleuropneumonia (CCPP) was first described in Africa in the late 1800s and remains an important disease in northern and western Africa, the Middle East, and the Indian subcontinent. The difficulty in isolating the causative agent in culture caused much confusion in the early literature, but the cause of CCPP is now known to be **Mycoplasma capricolum ssp. capripneumoniae**. Although other mycoplasmas may cause similar lesions, these are not considered CCPP. Classic CCPP caused massive outbreaks with high morbidity and mortality in naive goats of all ages. *Currently, CCPP, an OIE (World Organization for Animal Health) listed disease, causes endemic sporadic disease in some countries and intermittent epizootics in others.* Affected goats are lethargic, dyspneic, and febrile; have bouts of coughing; but may continue to eat. Young goats may be lame because of polyarthritis.

M. capricolum ssp. *capripneumoniae* (formerly *Mycoplasma* F38) is phylogenetically related to, but distinct from, *M.*

mycoides. The virulence factors of this pathogen have not been well defined. Subclinical carriers are important sources of infection, and are the usual source of introduction of the disease into naive herds. Stress may trigger shedding of organisms from subclinically infected animals. Individual goats are infected by inhalation of droplets through close contact with coughing goats. The infection is restricted to the respiratory tract. It mainly affects goats, although infection has been recently detected in wildlife.

Pulmonary lesions are often unilateral but may be bilateral. The pleura is covered by a thick layer of fibrin, and serous fluid fills the pleural cavity. Lobular areas of consolidation and purple-gray discoloration are present in the lung, either diffusely or forming focal lesions, and these may contain extensive areas of necrosis or have a dry granular texture. Fibrinous pericarditis is common. Chronic cases develop focal nodules of necrosis and mineralization with a fibrous capsule, or lung abscesses if secondary bacterial infection develops. However, in contrast to contagious bovine pleuropneumonia, *sequestra and interlobular edema are not features of the caprine disease.* Histologically, the exudate in alveoli and interlobular septa varies from serofibrinous to fibrinopurulent. Thrombosis and vasculitis are often present. With time, the fibrinous exudates organize to form a mass of fibrous tissue.

Gross lesions are suggestive, but not diagnostic. Other mycoplasmas, particularly *M. mycoides* ssp. *mycoides* (large colony type [LC]), and *M. mycoides* ssp. *capri*, may cause epidemics with similar lung lesions. Features that suggest CCPP rather than other mycoplasmas include the presence of both pneumonia and pleuritis, the absence of interlobular edema and inflammation, and the absence of mastitis, arthritis, or keratitis. Laboratory examination is required for definitive diagnosis.

M. capricolum ssp. *capripneumoniae* is an extremely difficult organism to propagate in culture, although it can often be recovered from the pleural fluid and consolidated lung of acutely ill animals. Detecting mycoplasmal nucleic acid using the PCR on samples of pleural fluid is a more rapid and sensitive method of diagnosis. Complement fixation and latex agglutination tests are effective methods of serodiagnosis.

Further reading

Nicholas R, Churchward C. Contagious caprine pleuropneumonia: new aspects of an old disease. Transbound Emerg Dis 2012;59: 189-196.

Other mycoplasmal pneumonias. Many mycoplasmas cause disease in sheep and goats throughout the world, including *M. ovipneumoniae*, *M. mycoides* ssp. *mycoides* LC, *M. mycoides* ssp. *capri*, *M. capricolum* ssp. *capricolum*, *M. putrfaciens*, and *M. agalactiae*. *M. capricolum* ssp. *capripneumoniae*, the cause of CCPP, is discussed earlier. *M. agalactiae* causes contagious agalactia of sheep and goats, but may also induce respiratory disease. Minimally pathogenic mycoplasmas in small ruminants include *M. arginini*, *M. auris*, *M. cottewi*, and *M. yeatsii*. Transmission requires close contact with infected animals. Young animals are often infected by ingestion or inhalation of contaminated milk.

These agents cause a diverse spectrum of clinical signs and lesions. *Mastitis and agalactia are common in adults, and may be accompanied by arthritis or keratitis. Kids and lambs more* commonly *develop pneumonia or pleuropneumonia, fibrinopurulent polyarthritis, or septicemia with fibrinous polyserositis and interstitial pneumonia.* The lung lesions may resemble those described previously for CCPP, but thickening of interlobular septa by edema and fibrin exudation is not typically present in CCPP. *M. mycoides* ssp. *mycoides* LC is particularly capable of causing pleuropneumonia, polyarthritis, and septicemia in goat kids and, to a lesser extent, in lambs; the worldwide distribution of this pathogen is in contrast to those of contagious caprine and bovine pleuropneumonia. *M. capricolum* principally causes fibrinopurulent polyarthritis in kids, but may also cause septicemia in kids and mastitis in does.

Chronic bronchopneumonia (chronic nonprogressive pneumonia) in lambs and kids is common, often subclinical, but reduces growth rates. Multiple etiologic agents are implicated, including *Mannheimia haemolytica*, *Mycoplasma ovipneumoniae*, parainfluenza-3 virus and respiratory syncytial virus. Of these agents, *M. ovipneumoniae* is isolated particularly frequently and probably plays an important causal role. Stress, poor air quality, and adverse weather conditions also contribute to development of disease.

Lesions typically affect the cranioventral lung, and include lymphoid hyperplasia around airways, neutrophil accumulation within airspaces, hyperplasia of bronchiolar and alveolar epithelium, bronchiolar mucous metaplasia, and a unique lesion of hyaline scars. The latter consist of nodular masses of fibrillar eosinophilic matrix and fibroblasts within the wall of bronchioles that bluntly compress the lumen, but do not form the intrabronchiolar polyps seen in bronchiolitis obliterans. The lesions do not indicate a specific etiology and *diagnosis requires culture of lesional lung tissue.*

Further reading

Sheehan M, et al. An aetiopathological study of chronic bronchopneumonia in lambs in Ireland. Vet J 2007;173:630-637.

Parasitic diseases

Oestrus ovis. *Oestrus ovis* (sheep bot fly) adult flies deposit first-stage larvae on the nares. The larvae molt twice as they *migrate through the nasal passages.* Larvae may become incarcerated in sinuses or recesses of turbinates as they grow, and eventually die there (eFig. 5-92). Development in the nasal passages can take up to 10 months, although larvae deposited early in summer are able to mature in that season. The full-grown larvae are about 3 cm long, with black oral hooks, dorsal dark transverse bands, and ventral rows of small spines. Pupation occurs on the ground.

The larvae attach to the mucous membrane by their mouthparts. They produce mucosal defects at the points of attachment and, because the cuticle is spinous, cause irritation as they wander. An immune response against excreted or secreted larval antigens, and the ensuing eosinophil and mast cell response, may also contribute to nasal inflammation and irritation. Affected sheep develop catarrhal rhinitis and sinusitis. Apart from persistent annoyance and the debility that this may cause, *there are seldom untoward effects of the parasitism.* Rarely, larvae penetrate the cranial cavity, or secondary bacterial infections spread from the olfactory mucosa to the meninges. Mild infestations of *O. ovis* occur in goats and dogs, as well as conjunctival infections in humans.

Table • 5-3

Major lungworms of sheep and goats

Lungworm	Gross features	Histologic features
Muellerius capillaris	Pale nodules Worms are microscopic	Adults and larvae mainly in alveoli Alveolar fibrosis ± granulomatous inflammation
Cystocaulus ocreatus	Dark nodules Hair-like worms	Adults and larvae in alveoli and small bronchioles
Dictyocaulus filaria	Focal atelectasis or consolidation ± emphysema Threadlike worms in bronchi	Bronchi and large bronchioles contain adult worms, lymphoplasmacytic or eosinophilic inflammation, and smooth muscle and epithelial hyperplasia
Protostrongylus rufescens and Neostrongylus linearis	Angular nodules Adults grossly visible in parenchyma and smallest bronchi	Adults in terminal bronchioles Granulomatous and/or eosinophilic bronchiolitis, with prominent peribronchiolar lymphofollicular cuffs

Further reading

Gomez-Puerta LA, et al. A case of nasal myiasis due to *Oestrus ovis* (Diptera: *Oestridae*) in a llama *(Lama glama)*. Rev Bras Parasitol Vet 2013;22:608-610.

Muellerius capillaris. *Muellerius capillaris is the most common and ubiquitous lungworm of sheep and goats* (Table 5-3). There is usually no clinical evidence of respiratory disease in sheep, although experimental infections may cause hyperpnea, impaired pulmonary gas exchange, and reduced weight gains. Heavy infestations are purported to predispose to bacterial and viral infections of the lung.

Muellerius capillaris, also known as the *small lungworm of sheep and goats*, is a nematode of the superfamily *Metastrongyloidea*, family *Protostrongylidae*. Adults, which are 12-24 mm long and threadlike, live in nodular lesions in the alveoli and rarely in bronchioles, but are usually not visible at autopsy. Eggs are laid and rapidly hatch, and first-stage larvae are coughed up, swallowed, and passed in the feces. In some cases, each nodule in the lung may contain adult worms of only one sex. The infection in such cases is sterile, and larvae will not be detected in feces. The intermediate hosts are various slugs and snails. The infective stage is reached after 2 molts in the intermediate host, and the life cycle is completed when sheep and goats swallow the intermediate hosts. The larvae migrate to the lungs, presumably via the lymphatics, and break out into the alveoli. As a consequence of this type of life cycle, infections are gradually acquired, and large worm burdens are seldom observed in animals <6 months of age. On the other hand, heavy infections are not common in old sheep and goats, as repeatedly infected animals become resistant.

The characteristic finding is multiple, subpleural nodules in the dorsal regions of the caudal lobes (Fig. 5-67). However, they may occur anywhere in the lung, and occasionally in the regional lymph nodes. The nodules are soft and hemorrhagic in the acute stages, corresponding to histologic lesions of hemorrhage and eosinophil infiltration. However, most cases represent chronic infestations with raised gray-pink or yellow nodules that may mineralize.

The nodules are formed by masses of adult worms, embryonated eggs, and coiled larvae (see Fig. 5-67). The adults have polymyarian-coelomyarian musculature, the intestine is composed of a few multinucleated cells with an indistinct brush border, and the uteri often contain thick-shelled embryonated eggs and larvae. The inflammatory response is often minimal, although alveolar septa may be thickened by fibrous tissue, lymphocytes, and smooth muscle hyperplasia (see Fig. 5-67, eFig. 5-93). In older animals or chronic infestations, presumably associated with developing resistance, the cellular reaction is more marked and targets the first-stage larvae and adults. Eosinophils aggregate around the larvae; the alveolar spaces contain macrophages, eosinophils, and giant cells. Larvae that escape into small bronchioles are enclosed in plugs of mucus and cellular debris. When larvae leave the nodules, the cellular reaction subsides, but thickening of the alveolar septa persists because of patchy or diffuse fibrosis. Adult worms incite a similar reaction of eosinophils, macrophages, and giant cells. *The cellular debris becomes mineralized, particularly when the worms die, and these mineralized nodules persist indefinitely as spherical masses of calcium salts surrounded by a fibrous capsule.*

The gross appearance of *Muellerius* infestation can closely resemble that of **Cystocaulus.** However, the nodules of *Cystocaulus* are darker and may be larger than those of *Muellerius*, the adult worms may be grossly visible, and bronchial epithelial hyperplasia is more likely in *Cystocaulus* infestation. In **Dictyocaulus** and **Protostrongylus** infections, the adult worms are located in large bronchioles/bronchi and the terminal bronchioles, respectively.

In **goats,** *Muellerius* infestation has been associated with severe diffuse interstitial pneumonia in the absence of nodular lesions. Histologic lesions included diffuse thickening of alveolar septa with mononuclear cells, and fibromuscular hyperplasia in alveolar septa; but the possibility that these lesions might have been caused by caprine arthritis encephalitis virus or *Mycoplasma* infection cannot be ruled out.

Further reading

Panayotova-Pencheva MS, Alexandrov MT. Some pathological features of lungs from domestic and wild ruminants with single and mixed protostrongylid infections. Vet Med Int 2010;2010:741062.

Protostrongylus rufescens. *Protostrongylus rufescens* is a nematode of the superfamily *Metastrongyloidea*, family

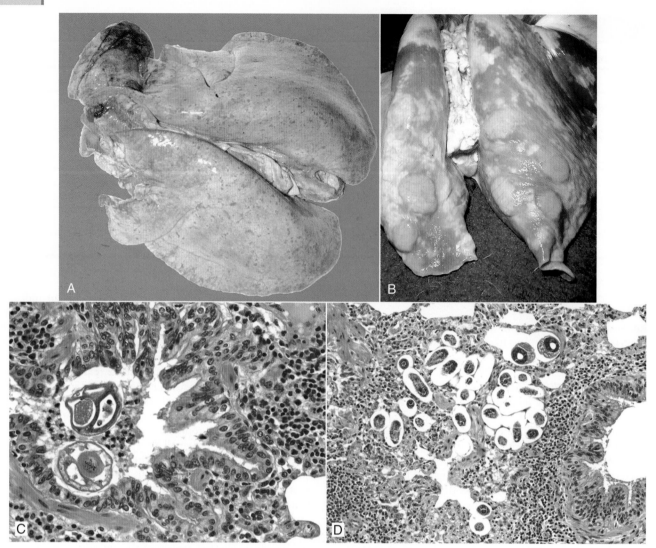

Figure 5-67 *Muellerius capillaris*. **A.** Tiny nodules mainly in the caudodorsal areas of lung in a sheep. **B.** Larger nodules with similar distribution, in a goat. (**A, B,** Courtesy University of Guelph.) **C.** Tiny adult nematodes are infrequent in the alveoli, or here in a bronchiole. **D.** More prominent are the nodular accumulations of embryonated ova and larva, accompanied by lymphocytic or granulomatous inflammation and smooth muscle metaplasia in alveolar septa.

Protostrongylidae, that infects sheep, goats, and deer. The adults are 16-35 mm in length, red, and mainly inhabit the terminal bronchioles. Eggs hatch to first-stage larvae in the lung, and are passed in the feces. They enter intermediate hosts, which are various genera of terrestrial snails, by boring through the foot. Two molts occur in the snail, and the infective third-stage larvae develop in 46-49 days. Sheep and goats eating the snails are infected by the larvae, which pass by way of the mesenteric lymphatics to the lungs.

Lesions consist of 2-4 cm diameter, angular, firm, tan nodules distributed throughout the lungs. The nodules are usually soft, in contrast to the firm texture of *Muellerius* nodules. Cross-sections may reveal fine white worms exuding from the parenchyma or occasionally leading to a small bronchus. Histologically, an eosinophilic inflammatory reaction targets adult worms, larvae, and eggs in the terminal bronchioles. Prominent lymphofollicular aggregates surround these airways. Smooth muscle hyperplasia is not a feature of *Protostrongylus* infestation.

Further reading

Berrag B, Cabaret J. Assessment of the severity of natural infections of kids and adult goats by small lungworms (*Protostrongylidae*, Nematoda) using macroscopic lesion scores. Vet Res 1997;28: 143-148.

Dictyocaulus filaria. Dictyocaulus filaria, the *large lungworm of sheep and goats*, is a slender, white, 3-10 cm long nematode that inhabits mainly the small bronchi. The life cycle and lesions are similar to those described for *D. viviparus*, which is described in detail with respiratory diseases of cattle. The lesions are localized, 3-4 cm diameter areas of atelectasis or consolidation that are most common in the dorsal aspects of the caudal lobes. Bronchi are prominently thickened by smooth muscle and cuffs of lymphocytes and granulocytes, and often contain adult threadlike worms (eFig. 5-94). A granulomatous alveolar reaction to aspirated eggs may occur.

Further reading

Panuska C. Lungworms of ruminants. Vet Clin North Am Food Anim Pract 2006;22:583-593.

Miscellaneous parasites. *Neostrongylus linearis,* a comparable nematode to *Protostrongylus rufescens,* is common in western Europe, the Middle East, and probably elsewhere. The adults are 5-15 mm long, and terrestrial gastropods are the intermediate hosts. The worms are contained within 1-4 mm diameter, red-violet or gray-pink nodules that are most numerous in the caudal lobes.

Cystocaulus ocreatus (*C. nigrescens*) reside in 5-20 mm diameter, dark, firm nodules in the caudodorsal lung. Cross-sections may reveal brown-black hairlike worms, which move when the lung section is immersed in saline. The life cycle resembles that of *Muellerius.*

Mammomonogamus (*Syngamus*) *nasicola* and *M. laryngeus* are nematodes of the nasal cavity and larynx. *Schistosoma nasalis* causes nasal granuloma in India. *Habronema* spp. are rare causes of fibrotic nodules adjacent to bronchioles. In sheep, the lung is a common site of hydatid cysts caused by *Echinococcus granulosus*; the cysts have multiple protoscolices within brood capsules (but these are apparent only in fertile cysts) surrounded by a thin layer of germinal epithelium, an eosinophilic PAS-positive noncellular laminated layer, and an outer adventitial layer that contains macrophages, lymphocytes, giant cells, and remnants of bronchiolar epithelium.

Further reading

Barnes TS, et al. Comparative pathology of pulmonary hydatid cysts in macropods and sheep. J Comp Pathol 2011;144: 113-122.

Kelly EJ, et al. Echinococcosis (hydatidosis) in a sheep. J Am Vet Med Assoc 2012;241:1449-1451.

Infectious respiratory diseases of horses

Viral diseases

Equine influenza. General features of influenza viruses are discussed previously (see Infectious respiratory diseases of swine). **Influenza A virus in horses** (colloquially, equine influenza virus, EIV) infection is widespread in most intensively managed horse populations. Outbreaks occur most commonly in the autumn and winter months in young immunologically naive horses. *Risk factors* for infection and disease include close confinement, transportation, training, and mixing of animals. These factors increase the chance of contact between naive and subclinically infected animals. *Antigenic drift is a feature of influenza viruses*; thus epizootics of influenza may occur even in vaccinated horses, when new antigenic variants of influenza viruses emerge.

EIV originated from avian influenza viruses and is placed within subgroup A based on the antigenicity of the nucleocapsid and matrix proteins. As with other influenza viruses, EIV can be identified by the hemagglutinin (H) and neuraminidase (N) surface glycoproteins. All currently circulating EIV belong to the H3N8 (formerly equi-2) subtype. H7N7 (formerly equi-1) influenza virus was an important cause of equine respiratory disease in the 1950s, but has been considered extinct since 1978.

Surface hemagglutinin is the immunodominant antigen, and inactivated vaccines induce short-lived protection that correlates with induction of antibody to this antigen. Vaccinated horses may be infected and shed virus, but have a milder and shorter clinical course. Horses that recover from natural infection have more prolonged resistance to disease, for at least 1 year, but in this case, resistance is not closely correlated to anti-hemagglutinin antibody titers.

As with influenza in swine and humans, *the disease in horses is usually characterized by high morbidity and low mortality, unless secondary bacterial pneumonia develops.* Most outbreaks spread rapidly through groups of horses, and are characterized by acute onset of fever of <4 days duration, severe nonproductive cough, mucopurulent nasal discharge, lethargy, and anorexia. Dependent edema is an uncommon finding. Although most clinical signs resolve within 1-2 weeks, coughing may persist for weeks or months. Occasionally, and rarely, introduction of certain strains of influenza virus into naive populations has caused outbreaks with nearly 100% morbidity and high mortality.

Infection with EIV is usually acquired by inhalation of infected aerosols. Viral replication is most extensive in epithelial cells of the upper respiratory tract and trachea, where infective viral particles bud from the plasma membrane within 2-4 days after infection. Influenza reduces mucociliary clearance both by impairing ciliary beating and by inducing necrosis of infected cells, and may also impair alveolar macrophage function; the ensuing bacterial pneumonia is responsible for many of the fatal cases. Epithelial repair following influenza may take up to 3 weeks, and affected horses may continue to cough well past the point of complete repair.

Gross and histologic lesions of uncomplicated EIV are not commonly seen as horses rarely die from such infections. *Gross lesions* of viral pneumonia occur mainly in foals, and consist of coalescent foci of consolidation separated by unaffected to hyperinflated lung; less commonly, diffuse lung consolidation is reported. Both foals and adult horses develop secondary bacterial bronchopneumonia (eFig. 5-95). Histologically, tracheitis is common, and foals may develop bronchointerstitial pneumonia with bronchitis and bronchiolitis characterized by epithelial necrosis as well as epithelial hyperplasia, and squamous metaplasia in the bronchi. Involvement of the alveolar parenchyma ranges from mild inflammation to severe necrosis, with hyaline membrane formation and type II pneumocyte hyperplasia. At all airway levels, inflammation consists primarily of a mix of neutrophils, lymphocytes, and plasma cells. Rarely, severe EIV infection affects the brain, heart, gastrointestinal tract, kidney, and other parenchymal organs.

The major differential diagnoses for nonfatal cases of upper respiratory infection include equid herpesviruses 1 and 4 and equine rhinitis A virus. In such cases, **diagnosis** is most commonly based on detection of virus by RT-PCR from nasal swabs. Isolation of influenza virus is less commonly used to diagnose disease and is most reliable during the phase of pyrexia in the first day or 2 of illness. In the rare cases that are acutely fatal, virus may be demonstrated in lung by RT-PCR, isolation, ELISA, or by immunohistochemistry. Serology is mainly used to follow animal exposure during EIV outbreaks, but is also of value for routine diagnosis.

Further reading

Begg AP, et al. Pathological changes in horses dying with equine influenza in Australia, 2007. Aust Vet J 2011;89(Suppl. 1):19-22.

Cullinane A, Newton JR. Equine influenza—a global perspective. Vet Microbiol 2013;167:205-214.

Patterson-Kane J, et al. The pathology of bronchointerstitial pneumonia in young foals associated with the first outbreak of equine influenza in Australia. Equine Vet J 2008;40:199-203.

Equid alphaherpesviruses. General features of herpesviruses are described above (see Infectious respiratory diseases of cattle). Equid alphaherpesviruses (EHV) cause upper respiratory infections, abortion, systemic disease of neonates, and neurologic disease. The latter 3 manifestations are described in more detail elsewhere. Systemic disease of yearling horses or adults is rare, but notable for the high mortality rates that may occur.

Upper respiratory infections of juvenile and adult horses may be caused by EHV-1 or EHV-4. Uncomplicated rhinitis elicited by these 2 viruses is clinically indistinguishable, with disease most common in foals <1 year of age. Affected animals are febrile with serous or mucopurulent nasal discharge. Both viruses readily infect nasal respiratory epithelial cells, causing local epithelial necrosis and inflammation that result in the aforementioned clinical signs. Less commonly, viral infection extends into the trachea, resulting in coughing in affected horses. Infection is rarely fatal, unless secondary bacterial pneumonia develops.

Viral replication occurs in the nasopharynx and associated lymphoid tissue, and the development of viremia is dependent on the strain of the virus and prior exposure of the host. Virus is shed from nasal secretions starting 2-10 days after infection. Viral shedding commonly occurs only during the phase of pyrexia, but is occasionally prolonged up to 3 weeks after infection. Latency for EHV-1 and EHV-4 is established within neuronal cells (e.g., trigeminal ganglion) and lymphocytes, as well as lung epithelial cells in the case of EHV-4. Seroconversion to both viruses is common, with nearly 100% of horses surveyed having seroconverted to EHV-4. Because of this, as well as the prevalence of vaccination for the viruses, serology is of limited use in diagnosing infection with these 2 viruses. Definitive **diagnosis** of EHV-1 or EHV-4 infection of the upper respiratory tract can be done using *virus-specific PCR* on material collected from nasal swabs or *isolation of virus* from such swabs.

EHV-1 causes systemic disease in live-born neonates. Lesions are similar to those in aborted foals (see Vol. 3, Female genital system) and include bronchointerstitial pneumonia; multifocal necrosis in liver, spleen, adrenal, and other tissues; prominent intranuclear inclusion bodies; and sometimes syncytial cells. The lungs are heavy with a diffuse rubbery-firm texture, and multiple white foci of necrosis may be present but inconspicuous (eFig. 5-96). EHV-1 occasionally causes systemic disease in yearling or adult horses. Lesions include pulmonary or systemic necrotizing vasculitis, pulmonary edema and hemorrhage, lymphoid necrosis, and encephalomyelitis with vasculitis.

Further reading

Lunn DP, et al. Equine herpesvirus-1 consensus statement. J Vet Intern Med 2009;23:450-461.

Equid gammaherpesviruses. Members of the subfamily *Gammaherpesvirinae* known to infect the respiratory tract of equids include *EHV-2 and EHV-5 in horses and 2 asinine herpesviruses (AHV-4 and AHV-5) in donkeys*. PCR-based detection of EHV-2 and EHV-5 is reportedly more common in surveys of nasal swabs and tracheal washes from horses with respiratory disease, but their role in the pathogenesis of upper respiratory tract disease in horses remains poorly defined. Lower respiratory tract disease is reported in horses and donkeys in association with infection with EHV-5, AHV-4, and AHV-5.

Equine multinodular pulmonary fibrosis *(EMPF) is a progressive fibrosing interstitial lung disease associated with lung infection with EHV-5.* EMPF is largely a disease of adult horses that is clinically characterized by low-grade fever, weight loss, and progressive exercise intolerance. The *gross pathology of EMPF* is restricted to the lungs and tracheobronchial lymph nodes. Within the lungs, there are variably sized nodular foci of fibrosis (Fig. 5-68). These vary from individual discrete nodules separated by relatively normal lung parenchyma to coalescent foci with little unaffected lung present. The tracheobronchial lymph nodes in cases of EMPF are often markedly enlarged. *Histologically,* the nodules are composed of abundant interstitial collagen accumulation, along with irregular alveolus-like spaces lined by cuboidal epithelial cells. Within the lumen of these spaces, there is a moderate inflammatory infiltrate of mostly neutrophils and macrophages. Occasional macrophages are enlarged and contain large eosinophilic intranuclear viral inclusion bodies (see Fig. 5-68).

The evidence for a link between lung infection with EHV-5 and the development of EMPF has been based on detection of virus by PCR as well as virus isolation, and co-localization of the virus with the lesions. The most compelling evidence for EHV-5 in the pathogenesis of EMPF comes from experimental infection of horses with EHV-5 isolates obtained from cases of EMPF. Nodular lung fibrosis with features similar to EMPF was induced in horses inoculated with these isolates of EHV-5, providing strong evidence that this gammaherpesvirus is the cause of EMPF.

Diagnosis of EMPF can be made using PCR to detect EHV-5 in lung from horses that develop the characteristic clinical disease and lesions. Isolation of EHV-5 can be challenging, as the gammaherpesvirus grows slowly in cells and may require multiple blind passages.

Interstitial pneumonia occurs in **donkeys** *in association with lung infection with AHV-4 and AHV-5.* The *gross lesions* in affected donkeys consist of lungs that fail to collapse, with patchy or multifocal firm lesions, most commonly in the cranioventral areas. *Histologically,* affected animals have a mix of bronchiolitis and interstitial pneumonia with the consistent presence of large multinucleated *syncytial cells.* Viral inclusion bodies are not present. Bronchiolar lesions range from mononuclear cell and neutrophil infiltrates around bronchioles, to necrosis of bronchiolar epithelium. Alveolar changes include similar leukocyte infiltrates, in some cases with extensive type II pneumocyte proliferation and interstitial fibrosis. *Diagnosis* is based on PCR testing to detect AHV-4 or AHV-5 in association with the characteristic histologic lesions.

Further reading

Fortier G, et al. Equine gammaherpesviruses: pathogenesis, epidemiology and diagnosis. Vet J 2010;186:148-156.

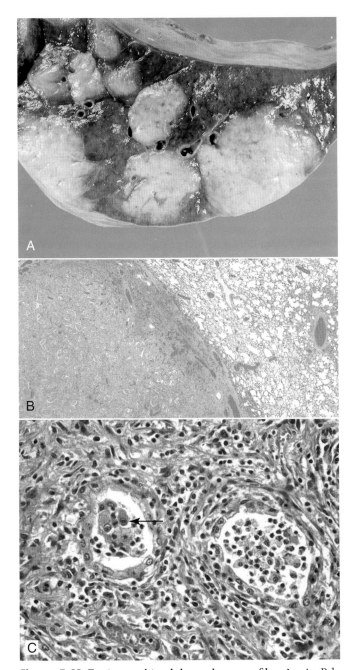

Figure 5-68 Equine multinodular pulmonary fibrosis. A. Pale well-demarcated nodules scattered throughout the lungs. **B.** The nodules have marked expansion of the interstitium by connective tissue, and type II pneumocytes line the alveoli. **C.** Macrophages fill the alveoli, and one contains an intranuclear inclusion (arrow).

Williams KJ. Gammaherpesviruses and pulmonary fibrosis: evidence from humans, horses, and rodents. Vet Pathol 2014;51:372-384.
Williams KJ, et al. Experimental induction of pulmonary fibrosis in horses with the gammaherpesvirus equine herpesvirus 5. PLoS ONE 2013;8:e77754.

Adenovirus. *Equine adenovirus 1* infection is widespread in horses, and is mainly associated with upper respiratory tract infections. Adenoviral pneumonia is a well-described complication of inherited combined immunodeficiency in young Arabian foals. This severe disease has become rare as this genetic immunodeficiency becomes less common. At autopsy, the *gross lesions* consist of a lobular or confluent pattern of atelectasis and/or consolidation primarily, but not exclusively, within cranioventral lung. In the early stage of severe infection, there is extensive necrosis and sloughing of bronchiolar epithelium. Later, bronchiolar epithelium is hyperplastic, and swollen superficial epithelial cells contain amphophilic intranuclear inclusion bodies. Occasionally, there are intranuclear inclusions in alveolar epithelial cells and increased numbers of macrophages and neutrophils. Secondary bacterial pneumonia or *Pneumocystis* pneumonia may also be present in these immunocompromised foals.

Further reading

Bell SA, et al. Equine adenovirus 1 infection of hospitalised and healthy foals and horses. Equine Vet J 2006;38:379-381.

Hendra virus. Hendra virus was first described as a cause of fatal pulmonary disease of horses in 1994 in Australia. Natural infections and disease have been reported in humans and horses and experimentally-induced in cats and guinea pigs. Fruit bats (flying foxes) in the genus *Pteropus* are the reservoir host for the virus, carrying the virus subclinically and serving as the source of infection for horses. Most human infections have occurred following contact with infected clinically ill horses. Hendra virus and the related Nipah virus are members of the genus *Henipavirus*, family *Paramyxoviridae*. *Hendra virus has tropism for endothelial cells, and many of the lesions arise from vascular injury.* Viral particles are detectable in the cytoplasm of endothelial cells. *Gross lesions* in horses reflect the viral vascular tropism, and include prominent *pulmonary edema and congestion* with dilation of subpleural lymphatic vessels, petechial hemorrhages, and abundant tracheal froth. The most prominent *histologic lesion* is serofibrinous fluid and increased numbers of macrophages in alveoli. Closer inspection reveals subtle vascular lesions in the lung, heart, glomeruli, and stomach, consisting of thrombi in capillaries and/or necrotic debris and hemorrhage in the walls of arterioles. The presence of syncytial cells in small vessels is a unique but inconsistent lesion. The *differential diagnosis* for massive pulmonary edema includes African horse sickness, heart failure, and anaphylaxis.

Further reading

Hazelton B, et al. Hendra virus: a one health tale of flying foxes, horses, and humans. Future Microbiol 2013;8:461-474.

Bacterial diseases

Rhodococcus equi. *Rhodococcus equi* (*Rhodococcus hoagii*, *Prescotella equi*) is an important cause of pneumonia and occasionally enteric disease in 1-6 month-old foals. The prevalence of the disease is highly variable between farms, and probably reflects the bacterial load within airborne dust, as soil is the important source of infection. Environmental factors favoring the disease include hot seasonal temperatures in temperate climates, neutral soil pH, and repetitive high-density stocking of dry paddocks. The clinical presentation may be either acute or insidiously progressive, although the infection and lesions are invariably chronic by the time clinical signs are noted. Thoracic ultrasound shows that most foals with lung abscesses do not develop clinical disease, and many recover without therapy. When clinical disease occurs, it is most frequent in the summer, with pyrexia, tachypnea, dyspnea, cough, and mucopurulent nasal discharge. *Because of the chronic nature of the disease, case fatality rates are high in untreated foals.* Animals with the *colonic form* of disease may have diarrhea, weight loss, ascites resulting from hypoproteinemia, and occasionally colic.

Foals with bronchointerstitial pneumonia, described previously, frequently have concurrent *R. equi* infection, yet the relationship between these conditions remains obscure. Foals with *R. equi* pneumonia occasionally have histologic evidence of *Pneumocystis carinii* infection of the lung.

R. equi is a gram-positive facultative intracellular pathogen, distantly related to mycobacteria, which grows well in soil and in horse manure. Neonatal foals have the greatest susceptibility to infection, compared to those 6 weeks of age. *Pulmonary infection results from inhalation of soil-borne bacteria*, and inhalation of greater numbers of bacteria is facilitated by the presence of a dusty, contaminated environment. Enteric infections may result from ingestion of soil-contaminated feed, or swallowing expectorated material from the lungs. Experimental studies indicate that hematogenous spread from enteric lesions is not a common route of pulmonary infection.

The bacterium is engulfed by macrophages but survives this encounter by preventing maturation of the phagosome and its fusion with the lysosome. Nevertheless, macrophages are able to kill *R. equi* when the bacteria are opsonized or when the macrophages are activated by lymphocyte-derived interferon-γ. Infection elicits a pyogranulomatous inflammatory response, presumably resulting from cytokines secreted by infected macrophages or responding lymphocytes.

The *virulence* of *R. equi* varies between isolates, and correlates closely with the presence of an 80-90 kb virulence-associated plasmid (pVAP). Species specificity for horses, pigs, or cattle is conferred by the presence of different host-adapted plasmids. The pVAP carries a pathogenicity island that contains the variety of genes (including *vapA*) needed by the bacteria to survive within macrophages following phagocytosis. The macrophage is the preferred cell type for replication of the bacterium, and central to the pathogenesis of disease. Other virulence factors of *R. equi* include glycolipids containing long-chain mycolic acids, capsular polysaccharide, the "equi factors" cholesterol oxidase and choline phosphohydrolase, and the iron-binding protein rhequichelin.

Immune responses to *R. equi* have been intensively investigated because of the interest in developing vaccines against this important disease of foals. The finding that passive immunization with hyperimmune plasma is effective in preventing disease indicates that humoral immunity is protective, probably because antibody-mediated opsonization augments phagocytosis and killing of *R. equi* by macrophages and neutrophils. In contrast to the role of humoral immunity in prevention of disease, T-helper-1 cellular immune responses are probably necessary for recovery from established infection. Both CD4+ and CD8+ T cells are important in clearing *R. equi* in mouse models of disease. CD4+ T cells produce IFN-γ, which activate macrophages to produce more bactericidal nitric oxide, oxygen radicals, and peroxynitrite; whereas CD8+ T cells induce lysis of infected macrophages.

The *pulmonary lesions* caused by *R. equi* are most constant in the cranioventral lung, but most of the lung may be affected in severe cases. *The most consistent lesion is pyogranulomatous bronchopneumonia*, in which 1-10 cm, white-tan, firm,

coalescing nodules develop in the infected lung (Fig. 5-69). Intervening areas of lung are reddened and firmer than normal. With time, the centers of the pyogranulomas become friable and caseous or liquefying. These may be mistaken for abscesses, but they generally lack a fibrous capsule. Pleuritis is uncommon. Bronchial lymph nodes are enlarged and may contain focal caseous necrosis.

Intestinal lesions are present in approximately half of the foals with pulmonary rhodococcosis; 5% of cases have lesions restricted to the intestine. The colon, cecum, and associated lymph nodes are most commonly affected, but small intestinal lesions may occur. Colonic lesions begin as focal mucosal ulcers that are centered on lymphoid follicles. The ulcer bed is reddened and covered with fibrin, and the borders of the ulcers are raised and pale because of pyogranulomatous infiltrates. Pyogranulomas or foci of caseous necrosis may extend through the wall of the intestine. The colonic lymph nodes are often enlarged, pale, and contain necrotic foci. The colonic pyogranulomas enlarge over time and develop central areas of caseation or liquefaction. Large abdominal abscesses may be the sole lesion in some cases.

The earliest histologic lesion following *R. equi* infection is suppurative bronchopneumonia. By 4 days after infection, alveoli and bronchioles are filled with macrophages, neutrophils, and fewer lymphocytes and plasma cells. *Macrophages are numerous in the well-developed lesions, but neutrophils may also be plentiful. Gram-positive bacteria are present in the cytoplasm of plump uninucleated or multinucleated macrophages amid this exudate*, and are particularly numerous within degenerating macrophages that have cytoplasmic eosinophilia and nuclear pyknosis (see Fig. 5-69). Areas of caseous necrosis, when present, usually contain cellular debris, many neutrophils and macrophages, fibrin, and edema.

In the intestine, the dome epithelium overlying lymphoid follicles is the primary route of infection. Macrophages underlying the dome epithelium contain intracytoplasmic bacilli, and neutrophils infiltrate the epithelium and exude into the lumen. With time, the lymphoid follicles are invaded by macrophages and neutrophils, and central areas of caseous necrosis eventually extend to the mucosal surface. In the developed lesions of ulcerative colitis, ulcers are filled with fibrinonecrotic debris and encompassed by neutrophils and macrophages, many of which contain bacteria.

About ⅓ of affected foals have *polyarthritis*. This may cause severe lameness, suppurative synovitis, and positive joint cultures, resulting from hematogenous spread of infection. In contrast, other foals have milder, probably *immune-mediated polyarthritis*. These are characterized by sterile joints, lymphoplasmacytic synovitis, mononuclear cells in joint fluid, and immunoglobulin deposits in synovium.

More widespread dissemination of infection in foals can occasionally give rise to abscesses in the mesenteric or mediastinal lymph nodes, liver, spleen, or skin; osteomyelitis affecting the vertebrae or metaphyses of long bones; and hypopyon. *R. equi* may also cause ulcerative lymphangitis, and has been associated with metritis and abortion in mares, metritis in cows, pneumonia in calves, and tubercle-like lesions in lymph nodes of pigs and cattle.

Lesions of cranioventral pyogranulomatous pneumonia or multifocal ulcerative colitis in foals are highly suggestive of *R. equi* infection. In most cases, the *diagnosis is easily confirmed by culture*, or by identifying intracytoplasmic gram-positive bacilli in macrophages on impression smears or tissue sections.

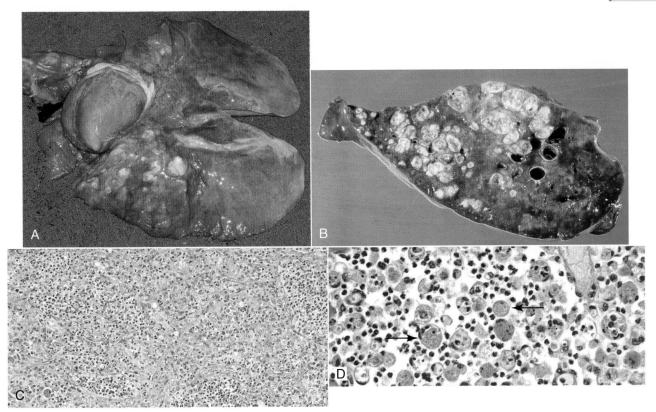

Figure 5-69 *Rhodococcus equi* **pneumonia in a foal. A.** Ventral view of the lungs, showing cranio-ventral consolidation with multiple pale bulging nodules. **B.** On cut section (a different case), the consolidated tissue contains multiple liquefying foci of pyogranulomatous inflammation. (Courtesy University of Guelph.) **C.** Infiltration of macrophages and neutrophils. **D.** Some macrophages are enlarged and contain visible bacteria in the cytoplasm (arrows).

Idiopathic bronchointerstitial pneumonia or *Pneumocystis carinii* infection may be present in foals with *R. equi* pneumonia.

Further reading

Giguere S, et al. *Rhodococcus equi*: clinical manifestations, virulence, and immunity. J Vet Intern Med 2011;25:1221-1230.

Muscatello G. *Rhodococcus equi* pneumonia in the foal—part 1: pathogenesis and epidemiology. Vet J 2012;192:20-26.

Opportunistic bacterial pathogens in foals. Pneumonia caused by opportunistic bacterial pathogens is common in 1-8 month-old foals, and is of similar pathogenesis as in other species. *Streptococcus equi* ssp. *zooepidemicus* is the most prevalent cause, with occasional cases resulting from infection with α-hemolytic streptococci, *Bordetella bronchiseptica*, *Staphylococcus epidermidis*, *Klebsiella pneumoniae*, *Actinobacillus equuli*, and others. Pneumonia in neonates is commonly caused by bacteria that cause septicemia, and the 2 processes may be concurrent; *E. coli*, *Streptococcus* spp., *A. equuli*, and *Klebsiella pneumoniae* are the most common isolates.

Further reading

Erol E, et al. Beta-hemolytic *Streptococcus* spp. from horses: a retrospective study (2000-2010). J Vet Diagn Invest 2012;24: 142-147.

Equine bacterial pneumonia and pleuropneumonia. *Pleuropneumonia is common in 2- to 4-year-olds*, and older horses may also be affected. Presenting signs include fever, depression, respiratory distress, and colic. Evidence of thoracic pain may be apparent at rest, with grunting respiration or abduction of the elbows, or be elicited by thoracic percussion. Horses with bacterial pneumonia develop fever, tachypnea, and coughing. Risk factors for the development of both pneumonia and pleuropneumonia include recent transportation, general anesthesia (probably leading to aspiration pneumonia), other stressful events, and viral infection.

Numerous opportunistic bacterial pathogens have been isolated from lesions of pleuropneumonia in horses, and *mixed infections are present in most cases*. Attempts to isolate bacteria may fail in cases that have been heavily treated with antibiotics. *Streptococcus equi* ssp. *zooepidemicus* is the most common isolate; others include *S. equisimilis*, *S. equi* ssp. *equi*, *Actinobacillus suis*–like bacteria, other streptococci, *Pasteurella* spp., *Bordetella bronchiseptica*, *E. coli*, *Bacteroides*, and *Fusobacterium*. *Mycoplasma felis* has been identified in a small number of horses with pleuritis, suggesting it should be considered as a differential diagnosis of cases of pleuritis without pneumonia.

Identification of a unilateral distribution of lesions and a mixed infection with aerobic and anaerobic bacteria imply that *many cases result from aspiration pneumonia*. The equine trachea at the thoracic inlet contains a pool of secretions contaminated by bacteria, the so-called *"tracheal puddle."* One frequent pathogenesis seems to involve transport of horses with the head held in an elevated position, thus predisposing to aspiration of these contaminated secretions into the lung.

The gross lesions of well-developed cases of pleuropneumonia are spectacular, and the lesions are often more chronic than suggested by the clinical history. Massive amounts of fibrin and malodorous serofibrinous exudate fill the pleural space, and may form cavitating masses encased in maturing fibrous tissue. Most cases of pleuritis in horses arise from underlying pulmonary lesions, although the lesions of pneumonia are overshadowed by the pleural exudate. Although often described as lung abscesses, the lung lesions are more usually localized areas of consolidation. Lesions in the lung are often unilateral, and the pleural exudate in these cases is also usually unilateral. Occasionally, pleuritis extends from bilateral lesions of bronchopneumonia, which may include localized areas of thrombosis and infarction.

Further reading

Erol E, et al. Beta-hemolytic *Streptococcus* spp. from horses: a retrospective study (2000-2010). J Vet Diagn Invest 2012;24: 142-147.

Strangles and *Streptococcus equi*. *Strangles is an acute contagious disease of horses characterized by inflammation of the upper respiratory tract and abscess formation in the regional lymph nodes.* The disease commonly occurs in young horses following exposure to carriers or diseased horses. Clinical signs may include purulent nasal discharge, inappetence, fever, depression, unilateral or bilateral swelling of the throat region, stertor, and dysphagia.

Strangles is caused by ***Streptococcus equi* ssp. *equi***, a Lancefield group C streptococcus closely related to *S. equi* ssp. *zooepidemicus*. Unlike *S. equi* spp. *zooepidemicus*, which may infect a variety of species, *S. equi* spp. *equi* only infects horses. A range of virulence factors has been described. The hyaluronic acid capsule is necessary for virulence, mediates binding of the bacterium to host cells, and confers resistance to phagocytosis. The M protein and a factor-H–binding protein bind fibrinogen and prevent deposition of complement factor C3b, thereby blocking recognition and phagocytosis by macrophages. Two endopeptidases cleave immunoglobulin G. Peptidoglycan activates complement by the alternative pathway, inciting recruitment of neutrophils to sites of infection. The fact that many of the recruited neutrophils rapidly undergo necrosis may be an effect of streptolysin-S and another cytotoxin.

Streptococcus equi in exudates can survive for many months in the external environment, and may be transmitted through contaminated drinking water or by fomites. The initial source of infection, however, is usually a carrier animal or one with active but not necessarily obvious clinical disease. The incubation period of strangles is 3-4 days, although it may be as short as 2 or as long as 15 days. The pathogenesis of the infection involves rapid transport of bacteria from the tonsil to local lymph nodes, within 3 hours after experimental infection. *S. equi* spp. *equi* only transiently colonizes nasopharyngeal epithelial cells; therefore attempts to culture the bacteria from nasopharyngeal samples can be fruitless in the face of an active infection. Following entry of the bacteria into regional lymph nodes, there is chemotaxis of neutrophils to the infected lymph nodes. The organism resists phagocytosis, leading to further increases in the number of neutrophils, neutrophil

lysis, and formation of intranodal abscesses. Recovery from strangles confers immunity in about 75% of horses, associated with IgA and IgG antibody produced locally in the nasopharynx. Although antibodies to M protein confer partial immunity, other protective antigens are not yet fully defined.

The submandibular and retropharyngeal nodes are the first and usually the most severely affected. The swollen lymph nodes are initially firm, but this swelling becomes fluctuant as the suppurative exudate liquefies. The typical and most favorable clinical outcome of the lymphadenitis is for the abscesses to rupture onto the skin 1-3 weeks after onset of infection, releasing creamy yellow-white pus containing numerous infective bacteria. Infection also often extends from retropharyngeal lymph nodes to involve the guttural pouches, and purulent exudates within these structures can inspissate to form so-called *chondroids*. Drainage from the guttural pouch into the nasal cavity is a major reason for suppurative nasal discharge.

Most cases of strangles recover quickly unless the enlarging lymph nodes obstruct the upper respiratory tract, but complications develop in 20% of clinically affected animals. This may involve extension of infection to adjacent structures, resulting in purulent sinusitis, guttural pouch empyema, periorbital abscess formation, facial cellulitis, or local damage to cranial nerves, resulting in laryngeal paralysis (roaring), facial nerve paralysis, or Horner's syndrome. Horses with guttural pouch empyema may remain infected, intermittently shed bacteria, and be an important source of infection for at least 8 months after resolution of the acute disease.

More serious complications include pneumonia or pleuropneumonia, myocarditis, mesenteric lymph node abscesses, and purpura hemorrhagica. Retropharyngeal abscesses may discharge into the pharynx, allowing pus to be aspirated into the lungs where localized areas of necrotizing pneumonia develop. Metastatic abscesses (*"bastard strangles"*) occasionally form in the liver, kidneys, synovium, and brain, but are most common in mediastinal and mesenteric lymph nodes. Abscesses in these lymph nodes tend to be very large and, although rupture is unusual, the suppurative process can extend to adjacent serous membranes and cause purulent pleuritis or peritonitis. Purpura hemorrhagica is a systemic leukocytoclastic vasculitis, and follows deposition of immune complexes of IgA or IgG with bacterial M protein in small blood vessels and glomeruli. Purpura hemorrhagica develops in 1-2% of cases, 2-4 weeks after the acute infection. There is edema of the head and limbs, petechial hemorrhages on mucosal and serosal surfaces and in muscles, and occasionally glomerulonephritis.

Because similar, but usually milder, lesions may be caused by *S. equi* spp. *zooepidemicus* or other bacteria, *definitive diagnosis relies on isolation of S. equi spp. equi from purulent exudate*. PCR assays are also available and are particularly useful in detecting chronically infected horses.

Further reading

Timoney JF, Kumar P. Early pathogenesis of equine *Streptococcus equi* infection (strangles). Equine Vet J 2008;40:637-642.

Waller AS, et al. *Streptococcus equi* a pathogen restricted to one host. J Med Microbiol 2011;60:1231-1240.

Waller AS, Robinson C. *Streptococcus zooepidemicus* and *Streptococcus equi* evolution: the role of CRISPRs. Biochem Soc Trans 2013;41: 1437-1443.

Glanders. Glanders is caused by ***Burkholderia mallei*** and typically affects horses, donkeys, and mules. It is now mostly of historic importance, having flourished when horses played a larger role in human transport and military campaigns and has disappeared from many countries, but still exists in Eastern Europe, Asia, and South America. Natural disease occurs in carnivores, sheep, and goats, whereas cattle and pigs are considered more resistant. Humans are susceptible, and glanders is a potential bioterrorist threat. *B. mallei* is sensitive to the external environment, and infection is acquired directly or indirectly from excretions and discharges of affected animals. In the absence of definitive information, it is assumed that the organisms traverse the pharyngeal mucosa, and perhaps the intestinal mucosa, and are conveyed to the lungs, where lesions almost always occur. From there, hematogenous spread is believed to result in nasal, cutaneous, and lymph node lesions.

Glanders is characterized by nodular lesions in the lungs, and ulcerative and nodular lesions of the skin and respiratory mucosa. Lung lesions are often present as generalized pinpoint to 2-cm diameter *pyogranulomatous nodules throughout the lung*, often with central areas of liquefactive necrosis. Histologically, the nodules are composed of a central core of neutrophils, often with necrosis of neutrophils and liquefaction of the tissue, and a peripheral rim of epithelioid macrophages and fibrosis. The relative proportions of neutrophils, macrophages, fibrosis, and mineralization are variable.

Nasal lesions are often unilateral, with copious, purulent, green-yellow exudate. Multiple small nodules in the submucosa each consist of an inner core of neutrophils and a periphery of macrophages. The core liquefies and the overlying mucosa may slough, leaving a crateriform ulcer that heals to form a white stellate scar. Similar pyogranulomatous ulcerative lesions line the pharynx, larynx, and trachea. Hematogenous metastases are common in the spleen and less common in other tissues. Enteric lesions are rare. *The cutaneous lesions of glanders are termed "farcy."* These consist of chains of nodules or ulcers that follow lymphatic vessels, and represent purulent lymphangitis with extensive leukocyte necrosis.

Further reading

Dvorak GD, Spickler AR. Glanders. J Am Vet Med Assoc 2008;233: 570-577.

Khan I, et al. Glanders in animals: a review on epidemiology, clinical presentation, diagnosis, and countermeasures. Transbound Emerg Dis 2013;60:204-221.

Mycoplasmal diseases

Mycoplasma **spp.** Although several mycoplasmas have been isolated from the respiratory tract of horses, particularly *Mycoplasma equirhinis* and *M. felis*, there have been no studies to determine whether they are capable of causing pneumonia. *M. felis* is an uncommon cause of fibrinous pleuritis without pneumonia, and lesions were reproduced by intrapleural inoculation of *M. felis*. *M. felis* has also been associated with outbreaks of lower respiratory tract disease in horses, based on seroconversion and isolation of the organism.

Further reading

Wood JL, et al. Association between respiratory disease and bacterial and viral infections in British racehorses. J Clin Microbiol 2005; 43:120-126.

Fungal diseases

Coccidioidomycosis, cryptococcosis, and **pneumocystosis** are described elsewhere. **Pulmonary aspergillosis** is an uncommon disease of horses, and usually represents hematogenous spread of fungal hyphae resulting from colitis, as a consequence both of neutropenia and disruption of the mucosal barrier. Lesions are multifocal embolic pneumonia, often centered on pulmonary vessels, and include neutrophil and fibrin exudate in alveoli, hemorrhage, necrosis, and leukocytoclastic vasculitis. Septate branching hyphae are most common at the periphery of foci of necrosis (Fig. 5-70).

Entomophthoromycosis (phycomycosis) is a chronic nasal or cutaneous disease of horses, sheep, and rarely of cattle caused by *Conidiobolus coronatus, C. lamprauges,* and *Basidiobolus haptosporus* (class Zygomycetes, order Entomophthorales), which are saprophytic fungi limited to tropical and subtropical climates. The nasal lesions are most common in the nostril, but can form larger masses obstructing the nasal cavity and invading adjacent tissues, including the retro-orbital space. The lesions in sheep are described to most consistently affect the ethmoid conchae. Lesions invade adjacent tissues, including the sinuses, retro-orbital space, or brain, and may spread to lung, brain, and other tissues. The masses consist of ulcerating and cavitating granulomas containing coral-shaped granules. Histologic evaluation reveals eosinophils, neutrophils, macrophages, and giant cells. Fungal hyphae are numerous mainly in the brightly eosinophilic amorphous granules (Splendore-Hoeppli phenomenon). The hyphae of *C. coronatus* and *C. haptosporus* appear with H&E stain as unstained filaments within the eosinophilic amorphous material; a silver stain reveals them to be nonpigmented, commonly septate,

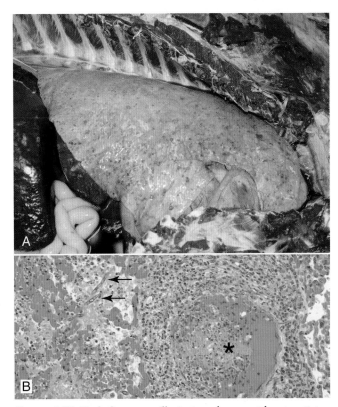

Figure 5-70 **Embolic aspergillosis** in a horse with necrotizing colitis. **A.** Multiple dark nodules in an embolic pattern throughout the lung. **B.** A blood vessel in the lung (asterisk) contains a fibrin thrombus, neutrophils and other leukocytes that extend to adjacent tissue, and fungal hyphae (arrows).

irregular in contour, 5-13 μm or 5-20 μm diameter, respectively, and irregularly branched. PAS stains are not considered useful. *Pythium insidiosum* (an aquatic fungus-like oomycete pathogen) induces a lesion in horses, cattle, and sheep that is similar to entomophthoromycosis, but eosinophils are numerous, and the hyphae are 2-7 μm diameter, thick walled, and infrequently septate. However, pythiosis and entomophthoromycosis are difficult to differentiate histologically, and definitive diagnosis requires culture, PCR testing, or immunohistochemistry. The *differential diagnoses* for eosinophilic cutaneous or nasal masses in horses include habronemiasis and mast cell tumor.

Further reading

Silva SM, et al. Conidiobolomycosis in sheep in Brazil. Vet Pathol 2007;44:314-319.

Ubiali DG, et al. Pathology of nasal infection caused by *Conidiobolus lamprauges* and *Pythium insidiosum* in sheep. J Comp Pathol 2013;149:137-145.

Parasitic diseases

Dictyocaulus arnfieldi is mainly a lungworm of donkeys, in which it survives for long periods with few clinical signs. *D. arnfieldi* is an occasional cause of chronic coughing in horses. Infection of adult horses often results in failure of the worm to develop to sexual maturity, and larvae cannot be detected in the feces of these animals. The worms can mature if horses or ponies are infected as young foals. The gross lesions are scattered wedge-shaped foci of overinflation, mostly in caudal lobes. In the center of the lesions are *small bronchi packed with coiled adult worms*. Histologically, the worms are associated with goblet cell hyperplasia and lymphocytic infiltrates. Adult worms cause relatively little luminal response, whereas first-stage larvae stimulate an intense mucopurulent reaction, or chronic catarrhal and eosinophilic bronchiolitis.

Parascaris equorum larval migration causes *nodular lesions in the lung*. The acute lesions are distinctive by virtue of the mass of eosinophils present and the occasional presence of ascarid larvae in bronchioles or alveoli. However, the chronic nodules consist of aggregates of lymphoid tissue with fibrosis and mineralization, and need to be differentiated from residual lesions of small abscesses or granulomas.

Echinococcus equinus causes cysts in the lung of horses in western Europe. The cysts have a characteristic histologic appearance, with an inner germinal membrane containing brood capsules, protoscolices, and mineralized corpuscles; a noncellular laminated middle layer; and an outer adventitial layer of fibrosis and chronic inflammation (eFigs. 5-97, 5-98).

Infection with amebae rarely causes encephalitis in horses. Multifocal granulomatous pneumonia with necrosis and thrombosis, with histologically visible trophozoites and cysts, are reported in those cases caused by *Acanthamoeba*.

Miscellaneous parasitisms include *Schistosoma nasalis*, a cause of nasal granuloma in India; hydatid cysts; and *Habronema* spp., a rare cause of fibrotic nodules adjacent to bronchioles.

Further reading

Blutke A, et al. Cystic echinococcosis due to *Echinococcus equinus* in a horse from southern Germany. J Vet Diagn Invest 2010;22: 458-462.

Infectious respiratory diseases of dogs

Canine infectious respiratory disease (CIRD) complex, also known as kennel cough or infectious tracheobronchitis, is important and common in dogs. The disease is most prevalent in dogs that have been brought into close contact with others at shelters, pet stores, kennels, and dog shows. The name recognizes that, as in cattle and swine, highly contagious respiratory disease occurs in dogs as a result of complex interactions among host factors and a variety of viruses and bacteria. The major bacterial causes include *Bordetella bronchiseptica*, *Streptococcus zooepidemicus*, and *Mycoplasma cynos*. Canine distemper virus, canine adenovirus 2, and canid herpesvirus 1 have been important in the past and still occur, but more frequent viral causes now include canine parainfluenza virus, canine respiratory coronavirus, and canine influenza virus. Other viruses of less certain significance include pantropic canine coronavirus, canine pneumovirus, canine bocavirus, and canine hepacivirus.

Further reading

Priestnall SL, et al. New and emerging pathogens in canine infectious respiratory disease. Vet Pathol 2014;51:492-504.

Schulz BS, et al. Detection of respiratory viruses and *Bordetella bronchiseptica* in dogs with acute respiratory tract infections. Vet J 2014;201:365-369.

Viral diseases

Canine distemper. Canine distemper is caused by a *Morbillivirus* (family *Paramyxoviridae*). Although now uncommon in countries with well-vaccinated dog populations, it continues to be a frequent and serious disease in many parts of the world. *Canine distemper virus (CDV) infects a wide range of terrestrial carnivores*, including *Canidae* (wild and domestic dogs), *Mustelidae* (ferrets, mink), and *Procyonidae* (raccoons); ferrets are particularly susceptible. Some species of seals are vulnerable to CDV infection, and distinct closely related phocid morbilliviruses are also important causes of distemper-like disease in these species.

As with the closely related morbilliviruses, measles virus and rinderpest virus, CDV is a large, 150-250 nm diameter, irregularly shaped virus composed of an outer lipoprotein envelope, an inner matrix, and a nucleocapsid containing single-strand negative-sense RNA. The envelope is studded with hemagglutinin glycoproteins that mediate viral attachment to host cells, and fusion glycoproteins that allow penetration of host cells and fusion of infected cells with uninfected cells.

Virus is shed in secretions of the respiratory tract, and to a lesser extent in other secretions. Infection is usually acquired by inhaling aerosols or by close contact with infected dogs. The virus infects macrophages of the upper respiratory tract or lungs, which convey it to local lymph nodes and tonsils during the first 24 hours. The virus replicates further in local lymphoid tissues, and by 2-5 days after exposure is present in lymphoid tissues throughout the body, including bone marrow, thymus, spleen, and intestinal lymphoid tissue.

Clinical signs of fever, depression, and anorexia develop about 5 days after infection. At this stage of viremia, virus particles are free in the plasma as well as within blood mononuclear cells. *Further development of the disease is highly dependent on the immune status of the host, the titer of antibodies to envelope glycoproteins, the age of the host, and the strain of virus.* Dogs with adequate humoral and cellular immunity are able to neutralize the virus and clear the infection by 14 days after infection, and may not shed virus from mucosal surfaces. In dogs with intermediate levels of cellular and humoral immunity, viremia leads to infection of mucosal epithelium and brain. Virus is shed in secretions, but clinical signs attributable to epithelial infection may be minor or absent, although neurologic disease may develop in these partially immune dogs. Dogs that fail to mount an adequate immune response develop systemic infection of epithelial tissues that evokes clinical signs of respiratory and enteric disease, infection of the central nervous system, and shedding of virus in respiratory secretions, feces, and urine.

Clinical disease in dogs is most common at 12-16 weeks of age, as puppies with waning passive immunity are exposed to subclinically infected dogs. *The infection is systemic, and clinical signs are often referable to the respiratory, gastrointestinal, and nervous systems.* Ocular disease, pustular and/or hyperkeratotic cutaneous lesions, dental defects, and abortion are other manifestations. In some cases, clinical signs are primarily caused by secondary infections that are a consequence of *virus-induced immunosuppression*, probably an effect of viral infection of lymphocytes and macrophages. Secondary infections include *Bordetella*, adenovirus, *Pneumocystis*, *Toxoplasma*, *Clostridium piliforme*, *Sarcocystis*, *Encephalitozoon*, and enteric infections with *Cryptosporidium* or attaching-and-effacing *E. coli.*

The systemic form of the disease often begins with fever and conjunctivitis, and rapid progression to coughing, depression, anorexia, vomiting, and diarrhea. Affected dogs may die at this stage, fully recover, or develop neurologic disease 1-4 weeks later. Neurologic disease may also be the primary clinical manifestation, particularly in animals with partial immunity. Neurologic manifestations are quite variable, depending on the anatomic location of the lesions, and include seizures, cerebellar or vestibular ataxia, paraparesis or paraplegia, and myoclonus.

The **histologic lesions** of canine distemper are fairly specific when the disease is well developed, particularly if inclusion bodies are apparent. However, *lesions in mild cases are nonspecific*, particularly in dogs with clinical signs limited to the upper respiratory tract. *Inclusion bodies are most numerous 10-14 days after infection*, but their numbers diminish rapidly by 5-6 weeks. *Inclusions are most obvious in brain and epithelial tissues*, and less easily identified in lymphoid tissues. Inclusion bodies can be found in the central nervous system before changes of encephalomyelitis are present, and they often persist in the neural tissue when they have disappeared from other sites. The inclusion bodies are eosinophilic and often intranuclear in nervous tissue but usually intracytoplasmic in other tissues.

Lymphopenia and lesions in lymphoid organs are regularly present. *Lymphoid lesions* may be inapparent on gross examination, or there may be either atrophy or edematous swelling. Thymic atrophy is a particularly common finding in CDV-infected puppies. The earliest lesions following experimental infection with CDV consist of depletion of lymphocytes in the cortical zone of the lymph nodes within 6 days of infection. By day 9, the lymph nodes and spleen contain lymphocytic necrosis and depletion, and infiltration of neutrophils. Syncytial cells may form in the lymph nodes, and these often contain inclusion bodies. Approximately 2 weeks after exposure, hyperplasia of histiocytic cells develops, but repopulation of the node by lymphocytes may be delayed for weeks or months. Thymic atrophy is due both to loss of cortical thymocytes as well as great reduction in the medulla.

Respiratory tract lesions are common. Grossly, serous, catarrhal, or mucopurulent exudate covers the nasopharynx. The lungs are edematous, and secondary bronchopneumonia is often present, particularly in subacute or chronic cases. *The specific lesion of canine distemper is bronchointerstitial pneumonia*, which usually appears as patchy, generalized, red-tan, rubbery lesions beneath the pleura and at the margins of the lung. Generalized diffuse reddening and consolidation is a less common manifestation. Histologically, bronchioles contain scant suppurative exudate, there is patchy necrosis and attenuation of bronchiolar epithelium, and lymphocytes are present around bronchioles. *Inclusion bodies are often most obvious in the cytoplasm of bronchial and bronchiolar epithelial cells* (eFig. 5-99). Alveoli contain protein-rich edema fluid, scant fibrin, mononuclear cells, and necrotic epithelial cells. Alveolar septa are thickened by mononuclear cells. Proliferation of type II pneumocytes, which occasionally contain cytoplasmic inclusions, may form a complete cuboidal lining to scattered groups of alveoli. Inclusion bodies are common in type II pneumocytes and alveolar macrophages, and *alveolar epithelial syncytial cells are a characteristic feature when present*. Chronic lesions in subpleural and peribronchiolar alveoli include macrophage accumulation, type II pneumocyte proliferation, and alveolar septal fibrosis. Inclusion bodies tend to persist in the bronchiolar and alveolar epithelium longer than in other non-neural tissues.

Intracytoplasmic and rarely intranuclear inclusion bodies are regularly found within swollen transitional epithelial cells of the *urinary bladder and renal pelvis* in the acute systemic disease. Inclusion bodies, mild degenerative changes, and mononuclear cell infiltrates may be present in a variety of other epithelia, including the gastric surface epithelium, chief and parietal cells of the stomach, cholangiolar epithelium in the liver, pancreatic ductular epithelium, epididymis, and testis.

In the *central nervous system*, the virus appears first in perivascular astrocytes and macrophages, but infection of the choroid plexus epithelium occurs early, and the cerebrospinal fluid contains large amounts of virus. Lesions in the white matter and grey matter differ histologically; these may occur concurrently or one may predominate. *Demyelination in white matter tracts* is most severe in the cerebellum, rostral medullary velum, optic tracts, spinal cord, and surrounding the fourth ventricle, and probably arises from distribution of virus through the cerebrospinal fluid. The lesions are multifocal or patchy in distribution, with vacuolation of the neuropil, loss of myelin (particularly notable with Luxol fast blue stain), and, in the early stages, preservation of axons. Astrocytes usually contain nuclear and, less frequently, cytoplasmic inclusions, and astrocyte-derived syncytia are present in a minority of cases. As the lesion progresses, gliosis and axonal degeneration may occur, and mononuclear cells infiltrate the lesion in low numbers; however, the early lesion is noninflammatory. Animals that survive may be left with sclerotic astrocytic foci and myelin loss.

Grey matter lesions, which are less frequent than those in white matter, often target the cerebral cortex, cerebellum, brainstem, and spinal cord. In early stages, inclusion bodies are usually present in the nucleus or occasionally in the cytoplasm of neurons; these neurons undergo necrosis, and mononuclear cells congregate around the dying neurons. With time, a non-suppurative inflammatory response develops, and mononuclear cells aggregate around blood vessels and infiltrate the neuropil. Nonsuppurative meningitis is usually mild.

Old dog encephalitis is a rare variant, possibly caused by infection with replication-defective virus. This syndrome is characterized by chronic progressive neurologic disease, widely distributed perivascular infiltrates of lymphocytes and plasma cells, and intranuclear inclusions in astrocytes and neurons. Viral antigen may be demonstrated by immunohistochemistry, but virus cannot be isolated from the brain. Canine distemper may occasionally result from administration of modified live CDV vaccines. Neurologic disease is the usual manifestation in these cases, and lesions in the grey matter include neuronal necrosis, intranuclear inclusions, and lymphocytic encephalitis.

Dental lesions follow infection of young animals with CDV. Necrosis and cystic degeneration of ameloblastic epithelium of the developing tooth, associated with syncytia and cytoplasmic inclusions, give rise to the *defective enamel* seen in animals that have recovered from infection. The defects vary from focal depressions to large, sharply demarcated areas of enamel hypoplasia.

Ocular lesions include conjunctivitis, keratitis, retinitis, and optic neuritis. Conjunctivitis is very common in the early stages of disease, and occasionally extends to the cornea to cause ulcerative keratitis. Retinal lesions, which are common following systemic infection, include intranuclear inclusions in ganglion cells and glia, degeneration of ganglion cells, photoreceptor loss, retinal edema, and perivascular cuffs of mononuclear cells. These lesions progress to neuronal loss, retinal scarring, and proliferation of retinal pigment epithelium in the chronic stages. Lesions in the optic nerve are inconstant, but papilledema may be observed in acute cases, and gliosis or demyelinating neuritis in chronic ones.

Cutaneous lesions of hyperkeratosis and parakeratosis may affect the footpad and nose, and rarely the haired skin. The epidermis may contain syncytial cells, and nuclear and cytoplasmic inclusion bodies. Pustular dermatitis caused by secondary pyoderma may be present. Experimentally infected dogs commonly develop *bone lesions*, with necrosis of osteoclasts and consequent persistence of the primary spongiosa. Pale streaks in the heart caused by multifocal *myocardial necrosis and mineralization* are described in association with canine distemper.

The histologic findings are characteristic if a spectrum of lesions is present and inclusion bodies are discovered. Rabies and poxviruses are the other causes of intracytoplasmic inclusions in dogs, but the clinical and pathologic findings in these diseases are usually distinct from canine distemper. Other viruses causing inclusion bodies in bronchiolar or airway epithelial cells include canine adenovirus 2, canid herpesvirus 1, and canine minute virus (canine parvovirus 1). Confirmation of the diagnosis benefits from a diversity of diagnostic options, including virus isolation, immunohistochemistry, indirect immunofluorescence, in situ hybridization, and PCR.

Further reading

Beineke A, et al. Pathogenesis and immunopathology of systemic and nervous canine distemper. Vet Immunol Immunopathol 2009;127: 1-18.
Martella V. Canine distemper virus. Vet Clin North Am Small Anim Pract 2008;38:787-797.
Vandevelde M. Demyelination in canine distemper virus infection: a review. Acta Neuropathol 2005;109:56-68.

Canine parainfluenza. *Canine parainfluenza virus* (CPIV) (genus *Rubulavirus*, family *Paramyxoviridae*) causes clinical signs 3-10 days after experimental infection, mainly of fever and hacking cough typical of infectious tracheobronchitis. Virus is shed in nasal secretions for about 8 days after infection. Lesions are of *tracheobronchitis and bronchiolitis*, with epithelial vacuolation and necrosis, mixed cellular inflammatory infiltrates, and submucosal edema. Subacute and chronic lesions include bronchitis and bronchiolitis with epithelial hyperplasia and occasionally bronchiolitis obliterans. The virus does not replicate in macrophages and does not induce significant bronchointerstitial pneumonia in immunocompetent dogs. Canine parainfluenza virus can act as a primary pathogen, but mainly causes disease in conjunction with *Bordetella* infection. In addition, CPIV-2 predisposes to bacterial pneumonia by impairing mucociliary clearance, and increases the bronchoconstrictive response to agonists such as histamine. Infection has been shown to impair olfaction in the absence of nasal lesions; the clinical significance of this intriguing phenomenon is unknown.

Further reading

Ellis JA, Krakowka GS. A review of canine parainfluenza virus infection in dogs. J Am Vet Med Assoc 2012;240:273-284.
Weese JS, Stull J. Respiratory disease outbreak in a veterinary hospital associated with canine parainfluenza virus infection. Can Vet J 2013;54:79-82.

Canine respiratory coronavirus. *Canine respiratory coronavirus* (CRCoV) infection was first identified as a cause of respiratory disease in 2003, and occurs mostly in situations of frequent contact with other dogs. The causative virus is in the genus *Betacoronavirus*, family *Coronaviridae*, and is thus related to bovine coronavirus. In contrast, enteric or pantropic canine coronavirus is an alphacoronavirus. CRCoV infections cause mild upper respiratory tract disease, leading to nonspecific clinical signs of coughing and nasal discharge. Following experimental infection with CRCoV, viral shedding from the oropharynx has been detected for up to 10 days using RT-PCR and by virus isolation for up to 6 days postinfection.

CRCoV preferentially infects canine respiratory epithelial cells, including ciliated cells and goblet cells in the trachea, bronchi, and bronchioles. The reported lesions include shortening or loss of cilia on ciliated cells and a modest inflammatory response, mainly in the upper respiratory tract, with only minor lesions in the lung. Diagnosis of CRCoV infection can be made using ELISA and immunofluorescence. Serology, using paired sera 2-3 weeks apart, is valuable to follow animals during an outbreak of CIRD.

Further reading

Mitchell JA, et al. Tropism and pathological findings associated with canine respiratory coronavirus (CRCoV). Vet Microbiol 2013;162:582-594.
Priestnall SL, et al. New and emerging pathogens in canine infectious respiratory disease. Vet Pathol 2014;51:492-504.

Canine influenza. H3N8 influenza A virus infection as a cause of respiratory disease in dogs was first recognized in 2004 in racing greyhounds, with subsequent identification in other populations of dogs. The virus has homology to and is thought to have arisen from equine influenza virus. The virus spreads readily among dogs, and thus is most common in animals involved in racing, shows, or frequent commingling with others. Rarely, dogs are infected with other influenza viruses, but inefficient transmission between dogs has so far limited their impact.

Clinically, canine influenza is usually a self-limiting upper respiratory tract disease that manifests as anorexia, oculonasal discharge, and coughing. Histologically, influenza virus infection causes tracheobronchial epithelial cell necrosis, hyperplasia, and infiltration of neutrophils, and a unique lesion that similarly affects the bronchial glands. Less frequent is involvement of the distal airways, with bronchiolar erosion or hyperplasia with neutrophil exudates in the lumen, and alveolar infection with neutrophils in alveolar lumens and subtle proliferation of type II pneumocytes. In racing greyhounds, influenza can cause severe peracute disease and death related to hemorrhagic pneumonia associated with bacterial infection; hemorrhage into the pleural cavity and mediastinum may also be present. Diagnosis of canine influenza is based on RT-PCR assays using samples collected from the upper airways of typically affected dogs. Influenza virus can also be isolated from upper airway—nasal or tracheal collected at autopsy.

Further reading

Castleman WL, et al. Canine H3N8 influenza virus infection in dogs and mice. Vet Pathol 2010;47:507-517.

Crawford PC, et al. Transmission of equine influenza virus to dogs. Science 2005;310:482-485.

Dubovi EJ. Canine influenza. Vet Clin North Am Small Anim Pract 2010;40:1063-1071.

Other canine respiratory viruses. Several viruses representing diverse taxonomic origins have recently been identified in respiratory tissues of dogs with mild respiratory disease. These viruses are **canine pneumovirus, canine hepacivirus, and canine bocavirus.** Their causal role in canine respiratory disease is thus far inconclusive. **Pantropic canine coronavirus,** an alphacoronavirus (related to feline coronaviruses and transmissible gastroenteritis virus, but more distantly to betacoronaviruses, including canine respiratory coronavirus) mainly causes enteric and neurologic disease but has been associated with necrotizing bronchiolitis and pulmonary vascular necrosis.

Canine adenovirus 2 (CAV-2) is serologically related to, but genetically distinct from, CAV-1, the cause of infectious canine hepatitis. The contribution of CAV-2 to CIRD complex is assumed to be similar to CPIV-2 discussed previously. Naturally occurring adenoviral pneumonia is rare in dogs, and is usually a consequence of immunosuppression. Gross lesions may be cranioventral or disseminated, lobular or confluent, and consist of atelectasis, reddening, edema, and mild firmness. *Amphophilic intranuclear inclusions* are present in alveolar macrophages, type II pneumocytes, and airway epithelium. Bronchioles contain necrotic epithelial cells and suppurative exudate, and macrophages, neutrophils, and fibrin are present in alveoli. Peribronchiolar and interstitial infiltrates of lymphocytes occur but are not prominent.

Canid herpesvirus 1 is occasionally isolated from dogs with *acute respiratory disease,* although systemic disease in neonatal puppies is a more common manifestation. Aerosol challenge of 12-week-old dogs caused necrotizing rhinitis, bronchointerstitial pneumonia, and multifocal alveolar necrosis with infrequent eosinophilic intranuclear inclusion bodies. Intraperitoneal inoculation of neonatal puppies with the same viral strain caused necrosis and hemorrhages in many organs, supporting the contention that the manifestation of disease is dependent on the route of exposure and the age of the host. Herpesviruses are infrequently isolated from dogs with kennel cough, either alone or with other infectious agents. The respiratory lesions are those to be expected from herpesviruses, namely necrotizing rhinotracheitis and possibly bronchopneumonia. Eosinophilic intranuclear inclusions can sometimes be found in epithelial cells in early lesions, particularly in nasal mucosa.

Further reading

Erles K, Brownlie J. Canine respiratory coronavirus: an emerging pathogen in the canine infectious respiratory disease complex. Vet Clin North Am Small Anim Pract 2008;38:815-825.

Kapoor A, et al. Characterization of novel canine bocaviruses and their association with respiratory disease. J Gen Virol 2012;3:341-346.

Renshaw RW, et al. Pneumovirus in dogs with acute respiratory disease. Emerg Infect Dis 2010;16:993-995.

Bacterial diseases

Pneumonia caused by opportunistic bacterial pathogens is moderately common in dogs. Because most of the pathogens involved are commonly isolated from healthy dogs, a diagnosis of bacterial pneumonia should prompt a search for predisposing causes. *Aspiration pneumonia* is frequent in dogs and may result from anesthesia, megaesophagus, myasthenia gravis, neurologic disease, laryngeal paralysis, or other causes of regurgitation or vomiting. Alternatively, bacterial pneumonia may arise as a consequence of *impaired respiratory defenses.* These include respiratory viral infections (reviewed previously); drugs that induce immunosuppression or neutropenia; concurrent disease conditions that impair immune responses or neutrophil function, including uremia, hyperadrenocorticism, diabetes mellitus, parvoviral enteritis, systemic mycoses, or primary immunodeficiencies; ciliary dyskinesia; and environmental and social stresses.

Multiple bacterial pathogens may be isolated from the lung of some dogs with bacterial pneumonia, as would be expected if the primary problem in these dogs is a failure of lung defenses. *Bordetella bronchiseptica, Streptococcus* spp., *Staphylococcus* spp., *Pasteurella multocida, E. coli, Klebsiella pneumoniae, Pseudomonas aeruginosa,* and *Acinetobacter* spp. are the most common isolates from transtracheal aspirates of dogs with pneumonia. *Bordetella, Streptococcus,* and extraintestinal pathogenic *E. coli* (ExPEC) are discussed more fully later. Other strains of *E. coli* are frequently associated with aspiration pneumonia; complications include bacteremia or disseminated intravascular coagulation.

The morphology of bacterial pneumonia in dogs does not usually suggest a specific infectious agent (see Bronchopneumonia, previously). Lesions may affect entire lobes or follow a lobular distribution. Unilateral or lobar pneumonia may suggest aspiration as the cause.

Streptococcus zooepidemicus (β-hemolytic, group C) is an opportunistic pathogen causing bronchopneumonia as described previously. It is also notable for causing outbreaks of fatal hemorrhagic pneumonia in dogs. Affected dogs have fever, depression, and dyspnea, with a rapidly progressive fatal course. The typical pathologic findings are acute hemorrhagic pneumonia, in some cases with bloody thoracic and mediastinal fluid. Gram-positive cocci are histologically visible, and thrombosis and fibrin exudation may be present; neutrophils can be few or many, presumably dependent on the rapidity of disease progression. Clusters of bacteria may also be observed in spleen and renal glomeruli. Exotoxins perhaps acting as superantigens are thought to play a role in development of disease, and the degree of host cytokine production may also be important.

ExPEC, which produces cytotoxic necrotizing factor-1, α-hemolysin, and other toxins, can be isolated from the lungs of dogs and cats following a very rapid clinical course that leads to death in 24-48 hours. In laboratory dogs, an association with recent arrival at the facility is described. Infection is thought to reach the lung by inhalation or via the blood, and does not apparently result from aspiration of gastrointestinal content. The gross distribution of ExPEC pneumonia may be bilateral, unilateral, or asymmetrical, and multifocal, diffuse, or patchy. The characteristic features are *extensive hemorrhage, coagulative necrosis, thrombosis, and aggregates of tiny coccobacilli*. Some lesions have very few leukocytes despite the presence of many bacteria, whereas others have more typical infiltration of neutrophils. Necrotizing lesions may be present in liver and other organs. Definitive diagnosis is based on identification of toxin genes in the bacterial isolate.

Bordetella bronchiseptica is a gram-negative coccobacillus that is commonly carried in the upper respiratory tract, but not the lungs, of healthy dogs, cats, and many other domestic animals. It can act as a primary pathogen, causing tracheobronchitis and occasionally pneumonia, but causes more frequent and more severe disease in polymicrobial infections with viruses, mycoplasmas, and other bacteria. Some animals are affected by tracheobronchitis and develop persistent, harsh, nonproductive or productive coughing, but are otherwise clinically normal. Most of these cases recover spontaneously, although signs can persist for 3 weeks or longer. Other cases develop bacterial pneumonia with lethargy and dyspnea; only half of affected dogs have fever or leukocytosis. The gross and histologic findings are similar to bronchopneumonia caused by other bacteria, with the unique finding of cilia-adherent bacteria in the large airways of some cases. These appear as a densely fibrillar layer covering the respiratory epithelium, and are highlighted by Warthin-Starry silver stain or Gram stain (Fig. 5-71).

There is considerable genetic diversity among strains of *B. bronchiseptica*, but the relation of genetic variation and virulence remains an area for exploration. The expression of virulence factors of *Bordetella* is dependent on environmental conditions, regulated by the *Bordetella virulence gene (bvg) operon*. In vitro, such virulence genes are repressed at 25° C or in the presence of sulfate or nicotinic acid, and activated at 37° C. After entering the host, a first wave of *bvg*-regulated genes expressed, including those encoding the adhesive proteins filamentous hemagglutinin (FHA) and pertactin, and fimbriae that allow *B. bronchiseptica* to attach to ciliated epithelial cells. Following attachment of bacteria to the mucosal surface, a second wave of *bvg*-regulated genes is expressed that

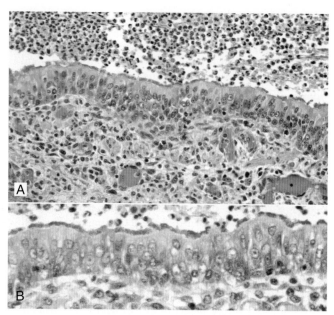

Figure 5-71 ***Bordetella bronchiseptica*** **pneumonia** in a dog. The lesions are typical of bronchopneumonia, with the unique feature of cilia-adherent bacteria in the large airways. **A.** An inflamed bronchus contains neutrophils in the lumen, and basophilic carpeting of the apical surface of the epithelial cells. **B.** Brown and Hopps stain highlights the cilia-adherent gram-negative bacteria.

mediate motility, iron scavenging, and urease and phosphatase activity.

Secreted toxins are important contributors to bordetellosis. The adenylate cyclase toxin (hemolysin) is an RTX toxin, like *Mannheimia haemolytica* leukotoxin and the Apx toxins of *Actinobacillus pleuropneumoniae*. The RTX domain of the toxin forms pores in target cell membranes that permit transfer of the adenylate cyclase component. Entry of this toxin into leukocytes causes increased cyclic AMP production that impairs phagocytosis and oxidative burst.

Other virulence factors that are not regulated by the *bvg* operon include a lipo-oligosaccharide with endotoxin activity and a soluble peptidoglycan-derived tracheal cytotoxin. The latter is not directly toxic to tracheal epithelium, but stimulates host cells to produce nitric oxide that in turn induces ciliostasis and apoptosis of ciliated epithelial cells.

B. bronchiseptica can adhere to macrophages and neutrophils, probably by binding of FHA to complement receptors on macrophages. Following adhesion, the bacteria are internalized and survive within macrophages without inciting an oxidative burst, and may induce apoptosis of these cells through secretion of the adenylate cyclase toxin. In addition, *Bordetella* is able to enter and survive within nonphagocytic cells, presumably affording protection from host defenses and a ready supply of nutrients.

Although mucosal antibody responses are detectable within 4 days of infection, and the duration of clinical illness is usually only 2-3 weeks, *Bordetella* infections often persist for 2-3 months, and infected dogs may remain a source of infection for others in the kennel. Immune responses to *B. bronchiseptica* confer partial protection against subsequent challenge. FHA and pertactin are immunodominant antigens, and mucosal antibody responses to these antigens are partially protective.

Further reading

Breitschwerdt EB, et al. Isolation of necrotoxigenic *Escherichia coli* from a dog with hemorrhagic pneumonia. J Am Vet Med Assoc 2005;226:2016-2019.

Handt LK, et al. Clinical and microbiologic characterization of hemorrhagic pneumonia due to extraintestinal pathogenic *Escherichia coli* in four young dogs. Comp Med 2003;53:663-670.

Kogan DA, et al. Clinical, clinicopathologic, and radiographic findings in dogs with aspiration pneumonia: 88 cases (2004-2006). J Am Vet Med Assoc 2008;233:1742-1747.

Lamm CG, et al. Streptococcal infection in dogs: a retrospective study of 393 cases. Vet Pathol 2010;47:387-395.

Pesavento PA, et al. A clonal outbreak of acute fatal hemorrhagic pneumonia in intensively housed (shelter) dogs caused by *Streptococcus equi* subsp. *zooepidemicus*. Vet Pathol 2008;45:51-53.

Radhakrishnan A, et al. Community-acquired infectious pneumonia in puppies: 65 cases (1993-2002). J Am Vet Med Assoc 2007;230:1493-1497.

Mycoplasmal diseases

Mycoplasmas that infect the respiratory tract of dogs include *Mycoplasma canis*, *M. cynos*, *M. bovigenitalium*, *M. spumans*, *M. edwardii*, *M. gateae*, *M. feliminutum*, and several unclassified species of *Mycoplasma*, *Ureaplasma*, and *Acholeplasma*. Mycoplasmas are present in the nasopharynx of most normal dogs, and can be isolated from tracheobronchial washes from about 30% of normal adult dogs and a similar percentage of those with pneumonia. Of the mycoplasmas, **M. cynos** is the most pathogenic. Experimental infection with *M. cynos* did not result in clinical signs of disease, but induced peribronchial infiltration of lymphocytes and plasma cells, exfoliation and hyperplasia of bronchiolar epithelium, and neutrophil exudation into bronchioles and alveoli. Its presence does seem to contribute to the polymicrobial respiratory disease that develops in animal shelters.

Other mycoplasmas appear to be minimally pathogenic. Experimental infection with *M. bovigenitalium* resulted in mild suppurative and lymphocytic bronchiolitis, but no clinical signs. Pathologic or clinical changes were not apparent in dogs challenged with *M. spumans*, *M. canis*, or *M. gateae*. Unclassified mycoplasmas have been associated with similar lesions and with chronic bronchitis and bronchiectasis in dogs.

Further reading

Hong S, Kim O. Molecular identification of *Mycoplasma cynos* from laboratory beagle dogs with respiratory disease. Lab Anim Res 2012;28:61-66.

Zeugswetter F, et al. Lethal bronchopneumonia caused by *Mycoplasma cynos* in a litter of golden retriever puppies. Vet Rec 2007;161:626-627.

Fungal diseases

Mycotic rhinitis. Mycotic rhinitis is common in dogs and occasionally diagnosed in other species. Cases may be presented with variable combinations of chronic sneezing, stertor, unilateral or bilateral mucopurulent nasal discharge, nasal hemorrhage, and nasal pain. Distortion of nasal bones may occur, and extension of infection to adjacent structures may rarely induce exophthalmos or neurologic disease.

Aspergillus fumigatus is the usual cause of mycotic rhinitis in dogs, although other species of *Aspergillus* or *Penicillium* are occasional causes of otherwise similar disease. These fungi are common in the environment and reach the nasal cavity of most normal animals by inhalation. It is not known whether disease results from exposure to higher numbers of inhaled fungi or from suppression of the normal nasal defenses, but immunosuppression or other predisposing causes have only rarely been identified in dogs with nasal aspergillosis.

Lesions are often focal within the nasal cavity or paranasal sinuses, and consist of yellow, green, or black plaque-like mats or masses of fungal growth (Fig. 5-72). The surrounding mucosa is hyperemic and edematous, and there is often purulent exudate, caseous debris, or hemorrhage throughout the nasal cavity. Destruction of turbinate bones is common, and remodeling of the nasal septum or nasal bones may occur. *Histologic diagnosis requires biopsy of the fungal plaques*, which may be very localized despite the presence of widespread exudate. The plaques consist entirely of fungal hyphae, and occasionally contain conidia (see Fig. 5-72). *Aspergillus* spp. hyphae are 5-7 μm diameter and have parallel sides, frequent septa, and branch dichotomously at 45°C. The infection is noninvasive, and hyphae are very rarely observed in biopsies of inflamed nasal tissue biopsies, but these tissues do have nonspecific lesions of suppurative or eosinophilic rhinitis. *Aspergillus* also causes chronic rhinitis and pulmonary fungus ball in German Shepherd dogs, described previously (see eFig. 5-45).

Further reading

Day MJ. Canine sino-nasal aspergillosis: parallels with human disease. Med Mycol 2009;47:S315-S323.

Sharman MJ, Mansfield CS. Sinonasal aspergillosis in dogs: a review. J Small Anim Pract 2012;53:434-444.

Rhinosporidiosis. Rhinosporidiosis is a disease of humans and dogs, and rarely of other domestic mammals and fowl. The disease is endemic in wet tropical and subtropical environments, uncommon in North America and Africa, and rare in Europe. It has been determined by molecular analyses that the causative agent, **Rhinosporidium seeberi**, is not a fungus, but is a member of the Mesomycetozoa or so-called "DRIP" *clade of aquatic protistan parasites*. The agent can be cultured only with specialized techniques. Infection results from exposure of nasal mucosa to contaminated water.

The typical lesion is a *single unilateral nasal polyp*, which is soft, pink, up to 3-cm diameter, and bleeds easily. Histologic investigation reveals epithelial hyperplasia, loose fibrous tissue, lymphoplasmacytic inflammation, and sporangia of *R. seeberi* (Fig. 5-73). Juvenile sporangia are 15-75 μm diameter, contain a single nucleus, and have a unilamellar PAS-positive wall. Mature sporangia, which may be visible grossly as pinpoint white foci, are 100-500 μm diameter with a bilamellar wall, and contain numerous 5-10 μm diameter endospores. The large size of the sporangia and the presence of endospores might only be mistaken for *Coccidioides*, and finding such structures in a nasal polyp is considered diagnostic.

Further reading

Burgess HJ, et al. Equine laryngeal rhinosporidiosis in western Canada. J Vet Diagn Invest 2012;24:777-780.

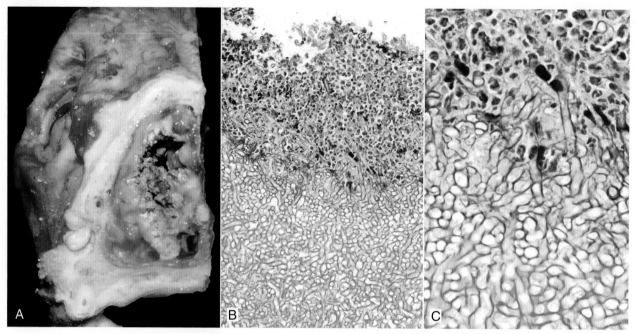

Figure 5-72 Nasal aspergillosis in a dog. **A.** Transverse section of nasal cavity, with unusually exuberant growth of green mold excavating the conchae. **B.** Fungal plaque formed by a mass of fungal hyphae but, as is typical, no recognizable host tissue. **C.** Higher magnification of the parallel-sided hyphae, with eosinophil accumulation at the surface.

Hill SA, et al. Nasal rhinosporidiosis in two dogs native to the upper Mississippi river valley region. J Am Anim Hosp Assoc 2010;46: 127-131.

Blastomycosis. *Blastomycosis is an infectious noncontagious disease primarily of dogs and humans,* with fewer cases in cats, horses, and other species. The disease occurs primarily in North America, with occasional cases in Africa, Europe, Asia, and Central America. Endemically infected areas in North America include the Mississippi, Ohio, and St. Lawrence River valleys, northern Ontario in Canada, and the mid-Atlantic States in the United States.

Blastomyces dermatitidis is a dimorphic fungus. At environmental temperatures, it grows as a mycelial form and produces spores that are infectious to animals. The ecologic source of the mycelial form is uncertain, but is associated with acidic sandy soils. *Recently disturbed soil* is a recognized factor in some outbreaks, and geographic clustering of cases is well documented. *At body temperatures, the fungus grows as a yeast form that is not contagious.* Although the potential exists for mycelial forms to grow in cooled tissue specimens, reports of infection acquired at autopsy are rare and have been caused by accidental penetrating wounds rather than inhalation.

Virulence factors of *B. dermatitidis* are poorly described. BAD-1 is a surface protein that mediates adhesion to host cells, may modulate the inflammatory response, and is an immunodominant antigen. Antibody responses to BAD-1 reduce disease severity, but are not completely protective. The cell-wall polysaccharide α-glucan is associated with virulence and may protect against killing by macrophages.

Infection is usually acquired by inhalation of spores into the lung, where they rapidly transform to the yeast form. Local inoculation may be the cause of the rare lesions that are restricted to the skin. Experimentally infected dogs develop a much higher prevalence of lesions than for other systemic

mycoses, although in most the disease is mild and resolves without treatment. Subclinically infected dogs are apparently rare. Yeast forms proliferate in the lungs and disseminate via the blood and lymphatic vessels. Naturally infected animals may have suppression of humoral and cellular immune responses but, as for other systemic mycoses, this probably represents an effect rather than a cause of the disease. Most animals do not have pre-existing immunosuppressive conditions. T-helper-1 immune responses have been associated with protection in mouse models, and immune responses target cell-wall components, including BAD-1.

The lung is the most consistently affected site. Grossly, there is generalized multifocal distribution of 3-mm to several-centimeter diameter, coalescing, grey-white nodules of granulomatous inflammation (Fig. 5-74, eFig. 5-100). Most pulmonary nodules are firm throughout, but some undergo central caseation and resemble abscesses. Such foci may fistulate into a bronchus or onto the pleura. Mineralization is minimal or absent. Microscopically, coalescing granulomas are formed by epithelioid macrophages, histiocytic giant cells and variable numbers of neutrophils, an outer layer of lymphocytes and less reactive macrophages, and often a peripheral rim of fibrous tissue (see Fig. 5-74). In some cases, there is extensive caseous necrosis in the centers of the granulomas, with merely a thin rim of macrophages. *Yeast bodies are quite variable in number and may be overlooked if only H&E-stained sections are examined;* in cases treated with antifungal drugs or with partial immunity, a diligent search of sections stained by the periodic acid–Schiff reaction or with methenamine silver may be required to reveal the fungi. The yeast forms are 5-15 μm (or occasionally up to 30 μm) diameter, round, non-encapsulated, with a distinct wall about 1-μm thick, and granular protoplasm completely or partly filling the center (see Fig. 5-74). The double contour of the wall that is well described in cytologic preparations or culture imprints is often

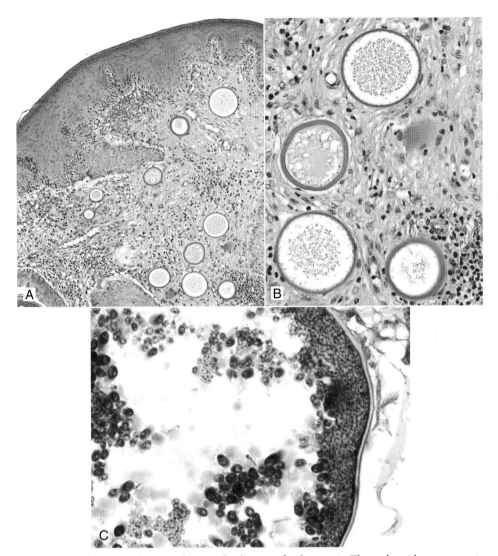

Figure 5-73 *Rhinosporidium seeberi* **in the larynx of a horse. A.** The polypoid mass contains juvenile sporangia, up to 100-μm diameter, in the lamina propria. **B.** Detail of juvenile sporangia. **C.** Mature sporangium with multiple endospores. (Courtesy H. Burgess.)

inapparent histologically. Occasional yeast display *broad-based budding* of single daughter cells. Filamentous or pseudohyphal forms and conidia are infrequently found in tissues, and are usually accompanied by yeast forms.

Disseminated lesions are common in lymph nodes, eyes, skin and subcutaneous tissues, bones, and joints. Testes, prostate, brain, heart, liver, spleen, kidneys, intestines, and other organs are less commonly affected. The lesions are either granulomas with numerous epithelioid and giant cells, or pyogranulomatous foci with central accumulation and necrosis of neutrophils and macrophages.

Demonstration of the yeast bodies in tissue section or in cytologic preparations is the usual method of diagnosis. Blastomyces is readily differentiated from other fungi in culture, but safety precautions must be in place because infection of laboratory personnel by the cultured mycelia is well documented. An immunoassay to detect *B. dermatitidis* galactomannan has become a widely used clinical test; the sensitivity to detect the fungal antigen was 94% for urine and 87% for serum. Serologic tests are available, but false negatives are common.

The *differential diagnosis* for multinodular lesions in lung and other organs includes other systemic mycoses and metastatic neoplasia. Examination of impression smears or histologic sections may be needed to distinguish neoplasia from mycoses. Morphologic features are usually adequate to differentiate *Blastomyces* from other fungi: *Cryptococcus neoformans* usually has a thick capsule and only a mild inflammatory response, *Histoplasma capsulatum* at 2-4 μm is much smaller and resides in the cytoplasm of macrophages, and *Coccidioides immitis* at 20-200 μm is much larger and often contains endospores. Mutants of *Cryptococcus* that lack the characteristic thick capsule may closely resemble *Blastomyces* and incite a similar granulomatous response, but the presence of narrow-based budding differentiates them from *Blastomyces* which divides by broad-based budding. *Blastomyces, Cryptococcus,* and *Histoplasma* are reliably differentiated in culture by the presence and morphology of mycelia, conidia, and yeast.

Further reading

Davies JL, et al. Prevalence and geographic distribution of canine and feline blastomycosis in the Canadian prairies. Can Vet J 2013;54: 753-760.

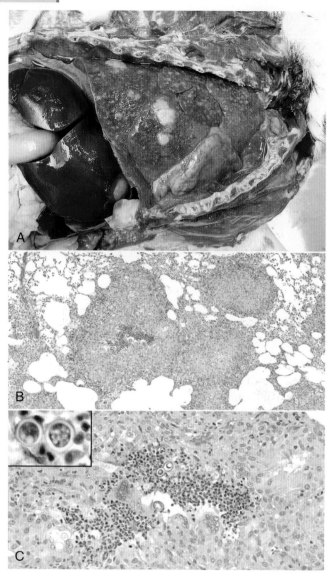

Figure 5-74 Blastomycosis. A. The lung contains multiple coalescing nodules. (Courtesy Michigan State University.) **B.** Coalescing granulomas. **C.** Pulmonary granuloma formed by epithelioid macrophages, giant cells, and central neutrophil accumulation with yeast bodies. Inset: higher magnification of thick-walled yeast bodies.

Werner A, Norton F. Blastomycosis. Compend Contin Educ Vet 2011; 33:E1-E4.

Cryptococcosis. Cryptococcosis is a mycotic disease of worldwide distribution caused by **Cryptococcus neoformans** or **Cryptococcus gatti**. *Cryptococcosis is the most common systemic mycotic disease of cats*, and it also affects dogs, horses, cattle, humans, and many other species. Disease is sporadic and, as is generally true for the systemic mycoses, the infection is apparently *neither contagious nor zoonotic. Many cases have chronic nasal disease*, with sneezing and serous or mucopurulent discharge. Other common manifestations include ulcerating cutaneous nodules, encephalitis, chorioretinitis or panophthalmitis, and pneumonia.

Cryptococcus spp. are basidiomycete yeast-like fungi. Unlike the dimorphic fungi *Blastomyces* and *Coccidioides*, the sexual mycelial phase of *Cryptococcus* does not occur under normal laboratory conditions. *Cryptococcus neoformans*, the usual cause of disease in temperate climates, is a saprophyte found in soil, pigeon or other avian guano, and decaying organic matter. *C. gatti* historically was found mainly in tropical climates, but is now considered to have a global distribution and is an important cause of disease in humans and dogs, especially in the Pacific Northwest of North America. *C. neoformans* and *C. gatti* exist in these environments in a filamentous form known as a teleomorph, with the name *Filobasidiella neoformans* and *F. bacillosporus*, respectively; this form of the organism undergoes both sexual as well as asexual reproduction in the environment. Based on genome sequence information *C. neoformans* is subdivided into types VNI, VNII, VNIII, and VNIV, and *C. gatti* is divided into VGI, VGII, VGIII, and VGIV. Where the agents fall in this classification scheme is of more than academic interest, as the pathogenicity and response to therapy varies by subtype of the organisms.

Dogs are primarily infected with *C. neoformans* (except in regions with high endemicity for *C. gatti*, i.e., the Pacific Northwest of North America), whereas *C. gatti* is more frequent in cats. *Most infected animals do not develop clinical disease*. Immune suppression, such as from corticosteroid therapy or pre-existing infections, often underlies *C. neoformans* infections, but *C. gatti* is a primary pathogen and may infect hosts without known immune deficiencies. Infection is usually acquired by inhalation of basidiospores or desiccated yeast from contaminated dust. These small forms are inhaled into alveoli, where replication can occur with subsequent spread hematogenously or locally to other organs, such as the brain, eyes, lymph nodes, skin, and other organs. Occasional cases of cutaneous cryptococcosis are probably the result of local inoculation, and *cryptococcal mastitis* in cows is an ascending rather than hematogenous infection.

The major virulence factors of Cryptococcus are the capsule and the production of melanin. The thick capsule, composed of glucuronoxylomannan and other mannose-rich polysaccharides, impairs phagocytosis, activates complement, and may suppress T-cell responses. The role of the capsule in concealing the yeast from the immune response is highlighted by uncommon strains of *Cryptococcus* that lack a capsule; these are readily phagocytosed, incite a strong granulomatous response, and are generally minimally pathogenic. Most strains consistently produce a capsule in tissues, but its thickness is variable in cultures. The ability to synthesize melanin when grown on specific substrates is associated with virulence, and attributed in part to the enzyme phenoloxidase (laccase). Melanin and/or phenoloxidase may scavenge oxygen radicals produced by activated macrophages, and modulate the host immunoinflammatory response. Other potential virulence factors include secretion of eicosanoids and mannose protein that modulate immune and inflammatory responses, and production of superoxide dismutase and laccase that augment resistance to oxidative killing.

Immunity to *Cryptococcus* is dependent on delayed-type hypersensitivity reactions, in which IFN-γ and other cytokines elicit and activate macrophages and perhaps neutrophils to kill the yeast by using reactive nitrogen and oxygen intermediates. In addition, cytotoxic T-cell responses may directly limit viability or proliferation of this pathogen.

Lesions take the form of gelatinous masses, granulomas, or ulcerating nodules. Facial swelling is a common feature of cryptococcal rhinitis of cats. Infection may spread locally from the nasal cavity to involve the skin, oral mucosa, eyes, or brain,

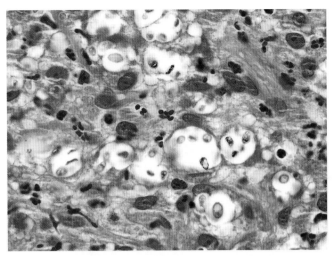

Figure 5-75 *Cryptococcus neoformans* **in the lung of a dog,** with characteristic thick mucoid capsule, small cell bodies, occasional melanization, and minimal inflammatory response.

and occasionally there is wider dissemination to local lymph nodes, lung, and other viscera. Skin lesions are often nodular and ulcerative. Visceral lesions consist of multifocal discrete white gelatinous lesions. Gross lesions in the brain are often subtle, but may include gelatinous material in meninges and ventricles.

The prominent histologic lesion is a mass of yeast, and the abundant nonstaining capsular material lends a "soap bubble" appearance to the lesion. In contrast to other mycotic infections, the granulomatous reaction is often quite minimal, presumably because the capsule masks the yeast from recognition by phagocytes. *C. neoformans* yeast bodies are 4-8 μm diameter, plus a capsule that varies from 1-30 μm thick (Fig. 5-75). Occasional yeast have single buds that are attached by a thin stalk; *this narrow-based budding differentiates Cryptococcus from Blastomyces.*

The *diagnosis* is usually based on identifying the yeast in histologic sections or cytologic smears. *The thick capsule is characteristic,* C. neoformans *being the only pathogenic fungus with a capsule,* and it can be further identified with mucicarmine. In wet mounts, the capsule can be identified by negative staining with India ink. The yeast bodies stain with periodic acid–Schiff or methenamine silver stains, and melanin production may be demonstrated with Masson-Fontana stain. Culture is required for definitive diagnosis. Detection of antibodies to capsular antigen in serum or cerebrospinal fluid is a useful method of clinical diagnosis.

Further reading

Lester SJ, et al. Cryptococcosis: update and emergence of *Cryptococcus gatti*. Vet Clin Pathol 2011;40:4-17.

Vorathavorn VI, et al. Cryptococcosis as an emerging systemic mycosis in dogs. J Vet Emerg Crit Care 2013;23:489-497.

Coccidioidomycosis. Coccidioidomycosis, caused by the dimorphic fungi **Coccidioides immitis** or **C. posadasii,** is endemic in the semiarid Lower Sonoran life zone of the southwestern United States, northern Mexico, and parts of Central and South America. The fungus can apparently infect all mammals, with reports of disease occurring in a variety of terrestrial and aquatic mammals; in addition, it is a persistent and serious health issue in humans living in these areas. In veterinary medicine, the disease primarily affects dogs, is less common in horses and cats, and may cause incidental pulmonary lesions in cattle and swine. Clinical manifestations in dogs include fever; chronic respiratory disease with coughing, weight loss, and eventual respiratory distress; visceral disease causing anorexia, weight loss, and malaise; draining cutaneous nodules; lameness resulting from osteomyelitis; ocular disease; and heart failure resulting from myocardial or pericardial lesions. Nodular skin disease is the most common presenting sign in cats. Clinical findings in horses include chronic weight loss, pulmonary disease, and lameness resulting from osteomyelitis.

Coccidioides is a geophilic dimorphic fungus. The mycelial form survives well in dry hot conditions, grows after periods of intense rainfall in soil containing fecal or other organic matter, and releases arthroconidia that are disseminated widely in wind-blown dust after the soil desiccates. *Inhalation of airborne arthroconidia is the usual route of infection;* local inoculation occasionally causes a cutaneous lesion that does not usually progress to systemic infection. *Although most animals in endemic areas probably become infected during their life, relatively few develop disease.* Following deposition in the lung, the arthroconidia transform into the yeast form. Immature *spherules* are 10-20 μm diameter; as they mature, the spherules (or sporangia) enlarge up to 200 μm diameter and develop numerous 2-5 μm *endospores* (Fig. 5-76). Mature spherules rupture, and the released endospores form either new spherules in tissue or mycelia if released to the environment. Infection of autopsy personnel has been attributed to inhalation of aerosolized tissue endospores, although the paucity of such cases suggests the risk is limited.

Lesions may be limited to the *lungs,* where they vary from nodular to miliary. The *pyogranulomas or granulomas* are greywhite nodules that often contain a caseous or liquefying center. Large nodules may be formed by a collection of small discrete granulomas separated by fibrous tissue. The initial reaction to the infectious forms—inhaled arthroconidia and endospores released from mature spherules—is primarily suppurative. The lesion forms a pyogranuloma or granuloma as it matures, with epithelioid macrophages, a few giant cells, lymphocytes, and neutrophils. In diagnostic cases, the lesions mainly appear as multifocal areas of necrosis with few spherules, and granulomatous or pyogranulomatous inflammation in the adjacent tissue. Formation of discrete granulomas is less frequent. In cattle, spherules are often enmeshed in eosinophilic material similar to the Splendore-Hoeppli phenomenon; this may reflect the higher level of resistance of this species.

Systemic lesions develop from hematogenous spread from the lung. Cases with systemic lesions that lack pulmonary involvement are thought to reflect resolution of the lung disease rather than an extrapulmonary route of infection. Tracheobronchial lymph nodes are often enlarged and reactive, but generalized lymphadenopathy is uncommon. Nodular lesions in the skin develop draining tracts or form fluctuating abscesses. Osteomyelitis often occurs late in the disease, with osteolytic granulomatous or cavitating masses surrounded by proliferating new bone tissue. Granulomatous lesions may be present in the pericardium or the heart and cause right-sided heart failure. Granulomas in the central nervous system are most common in cerebrum and midbrain. Ocular lesions

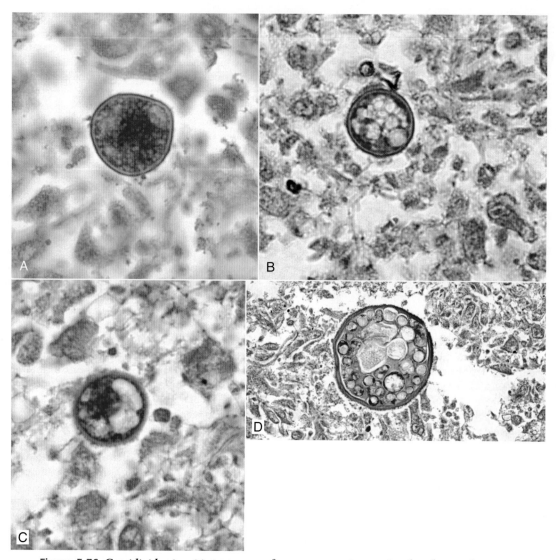

Figure 5-76 *Coccidioides immitis* in an area of caseous necrosis, associated with granulomatous inflammation in the lung of a dog. **A-C.** 10-20 μm uninucleate spherules. **D.** Mature spherule (sporangium) contains multiple endospores and may be up to 200-μm diameter. (Courtesy D. Wilson.)

include chorioretinitis, retinal detachment, anterior uveitis, and keratitis. Other organs affected include liver, spleen, kidney, and testes. Abortion and mastitis are described in horses.

The **diagnosis** is usually established by identifying the spherules in tissue sections, although they are usually present in low number. *The large size and endosporulation of the mature spherules is characteristic,* and can only be confused with *Rhinosporidium seeberi.* Culture is a useful method of definitive identification; safety precautions are essential because arthroconidia are easily detached from the mycelial form and are highly infectious for laboratory personnel. Serum antibodies to *Coccidioides immitis* can be detected in most cases, particularly in the acute stages of disease, and high titers suggest active disease.

Further reading

Graupmann-Kuzma A, et al. Coccidioidomycosis in dogs and cats: a review. J Am Anim Hosp Assoc 2008;44:226-235.

Shubitz LF, et al. T-lymphocyte predominance in lesions of canine coccidioidomycosis. Vet Pathol 2011;48:1008-1011.

Other fungal infections. Adiaspiromycosis is primarily a disease of wild rodents, but rarely affects domestic animals and humans. The causative agents, ***Emmonsia parva*** and ***E. crescens*** (formerly *Chrysosporium* spp.), are dimorphic fungi related to *Blastomyces.* Lesions are most common in the *lung* but occasionally involve local lymph nodes, and consist of *nodules of granulomatous inflammation.* The diagnosis is based on finding adiaspores—large, spherical, uninucleate conidia—in the nodules (Fig. 5-77). The adiaspores of *E. parva* are often 10-20 μm diameter, whereas those of *E. crescens* may be up to 300-μm diameter. Both have a thick (5 μm) PAS-positive wall. Their large size and thick wall might be mistaken for *Coccidioides,* but endosporulation is not a feature of *Emmonsia.*

Lycoperdon spp. (puffball mushrooms) release large numbers of spores to the environment, and inhalation of these spores by dogs incites a multifocal pyogranulomatous reaction

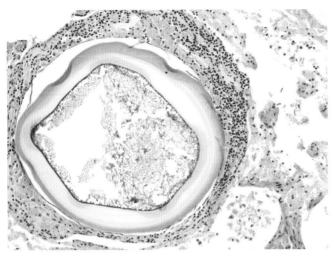

Figure 5-77 **Adiaspiromycosis** in the lung of a badger. Adiaspores of *Emmonsia* sp. are uninucleated and thick walled. (Courtesy D. Ni Bhuachalla.)

throughout the lung. Intracellular and extracellular 3-5 μm diameter spores are visible within the pyogranulomas and are highlighted by silver stains.

Further reading

Alenghat T, et al. Lycoperdonosis in two dogs. J Vet Diagn Invest 2010;22:1002-1005.

Koller LD, et al. Adiaspiromycosis in the lungs of a dog. J Am Vet Med Assoc 1976;169:1316-1317.

Parasitic diseases

***Pneumonyssoides caninum* is a parasitic mite of the nasal cavity and paranasal sinuses of dogs.** The prevalence is ~20% in Scandinavian dogs, but it appears to be less common in other areas. The female adult mite is motile, oval, light yellow, and 1-1.5 mm long. The mites are presumably transmitted by direct contact. They are usually an incidental finding, but clinical signs include sneezing, head shaking, and impaired olfaction. The mites induce catarrhal rhinitis and sinusitis with goblet cell hyperplasia, hyperemia, and infiltration of neutrophils, eosinophils, and lymphocytes. *Pneumonyssoides* is, in addition to allergic rhinitis, a consideration in cases of eosinophil-rich inflammation in the nasal mucosa.

Further reading

Gunnarsson LK, et al. Prevalence of *Pneumonyssoides caninum* infection in dogs in Sweden. J Am Anim Hosp Assoc 2001;37: 331-337.

***Linguatula serrata*: pentastomiasis.** *Linguatula serrata*, a parasitic arthropod, is of wide geographic distribution. Adult pentastomes are large, long-lived, specialized hematophagous parasites of the respiratory tracts of reptiles, amphibians, and carnivorous mammals. They are related to but distinct from the arthropods. The adults of *L. serrata* are transversely striated and tongue shaped (hence the name). Males are ~2 cm in length and females 1.0-1.2 cm. The definitive hosts are carnivores, but in aberrant parasitisms, herbivores and humans

may be host to the final stage. Herbivorous animals are the intermediate hosts. Carnivores are infected by eating the infected viscera of herbivores, and the nymphs migrate to the nasal passages, where they mature. The parasites may be found anywhere in the nasal cavity, and occasionally, they find their way into the paranasal sinuses or pass via the Eustachian tube to the inner ear. They lie on the surface of the nasal mucosa and induce nasal irritation and a catarrhal to lightly blood-stained exudate. The gravid females discharge a large number of eggs that are removed by sneezing.

The larvae of *Linguatula* or pentastomids of other species develop in the alimentary tract of the intermediate host and migrate to the mesenteric lymph nodes and other organs, where they develop into infective nymphs within cysts that are encircled by inflamed fibrous tissue. The nymphs have histologic features of arthropods: pseudosegmented body, a chitinous cuticle with sclerotized openings, striated muscle, and a body cavity, as well as numerous brightly eosinophilic glands, and prominent villi lining the cuboidal epithelial cells in the intestine.

Further reading

Brookins MD, et al. Massive visceral pentastomiasis caused by *Porocephalus crotali* in a dog. Vet Pathol 2009;46:460-463.

Eucoleus aerophilus. *Eucoleus aerophilus* (*Capillaria aerophila*) is a trichurid nematode (order Enoplida, superfamily *Trichuroidea*, family *Trichuridae*) that *parasitizes the trachea and bronchi of wild canids*, domestic dogs, and occasionally cats. The worms are slender, 2-3 cm long, and embedded in the airway mucosa. Histologic examination reveals characteristic features: bacillary bands, which are segmental thickenings of the hypodermis; a stichosome, which is a deeply basophilic gland encircling the esophagus; and the possible presence of embryonated eggs. The eggs are laid in the airways, move with mucus to the pharynx, are swallowed, and passed in the feces. The eggs are oval with characteristic bipolar plugs, and closely resemble those of *Trichuris vulpis* of the intestine or *Pearsonema* (*Capillaria*) *plica* of the urinary bladder. The larvae undergo initial development in the egg, and then progress to the infective stage within earthworms, which are a required intermediate host. Eggs also hatch in ~40 days under suitable environmental conditions, but the resulting larvae are apparently not infective. After ingestion of the earthworm, the larvae reach the lungs in ~1 week and are mature in the trachea in ~25 days. Most infestations of *E. aerophilus* are inapparent and provoke only mild catarrhal inflammation. Heavy infestations cause more severe irritation that may result in obstruction of the lumen of the airways. Chronic coughing and intermittent dyspnea may then be observed, and secondary bacterial bronchopneumonia may occur.

A related trichurid, ***Eucoleus* (*Capillaria*) *boehmi*,** is reported occasionally in the nasal cavity and sinuses of wild canids and rarely in domestic dogs.

Further reading

Traversa D, et al. Canine and feline cardiopulmonary parasitic nematodes in Europe: emerging and underestimated. Parasit Vectors 2010;3:62.

Oslerus osleri. *Oslerus (Filaroides) osleri* is of wide geographic distribution and is common in wild canids. The tracheal nodules are uncommonly encountered during bronchoscopy or autopsy of domestic dogs, and they rarely cause clinical signs of chronic coughing or dyspnea. Most infestations occur in dogs <1 year of age, and are acquired from the dam through grooming or regurgitative feeding.

O. osleri is a 5-15 mm long nematode of the superfamily *Metastrongyloidea*, family *Filaroididae*. The thin-walled embryonated eggs are coughed up and swallowed and many hatch before being passed as infective larvae in the feces. Unlike other metastrongyles, the *Filaroididae* do not require an intermediate host. The first-stage larvae of *O. osleri* are immediately infective, and pups are infected by ingestion of larvae in the saliva, tracheobronchial secretions, or feces of their dams. Larvae migrate from the gut through the blood to the lung. They develop into fifth-stage larvae by 5 weeks after infection, and the tracheal nodules are detectable at 10 weeks and well developed by 18 weeks. The caudal end of the gravid female protrudes through the epithelium, and the eggs are laid onto the tracheal surface.

The typical lesions are single or multiple, 1-10 mm diameter, firm, grey-pink, sessile or polypoid, submucosal nodules in the trachea and bronchi, often in the region of the tracheal bifurcation (Fig. 5-78). The larger masses are oval, with the long axis parallel to that of the trachea. On careful inspection, coiled worms are visible through the intact overlying mucosa.

The nodules are formed by coiled adult or fifth-stage larval nematodes lying in tissue spaces in the lamina propria, and the nodules are often encircled by fibrous tissue. The adults have coelomyarian musculature, a gut formed by a few multinucleated cells with indistinct microvilli, and larvae or embryonated eggs within the uterus. The live worms provoke little reaction apart from a few lymphocytes and plasma cells. Dead worms incite a foreign-body reaction with neutrophils and giant cells. Immature worms, probably still migrating toward the trachea, may be found in the pulmonary lymphatics and occasionally in the alveoli without significant tissue reaction. The *diagnosis* is based on identifying the adults in histologic or crush preparations of the tracheal nodules, or discovering larvae in smears of tracheal mucus or Baermann preparations of feces.

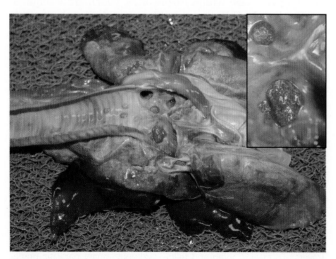

Figure 5-78 *Oslerus osleri* in a wolf. Tightly coiled adult nematodes (inset) form nodules near the tracheal bifurcation. (Courtesy D.G. Campbell.)

Further reading

Yao C, et al. *Filaroides olseri (Oslerus osleri):* two case reports and a review of canid infections in North America. Vet Parasitol 2011; 179:123-129.

Crenosoma vulpis. *Crenosoma vulpis* is a common lungworm of foxes, but also occurs in other canids, including domestic dogs, perhaps in mustelids, but not in cats. It is a nematode of the superfamily *Metastrongyloidea*, family *Crenosomatidae*, and snails and slugs are intermediate hosts. *Adult worms reside in bronchioles and small bronchi.* After a prepatent period of 18-21 days, adults produce larvae that are coughed up, swallowed, and passed in the feces. The usual gross lesions in dogs are gray consolidation of the caudodorsal lung. Histologically, the lesions caused by adult worms are catarrhal, eosinophilic bronchitis and bronchiolitis. Aspirated larvae may induce a granulomatous reaction in alveoli.

Further reading

Conboy G. Natural infections of *Crenosoma vulpis* and *Angiostrongylus vasorum* in dogs in Atlantic Canada and their treatment with milbemycin oxime. Vet Rec 2004;155:16-18.

Angiostrongylus vasorum. *Angiostrongylus vasorum* occurs in endemic foci in parts of Western Europe, and is also reported in Uganda, South America, Eastern Asia, and Atlantic Canada; reports suggest the prevalence is increasing in Europe. Clinical expression of angiostrongylosis varies from mild to severe respiratory disease; cor pulmonale may develop in response to chronic pulmonary vascular disease and lung fibrosis. Other less common clinical signs include neurologic signs referable to cerebral hemorrhage as a result of disseminated intravascular coagulation, as well as miscellaneous signs that reflect aberrant migration of larvae in a variety of organs.

A. vasorum is a nematode of the superfamily *Metastrongyloidea*, family *Angiostrongylidae*. *Adults inhabit the pulmonary arteries and right ventricle of dogs and foxes.* Eggs pass via the blood to the lungs, where the larvae hatch, penetrate into alveoli, are coughed up and passed in the feces. The prepatent period is 38-57 days. Snails and slugs serve as intermediate hosts, and frogs can be paratenic hosts.

Lesions during the prepatent period are mild. *Adult, 14-21 mm long worms are present in the pulmonary arteries,* and the lungs contain a few 1-2 mm red nodules, consisting of aggregates of eosinophils and mononuclear cells. The females have a "barber-pole" appearance because of the helically arranged red gut and white ovaries. *Angiostrongylus* can be differentiated from *Dirofilaria* by examination of intact adults, or by histologic examination. *Angiostrongylus* adults are 270-350 μm diameter with thin coelomyarian musculature, a large, strongylid intestine composed of few tall multinucleated cells, and eggs in the uterus. In contrast, *Dirofilaria* has well-developed coelomyarian musculature, a smaller intestine, and a uterus containing microfilariae.

More severe lesions develop at the time of patency, including proliferative endoarteritis in response to the adult worms in the pulmonary arteries, and eosinophilic and granulomatous pneumonia as a consequence of embolized eggs and larvae. Arterial lesions include thrombosis, thickening of the tunica intima by fibromuscular tissue and numerous eosinophils, medial hypertrophy, and lymphoplasmacytic aggregates in the adventitia. Pulmonary lesions consist of red or golden-brown, nodular or confluent areas of hemorrhage, edema, and firmness at the periphery of the lung. Histologically, *coalescing granulomas* are formed by macrophages, eosinophils, neutrophils, and giant cells, and are sometimes centered on parasite eggs and larvae. Larvae are about 10 μm wide, whereas eggs are about 100-μm diameter, and contain either basophilic and eosinophilic granular material or embryos (larvae). There is mild proliferation of type II pneumocytes, alveolar hemorrhage, hemosiderin-laden macrophages, and arteriolar thrombosis. Fibrosis and recanalization of arterial thrombi develop as the lesion ages. Similar granulomas are reported in brain, kidney, and other tissues.

Coagulation abnormalities are the second most common clinical manifestation associated with angiostrongylosis. The abnormalities are suggestive of disseminated intravascular coagulation, with increased prolonged activated partial thromboplastin time or prothrombin time, thrombocytopenia and increases in circulating D-dimer and fibrin degradation products in affected dogs. The pathogenesis of the coagulopathy is not well understood, but may represent thrombosis triggered by parasite proteins or endothelial damage from the adult and larval nematodes. Petechiae and ecchymoses may develop in tissues of such dogs; as noted above, a small percentage of dogs may have severe neurologic signs from intracerebral hemorrhage.

Further reading

Bourque AC, et al. Pathological findings in dogs naturally infected with *Angiostrongylus vasorum* in Newfoundland and Labrador, Canada. J Vet Diagn Invest 2008;20:11-20.

Koch J, Willesen JL. Canine pulmonary angiostrongylosis: an update. Vet J 2009;179:348-359.

Filaroides hirthi. Infection is mostly reported in colonies of laboratory beagles, but cases are described in pet dogs. Adult *Filaroides hirthi* are 6-10 mm long and contain larvae or embryonated eggs in the uterus. *The adults live in alveoli and respiratory bronchioles.* Like other members of the *Filaroididae*, *F. hirthi* has a direct life cycle, and infective first-stage larvae are passed in the feces. Many infections are probably acquired from the dam.

The lesions in most cases are incidental at autopsy, with grey-tan or black-green, 1-5 mm diameter nodules scattered widely in subpleural regions of the lung. Nodules may have clear cystic centers, or be white and firm. The lesions in fatal cases, which may occur in immunosuppressed dogs, are of severe generalized diffuse or miliary granulomatous pneumonia. Histologically, there is little response to living adult worms, but a severe granulomatous response with many eosinophils occurs around dead or degenerating worms. Killing the worms with an anthelmintic may incite a severe response. Larvae stimulate an acute neutrophilic reaction. Foci of granulomatous interstitial pneumonia can often be found in which worm remnants may no longer be identified. The **diagnosis** is based on discovery of larvae in smears of bronchial exudate, or identifying the adults in histologic sections of lung. Definitive diagnosis requires extraction of intact adults from the lungs, as the histologic appearance is similar to *Andersonstrongylus milksi*.

Further reading

Caro-Vadillo A, et al. Verminous pneumonia due to *Filaroides hirthi* in a Scottish terrier in Spain. Vet Rec 2005;157:586-589.

Andersonstrongylus milksi. *Andersonstrongylus milksi (Angiostrongylus milksi, Filaroides milksi)* is a metastrongylid nematode in the superfamily *Metastrongyloidea*, family *Angiostrongylidae*. The literature related to this parasite is confusing, because the diagnosis in many reports is exclusively based on histologic lesions. However, examination of intact worms, which are difficult to tease from the lung, is required to definitively differentiate *A. milksi* from *F. hirthi*. A molluscan intermediate host has been proposed, but the life cycle is unknown. *Adults inhabit the bronchioles and the alveoli*, and the gross and histologic lesions are similar to those caused by *Filaroides hirthi*. Larvae may also be found in the brain, abdominal viscera, and other organs.

Dirofilaria immitis is described elsewhere (see Vol. 3. Cardiovascular system). The microfilariae may be encountered as incidental findings in pulmonary vessels, or elicit thrombosis (Fig. 5-79) or eosinophilic and granulomatous pneumonia.

Infectious respiratory diseases of cats
Viral diseases

Influenza viruses adapted to cats have not been described, but cats are susceptible to disease arising from human H1N1 and avian H5N1 and H7N7 viruses. Inhalation results in similar lesions as in other species, with lesions mainly affecting the alveolar epithelium. Ingestion of H5N1-infected chicken liver induces systemic infection with targeting of endothelial cells, widespread hemorrhages, and multifocal necrosis in lymphoid tissues and many other organs. Similarly, cats infected with **severe acute respiratory syndrome (SARS) coronavirus** develop tracheobronchitis, necrosis and inflammation of tracheobronchial glands, and diffuse alveolar damage. **Cowpox virus** mainly causes skin lesions in cats, with rare cranial lung lesions containing necrosis, epithelial hyperplasia, syncytial

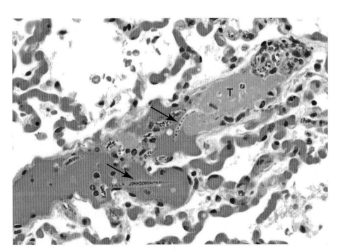

Figure 5-79 *Dirofilaria immitis* microfilaria (arrows) associated with thrombosis (T) of pulmonary venules in a dog. (Courtesy M.J. Hazlett.)

cells, and intracytoplasmic inclusion bodies in epithelial cells.

Further reading

Reperant LA, et al. Marked endotheliotropism of highly pathogenic avian influenza virus H5N1 following intestinal inoculation in cats. J Virol 2012;86:1158-1165.

Schoniger S, et al. Cowpox virus pneumonia in a domestic cat in Great Britain. Vet Rec 2007;160:522-523.

van den Brand JMA, et al. Pathology of experimental SARS coronavirus infection in cats and ferrets. Vet Pathol 2008;45:551-562.

Feline viral rhinotracheitis. *Felid herpesvirus 1 (FeHV-1) infection is widespread in most cat populations and is an important cause of acute and chronic upper respiratory tract disease.* Clinical signs are most common in kittens but occur regularly in adult cats, probably because of recrudescence of latent infections. Morbidity may be high in naive populations of kittens, but mortality is generally low, and most cats recover in 10-14 days. Clinical signs include fever, oculonasal discharge, sneezing, coughing, and anorexia. *Chronic rhinitis* and sinusitis is a frequent and serious sequela caused by intermittent reactivation of latent infections, loss of respiratory defenses caused by excavation of nasal conchae, or failure of drainage of sites of secondary bacterial infection in the sinuses.

General features of herpesviruses are described in the section Infectious bovine rhinotracheitis. FeHV-1, like other alphaherpesviruses, *causes cytolytic infections of mucosal epithelial cells and establishment of latency in the trigeminal ganglion, optic nerve, olfactory bulb, and cornea.* Reactivation of latent infection is often of unknown cause, but may be triggered by corticosteroid therapy, stresses associated with environmental changes, or parturition. The virus replicates optimally at temperatures <37° C; thus most infections are limited to the upper respiratory tract and conjunctiva.

FeHV-1 is transmitted by contact with infected nasal or ocular secretions, or by aerosol. Transmission by fomites may occur, but the virus survives for <18 hours under most environmental conditions. The host range is limited to felids, including a variety of species of wild cats. The incubation period is short, typically just 2-4 days. In most cases, infection is restricted to the nasal mucosa, nasopharynx, sinuses, and tonsils, with lesser viral replication in the conjunctiva and upper trachea. Viremia may occur in neonates, but is not common in older kittens. It is likely that most cats recovering from the disease remain latently infected, and perhaps 20-40% of these cats intermittently shed infective virus during periods of stress, such as following a change in housing, or during lactation; recrudescence may also be triggered by corticosteroid therapy.

The distribution of **gross lesions** corresponds to the predilection sites for viral replication—the epithelium of nasal passages, pharynx, soft palate, conjunctivae, tonsils, and to a lesser extent trachea. The initial serous inflammation becomes mucopurulent or fibrinous within a few days, and crusting is often present around the eyes and nares. Multifocal erosions of the nasal mucosa are covered by mucoid or mucopurulent exudate. The trachea may contain hemorrhage or fibrinous exudate. Tonsils are enlarged and contain petechiae or rare foci of necrosis. The regional lymph nodes are usually enlarged, reddened, and edematous. *Ulceration of the tongue is uncommon*

but does occur. This contrasts with the frequent finding of vesicular to ulcerative lesions on tongue, hard palate, or nostrils with feline calicivirus infection. Ocular involvement is usually limited to purulent conjunctivitis, but it can progress to ulcerative keratitis.

Microscopically, *large eosinophilic intranuclear inclusion bodies* are present in many virus-infected cells during the period of active viral replication from 2-7 days after infection (eFigs. 5-101, 5-102). They may be found in lesions from cats dying of the disease, but are rarely detected beyond 7 days after infection. Infected cells undergo hydropic change with cytoplasmic swelling and pallor. There is loss of epithelial organization, and the disrupted epithelium is soon eroded or ulcerated. An acute inflammatory reaction develops with exudation of fibrin and many neutrophils. Repair may be delayed for up to 17 days after infection, and the epithelial tissue undergoes squamous metaplasia as it repairs.

Resorption of nasal turbinate bones along with new bone formation and fibroplasia has been described in both natural and experimental infections, mainly in cats <6 months of age, and may lead to chronic nasal disease by impairing clearance of opportunistic pathogens. Focal necrosis accompanied by acute inflammation may be found in tonsils and local lymph nodes. Erosive lesions may occur in stratified squamous epithelium of the nares or the tongue.

Pulmonary involvement is uncommon except in fatal cases. In fulminant FeHV-1 infections, there is widespread multifocal necrotizing tracheitis, bronchitis, bronchiolitis, and diffuse alveolar damage, with extensive serofibrinous flooding of airspaces. Inclusion bodies are identified in airway epithelial cells. Necrosis of pulmonary blood vessels is rarely described, with viral antigen in the vessel wall. Secondary bacterial bronchopneumonia is a more common complication of FeHV-1 infection than is primary viral pneumonia.

Systemic disease is uncommon in FeHV-1 infection, in contrast to the analogous alphaherpesvirus infections of young calves and dogs. Ocular lesions are described elsewhere. Experimental infection of pregnant queens produces abortion and generalized neonatal disease, but this has been difficult to identify in natural outbreaks. Multifocal hepatic, pancreatic, and adrenocortical necrosis are the expected features of systemic disease. A syndrome of nasofacial ulcerative dermatitis and stomatitis with histologic lesions of eosinophilic inflammation and infrequent epithelial intranuclear inclusion bodies may be associated with corticosteroid therapy or crowding. Necrosis accompanied by inclusion bodies has also been found in sites of osteogenesis in a wide variety of bones of kittens after intravenous inoculation. Degeneration of olfactory nerve fibers and focal lymphocytic infiltration of the olfactory bulbs have occurred in experimentally infected, germ-free cats, but the extent of lesions in the brain has not been properly documented.

The major *differential diagnosis* for upper respiratory disease in cats is feline calicivirus infection. Other contributors of minor or uncertain significance include *Chlamydophila felis, Bordetella bronchiseptica*, and *Mycoplasma* spp. **Diagnosis** of FeHV-1 using PCR assays is a sensitive test to detect viral nucleic acid in tissues. If necessary, this diagnosis can be confirmed by *virus isolation*. Finding eosinophilic intranuclear inclusion bodies amid necrotizing lesions of respiratory epithelium is usually sufficient for diagnosis in postmortem samples, but as discussed previously, it is not uncommon to miss the period when viral inclusions are apparent. Several other techniques are applicable to tissues obtained at autopsy, including immunohistochemistry, in situ hybridization, and indirect immunofluorescence assays.

Further reading

Burns RE, et al. Histologic and molecular correlation in shelter cats with acute upper respiratory infection. J Clin Microbiol 2011;49:2454-2460.

Chvala-Mannsberger S, et al. Occurrence, morphological characterization and antigen localization of felid herpesvirus-induced pneumonia in cats: a retrospective study (2000-2006). J Comp Pathol 2009;141:163-169.

Pesavento PA, Murphy BG. Common and emerging infectious diseases in the animal shelter. Vet Pathol 2014;51:478-491.

Feline calicivirus. Feline calicivirus *(FCV) is a common cause of upper respiratory tract disease that can also cause oral ulcers, chronic stomatitis, pneumonia, systemic disease, or lameness.* Infection with FCV is widespread, with *15-25% of cats being subclinical carriers.* Morbidity is often high, particularly in kittens, but most cats recover from clinical disease. Clinical signs are variable and include serous or mucopurulent nasal and ocular discharge, *oral ulcers,* conjunctivitis, sneezing and coughing, anorexia, and fever. FCV is a non-enveloped, 35-40 nm, positive-sense, single-stranded RNA virus in the genus *Vesivirus,* family *Caliciviridae.* Open reading frames 1, 2, and 3 encode a helicase, a protease, and polymerase; the single capsid protein; and an RNA-associated structural protein, respectively. The capsid protein is the target of protective immune responses, but hypervariable regions in this gene confer antigenic variability that allows viral persistence in the face of a developing immune response.

Transmission is by direct contact with infected oronasal secretions, and fomites are a potential source of infection. The clinical manifestation of the disease likely depends on the strain of the virus, the immune status of the host, and the route of infection. The incubation period varies from 2-14 days, and many cats recover in 7-14 days after onset of illness. However, *viral infection persists despite resolution of clinical signs,* and 25% of infected cats continue to shed virus for months or years. These cats are important sources of infective virus for naive cats or those with immunity to other strains of calicivirus. Occasionally, these chronically infected cats develop chronic lymphoplasmacytic and/or ulcerative stomatitis that is refractory to therapy.

In addition to upper respiratory infections, *ulcerative stomatitis may occur.* The oral ulcers, which begin as vesicles that rapidly rupture, are most often present on the dorsal surface or lateral margins of the tongue and on the hard palate. Cutaneous ulcers may occur on the nares and the muzzle.

Caliciviral pneumonia is an uncommon occurrence. Pneumonia is more likely following aerosol rather than oronasal exposure, and specific strains of FCV may have tropism for the lungs. Gross lesions are irregularly distributed but often include the margins of the cranioventral lung. The virus causes lytic infection of type I pneumocytes, resulting in acute to subacute interstitial pneumonia. Hyaline membranes may be present, and the alveoli often contain serofibrinous exudate and neutrophils. As the lesion heals, type II pneumocytes proliferate and form a cuboidal lining of the alveoli, and alveolar septa are thickened by lymphocytes, plasma cells, and fibrous tissue in the later stages.

Virulent systemic feline calicivirus (VS-FCV) infection is a rare manifestation. VS-FCV occurs in individual cats or emerges as a localized epizootic. The disease is highly contagious and rapidly fatal, affecting both kittens and adult cats, even those previously vaccinated. Affected cats develop edema and ulcers, mainly on the head, limbs, footpads, and inguinal region. Subcutaneous edema, with foci of fat necrosis, pancreatitis with peripancreatic fat necrosis, disseminated intravascular coagulation, intestinal crypt necrosis, single-cell necrosis of hepatocytes, and interstitial pneumonia are all reported in VS-FCV infections. The disease has been experimentally reproduced, suggesting that viral factors are at least partly responsible for increased virulence, but this has not been correlated with specific genomic sequences.

The pathogenesis of VS-FCV is poorly understood. It is often impossible to distinguish FCV infection from other causes of upper respiratory tract infection in cats, particularly felid herpesvirus 1 and *Chlamydophila. The finding of oral ulcers is suggestive of calicivirus infection* although FeHV-1 can cause similar lesions. In contrast to the bronchointerstitial pneumonia caused by FeHV-1, airway lesions are usually not present in FCV infection. Toxoplasmosis, sepsis, and aspiration of gastric acid are additional causes of interstitial pneumonia in cats. The lesions are, in most cases, not etiologically specific, and *definitive diagnosis requires laboratory support.* PCR and virus isolation are widely used to detect FCV in tissues. and immunohistochemistry is useful to localize viral antigen in tissue sections.

Further reading

Pedersen NC, et al. An isolated epizootic of hemorrhagic-like fever in cats caused by a novel and highly virulent strain of feline calicivirus. Vet Microbiol 2000;73:281-300.

Pesavento PA, et al. Molecular virology of feline calicivirus. Vet Clin North Am Small Anim Pract 2008;38:775-786.

Bacterial diseases

Bacterial pneumonia is common in cats. The most frequent isolates are *Bordetella bronchiseptica* and *Pasteurella multocida.* These agents are carried in the nasopharynx of most healthy cats; as in other domestic species, the development of pulmonary infection probably requires that the normal lung defenses be impaired or overwhelmed by various "stressors" or antecedent viral infections such as FHV-1 or FCV. **B. bronchiseptica** is a minor zoonotic pathogen; several human cases of pneumonia have been described that appear to have been acquired from cats. **Streptococcus equi** ssp. **zooepidemicus** causes suppurative or necrosuppurative bronchopneumonia as in dogs. **Extraintestinal pathogenic E. coli** is associated with hemorrhagic and necrotizing pneumonia and fibrinous pleuritis similar to that described in dogs.

Further reading

Blum S, et al. Outbreak of *Streptococcus equi* subsp. *zooepidemicus* infections in cats. Vet Microbiol 2010;144:236-239.

Foster SF, et al. Lower respiratory tract infections in cats: 21 cases (1995-2000). J Feline Med Surg 2004;6:167-180.

Highland MA, et al. Extraintestinal pathogenic *Escherichia coli*-induced pneumonia in three kittens and fecal prevalence in a clinically healthy cohort population. J Vet Diagn Invest 2009;21:609-615.

Chlamydial diseases

Chlamydophila felis (formerly *Chlamydia psittaci*) is of most importance as a *cause of persistent conjunctivitis in cats*. PCR-based surveys of the feline upper respiratory tract suggest C. *felis* is a minor contributor to upper respiratory disease in cats and, despite the disease name "feline pneumonitis," does not apparently cause pulmonary infection or disease.

Further reading

Masubuchi K, et al. Experimental infection of cats with *Chlamydophila felis*. J Vet Med Sci 2002;64:1165-1168.

Mycoplasmal diseases

Mycoplasma felis, M. gateae, M. arginini, and *Acholeplasma laidlawii* often colonize the upper respiratory passages of cats. Most evidence suggests that mycoplasmas are not important primary causes of respiratory disease in cats. Mycoplasmas can be isolated from tracheobronchial washes of 20% of cats with pulmonary disease, but from few normal cats. As in dogs, the significance of this finding is complicated by the potential for mycoplasmas to secondarily colonize lungs that are diseased for other reasons. Kittens experimentally infected with *M. felis, M. gateae, and M. arginini* did not develop clinical signs of respiratory disease. Unclassified *Mycoplasma* spp. have been isolated from pulmonary abscesses and lesions of suppurative pleuritis in cats.

Further reading

Burns RE, et al. Histologic and molecular correlation in shelter cats with acute upper respiratory infection. J Clin Microbiol 2011;49:2454-2460.

Fungal diseases

Fungal diseases of cats are described with those of dogs (see Infectious respiratory diseases of dogs, previously).

Parasitic diseases

Toxoplasmosis. Toxoplasmosis is described more fully in the chapter on the gastrointestinal system (Vol. 2, Alimentary system and peritoneum). Lung lesions are most commonly identified in kittens, and grossly consist of numerous *pinpoint white foci scattered throughout the lung or diffuse interstitial pneumonia* (Fig. 5-80, eFig. 5-103), either alone or as a component of multisystemic disease. Histologically, there are multifocal to diffuse alveolar lesions, consisting of fibrin exudate or hyaline membranes, fibrinonecrotic debris in alveoli, proliferation of type II pneumocytes, necrosis of bronchiolar epithelium, and infiltration of neutrophils, mononuclear cells, variable numbers of eosinophils, and protozoal cysts (see Fig. 5-80, eFig. 5-103). *Diagnosis* can be made using PCR or immunohistochemistry to identify cysts within the lung.

Further reading

Jokelainen P, et al. Feline toxoplasmosis in Finland: cross-sectional epidemiological study and case series study. J Vet Diagn Invest 2012;24:1115-1124.

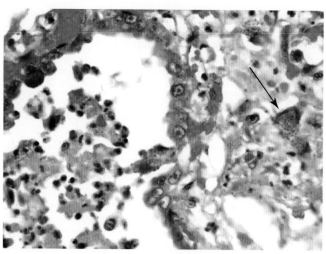

Figure 5-80 Pulmonary toxoplasmosis. In the lung of a cat, alveoli are lined by cuboidal type II pneumocytes with necrotic debris in the lumen, and *Toxoplasma* cysts are present in alveolar epithelial cells and in the interstitium (arrow).

Aelurostrongylus abstrusus. *Aelurostrongylus abstrusus* is a moderately common lungworm of cats. Cats may be subclinically infected and display no clinical signs, but heavy infections cause coughing or increased respiratory rate.

Aelurostrongylus abstrusus is a nematode of the superfamily *Metastrongyloidea*, family *Angiostrongylidae*. The adults, which are slender and up to 1 cm long, live in the terminal and respiratory bronchioles. The eggs form nodular deposits in alveoli, where they embryonate and hatch to release first-stage larvae. The larvae move to the airways, are coughed up and swallowed, and passed in the feces. Snails and slugs are intermediate hosts, whereas birds, rodents, frogs, and lizards are paratenic (transport) hosts. The life cycle can be completed if a cat eats either an intermediate host or a paratenic host. Infective larvae migrate to the lungs and reach maturity ~4-6 weeks after ingestion of the third-stage larvae.

Heavy infections in the prepatent period cause randomly distributed hemorrhages or white foci, which represent an eosinophilic and granulomatous reaction to the migrating larvae. *In the patent period, there are 1-10 mm diameter, firm, off-white to pale yellow, slightly raised nodules scattered throughout the lungs.* In severe infections, nodules may coalesce to form confluent areas of consolidation.

Microscopically, *the nodules are formed by masses of eggs and larvae in the alveoli and terminal bronchioles, with fewer adult worms* (eFigs. 5-104, 5-105). Eosinophils and neutrophils infiltrate the early lesions, but most cases are dominated by mononuclear cells and giant cells in the alveoli and around degenerating eggs and larvae. Alveoli are dilated, and alveolar septa may be disrupted. Necrosis and mineralization seldom occur. Lymphocytic nodules form around vessels and airways, and there is hypertrophy and hyperplasia of the smooth muscle in the walls of the bronchioles and alveolar ducts. The presence of adult worms, eggs, or larvae in the bronchioles is associated with chronic catarrhal and eosinophilic bronchiolitis; similar inflammation may be present within the tracheal mucosa, presumably in response to larvae moving up the trachea to be swallowed. In older lesions from which eggs and larvae have disappeared, alveoli remain epithelialized and septa are persistently thickened by fibrous tissue and smooth muscle (see eFig. 5-93). Bronchial glands and smooth muscle in the media of small pulmonary arteries and arterioles may be quite prominent in cats infected with *Aelurostrongylus*, but these changes are also common in clinically healthy cats that have no evidence of parasitism.

Further reading

Rolim VM, et al. *Aelurostrongylus* pneumonia in a cat. J Am Vet Med Assoc 2012;241:1587-1589.

Paragonimus kellicotti. Of the *trematodes*, the only genus that has its final habitat in the lungs is *Paragonimus. P. kellicotti* occurs in America, and ***P. westermanii*** in Asia. Mink and other fish-eating carnivores are the usual hosts of *P. kellicotti*, but it infects many other species. Among domestic animals, it is *most commonly found in cats* and occasionally in dogs. Clinical signs are usually absent in animals with paragonimiasis.

The life cycle of the parasite is typical of trematodes. The first intermediate hosts are small aquatic snails. The second intermediate host is a freshwater crab or crayfish. When the crayfish is eaten by the definitive host, the metacercariae are liberated in the intestine and migrate across the peritoneal and pleural cavities to the lungs. Their passage through the pleura is marked by multiple small hemorrhages and foci of eosinophilic and fibrinous pleuritis that heal as small umbilicated scars. Adult flukes are ovoid, red-brown, and up to 17 mm long. They are often found in pairs in inflammatory cavitations in the pulmonary parenchyma and occasionally in the bronchi. The cavitations frequently communicate with bronchioles, permitting liberation of eggs into the airways, expulsion to the nasopharynx, and passage in the feces.

The cavitations, which are more common in the caudal lobes, are spherical, 1-3 cm diameter, soft, and dark red-brown (Fig. 5-81, eFigs. 5-106 to 5-109). The cavitations contain intense eosinophilic and granulomatous inflammation, hemorrhage with numerous hemosiderin-laden macrophages, a fibrous capsule, and adult flukes. The adults exhibit characteristic features of trematodes: the body is filled with loose parenchyma, but there is no body cavity, paired ceca contain dark pigment, oral suckers are present in some sections, the tegument has surface spines, and vitellaria beneath the tegument contain eosinophilic globular yolk material. In patent infections, there are numerous 80-100 µm long, yellow-brown, operculate eggs, which persist as fractured shells in chronic lesions (eFig. 5-110; see Fig. 5-81, eFigs. 5-106 to 5-109). As cavitations mature and establish connections with bronchioles, they become partially lined by cuboidal epithelium to form *true cysts*. At this stage, bronchioles contain eggs and eosinophilic exudate, with hyperplasia of peribronchiolar glands and smooth muscle. Other lesions include chronic catarrhal eosinophilic bronchiolitis, granulomatous pleuritis, and pleural lymphangitis associated with the presence of eggs. Rupture of the cysts causes pneumothorax, which may lead to acute respiratory distress.

Further reading

Weina PJ, England DM. The American lung fluke, *Paragonimus kellicotti*, in a cat model. J Parasitol 1990;76:568-572.

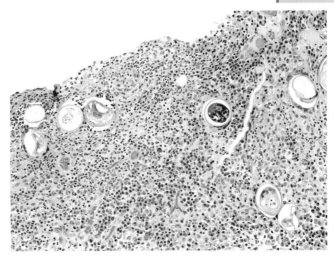

Figure 5-81 ***Paragonimus kellicotti*** infection in a cat. Parietal pleural with pyogranulomatous inflammation and pigmented ova. The cat died of respiratory distress, presumably from pneumothorax resulting from rupture of the bronchus-associated cyst, but the chronic inflammatory reaction in the parietal pleura suggests prior leakage of cyst contents.

Miscellaneous parasites. *Mammomonogamus* sp. nematodes are reported to infect cats. Depending on the species of nematode, infection may occur in the nasal sinuses, larynx, and trachea. Infection is mostly reported in cats in the Caribbean. ***Eucoleus aerophilus*** is described in the section Infectious respiratory diseases of dogs, previously. ***Oslerus rostratus*** is a viviparous parasite of cats that causes sinuous thickenings of the walls of large bronchi, formed by adult worms within cystic spaces. When the adults die, they provoke intense infiltration of neutrophils, with eventual mineralization and fibrosis.

Troglostrongylus brevior and **T. *subcrenatus*** are metastrongyloid *(Crenosomatidae)* nematodes that reside in the trachea and bronchi of cats. In heavily infected cats, clinical signs consist of dyspnea, tachypnea, and coughing. Catarrhal inflammation within the airways and bronchopneumonia may develop in response to the parasites. The lifecycle of this parasite is not completely known, but likely involves L1 larvae being passed in the feces of infected cats and infecting terrestrial molluscs, where they develop into L3 larvae to be consumed by cats or a variety of paratenic hosts.

Further reading

Brianti E, et al. *Troglostrongylus brevior* and *Troglostrongylus subcrenatus* (Strongylida: *Crenosomatidae*) as agents of bronchopulmonary infestation in domestic cats. Parasit Vectors 2012;5:178.

 For more information, please visit the companion site: PathologyofDomesticAnimals.com

INDEX

Entries followed by "*f*," "*b*," and "*t*" refer to figures and tables, respectively. The volume number of the entry is indicated in *italics* at the beginning of the page number.

A

Abdominal distention, *2*:44
Abdominal fat necrosis, *2*:76-77, *2*:249, *2*:249*f*
Abdominal trauma, *2*:246-247, *2*:246*f*
Abdominal wall, ventral hernia, *2*:80
Abdominally retained testis, *3*:470*f*
Aberdeen Angus cattle
  bovine familial convulsions and ataxia, *1*:319
  brachygnathia inferior, *2*:3
  hip dysplasia, *1*:135-136
Abiotrophy, *1*:265
  cerebellar, *1*:276, *1*:276*f*, *1*:318-326
Abomasal fistulae, *2*:49
Abomasal helminthosis, *2*:205-211, *2*:205*f*
Abomasitis, *2*:52
  associated with viral infection, *2*:54
  chemical, *2*:52
  mycotic, *2*:54, *2*:54*f*
Abomasum. *See* Stomach and abomasum
Abortion, *3*:395, *3*:398-440. *See also* Female genital system; Gestation
  bacterial causes of, *3*:402-417
  diagnosing infectious causes of, *3*:399-402
  epizootic bovine, *3*:419-420
  infectious causes of, *3*:399*b*
  in mares, *3*:417-418
  mycotic, *3*:418-419, *3*:418*f*-419*f*
  protozoal causes of, *3*:420-424
Abscess(es), *1*:636-637
  Brodie's, *1*:98, *1*:98*f*
  cerebral, *1*:358-362, *1*:358*f*, *1*:360*f*
  epidural/subdural, *1*:353-354, *1*:354*f*
  jowl, *3*:208-209, *3*:208*f*-209*f*
  liver, *2*:315-316, *2*:315*f*
  lung, *2*:520
  lymph node, *3*:203*f*, *3*:203.e1*f*
  meningitis, *1*:359*f*
  ovarian, *3*:371
  pancreatic, *2*:361
  pulmonary hemorrhage and, *2*:490
  splenic, *3*:183-184, *3*:184*f*
  subdural/intradural, *1*:354*f*
  uterine, *3*:390
Abyssinian cats
  atopic dermatitis, *1*:593
  feline ceruminous cystomatosis, *1*:507
  retinal degeneration, *1*:469-470
Acacia cambadgei, *3*:34
Acacia georginae, *3*:34
Acanthamoeba, *2*:574
Acanthocephalan infections, *2*:227
Acantholysis, *1*:518, *1*:518*f*
Acantholytic cells, *1*:518
Acantholytic dermatoses
  cattle, *1*:537-538
  dogs, *1*:537-538, *1*:537.e1*f*
Acanthomatous ameloblastomas, *2*:22-23, *2*:23*f*-24*f*
Acanthosis, *1*:518
Accessory adrenal cortical tissue, *3*:338, *3*:338*f*

Accessory cortical nodules, *3*:343
Accessory lung, *2*:484-485
Accessory pancreatic tissue, *2*:356
Accessory spleens, *3*:162-163, *3*:163*f*
Accessory thyroid tissue, *3*:310
Accreditation, laboratory, *1*:14
Acetaminophen, *2*:327
Acetylcholine, *2*:45
Acetylcholinesterase, *1*:170
Achalasia, esophageal, *2*:33
Achlorhydria, *2*:47
Achondroplasia, *1*:37*t*
Acid-base imbalance, *2*:384
Acidophil adenomas, *3*:286, *3*:286*f*
Acidosis, carbohydrate overload, *2*:40-43
Acid treatment, of hemoglobin, *2*:55-56
Acid urine, antibacterial effect of, *2*:459
Acinar cells, *2*:355
  necrosis, *2*:356
Acinic cell carcinomas, *2*:30
  nasal, *2*:478-479
Acne, *1*:549
Acorn poisoning, acute, *2*:85
Acoustic trauma, *1*:493
Acquired cysts, *2*:396
Acquired deafness, *1*:493
Acquired diaphragmatic hernia, *2*:246-247, *2*:246*f*
Acquired Fanconi syndrome, *2*:428
Acquired hyperpigmentation, *1*:554
Acquired hypopigmentation, *1*:557, *1*:557*f*
Acquired melanosis, *2*:270
Acquired platelet disorders, *3*:260
Acquired porphyria, *1*:59-60
Acquired portosystemic shunts
  liver, *2*:290, *2*:298-299, *2*:299*f*
  vascular, *2*:266*f*
Acquired thrombocytopenia, *3*:258
Acral lick dermatitis, *1*:561-562, *1*:561*f*-562*f*
Acrocyanosis, *3*:65
Acrodermatitis, lethal, *1*:533, *1*:533.e1*f*
Acromegaly, *3*:286, *3*:286*f*
Acromelanism, *1*:555
Actinic diseases of skin, *1*:575-580
Actinobacillosis, *2*:18-19, *2*:18*f*
Actinobacillus equuli, *2*:113-114, *2*:433, *2*:433*f*, *2*:452, *2*:543, *3*:417-418, *2*:433.e1*f*
  endocarditis and, *3*:30-31
  liver and, *2*:314-315
  myocarditis and, *3*:42
Actinobacillus pleuropneumoniae (APP), *2*:531-532, *2*:531*f*, *2*:543, *3*:69
Actinobacillus seminis, *3*:490
Actinobacillus suis, *2*:543
Actinobaculum, *2*:459
Actinobaculum suis, *2*:459
Actinomyces spp.
  cutaneous, *1*:637-639, *1*:638*f*
  inflammation in buccal cavity due to, *2*:13-14
  tonsillitis, *2*:20
  tooth decay and, *2*:9

Actinomyces weissii, *2*:19
Activated clotting time (ACT), *3*:263
Activated partial thromboplastin time (APTT)
  prolonged, *3*:263
Active hyperemia, *3*:169
Acute arthritis in cats, *1*:154
Acute bacterial endocarditis, *3*:32
Acute bovine liver disease, *2*:343-344, *2*:343.e1*f*
Acute eosinophilic (or acidophilic) degeneration, *1*:253-254, *1*:253*f*
Acute hepatitis, *2*:301
Acute intermittent porphyria, *1*:59
Acute interstitial lung disease in feedlot cattle, *2*:513*f*, *2*:513.e1
Acute kidney injury (AKI), *2*:398
Acute local peritonitis, *2*:39
Acute lymphadenitis, *3*:202-203
Acute lymphocytic-plasmacytic chorioretinitis, *1*:474
Acute lymphoid leukemia (ALL), *3*:132-133, *3*:133*f*
Acute myeloid leukemia (AML), *3*:129-134, *3*:130*f*-132*f*
Acute osteomyelitis, *1*:95, *1*:95*f*
Acute pancreatic necrosis, *2*:357-360, *2*:359*f*-360*f*
Acute pancreatitis, *2*:360
Acute polyradiculoneuritis, *1*:394
Acute renal failure (ARF), *2*:383-384, *2*:398, *2*:418
Acute rupture of chordae tendineae, *3*:27
Acute selenium toxicosis, *3*:36
Acute serous uveitis, *1*:448-449
Acute toxic hepatic injury, *2*:327, *2*:328*f*
Acute tubular injury (ATI), *2*:383, *2*:386, *2*:398, *2*:421-422
  epithelial injury, *2*:422*f*
Acute tubular necrosis (ATN), *2*:382, *2*:398, *2*:422
Addison's disease, *1*:225
Adenocarcinomas. *See* Carcinomas/adenocarcinomas
Adenohypophysis, *3*:276
  bacterial septicemia, *3*:289
  functional cytology, *3*:276-277
  hypothalamic control of, *3*:277, *3*:278*f*
  inflammation, *3*:289-290
Adenoid cystic carcinomas, *2*:478-479
Adenomas, *2*:462. *See also* Carcinomas/adenocarcinomas
  acidophil, *3*:286, *3*:286*f*
  adrenal cortex, *3*:344-345, *3*:345*f*
  aortic body, *3*:354-355, *3*:354*f*
  carotid body, *3*:355-356
  corticotroph (ACTH-secreting), *3*:281-282, *3*:281*f*, *3*:283*f*-284*f*
  endocrine gland, *3*:271
  exocrine pancreatic, *2*:366
  hepatocellular, *2*:346, *2*:346*f*
  lactotroph, *3*:286-287

Australian Kelpie dogs, globoid cell leukodystrophy in, *1*:339

Australian Shepherd dogs
choroidal hypoplasia, *1*:413
cobalamin deficiency, *3*:127
cochleosaccular degeneration, *1*:492
spindle cell tumor, *1*:486

Autoimmune dermatoses, *1*:600-607
pemphigus complex, *1*:518, *1*:600-603

Autolytic changes in retina after death, *1*:467

Autopsy. *See* Gross and histologic examinations

Autopsy-in-a-jar pathology, *1*:2

Autosomal recessive congenital ichthyoses (ARCI), *1*:530, *1*:531*f*

Autosomal recessive PKD (ARPKD), *2*:396

Autosomal recessive severe combined immunodeficiency, *3*:140-141

Avascular chorion, *3*:397

Avipoxvirus, *1*:616

AV node, *3*:2
heart examination and, *3*:13-14
impulse formation disturbances, *3*:5

Avocado poisoning, *3*:38

Axillary nodular necrosis, *1*:695

Axonal dystrophy, *1*:257-258, *1*:258*f*, *1*:324-325

Axonopathy, *1*:256, *1*:318-334
distal, *1*:257
peripheral, *1*:334-336
proximal, *1*:257, *1*:257*f*

Axons, *1*:255-258, *1*:256*f*
growth disorders, *1*:268-269

Ayrshire cattle, cropped and notched pinnae in, *1*:502

B

Babesia bigemina, *3*:119
Babesia bovis, *3*:118
Babesia caballi, *3*:119-120
Babesia canis, *1*:665, *3*:119, *3*:119.*e1f*
Babesia divergens, *3*:119
Babesia felis, *3*:120
Babesia gibsoni, *1*:665, *2*:412
Babesia major, *3*:119
Babesia rossi, *3*:119
Babesia spp., *1*:611, *3*:117-120, *3*:117*f*
differential diagnosis, *3*:119
splenic babesiosis, *3*:161, *3*:161*f*
Baccharis cordifolia, *2*:89
Baccharis megapotamica, *2*:89
Baccharis pteronioides, *2*:89
Bacillary angiomatosis, *1*:646
Bacillary hemoglobinuria, *2*:317, *2*:317*f*
Bacillus anthracis, *3*:171-174
Bacillus fragilis, *2*:113
Bacillus piliformis, *3*:42
Bacterial arthritis, *1*:148-154
Bacterial diseases, tooth surface, *2*:9
Bacterial endophthalmitis, *1*:449
Bacterial enterotoxin, *2*:71
Bacterial granulomas, *1*:637-642
Bacterial hemolysins, *3*:126
Bacterial infections
abortion and stillbirth due to, *3*:398, *3*:399*b*, *3*:402-417
alimentary tract, *2*:158-201
central nervous system, *1*:353-365
endocarditis, *3*:30-33, *3*:31*f*

Bacterial infections *(Continued)*
liver, *2*:314-318
lungs and, *2*:472-473
myocarditis, *3*:42
pneumonia, *2*:562-563, *2*:562*f*
respiratory system, *2*:531-532, *2*:531*f*
cats, *2*:589
cattle, *2*:542-551
dogs, *2*:577-579
horses, *2*:569-573
pigs, *2*:531-533
sheep and goats, *2*:562-563
skin, *1*:629-646
lesions in, *1*:645-646
teeth, *2*:9

Bacterial osteomyelitis, *1*:98-103, *1*:98*f*-99*f*
cats, *1*:99-100
cattle, *1*:99
dogs, *1*:99-100
horses, *1*:99, *1*:99*f*, *1*:101*f*

Bacterial overgrowth, small intestine, *2*:364

Bacterial pododermatitis of horses and ruminants, *1*:642-645

Bacterial pseudomycetoma, *1*:642, *1*:642*f*

Bacterial septicemia, *3*:289, *3*:290*f*

Bacteriology, *1*:10-11

Bacteroides fragilis, *2*:113, *2*:199

Bacteroides spp., *2*:9

Balanoposthitis, *3*:507

Balantidium, *2*:243-244, *2*:244*f*

Baldy calf syndrome, *1*:538

Bali cattle, Jembrana disease in, *3*:195-196, *3*:195*f*

Balloon cell malignant melanomas, *1*:722

Ballooning degeneration of epidermis, *1*:519, *1*:519*f*

Bandera's neonatal ataxia, *1*:318-319

Banzi virus, *1*:281

Barbados Blackbelly sheep, osteogenesis imperfecta in, *1*:50

Bartholin's glands, *3*:442

Bartonella, *1*:646
endocarditits and, *3*:30-31
liver and, *2*:318

Bartonella berkhoffi, *1*:646

Bartonella henselae, *3*:42

Bartonella vinsonii, *1*:99-100, *1*:646

Basal cell carcinomas, *1*:714

Basement membrane zone (BMZ), *1*:513-514

Basic multicellular unit (BMU), *1*:26

Basidiobolomycosis, *1*:660
granulomatous rhinitis and, *2*:476

Basilar membrane, *1*:489-490

Basophilia, *3*:111

Basophilic intranuclear viral inclusions, *2*:22

Basosquamous carcinomas, *1*:714

Basset Hound dogs
canine atopic dermatitis, *1*:591
degenerative diseases of cartilaginous joints, *1*:143-144
globoid cell leukodystrophy, *1*:339
granulomatous hepatitis, *2*:318
platelet dysfunction, *3*:259
seborrhea, *1*:548
severe combined immunodeficiency (SCID), *3*:139

Baylisascaris procyonis, *1*:390-391

B-cells
chronic lymphocytic leukemia/small lymphocytic lymphoma (B-CLL/SLL), *3*:219-220

B-cells *(Continued)*
diffuse large B-cell lymphomas, *3*:220-222, *3*:221*f*
follicular-derived B-cell lymphomas, *3*:222-226, *3*:223*f*
lymphoid hyperplasia, *3*:201
in masticatory myositis, *1*:226-227
Reed-Sternberg cell, *3*:219
T-cell-rich B-cell lymphoma, *3*:221-222, *3*:222*f*

Beagle dogs
chondrodysplasia, *1*:44, *1*:45*f*
cobalamin deficiency, *3*:127
Factor VII deficiency, *3*:264
globoid cell leukodystrophy, *1*:339
hypertrophy type 1 and 2, *1*:225
iatrogenic acromegaly, *3*:286*f*
lymphomas, *3*:238
osteogenesis imperfecta, *1*:50
osteoporosis, *1*:67
pain syndrome, *1*:158, *3*:70
peripheral vestibular disease, *1*:494
selective deficiencies of immunoglobulins, *3*:139

Beagle pain syndrome. *See* Steroid-responsive meningitis-arteritis

Beauceron dogs, canine atopic dermatitis in, *1*:591

Bedlington Terriers, *2*:303, *2*:303.*e1f*

Belgian Blue cattle
dermatosparaxis, *1*:48
osteopetrosis, *1*:51-52

Belgian Gorenendael Shepherd dogs, canine X-linked muscular dystrophy in, *1*:192

Belgian Malinois dogs, vitiligo in, *1*:556.*e1f*

Belgian Tervuren dogs
canine atopic dermatitis, *1*:591
vitiligo, *1*:555-556

Benign bone cysts, *1*:126

Benign cortical fibromas, *2*:447

Benign epithelial neoplasms, *2*:478-479, *2*:479*f*

Benign mammary neoplasms, *3*:460

Benign melanocytic tumors, *1*:721

Benign spindle cell tumors, *1*:722-723

Benign tumors of joints, *1*:160-162

Bergmann's glia, *1*:261

Bergmeister's papilla, *1*:417-419, *1*:418*f*

Bernese Mountain dogs
afibrinogenemia, *3*:265
Alexander disease, *1*:341
canine hypomyelinogenesis, *1*:338
degenerative radiculomyelopathy, *1*:330
vasculitis, *3*:70

Besnoitiosis, *1*:661-663, *1*:662*f*
granulomatous rhinitis and, *2*:476

Besnoitia spp., *2*:239

B-cells, endocrine pancreas, *2*:368

β-glucuronidase-deficient MPS, *1*:290

β-Mannosidosis, *1*:289, *1*:492

B_2-microglobulin, *2*:385

Betaherpesviruses, *2*:537

Bibersteinia trehalosi, *2*:543, *2*:562-563

Bichon Frise dogs, canine atopic dermatitis, *1*:591

Bilateral extraocular muscle myositis of dogs, *1*:228

Bilateral hypoplasia, *2*:392

Bile cast nephropathy, *2*:430

Bile peritonitis, *2*:250

Ehlers-Danlos syndrome (EDS), *1*:543-544
Ehrlichia canis, *2*:414, *2*:418, *3*:111
   platelet dysfunction, *3*:260
Ehrlichia platys, *3*:260
Ehrlichia ruminantium, *3*:80-82
Ehrlichiosis, *1*:449
Eimeria alabamensis, *2*:230-231
Eimeria apsheronica, *2*:233
Eimeria arloingi, *2*:232, *2*:232*f*
Eimeria auburnensis, *2*:230
Eimeria bareillyi, *2*:231
Eimeria bovis, *2*:229
Eimeria bukidnonensis, *2*:230-231
Eimeria caprina, *2*:231
Eimeria christenseni, *2*:231-232
Eimeria crandallis, *2*:233
Eimeria gilruthi, *2*:54-55
Eimeria leuckarti, *2*:233-234, *2*:233*f*
Eimeria ninakohlyakimovae, *2*:231
Eimeria ovinoidalis, *2*:231
Eimeria zuernii, *2*:229
Elaeophora bohmi, *3*:88
Elaeophora poeli, *3*:88, *3*:88.*e*1*f*
Elaeophora schneideri, *1*:390, *1*:451-452,
   3:88
Elaeophoriasis, *3*:88
Elaphostrongylus cervi, *1*:390
Elaphostrongylus panticola, *1*:390
Elaphostrongylus rangifera, *1*:390
Elastic fibers, dermal, *1*:514
   abnormalities of, *1*:545
Elbow hygroma, *1*:155, *1*:155*f*
Electrical burns, *2*:13
Electrolytes
   abnormalities and myopathies, *1*:225
   balance, *2*:384
Ellipsoids, *1*:256
Ellis van Creveld syndrome 2, *1*:39,
   1:39*f*
Elokomin fluke fever, *3*:149
Embolic pneumonia, *2*:520, *2*:520.*e*2*f*
Embolic suppurative myocarditis,
   3:42.*e*1*f*
Embolism
   arterial, *3*:63-66, *3*:63*f*-64*f*
   coronary, *3*:36
   pulmonary, *2*:489, *2*:490*f*
      fat, *2*:490
      septic, *2*:490
   septic, *1*:358-362, *1*:358*f*
Embryonal carcinoma, *3*:496
Embryonal rhabdomyosarcoma, *1*:241-243,
   1:243*f*
Embryonal tumors, *1*:401-403
Embryonic death, *3*:395
   with persistence of membranes, *3*:396
Embryonic stage of lung growth, *2*:484
Emmonsia crescens, *2*:584
Emmonsia parva, *2*:584
Emphysema
   fetal, *3*:396
   lymph node, *3*:199
   pulmonary, *2*:486-487, *2*:487*f*
Emphysematous cystitis, *2*:459, *2*:460*f*
Emphysematous pyelonephritis, *2*:440
Empyema, *1*:353-354
   of sinus, *2*:477, *2*:477*f*
Enamel, *2*:5
   hypoplasia, *2*:7*f*
   loss, *2*:10
Encephalitozoon, *1*:451

Encephalitozoon cuniculi, *1*:385-386, *2*:431,
   3:418
Encephalocele, *1*:267, *1*:267*f*
Encephalomalacia, *1*:307
   focal symmetrical, *1*:300-301, *1*:301*f*
   pigs, *1*:308-309
   nigropallidal, *1*:314, *1*:314*f*
Encephalomyelopathies, spongy, *1*:342*f*,
   1:345*f*, *1*:346-347
Encephalomyocarditis virus (EMCV), *3*:43
Enchondromatosis, *1*:116
Endoarteritis, *2*:84
Endocardiosis, *3*:27, *3*:28*f*-29*f*
Endocarditis, *3*:30-33, *3*:31*f*, *3*:31.*e*1*f*
Endocardium, *3*:3
   disease, *3*:27-33
      degenerative lesions, *3*:27-30
   mural and valvular, *3*:4
Endochondral ossification, *1*:22, *1*:22*f*
   rickets and, *1*:71-72
Endocrine cells, *2*:45
Endocrine pancreas, *2*:368-375
   diabetes mellitus, *2*:370-373, *2*:371*f*
      cats, *2*:372, *2*:373*f*
      cattle, *2*:372
      diabetic cataract, *1*:443
      dogs, *2*:373
      horses, *2*:372
      retinopathies, *1*:472
   hyperplastic and neoplastic diseases,
      2:373-375, *2*:374*f*
Endocrine system, *3*:269-357
   adrenal cortex, *3*:336-348
   adrenal medulla, *3*:348-354
   diseases/disorders, *2*:384-385
      atrophy of, *1*:178, *1*:178*f*
      mechanisms, *3*:272-276
      myopathies associated with, *1*:224-225
      of skin, *1*:587-590
   general considerations, *3*:270-276
   hormones
      calcium-regulating, *3*:291-310, *3*:291*f*
      catecholamine and iodothyronine, *3*:271
      steroid, *3*:271
      thyroid, *3*:311-312
      types, *3*:270-271
   multiple endocrine neoplasia (MEN),
      3:356-357
   paragangliomas, *3*:354-356
   parathyroid gland, *3*:292-295, *3*:292*f*
   pituitary gland, *3*:276-291
   proliferative lesions, *3*:271-272
   thyroid gland, *3*:310-336
   tumors, *3*:272
Endogenous anticoagulants, *3*:265-266
Endogenous lipid pneumonia, *2*:517
Endogenous protein, *2*:72-73
Endometritis, *3*:388-389, *3*:388*f*
Endolymph, *1*:489
Endometrial biopsy, *3*:393
Endometrial cups, *3*:394, *3*:394*f*
Endometrial polyps, *3*:385, *3*:386*f*
Endometritis, *3*:388-389, *3*:388*f*
   chronic, *3*:389-390
Endometrium, *3*:382-387, *3*:382*f*
   carcinoma, *3*:449-450
   cysts, postpartum, *3*:440
   endometritis, *3*:388-389, *3*:388*f*
Endophthalmitis, *1*:446
   bacterial, *1*:449
   mycotic, *1*:449-451

Endophthalmitis *(Continued)*
   parasitic, *1*:451-452
   protozoal, *1*:451
   viral, *1*:452
Endothelial cells
   hepatic, *2*:262-263
   sinusoidal, *2*:260
   vascular, *3*:55
      disorders, *3*:255-268
Endothelial protein C receptor (EPCR),
   3:265-266
Endothelium-mediated fibrinolysis, *3*:266
End-stage kidneys, *2*:377-378
English Bulldogs
   acne, *1*:549
   brachycephalic airway syndrome, *2*:482,
      2:482*f*
   demodectic mange, *1*:679
   factor VII deficiency, *3*:264
   hypothyroidism, *1*:587, *3*:315
   keratoconjunctivitis sicca, *1*:436
   recurrent flank alopecia, *1*:590
English Cocker Spaniel hereditary nephritis,
   2:416
English Pointer dogs
   chondrodysplasia, *1*:44
   motor neuron disease, *1*:331
   sensory and autonomic neuropathies,
      1:334
English Setter dogs, atopic dermatitis in,
   1:591
English Springer Spaniel dogs
   canine congenital myasthenia, *1*:209
   canine hypomyelinogenesis, *1*:337
   chronic hepatitis, *2*:304
   gangliosidosis, *1*:58-59
   lichenoid-psoriasiform dermatosis,
      1:552-553
   malignant hyperthermia, *1*:210
   persistent atrial standstill, *3*:51
   phosphofructokinase (PFK) deficiency,
      1:204-205
   polymyopathy, *1*:198
   prolonged APTT, *3*:263
   retinal folding, *1*:419
   seborrhea, *1*:548
   sensory and autonomic neuropathy,
      1:334
Enrofloxacin, *1*:472
Entamoeba histolytica, *2*:98-99, *2*:242
Enteric clostridial infections, *2*:183-194
Enteric coronaviral infections,
   2:146-151
Enteric disease, pathophysiology of, *2*:69-73,
   2:107
   anemia, *2*:73
   diarrhea, *2*:70-72
      increased intestinal motility, *2*:72
      increased permeability, *2*:71
      large-bowel, *2*:71
      malabsorptive, *2*:71
      secretory, *2*:71
      small-bowel, *2*:71
   inappetence/anorexia, *2*:69
   malassimilation, *2*:69-70
      assimilation of fat, *2*:70
      lipids, malabsorption of, *2*:70
      polysaccharides, maldigestion of,
         2:70
      protein maldigestion, *2*:70
   protein-energy malnutrition, *2*:69

Shorter-acting sulfonamides, crystalline
   nephropathy, 2:424
Shorthorn cattle
   bovine hypomyelinogenesis, 1:338-339
   lethal trait A46, 3:141
Shoulder joint, degenerative joint disease of,
   1:143
Shunted blood flow to heart, 3:6
   malformation causing, 3:16-18, 3:16f
Shunts, hepatic, 2:267, 2:267f, 2:267.e1f
   acquired portosystemic, 2:290, 2:298-299,
   2:299f
Shwartzman reaction, 2:398-399
Sialoadenitis, 2:29
Sialocele
   nasopharyngeal, 2:477.e4f
   salivary, 2:29
Siamese cats
   congenital hypotrichosis, 1:539
   congenital idiopathic megaesophagus, 2:34
   Maroteaux-Lamy syndrome, 1:58
   photosensitization, 1:579
   vitiligo, 1:556
Siberian Husky dogs
   alopecia X, 1:589-590
   canine uveodermatologic syndrome, 1:557
   degenerative radiculomyelopathy, 1:330
   motor neuropathy, 1:335
   oral eosinophilic granuloma, 2:16
   vitiligo, 1:555-556
   zinc-responsive dermatoses, 1:585-586
Sick sinus syndrome, 3:51
Siderocalcinosis, 3:61
Siderosis, 1:297, 1:298f
Sideritic pigmentation, 1:255
Siderotic plaques, splenic, 3:163, 3:164f,
   3:163.e2f
Signet ring cells, 2:101-102
Signet-ring malignant melanomas, 1:722
Silica calculi, 2:455
Silicate pneumoconiosis, 2:518
Silicates, 2:518
Silky Terrier dogs
   rabies vaccine-induced vasculitis and
   alopecia, 1:612
   spongy myelinopathy, 1:343-344
Silo gas, 2:518
Silver fox
   spongiform myelinopathy, 1:343f, 1:344
   status spongiosus, 1:342f
Simmental cattle
   epidermolysis bullosa simplex, 1:535
   inherited progressive spinal myelopathy,
   1:325
   osteopetrosis, 1:51
Simondsia spp., 2:54
Simple follicles, 1:515-516
Simple renal cysts, 2:394-395
Simple secretory epitrichial adenomas, 1:718
Sinus erythrocytosis, 3:199-200, 3:200f,
   3:200.e1f
Sinuses
   diseases, 2:477, 2:477f
   neoplasms, 2:478-480, 2:478f
   nonflammatory thrombosis of cranial dural,
   1:300
   non-neoplastic proliferative disorders,
   2:477-478
Sinus hairs, 1:517
Sinusitis, chronic suppurative, 2:477-478,
   2:477.e1f

Sinus node, 3:2
Sinusoidal domain, liver, 2:262
Sinusoidal endothelial cells, 2:260
Sinusoidal leukocytosis, 2:300-301
Sinusoidal lining cells necrosis, 2:285
Size-dependent barrier, 2:380
Skeletal dysplasias, 1:37t
   localized, 1:54-57, 1:54f
   osteochondromatosis, 1:54
Skeletal muscles, dermal, 1:515
Skeleton. *See also* Bone(s)
   genetic and congenital diseases of, 1:36-60,
   1:37t
   genetic diseases indirectly affecting,
   1:57-60
   manganese deficiency and, 1:80
   postmortem examination of, 1:28-30, 1:29f
Skin, 1:509-736
   actinic diseases of, 1:575-580
   algal diseases of, 1:665
   bacterial diseases of, 1:629-646
   basement membrane zone (BMZ),
   1:513-514
   canine cutaneous histiocytoma, 3:243-245,
   3:244f-245f, 3:244.e1f, 3:243.e1f
   canine juvenile cellutitis, 1:690-691, 1:691f
   canine reactive histiocytosis, 3:247-250,
   3:248f, 3:247.e1f
   congenital and hereditary diseases of,
   1:530-547
   dermal muscles, 1:515
   dermatohistopathology, 1:518-530
     gross terminology, 1:524
     histologic terms, 1:518-524
     pattern analysis, 1:524-530
   dermis, 1:514-515
   endocrine diseases of, 1:587-590
   epidermal differentiation disorders,
   1:547-554
   epidermis, 1:512-513
   fungal diseases of, 1:646-661
   general considerations, 1:511-518
   hair follicles, 1:515-517
   helminth diseases of, 1:685-690
   immune-mediated dermatoses, 1:590-615
     autoimmune dermatoses, 1:600-607
     drug eruptions, 1:607-608
     hypersensitivity, 1:590-600
   immunologic function, 1:515
   lesions with canine distemper virus,
   2:576
   lymphomas, 3:237, 3:237f, 3:239f,
   3:239.e1f
   neoplastic and reactive diseases, 1:703-736
   nutritional diseases of, 1:580-587
   paraneoplastic syndromes, 1:691-693
   perianal glands, 1:517
   physiochemical diseases of, 1:558-575
     chemical injury, 1:566-575
     physical injury, 1:559-566
   pigmentation disorders, 1:554-558
   protozoal diseases of, 1:661-665
   sebaceous glands, 1:517
   subcutis, 1:518
   sweat glands, 1:517-518
   tags, 1:722-723
   tumor-like lesions, 1:705
   viral diseases of, 1:615-628
Skin-associated lymphoid tissue (SALT),
   1:515
Skin-homing memory T-cells, 1:515

Skin immune system (SIS), 1:515
Skull bones, 1:21
   congenital abnormalities, 1:56, 1:56f
   craniomandibular osteopathy, 1:91-92,
   1:92f
   fractures, 1:302-303
   sutures, 1:128
Skye Terrier dogs, chronic hepatitis in, 2:304
Slaframine, 2:29
SLC2A9 gene, 2:457
SLC3A1 genes, 2:458
SLC7A9 genes, 2:458
Slipped epiphysis, 1:31
Sly syndrome, 1:58
Small-bowel diarrhea, 2:70-71
Small-cell carcinoma
   neuroendocrine, 2:497-498
   thyroid, 3:330-331
Small-cell lymphocytic villus lymphoma,
   2:107-108
Small intestinal bacterial overgrowth (SIBO),
   2:86, 2:364
Small intestine, 2:81, 2:82f
   cardinal finding, 2:92
   idiopathic inflammatory bowel disease,
   2:92
   lymphangiectasia, 2:90f
   mucosa, 2:124
     hypoplasia, 2:74
     vascular supply, 2:61
   obstruction, 2:76
     dogs, 2:75f
   pseudodiverticulosis of, 2:87
Small ruminant lentiviruses, 2:558-560,
   2:559f, 2:558.e1f
Smoke inhalation
   lung injury, 2:518
   trachea and, 2:483, 2:483f
Smooth Fox Terrier dogs
   canine congenital myasthenia, 1:209
   multisystem axonal degeneration, 1:325
Smooth muscle cells, lungs, 2:469
Smooth-surface caries, 2:10
Snakebite envenomation, 1:568
Snowshoe hare virus, 1:383
Snorter dwarfism, 1:39, 1:39f
Sodium absorption, 2:65-66
Sodium fluoroacetate, 3:37-38
Sodium iodide symporter (NIS), 3:311
Soemmering ring cataract, 1:444, 1:444f
Soft callus, 1:34-35
Soft tissue sarcomas, 1:245
Solanaceae, 2:331
Solanum glaucophyllum, 3:301-302,
   3:301f-302f
Solanum poisoning, 1:321-322
Solar dermatitis, 1:576, 1:576f
Solar elastosis, 1:577, 1:577f
Solar keratoses, 1:577
Solar radiation
   burns and, 1:566
   direct effect of, 1:575-577
Solid basal cell carcinoma, 1:714
Solid-cystic epitrichial adenomas, 1:718-719
Solid-cystic epitrichial carcinomas, 1:719
Solitary biliary cysts, 2:264
Solitary mucosal lymphoid nodules, 2:64
Somatostatin, 2:368
Somatostatinoma, 2:375
Somatotroph adenomas, 3:285-286,
   3:285f-286f